SURGICAL
PATHOLOGY
OF THE
HEAD AND NECK

VOLUME 3

SURGICAL PATHOLOGY OF THE HEAD AND NECK

Third Edition

EDITED BY

LEON BARNES

University of Pittsburgh Medical Center
Presbyterian-University Hospital
Pittsburgh, Pennsylvania, USA

informa
healthcare

Informa Healthcare USA, Inc.
52 Vanderbilt Avenue
New York, NY 10017

© 2009 by Informa Healthcare USA, Inc.
Informa Healthcare is an Informa business

No claim to original U.S. Government works
Printed in India by Replika Press Pvt. Ltd.
10 9 8 7 6 5 4 3 2 1

International Standard Book Number-10: 1-4200-9163-8 (V1; Hardcover)
International Standard Book Number-13: 978-1-4200-9163-2 (V1; Hardcover)
International Standard Book Number-10: 1-4200-9164-6 (V2; Hardcover)
International Standard Book Number-13: 978-1-4200-9164-9 (V2; Hardcover)
International Standard Book Number-10: 1-4200-9165-4 (V3; Hardcover)
International Standard Book Number-13: 978-1-4200-9165-6 (V3; Hardcover)
International Standard Book Number-10: 0-8493-9023-0 (Set; Hardcover)
International Standard Book Number-13: 978-0-8493-9023-4 (Set; Hardcover)

Library of Congress Cataloging-in-Publication Data

Surgical pathology of the head and neck / edited by Leon Barnes. – 3rd ed.
    p. ; cm.
  Includes bibliographical references and index.
  ISBN-13: 978-0-8493-9023-4 (hb : alk. paper)
  ISBN-10: 0-8493-9023-0 (hb : alk. paper)
  1. Head–Diseases–Diagnosis. 2. Neck–Diseases–Diagnosis. 3. Pathology, Surgical. 4. Head–Tumors–Diagnosis.
5. Neck–Tumors–Diagnosis. I. Barnes, Leon, 1941-
  [DNLM: 1. Head–pathology. 2. Neck–pathology. 3. Head–surgery. 4. Neck–surgery. 5. Pathology, Surgical.
WE 705 S961345 2008]
  RC936.S87 2008
  617.5′10754–dc22

                                     2008026087

For Corporate Sales and Reprint Permissions call 212-520-2700 or write to:
Sales Department, 52 Vanderbilt Avenue, 7th floor, New York, NY 10017.

Visit the Informa Web site at
www.informa.com

and the Informa Healthcare Web site at
www.informahealthcare.com

Preface to Third Edition

Seven years have elapsed since the second edition of *Surgical Pathology of the Head and Neck* was published. During this interval there has been an enormous amount of new information that impacts on the daily practice of surgical pathology. Nowhere is this more evident than in the area of molecular biology and genetics. Data derived from this new discipline, once considered to be of research interest only, have revolutionized the evaluation of hematolymphoid neoplasms and are now being applied, to a lesser extent, to the assessment of mesenchymal and epithelial tumors. While immunohistochemistry has been available for almost 30 years, it has not remained static. New antibodies are constantly being developed that expand our diagnostic and prognostic capabilities.

Although these new technologies are exciting, they only supplement and do not replace the "H&E slide," which is, and will continue to be, the foundation of surgical pathology and this book particularly. This edition has been revised to incorporate some of these new technologies that further our understanding of the pathobiology of disease and improve our diagnostic acumen, while at the same time retaining clinical and pathological features that are not new but remain useful and important.

Due to constraints of time and the expanse of new knowledge, it is almost impossible for a single individual to produce a book that adequately covers the pathology of the head and neck. I have been fortunate, however, to secure the aid of several new outstanding collaborators to assist in this endeavor and wish to extend to them my sincere thanks and appreciation for lending their time and expertise. In addition to new contributors, the illustrations have also been changed from black and white to color to enhance clarity and emphasize important features.

This edition has also witnessed changes in the publishing industry. The two previous editions were published by Marcel Dekker, Inc., which was subsequently acquired by Informa Healthcare, the current publisher. At Informa Healthcare, I have had the pleasure of working with many talented individuals, including Geoffrey Greenwood, Sandra Beberman, Alyssa Fried, Vanessa Sanchez, Mary Araneo, Daniel Falatko, and Joseph Stubenrauch. I am especially indebted to them for their guidance and patience.

I also wish to acknowledge the contributions of my secretary, Mrs. Donna Bowen, and my summer student, Ms. Shayna Cornell, for secretarial support and Ms. Linda Shab and Mr. Thomas Bauer for my illustrations. Lastly, this book would not have been possible without the continued unwavering support of my family, Carol, Christy, and Lori, who have endured yet another edition!

Leon Barnes

Contents

Contributors

Kristen A. Atkins   Department of Pathology, University of Virginia Health System, Charlottesville, Virginia, U.S.A.

Aaron Auerbach   Department of Hematopathology, Armed Forces Institute of Pathology, Washington D.C., U.S.A.

Leon Barnes   Department of Pathology, University of Pittsburgh Medical Center, Presbyterian-University Hospital, Pittsburgh, Pennsylvania, U.S.A.

Margaret Brandwein-Gensler   Department of Pathology, Albert Einstein College of Medicine, Montefiore Medical Center—Moses Division, Bronx, New York, U.S.A.

Harry H. Brown   Departments of Pathology and Ophthalmology, Harvey and Bernice Jones Eye Institute, University of Arkansas for Medical Sciences, Little Rock, Arkansas, U.S.A.

Steven D. Budnick   Emory University School of Medicine Atlanta, Georgia, U.S.A.

Alexander C. L. Chan   Department of Pathology, Queen Elizabeth Hospital, Hong Kong

John K. C. Chan   Department of Pathology, Queen Elizabeth Hospital, Hong Kong

Louis P. Dehner   Lauren V. Ackerman Laboratory of Surgical Pathology, Barnes-Jewish and St. Louis Children's Hospitals, Washington University Medical Center, Department of Pathology and Immunology, St. Louis, Missouri, U.S.A.

Samir K. El-Mofty   Department of Pathology and Immunology, Washington University, St. Louis, Missouri, U.S.A.

Samir K. El-Mofty   Lauren V. Ackerman Laboratory of Surgical Pathology, Barnes-Jewish and St. Louis Children's Hospitals, Washington University Medical Center, Department of Pathology and Immunology, St. Louis, Missouri, U.S.A.

Tarik M. Elsheikh   PA Labs, Ball Memorial Hospital, Muncie, Indiana, U.S.A.

Lori A. Erickson   Mayo Clinic College of Medicine, Rochester, Minnesota, U.S.A.

John Wallace Eveson   Department of Oral and Dental Science, Bristol Dental Hospital and School, Bristol, U.K.

Julie C. Fanburg-Smith   Department of Orthopaedic and Soft Tissue Pathology, Armed Forces Institute of Pathology, Washington D.C., U.S.A.

Robert D. Foss   Department of Oral and Maxillofacial Pathology, Armed Forces Institute of Pathology, Washington D.C., U.S.A.

Kim M. Hiatt   Department of Pathology, University of Arkansas for Medical Sciences, Little Rock, Arkansas, U.S.A.

William B. Laskin   Surgical Pathology, Northwestern Memorial Hospital, Feinberg School of Medicine, Northwestern University, Chicago, Illinois, U.S.A.

Jerzy Lasota Department of Orthopaedic and Soft Tissue Pathology, Armed Forces Institute of Pathology, Washington D.C., U.S.A.

James S. Lewis, Jr. Department of Pathology and Immunology, Washington University, St. Louis, Missouri, U.S.A.

Ricardo V. Lloyd Mayo Clinic College of Medicine, Rochester, Minnesota, U.S.A.

Mario A. Luna Department of Pathology, The University of Texas, M.D. Anderson Cancer Center, Houston, Texas, U.S.A.

Susan Müller Department of Pathology and Laboratory Medicine and Department of Otolaryngology-Head & Neck Surgery, Emory University School of Medicine, Atlanta, Georgia, U.S.A.

Panna Mahadevia Department of Pathology, Albert Einstein College of Medicine, Montefiore Medical Center—Moses Division, Bronx, New York, U.S.A.

Thijs A.W. Merkx Department of Oral and Maxillofacial Surgery, Radboud University Nijmegen Medical Center, Nijmegen, The Netherlands

Stacey E. Mills Department of Pathology, University of Virginia Health System, Charlottesville, Virginia, U.S.A.

Mark D. Murphey Department of Radiologic Pathology, Armed Forces Institute of Pathology, Washington D.C., U.S.A.

Toshitaka Nagao Department of Diagnostic Pathology, Tokyo Medical University, Tokyo, Japan

Daisuke Nonaka Department of Pathology, New York University School of Medicine, New York University Langone Medical Center, New York, New York, U.S.A.

Jennifer B. Ogilvie University of Pittsburgh Medical Center, Pittsburgh, Pennsylvania, U.S.A.

Shayesteh Pashaei Department of Pathology, University of Arkansas for Medical Sciences, Little Rock, Arkansas, U.S.A.

Finn Prætorius Department of Oral Pathology, University of Copenhagen, Copenhagen, Denmark

Robert A. Robinson Department of Pathology, The University of Iowa, Roy J. and Lucille A. Carver College of Medicine, Iowa City, Iowa, U.S.A.

Reda S. Saad Sunnybrook Hospital, University of Toronto, Toronto, Ontario, Canada

Raja R. Seethala University of Pittsburgh Medical Center, Pittsburgh, Pennsylvania, U.S.A.

Jan F. Silverman Department of Pathology and Laboratory Medicine, Allegheny General Hospital, and Drexel University College of Medicine, Pittsburgh, Pennsylvania, U.S.A.

Harsharan K. Singh University of North Carolina-Chapel Hill School of Medicine, Chapel Hill, North Carolina, U.S.A.

Pieter J. Slootweg Department of Pathology, Radboud University Nijmegen Medical Center, Nijmegen, The Netherlands

Bruce R. Smoller Department of Pathology, University of Arkansas for Medical Sciences, Little Rock, Arkansas, U.S.A.

Steven D. Vincent   Department of Oral Pathology, Oral Radiology and Oral Medicine, The University of Iowa College of Dentistry, Iowa City, Iowa, U.S.A.

Mohamed A. Virji   University of Pittsburgh Medical Center, Pittsburgh, Pennsylvania, U.S.A.

Beverly Y. Wang   Departments of Pathology and Otolaryngology, New York University School of Medicine, New York University Langone Medical Center, New York, New York, U.S.A.

Bruce M. Wenig   Department of Pathology and Laboratory Medicine, Beth Israel Medical Center, St. Luke's and Roosevelt Hospitals, New York, New York, U.S.A.

David Zagzag   Department of Neuropathology, New York University School of Medicine, Bellevue Hospital, New York, New York, U.S.A.

Odontogenic Tumors

Finn Prætorius
Department of Oral Pathology, University of Copenhagen, Copenhagen, Denmark

INTRODUCTION

The term "odontogenic tumors" comprises a group of neoplasms and hamartomatous lesions derived from cells of tissues involved in the formation of teeth or remnants of tissues that has been involved in the odontogenesis. Few of them are odontogenic in the sense that the formation of dental hard tissues takes place in them; it is primarily the case in the ameloblastic fibro-odontoma (AFOD), the odontomas, and the cementoblastoma (CEMBLA).

The tumors occur exclusively in three locations (*i*) intraosseous (centrally) in the jaws, (*ii*) extraosseous (peripherally) in the gingiva or alveolar mucosa overlying tooth bearing areas, and (*iii*) in the cranial base, as one of the variants of the craniopharyngioma, a tumor arising from cell rest derived from the hypophyseal stalk or Rathke's pouch. The craniopharyngioma occurs as subtypes, which resembles ameloblastoma, calcifying odontogenic cyst (COC) or AFOD with intracranial formation of tooth-like elements (1–4). The craniopharyngiomas are not further described in this chapter.

Odontogenic tumors are rare, with some of them being exceedingly rare. Our knowledge of these tumors is primarily based on published reports of cases, reviews of such cases, and reviews of cases from files from institutions. In the later years, the use of electron microscopy, immunohistochemistry, and molecular biological techniques has increased our knowledge of the biology of the tumors considerably (5). Development of experimental models of odontogenic tumors in animals have been tried, but with limited success; although it has been possible to breed animals that develop tumors resembling, e.g., ameloblastomas and odontomes (6,7), they are not true equivalents to odontogenic tumors in humans—their histology is similar, but their biological behavior is different (8). Tissue culture has been more successful and has primarily been used in studies of the molecular biology of the tumors.

The accumulated knowledge has led to numerous attempts at classification of odontogenic tumors, reviews of older classifications have been written by Gorlin et al. (9) and Baden (10), and valuable information about older references is found in these articles. A short, but more recent review, including the classifications issued by World Health Organization (WHO) in 1971, 1992, and 2005 has been published by Philipsen et al. (11). The description of the tumors in the present chapter in based on the WHO 2005 classification (12) (Table 1), apart from a diverging conception of the odontogenic ghost cell lesions and the inclusion of some very rare tumors, which were left out of the 2005 WHO classification as they were considered insufficiently defined.

The etiology of the odontogenic tumors is essentially unknown, apart from indications that genetic factors play a role as cofactor in some cases. The pathogenesis is incompletely understood, the subject has been discussed in several articles (13–17).

Since odontogenic tumors appear to develop from remnants of odontogenic tissues and many of the histomorphological and other biological features of the normal odontogenesis are retrieved in odontogenic tumors, particularly in the group consisting of odontogenic epithelium and odontogenic ectomesenchyme, with or without hard tissue formation, a certain knowledge of the normal odontogenesis is required to identify and understand the tissue changes observed. Apart from chapters in textbooks like *Oral Cells and Tissues* by Garant (18), shorter reviews have been published by Theslaff et al. (19), Peters et al. (20), Coubourne et al. (21), and Philipsen et al. (16).

The histomorphological variants of odontogenic tumors are numerous and cannot be fully illustrated in a single treatise. Additional photos in colors are accessible in the three publications by WHO (12,22,23), in Sciubba et al. (24) and Reichart et al. (25).

I. BENIGN ODONTOGENIC TUMORS

1. Tumors of Odontogenic Epithelium with Mature, Fibrous Stroma Without Odontogenic Ectomesenchyme

This group of tumors covers the following recognized entities: ameloblastoma, squamous odontogenic tumor (SOT), calcifying epithelial odontogenic tumor (CEOT), and adenomatoid odontogenic tumor (AOT).

Table 1 WHO Histological Classification of Odontogenic Tumors (2005)

Malignant Tumors	
Odontogenic carcinomas	
Metastasizing (malignant) ameloblastoma	
Ameloblastic carcinoma: primary type	9310/3
Ameloblastic carcinoma: secondary type (dedifferentiated), intraosseous	9270/3
Ameloblastic carcinoma: secondary type (dedifferentiated), peripheral	9270/3
Primary intraosseous squamous cell carcinoma: solid type	9270/3
Primary intraosseous squamous cell carcinoma derived from keratocystic odontogenic tumor	9279/3
Primary intraosseous squamous cell carcinoma derived from odontogenic cysts	9270/3
Clear cell odontogenic carcinoma	9270/3
Ghost cell odontogenic carcinoma	9341/3
Odontogenic sarcomas	9302/3
Ameloblastic fibrosarcoma	
Ameloblastic fibrodentino- and fibro-odontosarcoma	9330/3
Benign Tumors	9290/3
Odontogenic epithelium with mature, fibrous stroma without odontogenic ectomesenchyme	
Ameloblastoma solid/multicystic type	
Ameloblastoma, extraosseous (peripheral) type	9310/0
Ameloblastoma, desmoplastic type	9310/0
Ameloblastoma, unicystic type	9310/0
Squamous odontogenic tumor	9310/0
Calcifying epithelial odontogenic tumor	9312/0
Adenomatoid odontogenic tumor	9340/0
Keratocystic odontogenic tumor	9300/0
Odontogenic epithelium with odontogenic ectomesenchyme, with or without hard tissue formation	9270/0
Ameloblastic fibroma	
Ameloblastic fibrodentinoma	9330/0
Ameloblastic fibro-odontoma	9271/0
Odontoma	9290/0
Odontoma, complex type	9280/0
Odontoma, compound type	9282/0
Odonto-ameloblastoma	9281/0
Calcifying cystic odontogenic tumor	9311/0
Dentinogenic ghost cell tumor	9301/0
Mesenchyme and/or odontogenic ectomesenchyme, with or without odontogenic epithelium	9302/0
Odontogenic fibroma	
Odontogenic myxoma/myxofibroma	9321/0
Cementoblastoma	9320/0
	9273/0

Note: The numbers indicate the morphology code of the International Classification of Diseases for Oncology (ICD-O) and the Systematized Nomenclature of Medicine (http://snomed.org).
Behavior is coded /0 for benign tumors, /3 for malignant tumors, and /1 for borderline or uncertain behavior.
Source: From Ref. 12.

1.1 Ameloblastoma

1.1.1.1 Solid/Multicystic Ameloblastoma–Central.

Introduction. The central solid/multicystic ameloblastoma (s/mAM) is a slowly growing, locally invasive epithelial odontogenic neoplasm of the jaws with a high rate of recurrence but with a very low tendency to metastasize (26).

ICD—O 9310/0

Synonyms: Conventional ameloblastoma; classical intraosseous ameloblastoma.

Clinical Features. The prevalence and incidence of the s/mAM is unknown apart from two studies, both of which comprised all variants of ameloblastoma, not only the s/m. Shear et al. (27) calculated age-standardized incidence rates of the tumor in the population of the Witwatersrand region of South Africa from 1965 to 1974. The annual incidence rates, standardized against the standard world population, for all variants of ameloblastomas per million populations were 1.96, 1.20, 0.18, and 0.44 for black males, black females, white males, and white females, respectively. The figures show that ameloblastoma is very much more common in blacks than in whites in the population at risk. Gardner (28) recalculated the figures without separating the two genders and found the incidence rates to be 2.29 new cases each year per one million people for blacks and 0.31 for whites. It is unknown whether this marked difference is caused by genetic or environmental factors.

Another valuable study of the incidence of ameloblastomas was published by Larsson et al. (29). All cases of ameloblastoma reported to the Swedish Cancer Register in the period 1958–1971 (except the years 1966 and 1969) were reexamined histologically with criteria indicated in the 1971 WHO classification (22); 31 cases of ameloblastoma (peripheral and unicystic included) were accepted. The number of annual cases varied between 1 and 5, corresponding to 0.13 to 0.63

annual cases per one million people, and an average of 0.3 annual case per one million inhabitants. On the basis of the study of the files of two major hospitals, the authors estimated an under registration of about 50%. The true incidence was thus close to 0.6 cases each year per one million people, a figure which can be accepted as a reasonable estimate of the incidence of ameloblastoma in a Caucasian population.

The relative frequency of the tumor is known from several studies, it is the second most common odontogenic tumor after the odontomas. The relative frequency of the tumor in material received for histological diagnosis in services of diagnostic pathology in various countries for various amounts of years ranges from 11.0% to 73.3% in studies comprising more than 300 samples of odontogenic tumors. Except for one study [Buchner et al. (30)] subdivision in ameloblastoma variants (s/m, peripheral, desmoplastic, and unicystic) have not been made in these studies. The results are indicated as follows: number of odontogenic tumors/number of ameloblastomas/percentage. Regezzi et al., Michigan, U.S.A. (31): 706/78/11.0%, Günhan et al., Turkey (32): 409/149/36.4%, Daley et al., Canada (33): 392/53/13.5%, Mosqueda-Taylor et al., Mexico (34): 349/83/23.7%, Ochsenius et al., Chile (35): 362/74/20.4%, Adebayo et al., Nigeria (36): 318/233/73.3%, Fernandes et al., Brazil (37): 340/154/45.3%, Ladeinde et al., Nigeria (38): 319/201/63.0%, Buchner et al., California (30): 1088/127/11.7% [unicystic ameloblastoma (UNAM) 5.3%, solid/multicystic (s/m) 6.3%], Jones et al., England (2006, pooled figures from two studies)(39,40): 523/111/21.2%, Olgac et al., Turkey (41): 527/133/25.2%, and Jing et al., China (42): 1642/661/40.3%. The data are skewed, however, the figures reflect regional differences in type of lesions sent for histopathological confirmation rather than effects of genetical or environmental factors.

The most comprehensive review of ameloblastomas has been published by Reichart et al. (43) who evaluated 3677 cases published in various languages between 1960 and 1993, including 693 case reports and 2984 cases from reviews.

In this review, figures were reported for occurrence in the three major racial groups (Caucasoid, Mongoloid, Negroid), no conclusions can be drawn from this information. As pointed out by Gardner (28) the numbers do not reflect the occurrence of ameloblastomas in the three major racial groups but rather the number of published cases in those groups, and the number of published cases does not reflect the actual prevalence in a population.

Details for age (including peripheral and unicystic variants) were retrieved from 2280 cases (1630 from reviews, 650 from case reports) the age range at time of diagnosis was 4 to 92 years, and the median age was 35 years. The mean age from case reports was 37.4 years and from reviews 35.4 years. The figures for the individual variants were "hidden" in the review, but recalculated by Gardner (28) who estimated a mean age of 39 years for s/mAM, 51 years for peripheral, and 22 years for UNAMs. In comparison Ledesma-Montes (44) found (N = 163) that the mean

age was 41.4 years for s/mAM and 26.3 years for UNAM (p < 0.001).

The majority of ameloblastomas in Caucasian children, but not in African are unicystic. Ord et al. (45) reported 11 own cases of ameloblastoma in children (2 s/m AM and 9 unicystic) and reviewed the literature on ameloblastoma in children in Western reports (85 children) and reports from Africa (77 children). The mean age was 15.5, 14.3, and 14.7 years, respectively. UNAMs accounted for 76.5% of the Western and only for 19.5% of the African children. The pattern in African children seems to resemble the pattern of adults. These findings were confirmed by Arotiba et al. (46).

Reichart et al. (43) found the mean age of patients with tumors of the maxilla to be 47.0 years compared with tumors of the mandible with a mean age of 35.2 years. The difference may at least partly be explained by the fact that UNAMs are rare in the maxilla and about 30% of solid/multicystic ameloblastomas-peripheral (PERAMs) occur in the maxilla.

The gender distribution has varied in different reviews but is often close to 50:50; in the review by Reichart et al.(43) 53.5% were males and 46.7% were females (N = 3677).

The location of the tumor was recorded in the same review, but only for all variants combined. The ratio between maxillary (N = 185) and mandibular (N = 404) ameloblastomas was 1:2.2 when case reports were evaluated. If, however case reports and reviews were considered together (N = 1932) the ratio between maxillary and mandibular tumors was 1:5.8. The difference is presumably because ameloblastomas, as they are more unusual, are reported more often in case reports. The incisor region and ramus of the mandible were affected more often in females than in males. The premolar region and the maxillary sinus were affected more often in males than in females, whereas the molar region was affected equally in both genders. The predilection site is the posterior part of the mandible in which 44.4% of the tumors (all variants) were located. In the study by Ledesma-Montes et al. (44) 79.3% of the s/mAM were located in the mandible and 20.7% in the maxilla (N = 163). Forty percent were located in the mandibular molar area, 26.2% in the mandibular angle.

The tumor is slowly growing and with few symptoms apart from the swelling. Some published cases of mandibular ameloblastomas have been extremely large (25 cm or more), a huge tumor reported by Carlson et al. (47) had been present for 16 years. The duration of symptoms varied from half a year to 40 years (for all variants, N = 198) in the review by Reichart et al (43); the median duration was six-and-a-half months, and the mean duration time was 27 months. Ledesma-Montes et al. (44) reported a range of duration time from 1 to 39 years for s/mAM (N = 163), with a mean of 4.5 years. In this review, the most common clinical findings were swelling (97%), pain (34.4%), ulceration (12.5%), and tooth displacement (12.5%). Delayed tooth eruption and mobility of teeth has also been reported (43). In large tumors with expansion and resorption of the jawbone a crepitation

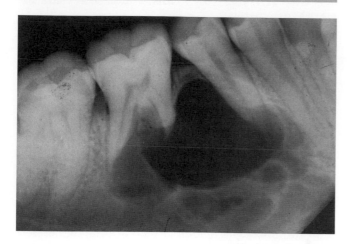

Figure 1 Radiogram of an ameloblastoma with soap bubble appearance in the right side of the mandible of a 25-year-old woman. There was a swelling of the mandible, which was noticed six months earlier and had reached the size of 3.5 cm. No other symptoms. Note the partial resorption of the roots of the first molar and the second premolar.

may be elicited, perforation of the cortical bone is a late feature, however. Paresthesia of the lower lip is a rare symptom (48).

Imaging. A radiolucent, often well-demarcated, sometimes corticated, multilocular radiolucency is a characteristic radiological appearance of the s/mAM, but it is not diagnostic (Fig. 1). The radiographic image may vary considerably. Among 55 cases reviewed by Ledesma-Montes et al. (44) 88.1% were radiolucent, 66.7% were unilocular, and 66.7% were well defined. The radiographic descriptions of 1234 cases (377 case reports and 857 cases from reviews) were evaluated by Reichart et al. (43), but were only reported for all four variants combined, 102 were of the unicystic type. The appearance was unilocular in 51.1%, and multilocular ("soap-bubble-like") in 48.9%. Embedded teeth were detected in 8.7%, root resorption of neighboring teeth in 3.8%, and undefined borderline in 3.6%. Embedded teeth were not surprisingly seen more often in younger patients. The size of the tumor was stated in 129 cases, the maximum size was 24 cm. The mean size was 4.3 cm, and the median size 3.0 cm. Ledesma-Montes et al. (44) reported ($N = 55$) a mean size of 6.7 cm for mandibular s/mAM and a mean size of 4.6 cm for the maxillary tumors.

Some s/mAM particularly those with a plexiform growth pattern show a highly vascular stroma, this feature may have an impact on the radiographic image making the lesion resemble a poorly-defined fibro-osseous lesion (49). In such cases, and in the diagnosis of ameloblastomas in general the use of computed tomography (CT) and magnetic resonance imaging (MRI) is highly recommended (47). Asaumi (50) demonstrated the quality of MRI and dynamic contrast-enhanced MRI in the study of 10 ameloblastomas. Solid and cystic portions of the tumor could be identified, mural nodules and thick walls could be

detected, and solid and fluid areas could be distinguished. No differences in the signal intensities between primary and recurrent cases were found.

Pathology. The etiology of the s/mAM is unknown. The pathogenesis is insufficiently understood. The tumor is believed to arise in remnants of odontogenic epithelium, primarily rests of the dental lamina, which however have been found primarily in the overlying gingiva or oral mucosa (14). The remnants of the epithelial root sheet (islands of Malassez) are usually not considered a likely source of ameloblastomas although some cases of early ameloblastoma in the periodontal area might suggest this as a possibility (51,52). Dentigerous cysts as a source of ameloblastoma cannot be excluded but it seems unlikely as discussed in the section on UNAM. It has some times been suggested that an ameloblastoma could develop from the basal cells of the overlying surface epithelium; it is well known that intraosseous ameloblastomas, which progress through the cortical bone and reaches contact with the surface epithelium may cause induction of the surface epithelium to produce ameloblastomatous proliferations. Since benign PERAMs do not invade the underlying bone, it is difficult to envision that intraosseous ameloblastomas should develop from the surface epithelium. Studies of cytokeratins (CK) (53) have also supported the hypothesis that ameloblastomas are of odontogenic origin and not direct derivates of basal cells of oral epithelium.

The macroscopical appearance of the operation specimen depends on the size of the tumor and the treatment modality. Resected tumors are surrounded by normal bone and may contain teeth. The tumor area is grayish and does not contain hard tissue apart from the border areas, it usually presents as a mixture of solid and multicystic areas, but some lesions are completely solid, and others are dominated by formation of cysts. The cysts are of varying size, usually most of them are small some are microscopic, but in large tumors several may be quite conspicuous. They are filled with a brownish fluid, which often is of low viscosity, but may be more gelatinous.

Microscopically the tumor consists of odontogenic epithelium growing in a relatively cell-poor collagenous stroma. Two growth patterns and four main cell types are recognized within the histopathological range of the entity (Table 2). The two growth patterns are named *follicular* and *plexiform*.

In the follicular pattern the tumor epithelium (Figs. 2, 3) primarily presents as islands of various size and shape (23,54). They usually consist of a

Table 2 Ameloblastoma Growth Patterns and Cell Types

Growth patterns
  Follicular growth pattern
  Plexiform growth pattern
Cell types
  Stellate reticulum-like cell type
  Acanthomatous (squamous cell) cell type
  Granular cell type
  Basal cell type

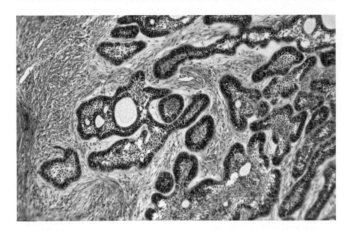

Figure 2 Solid/multicystic ameloblastoma with follicular growth pattern and stellate reticulum-like cells in the islands. Squamous metaplasia is seen in a few islands. Minor cysts are seen in the islands, as well as in the stroma. H&E stain.

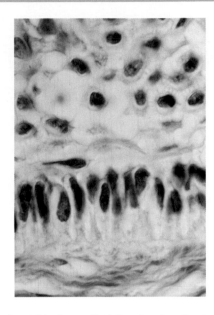

Figure 4 Ameloblastoma. Peripheral cells of a tumor island. The basal cells are palisaded and columnar with reverse polarity of the nucleus and show some morphological similarity to pre-ameloblasts. The suprabasal cells are stellate reticulum-like. van Gieson stain.

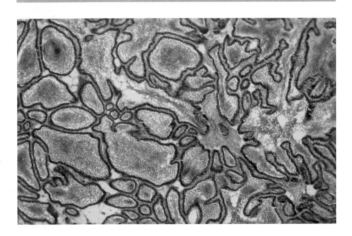

Figure 3 Solid/multicystic ameloblastoma with follicular growth pattern in a stroma consisting of narrow strands of collagenous connective tissue. H&E stain.

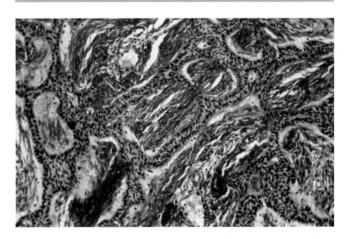

Figure 5 Solid/multicystic ameloblastoma with a plexiform growth pattern. van Gieson stain.

central mass of polyhedral or angular cells with prominent intercellular contact and conspicuous intercellular spaces. The morphology has some resemblance to the stellate reticulum of the normal enamel organ, but many details are different. The peripheral cells are palisaded, columnar, or cuboidal with dark nuclei. The columnar cells contain elongated nuclei, which may show reverse polarity and have a histomorphological likeness to preameloblasts (Fig. 4). Mitoses are absent or very infrequent. The term follicular alludes to a certain resemblance of the structure of the epithelial islands to enamel organs. The stellate reticulum-like cells may be replaced by squamous cells, granular cells, or basal cells (*vide infra*). If cysts develop, they arise in the center of the islands.

In the plexiform growth pattern (Fig. 5) the tumor epithelium is arranged as a network (plexus), which is bounded by a layer of cuboidal to columnar cells and includes stellate reticulum-like cells (23). The width of the epithelial cords in the network may vary considerably. Sometimes double row of columnar or cuboidal cells are lined up back to back. The peripheral cells are similar to those seen in the follicular pattern, although they are more often cuboidal and may even be squamous. In the plexiform type as well, but more rarely, the stellate reticulum-like cells may be replaced by squamous cells, granular cells, or basal

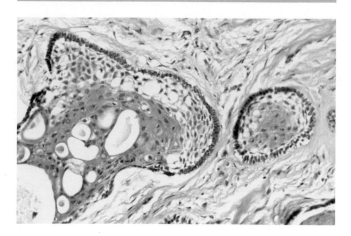

Figure 6 Islands of an ameloblastoma with follicular growth pattern. Squamous metaplasia is seen in the central areas. Ameloblastomas with extensive squamous metaplasia are termed acanthomatous. H&E stain.

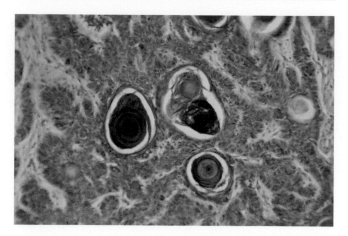

Figure 7 Unusual ameloblastoma with keratinization and calcification without conspicuous squamous metaplasia. The case was published by Pindborg et al. in 1958 (56). Periodic acid–Schiff stain. *Source*: Ref. 56.

cells. The stroma is generally looser than in the follicular pattern, and if cyst formation occurs, it is usually due to stromal degeneration rather than to a cystic change within the epithelium.

Each of the two growth patterns may be dominating in a s/mAM, but often both patterns are present in the same tumor. It is generally believed that the growth pattern is unrelated to the clinical behavior of the tumor, but some reports have suggested a higher tendency for recurrence in follicular than in plexiform ameloblastomas (55) and many molecular biological findings are different (5).

Squamous cell metaplasia of the central areas of the tumor epithelium is not unusual (Fig. 6), and is particularly seen in tumors with a follicular growth pattern. When extensive squamous metaplasia is seen, sometimes with keratin formation the term *acanthomatous ameloblastoma* is applied. This variant accounted for 12.1% of 397 cases reviewed by Reichart et al. (43). When cysts are formed in the epithelium, they are lined by squamous cells. The squamous cells are sometimes plump or fusiform and may exhibit few junctions.

Rarely an s/mAM shows formation of orthokeratinized or more often parakeratinized horn pearls in central areas of the tumor epithelium. It may even be seen in areas, which are not dominated by squamous cell metaplasia (Fig. 7). Very rarely calcifications are seen in these horn pearls (56).

The central stellate cells may be replaced by large eosinophilic rounded or polyhedral granular cells. The granules may be diastase resistant period acid–Schiff (PAS)-positive and they represent lysosomes. Most nuclei in these cells are placed at the periphery of the cells (Fig. 8). The granular cells may take up a complete epithelial island and then even the basal cells are granular. When a conspicuous part of the tumor or the entire tumor is composed of granular cells, the tumor is usually called a *granular cell ameloblastoma*.

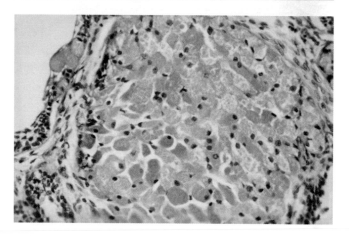

Figure 8 Granular cell ameloblastoma. The nuclei are placed in the periphery in most of the rounded cells. A few cuboidal basal cells are still seen. H&E stain.

Such tumors are infrequent, particularly those with a plexiform growth pattern (Fig. 9) (57,58).

Hartman (59) studied 20 cases of granular cell ameloblastom, which accounted for 5% of all ameloblastomas in their file and stated that they occurred predominantly in the posterior regions of the mandible (which is a predilection site for all s/mAMs). He observed that they had a marked tendency to recur after conservative treatment, but this behavior seems related to the treatment modality and not to the histology of the tumor.

Rarely, an ameloblastoma may show a predominantly basaloid pattern (Fig. 10), and this tumor is referred to as a *basal cell ameloblastoma*, or basaloid ameloblastoma (23). It is the least common of the cytological variants and accounted for 2% of the case reports reviewed by Reichart et al. (43). The epithelial

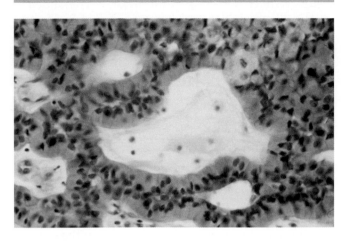

Figure 9 Granular cell ameloblastoma with plexiform growth pattern. H&E stain.

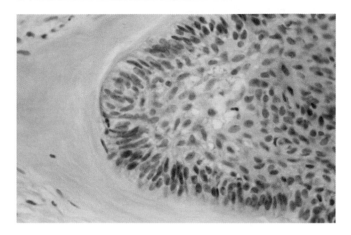

Figure 11 Ameloblastoma. Conspicuous stromal hyalinization is seen adjacent to a tumor island. H&E stain.

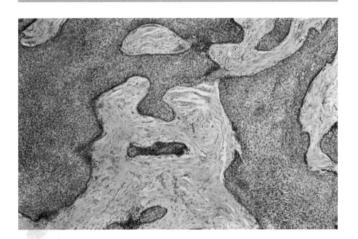

Figure 10 Basal cell type ameloblastoma from the posterior part of the maxilla of an 85-year-old man. The peripheral cells are primarily cuboidal. The tumor cell plates and islands show a highly increased cellular density. The cells are small with dark nuclei, and an elevated number of mitotic figures were found. H&E stain.

elements are composed almost exclusively of islands of plump cells with a high nucleus to cytoplasm ratio, and reticulum-like cells are few or absent (54). The periphery is dominated by cuboidal rather than columnar cells. Cystic changes in the epithelial component are infrequent.

Mucous cell metaplasia may be seen in the tumor epithelium, but is very rare (60,61).

Clear cells may be found in an s/mAM; if they occur in more than a few areas, a clear cell odontogenic carcinoma (CCOC) should be considered. The significance of clear cells is discussed in the section on that tumor.

Tumor cells containing melanin granules may be observed.

Various amounts of ghost cells may be seen, but they are not frequent (62). A dentinogenic ghost cell tumor (DGCT) should be considered, but the diagnosis requires that the tumor has formed dentinoid in the stroma adjacent to the epithelial tumor component.

The connective tissue stroma varies in amount, vascularity, and collagen content. No dental hard tissue is formed. The basement membrane may be thick and hyalinized, and this juxtaepithelial hyalinization may be conspicuous (Fig. 11). Few cells, if any are seen in the hyalinized zone. Scattered lymphocytes may be observed, but there is no inflammation, except caused by secondary factors.

In ameloblastomas with a plexiform growth pattern, a highly vascular stroma may be seen, and it may be in terms of several highly dilated vessels. The pattern should be considered within the spectrum of appearances of an ameloblastoma. Previously such cases were called hemangioameloblastoma (63).

Cystic degeneration of the stroma is not unusual in s/mAMs with a plexiform growth pattern. Residual capillaries may be found in these stromal cysts and cellular debris is a common finding in the cysts.

In a study of 31 cases of s/mAM Müller et al. (64) observed that infiltration of the surrounding spongy bone is frequent, but there was little tendency to invade cortical bone. They also found that periosteum largely prevented extension of the tumor. Gortzak et al. (65) studied five voluminous mandibular ameloblastomas after resection and confirmed the invasive growth pattern. Small tumor nests were found in the cancellous bone at a maximum distance of 5 mm from the bulk of the tumor (Fig. 12). Expansive and invasive growth in the Haversian canals was observed, but there was no invasion of the inferior alveolar nerve. The mucoperiosteal layer was invaded but not perforated, and no invasion was observed in the surrounding soft tissues of the periosteum and in the skin tissues. The authors stated that when the tumor is radiologically closer than 1 cm to the inferior border of the mandible, a continuity resection is mandatory.

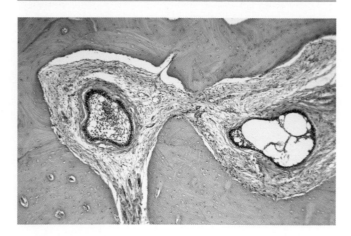

Figure 12 Solid/multicystic ameloblastoma. Invasion by tumor islands of the bone surrounding the tumor is the reason for excision with a margin of 1 to 1.5 cm. H&E stain.

Immunohistochemistry. Because ameloblastoma is one of the more common odontogenic tumors and because of the florid development of the immunohistochemical technique, the literature concerning immunohistochemical investigations of ameloblastomas is very extensive. Several investigators have used immunohistochemistry together with molecular biological methods to study a special subject, many of these reports published before the middle of 2005 were reviewed by Kumamoto in 2006 (5). These studies will primarily be reviewed in the section on molecular-genetic data.

The following summaries comprise primarily reports regarding cytofilaments, extracellular matrix proteins, basement associated molecules, protein kinases, and cell proliferation markers.

Heikinheimo et al. (53) studied the presence of CKs and vimentin in nine s/mAMs and three fetal human tooth germs at bell stage. They used eight antibodies against CKs, which individually or in combination could detect CK-4, CK-5, CK-6, CK-8, CK-10, CK-11, CK-13, CK-16, CK-17, CK-18, and CK-19. Most, but not all ameloblastomas lacked CKs typical of keratinization. CK-8 and CK-19 were expressed in all, and CK-18 in the epithelial component of most of the ameloblastomas, including the granular cell type, which expressed CK-8, CK-18, and CK-19 very distinctly. Vimentin was detected in the epithelial cells of all ameloblastomas except the granular cell type. The ameloblastomas and the human tooth germ epithelia shared a complex pattern of CK polypeptides together with the expression of vimentin. The authors concluded that the findings strongly supported that ameloblastomas are of odontogenic origin and not derived from basal cells of the gingiva or oral mucosa.

Crivelini et al. (66) performed a similar study on 10 ameloblastomas and four other types of odontogenic tumors. They used monoclonal antibodies against single CK types CK-7, CK-8, CK-10, CK-13, CK-14, CK-18, CK-19 and against vimentin. The results differed somewhat from those of Heikinheimo et al.; all ameloblastomas were CK-8, CK-18, and vimentin negative. They were all, including the granular cell type immunoreactive to CK-14. They also reacted to CK-13 and CK-19, but only in metaplastic squamous cells, central stellate cells and in the lining of cystic structures.

Extracellular matrix proteins and basement membrane associated molecules have been studied.

Ito et al. (67) detected versican, a large aggregating chondroitin sulfate proteoglycans in 17 ameloblastomas. All samples showed a positive reaction for versican in the connective tissues, whereas positive staining of epithelial nests was observed in only some samples.

Tenascin, an extracellular matrix glycoprotein was detected by Heikinheimo et al. (68) in the stromal component of all of 11 ameloblastomas. The epithelial component was negative. Nagai et al. (69) got very variable results in the study of 10 ameloblastomas. Hyalinized stroma was both positive and negative. Cystic stroma was negative. The basement membranes showed an irregular linear positive reaction with focal accumulation of tenascin. Mori et al. (70) on the other hand detected a strong reaction to tenascin in the interface around the epithelial component, although with frequent breaks. A positive reaction was found in stellate reticulum-like cells and granular epithelial cells as well.

Nadimi et al. (71) studied laminin in 29 ameloblastomas. An intense linear deposit was found in the basement areas of all of them. Heikinheimo et al. (68) confirmed these results.

Nadimi et al. (71) were unable to detect fibronectin except in areas with inflammation. Nagai et al. (69) got very variable results but detected an irregular linear immunoreaction in basement areas. Heikinheimo et al. (68) detected an extra domain sequence-A-containing form of fibronectin in the extracellular matrix of all ameloblastomas ($N = 11$), and an oncofetal domain containing form of fibronectin in most ameloblastomas. They studied collagen type VII as well; the immunoreaction was very similar to that of laminin: most ameloblastomas exhibited a continuous staining of the basement membranes.

Parikka et al. (72) detected collagen XVII, a hemidesmosomes transmembrane adhesion molecule, in the cytoplasm of basal and suprabasal cells in 11 s/mAMs and 2 UNAM using immunohistochemistry and in situ hybridization (ISH).

Poomsawat et al. (73) used antibodies against laminins 1 and 5, collagen type IV, and fibronectin on 14 ameloblastomas. An intense staining of laminin 1 and a weak to moderate intensity of laminin 5 were seen as continuous linear deposits at the basement membrane zone surrounding tumor islands. Collagen type IV showed irregular patterns; focal loss of staining was observed. A weak to moderate staining for fibronectin was occasionally present; fibronectin was also present in the fibrous stroma. The tumor cells also showed reaction to laminin 1 and 5, collagen type IV, and fibronectin. In general, laminin 1 showed moderate to strong intensity in the cytoplasm of both central and peripheral cells; collagen type IV was rarely observed. Laminin 5 was expressed in peripheral cells, but less often.

Collagen type IV was also studied by Nakano et al. (74) and Nagatsuka et al. (75). Nakano et al. found that ameloblastoma ($N = 2$) basement membranes expressed five of six genetically distinct forms of collagen IV: α1(IV), α2(IV), α5(IV), and α6(IV)—chains occurred as intense linear stainings without disruption around neoplastic epithelium. A similar study of 5 ameloblastomas by Nagatsuka et al. (75) gave the same results.

Integrin, a plasma membrane protein, which plays a role in the attachment of cell to cell and cell to the extracellular matrix, and as a signal transductor has been studied by Souza Andrada et al. (76). Integrin α2β1, α3β1, and α5β1 were detected in 20 s/mAMs, 10 UNAMs, and 12 AOT. The labeling intensity was considerably stronger in the ameloblastomas than in the AOTs, but no significant differences were found between the two variants of ameloblastoma. In s/mAMs the immunoreaction was detected in intercellular contacts and at the connective tissue interface.

Using immunohistochemistry, in situ hybridization, immunoprecipitation, and reverse transcriptase polymerase chain reaction (RT-PCR), Ida-Yonemochi et al. (77) detected basement-type heparan sulfate proteoglycan (HSPG), also known as Perlecan in the intercellular spaces of the epithelial component and in the stroma of 20 ameloblastomas and cultured ameloblastoma cells. The studies indicate that ameloblastoma cells synthesize HSPG.

The roles of mitogen-activated protein kinases (MAPKs) in oncogenesis and cytodifferentiation of odontogenic tumors were investigated by Kumamoto et al. (78), using antibodies against phosphorylated c-Jun NH$_2$-terminal kinase (p-JNK), phosphorylated p38 mitogen-activated protein kinases (p-p38 MAPK), and phosphorylated extracellular signal-regulated kinase 5 (p-ERK5) on 47 ameloblastomas (including 4 desmoplastic), 2 metastasizing ameloblastomas (METAMs), 3 ameloblastic carcinomas (AMCAs), and 10 human third molar tooth germs. Almost all s/mAMs were p-JNK negative. From 84% to 91% of the various histological types of ameloblastomas were moderately p-p38 MAPK positive. The basal cell ameloblastomas ($N = 3$), however, and the desmoplastic ameloblastomas (DESAMs) ($N = 4$) were 100% positive, three of six granular cell ameloblastomas were positive. Between 64% and 66% of the histological types of ameloblastoma were p-ERK5 positive, except basal cell and DESAM, which were 100% positive. The authors suggested that these MAPK signaling pathways contribute to cell proliferation, differentiation, or apoptosis in both normal and neoplastic odontogenic tissues.

Cell proliferation markers have been studied by several investigators. The results have been somewhat contradictory. Kim et al. (79) used antibodies against proliferating cell nuclear antigen (PCNA) on 25 s/mAMs and 13 unicystic types and a case of AMCA. There was no significant difference between the proliferating activities of the different histological types of s/mAM, but a recurrent ameloblastoma and the

AMCA showed remarkably higher PCNA activity. Funaoka et al. (80) measured the PCNA index in 23 s/mAMs, they found a higher, but not significantly higher index in follicular than in plexiform ameloblastomas. Interestingly, they found a remarkable difference in the index of biopsies of the same tumor taken at different times. Ong'uti et al. (81) measured the Ki-67 index in 54 s/mAMs, 24 follicular, and 30 plexiform. They found a significantly higher labeling index (L.I.) in ameloblastomas with a follicular growth pattern than in those with a plexiform pattern. They did not find any significant correlation between the Ki-67 L.I. and clinical features like age, gender, and tumor size.

Piattelli et al. (82) evaluated the proliferative activity of 22 ameloblastoma among which 13 were s/mAM by measuring the immunoreactivity of PCNA. Recurrent ameloblastoma ($N = 4$) presented higher PCNA positive cell counts than other types of ameloblastoma.

Sandra et al. (83) used antibodies against PCNA and Ki-67 on 25 s/mAMs, 5 unicystic, and 3 DESAMs, and measured the indices. There was a strong correlation between the PCNA and the Ki-67 labeling indices. Positively stained cells were primarily found in the peripheral layers. The basal cell types of ameloblastomas showed the highest L.I., but it was not significantly higher than that of follicular, plexiform, and acanthomatous types. It was significantly higher, however, than the labeling indices measured in unicystic and DESAMs. On the contrary, Meer et al. (84) found a statistically significantly higher PCNA and Ki-67 L.I. in unicystic ($N = 10$) than in the s/m variant ($N = 10$).

Thosaporn et al. (85) used antibodies against a novel cell proliferation marker, IPO-38 (N-L 116) on 10 ameloblastomas, 10 keratocystic odontogenic tumors (KCOTs), 7 orthokeratinized odontogenic cysts, and 8 dentigerous cysts. Positive nuclei were found in the peripheral cell layers of the ameloblastomas. The L.I. was similar to that of the KCOTs, but twice as high as that of the orthokeratinized odontogenic cysts and 14 times higher than that of the dentigerous cysts.

Payeras et al. (86) evaluated the proliferation activity in 11 cases of s/mAM by means of quantification of the argyrophilic nuclear organizer regions (AgNORs) and the pattern of immunohistochemical expression of the epidermal growth factor receptor (EGF-R). There was no significant statistical difference as per quantification of the AgNORs, the expression of the EGF-R on the epithelial islands of ameloblastoma was not uniform, and the location of the expression was also variable. The authors concluded that the tumor presents an irregular growth, and that smaller epithelial islands could be responsible for tumor infiltration since they are associated with a higher proliferation activity.

Granular cell ameloblastoma has been studied in particular by Kumamoto et al. (87). Granular cells were positive for CK, CD68, lysozyme, and alpha-1-antichymotrypsin, but negative for vimentin, desmin, S-100 protein, neuron-specific enolase (NSE) and CD 15, indicating epithelial origin and lysosomal aggregation. The authors suggested that the cytoplasmic granularity in granular cell ameloblastomas might be caused by increased apoptotic cell death of neoplastic cells and associated phagocytosis by neighboring neoplastic cells.

Electron Microscopy. Several studies have reported the ultrastructure of the ameloblastoma, Moe et al. (88), Sujaku et al. (89), Csiba et al. (90), Navarrette et al. (91) Lee et al. (92), Mincer et al. (93), Cutler et al. (94), Tandler et al. (95), Kim et al. (96), Matthiessen et al. (97), Rothouse et al. (98), Chomette et al. (99), Nasu et al. (100), Takeda et al. (101), Smith et al. (102), and Farman et al. (103). Some of the earlier studies concentrated on ultrastructural similarities between the columnar peripheral epithelial cells of the s/mAM and the preameloblasts of the normal enamel organ (88,89,92,93). Kim et al. (96) and Matthiessen et al. (97) confirmed this similarity and further observed that the stellate cells of the tumor epithelium were in many respects similar to the stellate reticulum of the normal enamel organ. They were joined by desmosomes and the nucleus occupied a central position within the cell. The perinuclear cytoplasm contained mitochondria, tonofilaments, endoplasmic reticulum, and dense granules. Some epithelial cells contained numerous lipid granules and mitochondria formed a network of cords. Matthiessen et al. (97) found that the low peripheral cells in s/mAM were very similar to the external enamel epithelium cells. The central cells of the islands had a certain resemblance to the stellate reticulum and stratum intermedium cells. The high peripheral cells of the s/mAM had no counterpart in the enamel organ. Unlike the enamel organ the ameloblastoma showed extremely few and small gap junctions.

The ultrastructural features of squamous epithelial cells were similar to those described for basal cells and lower prickle cells of the oral mucosa. The granular cells in particular were studied by Navarrette et al. (91) and Tandler et al. (95) and Nasu et al. (104). The granular cells commonly occur in the islands of ameloblastomas with a follicular growth pattern, in one of the cases reported by Nasu et al. (104), they were in a plexiform pattern. The cytoplasmic granules were identified as lysosomes, supported by the fact that they were intensively stained for acid phosphatase; no cytoplasmic components were found in the numerous lysosomes, they do not seem to be engaged in autophagy, their function is unknown. The occurrence of intracytoplasmic desmosomes was described by described by Cutler et al. (94) in an ameloblastom from the maxilla. Hyaline bodies, a structure that is relatively common in odontogenic cysts were observed by Takeda et al. (101), ultrastructurally they did not differ from those found in the epithelium of the wall of odontogenic cysts. Farman et al. (103) studied the interface between the tumor component and the stroma in seven ameloblastomas. All showed differing degrees of thickening of lamina densa by a granulofilamentous material having a range of width of approximately 80 to 800 nm. Fragmentation of the granulofilamentous material was seen in several instances. The resulting defects were less linear and

had more of a soap bubble appearance. The hyaline cell free zone, which may be seen adjacent to the epithelium, comprised relatively cell-free, normally banded, mature collagen. The stroma contains fibroblasts and collagen fibers. Multinucleated giant cells near the epithelial component were described by Kim et al. (96). Rothouse et al. (98) detected myofibroblasts in the stroma, a finding that was confirmed by Smith et al. (102) in a case of recurrent s/mAM.

Molecular-Genetic Data. It is not possible within the frame of this chapter to review all studies of the molecular pathology of the ameloblastoma. A comprehensive review of the molecular pathology of odontogenic tumors covering the literature till the middle of 2005 was published by Kumamoto (5), the majority of the studies deals with ameloblastomas. For the following summaries the same subheadings as used by Kumamoto have been used; the majority of articles have been selected because they were not mentioned in Kumamoto's review or were published subsequently.

1. Molecules Involved in Tumorigenesis and/or Cell Differentiation of Ameloblastomas.

a. *Oncogenes.* In ameloblastomas, $p21^{Ras}$ is expressed in the epithelial cells and overexpression has been detected (105). c-Myc oncoprotein is expressed predominantly in the tumor cells neighboring the basement membrane (106). On cDNA microarray and subsequent real-time reverse transcriptase RT-PCR overexpression of Fos has been detected (107).

b. *Gene Modifications.* Jääskeläinen et al. (108) used immunocytochemical staining with MIB-1 antibodies and comparative genomic hybridization (CGH) to study cell proliferation and chromosomal imbalances in 20 cases of ameloblastoma. CGH involved hybridization of FITC-dUTP-labeled tumor DNA with Texas-red-labeled normal DNA. The MIB-1 index was low for all tumors and was not correlated to the tendency to recur; it does not seem helpful in assessing future clinical behavior of the tumor. Chromosomal aberrations were only detected in 2 of 17 cases.

Carinci et al. (109) compared the expression profiles of three ameloblastomas and three malignant odontogenic tumors by hybridization to microarrays containing 19,200 cDNAs to identify genes, which were significantly differentially regulated when compared with nonneoplastic tissues. The investigators detected 43 cDNAs, which differentiated the three malignant tumors from the three ameloblastomas. The cancer specific genes included a range of functional activities like transcription, signaling transduction, cell-cycle regulation, apoptosis, differentiation, and angiogenesis. The authors suggested that the identified genes might help to better classify borderline odontogenic tumors.

A study for loss of heterozygosity of tumor suppressor genes in 12 ameloblastomas revealed that DNA damage in ameloblastomas seems to be sporadic and cumulative (110). The frequency of allelic loss and intratumoral heterogeneity did not correlate with age, gender, histological subtype, or prognosis.

In a study performed to identify possible genes involved in the development and progression of ameloblastomas the investigators used microarray analysis, semiquantitative RT-PCR and immunohistochemistry on selected genes (111). Tissue from dentigerous cysts was used as control. Overexpression of 73 genes was detected and 49 genes were underexpressed.

Mutations in microsatellite sequences have been studied in 24 ameloblastomas by DNA sequencing analysis (112) and supplied with an evaluation of the Ki67 L.I. of the tumors. The occurrence and the pattern of microsatellite alterations, in form of loss or length variation, was evaluated and correlated with the Ki67 L.I. and with other clinicopathological parameters. Alterations of at least one of the selected loci were observed in all (100%) the ameloblastomas with a mean of four altered microsatellites for each tumor. Microsatellite alterations were more frequent in tumors displaying a high Ki67 L.I., and in a univariate analysis, their occurrence was found to be a predictor of increased risk of recurrence, but no correlation was found to the patient's age or gender, or to tumor size, location and histology.

c. *Tumor Suppressor Genes.* Increased immunohistochemical reactivity for p53 has been detected in ameloblastomas (113,114), although it has been shown in several studies that p53 mutations are infrequent in ameloblastomas (115–117). Regulators of p53, murine double minute 2 (MDM2), and p14 (ARF), are also expressed in ameloblastomas, and overexpression has been detected (118,119).

Two members of theTP53 gene family, named p73 and p63, have been identified and analyzed by immunohistochemistry and RT-PCR in ameloblastomas. They seem to function differently from p53 in odontogenic tissue (120). Immunohistochemical reactivity for p63 was detected by Lo Muzio et al. (121) in 26 s/mAMs and several other benign and malignant odontogenic tumors. Benign odontogenic, locally aggressive tumors with a high risk of recurrence exhibited statistically higher p63 expression than benign odontogenic, nonaggressive tumors with a low risk of recurrence.

The immunohistochemical reactivity for the APC gene that inhibits cell proliferation was found to be lower in benign and malignant ameloblastomas than in tooth germs (122).

Retinoblastoma protein (RB) is a product of the *retinoblastoma (RB)* tumor suppressor gene, which acts as a signal transducer connecting the cell cycle with the transcription machinery. Kumamoto et al. (123) used antibodies against RB, E-2 promotor-binding-factor-1(E2F-1), and phosphorylated RB on 40 ameloblastomas (including 4 desmoplastic), 2 METAMs, 3 AMCAs, and 10 human tooth germs to clarify their roles in cell-cycle regulation in oncogenesis and cytodifferentiation of odontogenic tumors. Ki-67 antibody was used as a marker of cell proliferation. The levels of immunoreactivity for RB, E2F-1, phosphorylated RB, and Ki-67 were slightly higher in benign and malignant ameloblastomas than in tooth germs. Plexiform ameloblastomas showed significantly higher expression of RB than follicular ameloblastomas. Expression of RB, E2F-1, and phosphorylated RB was considered to be involved in cell proliferation and differentiation of odontogenic epithelium via control of the cell cycle.

d. *DNA-Repair Genes.* Errors during DNA replication or repair are maintained by DNA-repair genes belonging to the human DNA mismatch repair (hMMR) system. It is composed of at least six genes. The protein expression of two of the genes, hMSH2 and hMLH1 was studied by means of antibodies in 25 cases of ameloblastoma, including three peripheral and three unicystic (124). All ameloblastomas showed a nuclear expression of the proteins in the peripheral layers of the epithelial component. These data suggest that the development and progression of these tumors do not depend on a defect in the hMMR system.

e. *Oncoviruses.* Although several investigators have reported detection of human papillomavirus (HPV) (125–128) and Epstein–Barr virus (EBV) (129) in ameloblastomas the etiological role of the viruses remains controversial.

f. *Growth Factors.* Using ISH Heikinheimo et al. (130) detected EGF-R and transforming growth factor alpha (TGF-α) mRNA in 4 ameloblastomas; EGF transcripts was not found. The findings have been confirmed (131,132). The growth factors seem to be involved in the tumogenesis.

Transforming growth factor beta (TGF-β), a multifunctional growth factor has been demonstrated in ameloblastomas and has been attributed an important role in cell differentiation and matrix formation (133,134).

Hepatocyte growth factor (HGF), which has mitogenic, motogenic, and morphogenic functions, has been found in ameloblastomas (134).

Various types of fibroblast growth factors (FGF) and their receptors (FGFR) have been studied. FGF-1 and FGF-2 are mitogenic polypeptides that have been demonstrated to enhance cell growth in a dose dependent manner of cultered ameloblastoma epithelial cells (135). In tissue specimens, FGF-1 was localized in the epithelial component, whereas FGF-2 was primarily found in the basement membranes. In another study (136), ameloblastomas showed a weak and focal reaction for FGF-1 and FGFR3 in the tumor epithelium, while FGF-2 and FGFR2 exhibited significant cytoplasmic staining of all layers of the neoplastic epithelium.

Expression of platelet-derived endothelial cell growth factor/thymidine phosphorylase (PD-ECGF/TP) and of angiopoietins have been detected immunohistochemically in the stroma of ameloblastomas and in the ectomesenchymal cells of human tooth germs (137). The level of PD-ECGF/TP reactivity was significantly higher in ameloblastomas than in tooth germs. Granular cell ameloblastoma showed PD-ECGF/TP reactivity in granular neoplastic cells as well as in stromal cells. Immunoreactivity for angiopoietins-1 and -2 was detected predominantly in odontogenic epithelial cells near the basement membrane in tooth germs and in the ameloblastomas.

The authors suggested that these angiogenic factors participate in tooth development and odontogenic tumor progression by regulating angiogenesis.

The immunohistochemical expression of insulin-like growths factors (IGFs), platelet-derived growth factor (PDGF), and their receptors has been analyzed in 47 ameloblastomas and 10 human tooth germs (138) by use of antibodies against IGF-I, IGF-II, IGF-I receptor (IGF-IR), PDGF A-chain, PDGF B-chain, PDGF α-receptor, and PDGF β-receptor. The reactivity for IGFs, PDGF chains, and their receptors was detected predominantly in odontogenic epithelial cells near the basement membrane in tooth germs as well as in ameloblastomas. The expression levels of IGF-II and PDGF chains were significantly higher in the tumors than in the tooth germs, and the expression level of PDGF chains were significantly higher in follicular ameloblastomas than in plexiform ameloblastomas. DESAMs showed higher expression of IGFs and IGFIR when compared with other ameloblastoma subtypes. These growth factor signals thus contribute to cell proliferation or survival in both normal and neoplastic odontogenic tissues.

g. *Telomerase.* Ameloblastomas have been consistently positive for telomerase activity suggesting that telomerase activation is associated with the tumorigenesis of the neoplastic epithelium (139,140). Telomerase is a specialized reverse transcriptase that synthesizes telomeric DNA at the ends of chromosomes and compensates for its loss with each cell division, and is thus a participant in cell immortalization. The immunoreactivity for telomerase in ameloblastomas shows a similar distribution pattern to that of the c-Myc oncoprotein. This oncogenic protein is known to activate telomerase transcription directly, so it possibly induces telomerase activity in ameloblastomas.

h. *Cell Cycle Regulators.* The immunoreaction of cell cycle-related factors were examined by Kumamoto et al. (141) in 8 human tooth germs and 31 ameloblastomas by means of antibodies against cyclin D1, $p16^{INK4a}$, $p2^{WAF1/Cip1}$, $p27^{Kip1}$, and DNA topoisomerase IIα and by ISH of histoneH3 mRNA. Cyclin D1, p16 protein, p21, and p27 were all expressed in the epithelium of tooth germs and ameloblastomas, although p21 was not expressed in granular epithelial cells and keratinizing cells. It is suggested that the odontogenic epithelium is strictly controlled by these cell cycle regulators.

i. *Apoptosis-Related Factors.* Physiological cell death, apoptosis is mediated by two alternative apoptotic pathways, death by receptors or death by mitochondria. A commonly used method to detect apoptosis is called TUNEL (Terminal deoxynucleotidyl transferase biotin-dUTP-nick-end labeling). Other ways of detection of apoptotic cells and specific parts of the apoptotic pathway are detection of caspase, fas-ligand, and annexin V activity. TUNEL and single-stranded DNA (ssDNA), fas-ligand, and caspase-3 antibodies have been used to detect apoptotic cells in ameloblastomas and ghost cell odontogenic carcinoma (GCOC) (87,114,142–145). Death receptors

such as fas, tumor necrosis factor (TNF) receptor I, and TNF-related apoptosis-related ligand (TRAIL) 1 and 2 have been demonstrated in ameloblastomas, but expression of caspase-8, an apoptosis initiator has been extremely limited, suggesting that apoptotic cell death in ameloblastomas is minimally affected by signaling of death factors (144,146).

Bcl-2 and inhibitor of apoptosis (IAP) family proteins are modulators of the mitochondrial apoptotic pathway. In ameloblastomas, apoptosis inhibitory factors, such as Bcl-2, Bcl-x, surviving, and X chromosome–linked IAP (XIAP) are predominantly expressed, which may indicate that these apoptosis modulators are associated with survival and neoplastic transformation of the odontogenic epithelial cells (147–149).

Factors involved in the apoptosis signaling pathways mediated by mitochondria have been investigated in ameloblastomas and normal human tooth germs (150). Tissue specimens were examined by RT-PCR and antibodies against cytochrome c, apoptotic protease-activating factor-1 (APAF-1), caspase-9, and apoptosis-inducing factor (AIF). The mRNA expression of APAP-1, caspase-9, and AIF was detected in all samples and immunoreactivity for cytochrome c, APAP-1, caspase-9, and AIF was positive in all samples. The results suggest that the mitochondria-mediated apoptotic pathway has a role in apoptotic cell death of normal and neoplastic odontogenic epithelium.

Expressions of tumor-necrosis-factor-related apoptosis-inducing ligand (TRAIL/Apo2L), a potent ligand in inducing apoptosis, has been studied in 32 ameloblastomas and in AM-1 cells (an HPV-16 infected ameloblastoma cell line) together with death receptor 4 (DR4) and 5 (DR5). It was observed that TRAIL cleaved caspase-8, -9, and -3, lowered mitochondrial membrane potential and markedly induced apoptosis in AM-1 cells. The results suggested that TRAIL is a potent apoptosis-inducing ligand in ameloblastoma (151). Osteoprotegerin (OPG) is a receptor that is capable in inhibiting receptor activator of nuclear factor-κB ligand (RANKL) in inducing osteoclastogenesis. As mentioned above TRAIL is a potent apoptosis-inducing ligand in ameloblastomas. The expression of OPG in ameloblastomas has been investigated by immunohistochemistry, immunofluorescense, and Western blot (152), and was observed in tissue samples from 20 ameloblastomas as well as in cultured ameloblastoma cells (AM-1). An apoptosis assay was performed to investigate the potential of TNF-α, TRAIL, and RANKL in inducing apoptosis. It was found that TRAIL had the highest potential in inducing apoptosis compared with TNF-α and RANKL. A binding assay revealed that OPG preferably binds with RANKL, rather than with TRAIL. The results suggest that the binding of OPG to TRAIL might cause TRAIL to induce apoptosis in ameloblastomas.

TNF-α is involved in inducing cell survival, proliferation, differentiation, and apoptosis. Its expression has been studied in 24 ameloblastomas and in AM-1 cells, and TNF-α as well as its receptors (TNFR1 and TNFR2) were clearly observed in all ameloblastoma samples and in AM-1 cells.

TNF-α-induced Akt (protein kinase) and MAPK signals were studied as well (153). The results suggested that TNF-α can induce Akt and p44/42 MAPK activation through PI3K (phosphatidylinositol-3-OH kinase), which might later induce cell survival and proliferation in ameloblastoma. In a subsequent study (154), it was observed that prolonged treatment of AM-1 cells with TNF-α induced the cells into apoptosis.

j. *Regulators of Tooth Development.* Underexpression of *Sonic Hedgehog* (*SHH*) gene and of *Patched* (*PTCH*), a cell-surface transmembrane protein has been shown in ameloblastomas on cDNA microarray (107). *SHH* is involved in the morphogenesis and cytodifferentiation of teeth. *SHH* signals control cell-to-cell interactions and cell proliferation in tissue patterning of various organs, including teeth. By means of RT-PCR and immunohistochemistry, Kumamoto et al. (155) detected expressions of SHH, *PTCH*, Smoothened (SMO), a membrane bounded protein, and GLI1 (a zinc finger DNA–binding protein) in ameloblastomas. Expression of SHH, *PTCH*, and GLI1 was more evident in epithelial than in mesenchymal cells, whereas SMO reactivity was marked in both components. Keratinizing and granular cells showed no or little reactivity.

The Wnt signaling pathway is a complex network of proteins involved in embryogenesis (including odontogenesis) and oncogenesis. Wnt signaling is regulated by the levels of the protein β-catenin. Mutations of β-catenin are detected frequently in COCs but are rare in ameloblastomas (156,157). The β-catenin protein is expressed in the nuclei of the ameloblastomas (122).

The transmembrane heparan sulfate proteoglycan, Syndecan-1 (SDC-1), also known as CD 138 and Wingless type 1 glycoprotein (Wnt1), which belongs to a large family of 19 secreted signal transducers and promotes cell proliferation has been detected in 29 s/mAMs, but not consistently (158). Immunostaining of SDC-1 was observed in the epithelial component as well as in the stroma cells. Wnt1 was almost exclusively seen in the epithelial tumor cells. The authors suggested that SDC-1 is a critical factor for Wnt-induced carcinogenesis in the odontogenic epithelium.

k. *Hard Tissue-Related Proteins.* Immunohistochemical expression of enamel proteins, such as enamelin, enamelysin, and sheathlin could not be detected in ameloblastomas (159–161). Amelogenin, however has been demonstrated immunohistochemically (162,163) and by mRNA phenotyping in combination with Northern blot analysis and ISH analysis of mRNA (164). Ameloblastin (AMBN) gene mutations were detected in two s/mAMs, an exon 11 mutation in a follicular ameloblastoma and a compound exon 4 mutation in a follicular ameloblastoma (165). The expression pattern of X and Y amelogenin genes (AMGX and AMGY) was studied in 19 ameloblastomas (9 male and 10 female) by RT-PCR, ISH, immunohistochemistry, and restriction enzyme digestion (166). All tumor samples expressed amelogenin mRNA. An increased level of AMGY expression, higher than that of AMGX was detected in all male samples, in contrast to normal male tooth development,

where expression of AMGY is very much lower than that of AMGX.

Bone sialoprotein (BSP) has been detected in the neoplastic epithelial component of ameloblastoma, but not in the stroma using cRNA ISH and immunohistochemistry (167). BSP is synthesized and secreted by bone- dentine- and cementum-forming cells and is implicated in de novo formation of bone formation and mineralization, but seems also involved in oncogenesis.

Gao et al. (168) were unable to detect bone morphogenetic protein (BMP) in 20 ameloblastomas by means of antibodies. On the contrary, Kumamoto et al. (169) demonstrated BMP, bone morphogenetic protein receptor (BMPR), core-binding factor α1 (CBFA1) [also known as run-related protein 2 (RUNX2)], and osterix, a zinc finger–containing transcription factor in the epithelial component as well as in the stroma cells of 31 ameloblastomas; 6 granular cell ameloblastomas, however showed no reaction in the granular cells. Acanthomatous ameloblastomas exhibited increased reactivity of BMP-7 in keratinizing cells. The investigators used RT-PCR and immunohistochemistry.

2. Molecules Involved in Progression of Ameloblastomas.

l. *Cell Adhesion Molecules.* Ameloblastomas express vascular endothelium cell adhesion molecules such as the cellular adhesion receptors ICAM-1, E-selectin, and VCAM-1 suggesting that stromal blood vessels are activated in these tumors (170).

E-cadherin and its undercoat protein α-catenin were detected in 24 ameloblastomas by means of monoclonal antibodies (171). There was a loss of expression in keratinizing areas and reduction in granular cell clusters. Several integrin subunits, $α_2$, $α_3$, and $β_4$ and CD 44 exhibited immunoreaction in 22 ameloblastomas that were studied to clarify the role of these cell adhesion molecules in epithelial odontogenic tumors (172). CD 44 showed decreased expression in keratinizing areas in acanthomatous ameloblastomas. Integrins and CD 44 are both families of cell surface glycoproteins that mediate cell-cell and cell–extracellular matrix adhesion. In an immunohistochemical study of 14 ameloblastomas with antibodies against integrin subunits, $α_2$, $α_3$, $α_5$, αv, $β_1$, $β_3$, and $β_4$ all integrins were detected. The immunoreaction showed variations in distribution and staining intensity(173).

m. *Matrix-Degrading Proteinases.* The role of proteolytic enzymes in extracellular matrix degradation has been studied by several investigators (174–178). Matrix metalloproteinases (MMPs) and their tissue inhibitors (TIMPs) were found in 22 ameloblastomas by means of antibodies against MMP-1, MMP-2 and MMP-9, and TIMP-1, and TIMP-2 (174). Intense reactivity for these antibodies was found in the cytoplasm of stromal fibroblasts, a weak reaction for MMP-2, MMP-9, and TIMP-1was found in the tumor cells of some s/mAMs. A strong expression of TIMP-2 was found on the basement membrane and in the stromal cells. These results were essentially confirmed by Pinheiro et al. (175) using immunohistochemistry, zymography, and

Western blotting. They observed expression of latent and active forms of MMP-1, -2 and -9, and compared the results with AgNOR analysis, which was used simultaneously. They found a strong reaction for the MMPs in granular cells of ameloblastomas. The MMPs might digest bone matrix and release mitogenic factors. The hypothesis was supported by the finding of an increased proliferation index in tumor cells in the vicinity of the bone. In a study of matrix-degrading proteinases regulators the immunohistochemical expression of MMP, membrane type 1-matrix metalloproteinase (MT1-MMP), MMP inhibitor RECK (reversion-inducing cysteine-rich protein with Kazal motifs), and EMMPRIN (extracellular matrix metalloproteinase inducer) were detected in the majority of 40 ameloblastomas (176). The reactivity was seen predominantly in tumor cells near the basement membrane. Follicular ameloblastomas showed significantly lower expression of RECK than plexiform ameloblastomas.

Heparanase, an endo-glucuronidase enzyme that specifically cleaves heparan sulfate has been detected by immunohistochemistry and mRNA ISH in 23 ameloblastomas (177). The enzyme was strongly expressed in the tumor epithelium of all samples. A weak reaction was seen in stromal cells adjacent to tumor cells, a stronger reaction was seen in inflammatory cells and endothelial cells of small blood capillaries. Heparanase is believed to contribute in the local invasiveness of the tumor.

The roles of EMC-degrading serine proteinases in progression of ameloblastomas has been evaluated by studying the immunoexpression of urokinase-type plasminogen activator (uPA), uPA receptor (uPAR), plasminogen activator inhibitor 1 (PAI-1), and maspin (a serine proteinase inhibitor) in 45 ameloblastomas (178). The uPA was recognized predominantly in mesenchymal cells, uPAR was evident in epithelial cells, PAI-1 was found in both epithelial and mesenchymal cells, and maspin was expressed only in epithelial cells. The findings suggest that interactions among these molecules contribute to EMC degradation and cell migration during tumor progression.

n. *Angiogenic Factors.* The association between vascular endothelial growth factor (VEGF) immunohistochemical expression and tumor angiogenesis has been studied in 35 ameloblastomas (179). Increased expression of VEGF, which enhances angiogenesis and vascular permeability, was found in peripheral tumor cells and in stromal cells adjacent to these cells, which suggests that VEGF is an important mediator of tumor angiogenesis in ameloblastomas. Granular cell clusters in granular cell ameloblastomas showed low reactivity.

o. *Osteolytic Cytokines.* The balance between bone formation and bone resorption is regulated by a wide variety of hormones, growth factors, and cytokines. Synthesizing of inflammatory cytokines with osteolytic activity such as interleukin-1 (IL-1), interleukin-6 (IL-6), and TNF-α in ameloblastomas has been demonstrated by several investigators (146,170,180,181).

Osteoclast differentiation and activation is stimulated by binding of receptor activator of RANKL to its receptor RANK, which is expressed on osteoclast precursors. Osteoprotegerin (OPG) functions as a decoy receptor for RANKL and inhibits osteoclastogenesis and osteoclast activation. RANKL and OPG have been detected in ameloblastomas predominantly in the stromal cells rather than in the neoplastic cells (182,183). The secretion of RANKL and TNF-α in ameloblastomas and its role in osteoclastogenesis has been confirmed (184).

Differential Diagnosis. Ameloblastomas with a plexiform growth pattern may be difficult to distinguish from hyperplastic odontogenic epithelium so commonly seen in the walls of odontogenic cysts. At low-power microscopy, a network of epithelial strands embracing islands of loose connective tissue is seen in both cases. If the basal cells are cuboidal or squamous in stead of columnar this criteria is not very helpful, and if the suprabasal epithelial cells are squamous rather than reticulum cell-like it may lead to diagnostic confusion (54). Inflammation is usually seen in the cystic environment and is rare in ameloblastomas and may be a useful feature, and the clinical and radiographic features should be included in the diagnostic decision.

The acanthomatous ameloblastoma should be distinguished from the SOT. In the latter, the stroma is more abundant; in the tumor component all cells are squamous cells, no stellate reticulum-like cells are seen, cyst formation is absent, and the peripheral cells are flattened.

The granular cell type of the s/mAM may be confused with the granular cell odontogenic tumor (GCOT). The main difference is that the s/mAM is an epithelial tumor and that the granular cells are epithelial, while the tumor component of the granular cell tumor is ectomesenchymal and the granular cells of the same origin. Cords and islands of odontogenic epithelium are seen, but they are quite different from the proliferating epithelium of an ameloblastoma.

A dental papilla–like connective tissue is never seen in an ameloblastoma, if it is observed in the tumor together with odontogenic epithelium with the morphology of an ameloblastoma, the extremely rare odonto-ameloblastoma (O-A) should be considered. If dental hard tissue has been produced in the dental papilla–like areas, the diagnosis is more straightforward.

The intraosseous basal cell ameloblastoma should be differentiated from the AMCA. Although hypercellularity and hyperchromatic nuclei may be seen in a basal cell ameloblastoma, numerous mitoses, nuclear and cellular pleomorphia, vascular and neural invasion are signs of malignancy and not a feature of this tumor.

Treatment and Prognosis. There has been some difference of opinion about the preferable methods of treatment of the s/mAM, and there is still no consensus. Nakamura et al. (185) reported on a long-term follow-up of treatment of 27 unicystic, 21 multicystic, and 30 solid ameloblastomas. In spite of a recurrence rate of 33.3% after conservative surgery compared with 7.1% after radical surgery, the authors advocated for conservative treatment except when the tumor invades and destroys the inferior border of the mandible, or when the tumor infiltration is close to the scull base. Huang et al. (186) advocated for a conservative treatment of ameloblastomas of children on the basis of a study of 8 unicystic and 7 s/mAMs. They stated that recurrence is probably not the most important consideration in the treatment of ameloblastomas in children. Other investigators have strongly advocated for radical surgical procedures in the treatment of s/mAM (187). Hong et al. (55) reported on a long-term follow-up of the treatment of 305 ameloblastomas and concluded that recurrence of an ameloblastoma in large part reflects the inadequacy or failure of the primary surgical procedure. In a review of the literature, Carlson et al. (47) stated that conservative treatment has an unpredictable course and that the presumption that small foci of persistent disease can always be treated adequately is inaccurate. They studied 82 cases of resected s/mAMs and showed that the tumor extends with a range of 2 to 8 mm (mean 4.5 mm) beyond its radiographic demarcation on specimen radiographs. They recommended resection with 1 to 1.5 cm linear bone margin. Ghandhi et al. (188) compared 22 cases from West Scotland with 28 cases from San Francisco with very similar clinical features. Primary care by conservative treatment led to recurrence in approximately 80% of cases, including cases of UNAM. The recurrence rate following local enucleation and curettage was unacceptably high, and this included cases of UNAM as well. Gortzak et al. (65) advocated for radical surgery and recommended continuity resection of the mandible if the tumor is radiologically closer than 1 cm to the inferior border of the mandible. They did not consider removal of an excess of perimandibular soft tissue indicated, but the overlying attached mucosal surface should be excised together with the underlying bone.

Radiotherapy and chemotherapy is discouraged.

Recurrence may occur several years after surgical treatment. Demeulemeester et al. (189) reported five cases with multiple and extremely late recurrences, some were diagnosed 24 and 27 years after primary surgery. Hayward (190) reported a case, which recurred first 3 years and then 30 years after conservative treatment.

Chapelle et al. (191) recommended partial maxillectomy or marginal or segmental resection as the treatment of intraosseous ameloblastoma, independent of imaging (unilocular or multilocular) with subsequent yearly follow-up the first five years, and every two years thereafter, for at least 25 years.

1.1.1.2 Solid/Multicystic Ameloblastoma–Peripheral.

Introduction. The PERAM is a rare, benign, slowly growing, exophytic lesion occurring on the gingiva or the attached alveolar ridge mucosa in edentulous areas. Histologically it consists of an unencapsulated focal mass of neoplastic odontogenic epithelium, which may show any of the features characteristic of the intraosseous ameloblastoma.

ICD-O code 9310/0

Synonyms: Soft tissue ameloblastoma, ameloblastoma of mucosal origin, ameloblastoma of the gingiva.

Clinical Features. The prevalence and incidence of the PERAM is unknown; it is a rare tumor. In reviews of material received for histological diagnosis in services of diagnostic pathology, a subdivision of the ameloblastoma has not been made, so the relative frequency in such studies is unknown.

Philipsen et al. (192) reviewed published cases and cases from earlier reviews, mounting to 160 cases. Other cases have been published since then (110,193–205). The estimated number of published cases is 176.

On the basis of 135 cases reviewed by Philipsen et al. (192), the age range is 9–92 years, but the majority of patients are in the fourth to eighth decades, very few patients have been younger than 30 years and older than 80. The mean age was 52.1 years [compared with 37.4 years for intraosseous ameloblastoma (43)]. The mean age for men was slightly higher (52.9 years) than that of females (50.6 years).

The gender distribution ($N = 160$) was 104 males (65.0%) and 56 females (35.0%). The gender distribution for intraosseous ameloblastoma [Reichart et al. 1995 (43)] was 54.5% in males and 45.5% in females.

The majority of cases, 112 (70.9%) were located in the gingiva or alveolar mucosa of the mandible ($N = 158$), 46 (29.1%) were located in the maxilla. The most common site was the mandibular premolar region (32.6%) and the anterior mandibular region (20.7%), quite different from the posterior mandible predilection of the intraosseous ameloblastoma. The majority of PERAMs in the mandible were located on the lingual aspect of the gingiva. In the maxilla, the most common location was the soft, palatal tissue of the tuberosity area, accounting for 11.1% of all cases.

Multicentric occurrence of PERAM has been reported by Balfour et al. (206) and Hernandez et al. (207).

Six cases have been reported of PERAM occurring in nontooth-bearing areas of the mouth, buccal mucosa, and floor of the mouth, and have been reviewed by Yamanishi et al. (208). Since they are encapsulated in contrast to PERAMs, and occur in areas without any remnants of odontogenic epithelium they are more likely to be a rare type of benign salivary gland tumor, which mimic the histopathology of an ameloblastoma, as already suggested by Wesley et al. (209) and Moskow et al. (210).

Cases of basal cell carcinomas of the gingiva have been published, they are believed to be PERAMs (26,211), and have been included in most reviews (192). Basal cell carcinoma is derived from hairbearing epithelium and arises on hair-bearing skin exclusively.

The size of the PERAM varies; in a review by Buchner et al. (212), the majority of lesions were between 0.3 and 2.0 cm, but two lesions were 4 and 4.5 cm. The mean size was 1.3 cm. A review about a tumor that measured 5 cm in greatest extent was published by Scheffer et al. (213). Like other peripheral odontogenic tumors, the growth rate is slower than that of the intraosseous counterpart.

Buchner et al. (212) reported the duration of symptoms before diagnosis to be between one month and two years, in most cases with a mean

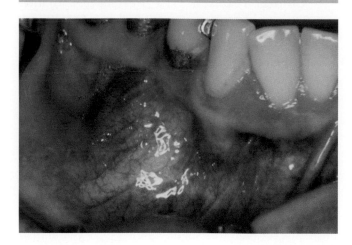

Figure 13 Peripheral ameloblastoma on the buccal side of the mandible of a middle-aged woman.

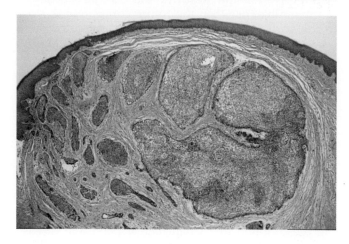

Figure 14 Peripheral ameloblastoma with follicular growth pattern. H&E stain. *Source*: Section by courtesy of Professor H. Strømme-Koppang, Oslo.

duration of one year. In some cases the duration has been up to five years (214). The lesions are generally painless; the exophytic growth is the main symptom. Some cases have given light symptoms (200,214). The clinical appearance varies considerably, most are sessile (Fig. 13), fewer are pedunculated, and the surface may be smooth, granular, nodular, papillary, or warty. The color varies from that of the surrounding normal mucosa to pink or dark red. Some become traumatized, which may lead to ulceration.

Since the PERAM is less common than many other types of hyperplastic growths on gingiva or alveolar mucosa and they may present with many different variations of color, morphology, and consistence, they are rarely diagnosed as ameloblastomas before they are examined histologically. The most common preoperative diagnoses are fibrous hyperplasia, teleangiectatic granuloma, peripheral giant cell granuloma, and papilloma. A few have been mistaken for squamous cell carcinoma (SCC) (212).

Imaging.   Generally the PERAM shows no radiological changes of the underlying bone (212). In a review of the literature Reichart et al. (43) found 73 cases of PERAM. Radiographic findings were reported in 36 cases, in 28 of these there were no radiographic findings, in 5 cases there was slight erosion ("saucerization") of the surface of the bone below the tumor. Cases have been published, however, where quite conspicuous erosion was detected (200,215) and even deeper invasion into the jaw bone (195,196); in such cases an AMCA should be suspected.

Pathology.   The etiology of the PERAM is unknown. Some lesions are clearly separated from the surface epithelium, they are supposed to arise in remnants of the dental lamina (14). In other cases there is continuity between the tumor epithelium and the surface epithelium (213,216,217), in such cases there is a possibility that the tumor may have arisen from the basal cells of the surface epithelium. It is difficult to prove, however, it is well known from

intraosseous ameloblastomas, which progress through the cortical bone and reaches contact with the surface epithelium that induction of the surface epithelium to ameloblastomatous proliferations may occur.

In a review of 27 cases by Buchner et al. (212), a band of connective tissue was found between the tumor and surface epithelium in 8 cases (30%) and a continuity was seen in 19 cases (70%); in 7 cases (26% of all cases) there was multiple areas of continuity.

Macroscopically the lesion presents as a firm to slightly spongy mass with an outline that partly depends on its clinical aspect (26). The cut surface may show minute cystic spaces.

Microscopically, the tumor is composed of a neoplastic odontogenic epithelium that shows the same growth patterns and cell types as the intraosseous solid/cystic ameloblastoma, although granular cells seems to be very rare or nonexisting. It is not encapsulated (Fig. 14). Many PERAMs display a follicular growth pattern with islands composed of a central area of stellate reticulum-like cells and a peripheral layer dominated by cuboidal and columnar cells (199–201). Some tumors exhibit more than one typical pattern. Many tumors are partly or totally acanthomatous with squamous cell metaplasia of the central areas. A minority of lesions are dominated by basal cells and may be histomorphologically indistinguishable from basal cell carcinoma (26). Clear cells (218) and ghost cells as well as calcifications, and formation of keratin pearls have been described (211). The stroma is composed of narrow strands of collagenous connective tissue with low cellularity.

Cases with cytological signs of malignancy have been described and should be considered AMCAs (195,219,220).

Immunohistochemistry.   In contrast to the s/m intraosseous ameloblastoma relatively few immunohistochemical studies have been performed on tissue from PERAM. The investigators have mainly concentrated on CKs in the neoplastic epithelium. Takeda et al. (221) used polyclonal antibodies against CK and found comparable reactions in the tumor and the gingival epithelium; the central cells of the tumor islands and the covering epithelium were positive, whereas the peripheral cells of the tumor islands and the elongated rete pegs were negative.

Yamamoto et al. (215) used four types of lectins, polyclonal antibodies ("total keratin," or TK) against 56 and 64 kDa CKs and monoclonal antibodies against 45 kDa and 56.6 kDa CK on a case of PERAM, 4 cases of intraosseous ameloblastoma and 3 cases of cutaneous basal cell carcinomas. No clear difference could be found in either lectins or keratins among the peripheral and central ameloblastomas and the basal cell carcinomas. Most tumors showed reaction to TK, but only one intraosseous ameloblastoma reacted to monoclonal keratin antibodies.

Lentini et al. (197) used antibodies against CK-19 and Ber-EP4 on a PERAM with basaloid features. Ber-EP4 is an antibody against a cell membrane glycoprotein, which has been detected in cutaneous basal cell carcinoma, trichoepithelioma, eccrine, and apocrine ducts and other epithelial tissues. The investigators found a diffuse immunoreaction for CK-19 in the neoplastic cells, in some areas more marked in the palisading peripheral cells. Some scattered positive areas were seen in the gingiva as well. Ber-EP4 was negative except some rare areas of faint reaction in basaloid cells. Since it has been reported in the literature that cutaneous basal cell carcinomas are negative for CK-19, and react positive to Ber-EP4, the authors suggest that the method might be useful in distinguishing basal cell carcinoma from PERAMs.

Lo Muzio et al. (121) studied the immunohistochemical expression of p63, a member of the Tp53 gene family, in the epithelial layers of four cases of PERAM, and in several other types of epithelial odontogenic tumors. Immunohistochemical reaction was detected in the epithelial cells of all odontogenic tumors and the positivity was only nuclear. P63 expression was found in both peripheral and central epithelial cells. Benign odontogenic locally aggressive tumors with a high risk of recurrence exhibited statistically significant higher p63 expression than benign odontogenic, nonaggressive tumors with low risk of recurrence.

Electron Microscopy. The ultrastructure of the PERAM has been studied by Greer et al. (222), Gould et al. (216), and Takeda et al. (221). In a case with continuity between the tumor epithelium and the surface epithelium, the latter showing extensions of rete pegs into the tumor area, the ultrastructural examination showed that the rete pegs gradually became transformed into double-stranded epithelial cords as they elongated deeply (221). The end of these cords gradually became transformed into tumor islands. The ultrastructure of the tumor islands was similar to that of intraosseous follicular ameloblastoma, but was different from that of cutaneous basal cell carcinoma.

Molecular-Genetic Data. Nodit et al. (110) studied 12 ameloblastomas (2 peripheral, 8 s/m, 2 mandibular UNAMs, and 3 AMCAs) for loss of heterozygosity of tumor suppressor genes on chromosomes 1p, 3p, 9p, 10q, and 17p (L-myc, hOGG1, p16, pten, and p53). L-myc (71% frequency of allelic loss) and pten (62% frequency of allelic loss) had the most frequent allelic loss. The overall frequency of allelic loss and intramural heterogeneity were higher in mandibular and in unicystic tumors, and lower in tumors that recurred/metastasized. There was no significant differences in rates of allelic loss between the benign and malignant tumors (46 vs. 52%, $p = 0.71$). The DNA damage in ameloblastomas and AMCAs seemed sporadic and cumulative and unrelated to aggressive growth.

Differential Diagnosis. As mentioned above the PERAM may exhibit a histomorphology which is similar to that of a basal cell carcinoma. When such a tumor appears on the gingiva or alveolar mucosa it is considered a PERAM. Some PERAMs are in intimate contact with the gingival surface epithelium. In such cases it is important to distinguish the tumor from an initial SCC from the gingival epithelium and from a peripheral AMCA. Cellular and nuclear pleomorphism and mitoses are not present in PERAM and suggest a malignant tumor (223). The cytology of an AMCA may vary, but peripheral palisading of tall columnar cells must be present in some areas, and inverted nuclear polarity may also be present (224). The differential diagnosis should also include adenoid cystic carcinoma and polymorphous low-grade adenocarcinoma, although these will be extensions of tumors in adjacent areas, since salivary glands are absent in the gingiva.

The *odontogenic gingival peripheral hamartoma,* or hamartoma of the dental lamina, rest is a rare epithelial lesion located to the gingiva and presenting as small nodules often at the lingual aspect of the oral mucosa (225). They were originally described by Baden et al. (226). They are foci of apparently inactive odontogenic epithelium and they are not hamartomas, since they do not develop during odontogenesis, which ceases about the age of 22 years. The term "hamartoma" indicates a tumor-like developmental anomaly and cannot be legitimately used for tumor-like lesions of odontogenic epithelium with self-limiting growth potential, which primarily occur in patients past the age of odontogenesis. It has been suggested that such lesions should be considered a variant of PERAM if they contain many epithelial islands with some although moderate proliferative activity (225,227). If they consist of a few islands of inactive odontogenic epithelium they are not PERAMs but rather related to the inactive proliferations of odontogenic epithelium, which may be found in the wall of dentigerous cysts (228).

Treatment and Prognosis. Apart from cases with invasive growth in the underlying bone with or without cytological signs of malignancy (195,196,223), lesions that should be considered AMCAs and treated radically, the PERAM does not exhibit invasive growth with destruction of bone. The lesion is adequately treated by conservative, supraperiosteal surgical excision with disease-free margins. Long-term follow-up is necessary, 10 years or more. Recurrence rates are much lower than for the intraosseous amelo-blastoma, which is a much more aggressive tumor. Buchner et al. reviewed 26 published cases of PERAM with follow-up information ranging from six months to eight years after treatment. There was no recurrence in 21 cases. In five cases (19%) recurrence developed, although the lesion was believed to be adequately removed. The recurrences were diagnosed after two months, one and a half years, five years (2 cases), and seven years, respectively.

1.1.2 Desmoplastic Ameloblastoma.

Introduction.   The DESAM is a rare, benign, but locally infiltrative, epithelial odontogenic tumor, which is considered a variant of ameloblastoma in spite of aberrant clinical, imaging, and histological features (26).

ICD-O code 9310/0

Synonym: Ameloblastoma with pronounced desmoplasia.

The special features of this tumor were first reported from Japan in 1981 and 1983 (229), but it was the article by Eversole et al. (230), which created more general awareness of this uncommon neoplasm, which is characterized by an epithelial neoplastic component surrounded by extensive, dense collage-nous stroma.

Clinical Features.   The prevalence and inci-dence of the DESAM is unknown. DESAM is a rare tumor; Philipsen et al. (231) reviewed 100 cases from the literature; since then about 21 cases have been published, accounting to 121. In reviews of material received for histological diagnosis in services of diag-nostic pathology a subdivision of the ameloblastoma has not been made. In five published series of DESAM the tumor has accounted for between 5.3% and 12.1% of all ameloblastomas, Waldron et al. (232): 12.1% (N = 116), Keszler et al. (233): 8.8% (N = 159), Lam et al. (234): 8.6% (N = 81), Takata et al. (235); 7.9% (N = 89), and Kishino et al. (236): 5.3% (N = 189).

The age, gender, and site distribution has varied somewhat in the reports of larger series of cases. Waldron et al. (232) reported 14 cases from United States, 7 males and 7 females with an age range of 21 to 68 years, mean age 45.5 years; 7 tumors were located in the maxilla (6 in the anterior region), and 7 in the mandible. Ng et al. (237) reported 17 cases from Malaysia, 5 males and 12 females with an age range of 21 to 60 years, mean age 36.6 years, median age 38 years; 7 lesions were in the maxilla, and 10 in the mandible, 14 were located in the anterior regions. Keszler et al. (233) reported 14 cases from Argentina, 2 males and 11 females; the age range was 19 to 62 years, the mean age 37.8 years; 2 were located in the maxilla and 10 in the mandible (N = 12). Kishino et al. (236) reported 10 cases from Japan, 9 males and 1 female. The age range was 17 to 58 years, mean age 44.7 years, median age 50 years. The site distribution was 4 in the maxilla and 6 in the mandible. Philipsen et al. (231) published a review of 100 cases from the literature. The gender distribution was equal M:F = 50:50, the age range (N = 63) was 17 to 72 years (21–68 for females), the mean age was 35.9 years (39.2 for males and 35.2 for females). The distribution in

decades showed two female peaks in the fourth and fifth decades, but a male peak in the sixth decade. Few patients were younger than 30 years or older than 59 years. In contrast to solid/multicystic ameloblas-toma (s/mAM) the site distribution (N = 76) was almost equal 39 tumors were located in the maxilla and 37 in the mandible. Seven cases occupied an entire maxillary quadrant, 15 cases crossed the mid-line (3 maxillary and 12 mandibular), 34 cases were located in the anterior regions, and only 4 cases (5.4%) were found in the mandibular molar region versus 39% of conventional ameloblastoma (43).

Generally the DESMA has a predilection for the anterior part of jaws, the distribution between the maxilla and the mandible is much more even than for the s/mAM, and there is no predilection for the posterior region of the mandible. Estimated from the reviews of the literature the mean age at the time of diagnosis seems to be about five years higher than for the s/mAM.

A single case of peripheral DESMA has been published by Smullin et al. (238). The tumor was an asymptomatic, nonulcerated slowly growing mass in the premolar area of the left hard palate of a 44-year-old female; it had begun to enlarge recently. It did not invade the underlying bone. The histology showed some similarity to the SOT.

A painless hard swelling that has been known for a long time—often for years—is the most common symptom reported. Occasional pain has been reported in very few cases (237,239).

Imaging.   In most cases the radiological picture of the DESAM differs from the picture usually seen in conventional ameloblastomas (26). Kaffe et al. (240) described the radiological features of 14 cases of DESAM reported in the literature and a case of their own. Among 13 of the cases one showed multilocular small unilocular lesions, 5 were unilocular, and 7 were not loculated. The borders of the lesion (N = 15) were well defined in 3 cases, poorly defined in 5 cases, and diffused in 7 cases. Three tumors developed in eden-tulous areas, among the remaining 12, tooth displace-ment was seen in 11 cases (92%), and root resorption of neighboring teeth in 4 cases (33%). Most lesions were larger than 3 cm. In the literature review by Philipsen et al. (231) the size varied from 1.0 to 8.5 cm at the longest diameter, and an association with an unerupted or impacted tooth was seen in only three cases (3.4%) compared with 8.7% among conventional ameloblastomas. An unusual finding is a single large cyst associated with the tumor. It was reported in the maxilla by Iida et al. (241) and in the mandible by Kawai et al. (242).

A mixed radiolucent–radiopaque pattern usually with ill-defined margins making the lesion more sug-gestive of a fibrous-osseous lesion than of ameloblas-toma was found in 53% of cases reviewed by Philipsen et al. (231) and in 60% of 17 cases reported by Ng et al. (237) and in 6 of 10 cases reported by Kishino et al. (236).

The ill-defined borders and the mixed pattern of the lesion are caused by bone resorption and bone formation at the margins of the lesion. Thompson et al. (243) demonstrated the value of CT and MRI in the diagnosis of DESMA. The information about the margins of the lesion is markedly improved and it was detected that the mixed fine and course trabecular pattern predominated at the periphery of the lesion.

Pathology. The etiology of the DESAM is unknown and the pathogenesis is poorly understood; it only occurs in the jaws and is believed to develop from remnants of odontogenic epithelium.

Macroscopically it presents as a white solid mass with gritty consistency on cross sectioning.

The histopathology was described in details by Eversole et al. (230) and Waldron et al. (232). The tumor resembles the conventional ameloblastoma in some aspects, and the SOT in other. It is composed of small islands and strands of tumor epithelium with high cellular density (Fig. 15). The epithelial cells are small, spindle-shaped or polygonal and sometimes arranged in a whorled pattern. The epithelium is lacking stellate reticulum cells and columnar basal cells, most of the latter are flattened or cuboidal (Fig. 16). Sometimes central squamous cell metaplasia and a few foci of keratinization is seen. There is a scant tendency in about 50% of the tumors (232) to form cystic or duct-like structures, which may fill out the whole island. Many islands, particularly the larger ones are very irregularly shaped with pointed extensions and long very narrow whipcord-like offshoots. The latter is composed of a single row of small cells with hyperchromatic nuclei. An occasional island may show columnar peripheral cells and a few islands with stellate reticulum-like cells in the center may be seen; Waldron et al. (232) detected such islands in 3 of 14 tumors. The stroma is conspicuously abundant

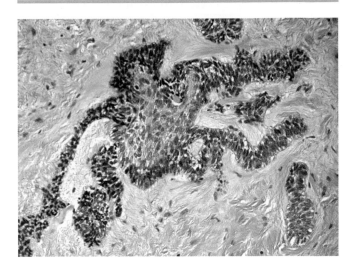

Figure 16 Desmoplastic ameloblastoma. Higher magnification shows cuboidal and columnar peripheral cells and fusiform and polygonal eosinophilic cells in the center. Hyalinized and myxomatous areas are seen around the tumor island. H&E stain.

with pronounced collagen formation and moderate cellularity. Oxytalan fibers, which are characteristic for periodontal membrane connective tissue, have been detected by Kawai et al. (242) and Kishino et al. (236). Acellular, amorphous, eosinophilic material may be seen adjacent to the epithelium, and quite often zones with myxomatous changes are seen around the epithelial islands. Spicules or trabeculae of mature laminar bone, resorption of bone trabeculae and new bone production around the resorbed trabeculae may be found about the periphery of the tumor, where invasion of tumor tissue into surrounding bone is seen some cases (232,236).

There are several clinical and pathological differences between DESAM and conventional ameloblastoma (Table 3), which raises the question if DESAM should be considered an entity of its own. The weightiest argument for considering the DESAM as a variant of the ameloblastoma and not as a separate entity is the existence of tumors that show the histopathological features of DESMA and of conventional intraosseous ameloblastoma simultaneously. About 10 such cases have been published, and have been called ''hybrid'' tumors (232,239,244–246).

Hirota et al. (247) reported a case of DESAM in the anterior maxilla of a 17-year-old woman who had symptoms for eight years. The tumor showed focal dedifferentiation with nuclear pleomorphism and mitoses. It is the only case of DESAM hitherto published with signs of malignancy. It was treated by maxillectomy and there was no recurrence after seven years.

Immunohistochemistry. Siar et al. (248) used antibodies against S-100 protein, keratin, desmin, and vimentin on sections of DESMA; the results were weak and variable apart from vimentin, a fibroblast marker, which was totally negative in the epithelium.

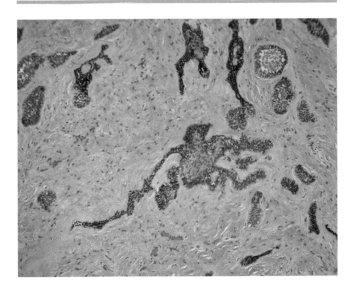

Figure 15 Desmoplastic ameloblastoma from a 36-year-old woman. Irregularly shaped tumor islands with pointed extensions and long, slender offshoots are seen in an abundant collagenous stroma. Myxomatous changes are seen around some of the tumor islands. In the upper part of the picture, a few islands with conventional ameloblastoma morphology are seen. H&E stain.

Table 3 Intraosseous Cystic/Solid Vs. Desmoplastic Ameloblastoma

	Intraosseous cystic/solid ameloblastoma	Desmoplastic ameloblastoma
Clinical features		
Average age	39 yr	43 yr
Male-female ratio	1:1	1:1
Maxilla-mandible ratio	1:5.4	1:0.9
Percent located to mandibular molar region	39%	5.4% (4 cases)
Radiology	Uni- or multilocular radiolucency with well-defined borders	Radiolucent: 47%
		Mixed radiolucent/radiopaque: 53%
		Well-defined borders: 7%
Association with unerupted or impacted tooth	8.7%	3.4% (3 cases)
Peripheral (extraosseous) variant	About 2–10% of all ameloblastomas	One doubtful case reported so far (among 121 cases)
Histology		
Growth pattern	Follicular (rounded shape) or plexiform	Narrow cords and islands with pointed extensions
Basal cell layer in islands	Columnar or cuboidal	Flat or cuboidal
Cell types	Stellate, acanthomatous, granular	Polygonal or fusiform keratinocytes
Cystic changes in epithelium	Development of cysts in tumour islands is very common. Cysts may become very large	Large cysts do not develop. Microcysts may be seen
Stroma	Mature collagenous fibrous tissue	Extensive stromal desmoplasia. Formation of bone in some cases
Collagen type VI	Not demonstrable	Strongly positive reaction
Transforming growth factor beta (cytokine)	Low production	Increased production
Tenascin	Immunopositive	Immunonegative

TGF-β immunoreactivity was studied by Takata et al. (249) in seven cases of DESAMs, including a hybrid lesion and compared with 10 cases of conventional follicular and plexiform ameloblastomas. TGF-β is one of the most potent local factors for modulating extracellular matrix formation. A marked immunoexpression was observed in both peripheral and central cells in tumor nests in all DESAMs except one. In the hybrid lesions TGF-β was detected in the DESAM areas, but not in areas of follicular ameloblastoma. The TGF-β produced by tumor cells is believed to play a part in the desmoplastic matrix formation.

Tenascin (an extracellular matrix protein), fibronectin (an extracellular matrix molecule), and collagen type I was studied by dos Santos et al. (246) in conventional ameloblastomas and hybrid DESAMs. There was a positive immunoreaction in fibrils of the conventional ameloblastoma, but the DESAMs were negative. There was a strong fibronectin positive immunoreaction from fibrils in the stroma of DESAMs with a linear marking along the interface between epithelium and connective tissue. There was a positive reaction in fibers of the stroma along the interface and an intense immunoreaction in the extracellular matrix.

Nagatsuka et al. (75) studied the presence of type IV collagen in three DESAMs, five solid/cystic ameloblastomas, and a number of other odontogenic tumors. Type IV collagen is the major component of basement membrane. The expression of α1(IV)/α2(IV) and α5(IV)/α6(IV) chains was stronger in desmoplastic than in conventional ameloblastomas. A marked immunoreactivity in the basement membrane presented as thin continued lines demarcating the tumor epithelium from the surrounding connective tissue stroma. A random intracellular staining of the tumor islands without differences in various cell types was seen. Collagen α4(IV) chains were not detected. Takata et al. (249) detected type IV collagen in the basement membrane of blood vessels in DESAMs, follicular, and plexiform ameloblastomas. No remarkable differences in the immunoreactivity between the types of ameloblastomas were found.

Philipsen et al. (239) detected an intense staining for collagen type VI in the stroma adjacent to tumor islands. Conventional ameloblastomas were negative.

Kumamoto et al. (178) investigated the immunoreaction of extracellular matrix-degrading serine proteinase in odontogenic tumors, and detected expression of uPA, uPAR, PAI-1, and maspin in four cases of DESAM.

To evaluate roles of the Akt-signaling pathway in oncogenesis and cytodifferentiation of odontogenic tumors Kumamoto et al. (250) investigated the expression of phosphorylated Akt, P13K, and PTEN in four cases of DESAM, which all reacted positive.

The roles of MAPKs in oncogenesis and cytodifferentiation of odontogenic tumors were investigated by Kumamoto et al. (78), who detected expression of p-p38 MAPK, and p-ERK5, but not p-JNK in four cases of DESAM.

Leocata et al. (158) studied the immunoreactivity of aberrant Wingless type 1 glycoprotein (Wnt1) and

SDC-1 in seven human tooth buds and 29 ameloblastomas, including four desmoplastic. A shift of SDC-1 expression from epithelial to stromal cells has been described in invasive nonodontogenic neoplasms. Wnt1-positive epithelial cells were mainly seen in follicular and acanthomatous intraosseous ameloblastomas, but was also found in some plexiform and desmoplastic ones. SDC-1 was not expressed in tumor epithelial cells of follicular and desmoplastic intraosseous ameloblastomas, but SDC-1 reactivity was variously observed in tumor stroma cells and the extracellular matrix of follicular, plexiform, acanthomatous, and desmoplastic intraosseous ameloblastomas.

Electron Microscopy. No data are available.

Molecular-Genetic Data. No data are available.

Differential Diagnosis. SOT is a very difficult differential diagnosis, both tumors show an abundant fibrous stroma, and some published cases of SOT are likely to be DESMA (251–253). The clinical picture of the two tumors may differ; lesions larger than 2 cm at longest diameter are unlikely to be SOT; the mixed radiolucent–radiopaque pattern often seen in DESMA is not seen in SOT; resorption of tooth roots is a common finding in DESAM and has not been reported in SOT. Histologically the DESAM may contain islands with ameloblastoma features, which are not found in SOT, like peripheral columnar cells with reverse nuclear polarization and central areas with stellate reticulum-like cells. If they are absent, attention must be drawn to other histomorphological differences. Although the epithelial islands of SOT may be irregular and show indentations, most of them are rounded or oval, while the islands of DESAM generally have a very irregular outline with pointed extensions, and show interconnecting cords between the islands, and long, ramifying whipcord-like offshoots of single layered epithelium, which are not a hallmark of the SOT. Both tumors are composed of squamous cells; in SOT they are larger, polygonal, and with a more abundant cytoplasm, in DESAM they are smaller, there is a higher cellular density, and the cells are spindle-shaped or polygonal and often arranged in a streaming pattern, which is not seen in the SOT. In DESAM the peripheral cells are more often cuboidal than flattened; the opposite is the case in SOT. Central cysts may be seen in the islands of the DESAM, sometimes filling the whole island, which is not a feature of SOT, where microcysts may be seen, which are about the size of a few epithelial cells. The stroma is abundant in both tumors, often myxoid changes are present in the juxtaepithelial stroma in DESAM, and they are not seen in SOT.

If nuclear pleomorphia and mitoses are observed an intraosseous SCC should be considered, these features should be not present in a DESAM.

Treatment and Prognosis. The treatment strategy for DESAM is the same at for the solid/cystic ameloblastoma. Resection with a 1 cm margin of spongy bone is recommended. Cortical bone may be resected more sparingly (254). Partial hemimaxillectomy may be necessary for larger maxillary tumors and partial mandibulectomy or semimandibulectomy may be required in the mandible. Curettage increases the risk of recurrence; Pillai et al. (255) reported a case of DESAM in the maxilla of a 24-year-old woman with involvement of antrum; two months after curettage a partial maxillectomy was required.

Recurrence rates are difficult to estimate because of limited information. One of the 17 cases reported by Ng et al. (237) recurred four years after "excision." One of seven cases reported by Takata et al. (235) recurred. Kishino et al. (236) reported 10 cases with a follow-up time between 5 and 23 years for nine of them. None of them recurred. Two smaller ones, one measuring 12 × 12 mm, the other one 30 × 26 mm had been enucleated, the remaining seven had been resected.

1.1.3 Unicystic Ameloblastoma.

Introduction. The UNAM is an odontogenic cystic neoplasm with a single often large lumen and development of an initial intralining or intraluminal or intramural ameloblastoma, or combinations of these. The accurate diagnosis and the character and the extent of the tumor cannot be made on the basis of an incisional biopsy; it requires microscopic examination of the entire specimen.

ICD-O code 9310/0

Synonym: Cystogenic ameloblastoma

The UNAM has been published under several other different diagnoses: plexiform UNAM, intracystic ameloblastoma, cystic ameloblastoma, unilocular ameloblastoma, extensive dentigerous cyst, and intracystic ameloblastic papilloma. The UNAM was proposed as an entity by Robinson and Martinez (256).

Clinical Features. The prevalence and incidence of the UNAM is unknown. In most reviews of material received for histological diagnosis in services of diagnostic pathology a subdivision of the ameloblastomas has not been made. Buchner et al. (30), however, subdivided the UNAM from other variants of ameloblastomas in a review of 1.088 odontogenic tumors from Northern California. Among these 127 were ameloblastomas, 69 were of the s/m variant and 58 were UNAMs that account for 5.3% of all the tumors, and 45.7% of the ameloblastomas. The relative frequency has varied in other reviews. The UNAM accounted for 15% ($N = 380$) of all cases of ameloblastoma reviewed by Ackermann et al. (257), for 18.9% ($N = 175$) in the review by Li et al. (258). In a comprehensive review of the literature Philipsen et al. (259) observed relative frequencies of UNAM varying between 5% and 22%.

Although the age range in some studies have included teenagers and young adults only (232,260,261), the age range in the study by Robinson et al. (256) was 10 to 79 years ($N = 20$), and in the Ackermann et al. study (257) 6 to 77 years ($N = 57$). The latter study consisted of 90% blacks, the mean age was 23.8 years (SD 14.9); 86% of the patients were in the second, third, and fourth decades. In 33 Chinese patients with UNAM (262) the age range was 8 to 60 years, with a mean age of 25.3 years, and a peak (70%) in the second and third decades. Waldron et al. (232) noted that the average age of 12 UNAMs among 116 ameloblastomas was 22 years compared with 45.5 years for all patients with ameloblastomas. This finding was confirmed by Philipsen et al. (259) in their review of the literature.

A large percentage of the UNAMs are associated with an uncrupted tooth, often a lower third molar (257,259,260,262). The association may simulate a dentigerous cyst; although it has not been possible to exclude the origin of an UNAM from a dentigerous cyst, it is considered highly unlikely by several investigators (257,262,263). In a review of 193 cases of UNAM from the literature, Philipsen et al. (259) observed that the mean age for patients with UNAM associated with a cyst (16.5 years) was considerably lower than the mean age for patients with UNAM not associated with a tooth (35.2 years). They also found a slightly different gender ratio in the two groups; the M:F ratio for the first group was 1.5:1 ($N = 90$) and for the latter 1:1.8 ($N = 101$). The age difference may at least in part be explained by the fact that more unerupted teeth are present in the jaws of patients below 22 years than past that age. If the UNAM develops in the posterior mandible before the eruption of the third molar there is an increased risk that it impedes the eruption of the tooth.

In most of the larger series published there have been a predominance of males, Gardner (264) 12 M:7 F, Eversole et al. (260) 20 M:13 F, Leider et al. (265) 20 M:13 F, and Ackermann et al. (257) 30 M:23 F. Some have found a female predominance, Rosenstein et al. (263) 10 M:11 F, and Lee et al. (266) 12 M:17 F.

All investigators have found a marked predominance for the mandible as to the UNAM and it is mostly seen in the posterior part of the mandible. Ackermann et al. (257) reported 3 tumors (6%) in the maxilla and 53 (92%) in the mandible. Li et al. (262) found 3 (9%) in the maxilla and 30 (91%) in the mandible. Among 31 cases reported by Leider et al. (265) all located in the mandible, 24 lesions (77.4%) were found in the ramus/molar area, 3 (9.7%) in the cuspid/premolar area, and 4 (12.9%) in the mandibular symphisis.

Larger lesions can produce jaw swellings and displace teeth. Swelling is the most common symptom. Many cases are found on radiograms taken for other purposes. Occasional pain, signs of lower lip numbness, and discharge or drainage in cases of secondary infection have been reported (259). In 21 cases reported by Olaitan et al. (267) all occurring in the mandible, swelling was present in all cases, and expansion of both cortical plates in 18 cases. The median age of onset of symptoms was 18 years, and the average time from onset of symptoms to presentation for clinical evaluation was four years.

Imaging. Although all lesions are unicystic histomorphologically, they do not necessarily present as a unilocular lesion on a radiogram, but most do present as well-corticated unilocular radiolucencies (Fig. 17). According to Eversole et al. (260), the predominant radiographic patterns of the UNAM include unilocular and scalloped or macromultilocular pericoronal, interradicular, or periapical expansile radiolucencies. Multilocularity is more often seen in older patients (263). Among the 33 cases reported by Li et al. (262) 22 were unilocular and 7 were multilocular. Seven

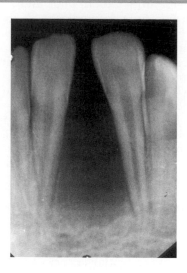

Figure 17 Unicystic ameloblastoma between the lower left incisors of a 9-year-old girl. Divergence but no resorption of the roots of the teeth is seen.

of the cases presented as pericoronal radiolucencies. Resorption of neighboring teeth was observed in 23 cases (70%). Root resorption has been reported in 40% to 70% of cases in published series (259).

In a review of 191 cases from the literature Philipsen et al. (259) noted that the UNAM in 90 cases (47%) were associated with an unerupted tooth. Among the 57 cases reviewed by Ackermann et al. (257) 11 (19%) were associated with an unerupted tooth, 5 of them (9%) were related to the crown in a true dentigerous cyst arrangement (histopathologically it was not possible to prove that they were dentigerous cysts), and 6 were displaced by the cyst.

In the same study the size of the lesion was recorded to be greater than 5 cm in 41 cases (75%), and more than 10 cm in greatest diameter in 20 cases (38%).

Konouchi et al. (268) showed that it was possible by means of contrast enhanced MRI to detect small intraluminal nodules in UNAM, which were undetectable by any other imaging method; the MRI scanning may thus be a very helpful tool. It must be remembered, however, that not all UNAMs show macroscopically visible nodules in the wall, and that the final diagnosis requires microscopic examination of the entire specimen.

Pathology. The etiology of the UNAM is unknown and the pathogenesis is poorly understood. In some cases the lesion simulates a dentigerous cyst, but it has not been possible to prove that a UNAM may arise in a dentigerous cyst (257,262), and Rosenstein et al. (263) observed that recurrent lesions appeared identical histologically to the original lesion, making the likelihood of development of these tumors from dentigerous cysts unlikely. They probably arise de novo from remnants of odontogenic epithelium.

Macroscopically the lesion presents as an encapsulated fluid-filled cyst, which may be in apparently

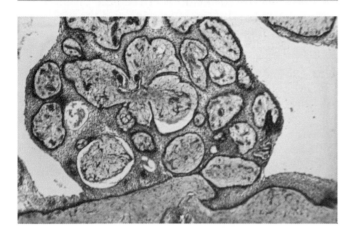

Figure 18 Unicystic ameloblastoma with intraluminal proliferations also called plexiform unicystic ameloblastoma. H&E stain.

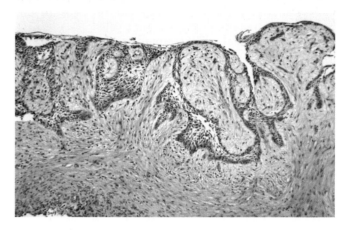

Figure 19 Unicystic ameloblastoma of the intramural (or mural) type. It is important to differentiate such neoplastic proliferations from the arcading rete epithelial hyperplasia so commonly seen in radicular cysts. H&E stain.

dentigerous relationship with a tooth, usually a lower third molar. The internal aspect may show a smooth surface or an exophytic extension into the lumen from the wall. In some cases it may almost fill the cyst lumen. If there are areas of mural thickening or if there are friable masses of intraluminal tissue present, these must be sampled extensively (269).

Three histological variants of the UNAM have been described by Ackermann et al. In the first, usually called *luminal* or *intralining* or *intraepithelial* type, the epithelial lining is inconspicuous except in focal areas where cuboidal or columnar basal cells with hyperchromatic nuclei are seen with nuclear palisading with reverse polarization, cytoplasmic vacuolization with intercellular spacing, and subepithelial hyalinization (23). Vickers et al. (270) described these histological changes as early histopathological features of ameloblastoma. The second variant is termed the "*intraluminal*" type (Fig. 18); it is sometimes referred to as the "*plexiform unicystic ameloblastoma*" (271). The lining is similar to that of the *interlining* type, but a localized nodule arises containing ameloblastomatous epithelium usually with a plexiform growth pattern. It may be an abundant intraluminal growth of hyperplastic, often inflamed, epithelium, which may not show the characteristic ameloblastoma criteria. The fibrous wall is devoid of neoplastic epithelium unless the lesion is a combination of more than one type. In the third type, which is referred to as the "*intramural*" (or *mural*) type (Fig. 19), some part of the connective tissue wall is infiltrated to a variable extent—from initial to extensive—with ameloblastoma growing in a plexiform or follicular pattern or both. Deeper extensions are sign of infiltrating ameloblastoma.

Combinations of these patterns are seen; the *intraluminal* and the *intramural* type often show simultaneous features of ameloblastoma in the epithelial lining, and some lesions may show the characteristics of all three types. In the review of 193 cases from the literature by Philipsen et al. (259) about two-thirds of

the cases were the *intramural* type, either alone or in combination with one or both the other types. The *intraluminal* type is seen more often in UNAM associated with an unerupted tooth.

The development of ameloblastoma is usually only present in focal areas, with remaining areas showing features that may be seen in a dentigerous or a radicular cyst.

The grouping into three types is related to treatment and prognosis.

Variations of minor importance have been described; granular cells like those seen in solid/cystic ameloblastoma have been described by Buchner (272) and Siar et al. (273), and ghost cells have been observed (274).

Immunohistochemistry. Calretinin, a 29-kDa calcium-binding protein, which is expressed widely in normal human tissue and is considered a marker for ameloblastic epithelium, has been studied by several investigators (275–277). Altini et al. (275) detected calretinin in 22 of 27 (81.5%) UNAMs and in 29 of 31 s/mAMs. The immunoreactivity presented as a diffuse, intense nuclear and cytoplasmic staining of several cell layers of the more superficial cells both in the characteristic and nondescript areas of the cyst linings in UNAMs. In a later study, Coleman et al. (276) investigated calretinin in 22 odontogenic keratocysts, 26 residual cysts and 20 dentigerous cysts; they were all negative. The authors suggested that calretinin could be considered an immunohistochemical marker for neoplastic ameloblastic epithelium. The results were partly confirmed by Piattelli et al. (277), who found a negative reaction to calretinin in 24 radicular cysts, 24 dentigerous cysts, and 10 orthokeratinized keratocysts. However, 8 of 12 parakeratinized keratocysts showed immunoreactivity for calretinin in the intermediate and parabasal layers. The findings still support the possibility of using calretinin as a marker for neoplastic ameloblastic epithelium, though.

The immunoreactivity of AgNOR, Ki-67, and PCNA in UNAM has been studied to measure the proliferative potential of the tumor cells.

Coleman et al. (278) counted the AgNOR activity in odontogenic keratocysts, residual cysts, dentigerous cysts, UNAMs, and solid/cystic ameloblastomas, 15 of each. The AgNOR count was significantly lower in the UNAM than in the dentigerous cysts. The authors concluded that AgNOR counts were of no diagnostic significance in distinguishing UNAMs from odontogenic cysts. The opposite conclusion was reached by Eslami et al. (279), but on basis of similar results. They found statistically significant differences in the AgNOR counts in four different lesions but not within each group, the coefficient of variation was 34 in dentigerous cysts, 28 in odontogenic keratocysts, 15 in UNAMs, and 13 in s/mAMs.

Antibodies against PCNA and/or Ki-67 have been used in four investigations to estimate the L.I. in UNAMs, s/mAMs, and dentigerous cysts (84,263,280,281). The results have been discrepant.

Li et al. (280) studied the expression of PCNA and Ki-67 in unicystic and s/mAMs. In UNAM the intramural, invading islands exhibited a significantly higher proliferating cell nuclear antigen labeling index (PCNA L.I.) than intraluminal nodules. The epithelial lining of UNAM had relatively few PCNA-positive cells, lower than invading islands and intraluminal nodules. The L.I.s in s/mAM were significantly higher than in any of the areas in UNAM. Similar results were found for Ki-67 expression except that no significant difference in L.I. in invading islands and intraluminal nodules in UNAM could be found. The authors suggested that the results indicated differences in proliferative potential between different areas of UNAM and between UNAM and s/mAM, which may be related to the biological behavior of the tumors.

Rosenstein et al. (263) used antibodies against Ki-67 on 10 dentigerous cysts, 10 UNAMs (7 of which had intramural proliferation), and 10 s/mAMs. They did not find a significantly different L.I. in the intramural proliferations and the epithelial lining in the UNAMs. The s/mAM showed the lowest L.I., and the dentigerous cysts the highest; the authors concluded that the biological aggressiveness of the UNAM may be related to other factors than increased cellular proliferation.

Piattelli et al. (281) used antibodies against Ki-67 on 8 dentigerous cysts, 5 UNAMs, and 3 s/mAM presumably developed from dentigerous cysts. They did not detect any significant differences in the L.I.s in the two types of ameloblastomas, but a significant difference between the L.I. of the ameloblastomas and the dentigerous cysts, which showed a considerably lower index.

Finally, Meer et al. (84) used antibodies against PCNA and Ki-67 on sections from 10 UNAMs and 10 s/mAMs and observed similar results with PCNA and Ki-67. The cellular proliferative activity varied within the ameloblastoma types, but the UNAMs showed statistically significantly higher PCNA and Ki-67 L.I.s than the s/mAM. The authors concluded

that there was no correlation between the proliferative activity as shown by these proteins and the biological behavior of the tumors.

Lo Muzio et al. (121) studied the immunohistochemical expression of p63, a member of the Tp53 gene family, in the epithelial layers of 13 cases of UNAM, 3 intralining, 4 intraluminal, and 6 intramural. They were all positive. The immunoexpression was found in cells in the basal cell layer and in two-thirds of the cases also in the superficial layer, signifying abnormal control of the cell cycle. The intensity was comparable to that of other odontogenic tumors with high risk of recurrence.

Electron Microscopy.   No data are available.

Molecular-Genetic Data.   Nodit et al. (110) studied 12 ameloblastomas (2 peripheral, 8 s/mAM and 2 mandibular UNAMs) and 3 AMCAs for loss of heterozygosity of tumor suppressor genes on chromosomes 1p, 3p, 9p, 10q, and 17p (L-myc, hOGG1, p16, pten, and p53). L-myc (71% frequency of allelic loss) and pten (62% frequency of allelic loss) had the most frequent allelic loss. The frequency of allelic loss (%) and intratumoral heterogeneity (%) was relatively high in the 2 UNAMs compared to most of the s/mAMs and the AMCAs. The overall frequency of allelic loss and intramural heterogeneity were higher in mandibular and in unicystic tumors, and lower in tumors that recurred/metastasized. The DNA damage in ameloblastomas and AMCAs seemed sporadic and cumulative and unrelated to aggressive growth.

Differential Diagnosis.   Although the diagnosis of an UNAM is made on basis of a combination of clinical, radiographic, and histological features, the diagnosis is made primarily histologically after examination of the entire lesion. The diagnosis cannot be predicted preoperatively on clinical or radiographic grounds, and many cases are diagnosed as UNAM only after removal by enucleation, the preoperative diagnosis having been a nonneoplastic odontogenic cyst (23,54). The differential diagnosis toward other ameloblastic odontogenic tumors is not particularly difficult, the essential problem is not to overlook the characteristics of the UNAM; they may be moderate and only seen in a few areas. It is important not only to look for intraluminal and intramural proliferations, but to inspect the lining of the cyst to exclude areas with changes compatible with initial development of ameloblastoma as described above. Since the changes may be present in a few areas only, adequate sampling is mandatory. A dentigerous cyst shows a flat basal cell layer, but may present inactive-looking islands of odontogenic epithelium in the connective tissue wall. A KCOT (odontogenic keratocyst) of the parakeratinizing type will show prominent palisaded columnar basal cells with dark staining nuclei, but no vacuolization or stellate reticulum-like cells, but rather small polygonal eosinophilic cells with large nuclei and a parakeratinized surface.

Treatment and Prognosis.   Unless the lesion has been suspected to be an ameloblastoma preoperatively, it is usually removed by enucleation and curettage as a nonneoplastic odontogenic cyst. Since the final diagnosis can only be made after histological examination of the entire specimen, the treatment strategy proposed by Chapelle et al. (191) is the most rational. Unilocular cystic lesions in the maxilla or mandibular body should be enucleated and submitted for histological examination. If the diagnosis is UNAM grade 1 (intralining) or grade 2 (intraluminal), no further treatment should be done immediately, but long-term follow-up (10–15 years) of the patient is required. If the diagnosis is UNAM grade 3 (intramural) or s/mAM, the treatment should be partial maxillectomy or marginal/segmental resection immediately after the primary surgery. In case of a unilocular cystic lesion in the retromolar trigon and ascending ramus of the mandible enucleation of the lesion and excision of the overlying mucosa should be done (14) possibly with supplementary treatment of the cavity with liquid nitrogen or chemical cauterization with Carnoy's solution (cave: risk of nerve damage). After histological examination the treatment strategy is the same as explained above.

The risk of recurrence is related to treatment method and histological type of UNAM. Li et al. (262) reported longtime follow-up for 29 patients with UNAM (3 maxillary and 26 mandibular). Six (35%) of the tumors recurred; all three maxillary UNAMs recurred. All recurrent tumors were diagnosed as nonspecific jaw cysts before surgery. Ameloblastoma was suspected in eight cases before surgery, seven of these were treated by marginal or segmental ostectomy, one with hemimandibulectomy; none of these recurred. None of the tumors recurred within the first four years after surgery; the range was 4 to 11 years, with a mean of seven years. The recurrence was related to histological subtype, 5 of 14 (35.7%) type 3 (intramural) UNAMs recurred, only 1 of 15 (6.7%) type 1 (intralining) or type 2 (intraluminal) UNAMs recurred.

Lau et al. (282) published an extensive review of cases with long-term follow-up reported in the literature. On the basis of strict criteria they selected 100 published cases from six acceptable articles (out of 61 chosen in a second round) for statistical analysis. There was no gender predilection in the material, the mean age was 25.9 years, and all 100 tumors were located in the mandible. The mean follow-up period was 6.57 years. There was no information about the histological type. Recurrence was 3.6% after resection, 30.5% after enucleation, 16.0% after enucleation, followed by cauterization with Carnoy's solution, and 18% after marsupialization, which must be considered treatment without knowing the exact diagnosis. The results from the latter group are controversial, seven cases that did not respond to marsupialization within a short time (all type 3) were treated with mandibulectomy (283).

1.1.4 Keratoameloblastoma.

Keratoameloblastoma is a very rare, slowly growing, benign, but nonencapsulated and locally invasive, epithelial odontogenic neoplasm with a unique histological pattern characterized by solid sheets, islands, and strands of epithelium with central para- or orthokeratin plugs and peripheral cuboidal to low columnar palisaded basal cell layer mixed with multiple variable sized cysts, with an epithelial lining suggestive of odontogenic keratocyst (KCOT).

ICD-O code: None

Synonyms: None

The neoplasm was mentioned in the second edition of the *WHO Histological Typing of Odontogenic Tumors* (23) as an ameloblastoma variant, but was left out in the *WHO Head and Neck Tumor* classification published in 2005 (12) because the lesion was considered insufficiently defined.

Six examples of this rare lesion have been published by Siar et al. (284), Norval et al. (285), and Said-al-Naief et al. (286). A similar case was published by Ide et al. (287); the primary tumor showed a histomorphology, which was undistinguishable from a keratoameloblastoma. Tissue from three following recurrences treated by curettage had essentially similar histological pattern. After a forth recurrence an en-bloc resection was made and the lesions presented now exclusively as multiple keratinizing cysts, for which reason the authors changed the diagnosis to a "solid-cystic variant of odontogenic keratocyst."

The six patients mentioned above were of various ethnic extractions, Caucasian, Afro-American, Malay, and Chinese. They were 3 men, 26-, 30-, and 35-years-old, respectively and 3 women, 26-, 35-, and 39-years-old, respectively. The age range was thus 26 to 39 years; mean age was 31.8 years, and median age 35 years.

Two of the lesions were located in the maxilla, and four in the mandible, in the anterior as well as in the posterior region.

The most common symptoms were a painless, slowly growing, hard swelling, which had been present for months or years. One was tender to palpation.

Radiography shows an often large radiolucent multilocular destruction of bone, some with distinct, others with indistinct borders. Encroachment of the maxillary sinus has been reported (286), and erosion of the buccal mandibular cortical plate was reported in one case (285). Resorption of roots of teeth has not been described.

The pathogenesis of the neoplasms is unknown. There can be little doubt that they are of odontogenic origin, they have only occurred in tooth-bearing regions and show histological similarities to the ameloblastoma and to the KCOT (odontogenic keratocyst).

The tumor must be distinguished from an ameloblastoma with keratinization in terms of horn pearls like the case published by Pindborg and Weinmann (56), it has a totally different histomorphology. The tumor presents as sheets, islands, and strands of an epithelium, which consists of stellate reticulum-like cells in the peripheral areas, and shows acanthomatous changes in the center with conspicuous para- or orthokeratinization (Fig. 20). Dystrophic calcification may be present in the keratin. Intermingled with these islands multiple smaller or larger keratinized cysts are seen resembling keratocysts, but without the uniform thickness of the wall and the tendency for separation of the epithelial lining from the underlying connective tissue, which is typically seen in a keratocyst. The stroma consists of mature connective tissue that may

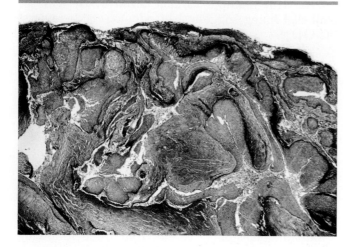

Figure 20 Keratoameloblastoma. The tumor occurred in the anterior maxilla of a 28-year-old man and consists of numerous cysts of varying size lined with a parakeratinizing squamous epithelium. The morphology is unique and distinctly different from the solid variant of the odontogenic keratocyst (solid keratocystic odontogenic tumor). H&E stain. *Source*: From Ref. 289 and by courtesy of Professor M. Shear, Cape Town.

show some degree of chronic nonspecific inflammation. The tumor is nonencapsulated and invades marrow spaces and erodes adjacent bone.

Siar et al. (284) studied their tumors immunohistochemically. TK polyclonal antibodies reacting with 41 to 64 kDa CKs yielded a strong expression in all epithelial cells. S-100 protein staining was focal and weak in the tumor cells, and was probably negative. Antibodies against desmin gave a similar result. Within the tumor elements there was no immunoreactivity with vimentin. A tumor in the anterior maxilla of a 45-year-old white man, published by Whitt et al. (288), showed many histomorphological similarities with other cases of keratoameloblastoma, but on top of these showed numerous Pacinian corpuscle-like stacks of lamellar parakeratin in the connective tissue without foreign body response. The epithelial tumor cells and the keratinized areas in this tumor reacted positively to pancytokeratin (AE1/AE3) antibodies. The authors used Ki-67 immunoreactivity to measure the proliferative index and found a high number of normal mitosis in the epithelium. Over two-thirds of the basal and parabasal cells were immunoreactive for Ki-67 with rare positive cells above this zone. The Ki-67 proliferative index was 22.8%.

The ultrastructure of the tumor has not been studied, and molecular-genetic data are not available.

The differential diagnosis may be difficult. The papilliferous keratoameloblastoma (*vide infra*) shows keratinizing cysts similar to those seen in the keratoameloblastoma, but consists mainly of cystic follicles lined with a papilliferous epithelium and lack the peripheral palisaded, columnar, or cuboidal cell layer. Lurie et al. (289) published a case named keratoameloblastoma, where the tumor consisted of relatively large islands of squamous epithelium with

slightly parakeratinized central clefts and a basal cell layer consisting of flat cells in some areas and well-oriented cuboidal cells with polarized nuclei in other areas. No similar neoplasm seems to have been published, and despite the title of the paper, the histomorphology is markedly different from other cases of keratoameloblastoma. Another important differential diagnosis, not for the surgeon, but for the pathologist is the so-called solid variant of odontogenic keratocyst published by Omura et al. (290) and by Vered et al. (291). The macroscopic appearance of these tumors is solid with multiple small cystic spaces. Microscopically they consist of multiple keratocysts of varying size, some with basal proliferation and budding, but with no evidence of follicles and islands resembling ameloblastoma. In the case published by Ide et al. (287), however, a case of keratoameloblastoma apparently converted into a solid variant of odontogenic keratocyst after several recurrences, so the relationship between the two lesions may be closer than believed.

The required treatment of the tumor is en-bloc resection with margins free of tumor. Curettage has lead to recurrences (286,287), except in the case published by Whitt et al. (288), but the follow-up time was only 10 months.

1.1.5 Papilliferous Keratoameloblastoma. Papilliferous keratoameloblastoma is an exceedingly rare, slowly growing, benign, but nonencapsulated and locally invasive, epithelial odontogenic neoplasm with a unique histological pattern characterized by multiple epithelial cysts of varying size. Some of the cysts resemble keratocysts and are filled with desquamated keratin, but the vast majority of the cysts are lined by a nonkeratinized papilliferous epithelium and filled with necrotic desquamated epithelial cells.

ICD-O code: None
Synonym: None

The neoplasm was mentioned and illustrated in the second edition of the *WHO Histological Typing of Odontogenic Tumors* (23) as an ameloblastoma variant, but was left out in the *WHO Head and Neck Tumor* classification published in 2005 (12) because the lesion was considered insufficiently defined.

Only two examples are known of this rare tumor. The first case was illustrated by Pindborg in a textbook (292). The tumor occurred in the left side of the mandible of a 57-years-old edentulous, Caucasian woman. She had experienced an increasing swelling of the area for the last two years. The radiogram showed a multilocular destruction from the second premolar area and included the entire ramus. It was treated by sectional mandibulectomy posterior to the canine. The case was distributed as IRC 6 by the International Reference Center to Collaborating Centers for preparation of the first WHO classification of odontogenic tumors, (22), and was later included as case No. 10 in the Slide Seminar on Odontogenic Tumours at the First scientific meeting of the International Association of Oral Pathologists in Gothenburg, Sweden, 1–4 June 1981. A second case was published by Altini et al. (293). It occurred in the right side of the mandible of a 76-years-old black edentulous woman

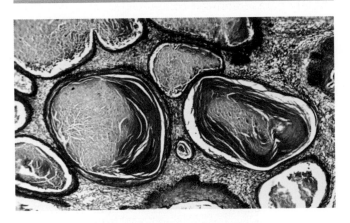

Figure 21 Papilliferous keratoameloblastoma. The tumor occurred in the mandible of a 57-year-old woman, and was described by Pindborg in 1970 (292), in some areas it consisted of multiple keratinizing cysts with a thin epithelial lining. This is the histologic pattern which has been described in most keratoameloblastomas. H&E stain. *Source*: From Ref. 292.

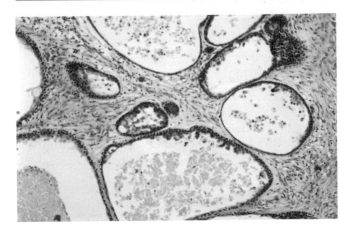

Figure 22 Papilliferous keratoameloblastoma. Same tumor as in Fig. 21. The majority of the tumor consisted of multiple cysts with a lining of a pseudo-papilliferous epithelium without keratinization. H&E stain.

who complained of a slowly enlarging swelling of one-year duration. The radiographic examination showed a large multilocular radiolucent lesion with scalloped margins extending from the right bicuspid area to the sigmoid notch. The coronoid process was completely destroyed. CT scans showed marked expansion of the mandible with perforation of the cortical plates, both buccally and lingually in several places. This is a rare finding in ameloblastomas. A hemimandibulectomy was done, and there was no recurrence after one year.

The histological findings were similar in the two cases. The tumor is nonencapsulated and consists of multiple cysts of varying size separated by rather narrow bands of fibrous connective tissue. Some of the cysts are lined with a parakeratinized stratified squamous epithelium and contain desquamated keratin (Fig. 21). The vast majority of the cysts are lined by a pseudopapilliferous epithelium 2 to 5 cells in thickness (Fig. 22), consisting of large rounded cells with centrally placed nuclei (Fig. 23) with prominent nucleoli (293). There is a loss of intercellular adherence in the surface layers, resulting in desquamation and necrosis of the cells. In some cysts true papillary projections into the lumen with connective tissue cores were seen covered with a similar epithelium. Both cases have lacked the peripheral palisaded columnar basal cell layer with polarization of the nuclei, subnuclear vacuolation, and stellate reticulum-like epithelium characteristic of ameloblastoma. For this reason the authors (293) question if the tumor is in fact a histological variant of the ameloblastoma or a separate, as yet unclassified odontogenic tumor.

No data on immunohistochemistry, ultrastructure, molecular biology, or genetics are available.

Because of the very characteristic histomorphology the differential diagnosis is uncomplicated. Only one case of odontogenic cystic tumor with papillary

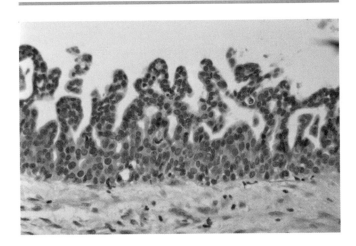

Figure 23 Papilliferous Keratoameloblastoma. Higher magnification of the pseudo-papilliferous epithelial lining seen in Figure 22. H&E stain.

proliferating keratinizing epithelium has been published (294). The tumor occurred in a 76-year-old Japanese man as a multilocular radiolucent lesion in the left side of the mandible extending from the left canine to the second molar area. Despite the papillary lining of the multiple cysts the histology was markedly different from that of the papillary keratoameloblastoma. The papillary projections were conspicuous and contained a core of connective tissue; they were keratinized on the surface, in some places with lamellar accumulation of keratin. The epithelial lining was broad, resembled stellate reticulum, and the basal cells were columnar and palisaded. Formation of hard tissue without relation to the odontogenic epithelium was seen in the stroma. A similar tumor has not been published.

Considering the destructive nature of the papilliferous keratoameloblastoma resection with tumor-free margins seems to be the required treatment.

1.2 Squamous Odontogenic Tumor.

Introduction. SOT is a rare, benign but locally infiltrative, odontogenic, epithelial neoplasm consisting of islands of well-differentiated squamous epithelium in a fibrous stroma (23,295).

ICD-O code 9312/0

The tumor was described as a new entity by Pullon et al. in 1975; they created the term (296).

Clinical Features. The prevalence and incidence of the tumor is unknown. The relative frequency of the tumor in material received for histological diagnosis in services of diagnostic pathology in various countries for various amounts of years ranges from 0.0% to 2.1% in studies comprising more than 300 samples of odontogenic tumors. The results are indicated as follows: number of odontogenic tumors/number of SOTs/%. Günhan et al., Turkey (32): 409/5/1.2%, Daley et al., Canada (33): 392/0/0.0%, Ochsenius et al., Chile (35): 362/2/0.6%, Adebayo et al., Nigeria (36): 318/1/0.3%, Fernandes et al., Brazil (37): 340/5/1.5%, Ladeinde et al., Nigeria (38): 319/6/1.9%, Buchner et al., California (30): 1088/3/0.3%, Jones et al., England (2006, pooled figures from two studies) (39,40): 523/1/0.2%, Olgac et al., Turkey (41): 527/11/2.1%, and Jing et al., China (42): 1642/3/0.2%.

Our knowledge of SOT is based on the publication of a little more than 40 cases of which 36 have been reviewed by Philipsen et al. (297). If dubious cases are excluded, i. e., cases that are more likely SOT-like proliferations, DESAMs or other lesions, the literature (1975–2005) contains 35 acceptable cases of SOT (296,298–318). Among these 35 cases 20 occurred in men and 15 in women; Caucasians, blacks, and Asians. The ratio men:women is thus 1:0.75. Most cases have been diagnosed in young adults or middle aged persons; 21 patients were between 22- and 46-years-old. The age range is 11 to 74 years. The mean age is 38 years (37.5 for men and 39 for women). The median age is 31 years (32 for men and 31 for women).

Multifocal and familial occurrences in three siblings have been reported (311), and another multicentric case has been described (306).

SOT usually develops intraosseously and often in proximity to a periodontal ligament. Some have been diagnosed in edentulous areas, and at least one case has developed in the follicle around the crown of an embedded lower third molar (318).

A few cases with extra osseous location have been published, some with a histology, which points more at PERAM or DESAM (319), but one case (314) appears convincing.

The tumor has been diagnosed in all regions of the jaws. Location was given in 34 of the accepted cases. Among the 34 cases 14 were located in the maxilla, 7 in the anterior, 5 in the posterior part, 1 of which was bilateral; 2 cases involved both the anterior and posterior part. Fourteen lesions were located in the mandible, five in the anterior and nine in the posterior area. Six cases were multicentric and included both the

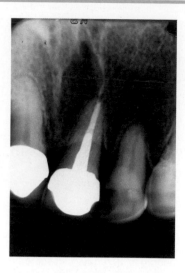

Figure 24 Squamous odontogenic tumor in proximity to the root of the left upper central incisor of a 45-year-old man. The lesion is well demarcated and no resorption of the root is seen.

maxilla and mandible, one was found in 2 quadrants, three in 3 quadrants, and two in 4.

Only a few cases have been associated with an impacted tooth (308,318).

Clinical signs are generally few. Some SOTs have caused bony enlargement and/or moderate pain. Mobility of the associated tooth/teeth has been described as well as sensivity to percussion. In about 25% of the cases the patient had no symptoms.

Imaging. On radiograms the typical lesion shows a triangular-shaped (pointing toward the marginal gingiva) or oval radiolucent defect between the diverging apices of the adjacent roots of teeth (Fig. 24). The lesions seldom exceed 1.5 cm at longest diameter. No periodontal ligament is visible between the lesion and the root of the tooth. In some instances vertical periodontal loss of bone has been seen, and erosion of the cortical plate of the mandible may be seen (320). The radiolucent area usually has a well-defined sclerotic margin, but may be somewhat ill defined. Resorption of adjacent roots of teeth has not been described. The minute calcifications found in some SOT are not visible on the radiograms. The diagnosis cannot be made on the basis of the radiogram alone.

Pathology. The etiology and pathogenesis of the SOT is unknown. Because of the close proximity of most SOTs to dental roots and periodontal tissue it is generally believed that they arise from remnants of the epithelial root sheet ("islands of Malassez"). At least one case (318) arose in the tissue covering the crown of an embedded mandibular molar.

Macroscopically the tissue is pink, firm, and rubbery, sometimes gristly in consistency with an irregular, smooth surface (296).

Histologically the SOT is composed of numerous islands of well-differentiated squamous epithelium, dispersed rather uniformly in an abundant fibrous connective tissue stroma with a moderate number of plumb, ovoid to spindle-shaped fibroblasts and sometimes with a light sprinkling of inflammatory cells (Fig. 25). The tumor is not encapsulated. Most of the epithelial islands are rounded or oval, but some may show indentations (Fig. 26). The islands may vary in size and shape, and some are narrow and elongated. A few of the larger islands may have pointed extensions (296,299,304,311,314).

The polygonal epithelial cells of the SOT have a uniform size and stainability with an abundant eosinophilic cytoplasm. Intercellular bridges (desmosomes) are numerous. There is virtually no mitotic activity. The islands are delineated by a flattened layer of basal

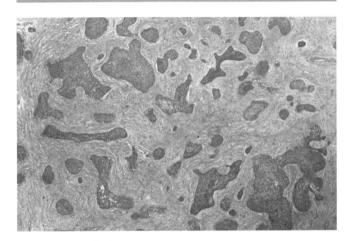

Figure 25 Squamous odontogenic tumor. Irregularly shaped and rounded islands of squamous epithelium are seen in a fibrous connective tissue stroma. The tumor was diagnosed in the maxillary premolar area of a 17-year-old woman. H&E stain. *Source*: From Ref. 317.

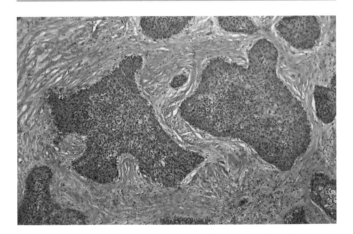

Figure 26 Squamous odontogenic tumor. Higher magnification of a part of the tumor seen in Figure 25. Tumor cells are small, uniformly sized, polyhedral and eosinophilic; the peripheral cells are flattened or cubic. Microcyst formation is seen in some areas. No stellate reticulum-like cells are seen in a SOT. H&E stain.

cells. No differentiation of central stellate reticulum and peripheral cylindrical basal cells is seen. Ghost cells have not, and clear cells have rarely been described. In some of the tumor islands, particularly the larger ones, small areas of microcystic vacuolization may be seen (300). Individual cell keratinization is a common feature and in some cases laminated, calcified bodies develop in the epithelial islands (304).

Hyperplastic islands of epithelium with morphology similar to those seen in SOT are sometimes seen in the wall of odontogenic cysts (321) and are not neoplastic. Several cases have been published in which conspicuous proliferation of SOT-like islands have been found in the mural connective tissue of odontogenic cysts (321–325). The term "squamous odontogenic hamartoid lesions" (SOHLs) have been suggested for such lesions (324). Apart from the extent of the proliferations no histological criteria exist to differentiate between SOHL and a genuine SOT. The question whether extensive SOT-like proliferations in a wall of an odontogenic cyst is in fact an initial neoplasm has not been solved.

Immunohistochemistry. No studies have detected any specific histochemical marker for the SOT, so the diagnosis is still based on histomorphology. The presence of CKs, involucrin, tumor suppressor gene products (p53), cell cycle regulators, amelogenin, and tenascin have been studied. In Tatemoto and coworkers' studies (251) of SOT (in tissue though with morphological resemblance to a DESAM), the tumor cells were negative for monoclonal PKK-1 detectable CK (40, 45 and 52, 5 kDa). Positive staining with monoclonal KL-1 (55–57 kDa CK) and polyclonal TK (41–65 kDa CK) was strong and confined to centrally located cells in tumor islands. Reichart and Philipsen (313) used monoclonal CK antibody ICN 8.12, which stains CK-13 (51 kDa) and CK-16 (48 kDa); tumor cells were strongly positive for both.

Yamada et al. (326) studied the presence of involucrin in SOT, and found a strong reaction in the center of the tumor islands. In the same study 31 of 40 ameloblastomas were negative and 9 faintly positive.

Tumor suppressor gene product p53 and cell cycle regulators PCNA and Ki-67 were studied by Ide et al. (315) on tissue from a recurrence of a SOT with initial SCC development. An overexpression of p53 was found in SCC cells, but SOT cells were negative. PCNA and Ki-67 was predominantly found in SCC cells. A weak reaction in some SOT islands was interpreted as related to beginning dysplastic changes.

The presence of amelogenin and tenascin was studied by Mori and coworkers (70,162). Moderate reaction for amelogenin was found in the epithelium of tumor islands; in centrally located, keratinized cells it was weak though. Tenascin (a multifunctional matrix glycoprotein, which can either promote or inhibit cell adhesion, depending on the cell type) was found in the interface (basement membrane) between tumor epithelium and the connective tissue, exclusively. Some areas were negative.

Electron Microscopy. No ultrastructural markers for SOT have been found. Studies (296,302,308) have shown tumor islands surrounded by a distinct basal lamina. The islands are composed of polyhedral epithelial cells of varying size and with irregular shape. Intercellular spaces are irregular, and in some areas edema is seen. The nuclei are large with many indentations. The chromatin is evenly distributed, nucleoli are few. In the cells of the center of some islands the nuclei are disintegrating. The cytoplasm contains few organelles: altered mitochondriae, some flattened cisternae of granular endoplasmic reticulum, a small Golgi apparatus, and glycogen granules, which are abundant in some cells and absent in others. Laminar structures (myelin bodies) have been described, but are few (296). Many cells have numerous tonofilaments in thick bundles. The connective tissue is striking (308); many fibroblasts exhibit an unusual shape with indented and convoluted nuclei and prominent endoplasmic reticulum. Often they are arranged concentrically around the epithelial islands. The fibrous component is very dense and often without clear typical periodic striation of collagen.

Molecular-Genetic Data. Leider et al. (311) reported one family with three affected siblings, each with multiple lesions. Mutations of the AMBN gene, which in humans maps to chromosome 4q21 have been detected in SOT, as well as in ameloblastoma and AOT (165), and were considered tumor-specific mutations. The SOT had a splicing mutation in exon 11 (IVS11-2A>G; A605G).

Differential Diagnosis. The most important differential diagnoses are: ameloblastoma (s/m, desmoplastic, and peripheral); SOHL in odontogenic cysts (324), pseudocarcinomatous hyperplasia in the gingival submucosa, and SCC.

Differentiation toward s/mAM and PERAM should not be difficult, even when they are acanthomatous. It is usually possible in some areas to find stellate reticulum-like epithelium and palisading, cylindrical basal cells with nuclei polarized away from the basement membrane, and sometimes a plexiform growth pattern can be seen as well; none of these features are seen in SOT. DESAM is a very difficult differential diagnosis; both tumors show an abundant fibrous stroma, and some published cases of SOT are likely to be DESAM (251–253). The clinical picture of the two tumors may differ; resorption of tooth roots is a common finding in DESAM. Histologically the DESAM may contain areas with ameloblastoma features (see above), if they are absent the most important differences found in DESAM are the many large and very irregular tumor islands with pointed extensions, interconnecting cords between the islands, presence of long, ramificating cords of single layered epithelium, and epithelial islands with increased cellular density with small sometimes spindle-shaped epithelial cells and cuboidal rather than flattened basal cells, as well as myxoid changes in the juxtaepithelial stroma. The SOT-like proliferations, which may be found (rarely) in an odontogenic cyst, have a morphology similar to that of the SOT. If they are extensive, a SOT should be considered and the follow-up of the patient adjusted accordingly. The most important differential diagnosis is intraosseous SCC. One convincing case of development of a SCC in a SOT in the lower left molar area of the mandible of a 53-year-old man has been published by Ide et al. (315). Norris et al. (306) published a case with bilateral maxillary SOT and a simultaneous mandibular SCC possibly arising in a SOT in a 26-year-old black man. In the former case cytological signs of epithelial dysplasia were evident in parts of the tumor. Benign SOT does not show cellular atypia.

Treatment and Prognosis. Conservative surgical procedures in terms of enucleation, curettage, or local excision are considered adequate (295). If one lesion is diagnosed it is important to remember that multifocal occurrence has been described. Recurrence has been described in two cases (296,316) and requires more extensive surgical excision. At least one case of SOT (315) has transformed into a carcinoma.

1.3 Calcifying Epithelial Odontogenic Tumor

Introduction. The CEOT is a slowly growing, benign, but nonencapsulated and locally invasive, epithelial, odontogenic neoplasm with a singular histomorphological pattern characterized by irregular sheets and islands of eosinophilic, polyhedral, and often pleomorphic cells, which eventually disintegrate into an eosinophilic, amorphous substance, which stains with amyloid markers and tend to calcify (327,328).

ICD-O code 9340/0

Synonyms: Pindborg tumor.

The tumor was defined as an entity by Pindborg in 1955 (329,330).

Clinical Features. The tumor is rare; no data about prevalence and incidence are available. The relative frequency of the tumor in material received for histological diagnosis in services of diagnostic pathology in various countries for various amounts of years ranges from 0.5% to 2.5% in studies comprising more than 300 samples of odontogenic tumors. The results are indicated as follows: number of odontogenic tumors/number of CEOTs/%. Regezzi et al., Michigan, U.S.A. (31): 706/6/0.8%, Günhan et al., Turkey (32): 409/6/1.5%, Daley et al., Canada (33): 392/5/1.3%, Mosqueda-Taylor et al., Mexico (34): 349/3/0.8%, Ochsenius et al., Chile (35): 362/2/0.6%, Adebayo et al., Nigeria (36): 318/3/1.0%, Fernandes et al., Brazil (37): 340/4/1.2%, Ladeinde et al., Nigeria (38): 319/5/1.6%, Buchner et al., California (30): 1088/5/0.5%, Jones et al., England (2006, pooled figures from two studies)(39,40): 523/13/2.5%, Olgac et al., Turkey (41): 527/5/0.9%, and Jing et al., China (42): 1642/10/0.6%.

The data are skewed; however, the figures reflect regional differences in type of lesions sent for histopathological confirmation rather than effects of genetical or environmental factors.

The number of published cases is close to 190. Major reviews of the literature have been published by Franklin et al. (331): 113 cases, Philipsen et al. (332): 181 cases, and Kaplan et al. (333): 67 cases.

Like most odontogenic tumors the CEOT occurs as an intraosseous and as a rarer and less aggressive extraosseous variant. The male:female ratio for the intraosseous variant is between 1:1 (332) and 1:1.5 (333), and for the extraosseous variant 1:0.8 (based on 11 cases only) (332).

The age range is between 8 and 92 years at the time of diagnosis, with a mean of 36.9 years for both topographic variants. The mean for the intraosseous variant is 38.9 years and for the extraosseous variant 34.4 years, which may be explained by the fact that the extraosseous variant presents as a gingival enlargement, which is likely to be diagnosed at an early stage. The age peak for men is in the third decade and for women in the fourth decade (332,334). The majority of intraosseous cases are diagnosed in patients between 20 and 60 years of age.

There is a predilection for peripheral (extraosseous) cases to occur in the anterior segment of the jaws (335). They present as a gingival swelling covered by mucosa of normal color (Fig. 27). The intraosseous tumors on the other hand occur primarily in the mandible and particularly in the premolar and molar regions. The mandible : maxilla ratio is 2:1 (332,333). Simultaneous occurrence of CEOT in more than one location has been described, but is exceedingly rare (336–338).

The growth rate is slow. The tumor is usually symptomless, apart from a slowly progressive swelling of the jaw. There are a few reports associated with pain, nasal obstruction, epistaxis, and proptosis (331). An unusual case of maxillary CEOT, which caused displacement of the eye in a 30-year-old woman, was published by Bridle et al. (339).

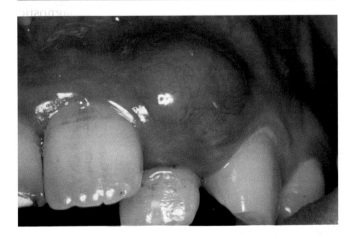

Figure 27 Peripheral calcifying epithelial odontogenic tumor in the upper left lateral incisor area of a 29-year-old woman. The lesion, which had existed for 5 years, was firm and symptom less apart from the swelling. There were no radiographic changes. *Source*: Ref. 348.

About 60% of the intraosseous tumors are associated with an unerupted permanent tooth, most often a mandibular molar (333).

Imaging. Radiograms of CEOTs may show a considerable variation; its appearance may range from a diffuse, poorly demarcated, or well-circumscribed unilocular radiolucency to a combined pattern of radiolucency and radiopacity with small intralesional septa producing a multilocular pattern. The pattern showing flecks of calcification scattered in an area of radiolucency has been called "driven snow." Early cases are radiolucent and resemble a dentigerous cyst or an ameloblastoma. With increasing calcification radio-opacities become visible and differential diagnoses are ossifying fibroma and odontogenic fibroma.

Kaplan et al. (333) have reviewed the radiographic features of 67 patients with CEOT (68 lesions), primarily from the literature. There were 27 males and 39 females in the group ($N = 66$) with an age range from 13 to 77 years (mean 43.5 years). The most frequent was a mixed radiolucent–radiopaque pattern, which was present in 44 (65%) of the lesions. Radiolucent lesions were present in 22 (32%) and radiopaque in two (3%). The mixed radiolucent–radiopaque type was nearly twice as prevalent as the radiolucent type in both jaws. Among 55 lesions 32 (58%) were unilocular; 15 (27%) were multilocular, and 8 (15%) were not loculated (diffuse).

The definition of the border of the tumor was described in 61 lesions, of which 12 (19.7%) had well defined or corticated borders, 36 (59%) had defined but not corticated borders, and 13 (21.3%) had diffuse borders.

In 41 cases (60%), one or more impacted teeth were involved. The specific tooth was indicated for 45 teeth: Three (7%) were incisors, five (11%) canines, seven (16%) premolars, 28 (62%) molars, and two (4%) were supernumerary or unidentified teeth. Among the molars 18 (40%) were first or second molars, and 10 (22%) were third molars. Cases with increased radiopacity close to the occlusal surface of an impacted molar ("coronal clustering") was described by Pindborg (330) and by others (Fig. 28). Coronal clustering was found in eight (12%) of the cases studied by Kaplan et al. (333). The driven snow pattern was clearly recognizable in only one case. Displacement of teeth was evident in 28 cases (41%), and root resorption in six (4%) cases.

The size of the lesions at time of surgery varied between 0.5 and 10 cm (mean 3.5 cm). Most of the small lesions (<3 cm) were radiolucent (89%) and none were mixed; most of the large lesions were mixed (74%) and only 21% were radiolucent.

Peripheral CEOTs usually contain little or no calcifications that is not detected on radiograms; some have shown superficial erosion of the underlying bone.

A clear-cell variant of the CEOT has been described and a more aggressive behavior has been attributed to them. Anavi et al. (340) reviewed 19 cases of this variant and found 12 central and 7 peripheral.

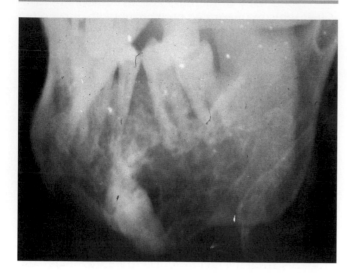

Figure 28 Calcifying epithelial odontogenic tumor in the right mandible of a 40-year-old man. The lesion is poorly demarcated and shows a honeycomb-like structure with a mixture of radiolucency and radiopacity. An embedded first molar is displaced to the base of the mandible. *Source*: From case No. 6 in Ref. 475.

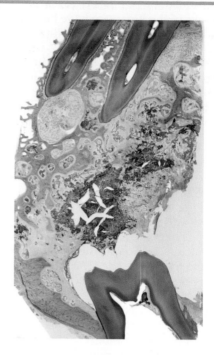

Figure 29 Calcifying epithelial odontogenic tumor. Section of the tumor seen in Figure 28, the tumor has destroyed the bone of the central area and is seen in the surrounding bone cavities. The heavily calcified tumor tissue close to the occlusal surface of the embedded molar is presumably the oldest part of the tumor, which may have developed from proliferations of odontogenic epithelium in the dental sac. Growth of the tumor takes place in the uncalcified areas primarily. H&E stain. *Source*: From Ref. 475.

The proportion of peripheral cases with clear cells is higher than in the conventional CEOT; they seem to have a greater tendency to develop on the gingiva. The radiographic picture of the central clear-cell variant differed in several ways. Of particular interest were a higher proportion of tumors with cortical perforation, 67% compared with 6.7% in conventional CEOT, which may indicate a more aggressive behavior.

Pathology.   The etiology and source of origin of the tumor is unknown. It was believed for a long time (17,330,341) that the tumor arises in the reduced enamel epithelium of an embedded tooth (Fig. 29). Since not all CEOTs develop in association with an embedded tooth, there must be other sources, and remnants of the dental lamina is an obvious candidate (16,342). Proliferating odontogenic epithelium at the top of the dental follicle of an unerupted tooth (343) at the lower orifice of the gubernaculum dentis is another possibility.

Although the tumor is in some cases relatively easily enucleated, it is nonencapsulated apart from focal areas in some tumors, and it resorbs and infiltrates the surrounding bone. Macroscopically it presents as a firm mass of varying color and at bisecting the specimen usually reveals calcified particles. There may be minute cystic spaces in the tissue, but only one case of unicystic lesion with the tumor developing apparently in the wall of a dentigerous cyst has been published (344).

The classic histological picture of an intraosseous CEOT as described by Pindborg (330) shows irregular sheets and islands often with many pointed extensions, which consist of polyhedral epithelial cells with abundant eosinophilic cytoplasm (Fig. 30), sharply defined cell borders, and well developed intercellular bridges (328). The nuclei are round and sometimes

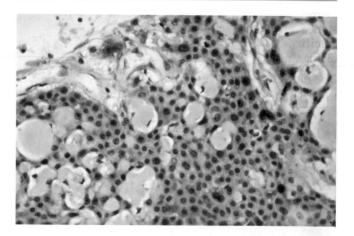

Figure 30 Calcifying epithelial odontogenic tumor. Polyhedral epithelial cells with abundant eosinophilic cytoplasm are seen. Many of them show various stages of disintegration with formation of homogeneous eosinophilic masses. Remnants of pycnotic nuclei are seen in several of the disintegrated cells. The intact tumor cells exhibit rounded nuclei with varying stainability and some pleomorphism. No mitoses are seen. H&E stain.

slightly lobulated, most of them are strongly basophilic, and they are frequently pleomorphic, but the number of pleomorphic nuclei differs from tumor to tumor. Mitotic figures are rarely encountered, and the nuclear pleomorphism is not a sign of malignancy. In a rare case of malignant transformation the number of mitoses is conspicuously increased, tumor cells are found within the vessels, and the Ki-67 index is considerably elevated (345–347). Double-nucleated cells may be seen, and the nucleoli may be prominent.

Within the sheets of tumor cells are various amounts of rounded, eosinophilic homogeneous masses (Fig. 30). The substance can be observed intracellularly in swollen epithelial cells with disintegrated nuclei displaced to the cellular border, which has lost its integrity (341,348–350) and presumably represents perished tumor cells, although it has also been interpreted as a secretion product (350), and even as enamel matrix (351,352). Most of the substance is found extracellularly and when it is distributed in foci within a tumor island the pattern is cribriform. Extensive amounts of the eosinophilic, homogeneous substance may be seen in the connective tissue at some distance from intact tumor islands. They may still represent areas of perished tumor cells, although they have been interpreted differently. Often small clusters of compressed cells remain in the areas.

Vickers et al. (353) demonstrated the substance to react positively to amyloid staining like Congo red and fluorescence with thioflavine T (Fig. 31). This finding has been confirmed by numerous later investigators (352,354–356). The eosinophilic, homogeneous, positive amyloid reacting substance eventually becomes calcified. Calcified foci are initially seen as tiny spots in small areas of the substance (Fig. 32). With increasing calcification they form spherules showing appositional basophilic concentric rings (Liesegang rings). Eventually the calcified areas coalesce, forming large calcified aggregates. Before calcification the homogeneous substance is faintly PAS-positive, but with progressive calcification the areas become more PAS-positive (355). Calcified spherules may also be seen scattered

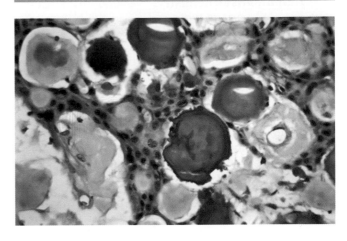

Figure 32 Calcifying epithelial odontogenic tumor. Calcification of the eosinophilic material is seen initially as tiny spots. With increasing calcification spherules with basophilic concentric rings are formed. H&E stain.

in the connective tissue without association to the homogeneous substance. In some tumors formation of rounded islands of hard tissue is seen; it is a cellular product that contains collagen and has morphology-like cementum.

There is a considerable histomorphological variation from tumor to tumor and within the individual tumors. Some are dominated by large irregular epithelial sheets, other show numerous small islands and strands of tumor epithelium in the connective tissue stroma, which always consist of mature collagenous connective tissue. Calcification may be sparse or conspicuous; extensive calcification is primarily seen in large tumors of long duration.

The extraosseous variant of CEOT shows principally the same histomorphology, but the tumors cells form rather strands and small islands than large sheets, and the amount of calcified material may be minimal or lacking. The extraosseous variants are undoubtedly diagnosed at an earlier stage than the intraosseous tumors.

In a few cases Langerhans cells have been described in the tumor (357,358); the cells were S-100 protein-positive and identified ultrastructurally on the finding of rod- and tennisracket-shaped Birckbeck's granules. Their function in the tumor is unknown.

The presence of numerous clear cells in CEOT is uncommon; Krolls and Pindborg (359) reported the first two examples of this rare tumor in 1974; Philipsen and Reichart reviewed 15 cases in 2000 (332), and further cases have been published (340,360,361). In some of the cases the clear cells component has been so dominating that the tumors are probably better classified as CCOC (340,362) with patterns of CEOT. Such CEOT patterns are also seen in AOTs. There is evidence that CEOTs with numerous clear cells are more aggressive than CEOTs without clear cells (340).

A hybrid tumor with areas showing the histomorphology of a CEOT and others with that of a typical s/mAM was published by Seim et al. (363).

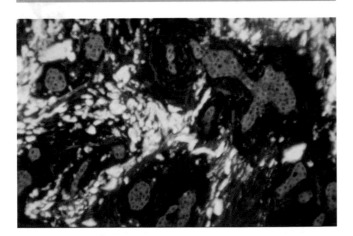

Figure 31 Calcifying epithelial odontogenic tumor. The eosinophilic homogeneous material reacts positively to amyloid staining. This section was stained with thioflavine T and observed in fluorescent light. An intense yellow light is emitted from the thioflavine positive material. Intact tumor islands with dark nuclei are faintly seen.

Immunohistochemistry. Several investigators have detected various types of CKs in the tumor cells. Broad spectred keratin antibodies and CK "cocktail" antibodies like KL-1, AE1/AE3, and TK have given consistently positive reaction particularly in strongly eosinophilic cells (352,360,362,364–366). Monoclonal antibodies against single CKs have given more controversial results (66,163,360,362,365). High molecular weight (mw) CKs, CK-1, CK-5, and CK-14 were detected by Kumamoto et al. (362); the finding of CK-14 were confirmed by others (66,360). The low mw CK-19 was detected in several studies, but not in all tumors (362) (66,320,365).

A CK antibody reaction was found in the amyloid-like material in two studies (352,367).

Epithelial membrane antigens (EMAs) have been detected in tumor cells (346,365) as well as filagrin (362). Vimentin (filaments) have been detected in a few studies (364,365).

Tenascin, an extracellular matrix protein has been found in the stroma and in moderate amount in tumor cells, particularly cells bordering amyloid-like substance (70,360).

Basement membrane–associated molecules have been studied by Sauk et al. (367) who detected laminin and type IV collagen in the amyloid-like deposits. Aviel-Ronen et al. (352) could not confirm these findings. Poomsawat et al. (366) detected laminin 1, laminin 5, and fibronectin in tumor cells, but they were collagen type IV negative.

Hard tissue–related proteins have been studied. BMP could not be detected (168), but BSP was clearly demonstrated by means of antibodies and ISH in calcified material and in tumor cells adjacent to calcified particles (167).

Enamel proteins are demonstrable in CEOTs. The results of the studies of amelogenin have been controversial. Mori et al. (162) found amelogenin in the amyloid-like substance in the periphery of well-calcified material, but not in the tumor cells. Saku et al. (159) detected amelogenin in small mineralized foci and in the tumor cells surrounding them. Kumamoto et al. (163) found amelogenin in tumor cells and in intercellular amyloid-like material, but not in the calcified tissue.

Enamelin has been demonstrated in small mineralized foci and in the tumor cells surrounding them (159).

Enamelysin (MMP-20) was detected by Takata et al. (160) at weak to moderate levels in amyloid-like material and in the adjacent tumor cells as well as in epithelial cells in the tumor islands. Some mineralized foci were positively stained.

The enzyme alkaline phosphatase, which is related to mineralization has been demonstrated in the tumor cells, particularly at the cell membrane by several investigators (368–370).

The amyloid-like material has been tested by means of antibodies against amyloid A, and was found negative in both studies (352,360).

Langerhans cells have been encountered in CEOT also within the tumor islands; they have been shown to be S-100 protein-positive (356,357,365,366).

Studies with the proliferation marker Ki-67 have shown that the index is low in benign CEOTs, but increased five times in tumors with signs of malignancy (346). In a case of malignant CEOT with metastases to the lung, Kawano et al. (371) assessed the proliferative activity with Ki-67 L.I. The Ki-67 index was significantly higher in the recurrent and the metastatic lesion than in the original lesion. An increase in KI-67 L.I. was associated with the appearance of histological features suggestive of malignancy.

Electron Microscopy. Ultrastructural studies of tumor cells have shown polyhedral epithelial cells with abundant cytoplasm with a large number of electron-dense bundles of tonofilaments (CKs) (355,358,368,370–373). The most peripheral part of the cytoplasm shows finer and less electron-dense filaments except at the desmosome junctions to which tonofilaments are attached. Some cells contain large numbers of mitochondria, a Golgi apparatus and pinocytotic vesicles, but no secretory vacuoles. The rough endoplasmic reticulum (RER) is generally poorly developed and free ribosomes are numerous in some cells, but sparse in others. Lysosomes of autophagic type are seen in some cells, and occasionally small clusters of glycogen are present. Most nuclei are large and rounded with foci of condensed heterochromatin. Nucleoli are prominent with a pronounced nucleolemma. Some nuclei have irregular outlines, and in between nuclei with very deep indentations are encountered. Tumor cells with more than one nucleus can be seen. A very conspicuous finding, which has been confirmed by all investigators is a large number of closely clustered delicate microvilli on the surface of the cells, only punctuated by the prominent desmosome connections between the cells. Lamina densa and hemidesmosomes are seen in the basal cells, and sometimes, replicated basal lamina is found around the peripheral cells.

Page et al. (372) reported that many cells within the tumor appeared to be in various stages of cellular necrosis and dissolution judged primarily from the irregular and pyknotic nuclear forms. Cells in an early stage showed light nuclear changes, loss of microvilli, and discontinuities in the outer cellular membrane. In later stages of dissolution pronounced karyorrhexis and dense nuclear pyknosis was observed, and the cytoplasm became divided in an inner almost empty area with few recognizable elements and an outer area with poorly formed electron-dense material arranged in laminar pattern. Neighboring tumor cells within the same field were well preserved.

Many investigators have studied the homogeneous amyloid-staining positive material (350,352,355, 358,370,374). Intracytoplasmic location of the substance has been observed by Mainwaring et al. (350), Chaudhry et al. (355), and Chomette et al. (370), but most studies have concentrated on the more abundant occurrence of the material extracellularly. It has been described as a granulofilamentous material with sheets of fine filaments measuring 10 to 12 nm (352,374). Numerous hypotheses have been forwarded regarding the formation and the nature of the substance; some have considered it a product from degeneration of the epithelial cells, some suggested it is a secretion product of the cells, and others have regarded it as a type of amyloid formed in the connective tissue. Studies of the molecular biology of the material has revealed it as a unique protein (375), but its pathogenesis is still poorly understood.

Some investigators have paid attention to other types of cells in the tumor. El-Labban et al. (373) observed myoepithelial cells peripheral and juxtaposed to the epithelial cells. Kumamoto et al. (362) described clear cells in CEOT and found abundant glycogen granules and a paucity of organelles in the cytoplasm.

Besides the calcifications in a CEOT some of them show varying amounts of islands of a hard tissue with cementum-like morphology (376,377). The outer layer of these consists of typical banded calcified collagen and has banded collagen fibers like Sharpey fibers arranged perpendicularly to the surface to the calcified lamellar bodies. Cells similar to cementoblasts or osteoblasts are seen in close association with the surface.

Molecular-Genetic Data.   The amyloid-reacting substance in CEOT has been studied by Solomon et al. (375). They used microanalytic techniques to characterize the protein nature of the CEOT-associated substance isolated from specimens obtained from three patients. As evidenced by the results of amino acid sequencing and mass spectrometry, the fibrils were found to be composed of a polypeptide of approximately 46 mer. This component was identical in sequence to the *N*-terminal portion of a hypothetical 153-residue protein encoded by the FLJ20513 gene cloned from the human KATO III cell line. That the amyloid protein was derived from this larger molecule was demonstrated by RT-PCR amplification of tumor cell RNA where a full-length FLJ20513 transcript was found. Furthermore, immunohistochemical analyses revealed that the amyloid within the CEOTs immunostained with antibodies prepared against a synthetic FLJ20513-related dodecapeptide. The authors claim that the studies provide unequivocal evidence that CEOT-associated amyloid consists of a unique and previously undescribed protein, which they designated APin in recognition of Dr. Jens J. Pindborg's initial reports of the tumor (330,348,354). Subsequently the name was changed to ODAM because the protein was detected in other odontogenic and non-odontogenic epithelial neoplasms (378).

Differential Diagnosis.   Microscopically the classic CEOT is quite distinctive and not too difficult to diagnose. In absence of calcification and presence of cellular pleomorphism a primary intraosseous squamous cell carcinoma (PIOSCC) or metastatic tumor should be ruled out. In contrast to these the CEOT is characterized by none or few mitotic figures and a low Ki-67 index.

In cases with a considerable amount of clear cells the differential diagnoses are CCOC, central mucoepidermoid carcinoma, central acinic cell carcinoma, and metastatic renal carcinoma.

Tumors consisting of short strands and small islands of epithelium in abundant fibrous connective

tissue stroma and with little or no eosinophilic, homogeneous, amyloid-staining positive substance or calcification may be difficult to distinguish from an epithelium-rich odontogenic fibroma. Both may show foci of calcified material and cementum-like hard tissue. As the connective tissue is the tumor component, it is conspicuously more cellular than the stroma of a CEOT. Amyloid staining (Congo red and fluorescent thioflavine T) in most cases will disclose minute areas of amyloid-positive homogeneous substance in a CEOT; it is not supposed to be present in an odontogenic fibroma. Dunlap (379) reported, however, two cases of what they considered epithelium-rich odontogenic fibromas, which both contained solitary or clustered eosinophilic hyaline droplets, which were weakly positive for amyloid staining. A similar case was published by Smith et al. (380) as a CEOT. In such atypical cases, particularly if the connective tissue component is moderately cellular, the differential diagnosis may be extremely difficult, but would have no consequence for the treatment.

Treatment and Prognosis.   Methods of treatment have varied from simple enucleation or curettage to hemimandibulectomy or hemimaxillectomy. Treatment is dictated to some extent by the location and the size of the tumor. Complete removal is necessary, so resection of the entire mass, with tumor-free surgical margins and long-term follow-up is indicated (24). Reports with longtime follow-up are not numerous. Franklin et al. (331) reviewed 17 cases with a follow-up of 10 years or more, and reported a recurrence rate of 14%, which was believed mostly to be due to inadequate treatment. There is a need for long-term follow-up; the longest period over which any CEOT has been reported to recur is 31 years (349). None of the peripheral cases have been reported to recur (332). Although the clear cell variant of CEOT can be considered more aggressive, it does not seem to recur more often with adequate treatment (340). Four cases of malignant transformation have been reported (345–347,371).

1.4   *Adenomatoid Odontogenic Tumor*

Introduction.   The AOT is a slowly growing, encapsulated, epithelial odontogenic tumor with a singular histomorphological pattern with whorled nodules of spindle cells, plexiform double cell strands and formation of microcystic or duct-like spaces. It has a limited growth potential, and generally it is not believed to be a neoplasm (23,334,381,382).

ICD-O code 9300/0

Synonyms: Adenoameloblastoma (obsolete).

Clinical Features.   The prevalence and incidence of the AOT is unknown. The relative frequency of the tumor in material received for histological diagnosis in services of diagnostic pathology in various countries for various amounts of years ranges from 1.7% to 7.5% in studies comprising more than 300 samples of odontogenic tumors. The results are indicated as follows: number of odontogenic tumors/ number of AOTs/%. Regezzi et al., Michigan, U.S.A.

(31): 706/22/3.1%, Günhan et al., Turkey (32): 409/11/2.7%, Daley et al., Canada (33): 392/13/3.3%, Mosqueda-Taylor et al., Mexico (34): 349/25/7.1%, Ochsenius et al., Chile (35): 362/24/6.6%, Adebayo et al., Nigeria (36): 318/9/2.8%, Fernandes et al., Brazil (37): 340/13/3.8%, Ladeinde et al., Nigeria (38): 319/24/7.5%, Buchner et al., California (30): 1088/19/1.7%, Jones et al., England (2006, pooled figures from two studies)(39),(40): 523/13/2.5%, Olgac et al., Turkey (41): 527/11/2.1%, and Jing et al., China (42): 1642/68/4.1%. The data are skewed; however, the figures reflect regional differences in type of lesions sent for histopathological confirmation rather than effects of genetical or environmental factors.

Although AOT is an uncommon lesion, more than 750 cases have been published (334), and it is the third or fourth most common odontogenic tumor in several of the studies after odontomas, ameloblastoma, and myxoma. In a review (383) comprising cases published to the end of 2005, cases collected from files in institutions in 12 different counties, and cases published in Chinese and Japanese languages 1082 cases were found.

Females are affected nearly twice as common as males. On the basis of a survey of more than 500 cases from the literature, the male-female ratio was 1:1.9 (334,384). The ratio was confirmed in the review of 1082 cases (383). An analysis of 67 cases from a Thai population (385) showed a ratio of 1:1.8. In the surveys from the oral pathology biopsy services mentioned above the ratio has varied from 1:0.8 to 1:2.7. It is uncertain if racial differences exist.

The age range has varied between 3 and 82 years, at the time of diagnosis (384). However, almost 70% of the tumors have been diagnosed in patients in their second decade of life and more than 50% in patients between 13- and 19-years-old (384). Few patients have been older than 30 years (383).

A peripheral (extra osseous) counterpart exists (386,387); Buchner et al. (212) reported six cases; a total about 20 cases have been published (384) and almost all have occurred in the anterior part of the maxilla. They are very rare in the mandible. Peripheral AOT presents as a pink gingival swelling. The mean age of 19 cases (range 3–21 years) was found to be 13.3 years (383).

More than 95% of all cases occur within the bone, however, and predominantly in the anterior regions. The maxilla is affected about twice as often as the mandible, ratio maxilla:mandible = 1:0.6 (383–385). The lower and particularly the upper canine area is a predilection site for development of the AOT (388), it occurs only rarely in the posterior regions. A total of 19 cases located to the third molar area have been reported (383).

The AOT is often asymptomatic; many of them are discovered during the course of a radiographic examination with the purpose of revealing the cause of a disturbance in tooth eruption. Larger lesions may cause painless expansion of the bone. The growth rate is slow.

Imaging. Since the majority of AOTs develop at an early age and often in the canine area, they easily become an obstacle in the way of eruption of the permanent canines. The consequence is that the eruption of the canines leads them in contact with the AOT, which wrap around the crown of the tooth or sometimes the entire tooth. This so-called "follicular" AOT simulates a dentigerous cyst (Fig. 33) and may be impossible to distinguish from a dentigerous cyst on a radiogram unless the radiolucency extends apically along the root past the cementoenamel junction. The tumor is well defined and unilocular; scattered fine radiopacities may be seen within the radiolucent area particularly on an intraoral film; they have been observed in between 50% and 75% of published cases (389,390). This follicular type is by far the most common and makes up about 70% of all AOTs (383,384,390). More rarely the AOT involves the second permanent incisor or the first permanent premolar. Involvement of other permanent teeth is rare and AOTs that surround deciduous teeth are exceedingly rare (385,391).

The intraosseous AOTs that are unrelated to an unerupted tooth ("extrafollicular" type) present as a well-delineated radiolucent lesion. Dependent on its location in relation to the teeth in the area the extrafollicular type can simulate a residual, a periapical radicular, a lateral radicular, or a lateral periodontal cyst. It may, however, also be located deep in the jaw without relation to any tooth (384,388). When situated adjacent to teeth, the tumor often causes displacement

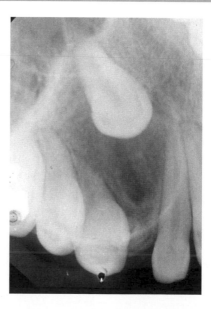

Figure 33 Adenomatoid odontogenic tumor in the maxillary canine area of a 12-year-old girl. On the radiogram the lesion simulates a dentigerous cyst around the crown of the canine and was diagnosed as such before removal.

of these. In isolated cases, root resorption (392–395), perforation of the bone corticals, and invasion of the maxillary sinus have been observed (388,390,396).

The size of the lesion has been between 1.5 and 3 cm in the vast majority of published cases (388). In a multicentric study including 39 cases, Leon et al. (390) found a range of size between 1 and 7 cm, with an average of 2.9 cm.

The peripheral type may occasionally show erosion ("saucerization") of the alveolar bone crest (397).

Pathology. The pathology and pathogenesis of the AOT is unknown. The most likely source of tumor development is residues of the dental lamina and proliferations of odontogenic epithelium adjacent to the reduced enamel epithelium of unerupted teeth.

Macroscopically the tumor is well circumscribed and usually encapsulated. Some present as a solid mass, those situated around the crown of a tooth are cystic or partly cystic (Fig. 34).

The histopathology of the AOT is unrelated to its location in the jaws; all types show the same pattern. Solid lesions consist of a proliferating epithelium surrounded by a well-defined fibrous capsule (Fig. 35). Various patterns are seen in the epithelium. In some areas, which are often dominating, spindle cells and polyhedral cells in a swirled pattern form ball of yarn-like nodules. Several nodules of various sizes are placed close together with narrow strands of more orderly arranged epithelial cells in between. The stromal tissue is minimal in these areas. Some epithelial cells are forming small nests ("rosettes") often enclosing droplets of an eosinophilic, PAS-positive diastase resistant substance, which is extracellular. Cystic spaces of different sizes may be seen between the nodules. They are usually referred to as "duct-like

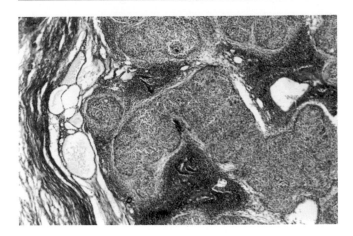

Figure 35 Adenomatoid odontogenic tumor. From the periphery of a tumor in the maxillary canine area of a 19-year-old woman. A capsule is clearly seen to the left. Tumor cells are seen in sheets and islands, they form ball of yarn-like structures in the less cell rich areas. Between these areas and the capsule, the tumor cells form loops of thin strands consisting of a single or two layers of cuboidal cells. The stroma within the loops has degenerated. van Gieson stain.

spaces" (334), but are globular, not tubular structures, irrespective of the direction in which they are cut. They are not present in all tumors and may be few in some of them. The lumen is lined by a layer of orderly arranged epithelial cells disposed radially. Around smaller cystic spaces the cells are columnar, around larger they are shorter or even cuboidal. The cytoplasm is lightly stained, and oval nuclei are polarized away from the lumen (381,398). Larger cystic spaces are lined by a cuboidal epithelium without polarization of the nuclei. In the lumen a wispy PAS-positive, diastase-resistant, eosinophilic material is often seen. Some of the cystic structures show invagination of part of the wall resulting in an almost horse-shoe formed structure with two layers of columnar cells separated by a narrow zone of PAS-positive, eosinophilic material and with the nuclei polarized away from that zone (Fig. 36).

There may be scattered foci of polyhedral squamous cells in the tumor. Another and conspicuous cellular pattern is characterized by long, narrow epithelial strands consisting of two layers or a single layer of cubic cells (Fig. 35). They form large loops, which are connected to each other in a plexiform pattern. The stroma inside the loop is often very loose and sometimes missing. This pattern is found in particular toward the periphery of the lesion. By some authors it is referred to as "cribriform" but most of the loops are large; they are not small apertures as in a sieve. A similar pattern is seen in O-As. In the stroma a perivascular hyalinization with concentric disposition of hyalinous layers in the surrounding connective tissue and degeneration of the endothelial layer is common finding (390,399).

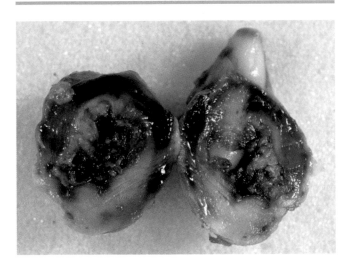

Figure 34 Adenomatoid odontogenic tumor. The macroscopic picture of the interior of the lesion seen in Figure 33 clearly shows that the cystic lesion is attached to the distal part of the root and not to the enamel-cementum border. The tooth has "erupted" into the lesion. Note the irregular surface of the cystic cavity.

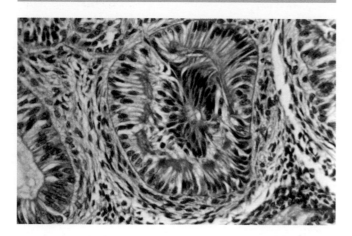

Figure 36 Adenomatoid odontogenic tumor. Higher magnification from the tumor in Figure 35. Part of a "duct"-like structure lined by palisaded columnar cells is seen to the left. In the middle a similar structure is seen with invagination of the wall and with two layers of columnar epithelial cells separated by a zone of PAS positive (diastase resistant) material. Periodic acid–Schiff—hemalun stain.

Calcified material in various amounts and sometimes dominating is seen in most of the tumors and often with a laminated pattern of concentric rings. The calcification takes place in the degenerated epithelium and in the extracellular, eosinophilic, PAS-positive material, which nature has been interpreted in many ways (400–402); the matter is not yet solved (334).

Eosinophilic, hyalinized, dentinoid material often with entrapped epithelium is seen in many cases (403), and part of it may be mineralized. During normal odontogenesis and in odontomes and ameloblastic fibro-odontomes the development of tubular dentin takes place only if a cellular, embryonic pulp-like odontogenic ectomesenchyme is present. Nevertheless a few cases of AOT with tubular dentin without such mesenchyme have been published (404,405).

A common feature in AOT is minor areas of tumor tissue showing a histomorphology similar to that of the CEOT (397,406–409). Careful study of such cases (410) including follow-up of the postoperative course has shown that the occurrence of such areas with structure of a CEOT does not change the behavior of the AOT, the capsule remains intact and recurrence is unlikely.

Very uncommon is the occurrence of AOT-like structures in lesions ("Adenomatoid dentinoma"), which must be interpreted as a kind of odontomes (411–414).

Mitotic figures may be found occasionally in AOT, but dysplasia has never been described. Melanin occurs sometimes in AOTs (415,416), as in many epithelial odontogenic tumors.

Like the solid AOT, the cystic, follicular variant has a thick fibrous capsule with a smooth surface. On section a large cystic cavity is seen, which is partially filled with solid tissue, and mineralized foci may be detected already macroscopically. In histological sections the tumor tissue is found on the inside and shows the same histomorphology as seen in the solid variant. Part of the luminal surface of the cystic lesion may be covered with a thin layer of squamous epithelium as seen in dental sacs and dentigerous cysts. If the tumor and the tooth were removed in toto it may be possible to see this layer in continuation with the reduced enamel epithelium of the dental sac.

Immunohistochemistry. A number of immunohistochemical studies with different types of antibodies have been published during the later years. AOT tumor cells are S-100 protein-negative (417,418). CK studies with AE1/AE3 (broad spectred CK antibodies) revealed a positive staining in epithelial tumor cells, primarily in nodular areas and in cells of the duct-like microcysts (390,419). The reaction to KL-1 was weaker (417). All epithelial cells in AOT react to pankeratin antibodies (159). Monoclonal antibodies against individual CKs were used by Leon et al. (390); the tumor cells reacted to the following type II CKs, CK-5, CK-7, and CK-8. CK-7 and CK-8 were mostly found in the loop forming narrow epithelial strands. Other investigators have been unable to detect CK-7 and CK-8 (66,420). Among the type I CKs, CK-10 and CK-13 are not expressed (66,390). Tumor cells have reacted strongly to CK-14 in several studies (66,390,420), Leon et al. (390) found, however, that columnar cell linings of the duct-like microcysts reacted negatively to CK-14, but positively to CK-19. Cells have been CK-18-negative in all studies (66,390,420,421). Crivelini et al. (420) could not detect CK-19 in AOTs.

Involucrin could not be detected (326).

Nestin, an intermediate filament of the cytoskeleton, which is related to tooth development and repair of dentin was detected by Fujita et al. (422), who found an intense expression in small nodular foci and rosette patterns and in whorled spindle cells.

Integrin, a plasma membrane protein plays a role in the attachment of a cell to the extracellular matrix and to other cells, and as a signal transductor has been studied by Souza Andrada et al. (76). Integrin α2β1, α3β1, and α5β1 were detected in ameloblastomas and AOTs. The labeling intensity was considerably stronger in the ameloblastomas than in the AOTs.

Surprisingly, vimentin, an intermediated filament protein characteristic of fibroblasts have been detected in the trabeculae and loop-forming strands areas and in the cuboidal cells peripheral to the nodules in 22 of 39 cases of AOT by Leon et al. (390). In other studies vimentin was not detected (417–421).

The presences of some growth factors have been studied. Kumamoto et al. (134) used antibodies against HGF, TGF-β, and their receptors C-Met and TβRs on sections from five AOTs. HGF expression was detected in tumor cells, and was especially prominent in pseudoglandular cells in duct-like structures. The reaction in the epithelium was moderate to strong for all four antibodies. The reaction in stroma cells to HGF and TGF-β was weak and to both receptors negative. Fibroblast growth factors FGF-1 and FGF-2 and receptors FGFR2 and FGFR3 were studied by So et al. in sections from three AOTs (136). FGF-2 and FGFR2 were detected in AOT epithelium, but reactions to FGF-1 and FGFR3 were negative.

Extracellular matrix proteins have been studied. Ito et al. (67) used antibodies against versican, a large chondroitin sulfate proteoglycan, and found a positive reaction in a few solid areas in the tumor cell nests and in calcified areas. Tenascin, a multifunctional glycoprotein involved in cell-to-cell and cell-extracellular matrix interactions during odontogenesis and several other functions was studied by Mori et al. (70). A positive staining was limited to the interface corresponding to the basement membrane of the pseudoglandular epitheliums of microcysts and the loop forming single/double cell layer strands.

Basement membrane–associated macromolecules like laminin, heparin sulfate proteoglycan, and fibronectin as well as collagen type IV and type V were studied by Murata et al. (402). Laminin, heparin sulfate proteoglycan, fibronectin, and type V collagen were localized in the luminal spaces of the duct-like microcysts and along the inner rim of the duct-like structures. They were also detected in the eosinophilic hyaline droplets and variously shaped inner stromal spaces of whorled or rosette-like foci. Crevelini et al studied laminin with similar results (420).

Hard tissue–related proteins have been studied by several groups. Gao et al. (168) did not find BMP in AOT. Kumamoto et al. (169) used RT-PCR analysis to identify expression of mRNA transcript for BMPs and their associated molecules and detected expression in three of six AOTs. A strong reaction to BMP-2, BMP-4, BMP-7, BMPRs, and CBFA1 was found in tumor spindle cells in whorled nodules and pseudoglandular cells in duct-like microcysts. A weak reaction was found in stromal cells.

Enamel protein has been detected by several investigators. Mori et al. (162) found amelogenin in epithelial cells surrounding pseudoductal microcysts. Saku et al. (159) detected amelogenin in hyaline droplets and a weaker concentration in the cells surrounding them. Amelogenin was also present in small mineralized foci and in the tumor cells surrounding them, as well as at the periphery of large mineralized material with homogeneous appearance.

Murata et al. (402) found amelogenin along the inner rim of duct-like microcysts and within their luminal space. The eosinophilic hyaline droplets showed basically the same staining pattern. Columnar cells around duct-like microcysts were positive for amelogenin, but the staining intensity decreased with flattening of the cells; cuboidal cells surrounding larger microcysts were negative.

Enamelin was demonstrated in hyaline droplets and cells surrounding them and in small mineralized foci and the cells surrounding them by Saku et al. (159). Similar results were obtained by Murata et al. (402). Like amelogenin, enamelin was recognized also at the periphery of large mineralized, homogeneous material.

In a study of sections from 23 cases of AOT Takata et al. (160) observed a distinct enamelysin immunostaining in small mineralized areas and hyaline droplets. Surrounding tumor cells were stained as well, but at a weaker intensity. Columnar cells around microcysts and low columnar cells forming rosettes or whorled arrangements were negative. A strong positive reaction for enamelysin was found in large calcified areas. Dysplastic dentin-like, hyaline material was negative.

Sheathlin, an enamel sheath protein was studied by Takata et al. (161). Distinct immunostaining was seen in the homogeneous, eosinophilic substance in tumor cell nests. Mineralized foci within the eosinophilic material were negative. Tumor cells facing the substance usually expressed sheathlin in their cytoplasm. Columnar cells in duct-like microcysts and small polygonal cells between the duct-like cysts were negative. Dysplastic dentin-like material (dentinoid) in the stroma was negative.

Neither wild type nor mutant p53 protein, a product of the tumor suppressor gene Tp53, or MDM2, an oncogene product was detected in eight cases of AOT (119), in contrast to KCOT, ameloblastoma and CCOC, which were all positive.

Moderate expression of the Tp 63 gene, a member of the Tp 53 family was detected in epithelial cells in one case of AOT by Lo Muzio et al. (121) and by Vera Sempere et al. (419), who also detected Ki-67, a proliferation marker, but only in 2% to 3% of the cells and primarily in nodules of fusiform cells. Leon et al. (390) found the mean percentage of Ki-67 positive cells in AOT to be 1.66% (± 0.78 SD), ranging from 0.5% to 4.6% of the cells. PCNA was detected in tumor cells by Crivelini et al. (420).

Electron Microscopy. The epithelial nature of the tumor cells has been confirmed in several studies. Well-developed gap junctions, desmosomes, desmosome-like junctions, and tonofilaments have been described (423). The great variation in morphology of tumor cells seen in the light microscope is also cognizable at the ultrastructural level and has given rise to subclassification into two (424,425), three (423), or four cell types (426). Polygonal, cuboidal, and columnar cells show abundant ribosomes, a relatively sparse endoplasmatic reticulum and mitochondria with few cristae; lysosomes, some coated vesicles, and some tonofilaments are seen. Occasionally a Golgi complex can be detected, but it is often ill defined (401,423). The small spindled cells have a dense cytoplasm and contain many organelles. Tonofilaments are prominent and seen in thick bundles, many well-developed desmosomes are found, and lysosomes are present in great numbers. Endoplasmic reticulum, Golgi complexes, and occasional glycogen particles can be detected. The nuclei are small and have a condensed nucleoplasm (423). Squamous cells show the ultrastructural characteristics of spinous cells in a stratified squamous epithelium, with bundles of tonofilaments, well-developed desmosomes, and keratinosomes.

Many investigations have concentrated on the ultrastructure of the eosinophilic droplets and the eosinophilic material in the duct-like microcysts (374,401,423,427). The conclusions have been controversial, some put attention to a similarity to amyloid (428), others compared the structure to developing enamel (401,423) or degenerated collagen (429), the latter on the basis of the finding of three different types of fibrils, thin collagen fibrils, electron-dense fibrils, and amyloid filaments. Electron-dense polymorphous plaques have been observed in the tumor droplets, which show a variety of shapes and internal structures including tubular structures, which may be coated with a fine granular material (423). El-Labban and Lee (399) found degenerative changes in 70% to 90% of the blood vessels in the stroma affecting both the endothelial lining and the perivascular connective tissue.

Molecular-Genetic Data. Mutation of the AMBN, which in humans maps to chromosome 4q21 has been detected in one case of AOT (165) and was considered a tumor-specific mutation. The AOT had a 334G>T transversion, causing a R90W amino acid change.

Differential Diagnosis. Although a considerable amount of AOTs has been misdiagnosed before removal, the histopathological diagnosis is simple because of the tumor's unique histomorphological pattern. If the lesion is small and found in the wall of a dentigerous cyst, it may be overlooked. The presence of a large amount of calcified material may confuse the pathologist.

Treatment and Prognosis. Enucleation of the tumor followed by curettage is the treatment of choice. The thick connective tissue capsule facilitates the enucleation from the bone. Although few cases have been published with a follow-up period of five years or more, the risk of recurrence is considered extremely low, only four cases have been reported, one recurred as late as 12 years after curettage (391,395,430). Malignant transformation has never been described.

Many authors consider the AOT a hamartoma. Although it is beyond doubt that the growth rate of the AOT is very slow, nobody has proved that the lesion stops growing at any time, and some lesions have reached a size of 6 to 7 cm (390,396,431), and in one case extension into the intracranial space of a recurrent tumor has been reported (334).

Removal of follicular or large AOTs may require removal of involved teeth. Impacted teeth do not necessarily need to be removed, though; in appropriate circumstances they can be preserved (432).

1.5   Keratocystic Odontogenic Tumor

At the editorial and consensus conference in Lyon, July 2003, in association with the preparation of the WHO volume *Pathology and Genetics of Head and Neck Tumours* (12), there was consensus that sufficient data about the neoplastic potential of the "odontogenic keratocyst" had been published to justify a change of its name into "keratocystic odontogenic tumour." Since it clinically presents as a cyst, it is described in chapter 18. An extensive and up-to-date review of the lesion is published as Chapter 3 "Odontogenic Keratocyst" in the book *Cysts of the Oral and Maxillofacial Regions* by Shear and Speight (228).

2.   Tumors of Odontogenic Epithelium with Odontogenic Ectomesenchyme with or without Hard-Tissue Formation

This group of tumors comprises three neoplasms and two hamartomas (15), which are truly odontogenic in the sense that they are composed of odontogenic epithelium and odontogenic ectomesenchyme, which under certain conditions are able to produce the dental hard tissues, dentin and enamel similar to what takes place during the normal odontogenesis. Because they are composed of tissue derived from two germ layers, ectoderm and mesoderm, they are sometimes called "mixed" (433). The histomorphology of the entities in this group reflects various stages of the odontogenesis differing in potential for proliferation, histodifferentiation, and morphodifferentiation. To understand the nature of these tumors certain knowledge is required of the sequential and reciprocal mechanisms of the epithelial-ectomesenchymal interactions, which take place during odontogenesis. Many reviews have been written on the subject, among others those by Slavkin (434), Thesleff et al. (19), Peters et al. (20), Tucker et al. (435), Sharpe (436), and Cobourne et al. (21).

Briefly, the first evidence of tooth formation in humans is observed in fetuses at the age of one month as a thickening of the oral epithelium in the mandibular, maxillary, and medial nasal processes. The early-stage oral epithelium is capable of inducing tooth development in nonoral ectomesenchyme. At a slightly later stage the epithelial cord becomes lengthened and broadened as it migrates into the adjacent ectomesenchyme (434). At specific sites the epithelium proliferates to form enamel organs, which develop through a bud stage and a cap stage to a bell stage with a convex outer surface and a concave inner surface. The bell-shaped enamel organ embraces a very cell-rich part of the ectomesenchyme, the dental papilla, which is the primordium of the later dental pulp. The dental papilla controls the shape of the tooth. The cell-dense ectomesenchyme continues around the enamel organ and forms the dental sac. At this stage the dental papilla is capable of inducing an enamel organ with following tooth formation in a nonodontogenic epithelium, such as skin. At the interface between the enamel organ and the dental papilla, the dentin-producing cells, odontoblasts develop from the ectomesenchyme, and the enamel-producing cells, ameloblasts develop from the enamel organ. These highly specialized cells are mutual dependent and controlled by an alternative flux of biological information between ectomesenchymal and epithelial cells. The odontoblasts do not develop from the ectomesenchyme unless in contact with the inner enamel epithelium of the enamel organ, and ameloblasts capable of producing enamel do not develop till an initial mineralization of the adjacent dentine formed by the odontoblasts has taken place. Over time the dentin and the enamel of the dental crown is produced and after the crown of the tooth is formed, root formation is initiated (433).

These reciprocal inductive influences of one tissue on the other play a similar role in this group of tumors consisting of odontogenic epithelium and odontogenic ectomesenchyme. Formation of dentin only takes place where the odontogenic epithelium has developed preameloblasts, which are capable of inducing odontoblasts formation in the adjacent ectomesenchyme, and enamel is only formed where odontogenic epithelium is in contact with dentin, which shows an initial mineralization. These requirements were observed already by Pflüger et al. in 1931 (1).

In the tumors three histomorphological patterns may bee seen: (*i*) A tumor consisting of strand and nests of odontogenic epithelium resembling the dental lamina and initial enamel organs, growing in a cellular odontogenic ectomesenchyme, and with no presence of dentine or enamel is called ameloblastic fibroma (AMF); (*ii*) A tumor showing various amount of dysplastic or more rarely tubular dentin besides the components found in the AMF is called ameloblastic fibrodentinoma (AFD); (*iii*) A tumor that furthermore contains various amount of regular or dysplastic enamel is termed "ameloblastic fibro-odontoma" (AFOD). All three tumors are considered neoplasms; they will grow continuously if not removed. An AMF does not differentiate into an AFD or an AFOD, and an AFD does not differentiate into an AFOD (13,433,437,438). At an initial stage of the development of an AFD or the AFOD, however, before the formation of the dental hard tissues the three variants will show a similar histomorphology. Two other lesions in the group are considered hamartomas. They consist of the same components as the AFOD but grow more slowly and eventually are made up primarily of the dental hard tissues with only a narrow peripheral rim with some soft tissue components. The growth abates. They are called odontomas. By and large they occur as two variants with a different level of morphodifferentiation. In the complex odontoma (ODTx) the dentin and enamel is organized in a nontooth-shaped pattern. In the compound odontoma (ODTp) tooth-like structures are formed. A developing odontoma will resemble the AMF or AFD or AFOD during its stages of maturational development and this fact causes diagnostic problems, which will be discussed under the individual lesions. Some authors (31,381) prefer to pool the AMF, the AFD, and the AFOD into one group of neoplasms and the two variants of odontomas into one group of hamartomas. If treatment is the only concern this makes sense, apart from the fact that the AMF has been reported to recur more often than the AFD and the AFOD (439,440). For scientific purposes it is an advantage to keep the entities separated (440,441).

In the WHO classifications of odontogenic tumors the way of classifying the neoplasms has varied. In the 1971 edition (22) the AMF, AFD, and AFOD were kept separately; the AFD was called "dentinoma" at that time. In the 1992 edition (23) the AFD and the AFOD were pooled together and in the 2005 edition the AMF and the AFD were pooled together.

2.1 Ameloblastic Fibroma

Introduction. The AMF is a rare, benign odontogenic neoplasm consisting of an odontogenic epithelium, which resembles the dental lamina and primordial enamel organs. The epithelium is growing in an abundant and cell-rich ectomesenchymal tissue, which resembles the dental papilla. No formation of the dental hard tissue is seen.

ICD-O code 9330/0

Synonyms: None, but in the past the tumor has been published under various obsolete terms like "soft odontoma."

Clinical Features. The differential diagnostic problems mentioned above have had an impact on the results of the surveys made of the tumor. Surveys and reviews may include cases of early odontomas, which have been diagnosed as AMFs. When diagnosing these tumors it is important to correlate the histological features with the clinical and radiographic findings.

The prevalence and incidence of the tumor is unknown. The relative frequency of the tumor in material received for histological diagnosis in services of diagnostic pathology in various countries for various amount of years ranges from 0.6% to 4.5% in studies comprising more than 300 samples of odontogenic tumors. In most of the surveys the percentage has been between 1.2% and 1.8%. The results are indicated as follows: number of odontogenic tumors/number of AMFs/%. Regezzi et al., Michigan, U.S.A. (31): 706/15/2.1%, Günhan et al., Turkey (32): 409/18/4.5%, Daley et al., Canada (33): 392/7/1.5%, Mosqueda-Taylor et al., Mexico (34): 349/5/1.4%, Ochsenius et al., Chile (35): 362/2/0.6%, Adebayo et al., Nigeria (36): 318/4/1.2%, Fernandes et al., Brazil (37): 340/6/1.8%, Ladeinde et al., Nigeria (38): 319/6/1.8%, Buchner et al., California (30): 1088/17/1.6%, Jones et al., England (2006, pooled figures from two studies)(39,40): 523/8/1.5%, Olgac et al., Turkey (41): 527/8/1.5%, and Jing et al., China (42): 1642/19/1.2%. The data are skewed; however, the figures reflect regional differences in type of lesions sent for histopathological confirmation rather than effects of genetical or environmental factors.

The total number of published cases of AMF is between 150 and 200. Comprehensive reviews have been written by Slootweg (437) and Philipsen et al. (441). In a study of 55 cases Slootweg found an age range from 6 months to 47 years. The mean age at time of diagnosis was 14.6 years. The gender distribution was 29 males and 26 females, the ratio was thus

M:F = 1.1:1. The tumor was located in the maxilla in 9 cases (1 anterior, 8 posterior) and in the mandible in 45 cases (5 anterior, 40 posterior), making the ratio maxilla:mandible = 1:5. Philipsen et al. included the cases reviewed by Slootweg; they covered the period 1946 to 1978. They added another 40 cases from the literature and analyzed a total of 122 cases. The gender rate and particularly the location came out differently. The age range was 6 months to 62 years, but only two cases were older than 49 years. The mean age at time of diagnosis was 14.8 years. The gender rate of M:F was 1.4:1; 71 tumors were diagnosed in men, and 50 in women. The location was somewhat different from the findings by Slootweg, 33 tumors were located in the maxilla and 90 in the mandible, the ratio maxilla:mandible was thus 1:2.7. In both studies the majority of tumors were diagnosed in the posterior part of the mandible, 74.1% in Slootweg's study and 68.9% in Philipsen et al.'s study, including eight cases, which covered more than one region. More recently Lu et al. (442) published 14 own cases, 6 in males and 8 in females. The mean age at time of diagnosis was 23.9 years. Four tumors were located in the maxilla (1 anterior, 3 posterior), 10 were located in the mandible (5 anterior, 5 posterior), the maxilla:mandible ratio was 1:2.5. Chen et al. (440) reported 13 cases of AMF from their own files. The patients were between 6 and 51 years (mean: 26 years). Seven patients were males and six, females. All tumors occurred in the mandible, with 10 in the posterior part, and 3 involving both the anterior and posterior part. Jing et al. (42) reported an additional five cases of AMF to those reported by Lu et al. (442). The 19 tumors were diagnosed in 9 males and 10 females. The mean age was 10 years lower: 19.6 years. The location distribution was about the same five AMF in the maxilla (2 anterior, 3 posterior), and 14 in the mandible (5 anterior, 9 posterior), ratio maxilla:mandible = 1:2.8.

In a study of 123 cases from the literature selected on the basis of well-documented follow-up data, Chen et al. (438) found the age at time of first presentation to range from 7 weeks to 54 years with a mean age of 15.9 years and a median age of 13 years. Only 30 patients were older than 22 years. The male:female ratio was 1.26:1 (68:54). The location of the tumors: 24 cases in the maxilla, 99 cases in the mandible, ratio maxilla:mandible = 4:1.1. The majority, 75 of 102 AMFs (73, 5%) were found in the posterior region of the mandible.

A single case of peripheral AMF has been published by Kusama et al. (443). It was a pedunculated tumor on the gingiva in the lower right premolar region of a 40-year-old woman. The histopathology of the tumor had a certain similarity to the AMF, but it showed features of an epithelium-rich and cell-rich odontogenic fibroma, a much more common lesion (444,445) and it is probably better classified as such. Ide (446) commented on two cases published in Japanese. They both presented as gingival hyperplasia, but the histological documentation showed they were AMF-like proliferations in opercula. No other case of extraosseous AMF has been published.

The AMF is usually painless; pain was recorded in 3 of the 24 cases reported by Trodahl (439) and in a single case reported by Chen et al. (440). The most common symptom is swelling, which is found in almost all cases (439–441). Chen et al. (438) registered the finding in 71.8% of 103 cases. Because of the insignificant symptoms about 20% of the tumors are discovered accidentally on radiograms (438). Unerupted teeth are associated with the tumors in three out of four cases (441).

Although the growth rate is slow, many of the tumors reach a considerable size. It varies between 0.5 and 16 cm; 9 out of 16 lesions reported by Trodahl (439) were larger than 4 cm, and 9 out 13 lesions reported by Chen et al. (440) were 4 cm or larger in greatest extent. In 39 cases from the literature the largest diameter of the tumor ranged from 0.7 to 16 cm, with a mean of 4.05 cm.

Imaging. Radiologically, the tumor appears as a well-defined, uni- or multilocular radiolucency, often with a radiopaque border. The multilocular appearance is particularly seen in larger lesions, which present with a swelling (438). In 8 of 10 lesions reported by Chen et al. (440), the radiolucency was multilocular; in 2 cases measuring 3 × 2 cm and 4.5 × 2 cm it was unilocular. Among 38 cases from the literature Chen et al (438) recorded 23 multilocular and 15 unilocular cases. The asymptomatic cases tended to show unilocular radiolucency.

In about 75% of the cases the tumors are related to an unerupted tooth. In the maxilla the AMF may encroach the maxillary sinus.

A CT scanning is recommended, particularly for large tumors; it improves the information about the outline of the tumor.

Pathology. The etiology of the tumor is unknown. It is interesting that four out of nine cases reported by Schmidt-Westhausen et al. (447) developed in areas of congenitally missing teeth. The tumor is supposed to arise from residues of odontogenic epithelium in the jaws. Since three out of four tumors are associated with an unerupted tooth and Philipsen et al. (448) have shown that in the opercula of 74 cases of unerupted first and second permanent molars 7 lesions were detected with a histopathology similar to the AMF, it is tempting to speculate that such proliferations of odontogenic tissue may be the source of origin in some cases.

Macroscopically, the tumor presents as a gray or whitish, rounded or oval soft mass with a lobular configuration and a smooth surface that seems covered with a thin capsule-like tissue. The cut surface is uniform; cystic changes are absent or inconspicuous, apart from the very unusual cases, where the tumor develops in the wall of a cyst, Pflüger (449) case 2, Nilsen et al. (450) case 2, and Edwards et al. (451).

Microscopically, the tumor is composed of strands and islands of odontogenic epithelium growing in a cell-rich mesenchymal tissue with a histomorphology similar to that of the dental papilla (Fig. 37). The periphery of the tumor is well demarcated, a thin capsule has been described in cases, which might

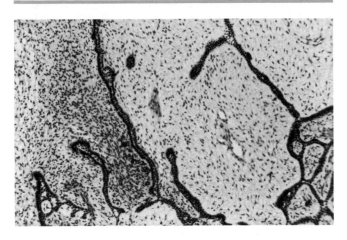

Figure 37 Ameloblastic fibroma. Section of a tumor from the molar and retromolar area of the left mandible of a 9-year-old boy. Ramified thin dental lamina-like strands of odontogenic epithelium are seen in a dental papilla-like ectomesenchyme, which exhibits variations in cellular density. The vascularity is low. H&E stain.

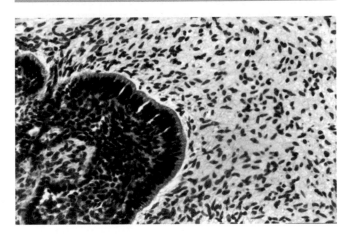

Figure 39 Ameloblastic fibroma. Higher magnification of the tumor in Figure 37. A bulbous thickening of the epithelium is seen which resembles an early stage of an enamel organ. The peripheral cells exhibit reverse polarity of the nuclei. Note the narrow cell free zone along the epithelial-ectomesenchymal interface. H&E stain.

rather be early stages of an odontoma (452). The amount and density of epithelium varies from tumor to tumor and may vary considerably from area to area within the same tumor. The strands are usually composed of a double layer of cuboidal cells and resemble the dental lamina. In some areas the strands are broader and the central area occupied by stellate cells (Fig. 38). The strands are ramificating, a pattern that may be more or less conspicuous. Buds of varying

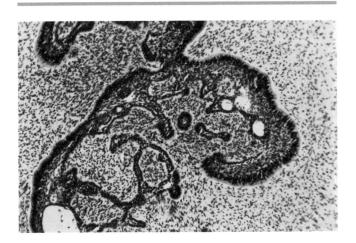

Figure 38 Ameloblastic fibroma. Higher magnification of the tumor in Figure 37. In this area the epithelial strands are broader with formation of some stellate reticulum-like cells and differentiation of preameloblasts-like cells along one side of the strands. The cellularity of the ectomesenchyme is reduced in the vicinity of these cells. H&E stain.

sizes develop from the epithelial strands; they are composed of stellate cells bordered by a basal layer of cylindrical cells with a reverse nuclear polarity and morphology-like preameloblasts (Fig. 39). These bulbous thickenings resemble early stages of enamel organs. Cyst formation within the epithelium is very uncommon, and the cysts remain small. Artefactual splits along the plane between the layers of the bilaminar epithelial strands are not unusual. Acanthomatous changes are rare (54). Islands of tumor epithelium may be found in the adjacent connective tissue and might represent a growth pattern (453). The ectomesenchymal tumor component is highly cellular and shows a striking similarity to the dental papilla. The morphology of the cells varies, most are stellate with fine cytoplasmic processes and angular nuclei, others are plumb, and fibroblast-like cells may also be seen. The matrix is myxoid and contains fine, fibrillar collagen. The cellularity and matrix composition may vary from tumor to tumor and within a given tumor (54), more mature collagenous fibers may be present in some areas. The vascularity is modest. Adjacent to the epithelial strands and particularly the bulbous extensions narrow, eosinophilic cell–free zones may be seen. More pronounced changes in terms of eosinophilic, hyalinized matrix is seen in some tumors. Such structural alterations are interpreted as the result of aberrant epithelial–ectomesenchymal inductive effects. Other types of reaction zones have been described. In some tumors enclaves of ramified strands of epithelium surrounded by broad zones of ectomesenchyme characterized by moderate cellularity are separated by plexiform strands of ectomesenchyme with high cellularity (449).

Mitoses with normal morphology may be found in the epithelium as well as in the ectomesenchyme.

Together with a high cellularity it may provoke suspicion of malignancy. If more than a few scattered mitoses are present and particularly in case of nuclear atypia this possibility must be taken in consideration (454).

Cases of "granular cell ameloblastic fibroma" have been published (455–457). The granular cells show a finely granular, eosinophilic cytoplasm and small, round, or oval nuclei, which are often eccentrically located. They are seen in the connective tissue and may be the dominating cell type. These tumors are clinically distinct from the AMF and are better classified as GCOTs (458).

Immunohistochemistry. CKs were studied by Tatemoto et al. (459) in four cases of AMF. They used polyclonal TK antiserum-detecting 41 to 65 kDa keratins, and monoclonal antibodies KL-1-detecting 55 to 57 kDa keratins, as well as monoclonal PKK-1-detecting CK-8, CK-18, and CK-19. PKK-1 bound slightly or not at all. Dental lamina–like epithelium showed a relatively stronger staining with TK, KL-1, and PKK-1 compared with ameloblastic epithelial islands with peripherally located columnar cells. The ectomesenchymal cells, which were strongly positive for vimentin, showed some coexpression of keratin. Yamamoto et al. (417) also detected reactions to KL-1 CKs (broad spectred antibodies) in the dental lamina–like epithelial strands and the stellate reticulum of an AMF. Crivelini et al. (66) investigated CKs in five AMFs with monoclonal antibodies against CK-7, CK-8, CK-10, CK-13, CK-14, CK-18, and CK-19. Reaction to CK-7, CK-13, and CK-14 was detected. CK-14 was found in all types of epithelial tumor cells. CK-13 was seen in cords and stellate reticulum, but not in cylindrical peripheral cells; reaction to CK-13 is not found in the stellate reticulum of normal tooth germs. CK-7 was found in one tumor only.

Nestin was detected by Fujita et al. (422) in focal areas of the ectomesenchyme particularly near the epithelial elements in two cases of AMF; the reaction was strong. Nestin was found to be upregulated in AMFs compared with normal tooth germs and was considered a marker of odontogenic ectomesenchyme in odontogenic tumors.

Vimentin has been studied by several investigators (459,460,417,461). All except Crivelini et al. (66) detected a positive reaction in the ectomesenchymal tumor cells.

No staining for desmin could be found in AMFs by Tatemoto et al. (459).

Neural tissue markers were used by Yamamoto et al. (417) and Takeda et al. (462). NSE and glial fibrillary acidic protein could not be detected (462). In both studies S-100 protein were detected in a few scattered cells of the epithelial component. The ectomesenchyme was negative in one study (417), while the dendritic and spindle-shaped cells were positive in the other.

So et al. (136) studied the immunohistochemical localization of fibroblast growth factors FGF-1 and FGF-2, and receptors FGFR2 and FGFR3 in three AMFs and other odontogenic tumors and cysts. Immunoreaction to FGF-2 (some nuclear reaction)

and to FGFR2, but not to FGF-1 and FGFR3 was found in the epithelium of the AMFs. The authors suggested that FGF-2 might be involved in directing nuclear activity at the histodifferentiation stage of odontogenesis.

Extracellular matrix proteins in AMFs have been studied. Ito et al. (67) detected versican, a large chondroitin sulfate proteoglycan in the ectomesenchymal tumor component in two cases of AMFs. Heikinheimo et al. (68) studied the immunohistochemical localization of two cellular fibronectins, tenascin, laminin, as well as type VII collagen in three AMFs. In two AMFs there was a notably weak immunoreactivity to an extradomain sequence-A-containing form of cellular fibronectin in the ectomesenchyme, the third tumor was bright-positive. A form of cellular fibronectin containing an oncofetal domain, which is found in carcinomas and ameloblastomas could not be detected. Tenascin was found in the ectomesenchymal component in all cases, the basement membrane bordering the tumor epithelium was clearly outlined. Laminin and type VII collagen had almost identical distributions; the basement membrane of the epithelial strands and islands of all AMFs exhibited an intense positive, linear staining with both antibodies. Mori et al. (70) and Yamamoto et al. (417) confirmed the findings of tenascin in AMFs.

The distribution of collagens type I, IV, and VI, procollagen type III, and undulin was studied in four cases of AMFs by Becker et al. (453). An excessive accumulation of collagen type VI was detected in the extracellular matrix of the ectomesenchymal tumor component showing a clear distinction to the connective tissue surrounding the tumor, while collagen type I, procollagen type III, and undulin showed a weak and amorphous distribution. Pronounced staining for collagen type I and IV was found in areas with high cellularity, though. The hyaline matrix seen around the epithelium in some areas showed a weak reaction for collagen type I, but was negative for type III, IV, and VI. This finding is in contrast to normal predentin and dentin, which is composed of collagens type I, III, and VI in a typical distribution. The author concluded that the ectomesenchyme of AMF represents an undifferentiated extracellular matrix.

Nagatsuka et al. (75) examined the distribution of collagen IV $\alpha1$ to $\alpha6$ chains in three cases of AMF. In the tumor areas $\alpha1(IV)/\alpha2(IV)$, $\alpha4(IV)$, and $\alpha5(IV)/\alpha6$ (IV) chains occurred as linear continuous patterns that clearly separated the epithelial islands and strands from the surrounding dental papilla–like ectomesenchyme.

Hard tissue–related proteins have been studied. Mori et al. (162) detected amelogenins in the tumor epithelium of four AMFs; the ectomesenchyme was negative.

PCNA was studied in a case of AMF by Yamamota et al. (417) who detected scattered PCNA-positive cells in the dental lamina–like epithelium and in the ectomesenchymal tumor component.

Sano et al. (463) assessed the growth potential of AMF by means MIB-1 immunohistochemistry, which recognizes the epitope of the Ki-67 antigen. In an AMF in a 16-year-old woman the index was 2.9% in the epithelial component and 2.9% in the ectomesenchymal. In a recurrent AMF in a 26-year-old man the index was 7.5% and 9.8%, respectively. In an ameloblastic fibrosarcoma (AFS) in a 38-year-old woman the index was 5.1% and 13.5%, respectively. The results suggest that the index can be used to assess the aggressiveness of the AMF.

The expression of the p21(ras) protein, a product of a RAS proto oncogene was measured in two cases of AMF and compared to findings in ameloblastomas and odontogenic myxomas (ODOMYXs). The AMFs showed an overexpression of p21(ras) and an almost identical staining pattern. Percentage of immunoreactive cells were 75% to 100% in the epithelial cells and 5% to 25% in the ectomesenchyme of one tumor and less than 5% in the other. The staining was somewhat more intense in the ectomesenchymal cells. The level was equal to that of some of the ameloblastomas and one of the myxomas.

Electron Microscopy. Csiba et al. (464) studied the ultrastructure of an AMF—the size of a hen's egg—in the posterior part of the mandible of a 15-year-old boy. The cells of the small epithelial islands were oval or polygonal. The basement membrane was intact; the basal cells were connected to it with hemidesmosomes. They were connected to each other with desmosomes; the intercellular spaces were very narrow. The nuclei were large and oval with dispersed chromatin, but much of the chromatin was arranged along the inner nuclear membrane. Nucleoli were seen. The cytoplasm contained free ribosomes, a moderately developed endoplasmic reticulum, some vesicles, some mitochondriae, and abundant tonofilaments. A Golgi apparatus could be seen but it was usually small. In the central area of the epithelial islands the intercellular spaces were large. The cells contained dense deposits of glycogen, which was arranged in a rim around the nucleus. Some of the centrally placed cells showed cytoplasmic extensions, which reached the basement membrane. The cells of the connective tissue resembled fibroblasts but had very voluminous and irregularly shaped nuclei with indentations and conspicuous cytoplasmic invaginations. Few organelles were seen, sporadically a less well-developed endoplasmic reticulum could be found, some vesicles and a few large mitochondriae. The eosinophilic homogeneous zone, which may be seen adjacent to the epithelium in the light microscope was ultrastructurally heterogeneous. It contained residues of cells and a granular amorphous substance, which resembled the basement membrane together with collagenous fibrils without any specific orientation.

Farman et al. (103) investigated the ultrastructure of an AMF, which was removed from the posterior region of the maxilla in a five-year-old boy. The tumor had expanded the bone; it recurred two years after curettage. The basement membrane around the epithelial islands consisted of a regular bilamellar structure to which a varying number of hemidesmosomes were attached. Elsewhere there was a thickening of the lamina densa by a granulofilamentous

material similar to what may be seen in ameloblastomas. In some of the epithelial cells there was a loss of definition of the basal lamina associated with a "hair on end" arrangement of aperiodic fibrils running perpendicular to the basal lamina. The adjacent hyaline material seen in the light microscope proved to be dense regular mature collagen.

Molecular-Genetic Data. Heikinheimo et al. (460) used in situ and Northern hybridization to study CK-1, CK-4, CK-8, CK-18, and CK-19 and vimentin gene expression in 13- to 24-week-old human fetal tooth germs, including overlying oral epithelium and six odontogenic tumors (ameloblastomas and AMFs). The results were compared with immunohistochemistry using monoclonal antibodies. The normal and neoplastic epithelia revealed a relatively strong expression of simple epitelial CK-19 mRNA, and a low, but significant expression of CK-8 and CK-18 mRNAs. The ectomesenchymal cells of AMF expressed low amount of simple epithelial CK-8, CK-18, and CK-19 as well as vimentin. The results indicate that the differentiation and cytoskeletal gene expression programs of odontogenic epithelia upon neoplastic transformation are not fully retained.

EGF and TGF-α, which regulate cell proliferation and functional maturation through the EGF-R, was investigated in two AMFs by Heikinheimo et al. (130) by Northern analysis, Southern blotting, ISH, and immunohistochemistry. Human fetal teeth in cap stage to early hard tissue formation were included for comparison. EGF-R mRNA and immunoreactivity were confined to neoplastic epithelium. Transcripts for TGF-α but not for EGF were detected in the tumors. It was concluded that regulation of EGF-R expression is developmentally regulated in human odontogenesis and may also be involved in odontogenic tumorigenesis.

By means of ISH Papagerakis et al. (461) studied the expression of osteocalcin and collagen type III RNA in normally developing postnatal teeth and five odontogenic tumors comprising AMF, AFOD, and ODTx. The study was combined with immunostaining with antibodies against human keratins (KL-1), vimentin, collagen type IV, fibronectin, osteonectin, osteocalcin, and bovine amelogenins. Abnormal expression of osteocalcin mRNA was observed in the high columnar epithelial cells of the odontogenic tumors. The mRNAs coding the α1 chain of collagen type III were found only in the ectomesenchymal cells of the tumors. Detection of keratin as well as vimentin in the epithelial cells of the tumors made the authors suggest that the level of differentiation corresponded to the cap and/or the bell stages of normal tooth development.

Differential Diagnosis. The main differential diagnoses are from ameloblastoma, AFD, AFOD, developing odontomes, AFSs, and epithelium-rich odontogenic fibroma.

In contrast to ameloblastomas the epithelium in the AMF forms bilaminar strands with buds rather than broad strands and large islands with a tendency for acanthomatous changes and formation of cysts. The amount of stellate reticulum-like epithelium is more pronounced in the ameloblastoma. The connective tissue component is very different. In the ameloblastoma it is a collagenous connective tissue stroma with vascularization, and moderate cellularity. In the AMF there is no stroma; the connective tissue is an equal component of the neoplasm with a histomorphology like the dental papilla.

In contrast to the AFD and the AFOD the AMF does not contain the dental hard tissues, dentin and enamel. It may require extensive sampling to find the hard dental tissue. Some investigators do not consider the finding of dentinoid or dentin or even enamel to be very important. Sciubba (381) considered the AFOD to be a variant of AMF. Odell et al. (54) considered the presence of dentin as part of the spectrum of ameloblastic fibro-odontomes. In the 1992 WHO classification the AFD was categorized together with the AFOD. In the 2005 WHO classification the AMF and the AFD were categorized together. Regarding the AMF a certain tendency for recurrence and even malignant transformation has been documented (*vide infra*), which does not seem to be the case or at least to a lower degree for the two dental hard tissue–producing variants. The presence of dental hard tissue might not be without importance for the prognosis.

At an early stage a developing ODTx may be histologically indistinguishable from an AMF. There is no known histochemical or other kind of marker to separate them. A developing odontoma is probably more often diagnosed as an AMF than vice versa. The amount of epithelium in proportion to the connective tissue is greater in an early odontoma and there are more large bulbous extensions with stellate reticulum. A more orderly arrangement of the epithelium also points toward an odontoma. Clinical information is important; a tumor with AMF features developed in a patient who is 22 years or older and therefore past the period of normal odontogenesis is likely to be an AMF. A small globular tumor in a young child is likely to represent the early stage of a developing odontoma.

The most important differential diagnosis is toward the AFS. Malignant transformation is an uncommon, but well-documented possibility. The sarcomatous transformation takes place in the ectomesenchymal component, which shows hypercellularity, frequent and abnormal mitoses, as well as nuclear and cellular pleomorphism. Only a few scattered normal mitoses may be seen in a benign AMF. The amount of epithelium is reduced in the AFS and may eventually disappear all together. Clinical features like sudden rapid growth and indistinct margins of the tumor on the radiogram are indicative, and malignant transformation is significantly more common in patients older than 22 years (438). In resection specimens the presence of infiltration of bone marrow spaces supports the impression of malignancy.

The differential diagnosis toward an epithelium-rich odontogenic fibroma may be difficult, particularly in case of the uncommon ameloblastomatoid central odontogenic fibroma (COF), which furthermore shows an increased cellularity of the connective tissue (465). The epithelium of the odontogenic fibroma has a different morphology; however, the strands are more irregular and their thickness varies from area to area, the center of the islands do not contain stellate reticulum-like cells. The peripheral cells may be cylindrical in some areas and even show reverse nuclear polarity, but in other areas they may be cuboidal or flattened. The cells in the connective tissue are generally more fibroblast-like and the content of collagenous fibers is higher in the odontogenic fibroma.

Treatment and Prognosis. AMF has been treated with conservative as well as radical surgery. For many years it has been known that the AMF is capable of recurrence (439), and sometimes even twice (466). In some cases it was a question of residual tumor after incomplete excision. In a few cases the recurrence has shown a higher differentiation with formation of dentin or even enamel indicating that perhaps the primary tumor was not a genuine AMF, but rather an early stage of AFOD. In more than 90% of the cases the recurrence show the same or a lower differentiation (438), and in some the recurrence show transformation into an AFS (467). Chen et al. (438) reviewed the available English language literature since 1891 and selected 123 cases of AMF with well-documented follow-up data to evaluate the clinical, pathological, and behavioral aspects of this tumor. The treatment was recorded as conservative (enucleation, curettage, simple excision) or radical (marginal resection, segmental resection, semiresection of the jaw). The treatment mode was detailed in 118 cases. Over 90% (108 cases) of the patients were primarily treated by conservative procedures; 10 patients were treated radically due to the extensive size of the tumor. Recurrence was reported in 41 cases (33.3%). The period of follow-up was stated in 94 cases. The 5-year and 10-year recurrence rate was 41.6% and 69.2%, respectively. Recurrence-free period ranged from 1 month to 96 months, with a mean of 33.2 months. A univariate analysis of all the data showed that only treatment mode of the patients was significantly related to recurrence. The recurrence-free period was significantly longer in patients treated with radical procedures. Malignant transformation was reported in 14 recurrent cases (11.4%). The 5-year and 10-year malignant transformation rate was 10.2% and 22.2%, respectively. The malignant transformation-free period ranged from 9 months to 264 months, with a mean of 79.0 months. In 11 cases, follow-up after the treatment of the malignant tumor was recorded; five patients were alive with no signs of recurrence, the other six cases recurred following surgery. Only one had extensive distal metastasis. Of the six recurrent cases, two died of disease. A statistical analysis of the recorded data showed that only the age of the patient at the first presentation was significantly related to the malignant transformation of AMF. Patients younger than 22 years were unlikely to develop malignant transformation in comparison with patients older than 22 years. It could be argued that the rates of recurrence and malignant transformation were overestimated because such cases are more likely to be documented. However, in two series with more than 10 cases reported, the recurrence rate was 36.4% (440)

and 45.5% (439), respectively, and the rate of malignant transformation in a series of 11 cases was even higher, 18.2%.

It was concluded that it is reasonable to treat patients younger than 22 years by conservative surgeries, and to apply a step-wise treatment principle to patients with multiple recurrences whose age was younger than 22 years. In patients older than 22 years, a radical surgery should be considered when the tumor is massive in size or when the tumor recurred more than once.

2.2 Ameloblastic Fibrodentinoma

Introduction. The AFD is a benign odontogenic tumor consisting of odontogenic ectomesenchyme resembling the dental papilla and epithelial strands and nests resembling dental lamina and enamel organ. Some formation of dentinoid and more rarely tubular dentine is seen in the tumor.

In the 2005 WHO classification of odontogenic tumors the AFD was categorized with the AMF (454); in the 1992 WHO classification it was categorized with the AFOD (23).

Already Gorlin (63) questioned the existence of the AFD as an independent entity, he suspected that many if not all were examples of odontomas prior to enamel formation. Cases have been published, however, with formation of mineralized and unmineralized dentin, which could not be expected to mature as odontomas (462,468–470), including a case of AMF in a six-year-old boy who recurred 21 after surgery as an AFD (440). Gardner (471) required evidence that the AFD had a different biological behavior than the AMF; otherwise their designation as a separate entity was not justified. Philipsen et al. and Reichart and Philipsen reviewed the cases published as AFD and stated that no case of recurrence has been published, a significant difference from the AMF.

The histopathological differences between the cases published as immature dentinoma and AFD has been discussed by Takeda (472).

ICD-O code 9271/0

Synonyms: Dentinoma, immature dentinoma (obsolete)

Clinical Features. The AFD is an exceedingly rare tumor. Reichart and Philipsen (25) reviewed 28 cases, and another 3 cases have been published by Chen (440). Some of the cases reviewed showed clinical and histological features, which differed somewhat from the definition of the lesions, the mesenchymal component being cell-rich, but not embryonic pulp-like (473). Among the 31 cases, 23 were diagnosed in males, and 8 in females, the ratio M:F is 1:0.3. The age ranged from 4 to 63 year, but 90% of the patients were younger than 30 years. Fourteen were found in the first decade (11M + 3F), nine in the second decade (7M + 2F), five in the third decade (4M + 1F), and one female in the fourth decade. Two patients were in the seventh decade, a 60-year-old man (474) and a 63-year-old woman (475). The histology was characteristic in the former case, but atypical in the second.

The majority (74%) of AFDs have been located in the posterior part of the mandible. Seven have been diagnosed in the maxilla (4 anterior, 3 posterior) and 24 in the mandible (1 anterior, 22 posterior, 1 anterior and posterior). Two cases of peripheral AFD have been described (476,477). The histology of the former case did not show typical embryonic pulp-like tissue, it is probably better classified as one of the much more common peripheral odontogenic fibroma with odontogenic epithelium and hard tissue formation. The second one exhibited dental papilla–like connective tissue and tubular dentin; it is likely to be an initial peripheral odontoma.

The AFD has been described as a slow-growing painless tumor, which may become quite large and cause swelling of the jaw (478). Some cases have been associated with unerupted teeth.

Imaging. The AFD has been described as a well-delineated sometimes multilocular radiolucency often with scalloped borders (468,473). Depending on the amount of dentin in the tumor varying degrees of irregular radiopacities may be seen. The size has varied from 1.5 to 6.5 cm in greatest extent. In cases where the tumor is associated with an embedded tooth it is usually located close to the crown of the tooth.

Pathology. The etiology is unknown. The pathogenesis is poorly understood, one case represented the recurrence of an AMF (440). The characteristic histopathological pattern shows an embryonic pulp-like ectomesenchyme with high cellularity in which strands of odontogenic epithelium with bulbous extensions are seen similar to what is seen in an AMF. Various amounts of dentinoid (dysplastic dentin) is seen adjacent to the odontogenic epithelium (Fig. 40). The dentinoid often contains entrapped cells.

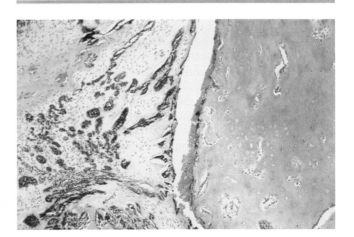

Figure 40 Ameloblastic fibrodentinoma. Section of a tumor in the frontal maxillary area of a 9-year-old girl. Strands and islands of odontogenic epithelium in dental papilla-like ectomesenchyme are seen to the left. To the right and near the lower border formation of nontubular dentin is seen with inclusions of cells. No enamel was found in this tumor.

Some cases have shown a different histology with a less cell-rich and more fibrous connective tissue, which is unlike the embryonic pulp-like ectomesenchymal tissue (473,479). Tubular dentin has been observed in some cases, and part of the dentin may be mineralized. Mitoses are not seen.

Immunohistochemistry. Nestin, an intermediate filament of the cytoskeleton and considered a marker of neural stem cells or progenitor cells, was studied by Fujita et al. (422) in a variety of odontogenic tumors. The findings in AFD showed similarities to the findings in AMFs, AFODs, and odontomas. A strong reaction was detected in focal areas of the ectomesenchymal component, particularly near the epithelial elements. Immunoreaction was seen in some epithelial cells as well.

Neural tissue markers (NSE, glial fibrillary acidic protein, S-100 protein) were studied in three cases of AFD and three cases of AMFs by Takeda et al. (422). Dendritic or spindle cells in the ectomesenchyme were S-100-positive in some areas of AFD and AMF. Positive staining for glial fibrillar acidic protein was only observed in juxtaepithelial mesenchymal tissue in the formation stage of immature dentin with various numbers of entrapped cells. NSE was not detected in AMFs and not in the ectomesenchyme, but was seen in the stellate reticulum-like cells, and more weakly in the peripheral cylindrical cells of the epithelial components that were surrounded by a cell-free zone or by an immature or mature dentin layer.

Gao et al. (168) detected BMP in the cytoplasm of odontoblasts-like tumor cells, and in unmineralized dentin-like matrix in three cases of "dentinomas" (AFDs). No BMP was found in mineralized dentin-like matrix.

Electron Microscopy. The ultrastructure of the AFD was studied by Hietanen et al. (468) and van Wyk et al. (469). Hietanen et al. found that the central cells of the epithelial tumor islands showed an ultrastructure similar to the stratum intermedium of the normal enamel organ. The hyaline areas of the ectomesenchyme were composed of a dense network of collagen fibers and aggregates of granular intercellular material. Van Wyk et al. did not find enamel organs mimicking islands of epithelium in an AFD, the ectomesenchymal component of the tumor consisted of numerous fibroblast-like cells embedded in a very fine reticulum-like matrix, which contained a few collagen-like fibers. More fibrous areas of the tumor had few cells, but many more collagen-like fibers. The authors noticed similarities to the normal odontogenesis, areas with cellular epithelial-connective interface corresponded to bud-cap stages; areas with cell-free zones surrounding the epithelium resembled the bud-cap stage as well. Areas with amorphous layers adjacent to the epithelium resembled the "intermediate bell" stage, whereas the interface with dentinoid materials had all the features of the "late bell" stage, except for the absence of calcification.

Molecular-Genetic Data. No data are available.

Differential Diagnosis. Many of the considerations discussed in the section on the differential diagnosis of the AMF also apply to the AFD. The main difference is the presence of dysplastic dentin (not just hyalinized areas) and sometimes even tubular dentin in the AFD. In some cases extensive sampling is necessary to find the areas with hard tissue; radiograms of the operation specimen may be helpful. If enamel stroma is found the tumor should be diagnosed as an AFOD. The correct differential diagnosis of the AFD toward the AMF and the AFOD has no therapeutical consequences, but the prognosis seems to differ. A relatively high recurrence rate has been found for AMFs (438), but not for AFD and AFOD, although cases of recurrent AFOD have been reported (480). Since the AFD, which is very rare, shares the ability to form dental hard tissue with the AFOD, and has the same low recurrence rate, it seems more meaningful to categorize the AFD together with the AFOD, as it was done in the WHO 1992 classification of odontogenic tumors (23), than to categorize it with the AMF (454). If the tumor is large and mainly consists of a hypercellular ectomesenchymal component with limited amount of odontogenic epithelium and a few scattered areas with dentinoid, it may be quite aggressive and should be treated like an AMF.

A cell-rich odontogenic fibroma with odontogenic epithelium and formation of hard tissue may be mistaken for an AFD. They occur in different age groups, the odontogenic fibroma contains much more collagen, the hard tissue is generally not in close contact with the epithelium, and the epithelium has a different morphology, it does not form ramificating bilaminar strands with bud formation.

Treatment and Prognosis. Surgical excision is the recommended treatment of AFD, and no recurrences have been reported. The literature is limited, however.

2.3 Ameloblastic Fibro-Odontoma

Introduction. The AFOD is a rare, benign, and noninvasively growing tumor, which almost exclusively occurs in children and young adults. It is composed of all the elements seen in odontogenesis: odontogenic epithelium, embryonic pulp-like ectomesenchyme, dentin, enamel, and now and then cementum. The AFOD is difficult, sometimes impossible to differentiate from an early stage of a large developing odontoma.

ICD-O code 9290/0
Synonyms: Ameloblastic odontoma (obsolete)

Clinical Features. Because a distinction between AFOD and early stages of odontomes has not been made in many previous publications, reviews and surveys often include both categories. The lesions share many biological features, but AFOD is a continuously growing neoplasm, while an odontoma is a hamartoma, which although it may in some cases become monstrous, it will gradually mature into dental hard tissues and stop growing.

The relative frequency of the tumor as diagnosed in material received for histological diagnosis in services of diagnostic pathology in various countries for various amounts of years ranges from 0.0% to 3.1% in reviews comprising more than 300 samples of odontogenic tumors. In 8 of the 12 reviews the frequency was 1, 3% or lower. The results are indicated as follows: number of odontogenic tumors/number of AFOD/%. Regezzi et al. Michigan, U.S.A. (31): 706/11/1.6%, Günhan et al., Turkey (32): 409/3/0.7%, Daley et al., Canada (33): 392/12/3.1%, Mosqueda-Taylor et al., Mexico (34): 349/3/0.8%, Ochsenius et al., Chile (35): 362/6/1.7%, Adebayo et al., Nigeria (36): 318/1/0.3%, Fernandes et al., Brazil (37): 340/1/0.3%, Ladeinde et al., Nigeria (38): 319/0/0.0%, Buchner et al., California (30): 1088/19/1.7%, Jones et al., England (2006, pooled figures from two studies) (39,40): 523/6/1.1%, Olgac et al., Turkey (41): 527/7/1.3%, and Jing et al., China (42): 1642/4/0.2%. The data are skewed; however, the figures reflect regional differences in type of lesions sent for histopathological confirmation rather than effects of genetical or environmental factors.

Less than 100 cases have been published. Philipsen et al. (441) reviewed the literature and included cases reviewed by Slootweg (437), a total of 86 cases were found. If suspected immature odontomas are discarded then the following further cases have been published by Sekine (481), Favia et al. (482), Ozer et al. (483), Yagishita et al. (484), Chang et al. (485), Fantasia et al. (486), Reichart et al. (487), and Oghli et al. (488).

In the review by Philipsen et al. the age range was found to be 1 to 22 years ($N = 86$), only one case was older than 20 years; the mean age was 9 years. Cases in patients older than 22 years have been reported, though (480,484). The AFOD was more common in males (54) than in females (37), the ratio M:F was 1.3:1. The majority (54%) of the AFODs were located in the posterior part of the mandible. Thirty cases were diagnosed in the maxilla (12 anterior, 18 posterior, 1 anterior and posterior), 55 tumors were located in the mandible (9 anterior, 46 posterior), the ratio maxilla:mandible was 1:1.8.

The AFOD is usually a painless, slowly growing, expanding tumor. Swelling of the jaw or an unerupted tooth in the area may lead to the diagnosis (440). The size has varied considerably; small ball-shaped tumors with little formation of dentin and enamel are usually impossible to differentiate from immature odontomas, but it has no consequences for the treatment. A considerable amount of the cases published have been quite large. AFOD is an expanding tumor; there is no bony infiltration.

Peripheral AFOD has not been described.

Imaging. Radiographically the AFOD presents as a unilocular or multilocular radiolucency with well-defined hyperostotic borders (54,54,440,441). Radiopacities are seen in foci scattered in the lesion (Fig. 41), mainly in the central area (488). If they are small and few, they may not be visible on the radiogram. Tumors that present with a rounded, regular radiopaque center surrounded by a wide ball-shaped or oval radiolucency are likely to be immature odontomas (489). Small ball-shaped lesions located at the occlusal surface of an unerupted molar are almost certain to be immature odontomas. Displaced and

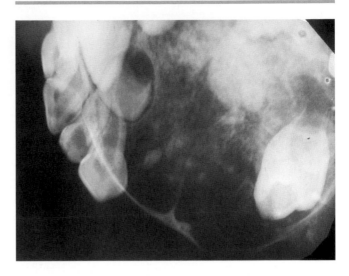

Figure 41 Ameloblastic fibro-odontoma. A large well-delineated radiolucent lesion in the right maxilla of a 5-years-old child. Scattered radiopacities are seen which represent formation of dental hard tissue.

impacted teeth may be seen, but root resorption is rarely found (484). In the mandible a tooth is sometimes missing in the area. Large tumors in the maxilla may encroach the maxillary sinus (482). CT scanning reveals details about the borders of larger lesion and facilitates the planning of treatment.

Pathology. The etiology of the tumor is unknown. There are indications, however, of causal relation to genetics. AFODs have been described as part of some rare syndromes. Savage et al. (490) described the simultaneous occurrence of a mandibular AFOD and a maxillary ODTp in a three-year-old boy with the neurocutaneous syndrome encephalocraniocutaneous lipomatosis. Herrmann (491,492) and Schmidseder et al. (493) described a father and his three children who all developed extensive AFODs bilaterally in the maxilla and mandible shortly after birth. The tumors were part of a possibly autosomal-dominant syndrome, which also included esophageal stenosis, pulmonary stenosis and hepatopathy, and other symptoms. It may be argued that the tumors were odontomes since they produced a high amount of dental hard tissues, even with high morphodifferentiation; they contained hundreds of small tooth-like elements (odontoids). Their potential for proliferation and the extension of their destruction of the jaws seems to indicate, however, that they were AFODs.

Macroscopically, the AFOD shows a solid mass with a smooth surface that is white to tan. On the cut surface the mineralized components are seen as granules or hard nodules dependent on the degree of formation of dental hard tissue.

Microscopically the AFOD is dominated by a cell-rich myxoid connective tissue of ectomesenchymal origin. Histomorphologically it is similar to the embryonic dental papilla. Branching strands of

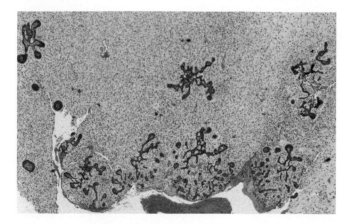

Figure 42 Ameloblastic fibro-odontoma. Section of the soft tissue part of a tumor in a 16-year-old boy. The histology of this area is similar to that of an ameloblastic fibroma. H&E stain.

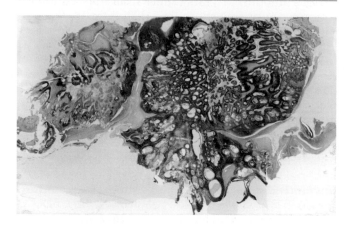

Figure 43 Ameloblastic fibro-odontoma. An area with complex odontome-like formation of dentin and enamel in the center of a large tumor in the right maxilla of a two-and-a-half-year-old-boy. The tumor consisted primarily of soft tissue. *Source*: From case No. 12 in Ref. 475.

odontogenic epithelium are seen in the ectomesenchymal tissue forming buds and more bulbous extensions (Fig. 42). The strands are primarily composed of bilaminar layers of cubic cells. The peripheral layer of the more voluminous extensions consists of palisading cylindrical cells with reversely polarized nuclei, the central cells are stellate; such structures mimic enamel organs at various initial stages (484). This part of the tumor's morphology is undistinguishable from that of the AMF apart from a higher tendency for formation of enamel organ–like extensions. The surface of the tumor is smooth and sometimes bordered by a thin capsule (484), epithelial nests may be embedded inside the capsule. Scattered in the tumor dentin and enamel is seen, mostly in the central areas, and often as irregular structures (Fig. 43), and only rarely a higher morphodifferentiation in terms of odontoids is seen. The sponge-like structure of dental hard tissue typically seen in an ODTx is only found in minor areas, not as a single large element. In cases of limited dental hard-tissue formation extensive sampling may be necessary; a radiogram of the pathological specimen will facilitate the orientation. Cementum is usually only seen on the root surface of odontoids. The morphodifferentiation of the dentine may vary from dentinoid, a form of dysplastic dentine, which may contain entrapped mesenchymal cells to regular tubular dentine with or without mineralization. Enamel is only seen in contact with mineralized dysplastic or tubular dentine (Fig. 44).

Some AFODs have shown the presence of aggregations of melanophages (494).

The AFOD may develop in association with a calcifying cystic odontogenic tumor (CCOT) (495).

Immunohistochemistry. Yamamoto et al. detected CK in the epithelial component of two AFODs by means of KL-1 antibodies, which react with CK-1, CK-2, CK-5-8, CK-11, CK-14, and CK-16-18.

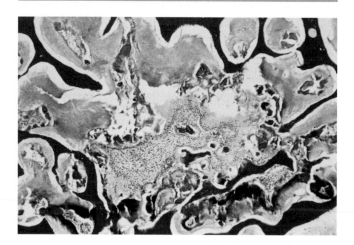

Figure 44 Ameloblastic fibro-odontoma. Detail from a dental hard tissue–producing area. Trabeculae of dentin (*red*) are seen at the periphery. Attached to the surface of the dentin enamel matrix is seen produced by the enamel epithelium placed in the middle. The youngest enamel with the lowest mineral content stains brown, enamel with somewhat higher mineral content stains grayish. van Gieson stain.

To investigate the presence of CK in an AFOD in the mandible of a three-year-old boy Miyauchi et al. (496) used KL-1, PKK-1 (which detects low mw CK-8, CK-18, and CK-19), and monoclonal antibodies against CK-4, CK-7, CK-8, CK-13, CK-13 + 16, CK-14, CK-18, and CK-19. There was no immunoreaction to CK-4, CK-7, and CK-13. The epithelial component showed a strong reaction to CK-16, CK-19, and KL-1 and PKK-1. There was a weak or partially positive reaction to

CK-8, CK-14, and CK-18. There was no difference between the reaction of the epithelium in the soft tissue areas and in the areas with dental hard-tissue formation.

Nestin, an intermediate filament of the cytoskeleton was detected by Fujita et al. (422) in focal areas of the ectomesenchymal component, particularly near the epithelial elements with a strong activity. Some reaction was also found in the epithelial elements. The localization of nestin showed the same pattern in AMFs, AFDs, AFODs, and odontomas.

Vimentin showed a strong reaction in the ectomesenchymal component of two AFODs investigated by Yamamoto et al. (417). These findings were confirmed by Miyauchi et al. (496) who also detected some immunoreactivity in the basal portion of the peripheral epithelial cells in the areas with soft tissue, but not in areas with formation of dental hard tissue.

S-100 protein could not be detected in the tumor cells by Yamamoto et al. (417).

Growth factors were studied by So et al. (136), who used antibodies against the acidic FGF-1, basic FGF-2, and fibroblast growth factor receptors (FGFR2 and FGFR3) on sections from three AFODs and other odontogenic tumors. The staining pattern was similar to that of the AMF. A significant immunoreaction to FGF-2 and FGFR2, but not FGF-1 and FGFR3 was found in the cytoplasm of the epithelial component, and nuclear staining was seen in some epithelial cells sharing interface with the mesenchymal component. The authors concluded that the staining patters in general were related to odontogenic differentiation rather than pathogenesis.

Mori et al. (70) detected an intense linear band-like immunostaining of the extracellular matrix protein, tenascin beneath the basement membrane of the odontogenic epithelium in two cases of AFOD. The odontogenic ectomesenchyme showed a weak diffuse staining. No reaction was found in calcified substance. Yamamoto et al. (417) found similar results in two cases of AFOD, but also observed that myxomatoid areas in the ectomesenchyme were negative for tenascin.

The presence of enamel proteins in AFODs has been investigated. Yagishita et al. (484) showed an intracellular immunoreaction to amelogenins exclusively in tumor epithelial cells, namely the cuboidal cells of tooth bud–like projections and the stellate reticulum-like cells inside the epithelial islands. In contrast, no positive staining was discernible in the cytoplasm of the columnar ameloblast-like cells, and there was no evidence for the massive secretion of amelogenins beyond the epithelial-mesenchymal junction into the ectomesenchymal tumor component, except for the restricted sites of enamel and dentinoid formation.

Takata et al. (160) observed an intense staining for enamelysin in immature enamel in four cases of AFOD. The dentine was negative. Neither the slender strands or islands of odontogenic epithelium nor the cellular mesenchymal dental papilla–like component showed immunoexpression of enamelysin.

Sheathlin was detected in the areas where inductive hard tissue formation occurred, immature enamel and neighboring ameloblastic cells in four cases of AFOD by Takata et al. (161). Neither the epithelial nor the ectomesenchymal tumor component showed immunoexpression of sheathlin.

Yamamoto et al. (417) estimated the number of PCNA-positive cells in two cases of AFOD and compared the findings with those in an AMF. While positive cells were frequent in the latter, very few PCNA-positive cells were found in the AFODs. Sekine et al. (481) used bromodeoxyuridine (BrdU) and PCNA immunohistochemistry to investigate the cell kinetics in case of AFOD. The L.I. for BrdU was 0.9% in the epithelial component and 2.1% in the ectomesenchymal component, for PCNA it was 2.2% and 7.7%, respectively. The authors suggested that the ectomesenchymal component was more proliferative than the epithelial component.

MIB-1 antibody, which recognizes the epitope of the Ki-67 antigen, was used by Sano et al. (463) on sections of two cases of AFOD, two AMFs, and one AFS to calculate the L.I. In the epithelial component of the two AFODs the L.I. was 3.3% and 4.6%, respectively compared with 2.9% in an AMF, 7.5% in a recurrent AMF, and 5.1% in the AFS. In the ectomesenchymal component the L.I. was 1.5% and 1.9% in the two AFODs compared with 2.9% in the AMF, 9.8% in the recurrent AMF, and 13.5% in the AFS. Thus the growth potential of the AFODs was relatively moderate, and the findings suggested that the method is valuable for estimating the aggressiveness in this group of odontogenic tumors.

Electron Microscopy. The ultrastructure of the AFOD was studied by Hanna et al. (497) who found that the ultrastructural features supported the light microscopic observations. The bilaminar epithelial strands consisted of cells with large indented nuclei. Intercellular spaces were found with microvilli that extended from the surface of the cells. Desmosomes were abundant between the cells and hemidesmosomes connected to the basal lamina. The cytoplasm contained few mitochondria and a poorly developed rough, endoplasmatic reticulum and Golgi apparatus. Tonofilaments were seen as dense bundles. In the ectomesenchymal component collagen fibers were randomly distributed, the density varied from area to area. The cells were stellate or elongated with an irregularly shaped nucleus. Mitochondriae were obvious, and RER was usually well developed. Some cells displayed few organelles and a poorly developed endoplasmic reticulum. The ectomesenchymal component seemed to be more active than the epithelial component.

Josephsen et al. (498) essentially confirmed these findings but concentrated on the ultrastructure of the epithelial–mesenchymal interface. The tumor tissue differed from that observed during normal odontogenesis by lacking matrix vesicles like those seen in the early formed predentin. The tumor cells were thus lacking the functional characteristics of developing odontoblasts. Enamel-like tissue was found in relation to an organic matrix of either a tubular or a fine granular texture. Only the tubular type of matrix was seen in direct contact with the epithelial cells, it was believed that the tubular structures were secretory products of the epithelial cells. Unlike normal odontogenesis focal areas of enamel-like tissue were found without direct contact with dentin and apparently confined within small islands of epithelium.

Other ultrastructural studies have been performed by Slootweg (499), Reich et al. (500), and Reichart et al. (487). Slootweg (499) studied the ultrastructure of five cases of AFOD that lacked formation of tubular dentin. One of the conclusions of the study was that the failure of odontoblasts and preameloblasts to make contact was a consequence of arrest of differentiation of the cells. Reich et al. (500) confirmed the previous findings. Reichart et al. (487) observed a cementoid-like material that revealed a mineralized matrix with formation of tubules reminiscent of dentin tubules.

Molecular-Genetic Data. Papagerakis et al. (461) used ISH to study the presence of osteocalcin mRNA and collagen III mRNA in AFOD and other "mixed" odontogenic tumors. Osteocalcin transcripts were found in the peripheral columnar epithelial cells and collagen III transcripts in the ectomesenchymal cells. The findings were confirmed by immunohistochemical studies.

Differential Diagnosis. Differentiation toward an ameloblastoma should be easy. The AFOD is noninvasive, shows a cell-rich, embryonic dental papilla–like connective tissue component and presence of dental hard tissues in contrast to the ameloblastoma. More difficult is the differentiation toward the AFD and the AMF, since the AFOD undergoes progressive histo- and morphodifferentiation and therefore at an early stage is histomorphologically undistinguishable from an AMF and later from an AFD. The latter situation has no therapeutical consequences. The AMF, however, has been shown to have a higher tendency to recur (438). It is probable that more AFODs are misdiagnosed as AMFs rather than the converse. As pointed out by Odell et al. (54) extensive well-formed stellate reticulum suggests progression toward hard tissue formation and is sparse in AMF, and the amount of epithelium is higher in an AFOD than in AMF. It is important to include clinical information in the differential diagnosis, a tumor with the features of an AMF in a person older that 22 years is almost certain to be an AMF.

The differentiation toward an immature ODTx is discussed in the section on odontomas.

Treatment and Prognosis. Enucleation followed by careful and thorough curettage is the recommended treatment. The tumor usually shells out easily. If an unerupted tooth with eruptive potential is present, it may be spared. A large tumor, which fills out most of the posterior part of the mandible or has destroyed the cortex or has encroached the maxillary sinus may complicate surgery considerably, particularly in small children. Initial conservative treatment should be attempted with close follow-up. In case of recurrence and especially if it shows a lower

histodifferentiation, marginal resection should be considered. Recurrence is unusual. Malignant transformation is rare, but has been reported in an 18-year-old woman, a 36-year-old man, and in a 14-year-old girl, respectively (480,501); in the latter case metastases to regional lymphnodes were found.

2.4   Odontomas, Complex and Compound

Introduction. Odontomas are tumor-like but nonneoplastic developmental anomalies (hamartomas) (15) composed of developed malformed teeth or tooth-like masses. They represent the most highly differentiated neoformations within the group of tumors composed of odontogenic epithelium and odontogenic ectomesenchyme. Two variants are recognized, complex and compound odontoma; the division is made according to the tumor's degree of morphodifferentiation; the former shows a complex pattern of dentin and enamel, the latter consists of tooth-like structures (odontoides). The distinction is arbitrary; although most odontomas show a preponderance of one of the patterns, many but not all lesions show elements of both patterns.

ICD-O code 9280/0

2.4.1 Complex Odontoma.
The ODTx is a hamartoma composed of a mass of intermixed enamel, dentin, and sometimes cementum with no morphological resemblance to teeth, either normal or miniaturized (433,502). Some lesions look poorly organized; larger tumors usually have a sponge-like structure.

ICD-O code 9282/0

Synonym: Complex composite odontoma

Clinical Features. The true prevalence and incidence of the ODTx is not known. The relative frequency has been reported by several authors, but it is obvious that the stimulus to submit an odontoma for histological examination varies considerably from place to place. The relative frequency of the ODTx in material received for histological diagnosis in services of diagnostic pathology in various countries for various amounts of years ranges from 3.3% to 30.3% in studies comprising more than 300 samples of odontogenic tumors. The results are indicated as follows: number of odontogenic tumors/number of ODTx/%. Regezzi et al., Michigan, U.S.A. (31): 706/214/30.3%, Günhan et al., Turkey (32): 409/38/9.3%, Daley et al., Canada (33): 392/74/18.9%, Mosqueda-Taylor et al., Mexico (34): 333/49/14.7%, Ochsenius et al., Chile (35): 362/91/25.1%, Fernandes et al., Brazil (37): 340/52/15.3%, Jones et al., England (2006, pooled figures from two studies) (39,40): 523/121/23.1%, Olgac et al., Turkey (41): 527/67/12.7%, and Jing et al., China (42): 1642/58/3.5%.

The data are skewed; however, the figures reflect regional differences in type of lesions sent for histopathological confirmation rather than effects of genetical or environmental factors.

In a review, which included an earlier review by Slootweg (437), Philipsen et al. (441) found the age range of 139 ODTx to be 2 to 74 years. The mean age was 19.9 years. The mean age was somewhat higher in other reviews of larger material, Ochsenius et al. (35): 20.8 years (N = 91), Fernandes et al. (37): 22.2 years (N = 52), and Hisatomi et al. (503): 23.0 years (N = 41).

The gender ratio has differed in the reviews published. In six reviews of more than fifty cases of ODTx there was a slight predominance of males in three (37,42,441) and of females in three others (35,41,504). In none of the cases were the differences statistically significant; there seems to be no gender predilection.

The location of the lesion has been studied in several reviews and some have found a predominant occurrence in the maxilla others in the mandible. In four reviews of more than 60 cases the distribution has been the following: Budnick et al. 1976 (505) maxilla:37, mandible: 25; O'Grady et al. (504) maxilla: 39, mandible: 37; Ochsenius et al. (35) maxilla: 46, mandible: 40, and Olgac et al. maxilla: 17, mandible: 50. The ODTx may occur anywhere in the tooth-bearing areas of the jaws. In the majority of the reviews it has been revealed that within the maxilla the ODTx occurs primarily in the anterior region, and within the mandible it is most common in the posterior region (34,35,41,503–505).

Extraosseous odontomas are very rare and are more often of the compound type. Some diminutive lesions have been found in operculae as described by Philipsen et al. (448). Location of odontomas in the maxillary sinus (506) has been described, and one has been diagnosed in nasopharynx (507). A retrotympanic odontoma has been published (508), as well as a case in the middle ear (509).

Multiple odontomas have been described and often termed odontomatosis (510,511). They present more often as ODTps than as ODTxs.

The growth rate of the ODTx is very slow. Symptoms are usually rare. Pain has been reported in some cases (512,513) but usually in relation to inflammation. Altered pattern of tooth eruption or impaction is a common symptom, which was found in 27 of 41 cases by Hisatomi et al. (503). If the lesion becomes sufficiently large, and some exceeds the size of a walnut, it causes expansion of bone; swelling was found in 19 of 33 cases by Chen et al. (440). In a few cases the odontoma has erupted into the oral cavity (513).

Imaging. Depending on the developmental stage and degree of mineralization the radiographic appearance of the ODTx ranges from a radiolucent well-demarcated area, via a radiolucent peripheral zone of variable width with a central core of densely opaque masses to a radiopaque mass of hard dental tissues surrounded by a thin radiolucent zone (514). Some show a pattern of irradiating radiopaque lines caused by the sponge-like architecture of the lesion. The majority of ODTx are diagnosed when they are in a late mature stage. They are often located above an unerupted tooth. Immature stages of large odontomas have been diagnosed as ameloblastic fibro-odontomes in some cases, Clausen (515) case 2, 3, and 4, Pantoja (516), Reich et al. (500), Hawkins (489), and Chen et al. (440) case 17 and 18. Unerupted teeth are a very

common finding (517,518), and agenesis of the permanent tooth in the area may be encountered (512,513). In contrast to odontoma-associated calcifying cystic odontogenic tumor (OaCCOT), resorption of neighboring teeth is a very rare finding.

The size of the tumor varies from a lesion that is only detectable in the microscope (519) to one that is 7 to 8 cm at the longest diameter (520–523). Amado-Cuesta et al. measured the size of 23 ODTx; the range of size at longest diameter was 10 to 60 mm (513).

Pathology. The etiology of the ODTx is unknown, but there are strong indications that genetic influence is an important etiological cofactor. Some laboratory animal strains develop odontoma-like lesions, and odontomas occur as part of Gardner's syndrome (524) and other hereditary syndromes (525,528).

The tumor is primarily found in children and young adults and is believed to arise in remnant of odontogenic epithelium in the jaws from the dental lamina and from proliferations of odontogenic epithelium and ectomesenchyme close to the outer enamel epithelium in a dental sac (17) as it is seen in operculae (448,519).

Macroscopically the mature ODTx is covered with a smooth, white fibrous capsule, which veils the rounded and lobulated contour of the hard substance. If the soft tissue is removed the sponge-like architecture of the ODTx is clearly seen (Fig. 45). An immature odontoma is covered by a thick layer of soft tissue and a thin fibrous capsule at the periphery.

Histologically, the ODTx has a sponge-like architecture. The skeleton of the "sponge" is composed of thin tortuous walls of dentin, which irradiate from the center from which the ODTx started to grow (Fig. 46).

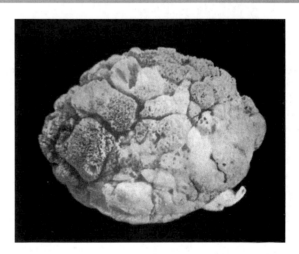

Figure 45 Complex odontoma. The lesion developed in the molar and retromolar area of the right mandible of a 13-year-old girl. The tips of the roots of an embedded second molar are seen in the right lower area. The outer layer of soft tissue was removed before photography; the sponge-like architecture of the dental hard tissue is clearly seen.
Source: From Ref. 527.

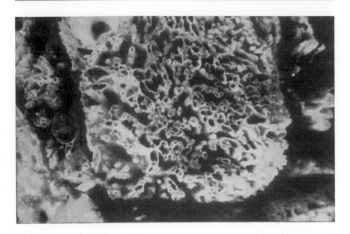

Figure 46 Complex odontoma. Closer view of the surface which reveals the pattern of tortuous walls of dental hard tissue which run from the center of the lesion to the periphery. *Source:* From Ref. 527.

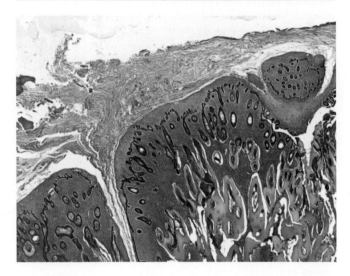

Figure 48 Complex odontoma. Low power view of the periphery of an immature complex odontoma. On the surface, a capsule of mature connective tissue is seen. The soft part of the tumor consists of organized laminae of odontogenic epithelium growing in a highly cellular ectomesenchyme. Deeper in the lesion the initial formation of the dentin walls are seen. H&E stain. *Source*: Section by courtesy of Professor P. A. Reichart, Berlin.

The walls of dentin contain a central pulpal space, which is slit formed and contains dental pulp-like ectomesenchyme. The walls are separated by narrow tortuous spaces, and enamel is formed on the surface of the walls, and in these spaces enamel epithelium, active or reduced is seen, and connective tissue with vessels are found (Fig. 47). At the periphery of the

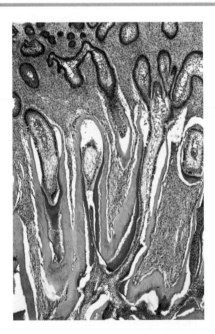

Figure 47 Complex odontoma. Detail from the peripheral zone of soft tissue covering an immature complex odontoma. The tortuous dental hard tissue walls are longitudinally cut. To one side they face the dental pulp tissue, which is responsible for the formation of the dentin, and to the other side they are covered by a layer of enamel matrix, which is produced by the ameloblasts of the enamel epithelium that covers the enamel. H&E stain. *Source*: Section by courtesy of Professor P. A. Reichart, Berlin.

tumor various amount of soft tissue is observed depending on the developmental stage of the ODTx (Fig. 48). This tissue resembles the tissue of an AMF, but the strands of epithelium show a more organized pattern and can in some places be followed down in the ectomesenchyme in the clefts between the dentin walls. At the surface of the lesion a thin capsule of connective tissue is seen. It is difficult to envision this pattern from the study of two-dimensional histological sections. Only in areas where the clefts are cut longitudinally is the structure evident. In cross or tangentially cut areas the lesion presents as a mass of primarily tubular dentin with numerous oval or circular "holes," some of which contain pulpal connective tissue (Fig. 49), while others show a coat of enamel on the surface of the dentin and contain enamel organ–like epithelium and strands of connective tissue with vessels in the center. If the ODTx is studied after decalcification—which is usually the case—empty spaces or enamel matrix is seen instead of enamel. Areas with tooth-like shapes, where the dentin has formed a root-like structure, which embraces a pulpal tissue and is covered by a crescent cap of enamel may be found mixed with the typical structure of the ODTx. Some odontomas show a less developed structure and present with a more irregular structure. The histology shows numerous variable details, areas of dentinoid (528,529) and dysplastic enamel (530,531) is usually found. Cementum is sparse in an ODTx, if tooth-like structures are seen it is found on the surface of the roots of these, but it may also be seen in

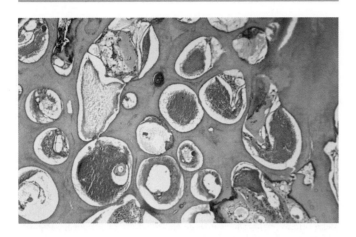

Figure 49 Complex odontoma. Section of a mature complex odontoma after demineralization. The lesion presents as a grid of dentin with holes, which contain enamel matrix and enamel epithelium and some stroma. Most of the canals that contained dental pulp are very narrow after the termination of the formation of dentin. H&E stain.

nontooth-like areas on the surface of the dentin where it is not covered by enamel. At the periphery of the hard tissue part of the lesion dentin and enamel may still be formed and the histological, but not morphological patterns, which characterize the normal odontogenesis are found. In the soft tissue in the clefts near the center of the lesion where enamel formation is completed reduced enamel epithelium is seen often with calcifications. Ghost cells may be found (532,533); Sedano et al. (534) detected ghost cells in 8 of 44 ODTx. Several authors reported ghost cells to be more common in complex than in ODTps, but Tanaka et al. (535) found ghost cells in 78.8% of 52 ODTps and in 29.4% of 17 ODTxs. If the odontoma has developed associated with a CCOT, it is located in the wall of a cyst covered with the epithelium, which shows the characteristics for that lesion.

Sometimes hyaline deposits (536), or amyloid-like material as seen in the CEOT or small duct-like structures similar to those in the AOT are seen.

2.4.2 Compound Odontoma.

The ODTp is a hamartoma composed of varying numbers of tooth-like elements (odontoides) (537).

ICD-O code 9281/0

Synonyms: Compound composite odontoma.

Clinical Features. The prevalence and incidens of the ODTp is not known. It is well-known fact that they are often diagnosed macroscopically by the oral surgeon and not submitted for histological examination or only the surrounding dental sac-like soft tissue is submitted.

The relative frequency of the tumor in material received for histological diagnosis in services of diagnostic pathology in various countries for various amounts of years ranges from 1.2% to 36.7% in studies

comprising more than 300 samples of odontogenic tumors. The results are indicated as follows: number of odontogenic tumors/number of ODTp/%. Regezzi et al., Michigan, U.S.A. (31): 706/37/36.7%, Günhan et al., Turkey (32): 409/36/8.9%, Daley et al., Canada (33): 392/128/32.7%, Mosqueda-Taylor et al., Mexico (34): 333/63/18.9%, Ochsenius et al., Chile (35): 362/71/19.6%, Fernandes et al., Brazil (37): 340/33/9.7%, Jones et al., England (2006, pooled figures from two studies) (39,40): 523/91/17.4%, Olgac et al., Turkey (41): 527/42/8.0%, and Jing et al., China (42): 1642/20/1.2%. The discrepancies in the figures are most likely due to a variation in incentive to submit the lesion for microscopy.

In a review, which included an earlier review by Slootweg (437), Philipsen et al. (441) found the age range of 143 ODTp to be 6 months to 73 years. The mean age at time of diagnosis was 17.2 years. The mean age was about the same in a review by Ochsenius et al. (35): 17.0 years ($N = 71$), but somewhat higher in two other studies Hisatomi et al. (503): 19.9 years ($N = 62$), and Fernandes et al. (37): 20.5 years ($N = 33$).

The gender ratio, males:females in three reviews of more than 50 cases has been almost 1:1, Philipsen et al. : 73:67 ($N = 140$), Hisatomi et al. : 33:29 ($N = 62$), and Ochsenius et al. : 35:36 ($N = 71$). If the two studies by Jones et al. (39,40) are pooled, however the gender ratio was M:F = 39:51 ($N = 91$). In several reviews of smaller material the occurrence was equal in the two genders; so it is doubtful whether any difference exists.

The location of the ODTp has been studied in several reviews, and in all studies a predominant occurrence in the maxilla was found. In four reviews of more than 60 cases the distribution has been the following: Budnick et al. (505) maxilla: 48, mandible: 17; Mosqueda-Taylor et al. (34) maxilla: 46, mandible: 17; Ochsenius et al. (35) maxilla: 48, mandible: 22; and Hisatomo et al. (503) maxilla: 32, mandible: 30. The ODTp may occur anywhere in the tooth-bearing regions of the jaws. In the majority of the reviews it has been revealed that within the maxilla the ODTp occurs primarily in the anterior region, and within the mandible it is most common in the anterior region as well (32,34,35,37,41,440,503–505).

Peripheral odontomas are very rare, but has been reported by Castro et al. (538) and Ledesma-Montes (539).

Multiple ODTps have been reported (510,511, 540–543), and have sometimes been termed odontomatosis. In the majority of cases they have been part of a syndrome.

The growth rate is slow and symptoms are rare, most compound odontomes are mature when they are diagnosed. Jacobs (544) reported five cases of ODTp in the mandible in three males and two females within an age range of 12 to 15.5 years. In all cases it was possible to retrieve previous orthopantograms taken at a time where there was no sign of the odontome. The radiograms were taken approximately 2, 3, 4, 5, and 5.5 years earlier. Although it was not possible to measure the exact time for the development of the odontomas, one of the cases suggested that an ODTp may grow from a size where it is invisible on the radiogram to a size of about 1 cm at the longest diameter in less than two years. In all cases the patients reached the late mixed dentition stage before the lesions were diagnosed.

Clinical symptoms are similar to those of the ODTx, and in many reviews no subdivision of the odontomes has been made. In four studies the number of impacted teeth was considerably higher in the ODTp group than in the ODTx group (440,503, 512,517). Swelling and pain is less common in the ODTp variant (440).

In rare cases the ODTp may erupt into the oral cavity (545).

Imaging. Radiographically the ODTp presents as a densely opaque mass of small tooth-like structures (odontoides) surrounded by a narrow radiolucent rim within a hyperostotic linear border (Fig. 50). The odontoides are not always recognizable on the radiogram. Smaller ODTp may be situated between the roots of erupted teeth. Unerupted teeth are often seen; in a review of 62 cases of ODTp, Hisatomo et al. (503) found an unerupted tooth in 49 cases, a missing tooth in the region in five cases, and a supernumerary tooth in two cases. Resorption of neighboring roots was not seen. ODTp is almost never diagnosed at an immature stage (537).

Pathology. The etiology of the ODTp is unknown, but like the ODTx there are strong indications that genetic influence is an important etiological cofactor. Hereditary cases have been published (493,525).

The ODTp is primarily found in children and young adults and is believed to arise in remnant of odontogenic epithelium in the jaws from the dental lamina and from proliferations of odontogenic epithelium and ectomesenchyme close to the outer enamel epithelium in a dental sac (17), as it is seen in operculae (448,519). The tumors develop primarily in the

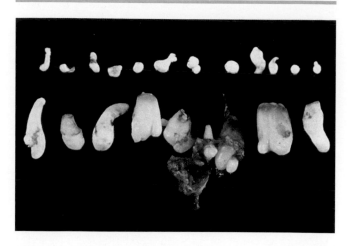

Figure 51 Compound odontoma. Macroscopic view of the odontoids and the capsule which surrounded them. The lesion was located in the canine area of the right mandible of a 16-year-old girl.

odontogenic period (544), and it is likely that lesions diagnosed later in life have been present in the jaws for many years because of lack of symptoms.

Macroscopically the tumor presents as a number of miniature and/or misshapen teeth (odontoides), which may be fused into larger masses. They are all found within a single dental sac, which is thin if the ODTp has matured (Fig. 51). In most cases the final diagnosis can be made on the basis of macroscopic examination. The size and number of odontoides varies considerably, in a case reported by de Visscher (546) 112 odontoides were counted. The odontoides may be drop-shaped, irregular, or resemble a normal tooth; they rarely exhibit more than one root. The differentiation between an ODTp and supernumerary teeth is arbitrary, more than two odontoides within the same dental sac is usually considered an ODTp. Not all the elements in an ODTp are necessarily tooth-shaped; a few or many may be irregular and resemble the elements of an ODTx.

Sections of immature, developing ODTps show several dysmorphic tooth germs in a loosely textured connective tissue with cords and islands of odontogenic epithelium (22,537,547). Much of the enamel matrix is preserved in spite of decalcification.

2.4.3 Complex and Compound Odontomas.

Immunohistochemistry. In some of the immunohistochemical studies it has not been stated which type of odontomas was studied. Apparently no difference in immunoreaction has been found in the two types of odontomas.

Keratins were studied by Crevelini et al. (66) in three compound odontomes using monoclonal antibodies against CK-7, CK-8, CK-10, CK-13, CK-14, CK-18, and CK-19. Only CK-7 and CK-14 were detected. CK-7 and CK-14 were found in parts of the

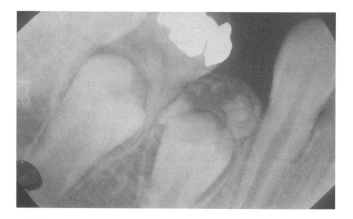

Figure 50 Compound odontoma in the premolar area of the right mandible of a 9-year-old girl. The odontoma was immature, which explains the mixed radiolucent/radiopaque structure.

epithelial strands and in stellate reticulum. CK-14 was negative in secretory ameloblasts. Also antibodies against vimentin was used, but with negative result.

Fujita et al. (422) studied the presence of nestin in 22 ODTx and 40 ODTps. Nestin is an intermediate filament of the cytoskeleton. Immunoreactivity was found in the odontoblasts adjacent to the dentin matrix, particularly in the compound odontomes. The dentinal fibers in the tubules of the dentin also showed immunoreactivity, and the pulp cells adjacent to the odontoblasts were positive in some cases. In ODTxs sparse flat cells adhering to the dentin and their processes were positive. A positive reaction was found in 16 of the ODTx and in 33 of the ODTps.

Growth factors were studied by So et al. (136), who used antibodies against the acidic FGF-1, basic FGF-2, and fibroblast growth factor receptors (FGFR2 and FGFR3) on sections from three AFODs and other odontogenic tumors. The staining pattern was similar to that of the AFOD. A significant immunoreaction to FGF-2 and FGFR2, but not FGF-1 and FGFR3 was found in the cytoplasm of the epithelial component and nuclear staining was seen in some epithelial cells sharing interface with the mesenchymal component. An intense staining for FGF-1 was found in amelo-blasts. The authors concluded that the staining patters in general were related to odontogenic differentiation rather than pathogenesis.

Tenascin, an extracellular matrix protein was detected in five ODTps by Mori et al. (70). A strong positive immunoreactivity was found in condensed connective tissue fibers, and was markedly concentrated in pulp-like tissue and odontoblasts, as well as in unmineralized dentinoid. No reactivity was found in calcified material.

The immunoreactivity to BMPs was investigated in two ODTps by Gao et al. (168). The reaction pattern was similar to that of normal tooth germs. Odonto-genic epithelium including ameloblasts showed a strong positive reactivity. Predentin and odonto-blasts-like cells showed a weak positive reaction. Calcified material and dental pulp was negative. Fibrous tissue around the tooth-like structures was positive.

Enamel proteins have been studied. A strong expression for amelogenin was found in the enamel matrices in ODTxs by Abiko et al. (548). Well-calcified materials, such as enamel-, dentin-, and cementum-like structures did not show a positive reaction.

Takata et al. (160) found a strong positive reaction for enamelysin in immature enamel in odontomas, whereas dentinoid, dentin, and cementum as well as pulpal tissue were devoid of immunoreactivity. Ameloblasts adjacent to enamel matrix showed moderate immunoreactivity. Ghost cells were found in some of the odontomas, and some of them were positive, especially in the periphery of clusters of ghost cells.

The presence of sheathlin was studied in 10 odontomas by Takata et al. (161). Immature enamel was strongly positive; dentin, cementum, and pulpal tissue were devoid of immunoreactivity. Cementum

deposits on the surface of sheathlin-positive enamel were a common finding.

Tanaka et al. (535) used antibodies against human hair protein, β-catenin and lymphoid enhancer factor 1(Lef-1) to study the presence of ghost cells, and the Wnt signaling pathway in 96 cases of odontomas, 17 complex and 52 compound. ODTps (78.8%) showed a higher incidence of ghost cells than ODTxs (29.4%). Human hair proteins are composed of hard keratins and matrix proteins, and it is believed that the Wnt-β-catenin-T cell factor/Lef pathway is involved in the expression of hard keratins. Expression of hard keratins was found only in the cytoplasm of ghost cells in 46 (66.7%) of the 69 odontomas. Expression of β-catenin and Lef-1 was observed in the cytoplasm and nucleus of odontogenic epithelial cells adjacent to the ghost cells in immature odonto-mas. According to the authors the findings suggested that odontoma is a hard keratin-expressing tumor-like lesion, and that the Wnt-signaling pathway may be involved in the formation of ghost cells in odontomas.

Papagerakis et al. (461) studied late phenotype markers of ameloblasts and odontoblasts, such as amelogenin, keratins, collagen types III and IV, vimentin, fibronectin, osteonectin, and osteocalcin in odontomas and other odontogenic tumors. The patterns found in ODTxs showed similarities to those found in normal developing teeth. The authors suggested that the epithelial cells in the lesion are recapitulating genetic programs expressed during normal odontogenesis, but exhibit abnormal expression patterns for these genes.

Electron Microscopy. Sapp et al. (549) studied the ultrastructure of calcifications in COCs and odontomas, and found that spherical calcifications in the two lesions had a different ultrastructure although they appear similar in the light microscope. The epithelial cells in odontomas were separated from the calcifications by a basement membrane exhibiting a prominent lamina densa and lamina lucida and containing hemidesmosomes. In the peripheral cytoplasm of epithelial cells adjacent to calcifications prominent microvesicular activity was seen.

Marchetti et al. (531) investigated the enamel of decalcified samples of ODTxs using light microscopy and transmission electron microscopy and undecalcified samples using transmission electron microscopy. Simultaneous presence of prismatic enamel at varying maturing stages with different structural characteristics was observed. In some sites, the enamel did not present a prismatic structure, but appeared as clusters of unstructured material with abundant organic component.

Molecular-Genetic Data. No data are available.

Differential Diagnosis. As it is the case with any intrabony jaw lesion it is important that the pathologist gets access to the radiograms or other imaging of the tumor. The features of the border, the shape and the structure of the lesion often reveal important information. Differential diagnosis between an odontoma and an ameloblastoma, even in cases of an immature odontoma dominated by soft tissue, should not be difficult. The presence of dental hard tissues and a dental papilla–like connective tissue instead of a mature fibrous stroma excludes an ameloblastoma. If the epithelium of the odontoma is inflamed, in some areas a proliferation of the epithelium may be seen, which show some similarity to that of an ameloblastoma, but lacks stellate reticulum-like cells and the elongated peripheral cells with reverse nuclear polarity.

If the odontoma-like structure, complex or (more often) compound, is seen in the wall of a cyst, which exhibits the histomorphology of a COC, it should be classified as an OaCCOT.

Odontoma-like structures are seen in the exceedingly rare O-A. In the solid type of that tumor the dental hard tissue is found in minor areas scattered in the tumor. In the unicystic type of the tumor it is found in enclaves in various locations in the cyst wall in relation to dental papilla–like ectomesenchyme and dental lamina–like epithelium. The remaining part of the cyst is covered by an ameloblastoma-like epithelium, which, however, may exhibit many bilaminar epithelial strands, which are not usually seen in ameloblastomas.

The most difficult diagnostic problem is to distinguish an immature odontoma from AMF, AFD, and AFOD. Initially the odontoma shows a histomorphology similar to that of an AMF (514). At a later stage the dental hard tissues have been formed and in cases where the lesion, particularly in a case of developing ODTx, is surrounded by a thick coat of soft tumor tissue, the differential diagnosis towards an AFOD may be difficult or even impossible. As indicated by Odell et al. (54) factors favoring one of the odontomas are a young (child) patient, a well-defined, often ball-shaped, unilocular lesion and a site overlying an unerupted tooth or replacing a tooth. Factors favoring AMF are a slightly older child or young adult, particularly if the patient is older than 22 years, and a multilocular lesion with progressive growth and displacement of teeth. The differential diagnosis between an AFOD and a large immature ODTx is particularly difficult. Factors favoring the AFOD are an irregularly shaped lesion with minor areas of irregularly shaped dental hard tissue scattered in the tumor, and indication of progressive growth. Factors favoring an immature odontoma are an oval or ball-shaped lesion, which contains a single mass of hard dental tissue in the center with irradiating radiopaque lines and is related to the occlusal surface of an impacted tooth. The irradiating structure is recognized in the microscope, as described above. Mature odontomas should not cause diagnostic problems; the ODTp in particular is often diagnosed macroscopically. The differentiation toward supernumerary teeth is arbitrary, more than two odontoides within the same dental sac is usually considered a ODTp. In the rare cases of multiple odontomas, and they are most often of the compound type, there is a high possibility that the odontomas are part of a syndrome.

Treatment and Prognosis. Conservative enucleation is adequate treatment for both types of odontomes, they usually cleave easily from the smooth surface of the bony cavity in which they are situated. The prognosis is excellent. Large odontomes may require special surgical considerations (550). Very often an impacted tooth is found below the odontome and in a large number of cases it is possible to save the tooth and bring it in situ by orthodontic management (551). Morning (517) reported follow-up of 42 cases of impacted teeth in relation to odontomas. The morphology of the impacted tooth was normal in 62% (26/42), in the remaining cases there was some root deviation. After removal of the odontoma the impacted tooth erupted in 45% (19/42) of the cases, 77% (13/17) of the remaining teeth erupted after a second operation. Overall, about three out of four of the impacted teeth erupted after removal of the odontoma. Recurrences are very rare and are probably only seen in cases of incomplete removal of immature odontomes (552,553).

2.5 Odonto-Ameloblastoma

Introduction. This rare composite tumor includes areas that resemble an ameloblastoma together with areas that correspond to AFOD or an immature odontoma (381,554).

ICD-O code 9311/0

Synonyms: Ameloblastic odontoma

Clinical Features. Little more than 12 cases of O-A have been published with sufficient documentation to prove that the description of the tumor complies with the diagnostic criteria suggested by the WHO working group (554).

Epidemiological data are thus unavailable. Among 13 well-documented cases (417,555–562) [including two unpublished cases, IRC-226 and IRC-296 distributed by the International Reference Centre to Collaborating Centres for preparation of the first WHO classification of odontogenic tumors (22))] 4 were diagnosed in females and 9 in males. Age range was 2 to 53 years; mean age: 19.3 years; median age: 15 years. Three of the patients were in the first decade, six in the second, two were 25 years old, and one was 42, and one, 53 years old.

In six cases the tumor was located in the maxilla, and in seven cases, in the mandible. The anterior region was involved in one case, the anterior and posterior in one case, the remaining tumors were located posterior to the canine area, and some involved the mandibular ramus.

The size has varied from 1.5 to 7 to 8 cm at longest diameter; most have been large—between 4 and 6 cm at longest diameter.

The growth rate is difficult to estimate because of paucity of symptoms. A few patients have indicated pain and soreness, but in the majority of cases enlargement of the jaw caused by bony expansion has been the only symptom. Most patients have noticed the swelling for two to four months. In a few cases, however, it has been possible to trace the lesion almost from the beginning, and the growth rate seems to be slow; the large lesions have existed for several years.

Imaging. Radiographically, the O-A has appeared as a unilocular radiolucency with a well-defined corticated margin unlike the conventional ameloblastoma. Often the lesion is less well demarcated in some areas, though. In some cases the dental hard tissue formed in the tumor has been so discrete that is was undetectable on the radiogram. In most cases the lesion presented itself as a large radiolucent lesion with minor irregular radiopacities in the center or along the periphery. A few O-As showed abundant irregular radiopaque masses surrounded by a radiolucent zone. No "honeycombing" pattern as seen in ameloblastomas has been described. Better than radiograms, CT scans give detailed information about the border of the tumor.

Displacement of teeth has been observed in several cases (555,557,562), as well as resorption of roots of adjacent teeth (558,562,561).

Pathology. The etiology of the O-A is unknown. The most likely sources of tumor development are residues of the dental lamina and proliferations of odontogenic epithelium and ectomesenchyme adjacent to reduced enamel epithelium of unerupted teeth.

In six cases the removed specimen was a cystic lesion (Fig. 52) with a marked thickening of the wall and proliferation of tumor epithelium in various areas of the wall (555,557,558,560,561), including case ICR 226 contributed to the International Reference Center by Dr. Ishikawa, Tokyo, and illustrated in Figures 37 and 38, in the first WHO classification of odontogenic tumors by Pindborg and Kramer (22). It was a tumor

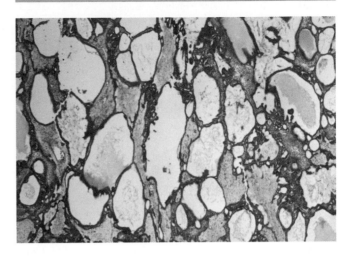

Figure 53 Odonto-ameloblastoma. Higher power of the tumor in Figure 52 showing the area with plexiform ameloblastoma. Degeneration with cystic change of the stroma is prominent. H&E stain. *Source*: Section by courtesy of Professor G. Ishikawa, Tokyo.

in the left side of the mandible in a 13-year-old boy; it had been known for 10 years. In other cases an abundant amount of hard tissues has been more dominating.

Microscopically, the tumor consists of an ameloblastoma component admixed with an AFOD/immature odontoma component (555,557,561,562). Areas that are indistinguishable from ameloblastoma are seen (Fig. 53), demonstrating follicular and in particular plexiform growth pattern of odontogenic epithelium in a fibrous connective tissue stroma. In other areas several O-As have shown a different odontogenic epithelium, which looks somewhat like a plexiform ameloblastoma, but the strands are long and narrow (Fig. 54) and consist of only two layers of basal cells without stellate reticulum cells between them. The strands form loops and are intermingled with plates of epithelium consisting of small cells with sparse cytoplasm and round nuclei. These cells form "ball of yarn"-like nodules within the sheets. The pattern is very similar to that seen as part of the histomorphology of an AOT and is well illustrated by Matsumoto et al. (561) in Figures 2 and 4 and Jacobsohn et al. (557) in Figure 5. Groups of ghost cells may be encountered particularly in areas where dental hard tissue is seen. The dental hard tissue forming areas are in close contact with areas with ameloblastoma and AOT morphology (Fig. 55). They may be a minor or a more dominant part of the tumor. They show the pattern of an immature, complex (560) or, more often, compound odontoma with formation of many tooth-like elements (odontoids) (555,557,559). Sometimes only dentin and no enamel had been found (558,560,561). The soft tissue part involved in the formation of hard tissue has a morphology similar

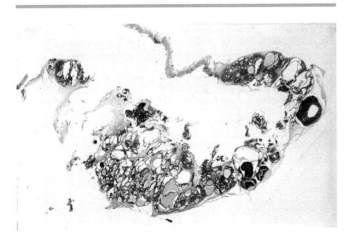

Figure 52 Odonto-ameloblastoma. Low power view of a unicystic type of the tumor which occurred in the left mandible of a 13-year-old boy. The radiogram of the lesion was published as Figure 37 in the 1971 edition of the WHO classification of odontogenic tumors. The thicker areas of the cystic lesion represent the ameloblastoma part; the immature odontoids are the seen in the right part of the lesion. H&E stain. *Source*: From Ref. 22 and section by courtesy of Professor G. Ishikawa, Tokyo.

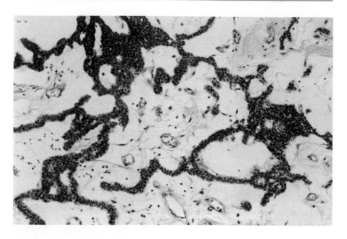

Figure 54 Odonto-ameloblastoma. Higher power of the tumor in Figure 52 showing an area with long narrow loop forming bicellular strands of epithelium that are uncommon in conventional ameloblastomas but have been described in several odonto-ameloblastomas and resemble those seen in adenomatoid odontogenic tumors. No stellate reticulum-like cells are seen in this area. H&E stain. *Source*: Section by courtesy of Professor G. Ishikawa, Tokyo.

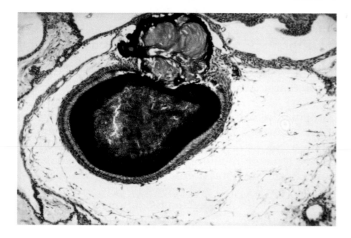

Figure 55 Odonto-ameloblastoma. Higher power of an island of enamel matrix surrounded by ameloblasts. The enamel is in contact with a cluster of partly mineralized ghost cells. No dentin is seen in this part of the section. H&E stain. *Source*: Section by courtesy of Professor G. Ishikawa, Tokyo.

to that found in an immature odontoma, and in some cases it is seen in such quantities compared with the hard tissue that it simulates an AFOD. Groups of ghost cells may be seen in several areas, particularly where the dental hard tissue is found (Fig. 55). In several of the cases consisting of one large cyst with proliferation of tumor tissue in various locations in the cystic wall, the border between the fibrous part of the cystic wall and the surrounding bone was well defined (555,557,558,560,561).

Immunohistochemistry. Only a single study has been published (417). The dental lamina–like epithelium in the soft part of the dental hard tissue forming areas reacted strongly to KL-1, a monoclonal marker for CKs-1, CK-2, CK-5-8, CK-11, CK-14, and CK-16-18 (563). The stellate reticulum-like epithelium reacted more weakly. The immature dental papilla–like ectomesenchyme around this epithelium was positive for tenascin and vimentin, while mesenchymal tissue showing myxomatous changes, and fibrous connective tissue was negative for tenascin, S-100 protein, and PCNA. A moderate amount of PCNA-positive cells were found in the dental lamina–like epithelium.

Electron Microscopy. No data have been published.

Molecular-Genetic Data. No data have been published.

Differential Diagnosis. Some authors (564) have found it impossible to distinguish between O-As and AFODs, but they concentrated primarily on clinical features. The diagnosis O-A should only be used for odontogenic tumors showing combined features of ameloblastoma and those of an immature odontoma or AFOD. Areas with loop-forming basal cell strands of epithelium and nodules with a swirling pattern like those seen as a part of the morphology of an AOT are also an important histomorphological hallmark. Such areas and those with ameloblastoma morphology are not seen in ameloblastic fibro-odontomes, which are the most important differential diagnosis.

Treatment and Prognosis. Most of the published cases were treated by curettage (417,555–562). In those with a unicystic appearance the tumor is found in a cavity with smooth walls. In one case hemimaxillectomy was done (558), other cases were treated by wide surgical resection and en-bloc resection (562). Follow-up for five years or longer has unfortunately only been reported in one case (555). The patient's lesion appeared cystic and was treated by curettage; it recurred twice and both times as an ameloblastoma. The second time it was treated by en-bloc resection; the reported follow-up there after was only for 1 and a half years. Since the lesion possess the biological potential of an ameloblastoma, and recurrences have been reported after local curettage alone (555,565,561) the recommended treatment is excision in form of a marginal or bloc resection with long-term (at least 15 years) follow-up (381).

2.6 Odontogenic Ghost Cell Lesions

The term-odontogenic ghost cell lesions embraces a heterogeneous group of odontogenic lesions that histopathologically are cysts, solid benign neoplasms, solid malignant neoplasms, or a combination of these. They may be intraosseous or extraosseous. They share cytological and histomorphological features in terms of an epithelium, which is histomorphologically similar to that seen in s/mAM and UNAMs, but in contrast with ameloblastomas they show a conspicuous presence of ghost cells with tendency for calcification and they show formation of dentinoid (dysplastic dentin) in the juxtaepithelial connective tissue.

Although cases of odontogenic ghost cell lesions had been published under various titles since 1932 by Rywkin (566), Boss (567), Spirgi (568), and Lurie (569), it was not till 1962 that the lesion was recognized as a new entity by Gorlin et al. (570). It was described on the basis of 11 own cases and 4 from the literature. They were all cystic lesions; one of them was associated with an ODTx. The authors stressed their peculiar histological features that distinguish them from the CEOTs for which they were often mistaken. The similarities to the cutaneous calcifying epithelioma of Malherbe (pilomatrixoma) were also drawn attention to. For the lesion, the name " 'calcifying odontogenic cyst (COC)' was chosen, at least until its nature is clarified."

Further cases were published in the following years by Gold (571), Gorlin et al. (572), Abrams et al. (573), Chaves (574), Jones et al. (575), Ulmansky et al. (576), and Fejerskov et al. (577) among others. It became apparent that not all the COCs are cystic. The two cases published by Fejerskov et al. were a solid extraosseous tumor in the palatal gingiva and an intraosseous cystic lesion associated with an odontoma. The authors suggested that the name of the lesion be changed to "calcifying ghost cell odontogenic tumor."

The COC was recognized in the first WHO classification of Odontogenic Tumours and Cysts (22) as a cystic nonneoplastic lesion, but classified among the benign odontogenic tumors. A malignant variant was recognized and illustrated in Figure 74 in the book as a carcinoma arising in a COC. The microphoto was taken from a case (IRC 58) contributed to the WHO International Reference Center for classification of Odontogenic Tumours by Dr. J. N. Astacio, El Salvador; it had been published in 1965 as a CEOT (578).

In the 1992 revision of the WHO classification (23) the COC was still classified among the benign odontogenic tumors. The contradictory term "nonneoplastic" was deleted. As pointed out by Li et al. (579), this classification implied that all COCs are neoplastic in nature, even though the majority may appear cystic and nonneoplastic. It was mentioned in the text of the classification that solid tumors had been described and termed "dentinogenic ghost cell tumor" (580) and "odontogenic ghost cell tumor" (581,582), but COC was still used as the general term to include all cystic and benign neoplastic variants. Consequently the term "calcifying odontogenic cyst" has been used in a number of publications in the last four decenniums as a common term to describe all the various variants of odontogenic ghost cell lesions (583–592), including two extensive reviews of the literature by Buchner et al. (593,594).

Prætorius et al. (580) suggested a classification, which classified cysts and neoplasms as two different entities. Hong et al. (582) studied 92 cases of COC from the files of Armed Forces Institute of Pathology (AFIP), Washington, DC, U.S.A., and found many variants that did not fit into the classification of Prætorius et al.; they suggested a classification with a main division in cystic and neoplastic lesions but with a more elaborated subdivision. Buchner et al. (594) in a review of 215 intraosseous cases from the literature suggested a classification with a main division of the lesions into extraosseous and intraosseous lesions and a subdivision into cystic and neoplastic lesions. Toida (595) reviewed the published classifications and suggested a classification dividing the lesions into cysts, neoplasms (benign and malignant), and combined lesions. In a study of 21 cases of odontogenic ghost cell lesions Li et al. (579) reviewed earlier classifications and suggested a revision. They divided the lesions into three groups: (i) developmental odontogenic cysts, (ii) benign odontogenic neoplasms, and (iii) odontogenic carcinomas (odontogenic ghost cell carcinoma). In the cyst group they placed the cystic COC with or without odontoma. The benign odontogenic neoplasm group was divided into odontogenic ghost cell tumor and combined lesions.

In the WHO classification of head and neck tumors published in 2005 (12), the benign and the malignant neoplasm was recognized as entities and named "dentinogenic ghost cell tumour" (596) and "ghost cell odontogenic carcinoma" (597), respectively. Cysts were excluded from the classification a priori, but with a view to the neoplastic potential of some COCs, the simple cysts and the cysts with a neoplastic potential were grouped together under the term "calcifying cystic odontogenic tumour" (598).

There are many good reasons (579), however, to keep the simple cysts separated from the cysts associated with odontomas or benign odontogenic neoplasms since many cystic lesions are nonneoplastic. It is therefore suggested to revise the classification of Toida and Li et al., as indicated in Table 4, where the terms accepted by WHO have been used and the lesions have been separated into simple cysts, combined lesions, benign neoplasms, and malignant

Table 4 Suggested Classification of Odontogenic Ghost Cell Lesions

Group 1. "Simple" cysts with or without limited proliferation of odontogenic epithelium in the cyst wall:
Calcifying odontogenic cyst (COC)

Group 2. Cysts associated with odontogenic hamartomas or benign neoplasms:
Calcifying cystic odontogenic tumor (CCOT)
The following combinations have been published:
Solid/multicystic ameloblastoma associated CCOT
Unicystic ameloblastoma associated CCOT
Adenomatoid odontogenic tumor associated CCOT
Ameloblastic fibroma associated CCOT
Ameloblastic fibro-odontoma associated CCOT
Odonto-ameloblastoma associated CCOT
Odontoma associated CCOT
Odontogenic myxofibroma associated CCOT

Group 3. Solid benign odontogenic neoplasms with similar cell morphology to that in the COC, and with dentinoid formation:
Dentinogenic ghost cell tumor (DGCT)

Group 4. Malignant odontogenic neoplasms with features similar to those of the dentinogenic ghost cell tumor:
Ghost cell odontogenic carcinoma (GCOC)

neoplasms. This classification has served as a basis for the description of the various entities in the following.

2.6.1 Calcifying Odontogenic Cyst

Introduction. The COC is a developmental cyst with a particular epithelial lining that resembles the lining of a UNAM with a basal layer of columnar cells, and an overlying layer that resembles a stellate reticulum. Groups of epithelial ghost cells are seen in the epithelial lining or in the epithelial strands and islands in the fibrous capsule. Dysplastic dentin is often laid down adjacent to the basal layer of the cystic lining or of the epithelial islands in the capsule.

Synonyms: Calcifying ghost cell odontogenic cyst, which may be a more precise term, but the term "calcifying odontogenic cyst" has been generally accepted for several decenniums.

Clinical Features. The prevalence and incidence of COC is unknown. The relative frequency of the tumor in material received for histological diagnosis in services of diagnostic pathology in various countries for various amounts of years ranges from 1.0% to 7.2% in studies comprising more than 300 samples of odontogenic tumors. The results are indicated as follows: number of odontogenic tumors/number of COCs/%. Regezzi et al., Michigan, U.S.A. (31): 706/15/2.1%, Günhan et al., Turkey (32): 409/4/1.0%, Daley et al., Canada (33): 392/18/4.6%, Mosqueda-Taylor et al., Mexico (34): 349/24/6.8%, Ochsenius et al., Chile (35): 362/26/7.2%, Adebayo et al., Nigeria (36): 318/8/2.5%, Fernandes et al., Brazil (37): 340/12/3.5%, Ladeinde et al., Nigeria (38): 319/17/5.3%, Buchner et al., California (30): 1088/17/1.6%, Jones et al., England (2006, pooled figures from two studies) (39,40): 523/21/4.0%, Olgac et al., Turkey (41): 527/29/5.5%, and Jing et al., China (42): 1642/36/2.2%. All these studies suffer from the bias that all benign variants of odontogenic ghost cell lesions have been pooled together. In all these series, however, the "simple" cyst, COC has accounted for the majority of cases. The percentage has been counted as the percent of odontogenic tumors, not of odontogenic cysts.

Shear (228) reported that only 30 examples accessioned as COCs were recorded in the archives of the University of the Witwatersrand, Department of Oral Pathology, South Africa, representing 0.9% of 3498 jaw cysts documented during the period 1958 to 2004 (46 years).

The age distribution of the COC is difficult to assess, again because other types of ghost cell lesions have been included in the surveys published. The OaCCOTs occur primarily in the second decennium and are very rare in patients older than 40 years. When this group is included, the age peak is moved markedly toward the younger age groups.

The line graph of ages of patients with COC without epithelial proliferations in the cyst wall ($N = 35$) in the study by Hong et al. (582) showed an age peak in the second and the eighth decade, the graph for COCs with epithelial proliferations in the cyst wall ($N = 17$) showed an even distribution over all decades. The mean age for all cystic variants was 33 years.

In the review by Buchner (594) of 144 published cases of COC the age range was 5 to 82 years, 50 cases occurred in the second and 25 cases in the third decennium, making up 52% of the cases.

The COC does not seem to have any gender predilection. In a review of 88 published cases Shear et al. (228) reported a gender distribution of 44 COCs in men and 44 in women. In Buchner's survey 105 patients were men and 110 women, but in the study by Hong et al., 47 were men and 31 women. These surveys all contain some cases, which are not simple cystic.

There seem to be an even distribution between COCs located in the maxilla and in the mandible. In Buchner's survey of all intraosseous histological variants 111 were in the maxilla and 104 in the mandible. The most common site of occurrence was the anterior parts of the jaws. Among 131 cystic lesions 62 were in the maxilla and 69 in the mandible. In the maxilla 71% were located in the incisor-canine region; in the mandible 55% were located in the incisor-canine region. Among 77 cases in the study by Hong et al., 67 occurred intraosseously, 30 in the maxilla, and 37 in the mandible. Ten cystic lesions were located extraosseously in the gingiva and were distributed evenly between maxilla and mandible. There was no significant preference for either maxilla or mandible among the cystic COCs except in the "ameloblastomatous" type, in which 9 of 11 cases occurred in the mandible. The "ameloblastomatous" type showed unifocal or multifocal intraluminal proliferative activity that resembled ameloblastoma, and thus resembled a UNAM. It corresponds to the "unicystic ameloblastoma-associated CCOT" in Table 4.

Clinically the extraosseous cases occur as firm or soft circumscribed, smooth-surfaced elevated masses on the gingiva or alveolar mucosa according to Buchner (593). The color is usually normal except for some lesions that are reddish. The size ranges from 0.5 to 4.0 cm, but most lesions are in the range from 0.5 to 1.1 cm in their greatest diameter. They are usually asymptomatic and detected during routine oral examination. The duration of the lesion has varied from 1 month to 15 years, but in half of the cases it ranged from one to eight months. Displacement of adjacent teeth has been reported.

In the review of 215 intraosseous ghost cell lesions by Buchner (594), which contained 72% COCs, 26% OaCCOTs, and 2% DGCTs, the lesions appeared as painless hard swellings. Expansion was recorded in 133 cases and perforation of bone in 10 cases. Early lesions did not exhibit expansion and were detected following radiographic examination, usually for the failure of tooth eruption. A few patients complained of tenderness or pain usually in association with a secondary infection. The time between the patient's awareness of the lesion and consultation for treatment was recorded in 54 cases and ranged from three days to 9 years; the median duration was six months.

Imaging. The peripheral cases sometimes show a superficial resorption of the underlying bone, which is noted at surgery. In a few cases the resorption is so marked that it is visible in preoperative radiograms (593).

In Buchner's review of intraosseous lesions (594) most of the lesions (156 cases) appeared radiographically as unilocular radiolucencies, only 12 cases were multilocular. The COCs usually have well-circumscribed borders, only in 10 cases they were poorly demarcated. The radiolucent lesion may show varying degree of scattered radiopaque material, ranging from tiny flecks to conspicuous masses, depending on the degree of calcification of the ghost cells in the lesion. Some of the maxillary COCs show antral involvement from encroachment to complete obliteration. Resorption of roots of teeth adjacent to the cyst has been reported in several cases (584,585), root diversion is less common (599). About one-third of the lesions are associated with unerupted teeth (Fig. 56), more common in the maxilla than in the mandible, in a few cases the cyst was associated with more than one unerupted tooth. The size of the cyst was known in 58 cases. It ranged from 0.5 to 12 cm. Almost 60% of the lesions were between 2 and 3.9 cm. The mean size was 3.3 cm.

In a study by Yoshiura et al. (600) it was shown that conventional radiography was adequate in most instances, but CT was useful as a means of identifying both desquamated keratin and peripheral calcification in COC.

Pathology. The etiology of the COCs is unknown. The peripheral cysts in the gingiva are believed to originate from remnants of the dental lamina and, less likely from the basal cells of the surface epithelium. The intraosseous cysts are believed to develop from reduced enamel epithelium of unerupted teeth or remnants of the dental lamina in

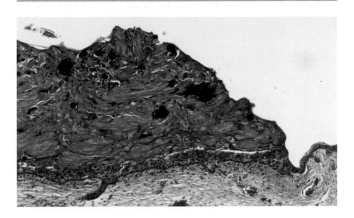

Figure 57 Calcifying odontogenic cyst. Extensive formation of ghost cells is seen in the epithelial lining to the left. Some ghost cells show calcification. Apart from a few cells, the basal cell layer is still unchanged. Note to the right that parts of the cystic lining may be without any formation of ghost cells. H&E stain.

terms of proliferating epithelium on the top of a dental follicle of an unerupted tooth.

On histological examination the lesion is characterized by a unicystic structure (23,54,228,570,601). Tangential sections of folded cysts may give a false impression of more that one lumen. However cases have been published in which, even on gross examination, the lesion appeared to be multicystic (594). The thickness and the morphology of the epithelial lining may vary from area to area, but at least in some areas the epithelium resembles that of an ameloblastoma with a well-defined basal layer of columnar cells with nuclei polarized away from the basal membrane (Fig. 57). Mitoses are rare. Generally the interface is flat without rete ridge formation. The overlying epithelium resembles the stellate reticulum of the enamel organ. Melanin is sometimes present in the epithelium, particularly in the stellate cells (602). Individual or more often clusters of ghost cells are seen in the epithelium (Fig. 58). They present as large, pale eosinophilic cells with a distinct outline and are considerably larger than the epithelial cells from which they seem to originate (Fig. 57). Some may contain remnants of the nucleus, but most cells show a well-defined, central empty space instead of a nucleus. Ghost cells are easily detected by means of trichrome staining (Fig. 59) or staining with rhodamine B and observed in fluorescent light (22,603,604). Some areas may show a flattened epithelium without ghost cells and with inconspicuous basal cells, others may show a narrow suprabasal epithelium with cuboidal basal cells with dark nuclei without polarization, and little or no stellate reticulum-like cells. Because of the size of the ghost cells the epithelium in areas with many ghost cells appear thicker than in other areas (Fig. 57). Most ghost cells are found in the upper layer of the epithelium. In areas where basal cells are transformed into ghost cells there is no distinct limit between the epithelium and the underlying connective tissue, and

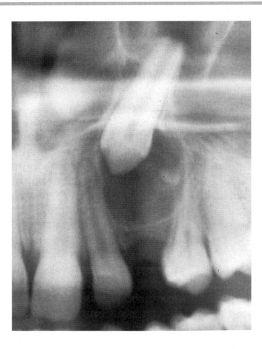

Figure 56 Calcifying odontogenic cyst. Radiograph of a COC simulating a dentigerous cyst around the crown of a left maxillary canine in a 14-year-old boy.

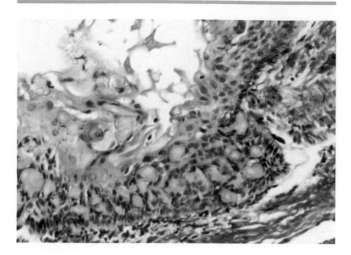

Figure 58 Calcifying odontogenic cyst. Higher magnification, which shows scattered ghost cells and the typical columnar palisading basal cells. van Gieson stain.

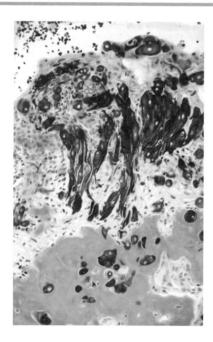

Figure 59 Calcifying odontogenic cyst. Ghost cells (*red*) and dentinoid (*turquoise blue*) are more clearly distinguished in a trichrome or van Gieson stained section than in a H&E stain stained one. Note the entrapped ghost cells in the dentinoid and the disintegration of the basement membrane in areas where basal cells have been transformed into ghost cells. Masson trichrome stain.

foreign body giant cells can be seen between the epithelial cells and in particular around ghost cells in the connective tissue. The ghost cells show an affinity for calcification (Fig. 57), initially as fine or course

basophilic granules, but stacks of mineralized ghost cells may present as calcified sheets, which may be visible on a radiogram. Some epithelial budding may be seen from the basal cells and formation of individual strands or islands of epithelium or small daughter cysts in the adjacent connective tissue. They vary from a few strands to extensive proliferation (605). In their study of 79 COCs, Hong et al. (582) found 17 cases with marked proliferation of the cyst-lining epithelium and multiple daughter cysts of variable size. Some authors prefer to subdivide the COCs into nonproliferative and proliferative variants (582,606,607). Yoshida et al. (606) demonstrated that the mean Ki-67 L.I. was slightly greater in COCs and OaCCOTs with proliferative-type lining epithelium (*vide infra*). Cases with unifocal or multifocal intraluminal proliferative activity resembling UNAM are better classified as UNAM-associated CCOT (Table 4). Atubular dentinoid is often found in close contact with the epithelial lining (Fig. 59) or the epithelial islands (601). It is osteoid-like, but called dentinoid because it is only seen in contact with the odontogenic epithelium and resembles the dentin, which may be formed in teeth traumatized during development. The connective tissue is fibrous (Fig. 58); no cellular embryonal pulp-like odontogenic ectomesenchyme is seen, not even in areas with dentinoid formation. The dentinoid may contain entrapped cells including ghost cells (Fig. 59). Slight nonspecific inflammation may be seen in the connective tissue. A single case of COC with clear cells has been described by Ng et al. (608); the cells were located in the subepithelial connective tissue and may not be epithelia cells; the significance is unknown.

Immunohistochemistry. Immunohistochemical studies have usually been made on materials from COCs, OaCOCs, and DGCTs without a clear distinction between the entities.

CKs have been studied by several authors (582,606,607,609–613). The results have been partly controversial.

Antibodies against CK-19, which has been detected frequently in odontogenic epithelium, were used by Kakadu et al. (610), Yoshida et al. (606), and Fregnani et al. (607), with comparable results. A positive immunoreaction was found in the upper intermediate and superficial cell layers of the lining epithelium, but not in the basal layer, except the study of Fregnani et al. (607) who found a positive reaction in the basal cell layer in 6 of 10 cases. Murakami et al. (612) using monoclonal antibodies against CK-19 found a positive reaction in the basal layers, but negative in the suprabasal layers. In contrast, Yamamoto et al. (609) using PKK-1 against CK-8, CK-18, and CK-19 found essentially no reaction in the epithelium. They also used KL-1, a broad-spectred antibody against CK-1, CK-2, CK-5-8, CK-11, CK-14, and CK-16-18 and found a slightly positive reaction in the basal and suprabasal epithelium. Using the same antigens Kakudo et al. (610) found a positive reaction exclusively in the upper intermediate and the superficial layers. Fregnani et al. (607) detected expression of broadspectred AE1/AE3 and 34βE12 (CK-1, CK-5, CK-10, CK-14) as well as monoclonal CK-8, CK-4, and CK-19 in the suprabasal cells of the lining epithelium in all 10 of their cases, and they found CK-14 and AE1/AE3 keratins expressed in the basal cells in all cases.

Ghost cells gave a negative response to broad-spectred antibodies (TK, KL-1, AE1/AE3) in the studies by Yamamoto et al. (609), Kakudo et al. (610), Hong et al. (582), and Gordeeff et al. (611). Monteil et al. (604), however, detected a weak reaction to the antibody Dako K518, and Murakami et al. (612) detected a positive reaction to CK-13. Fregnani et al. (607) found immunoreactivity of ghost cells to 34βE12 in 4 of 10 cases and to AE1/AE3 in 8 of 10 cases. Kusama et al. (613) raised three kinds of antibodies against hard α-keratins in human hair and used them to investigate ghost cells in pilomatrixomas, craniopharyngiomas and 14 cases of COC. Positive reaction was found in all cases and in ghost cells exclusively. The CKs of ghost cells thus seem to be closely related to hard α-keratins.

Involucrin was studied by Yamamoto et al. (609) who found that only few epithelial cells were positive. Kakudo et al. (610) detected involucrin in the upper intermediate cell layers exclusively. They studied filaggrin as well, only few epithelial cells reacted positively. Immunoreaction to vimentin in epithelial cells was moderate and only seen in individual cells.

HGF, TGF-β, and their receptors were studied by Kumamoto et al. (134) in six cases of COC. The epithelial cells of COC showed reactivity for HGF, TGF-β and their receptors. High expression of receptors was noted in ghost cells. The authors concluded that the findings support the hypothesis that HGF and TGF-β act on epithelial cells via paracrine and autocrine mechanisms.

Tenascin, a multifunctional extracellular matrix glycoprotein, was investigated in four cases of COC by Mori et al. (70). Positive reaction was found exclusively in the connective tissue along the basement membrane of the epithelial cells.

Chen et al. (167) used ISH and immunohistochemistry on a case of COC to study BSP, a major noncollagenous protein synthesized and secreted by bone-, dentine-, and cementum-forming cells. Strong BSP signals were seen in epithelial cells surrounding nests of ghost cells with both methods.

Versican, a large chondroitin sulfate proteoglycan in extracellular matrix, was studied by Ito et al. (67) in one case of COC and several cases of other odontogenic tumors. Ghost cells and calcified matrix in COC were positive; the connective tissue was essentially negative.

The presence of enamel proteins (amelogenin, enamelin, sheathlin, and enamelysin) have been studied by several investigators (159–162,548,606,614).

Amelogenin was detected by Mori et al. (162) in eight COCs. The epithelial cells of the cysts were almost devoid of amelogenin staining, the ghost cells showed immunoreactivity at varying intensity; calcified ghost cells were negative. The results by Saku et al. (159) from a study of three COCs were different; they found a weak, diffuse reaction in the epithelial cells, no reaction in the ghost cells, and a strong reaction in the calcified globules. Takata et al. (614)

studied the presence of amelogenin in ghost cells in six cases of COCs and three cases of pilomatrixoma. They found amelogenin located particularly to clusters of ghost cells, and sometimes exclusively to the periphery of the clusters. No amelogenin was present in the ghost cells of pilomatrixomas. In a study of two COCs Abiko et al. (548) confirmed that some ghost cells in the lining epithelium were strongly stained. Similar results were achieved by Yoshida et al. (606) in a study of 16 COCs among which 12 were OaCCOTs; amelogenin was expressed in the ghost cells, but not in the lining epithelial cells.

Enamelin was studied by Saku et al. (159) in three cases of COC. The reactivity was similar to that of amelogenin; in the lining epithelial layer, round mineralized material was diffusely positive for enamelin. The epithelial cells of the upper layers showed mild and diffuse immunoreaction in the cytoplasm. In the study of Takata et al. (614) enamelin was mainly expressed at the periphery of ghost cell clusters and not in centrally situated cells. The staining pattern in the individual ghost cell was often seen as linear fragments along the cytoplasmic membrane.

Sheathlin was studied in the same six cases of COC as mentioned above by Takata et al. (614) and a second time in 10 cases of COC (160). Although epithelial cells were generally negative for sheathlin, ghost cells in the epithelial lining showed distinct immunoreactivity, which was the most distinctive and frequent among the four enamel-related proteins examined. Dysplastic dentin was negative.

Enamelysin was studied in six COCs (614) and in 10 COCs (160) by Takata et al. by means of a monoclonal antibody (203-1C7). Although the epithelial cells surrounding the cysts were generally negative for enamelysin expression, selected ghost cells in the epithelial lining or in the connective tissue showed obvious immunoreactivity, especially at the peripheral areas of these cell clusters. Dysplastic dentin was negative.

The PCNA L.I. was assessed immunohistochemically in 12 cases of cystic COC and 9 cases of OaCCOT and compared to the index in ameloblastomas by Takata et al. (615). The COCs were divided into nonproliferative and proliferative according to the amount of epithelial proliferations in the connective tissue wall. The proliferative cystic COCs ($N = 8$) showed a higher PCNA L.I. (mean 17.2 ± 11.2, range 5.7–37.1) than the nonproliferative (mean 6.8 ± 2.8, range 3.2–9.6). The PCNA L.I. for the proliferative COCs was almost equivalent to that of ameloblastoma (mean 18.3 ± 13.3, range 5.1–40.8). Freganani et al. (607) confirmed these results in a study of 10 cases, which consisted of five central cystic COCs, three OaCCOTs, and two peripheral DGCTs, which they considered "nonproliferative." They found a mean L.I. of 10 (range <1–20) in the nonproliferative and a mean L.I. of 25 (range 10–50) in the proliferative. The L.I. for the five cystic COC (2 nonproliferative and 3 proliferative) was 20 (range <1–50).

Proteins produced by the proto-oncogene Bcl-2 suppress apoptosis. The protein was detected by Yoshida et al. (606) in a pool of 16 cases consisting of four cystic COCs and 12 OaCCOTs. Bcl-2 was absent in two and present in two of the COCs. In the above-mentioned study by Fregnani et al. (607) all 10 cases expressed Bcl-2 in the basal and suprabasal cells, but ghost cells were negative in all cases.

An assessment of the Ki-67 L.I. was made by the same investigators as part of the study mentioned above (606,607). Yoshida et al. (606) found a mean Ki-67 L.I. of 1.45 ± 0.50 for the four cystic COCs. Ki-67-labeled cells were found in nuclei of lining epithelial cells, but not in the ghost cells. Among the five cystic COCs four expressed Ki-67 and one was negative. The mean L.I. was 2 (range <1–4). In the entire group the lesions with epithelial proliferations showed a three times higher L.I. than the nonproliferative.

Mel-CAM, a multifunctional heterophilic cell-to-cell adhesion transmembrane glycoprotein, was investigated by Fregnani et al. (607) in the same study where PCNA, Bcl-2, and Ki-67 were investigated. Mel-CAM was frequently expressed in suprabasal and ghost cells, but was practically absent in the basal-lining cells.

Mutations of β-catenin, a transcriptional activator of the Wnt-signaling pathway was studied by Sekine et al. (156) in 20 cases of ameloblastoma and 10 simple cystic COCs by means of immunohistochemistry and genetic analysis. The results of the latter are discussed below. Monoclonal anti-β-catenin was used for immunohistochemical staining. All cases including two in which mutations were not identified showed similar β-catenin expression. The lining epithelium showed weak to moderate cytoplasmic staining. Cells around ghost cells tended to exhibit stronger nuclear accumulation. Peripherally palisading columnar cells showed somewhat stronger β-catenin expression in both the cytoplasm and the membrane. The study by Hassanein et al. (616) essentially confirmed these results. They found a strong nuclear and cytoplasmic staining in six of six COCs. The cytoplasmic staining was found in the basaloid and transitional cells. Ghost cells were negative in all cases.

Electron Microscopy. Donath et al. (617) published a detailed description of the ultrastructure of the COC. Basal cells were elongated and bordered on a conspicuous basement membrane. Desmosomes were seen and in the cytoplasm, a moderate number of tonofilaments, rough endoplasmatic reticulum, free ribosomes, mitochondria, and a small Golgi apparatus were detected. The nucleus was elongated and oval, had a small nucleolus and heterochromatin distributed at the periphery.

The spinal cells had narrow intercellular spaces and abundant desmosomes. Intracytoplasmic tonofilaments irradiating from the desmosomes were poorly developed. Free ribosomes, RER, a well-developed Golgi apparatus, and enlarged cisternae were seen. Cells in the stellate reticulum-like areas showed large intercellular spaces partly empty and partly filled with fine granula and small vesicles. The cytoplasm exhibited laciniated extensions with desmosomes. The ultrastructure of the cytoplasm was similar to that of the spinal cells except that some cells contained lipid droplets, myelin figures, and large vacuoles.

Many variations in shape and size were seen in the ghost cells, they were generally larger than basal and spinal cells. The cytoplasm was packed with parallel bundles of tonofilaments with intermediate vesicles some of which were empty, and some filled with granular material. Cells were seen with RER, remnants of mitochondriae, and osmiophilic membranes or granula packed around the nucleus or along the periphery of the cell. Heterochromatin was irregularly dispersed along the inner nuclear membrane. Only few fragments of cellular membranes with desmosomes were seen, but clusters of disintegrated desmosomes were found. Membranes of spinal cells adjacent to ghost cells exhibited disintegration and vesicular transformation. In areas with coalescence of ghost cells two types of changes of tonofilaments were found, some were fused, and others—less frequently—were fragmented. Between the ghost cells remnants of cell organelles with needle-shaped calcifications were found. Completely calcified ghost cells were divided in zones.

Dentinoid (dysplastic dentin) showed a grid of filaments, which had an increased osmiophilia at the periphery. Embedded ghost cells were detected. Collagen fibrils could only be found in areas adjacent to fibroblasts.

Abaza (618) confirmed most of these findings and described a cell type, which unlike the ghost cells with thick uniform fibrils contained moderately densely packed and evenly distributed tonofilaments oriented in different directions and occasionally residue of organelles. Similar cells had been described by Chen et al. (619) in DGCTs and have been called "hornified cells."

Mimura et al. (620) confirmed many of these findings and they also detected needle-like crystals around the epithelial cells. Many calcifications exhibited a distinctive ring formation around the periphery of an amorphous central core with no evidence of ghost cells. These calcifications were observed with necrotic remnants of nuclear material and many identifiable mitochondria, thin fibers, and epithelial cells. The cytoplasm of the ghost cells consisted of numerous short electron-dense tonofilaments bundles. In these calcification was observed. The needle-like structures were shown by X-ray diffraction analysis to be hydroxyapatite.

Molecular-Genetic Data. Somatic β-catenin mutations were found in 9 of 10 COCs analyzed successfully by Sekine et al. (156). All of the mutations caused amino acid substitution of serine/threonine residues of GSK-3β phosphorylation sites or residues flanking the first serine residue of the phosphorylation sites. The authors suggested that the results indicate that COC is caused by an activating mutation of β-catenin. Interestingly only 1 of 20 ameloblastomas showed β-catenin mutation, indicating that COC and ameloblastoma are two genetically distinct lesions, despite their histological resemblance.

Differential Diagnosis. If typical areas are present in the sample, differential diagnosis is usually not a problem. Ghost cells have been described in eruption cysts, ameloblastomas, AMFs, ameloblastic fibro-odontomes, and particularly in odontomes, although usually in moderate amounts (534). The mere presence of ghost cells is therefore an insufficient criterion for the diagnosis of COC; stellate reticulum-like areas and elongated basal cells must be present. Differential diagnosis between COC and CCOT associated with odontoma or odontogenic tumors is not difficult if sufficient sampling and clinical information is available, except cases with marked proliferation of epithelium in the connective tissue wall. Some degree of epithelial proliferation is acceptable within the spectrum of COC, but in case of extensive luminal or mural proliferation, the lesion is better classified as UNAM-associated CCOT (Table 4). Borderline cases are difficult and the decision is arbitrary. It is important of course to distinguish the COC from the GCOC. The malignant tumor may have arisen in a COC and there may be benign areas in the operation specimen besides the carcinoma. While mitoses are very rare in COCs, they are numerous in the GCOC, which also show increased cellularity, some degree of pleomorphism, and areas with necrosis.

Treatment and Prognosis. The COCs are effectively treated by enucleation in most cases. Recurrence is rare, but has been recorded (570,585,617,621–625); according to Buchner (594) nine cases of recurrences have been reported, but among these DGCTs may be included. The case reported by Slootweg et al. (622) was a COC in the mandible, which recurred seven years after enucleation. One of the two cases of recurrence reported by McGowan et al. (585) recurred after four years, and the one by Daniels et al. (625) after eight years. A follow-up time of about 10 years seems required. Cystotomy is not recommended; case 3 reported by Donath et al. (617) recurred after cystotomy, and case reported by Prætorius et al. (580) was treated by cystotomy, with the consequence that the entire lumen became filled with COC tissue within the following months and protruded through the surgical window. Malignant transformation has been reported, the subject is discussed in the section "Ghost cell odontogenic carcinoma."

2.6.2 Calcifying Cystic Odontogenic Tumor (Associated with Other Types of Odontogenic Tumors)

Introduction. As indicated above, the term "calcifying cystic odontogenic tumor (CCOT)" is used in this survey to designate a group of ghost cell lesions, which present as a calcified odontogenic cyst associated with an odontogenic neoplasm or an odontoma (Table 4). In rare cases, the cyst is associated with a malignant ghost cell containing tumor (581,626–631); these are called GCOCs and are discussed below under the heading Malignant Epithelial Odontogenic Tumors. ICD-O code 9301/0

The OaCCOT has been described in many reports, but only few cases of the other combinations are known. It is very unlikely that all these COC-associated tumors are collision lesions. It is far more plausible that the epithelial cells of the COC harbor genes that under favorable conditions initiate the

development of an odontogenic tumor. Numerous COCs have shown various amounts of islands and strands of epithelium in the connective tissue wall, the differential diagnosis between extensive proliferations and an initial ameloblastoma may be arbitrary. The so-called "Vickers – Gorlin criterions" (270) are a useful guideline, but not a distinguishing mark; it must be borne in mind that many areas in a genuine solid/cystic ameloblastoma do not fulfill these criterions.

The question whether the cyst develops from a preexisting odontogenic tumor in a CCOT associated with an odontogenic tumor or the tumor develops from the wall of the cyst has been debated in the literature (228,580,605). There are convincing indications that the cyst is the primary lesion and the tumor develops from the cyst since the proliferations of the odontogenic epithelium in the wall of the cyst displays such a vast spectrum, and many OaCCOTs have been published, which have shown a scale of development from small areas of formation of hard dental tissue in the wall of the cyst to large odontomas that fills most of the cystic space.

2.6.2.1 Solid/Multicystic Ameloblastoma–Associated CCOT. Three cases have been published of this variant. Hong et al. (582) described two cases. They occurred in a 10-year-old girl and in a 59-year-old man. Both tumors occurred in the posterior of the mandible and appeared as intraosseous, well-defined radiolucent lesions that produced progressive swelling. Few ghost cells and no dentinoid was seen in the ameloblastoma areas. Tajima et al. (632) reported a case in a 35-year-old man, which presented as a well-demarcated cystic lesion in the mandibular symphisis with slight enlargement of the overlying gingiva. Root resorption of the anterior teeth was observed. Besides the ameloblastoma-like appearance, the tumor contained dentinoid, and the epithelium showed a cribriform architecture, which is not usually seen in ameloblastomas. These cases should be treated as ameloblastomas.

2.6.2.2 Unicystic Ameloblastoma–Associated CCOT. Hong et al. (582) reported 11 cases of "ameloblastomatous calcifying odontogenic cyst." The term is not felicitous since the epithelium of all COCs resemble that of an ameloblastoma, but the authors also described the lesions as resembling UNAMs except for the ghost cells and calcification within the proliferative epithelium. The tumor developed primarily in age groups between the second and sixth decennium, and 9 of the 11 lesions occurred in the mandible. Li et al. (579) reported a similar case (case 3) in the mandible of a 50-year-old woman. The tumor presented as a multilocular radiolucency from the right premolar to the left second incisor. It was treated by enucleation, and there was no sign of recurrence after six years. The authors mentioned that fewer ghost cells and less dentinoid were found in the ameloblastoma-like proliferations than in the cystic part of the lesion. Aithal et al. (633) reported a case in the left posterior region of the mandible of a 28-year-old woman. It presented as a well-defined, hard, nontender swelling, which on the radiogram disclosed a multilocular radio-lucency extending from the canine to the second molar. The case reported by Iida et al. (592) was diagnosed in a 17-year-old Japanese man who had a painful swelling (due to trauma) of the right mandibular body. The tumor showed a well-defined multilocular radiolucen-cy from the right second molar to the right ramus with remarkable bony expansion toward buccal and lingual sides. It was treated with extirpation and curettage; there was no sign of recurrence after 13 years. Ide et al. (634) published a case, which was diagnosed in an edentulous posterior region of the right side of the mandible in a 79-year-old man. Radiograms showed a well-demarcated, multilocular mixed radiolucent–radiodense lesion; it was enucleated and no recurrence was recorded after five years. The lining showed typical COC features with dentinoid formation. Within the thick fibrous wall were many large follicles of amelo-blastoma without formation of ghost cells or dentinoid.

The majority of these lesions seem to develop in the mandible. The same treatment modalities, which are used in the treatment of UNAMs should be considered in these cases.

2.6.2.3 Adenomatoid Odontogenic Tumor-Associated CCOT. No case of CCOT associated with a fully developed AOT has been published, but five cases have been described in which limited areas of the cystic wall or the epithelial proliferations show the architecture of an AOT. Freedman et al. (584) published a case (case 1 of 6) of COC in the molar region of the mandible of a 15-year-old girl. An area of the epithelium in the wall resembled an AOT (Fig. 8 in the report). A similar architecture with loop forming two-cell-layered strands is found in O-As. In a large COC from the right to the left premolar area in the mandible of a 35-old-man Zeitoun et al. (635) found a minor area with pseudo-tubular structure characteristic of an AOT. Lukinmaa et al. (636) described a case with AOT-like areas in the lining of an otherwise simple cystic COC in the angle and ramus of the left side of the mandible in a 12-year-old boy. Furthermore there were minor areas in the wall, which were structured as an AMF. Buch et al. (637) found more extensive areas with AOT histomorphology in a CCOT in the premolar area of the mandible of an 11-year-old girl. In an AMF-associated CCOT, which occurred in the premolar–molar area of a six-year-old girl Lin et al. (638) observed sheet-like areas containing whorled masses of spindle-shaped cells and occasional duct-like structures, reminiscent of AOT.

The presence of AOT-like areas in a CCOT has no impact on the treatment.

2.6.2.4 Ameloblastic Fibroma-Associated CCOT. Four cases have been published of this rare lesion apart from the case (*vide supra*) published by Lukinmaa et al (636). Lin et al. (638) reported three cases. The first case was a six-year-old girl with a 3.8 × 2.0 cm cystic lesion in the right mandibular body. Some areas of the cystic wall were thickened and contained three nodules measuring up to 1.3 × 0.6 cm, which showed the histomorphology of an AMF. The lesion was enucleated and there was no sign of recurrence after

20 months. The second case was a 13-year-old boy with a large cystic lesion in the posterior area of the left side of the maxilla. One area of the wall was thickened and showed a rather large area in close contact with the lining epithelium with the histomorphology of an AMF. The lesion was excises through a Le Fort I osteotomy approach. The patient failed to return for follow-up. The third case was a cystic lesion around the crown of an impacted right third molar in a 22-year-old man. Slight nodular elevations were seen in the wall. The lining showed typical COC features in some areas and AOT-like structure in others, as mentioned above. In some of the nodular areas AMF-like structure was seen adjacent to the epithelial lining. The lesion was curetted; the patient did not show for follow-up. In all three cases the areas with AMF morphology were relatively large and without any sign of hard dental tissue formation, it is thus unlikely that they should represent initial odontoma formation. Yoon et al. (639) reported a case of cystic tumor, 3 cm in diameter in the right posterior maxilla of a 22-year-old woman. The cystic portion showed features characteristic of a COC with ghost cells and dentinoid. A solid portion of the tumor had characteristic features of AMF. Ghost cell masses were found in these areas as well. The lesion was excised, and no recurrence was observed at one-year follow-up.

It is not possible on the basis of these few cases with short time or no follow-up to draw any conclusions regarding treatment and prognosis. Enucleation may be adequate, but long-time follow-up is recommended bearing in mind the tendency for recurrence and even malignant transformation of some AMFs.

2.6.2.5 Ameloblastic Fibro-Odontoma-Associated CCOT. Only two cases are known of this rare lesion. A case was included in a review by Prætorius et al. (580) and discussed by Shear et al. (228); it was a tumor, which presented as a multilocular lesion, which occupied almost the entire left side of the mandible of a 17-year-old man (Fig. 60). The tumor contained a single large cyst with a COC lining, and the remaining part was structured as an AMF apart from clusters of ghost cells and deposits of dentinoid (Fig. 61). In a few minor areas enamel was present adjacent to ghost cells (Fig. 62). Hemimandibulectomy was performed; no information on follow-up was available. A second case was reported by Matsuzaka et al. (495). The patient was a 23-year-old-man with a partly radiolucent, partly radiopaque lesion, which occupied the entire left mandibular ramus and the region around the third molar. It consisted of a cyst the size of a hen's egg and covered with a typical COC lining; a thick wall was found on the outside, with the histomorphology of an AFOD. A segmental resection was done, there was no information on follow-up. The case was studied immunohisto-chemically with antibodies against CK-19, osteopontin, and osteocalcin. CK-19 was strongly immunoreactive in the epithelium of the lesion; osteopontin and osteocalcin reacted in the mesenchymal cells and weakly in the epithelial elements of the tumor.

Farman et al. (640) reported a case of "calcifying odontogenic cyst with ameloblastic fibro-odontome."

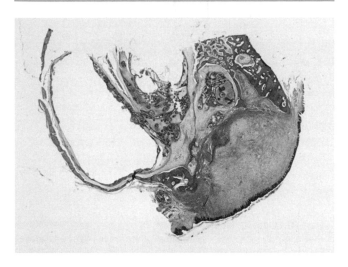

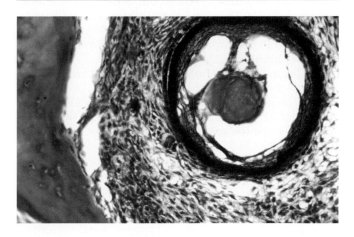

Figure 60 Ameloblastic fibro-odontoma-associated CCOT. A cross section of part of the left mandible of an 18-year-old man with a tumor, which measured 5 cm at greatest extent. To the left a large cyst is seen which shows the characteristics of a calcifying odontogenic cyst. The majority of the remaining part of the lesion consisted of an ameloblastic fibro-odontoma with limited formation of dentin and enamel. See also Figure 8.8 in Shear et al. (2007) (228). H&E stain. *Abbreviation*: CCOT, calcifying cystic odontogenic tumor.

Figure 62 Ameloblastic fibro-odontoma-associated CCOT. Higher magnification of one of the few areas of the tumor in Figure 60 where enamel matrix was found. Note the formation of enamel around a cluster of ghost cells. Dentinoid is seen to the left, but no dentinoid is seen in contact with the enamel in this section. H&E stain. *Abbreviation*: CCOT, calcifying cystic odontogenic tumor.

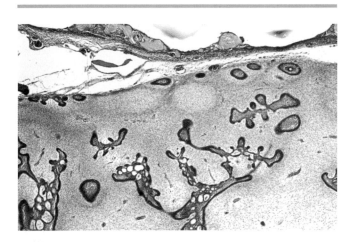

Figure 61 Ameloblastic fibro-odontoma-associated CCOT. The interface area between the cyst and the tumor seen in Figure 60 is shown. The lining of the cyst in seen in the upper part. The ameloblastic fibroma-like tissue dominates the lower part. The clefts in between the two components are artifacts. H&E stain. *Abbreviation*: CCOT, calcifying cystic odontogenic tumor.

The areas with AFOD-like features were very limited; the lesion is probably better classified as a CCOT with initial odontoma formation.

2.6.2.6 Odonto-Ameloblastoma-Associated CCOT. This entity was reported briefly by Ledesma-Montes (641). It was diagnosed in the anterior maxilla of a 21-year-old man. It measured 4 cm at longest diameter and was clinically diagnosed as a dentigerous cyst.

2.6.2.7 Odontogenic Fibromyxoma-Associated CCOT. A single case has been reported of this combination. Li et al. (579) described a tumor in the molar and ramus region of the right side of the mandible of a 15-year-old girl. The radiogram showed a large well-defined unilocular radiolucency associated with an unerupted third molar. The lesion consisted of a cyst with typical COC lining; adjacent to the cyst a tumor was seen with the histomorphology of an odontogenic fibromyxoma. The tumor made up the majority of the lesion. It was removed by enucleation, and there was no recurrence after one year.

2.6.2.8 Odontoma-Associated CCOT. This combination is much more common than any of the other CCOT variants.

As mentioned above, most surveys of COC have included more than one variant without clear distinction between them. From 17% to 75% of the published cases of COC have been associated with an odontoma in the reviews published with 10 cases or more, but in most reviews about 30% of the cases were odontoma associated (579,580,582,594,601,606,607,615,642).

Clinical Features. Hirshberg et al. (643) published a review of 52 OaCCOTs retrieved from the English language literature. It is the only review with focus on OaCCOTs exclusively. The authors suggested the name of the lesion changed to odontocalcifying odontogenic cyst.

The results of the review are basis for the following survey.

The age range was between 5 and 39 years, with a mean age of 16 years. The mean age at diagnosis is lower than that of the simple cystic COC (34.3 years), and very few cases have been diagnosed in persons older than 30 years (594). About 60% were in their second decade. The gender ratio was 1:1.9; 18 were males and 34 females. A female predominance has not been found in the simple cystic COC where the gender ratio was about 1:1(228,594).

The most common location was the maxilla (32 cases; 61.5%), of which 24 (75%) were in anterior region (incisor-canine region), and 5 (15.6%) were in the posterior region. In three cases (9.4%), the lesion occupied both the anterior and the posterior regions. Twenty cases (38.5%) were located in the mandible, of which 11 (55%) were in the anterior region and 4 (20%) were in the posterior region. In five cases (25%), both regions were involved. The distribution of the simple cystic COCs is different, among 131 intraosseous cystic COC reviewed by Buchner et al. (594), the ratio between the maxilla and the mandible was more even, 62 cysts (47%) were located in the maxilla and 69 (53%) in the mandible. In the maxilla, 44 cases were found in the anterior and 18 in the posterior region. In the mandible, 38 cysts were found in the anterior and 31 in the posterior region.

A case of extraosseous OaCCOT has been published by Ledesma-Montes et al. (539).

The most common symptoms of the OaCCOTs were swelling (52%) and unerupted teeth (13.5%). Pain was noticed in 9.6% of the cases, and tenderness of the region caused by secondary infection was observed in 9.6% of the cases. In 19% of the patients the lesion was accidentally discovered during routine radiographic examination. The growth rate of the OaCCOTs is slow.

Imaging. In 29 of 36 cases (80.6%) the lesion was well-defined on the radiograms with a mixed radiolucent–radiopaque appearance (643). The radiopacities varied from minor flecks to well-defined tooth-like structures, which in a few cases dominated the lesion. In several cases the radiopaque particles are located at the periphery of the lesion. In four cases the development of the odontoma was initial and not visible on the radiogram. Impaction of teeth was observed in 20 cases (38.5%), most frequently the canine (11 cases) followed by the incisors (5 cases). Impaction of more than one tooth was observed in five cases.

Divergence of teeth is common (599) and resorption of the root of adjacent teeth has been reported in a number of cases (572,599,601,642,644–648). Exact figures are not available, because most reviews have not separated the various variants. Martin-Duverneuil et al. (648) showed the increase of information about the lesions, which is obtained if CT and MRI are applied.

Pathology. The etiology is unknown. Pathogenetically the dental hard tissue seems to develop from an odontogenic activity in the lining of a single large cyst with typical COC structure, as described above (Fig. 63). Various stages of odontogenesis may be seen from areas with embryonic pulp-like ectomesenchyme and dental lamina and enamel organ–shaped odontogenic epithelium to fully developed and mineralized tooth-like structures (odontoides) (579,580,606,636,649). When the formation of odontoides is more extensive, they protrude into the

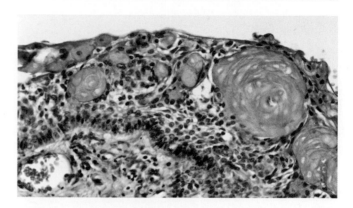

Figure 63 Odontoma-associated CCOT. High-power view of part of the lining of the cystic lesion. Palisaded columnar basal cells, stellate reticulum-like cells and scattered clusters of ghost cells are seen. The histology is similar to that of the lining of a calcifying odontogenic cyst. H&E stain. *Abbreviation*: CCOT, calcifying cystic odontogenic tumor.

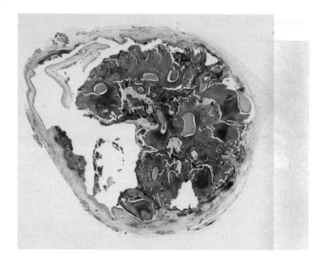

Figure 64 Odontoma associated CCOT. The cystic lumen to the left is partly collapsed. It is lined by an epithelium similar to that of a calcifying odontogenic cyst. The major part of the lumen is filled with an odontoma attached to the wall of the cyst and consisting primarily of fused odontoids. Immature odontoids are found in the wall of the cyst. H&E stain. *Abbreviation*: CCOT, calcifying cystic odontogenic tumor.

lumen of the cyst (Fig. 64), and in some cases fill out the cystic lumen completely. The structure of the dental hard tissue may be quite irregular, but in many cases it takes the shape of an ODTx (579,599,650) or apparently more often (Fig. 65) an ODTp (579,580,615,644,651,652,653). In some cases both morphologies are seen in the same tumor (599). The dental hard tissue formation is seen in close contact with the lining epithelium or deeper in the connective tissue. Variable amounts of dentinoid and

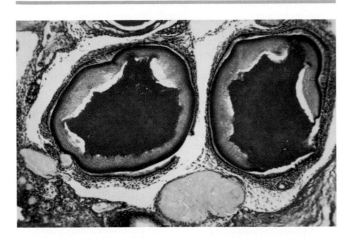

Figure 65 Odontoma-associated CCOT. Higher magnification of immature odontoids in the lesion seen in Figure 64. Formation of immature enamel is seen around two cores of tubular dentin. A cluster of ghost cells is seen in the adjacent enamel epithelium. van Gieson stain. *Abbreviation*: CCOT, calcifying cystic odontogenic tumor.

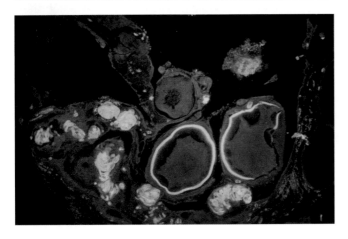

Figure 66 Odontoma-associated CCOT. In a rhodamine B stained section viewed in fluorescent light the ghost cells stand out particularly well, and the youngest enamel in the two immature odontoids is seen as two bright yellow rings. *Abbreviation*: CCOT, calcifying cystic odontogenic tumor.

cluster of ghost cells with or without calcification may be seen (Fig. 66).

Immunohistochemistry. Most of the immunohistochemically studies on odontogenic ghost cell lesions have been performed on material, which have been a mixture of the variants, mostly COCs, OaCCOTs, and DGCTs. Possible differences in the findings in the variants have rarely been reported, so the results reviewed above for the COC are also valid for the OaCCOT, apart from obvious differences between lesions with and without embryonic pulp-like ectomesenchyme. In the study by Lukinmaa et al. (636) the expression of the glycoprotein tenascin-C was concen-

trated to the dental papilla–like regions and the pulp tissue of the odontoides. In a few cases differences have been stressed; Yoshida et al. (606) reported that Bcl-2 expression and the mean Ki-67 L.I. in OaCCOTs were slightly higher than in simple cystic COC. However, these differences did not reach statistical significance.

Electron Microscopy. Fejerskov et al. (577) studied the ultrastructure of an OaCCOT in the maxilla of a 16-year-old female, and found that most ghost cells contained very thick electron-dense fiber bundles of relatively uniform size, which were sharply defined against large empty spaces in the cytoplasm unlike the even distribution of fine tonofilaments present in keratinizing cells of oral surface epithelia. Organelles could not be found in ghost cells.

In a study of the ultrastructure of two cases of OaCCOT, Eda et al. (654) observed that ghost cells contained abundant bundles of tonofilaments and that calcification seemed to start from the peripheries of the bundles. The calcified matrices had no clear structures. Sapp et al. (549) focused on the ultrastructure of the calcifications in OaCCOT. They observed three different types: (*i*) spherical calcifications, which form on ghost cells and which they interpreted as dystrophic; (*ii*) spherical calcifications, which appeared to be dysplastic enamel; and (*iii*) irregularly shaped, diffuse calcifications, which form on a collagenous matrix and appeared to be dysplastic dentin or cementum.

Satomura et al. (646) identified four types of cells in the epithelial layer of an OaCCOT. The basal cells were low columnar in shape and contained some intracellular organelles. Desmosomes attached to neighboring cells were seen on the cellular membranes, the basal cell layer resembled the inner enamel epithelium of the normal enamel organ. In the stellate reticulum-like layer the cells were polygonal and possessed desmosomes and many cytoplasmic projections. Some intracellular organelles and a few bundles of tonofilaments were observed in the cytoplasm. Cells in the vicinity of focal accumulations of ghost cells showed cell membranes that were discontinuous in parts and contained dilated membranous organelles and evenly distributed tonofilaments. In spite of discontinuous cell membranes the ghost cells, the fourth cell type, were attached to each other by means of desmosomes. The ghost cells contained many bundles of tonofilaments that were 60 to 240 nm in diameter and arranged in various directions. The cytoplasm did not contain intact intracellular organelles. A variety of vesicles, 90 to 450 nm in diameter, were scattered among the tonofilaments bundles. Some of the vesicles contained needle-like crystals, which were interpreted as initial calcification sites. These vesicles resembled matrix vesicles, and the authors suggested that matrix vesicle-like structures might be involved in the initiation of calcification of the ghost cells.

Molecular-Genetic Data. No data are available.

Differential Diagnosis. Previously the CEOT was sometimes confounded with the COC, CCOT, or DGCT (570). With the accessibility of more precise definitions and descriptions (328,596,598) these differentiation difficulties are hopefully reduced. Cases of OaCCOT should be easy to diagnose if sufficient clinical and radiological information is available together with adequate sampling of the lesion.

The rare cases of CCOTs associated with other types of odontogenic tumors may cause problems. In presence of conspicuous proliferation of odontogenic epithelium and absence of dental hard tissues it is necessary to decide if the morphology of the lesion falls within the spectrum of appearances of COC or the lesion should be interpreted as UNAM-associated CCOT or s/mAM-associated CCOT. It has an impact on the choice of treatment and time of follow-up. Most important is to distinguish between the benign variants of ghost lesions and the GCOC (597). The carcinoma may develop from a benign variant, and in such a case malignant and benign areas may be present in the same tumor.

Treatment and Prognosis. Simple enucleation is an adequate treatment of an OaCCOT, and prognosis is good. Yoshida et al. (606) reported several cases with long-term follow-up. In six cases there was no recurrence following enucleation after 9, 9, 13, 14, 15 and 21 years, respectively. Recurrences are rare, but have been reported (606,655). The case of OaCCOT reported by Wright et al. (655) recurred after five years, there was no dental hard tissue formation in the recurrence. Long-term follow-up is recommended.

2.6.3 Dentinogenic Ghost Cell Tumor

Introduction. The DGCT is a slowly growing benign, but nonencapsulated and locally invasive, epithelial odontogenic tumor characterized by ameloblastoma-like islands in a fibrous connective tissue stroma. Clusters of ghost cells are seen in the epithelial islands and sometimes in the connective tissue. Various amounts of dentinoid (dysplastic dentin) are seen adjacent to the epithelium. Tumors without presence of dentinoid and with a limited amount of ghost cells are better classified as s/m ameloblastom with ghost cells (596).

ICD-O code 9302/0

Synonyms: Odontogenic ghost cell tumor, calcifying ghost cell odontogenic tumor, epithelial odontogenic ghost cell tumor, dentinoameloblastoma, dentinogenic ghost cell ameloblastoma.

Formerly DGCT was often called solid variant of the COC (579,580,582,594,656,657).

Clinical Features. Like most odontogenic tumors the DGCT occurs as an intraosseous and a less aggressive extraosseous variant. Judged from the published cases the extraosseous variant is far more common than the intraosseous. About 32 acceptable extraosseous cases have been published (570,577,580, 582,585,588,591,593,607,636,658–668) and 14 intraosseous cases (579,580,582,669–676).

Among the 32 extraosseous cases the age range was 10 to 92 years, the mean age 57.6 years, and the median age 61 year. Apart from three patients who were 10 years old, all other patients were 33 years or older. It is tempting to speculate if the tumor in the three patients contained not only dentinoid, but also tubular dentin and were in fact initial OaCCOTs, rather than DGCTs. The gender ratio was almost equal, 18 males and 14 females. The age range in males was 10 to 82 years, mean age 53.0 years, and median age 57 years. In females, the age range was 10 to 92 years, the mean age 63.4 years, and median age 70 years.

The location was reported in 31 cases. The peripheral DGCT is more common in the mandible. Eight tumors were located in the maxilla, seven in the anterior region, one unspecified. Twenty-three tumors were located in the mandible; five in the anterior region, nine in the posterior, one in the anterior and posterior region, and eight unspecified.

It was reported in 18 cases that the tumor developed in an edentulous jaw or area, and several authors have suggested that traumatic influence from ill-fitting dentures could be an etiological cofactor (656). The lesions present as sessile, sometimes pedunculated nodules or irregular hyperplasias of the gingival or alveolar mucosa. They are usually slowly growing, have been observed for months or years, but in some cases recent rapid growth has been reported (658). Teeth in the affected area may be displaced. The tumors are otherwise symptomless, except when they become traumatized. The size was reported in 20 cases, it varied from 0.4 to 4 cm, but 14 of them measured 1 cm or less at longest diameter.

For the 14 intraosseous DGCTs the age range was 12 to 79 years, mean age 47.7 years, and median age 59 years. The gender ratio M:F was 1:0.3 (11 males and 3 females), there might be a male predilection, but the numbers are small. The age range for males was 12 to 79 years, mean age 50.9 years, and median age 59 years. The three females were 21, 24, and 63 years, respectively. The tumor was more common in the mandible; one was unspecified, but three were diagnosed in the maxilla, all in the posterior regions, and 10 in the mandible, two in the anterior, and seven in the posterior regions; the region was unspecified in one case. The most common symptom is bony expansion presenting as a slowly growing firm swelling, which may be soft in areas where the tumor has eroded the cortex and invaded the adjacent soft tissue (672,673,676). Tumors in the maxilla may obliterate the maxillary sinus. Pain is a rare symptom (669,670,672).

Imaging. The extraosseous DGCT may cause erosion of the underlying bone varying from a hardly visible change to a conspicuous bowl-shaped defect usually with well-defined smooth border. Several cases have been reported to be without bone involvement.

The intraosseous DGCT show a varying picture. Some have been radiolucent, unilocular, and well-defined (580). One was radiolucent with ill-defined borders; it had a rapid growth (671). Others have been described as radiolucent, multilocular, and ill defined (579,676). In three cases cortical erosion with tumor invasion of adjacent soft tissue was seen (673,675,676), a feature that is uncommon in solid/cystic ameloblastomas. Various amounts of scattered radiopaque material have been seen in the radiolucent areas in several cases. Teeth adjacent to the lesions may show root resorption (670), as it is seen in the COC and CCOT. In some cases impaction of teeth is seen. Tumors in the maxilla may encroach the maxillary sinus (582,673). CT scanning has been used in several cases and ameliorates the information on the borders of the tumor, particularly in cases with erosion of the cortical plates.

The size of the tumor has varied from 2 cm at longest diameter to a size where it has destroyed about 50% of or the entire mandible (579). The majority have been within the range of 6 to 7 cm at longest diameter.

Pathology. The etiology of the DGCT is unknown. The extraosseous variant has been found in edentulous areas so often that is has raised the question whether a local trauma from ill-fitting dentures could be a cofactor. Pathogenetically the extraosseous lesions are supposed to arise in remnants of dental lamina in the gingiva.

The central tumors are likely to arise in reduced enamel epithelium or proliferation of remnants of odontogenic epithelium in the jaw.

Macroscopically the lesion has been described as a grayish mass with firm consistency (665) often with scattered foci of calcification. Some contain small multiple cystic cavities (673).

The overall microscopic impression of the DGCT is a tumor, which resembles the solid, intraosseous ameloblastoma in several aspects. The main difference is the presence of many clusters of ghost cells and of dentinoid in DGCTs (Fig. 67). The tumor is nonencapsulated. It presents as nests and sheets of odontogenic epithelium in a fibrous connective tissue stroma (596). The peripheral cells are cuboidal to columnar, with a central or reversely polarized nucleus, which is round or elongated. Mitoses are unusual and generally not present. The majority of the cells in the sheets and islands are stellate and morphologically similar to the cells in an ameloblastoma. The cytoplasm is pale eosinophilic. In some tumors foci of epidermoid differentiation with intercellular bridges may be encountered and in rare cases there may be keratinized foci in terms of horn pearls (670,674). Minor cysts may be seen in the epithelial islands, but no large unicystic structure unless the DGCT has developed from a COC. The most conspicuous cell type is the ghost cells. They are enlarged lightly eosinophilic epithelial cells, which may occur individually or more common in clusters. They seem to develop from the stellate cells. Some of them may contain central nuclear remnants, but most of them show a sharply defined empty space where the former nucleus was placed. Outlines of the individual ghost cells may be discerned. Where basal cells are transformed into ghost cells, the basement membrane disappears, and ghost cells extrude into the fibrous connective tissue and evoke a foreign body reaction. The ghost cells show a tendency for calcification, which appears as basophilic granules. The extent of calcification varies from tumor to tumor and may be related to the age of the lesion. Dentinoid is seen in the connective tissue stroma in intimate association with the epithelial islands (596,656) and is a hallmark, which separates the tumor from a conventional ameloblastoma (Fig. 68). It lacks the tubular structure of normal dentin; it resembles the dentin, which can be seen in teeth, which have been traumatized during development. It occurs as small or large irregularly shaped eosinophilic masses, which react as collagen with trichrome staining. It usually contains a few cells and some of them may be entrapped ghost cells. There may be some mineralization of the dentinoid. The stroma is composed of fibrous connective tissue; no embryonic pulp-like tissue is seen in relation to the dentinoid, as it may be the case in OaCCOTs.

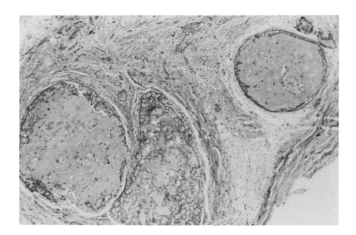

Figure 67 Dentinogenic ghost cell tumor (DGCT). Segment of peripheral DGCT in the palatal gingiva of a 52 year-old man. Nearly all tumor cells are transformed into ghost cells. H&E stain.

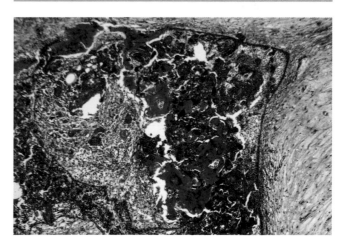

Figure 68 Dentinogenic ghost cell tumor. From an intraosseous tumor in the posterior part of the mandible of a 63-year-old woman. For details see case No. 11 of Ref. 475. Numerous ghost cells (*red*) are seen in the irregular islands of tumor epithelium. Dentinoid (*blue*) is formed in the stroma in close contact to the epithelium. Masson trichrome.

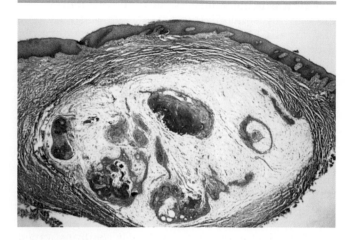

Figure 69 Dentinogenic ghost cell tumor. Peripheral tumor in the mandibular alveolus (premolar area) of an 82 year-old woman. Ghost cells (*yellowish*) and dentinoid (*red*) is clearly seen. Note the myxoid changes in the surrounding stroma. van Gieson–alcian blue stain. *Source*: Section by courtesy of Professor J. Hille, Cape Town.

In the peripheral DGCT (Fig. 69) the proliferation of the tumor epithelium may or may not be in continuity with the gingival or palatal surface stratified squamous epithelium, which seems stimulated to proliferate. Whether the tumor in some cases may arise from the basal cell layer of the surface epithelium is an unsolved question.

A single case has been published of an intra-osseous DGCT with a conspicuous component of clear cells. The tumor caused destruction of the anterior part of the mandible and extended into the floor of the mouth (675). The presence of a prominent number of clear cells in an odontogenic tumor is considered a sign of malignancy (677). It is unknown how many clear cells are needed to create an impact on the prognosis of the tumor. The tumor had been growing slowly; it was treated by marginal mandibulectomy followed by an iliac bone graft. There was no evidence of recurrence or metastasis for three years and two months after surgery, but a follow-up of 15 to 20 years is needed for conclusions.

Immunohistochemistry. Several investigators have studied CK in DGCTs, extraosseous as well as intraosseous (607,636,666,668,673,675,676,678). The results from use of broad-spectred CK-antibodies have been somewhat contradicting; Günhan et al. (678) used DAKO K-528 and detected a strong reaction from fragment of cells around ghost cells, and a questionable reaction in ghost cells. López-Tarruella et al. (673) used AE1/AE3 and tested CK-8 as well; all ghost cells were negative. All other investigators who used AE1/AE3 (607,666,668,675,676) found a strong, although not always homogeneous immunoreaction in tumor epithelium and a positive reaction from ghost cells in most cases.

Lukinmaa et al. (636) used high mw CK antibodies, 34βE12, and found a strong reaction in the tumor epithelium, while all ghost cells were negative;

using the same antibodies on two peripheral DGCTs, five COCs, and three OaCCOTs, Fregnani et al. (607) confirmed the findings in the tumor epithelium but found positive reaction in ghost cells in some cases (the variants were unspecified).

Kusama et al. (613) created antibodies against hard α-keratins and tested pilomatrixomas, craniopharyngiomas, and COCs and detected consistent and strong reactions from all types of ghost cells. The fact that antibodies to most other CKs have been raised against soft keratins may explain the previous inconsistent results.

Antibodies against low mw CKs have been used in three studies (607,636,675). Lukinmaa et al. (636) used PKK-1 (CK-8, CK-18, CK-19); the reaction was strong in the tumor epithelium except ghost cells, which were negative as expected. Fregnani et al. (607) used several types of monoclonal antibodies against CKs. Tumor cells reacted positively to CK-8, CK-14, and CK-19 in all cases. Yoon et al. (675) confirmed the latter findings—a positive reaction was found in ameloblastic as well as in the clear cells, which were present in that particular tumor.

EMA and carcinoembryonic antigen (CEA) was studied by Mascrès et al. (588), with negative results. Günhan et al. (678) studied the same antigens and detected immunoreaction for both antigens in laminated fragments around ghost cell.

Studies of S-100 protein have yielded contradicting results. Günhan et al. (678) found a strong reaction in ghost cells; Yoon et al. (675) did not find any reaction from S-100 in tumor epithelium, including ghost cells.

Lukinmaa et al. (636) detected a prominent staining for tenascin in the connective tissue in a peripheral DGCT; the walls of the blood vessels were positive, the staining in the tumor epithelium was weak.

PCNA L.I. and Ki-67 L.I. were studied by Fregnani et al. (607) in two cases of extraosseous DGCT. One case was totally negative; in the other case the L.I. was low, about four times lower than in intraosseous COC. The PCNA L.I. (mean and range, %) was 5 (<1–10) and the Ki-67 L.I. (mean and range, %) was 0.5 (<1–1). Piattelli et al. (666) using Mib-1 reported a strong positive reaction (30–40%) in the basal and parabasal cell layers of the tumor islands of an extraosseous DGCT, and some reaction in the stellate cells (5%). Ghost cells and dentinoid was negative. Iezzi et al. (668) confirmed these results without indicating any L.I.

The antiapoptotic protein Bcl-2 was studied in four investigations (607,666,668,676). Piattelli et al. (666) detected a strong immunoreactivity in the basal and suprabasal cells and cells adjacent to ghost cells of tumor epithelium. Ghost cells and dentinoid were negative. These findings were confirmed by Fregnani et al. (607) and Iezzi et al. (668). Kim et al. (676), however, did not find any reaction to Bcl-2 antibodies in an intraosseous DGCT.

In the same studies mentioned above Piattelli et al. (666) and Iezzi et al. (668) investigated p53 proteins. In the former study a few positive cells were found between the odontogenic epithelium and the dentinoid. Ghost cells and dentinoid were negative. Iezzi et al. could confirm the latter findings, but detected a few positive cells in the tumor islands and in the dentinoid.

Kim et al. (676) studied β-catenin in an intraosseous DGCT by means of immunohistochemistry, TUNEL assay, and gene mutation analysis. A missense mutation of β-catenin was found (*vide infra*) and the TUNEL assay, which discloses fragmented DNA ends of apoptotic cells, showed positive signals in nucleated cells adjacent to the ghost cells. Immunohistochemistry showed nuclear, cytoplasmic, and membranous accumulation of β-catenin in the tumor cells.

Electron Microscopy. Chen et al. (619) studied the ultrastructure of an extraosseous DGCT in details. The basal cells were cuboidal or low columnar; they were attached to neighboring cells by a few desmosomes and to lamina densa by hemidesmosomes. At the interface toward the stroma a lamina lucida and a lamina densa was seen. Individual or small bundles of tonofilaments were seen in the cytoplasm, scattered or attached to desmosomes or hemidesmosomes. A moderate number of organelles in shape of mitochondria, RER, and ribosomes were present. The nuclei were irregularly ovoid with irregular clumped chromatin along the inner nuclear membrane. Nucleoli were small. The cells of the stellate reticulum-like layer were polygonal and had more desmosomes and more villous-like cytoplasmic projections than the basal cells. They were surrounded by prominently expanded intercellular spaces. Bundles of tonofilaments were scattered in the cytoplasm; and a few keratohyaline granules could be found and an infrequent Golgi apparatus. Ribosomes were clustered as polysomes; mitochondria and endoplasmatic reticulum were moderately dilated. The nuclei were irregular circular with slightly condensed chromatin and a small nucleolus. The ghost cells were mostly anuclear and much enlarged compared with the stellate cells. Some contained pyknotic nuclei and residues of chromatin in the nuclear zone. Thick electron-dense fibrils of uniform size were found in the cytoplasm outside the large empty space previously occupied by the nucleus. Small needle-like crystals could be found in the ghost cells. In most of the cells the desmosomes and the villous-like projections had disappeared, and some of them had plasma membranes, which were thickened and irregularly disrupted. A fourth cell type was described, the "hornified cells," which in contrast to ghost cell contained evenly distributed tonofilaments oriented in different directions and occasional residues of markedly dilated organelles. The plasma membrane was thickened. These cells resembled those found in keratinized oral surface epithelium. They were seen scattered between ghost cells and stellate cells. Focal accumulations of ghost cells and hornified cells in the connective tissue were a frequent finding as well. Mineral crystals were deposited on bundles of tonofilaments of the ghost cells in the epithelium as well as in the connective tissue.

Molecular-Genetic Data. Kim et al. (676) investigated the β-catenin gene in a case of intraosseous DGCT with extensive destruction of the mandi-ble and extension into the floor of the mouth. The tumor contained a missense mutation on codon 3 ($\underline{A}CT \rightarrow \underline{T}CT$) of the β-catenin gene. Immunohistochemistry and a TUNEL assay were performed on the same tumor (*vide supra*). Mutations of the β-catenin gene were also found in COCs by Sekine et al. (156) but were rare in solid/cystic ameloblastomas.

Differential Diagnosis. The histomorphological pattern of the peripheral DGCT may resemble that of the PERAM, but the presence of clusters of ghost cells and dentinoid differentiates the DGCT from the ameloblastoma. The most difficult differential diagnosis may be the rare cases of multicystic COCs with some proliferation of odontogenic epithelium in the connective tissue. Sufficient information about clinical and radiographic features is crucial, particularly in case of intraosseous lesions. A COC is characterized by a rounded unicystic well-defined radiolucency. Microscopically the diagnosis of a DGCT requires a conspicuous amount of noncystic epithelial islands. The most important differential diagnosis is toward the GCOC. The clinical course of the GCOC is more aggressive. Microscopically the GCOC shows increased cellular density of small cells with sparse cytoplasm, darkly stained nuclei, and many mitoses as well as areas with necrosis. Mitoses are extremely rare in the DGCT. A GCOC may arise in a COC or DGCT, in such cases adequate sampling is extremely important since the lesion may contain benign-looking as well as malignant areas. The presence of islands of clear cells have been described (675). This cell type is considered a sign of malignancy when encountered in ameloblastomas (677), and may have a similar impact in a DGCT.

Treatment and Prognosis. Excision is an adequate treatment of peripheral DGCTs, recurrence has not been reported. Intraosseous DGCTs require wide marginal resection. Tumors that have been treated by enucleation have recurred, although it may take some years before the recurrence is evident. Li et al. (579) reported two cases, which were enucleated twice before they were resected. Both recurred twice. One case has been reported to recur five years after segmental resection. No other case has recurred after wide marginal resection, but the follow-up time has been limited in most cases. The longest have been 10 years (671), 4 years (674), and 3 years (675). A post-surgical follow-up time of 15 to 20 years is recommended.

Malignant transformation is a possibility, but seems to be extremely rare, although the number of published cases of GCOCs exceeds the number of DGCTs.

3. Tumors of Odontogenic Ectomesenchyme With or Without Included Odontogenic Epithelium

This group of tumors covers the following recognized entities: odontogenic fibroma, GCOT (or fibroma), ODOMYX/myxofibroma, and CEMBLA. None of them occur outside the jaws; they are believed to arise from odontogenic ectomesenchyme.

3.1 Odontogenic Fibroma

Introduction. The odontogenic fibroma is a rare, benign, expansively slowly growing, noninfiltrating odontogenic tumor composed of proliferating fibrous tissue containing various amounts of more or less inactive-appearing odontogenic epithelium.

It is the most ill defined and least understood of the neoplasms of odontogenic origin. In the 1992 edition of the WHO classification of odontogenic tumors (23) it was stated: "further subdivision of this group may become necessary, but at present criteria have not been agreed and differences in behavior have not been established." Unequivocal criteria for the diagnosis of the lesion have still not been established, so the following description comprises tumors, which vary from radiologically rather ill-defined lesions to well-defined with a radiolucent border, from encapsulated to nonencapsulated lesions, from hypercellular fibrous tumors to some with moderate cellularity, from lesions with no odontogenic epithelium via some with moderate amounts of epithelium to tumors dominated by proliferating odontogenic epithelium.

In the WHO classification of 2005 (12), the tumor has been divided into two subtypes: epithelium poor type and epithelium rich type.

ICD-O code 9321/0

Synonyms: odontogenic fibroma simple type (without epithelium), odontogenic fibroma complex type, also called WHO-type (with epithelium). These terms are obsolete.

Like most odontogenic tumors the odontogenic tumor occurs as an intraosseous/central variant and an extraosseous/peripheral variant.

3.1.1 Central Odontogenic Fibroma.

Clinical Features. The prevalence and incidence of the tumor is unknown. The relative frequency of the tumor in material received for histological diagnosis in services of diagnostic pathology in various countries for various amounts of years ranges from 1.4% to 4.9% in studies comprising more than 300 samples of odontogenic tumors. The reviews cited in the following are the few in which a subdivision between central and peripheral odontogenic fibromas has been made. The results are indicated as follows: number of odontogenic tumors/number of COFs/%. Daley et al., Canada (33): 392/19/4.9%, Mosqueda-Taylor et al., Mexico (34): 349/5/1.4%, Buchner et al., California (30): 1088/16/1.5%.

Approximately 60 cases of the COF have been published. The most recent reviews of the rare tumor have been published by Handlers et al. (679) and Kaffe et al. (680). Handlers et al. reviewed 39 cases, 19 from own files and 20 from the literature, Kaffe et al. reviewed 51 cases, 5 from own files and 46 from the literature, and focused on the radiology of the lesion. The COF may be seen at any age, but is discovered most frequently in the second to fourth decades. The age range among the 51 patients (680) was 4 to 80 years, with 55% of the patients between 11 and 39 years. The mean age was 34.4 years (33.5 years for males, and 33.8 years for females);

the median age was 30 years (28 years for males, 33 years for females).

The tumor is primarily seen in females. Thirty-five (68.6%) of the tumors were diagnosed in females and 16 (31.4%) in males. The gender ratio M:F is thus 1:2.2.

The distribution between the jaws is almost equal. In the review by Kaffe et al., 23 (45%) were found in the maxilla and 28 (55%) in the mandible. In the maxilla the COF occurred mostly in the anterior area (65%), in the mandible it is most common in the premolar (32%) and the molar (54%) regions.

COF is a slowly growing tumor. Heimdal et al. 1980 (681) reported a case of recurrent COF in the mandible, where the recurrence was overlooked on a radiogram four years after removal, when it measured 7 × 7 mm; it was diagnosed five years later when it measured 25 × 25 mm; it thus took nine years to reach that size. Dahl et al. reported a case of a large COF in the posterior mandible of an 80-year-old man. The tumor was not removed because of the age of the patient. The tumor exhibited limited growth and few symptoms till the patient died four years later for other reasons.

Handlers et al. (679) reported the symptoms from a review of 39 cases. In 36 cases the tumor was asymptomatic, three patients experienced slight sensitivity, and in five cases—but none of them in the anterior regions—the tumor was associated with an unerupted tooth. Kaffe et al. (680) observed bone enlargement in 28 (55%) of 51 cases.

Three cases of a rare syndrome with multiple COF-like lesions combined with enamel dysplasia have been published (682).

Imaging. The COF exhibits a great variation in radiological appearance. Some are small and unilocular (Fig. 70), others are large and multilocular; the latter

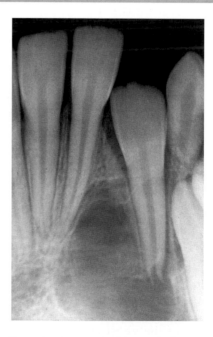

Figure 70 Central odontogenic fibroma between the first and second left mandibular incisor in a 9-year-old boy. The tumor was well delineated.

may resemble ameloblastomas or myxomas (683). Kaffe et al. (680) reviewed the radiographic features of 51 cases. The majority of COFs were unilocular with well defined, sometimes sclerotic borders, some were multilocular, some had poorly defined and some had diffuse borders. A few exhibited some radiopacity. The size varied from less than 1 cm to more than 5 cm at longest diameter. The unilocular tumors were below 4 cm, most were below 3 cm. A few of the multilocular were small (1–2 cm), but most were more than 3 cm. The tumor was radiolucent in 45 of 51 cases; 6 (3 in the maxilla, 3 in the mandible) showed a mixed radiolucent–radiopaque appearance. Border definition was mentioned in 45 cases, 33 were well defined, 5 were poorly defined, and 7 were diffuse. Among the 51 cases, the COF was associated with the crown of an unerupted tooth in 14 cases (27%), usually the incisors in the maxilla, and the third molars in the mandible. In six cases (12%) the tumor was found associated with roots of teeth, and in five cases (10%) it presented as a periapical lesion. Further more 15 (29%) were not tooth associated and 3 (6%) were located in edentulous areas. Tooth displacement was found in 25 of 45 cases and root resorption of adjacent teeth in 13 of 45 cases.

Pathology. The etiology of the COF is unknown. It is believed to arise from odontogenic ectomesenchyme, from the periodontal membrane in the cases that develop around the roots of teeth, and possibly from the dental sac in cases where the tumor is associated with the crown of an unerupted tooth. Wright et al. (684) demonstrated oxytalan fibers in the calcified material of periapical odontogenic fibromas, which supports the assumption that these lesions are of periodontal ligament origin.

Macroscopically, the COF is tan (685) or white, homogeneous, and glistening (686) in color and has a rubbery texture and a slightly hemorrhagic appearance. The cut surface may have a gritty consistency.

The WHO 2005 classification of odontogenic tumors (12) recognized two histological variants of COF, an epithelium-poor type and an epithelium-rich type. Variants of COFs exist, however, which exhibit a very well-demarcated, smooth surface covered with a thin fibrous capsule and contain no odontogenic epithelium at all (Figs. 71, 72). They exhibit a connective tissue with moderate cellularity; the fibroblast are seen in clusters surrounded by bundles of collagen with a slightly whorled and interlacing pattern. Such a tumor should not be classified as myxofibroma, which is an invasively growing tumor and requires more radical surgery. The histopathology of the epithelium-poor type (687) resembles that of a dental follicle. Moderate cellularity is seen, fibroblasts with primarily ovoid nuclei exhibiting finely dispersed chromatin, and distinct small nuclei are uniformly distributed between delicate collagen fibers and a considerable amount of ground substance. The nuclei may be plump and stellate. There is no mitotic activity. Scattered inactively-looking islands of odontogenic epithelium with various shapes are seen (Fig. 73). They do not exhibit peripheral cylindrical and palisading cells nor do they contain stellate reticulum-like cells. Various forms of calcifications may be seen.

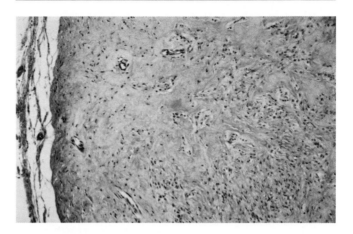

Figure 71 Central odontogenic fibroma, epithelium poor type. Section of the tumor seen in Figure 70. The tumor was completely encapsulated; part of the capsule is seen to the left. It was dominated by fibrous connective tissue, the cellularity varied from area to area. H&E stain.

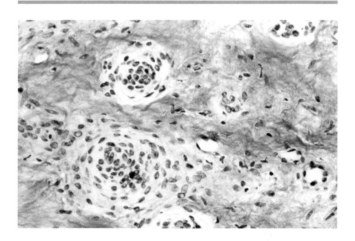

Figure 72 Central odontogenic fibroma, epithelium poor type. Higher magnification of the tumor seen in Figure 71. The fibroblasts were mainly assembled in clusters with high cellularity. No epithelium was found in this tumor. van Gieson stain.

The epithelium-rich type (687) is characterized by a cellular fibroblastic connective tissue interwoven with less cellular and often vascular areas. Some have a "pushing border," but many show an irregular border. The fibroblasts are elongated, spindle-shaped with dense nuclei. The cytoplasmic membranes are indistinct. There is no mitotic activity. The collagen is organized in parallel bundles of fibers, which show an interlacing pattern, and sometimes form a "herringbone pattern" (22). Islands and strands of inactive-looking odontogenic epithelium are an integral component. They contain cuboidal cells with uniformly stained predominantly round, but sometimes polygonal nuclei. In some tumors the epithelium exhibits long narrow strands of cells with a lightly stained

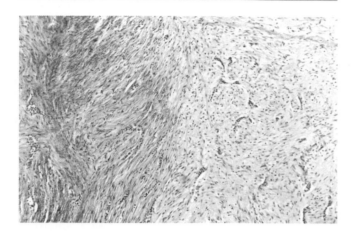

Figure 73 Central odontogenic fibroma, epithelium rich type. Section from a large tumor in the posterior maxilla of a 27-year-old man. The majority of the epithelial islands are small, narrow and elongated and consist of small polyhedral or cubic cells. Myxoid changes (*right*) were seen in many areas, the tumor could be termed myxofibroma. van Gieson–alcian blue stain.

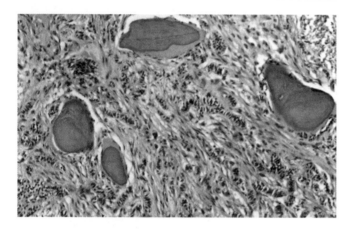

Figure 74 Central odontogenic fibroma, epithelium rich type with hard tissue formation. Section of another tumor. The morphology of the epithelial islands is different from the one seen in Figure 73. The hard tissue is mostly acellular and is probably cementum. H&E stain.

cytoplasm (679). Periepithelial hyalinization is usually not seen. Foci of calcified material is often seen with varying histomorphology resembling dysplastic cementum (Fig. 74), osteoid or dentinoid, the latter in particular is seen in close contact with the odontogenic epithelium. The epithelial component may be so abundant that it is tempting to consider the lesion an epithelial tumor. The demonstration of abundant proliferating epithelium and the induction of dentinoid suggest that the epithelium has more than a casual role (688). Ide et al. (465) published two cases of this variant, which they called ameloblastomatoid, central odontogenic fibroma. One of them contained a markedly cellular fibromatous connective tissue with

numerous strands and islands of active-looking odontogenic epithelium (Fig. 75). The connective tissue had no similarity to the dental papilla. No mineralized matrix was seen. Large epithelial sheets exhibited palisading of the peripheral cells, with the nuclei showing reversed polarity and apical vacuolization. In the larger islands many glycogen containing clear cells were seen. A hyalinized cuffing was present adjacent to the epithelium. The epithelium thus showed some features common with an ameloblastoma, but at the same time showed a tumor-like highly cellular connective tissue. It is difficult to consider such a tumor a variant of a COF.

Allen et al. (689) reported three cases of epithelial-rich COF with features of a central giant cell granuloma. Fowler et al. (690) reported three additional cases, and Odell et al. (691) published eight cases of this variant, two of which recurred after curettage, one case with cortical perforation. The recurrent lesion showed the same hybrid pattern as the initial lesion. The behavior of this variant is thus more like a central giant cell granuloma than like that of a COF.

Immunohistochemistry. Few histochemical studies of the tumor have been performed. Gao et al. (168) used antibodies against morphogenetic proteins in two cases of COF. The cells of the tumor were almost negative, except for some weak positive reaction in some odontogenic epithelial cells. In the unusual ameloblastomatoid cases of COF published by Ide et al. (465), the epithelial cells were strongly positive for broad spectred CK (AE1/AE3) and focally positive for CK-19.

Electron Microscopy. The ultrastructure of the COF was studied by Wesley et al. (686) and Watt-Smith et al. (692). Wesley et al. found fibroblast-like cells surrounded by numerous wavy collagen bundles. The cells were elongated with large central nuclei with an irregular nuclear membrane and a narrow band of peripherally clumped heterochromatin and uniformly distributed euchromatin. Dense small intranuclear inclusions were seen in some cells. The cytoplasm exhibited a prominent Golgi complex and large number of microfilaments. No tonofilaments were seen. Small amounts of RER were seen, some with dilated cisternae containing amorphous material. Small numbers of free ribosomes, empty vacuoles, and occasional lysosomes were present as well. Watt-Smith et al. (692) found that the fibroblastic cells exhibited features of myofibroblasts, they showed characteristics of both smooth muscle cells and fibroblasts.

Molecular-Genetic Data. No data are available.

Differential Diagnosis. The differential diagnosis is difficult and depends primarily on exclusion of other lesions (54). The diagnosis should be based on the overall histomorphology combined with the radiographic appearance of the lesion.

If the tumor does not contain odontogenic epithelium the following differential diagnoses should be considered: hyperplastic dental follicles, ODOMYX/myxofibroma, desmoplastic fibroma, (cemento-) ossifying fibroma, neurofibroma, and low-grade histiocytical sarcoma. In absence of odontogenic epithelium

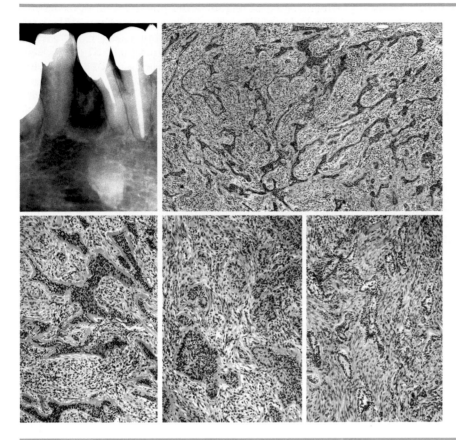

Figure 75 Ameloblastomatoid, central odontogenic fibroma. The tumor occurred in the premolar area of the mandible in a 74-year-old woman. The mesodermal component is hypercellular as expected in an odontogenic fibroma, but the epithelial component is so prominent and some of the islands so large and ameloblastoma-like that it cannot be regarded "inactive." The nature of this tumor is poorly understood, it evidently consists of an odontogenic epithelial as well as an ectomesenchymal component and seems unrelated to the ameloblastic fibroma. Note the hyaline cuffing. H&E stain. *Sources*: Image courtesy of Professor F. Ide, Saitama, Japan, and Ref. 465.

the diagnosis of COF should be made with caution (23). Lack of odontogenic epithelium does not preclude the diagnosis of odontogenic fibroma, but if the tumor does not have a rim of reactive bone at the border or exhibits a capsule, the diagnosis is likely not to be COF.

Hyperplastic dental follicles show a histomorphology, which may be indistinguishable from a COF. Evaluation of the size, location, and radiographic features should make it easy to exclude dental follicles.

The myxoma is characterized by a conspicuous myxoid component with scattered spindle, stellate, or rounded fibroblasts in contrast to the fibrous component of the COF. The myxofibroma is more fibrous and may be more cellular in areas, but show marked myxoid areas, which are not seen in the COF. Since both these tumors are growing invasively it is important to include the radiographic or other imaging features in the diagnosis.

The desmoplastic fibroma contains neither odontogenic epithelium nor hard tissue formation. It is characterized by mature fibroblasts exhibiting plump ovoid or long slender nuclei and prominent collagen-whorled bands, often broad bands. Like the COF it may resorb the roots of neighboring teeth. It is an invasively growing tumor. Few COFs are highly collagenous.

The (cemento-) ossifying fibroma shows a prominent hard tissue formation, which matures toward the center of the lesion.

The neurofibroma, the myxofibroma, and the low-grade histiocytic sarcoma should be differentiated on their histological features and immunohistochemical reactions.

If epithelium is present the following lesions must be excluded: hyperplastic dental follicles, myxoma/myxofibroma, AMF, AFD, and ameloblastoma.

The dental follicles may contain reduced enamel epithelium and hyperplastic odontogenic epithelium besides a histomorphology similar to that of COF. The size, location, and radiographic features of the lesion should make it easy to exclude a dental follicle.

A few scattered islands of odontogenic epithelium may be seen in myxomas and myxofibromas. The differential diagnosis is made on basis of a combined evaluation of the radiograms and the mesenchymal component of the tumor.

The epithelial component of the AMF and the AFD differs from that of the COF by forming bilaminar ramifying strands with formation of buds, which show cylindrical basal cells and may contain stellate reticulum-like cells. The ectomesenchymal component may focally be slightly fibrous, but overall it resembles the dental papilla.

Apart from the above-mentioned rare cases of ameloblastomatoid COFs the differential diagnosis toward the invasively growing ameloblastoma should be straight forward. The ameloblastoma always exhibits a fibrous, vascular stroma with moderate cellularity.

Treatment and Prognosis. The required treatment is enucleation and vigorous curettage and the prognosis is very good. Dunlap et al. (693) reported two cases, which were followed for 9 and 10 years without recurrence. Recurrence has been reported in a few cases (681,694). Kinney et al. (685) reported a thought-provoking case of aggressive epithelium-rich COF with ill-defined margins around the roots of a mandibular right second molar. It measured 2.5 cm and was asymptomatic apart from a slight buccal expansion. It was enucleated and separated easily from the adjacent bone. Histology was compatible with a COF, no clear cells were observed in the epithelium. One year later it recurred with marked expansion, painful swelling, and paresthesia of the lower right lip and chin. The lesion encompassed the entire right mandible with buccal and lingual erosion and perforation. Histological examination showed CCOC.

3.1.2 Peripheral Odontogenic Fibroma.

Introduction. The peripheral odontogenic fibroma (POF) is a benign, slowly growing, exophytic lesion occurring on the gingiva or the attached alveolar ridge mucosa in edentulous areas. Histologically it consists of an unencapsulated, focal mass of hypercellular fibrous and sometimes myxoid connective tissue that contains varying numbers of odontogenic epithelial islands or strands (444,695). The tumor was recognized in the 1971 and the 1992 WHO classification of odontogenic tumors (22,23), but only digressively mentioned in the 2005 edition (687).

ICD-O code 9322/0

Synonyms: There are no synonyms, but cases have been published under diagnoses like "odontogenic gingival epithelial hamartomas," "hamartoma of the dental lamina," "peripheral ameloblastic fibrodentinoma," and "peripheral ameloblastoma" (695). The term "hamartoma" was introduced to designate a tumor-like but nonneoplastic malformation or inborn error of tissue development characterized by an abnormal mixture of tissues indigenous to the part with excess of one or more of these tissues (15). Odontomes are hamartomas, they develop during the odontogenic period, which ceases about the age of 22 years, but the term cannot be legitimately used for tumor-like lesions of odontogenic tissue with self-limiting growth potential, which primarily occur in patients past that age.

Clinical Features. The prevalence and incidence of the POF is unknown. The relative frequency of the tumor in material received for histological diagnosis in services of diagnostic pathology in various countries for various amounts of years was 3.1% and 8.9% in two studies comprising more than 300 samples of odontogenic tumors and in which a subdivision between the central and the peripheral odontogenic fibroma has been made. The results are indicated as follows: number of odontogenic tumors/number of POFs/%. Daley et al., Canada (33): 392/35/8.9%, Mosqueda-Taylor et al., Mexico (34): 349/11/3.1%.

The POF seems far more common than the COF. Somewhat more than 120 cases have been reported.

Several reviews have been published (212,444,688,695–697). Daley et al. reviewed 36 cases from own files and 73 from the literature including cases from earlier reviews; operculae were not included. The age was indicated in 103 cases; the age range was 2 to 80 years, but there were few children below 10 years and few adults over 70 years. There was an age peak in the third decade and a somewhat lower, but almost equal number of patients in the fourth, fifth, sixth, and seventh decades. Siar et al. (696) reported 46 cases in Malaysians and calculated the mean age to be 32 years.

The gender distribution in the review by Daley et al. was quite different from that of the COF; the ratio was more balanced, among 107 cases 48 were males and 59 females.

In the same review the anatomic site of the lesion was stated in 59 cases. All sites and both buccal and lingual gingiva were affected. In the maxilla there was a predilection for the anterior region, in the mandible there was a predilection for the cuspid/premolar region. Garcia et al. (697) reported 17 cases of which 68% was found in the posterior region of the mandible.

Clinically the POF usually presents as a pedunculated or sessile, firm, nontender gingival mass of normal color. The size varies from 0.3 to 2.0 cm, with mean size of 1.0 cm (695). Occasionally displacement of teeth is seen. If traumatized by occluding teeth, the lesion may be inflamed or even ulcerated. Bleeding on tooth brushing was reported in 13 of 46 cases (28%) by Siar et al. (696). In the same review duration of symptoms in general ranged from one week to 10 years.

Imaging. De Villiers Slabbert et al. (688) reviewed 30 cases of POF from own files and reported that radiograms frequently showed calcified material inside the COFs.

Pathology. The COF shows a wide histological spectrum (688). All are nonencapsulated and most are poorly delineated. In all of them odontogenic epithelium is present (Fig. 76). In a review of 30 cases from

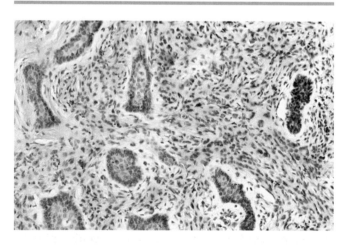

Figure 76 Peripheral odontogenic fibroma. The mesenchymal component is hypercellular and the islands of odontogenic epithelium are abundant, but small and without stellate reticulum-like cells. H&E stain.

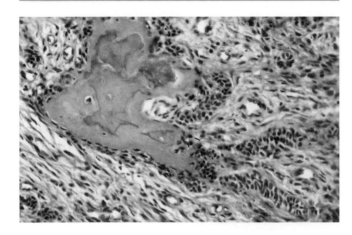

Figure 77 Peripheral odontogenic fibroma with hard tissue formation. Numerous strands and islands of odontogenic epithelium as seen in a cellular mesenchymal connective tissue. The hard tissue is formed in close contact with the epithelium, histomophologically it resembles cementum. H&E stain.

own files, de Villiers Slabbert et al. (688) found that the odontogenic epithelium was sparse in 15 cases, in 9 it was moderate, and in 6 it was exceptionally abundant, with little fibrous tissue between the islets. Most epithelial islands were small. In a few cases the odontogenic epithelium was intimately associated with hard tissue, which was recognized as dentinoid on basis of its histomorphology (Fig. 77). The connective tissue component varied; in most cases it presented as a cellular fibrous tissue with streaming and whirling, in some cases it was relatively acellular with abundant collagen. Myxomatous areas could be encountered. Buchner (695) described a pattern of markedly cellular strands of mesenchymal tissue interwoven with less cellular areas and occasionally observed cuffing of epithelial cells around mineralized material. In the review of POF he reported mineralized or unmineralized hard tissue in 20 (57%) of 35 cases; it was absent in 15 lesions. De Villiers Slabbert et al. (688) observed calcified material with great morphological diversity in 22 (73%) of 30 cases. They also noticed elongated rete ridges from the surface epithelium in 8 cases (27%) and inflammation due to trauma in all 30 cases.

Immunohistochemistry. Daley et al. (444) used high and low mw CK antibodies and detected a positive reaction in the odontogenic epithelium. Immunohistochemical studies have mainly concentrated on POFs with granular cells, which are discussed in the section on GCOT.

Electron Microscopy. The ultrastructure of the POF has been studied by Daley et al. (444) in two cases with a moderate cellular connective tissue and numerous islands and thin strands of odontogenic epithelium with hyaline cuffing. The epithelial cells exhibited desmosomes and tonofilaments that were focally prominent. The cytoplasm contained numerous polyribosomes, but a poorly developed endoplasmatic reticulum. The nuclei were round to oval; frequently

they showed indentations and often a well-developed nucleolus. Occasionally epithelial cells with clear cytoplasm was seen, they had an organelle-poor cytoplasm. The fibroblastic cells were spindle- to kite-shaped and had oval nuclei. The cytoplasm contained a RER, which was more developed than in the epithelial cells. Collagen fiber bundles were seen in the extracellular matrix but they were not abundant. The hyaline cuffing adjacent to the epithelial islands consisted of condensations of collagen fibers, which were orientated more or less parallel to the cell membrane.

Molecular-Genetic Data. No data are available.

Differential Diagnosis. Several so-called peripheral ossifying fibromas have been misdiagnosed as POF. It is a totally different lesion. It is unrelated to the central ossifying fibroma and is probably better termed "peripheral granuloma with ossification/calcification" or "calcifying fibroblastic granuloma." The main histological difference is that it is highly cellular, does not contain odontogenic epithelium, and does not exhibit a pattern of cellular areas interwoven with relatively less cellular areas.

POFs should be differentiated from peripheral AMF and peripheral AFD; both these neoplasms seem to develop as intraosseous lesions exclusively. A case reported as a peripheral AMF in a 40-year-old women (443) did not contain dental papilla–like connective tissue and is better classified as a POF. A case published as peripheral AFD (476) should also be considered a POF for the same reasons.

Differential diagnosis toward PERAM may be very difficult. The connective tissue in the ameloblastoma is a fibrous vascularized stroma with relatively few cells and the morphology of the epithelium is different and shows at least in some areas cylindrical peripheral cells with hyperchromatic nuclei with reversed polarity and a cytoplasm with vacuoles. The stroma of the ameloblastoma has a much lower cellularity than the connective tissue component of the POF.

The POF should also be differentiated from peripheral CEOT, which is characterized by islands composed of strongly eosinophilic polygonal cells and presence of hyalinized material, which stains positively with stainings for amyloid.

Treatment and Prognosis. The adequate treatment is local surgical excision. Recurrences are not uncommon. Among 30 cases de Villiers Slabbert et al. (688) reported a case of a 1.5 cm POF in the palatal gingiva in a 44-years-old man, which recurred after 14 months. Among 18 cases with sufficient follow-up information Daley et al. (444) reported recurrence in seven cases. Two cases recurred within a year, five cases recurred one to four years after treatment. The follow-up period in the 11 cases that did not recur was 10 months to 11 years. Malignant transformation has not been reported.

3.2 Granular Cell Odontogenic Tumor

Introduction. The GCOT is a rare, benign, slowly growing, noninvasive, but unencapsulated odontogenic neoplasm composed of connective tissue with varying cellularity and a varying amount of odontogenic epithelium. Most characteristic are clusters of granular cells in the connective tissue. The tumor shares clinicopathological features with the odontogenic fibroma, but there are indications that the granular cells do not derive from fibroblasts, but rather from a histiocytic cell line.

ICD-O code: None; the tumor was described briefly in the 1992 WHO classification (23) as a variant of the odontogenic fibroma. It was disregarded in the 2005 edition (687).

Synonyms: Granular cell odontogenic fibroma, granular cell tumor of the jaw.

Clinical Features.   The tumor is rare. The prevalence, incidence, and relative frequency is unknown.

Brannon et al. (698) published a review of 30 cases of central GCOT. Since then two cases of central GCOT (699,700) and one case of peripheral GCOT (701) have been published. In the review by Brannon et al. the age range was 16 to 77 years ($N = 30$), the mean age for both gender was 45.4 years; 53.3% of the patients were in the sixth decade. The patients were thus generally older than the patients with COF.

Like the COF the gender ratio showed female dominance. Among 29 cases 7 (26.7%) were males and 22 (73.3%) were females.

The site of the tumor was reported in 29 cases, 7 GCOTs were located in the maxilla and 23 in the mandible, and they were most common in the premolar and molar region.

The duration of symptoms varied from 5 months to 19 years ($N = 4$). Expansion of bone was recorded in nine cases ($N = 22$). Facial swelling, intraoral ulceration, maxillary sinus involvement, and cortical perforation were seen (1 case each).

Four peripheral (gingival) lesions have been published. They all occurred in women. The patients were 16-years-old (site not specified) (444), 34-years-old (maxillary premolar area) (457), 40-years-old (maxillary third molar area) (702), and 58-years-old (mandibular incisor area) (701), respectively.

Imaging.   In the review by Brannon et al. (698) radiological features were recorded in 22 cases, among these 19 were radiolucent, 2 had mixed density, and 1 was radiopaque. The patterns ranged from unilocular to multilocular, often with sclerotic border. Displacement of teeth was seen in two cases, and displacement of the mandibular canal in one case. The size ($N = 12$) varied from 0.5 to 8.0 cm, the average was 2.8 cm.

Pathology.   The etiology of the tumor is unknown. The pathogenesis is poorly understood, and the nature of the granular cells has not been established with certainty.

The histopathology resembles the odontogenic fibroma apart from sheets and clusters of round to polygonal cells with abundant eosinophilic, finely granular, lightly PAS-positive diastase-resistant cytoplasm (Fig. 78) and an eccentric round to ovoid nucleus (698). The size of the cells ranges from 20 to 50 μm. No mitoses are seen. Lobules of granular cells are separated by thin, fibrous connective tissue septae containing small thin-walled vessels. Cords and islands of odontogenic epithelium are seen scattered in the connective tissue and bordered with low columnar or

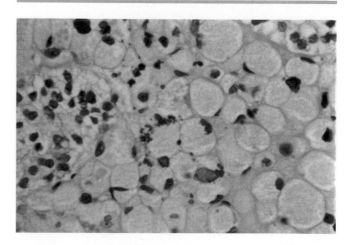

Figure 78 Granular cell odontogenic tumor. High-power view of the granular cells, which are found in the mesenchymal component of the tumor. Note that in the majority of the cells the nucleus is situated in the periphery of the cell. H&E stain.

cuboidal basal cells. No stellate reticulum-like cells are seen in the islands. Epithelial cells with clear cytoplasm are not unusual (698). If the pattern is lobular the epithelium is usually found in the center of each lobule (54). Small oval, basophilic islands of cementum-like tissue are often seen, and dystrophic calcifications may be seen, some with a concentric pattern. Calcifications may be intimately associated with granular cells (698). The periphery of the tumor is generally well demarcated, and in some cases a pseudocapsule is seen.

Two cases of malignant central GCOT (granular cell odontogenic sarcoma) have been published (109,703). The tumor described by Piattelli et al. (703) occurred in the maxilla of a 40-year-old man where it encroached the maxillary sinus and protruded toward the oral cavity. Strands of benign inactive-looking epithelium were scattered in the neoplastic component, which consisted of fibroblast-like spindle cells with slight nuclear pleomorphism and hyperchromatic and pleomorphic granular cells with frequent mitoses. Necrosis was absent.

The peripheral tumors show a similar histopathology. The tumor may extend to the covering gingival epithelium, and extensions from the basal layer of that epithelium may be seen in the tumor as double-stranded prolongations with morphology-like the epithelium deeper in the lesion (457,702).

Immunohistochemistry.   Several investigators have tried to disclose the function of the granular cells by immunohistochemical technique on sections of central and peripheral GCOT (698–700,704–711) as well as peripheral GCOT (444,701).

Broad spectred CK antibodies (AE1/AE3) yielded a positive immunoreaction in the cells of the odontogenic epithelium (444,698,701); a strong reaction to CK-14 was detected by Machado de Sousa et al. (711). Meer et al. (700) detected immunoreactivity to CK-marker MNF116 in the epithelial cells. The granular cells are nonepithelial, they were negative to CK antibodies in all assays (698,700,701,704–706,710,711).

Granular cells were vimentin-positive in most investigations (444,698,700,701,705,706,710,711). Epithelial cells have been invariably negative.

A negative immunoreaction to antibodies against S-100 protein was found in all investigations (444,698–701,705,707,709,710).

Granular cells have also been detected negative to actin, desmin, muscle-specific antigen, neurafilaments, and NSE (700,705,707,709,710).

CD1a, a marker for Langerhans cells could not be detected in granular cells by Brannon et al. (698) and Meer et al. (700). The cells have been tested positive for lysozyme/muramidase, α-1-antitrypsin, α-1-antichymotrypsin, carcinogenic embryonic antigen, and CD68. The latter is a marker for macrophages.

Meer et al. (700) used antibodies against the proliferation marker Ki-67, and the antiapoptotic protein Bcl-2. Granular cells as well as the cells of the odontogenic epithelium were tested negative for Ki-67. Both cell types were positive for Bcl-2.

The immunohistochemical results suggest that the granular cells are mesenchymal in origin and derived from a histiocytic cell line (700).

Piattelli et al. (703) studied a case of malignant central granular cell tumor. The tumor cells exhibited vimentin and CD 68 immunoreactivity and showed a high Ki-67 L.I. (21%) compared to less than 1% for the epithelial odontogenic cells. The tumor cells were negative for CKs.

Electron Microscopy. The ultrastructure of the GCOT has been studied by Wesley et al. (686), Mirchandani et al. (706), Chen et al. (708), Yih et al. (710), Brannon et al. (698), and Meer et al. (700). The peripheral variant has been studied by Takeda et al. (457). Epithelial cells are attached to each other by desmosomes. Tonofilaments, ribosomes, and mitochondriae are scattered in the cytoplasm. The Golgi apparatus is observed in small numbers. Numerous glycogen particles are found. Abundant intercellular collagen fibers are present. The granular cells are large cells with an irregularly curved cell membrane. No desmosomes are seen. The nucleus is ovoid in most cells with an irregularly indented nuclear membrane. The chromatin is evenly distributed in the nucleus, the nucleolus is moderately large (700,708). Well-preserved mitochondriae and profiles of RER are seen in most cells. The granular cells contain many primary lysosomes, autophagic vacuoles, and phagocytic vacuoles. Numerous intermediate filaments are scattered throughout the cytoplasm, and microtubules are frequently observed (710). Phygocytosis of collagen fibrils have been observed. No Birbeck's granules have been found, nevertheless it was stated by Chen et al. (708) that the granular cells resembled Langerhans cells more than macrophages and that they were distinct from myofibroblasts and fibroblasts morphologically. They suggested that the granular cells may be immediate precursors of Langerhans cells. Meer et al. (700) found that the ultrastructural findings supported the hypothesis that the granular cells of the central GCOT are of mesenchymal origin with a possible histiocytic cell lineage, and they expressed the opinion that both ultrastructural and immunohistochemical evidence suggest a phagocytic function for the granular cells.

The ultrastructure of the peripheral GCOT was similar to that of the central variant (457).

Molecular-Genetic Data. No data are available for benign GCOT. The genetic portrait of a malignant GCOT (granular cell odontogenic sarcoma) was studied by Carinci et al. (109). By using cDNA microarray they identified several genes, which were significantly differentially regulated when compared with nonneoplastic tissues. The cancer-specific genes included a range of functional activities like transcription, signaling transduction, cell-cycle regulation, apoptosis, differentiation, and angiogenesis.

Differential Diagnosis. The differential diagnosis must include the granular cell type of the s/mAM. The granular cells in ameloblastomas are epithelial. The epithelial islands are much larger, are a dominant component of the neoplasm, and in most cases some of them will show stellate reticulum-like cells in the center and cylindrical peripheral cells with hyperchromatic nuclei with reverse polarization and intracytoplasmic vacuoles. The connective tissue in ameloblastomas is a fibrous vascularized stroma with moderate cellularity.

In some GCOTs the granular cells are so sparse that they are easily overlooked, or it seems more reasonable to use the term "epithelium-rich odontogenic fibroma with granular cells." In neither case does it have any impact on the treatment and prognosis.

Treatment and Prognosis. The central GCOT is easily enucleated and has a tendency to encapsulate. Most tumors have been treated by conservative surgical removal, mostly enucleation and curettage. The peripheral GCOT is adequately removed by surgical excision. The prognosis is good. The cases reported have been entirely benign, except for a case in the maxilla of a 40-year-old man reported by Piattelli et al. (703), and the one studied by Carinci et al. (109). Recurrence is rare and metastases have not been reported (700).

Brannon et al. (698) reviewed 12 cases with adequate follow-up data; in 11 cases with follow-up from 2 to 15 years there was no recurrence. One case in the posterior maxilla of a 19-year-old woman recurred 13 years after curettage, it had increased in size; it showed the same histological features as the primary tumor, except that the granular cell component encompassed numerous medium-sized peripheral nerves.

3.3 Odontogenic Myxoma and Myxofibroma

Introduction. The ODOMYX is a benign, but locally invasive intraosseous neoplasm characterized by spindle, rounded or stellate cells embedded in an abundant myxoid or mucoid extracellular matrix. When a relatively greater amount of collagen is evident, the term myxofibroma may be used (712).

ICD-O code 9320/0.

Synonyms: Odontogenic fibromyxoma

Clinical Features. The prevalence of ODOMYX is unknown. A prospective study over a four-year period was carried out in Tanzania by Simon et al. (713) who calculated the annual incidence to be 0.07/million. Although it is a rare tumor, it is the third-most common odontogenic tumor after the odontomes and the ameloblastomas in most surveys. The relative frequency of the tumor in material received for histological diagnosis in services of diagnostic pathology in various countries for various amounts of years ranges from 2.2% to 17.7% in studies comprising more than 300 samples of odontogenic tumors. In the following the results are indicated as follows: number of odontogenic tumors/number of myxomas/% of all cases. Regezzi, Michigan, U.S.A. (31): 706/20/2.8%, Günhan, Turkey (32): 409/20/5.6%, Daley, Canada (33): 392/24/5.1%, Mosqueda-Taylor, Mexico (34): 349/62/17.7%, Ochsenius, Chile (35): 362/32/8.8%, Adebayo, Nigeria (36): 318/38/11.9%, Fernandes, Brazil (37): 340/31/9.1%, Ladeinde, Nigeria (38): 319/21/6.5%, Buchner, California (30): 1088/24/2.2%, Jones, England (2006, pooled figures from two studies) (39,40): 574/25/4.4%, Olgac, Turkey (41): 527/83/15.7%, and Jing, China (42): 1642/76/4.6%. The differences in frequency are conspicuous, but may only reflect differences in the type of lesions, which are considered necessary to send for histological diagnosis.

The age range is difficult to estimate because in a number of studies the age is indicated as the number of patients in decennia only. The range seems to be about 5 to 72 years, if the cases of infantile extraosseous paranasal myxomas are excluded (714). A number of such cases have been published as maxillary myxoma (715–719); they are not odontogenic. Jing et al. (42) found a mean age of 25.3 ± 13.2 years in 76 patients. Ochsenius et al. (35) found a mean age of 24.3 ± 14.5 in 32 patients. The mean age of 448 cases from the literature was 28.9 years (720). In most studies the majority of patients occur in the second and third decennium. Kaffe et al. (721) found 75% of 164 patients in the age groups between 11 and 40 years, and 49% between 20 and 39 years, other findings for the latter age groups have been 53.1% (442), 54.2% (41), and 44.7% (42).

The gender ratio has varied in the studies published; but in most cases it has been close to 1:1. In 213 cases from the literature, Farman et al. (722) found an M:F ratio of 1:1.3, Kaffe et al. (721) found an M:F ratio of 1:1.5 (*N* = 164), and MacDonald-Jankowski et al. (720) found 229 males and 335 females in 564 reported cases giving a ratio of 1:1.5. In four publications, which comprise more than 50 cases of ODOMYX the M:F ratio has been as follows: an exceptional 1:2.1 in a study of 61 cases from Mexico by Mosqueda-Taylor et al. (34); 1:1.1 (*N* = 83) in a study from Turkey(41), and 1:1.1 (*N* = 76) in a study from China (42). In general ODOMYX seems to be a slightly more common in women than in men.

ODOMYX may be present in any area of the jaws. It is striking that tumors are more common in the mandible than in the maxilla in three studies, which are mainly based on collected cases from the literature than in four studies based on cases from the

archives of one or a few diagnostic services. Farman et al. (722) found a maxilla:mandible ratio of 1:1.6 in 176 cases from the literature, Kaffe et al. (721) found 55 in the maxilla and 109 in the mandible, a ratio of 1:2 in 164 cases, and MacDonald-Jankowski et al. (720) a ratio of 1:1.3 in 536 cases.

In the studies from the diagnostic services the ratios were 1:1 (*N* = 50) (34), 1:1.1 (*N* = 64) (442), 1:1 (*N* = 83) (41), indicating an almost equal occurrence in the two jaws.

In most studies the majority of ODOMYXs have been located in the posterior part (including the premolar area) of the maxilla or the mandible with very few cases located in the anterior areas (34,42,442). Large tumors often comprise the posterior as well as the anterior region (720).

A few cases of peripheral ODOMYXs have been published. Some of these are better diagnosed as oral focal mucinosis (723,724). Others are myxomas, which present with a gingival swelling together with a conspicuous destruction of the underlying bone making it difficult to decide if the center of origin was intra- or extraosseous (725). No case of extraosseous myxoma in a tooth-bearing area with only slight erosion of the underlying bone has been published.

The rate of growth is generally slow, but unpredictable. Some undergo periods of rapid growth where they give rise to suspicion of malignancy, while others remain almost static in size despite repeated recurrence (720). Lesions of the maxilla, which involve the maxillary antrum, show a tendency for rapid growth (54).

Small ODOMYXs are asymptomatic; eventually they cause progressive swelling. MacDonald-Jankowski et al. (720) made a systematic review of the literature and found that only about one-third of the reports presented clinical details. The mean duration of symptoms before diagnosis was 2.0 years. In 5 of 14 cases (36%) where the information was given the tumor was symptom free or found incidentally. Swelling was reported in 76% of 155 cases, signs of pain in 14% of 159 cases, loosening of teeth in 22% of 41 cases, and displaced teeth in 53% of 49 cases. Tumors in the maxilla with encroachment on the maxillary sinus may cause nasal obstruction or exophthalmus. Paresthesia has been reported in a few cases of ODOMYX in the lower jaw (713). Ulceration of the overlying oral mucosa is seen when the swelling of the tumor brings the surface in contact with teeth.

Imaging. The radiographic appearance of ODOMYX varies and ranges from small unilocular lesions between roots of teeth and large multilocular tumors, which may displace teeth and less frequently resorb roots of teeth (726). The borders of the lesion may be well defined with sclerotic margins or ill defined with diffuse margins (Fig. 79). The interpretation of the radiogram is challenging, because the radiographic features overlap with those of other benign and malignant neoplasms like ameloblastoma, central giant cell granuloma, central hemangioma, aneurismal bone cyst, and metastatic lesions to the jaws (727). An analysis by MacDonald-Jankowski et al.

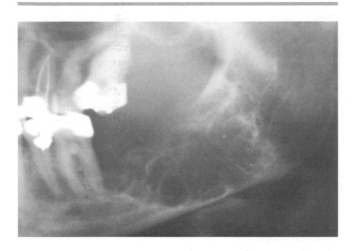

Figure 79 Odontogenic myxoma. Large, mostly poorly delineated tumor in the posterior part of the left mandible of a 39-year-old woman. A tennis racket appearance is seen in some areas.

(720) of the radiological features of reported cases revealed that among 55 cases 47% were unilocular and 53% multilocular, among 117 cases 55% had margins with good definition, and 45% with poor definition. Kaffe et al. (721) found 34 (35.4%) unilocular, 53 (55.2%) multilocular, and 9 (9.4%) not loculated myxomas among 96 cases; regarding borders 63 (65.6%) were well defined, 16 (16.7%) were poorly defined, and 17 (17.7%) were diffuse.

Noffke et al. (727) have published a detailed analysis with well-defined criteria of radiograms from 30 cases of ODOMYX, 11 from the maxilla, and 19 from the mandible. They found expansion of the mandible in 18 cases, and perforation of the mandibular cortex in 7 cases. In 11 of the maxillary cases invasion of the sinus was detected, and in two of these the tumor had also invaded the nasal cavity. They defined a unilocular lesion as a single radiolucent lesion that could include internal calcifications but no compartments. Unilocular lesions were small; they varied from 30 to 55 mm (mean, 42.5 mm). The presence of locules was indicative of septa. The term *multilocular* was used if the septa divided the radiolucent internal structure into at least two compartments. Multilocular lesions varied in size from 15 to 130 mm (mean, 70.7 mm). To describe the radiographic patterns created by the septa the following terms were used: *soap bubble* appearance represented large spaces surrounded by round or curved bony septa, *honeycomb* appearance represented small angular spaces, *tennis racket* appearance was represented by crossed straight septa resembling the strings of a tennis racket, and *ground glass* appearance described the visual effect of many, fine, poorly calcified trabeculations being superimposed on each other and without organized arrangement. Among the 30 tumors 6 were unilocular and 24 multilocular; 7 showed soap bubble, 13 tennis racket, 4 honeycomb, and 2 ground glass appearance. Calcifications were found in nine cases.

When the radiographic pattern of the septa was compared with the histomorphology of the tumor it could be shown that the coarse well-defined peripheral septa were reorientated residual lamellar cortical bone, while most of the delicate internal septa were found to be dense fibrous partitions that divided the tumor in myxomatous lobules. Impaction of teeth was found in 3 cases, extrusion and mobile teeth in 9 cases, tooth displacement in 22 cases, and root resorption in 13 cases. In two cases a widening of the periodontal ligament space was seen, mimicking an osteogenic malignancy. In other studies a few tumors have demonstrated a sunray or sunburst appearance mimicking an osteosarcoma (728,729).

It has been demonstrated that while tooth displacement and root resorption is better observed on conventional radiographs, the use of CT and MRI is superior when establishing the intraosseous extent of the tumor, cortical perforation and soft tissue involvement, and the extent of the tumor (720,727,730–733).

Pathology. The etiology of the ODOMYX is unknown. The tissue of origin is believed to be the odontogenic ectomesenchyme of a developing tooth or undifferentiated mesenchymal cells of the periodontal ligament. The odontogenic origin of the neoplasm is supported by some histological similarity to embryonic pulpal ectomesenchyme and particularly to the dental follicle, its rarity in nontooth-bearing areas although it does occur in the upper part of the mandibular ramus, its frequent occurrence in adolescence, its association with missing and unerupted teeth, and the sporadic presence of nonproliferating odontogenic epithelium within the neoplastic, myxomatous tissue.

Macroscopically the margins of the ODOMYX may be lobulated and well defined in some cases, but are usually ill defined. On cut section the surface may be homogeneous and slightly translucent. Gelatinous tumors tend to collapse or become fragmented; more heavily collagenous lesions tend to be firm and cohesive (24).

Histologically the tumor is nonencapsulated and composed of randomly orientated stellate, spindle-shaped, and round cells (Fig. 80) with long, fine, anastomozing pale or slightly eosinophilic processes extending from the centrally placed nucleus (712). The cellularity is relatively low. The tumor cells, which have been called myxoblasts (726,734) are almost evenly dispersed in an abundant myxoid stroma that contains only a few fine collagen fibers (Fig. 81). The amount of collagen may vary within a tumor and may be more prominent in some tumors, which are then usually called fibromyxomas, when the myxomatous part is dominating, and myxofibromas, when the collagenous part is dominating. In some tumors collagen is very scarce (735). Binucleated cells, mild pleomorphism (Fig. 80), and mitotic figures may occur (736). Areas with increased cellularity may be found. Nests or islands of odontogenic epithelium may be present, but is rarely seen (735,737,738) and are not necessary for the diagnosis (726); they may be surrounded by a hyalinized zone. Vascularity is generally minimal and inconspicuous (738) but some tumors may exhibit delicate capillaries (737).

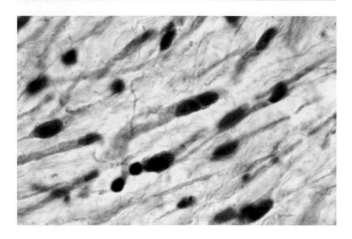

Figure 80 Odontogenic myxoma. High-power view of the neo-plastic cells (myxoblasts) which are spindle shaped in this area. Binuclear cells are seen. H&E stain.

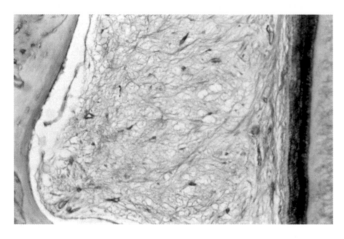

Figure 81 Odontogenic myxoma. Tumor tissue is seen between a bone trabecula and the surface of a root of a tooth. The cellularity is low; the histology is dominated by an abundant myxoid tissue with fine fibrils. Stellate as well as spindle shaped tumor cells are seen. Toluidin blue.

The intercellular matrix contains acid mucopo-lysaccarides, primarily hyaluronic acid and to a lesser degree hyaluronic acid (739). It stains strongly with alcian blue pH 2.5 (738) and reacts metachromatically to toluidin blue (Fig. 81). It usually stains faintly with periodic acid–Schiff reagent or not at all (740). Mori et al. (741) detected a high alkaline phosphatase activity in the anastomozing processes of the tumor cells, but the ground substance was devoid of activity.

Immunohistochemistry. CK has been demon-strated with broad spectred antibodies (AE1/AE3), and CK-19 was detected in the epithelial islands found in two myxomas by Li et al. (738); no other cells contained CK. CK-19 is often found in odonto-genic epithelium.

Fujita et al. (422) studied the immunoreactivity to nestin antibodies in nine cases of ODOMYX. Four of the nine cases displayed round, angular, or reticular neoplastic cells that were positive for nestin. Tumor cells were homogeneously stained in positive cases.

Vimentin has been detected in the tumor cells by several investigators (738,742–746).

Muscle specific actin was found by Moshiri et al. (745), Lo Muzio et al. (746), and Li et al. (738), but only in a fraction of the tumor cells. On the basis of such findings and results from ultrastructural studies (*vide infra*) it has been suggested that the majority of tumor cells are myofibroblasts (745,746).

Desmin could not be detected (738,744).

S-100 protein-positive tumor cells were found in ODOMYX in two investigations (742,743), but these findings could not be confirmed by others (738,744–746).

The presence of growth factors have been stud-ied by Heikinheimo et al. (130,133). The expression of EGF, TGF-α, and EGF-R was studied by means of RT-PCR and Southern blotting, ISH, and immunocyto-chemistry in two cases of ODOMYX. TGF-α and EGF-R are overexpressed in several neoplasms. No EGF-R transcripts were detected by ISH nor was immunore-activity observed. A low number of TGF-α mRNA was observed in the mesenchymal tissue. Spindle-shaped tumor cells and capillaries were immunopositive for TGA-α (130).

TGF-β2, a modulator of cell growth and differ-entiation, was studied by means of RNA extraction and Northern blotting, RT-PCR and Southern blotting, ISH, and immunocytochemistry in two cases of ODO-MYX (133). None of the tumors were associated with TGF-β2 mRNA and protein expression.

The immunoreactivity of some extracellular matrix proteins, collagen type I, procollagen type III, collagen type VI, undulin, tenascin, and fibronectin in tissue from four cases of ODOMYX was studied by Schmidt-Westhausen et al. (747). The tumor stroma showed a pronounced reaction for collagen type I. The myxoblasts displayed an intense intracytoplasmatic reaction for procollagen type III and collagen type I, which was not found in the fibroblasts of the adjacent normal oral mucosa. In contrast to the surrounding connective tissue, label for collagen type VI was weak, as was the reaction for fibronectin and tenascin. Undulin was almost undetectable.

Glycosaminoglycans in the extracellular matrix of a jaw myxoma were analyzed biochemically by Slootweg et al. (748) and compared with known data on glycosaminoglycans from the normal dental pulp and periodontal ligament. Glycosaminoglycans formed approximately 1% of the total tumor weight and 17% of the dry weight. Hyaluronic acid formed 72.4% of the glycosaminoglycans fraction. Neither the high glycosaminoglycans-content nor the high frac-tion of hyaluronic acid was found in the normal dental tissues.

Martins et al. (736) determined the cell-prolifer-ating index in 10 cases of ODOMYX and 6 cases of AMF by means of the AgNOR technique. The mean AgNOR counts were higher in the epithelium and mesenchyme of the AMF than in the mesenchyme of the ODOMYX; the differences between the mesenchymal components of the two tumors were statistically significant ($p < 0.05$).

Bast et al. (749) studied the expression of apoptotic proteins and matrix metalloproteinases in tissue from 26 ODOMYXs. They evaluated the expression of cell cycle protein Ki-67, apoptosis-regulating proteins Bcl-2, Bcl-XL, Bak, and Bax, and matrix metalloproteinases MMP-2, MMP-3, and MMP-9. The myxoblasts did not show an increase in cell division. Less than 1% of tumor and control cells were positive for Ki-67. The myxoblasts showed increased expression of antiapoptotic proteins (Bcl-2 and Bcl-XL) and the matrix metalloproteinase MMP-2. The tumor cells were negative for the proapoptotic proteins (Bak and Bax) and for the matrix metalloproteinases MMP-3 and MMP-9. The authors suggest that the production of antiapoptotic proteins and the secretion of matrix metalloproteinases are involved in progression of the disease.

Activated *RAS* genes have been found in both benign and malignant tumors. Using an immunohistochemical assay Sandros et al. (105) evaluated the expression of the *HRAS*- and *KRAS*-encoded gene products p21(ras) in two cases of ODOMYX and compared the findings with those in ameloblastomas, AMFs, and normal human developing teeth. The epithelium of the ameloblastomas and the AMFs showed the highest immunoreactivity. The two myxomas displayed different staining patterns. In one of them nearly all the tumor cells stained weakly positive for p21, while in the other tumor less than 5% of the cells were positive. The immunoreactive cells were evenly distributed throughout the tissue sections. The sparse amounts of odontogenic epithelium present in both cases were negative.

Electron Microscopy. The ultrastructure of the myxoma has been studied by several investigators (734,745,746,748,750–754,618). The main tumor cell type has been described as elongated and spindle-shaped or triangular with an irregular cellular outline with several invaginations and surface projections (734,745,746,748,753) and has been characterized as fibroblastic. The cell is round in cross sections. The nuclei are prominent with irregular contour, pores in the nuclear membrane, margination of condensed heterochromatin, and with one to two nucleoli. The cytoplasm is rich in organelles. The RER is well developed; a Golgi complex is invariably present. Mitochondria, glycogen particles, lipid vacuoles, vesicles, and polysomes are seen. Dense packed microfilaments are found throughout the whole cytoplasm. Goldblatt (734) identified two cell types. Type I was a spindle cell identical to the one described above; the author considered it a secretory cell. Type II was generally a round to ovoid cell with an abundant granular matrix, which was virtually devoid of RER, but contained free ribosomes. A few mitochondria were noted, but Golgi complex, if present, was inconspicuous. The nucleus was round, with mainly peripherally disposed heterochromatin and a less prominent nucleolus. Cell type II was considered nonsecretory. Lo Muzio et al. (746) identified cells

with several morphological variations, but considered them one cell type. Like Moshiri et al. (745) they found that several of the cells were very similar to myofibroblasts, a suggestion that was supported by immunoreaction to muscle-specific antigen in many of the cells (*vide supra*).

The matrix background has been described as fine granular with sparse collagen fibers.

Molecular-Genetic Data. To investigate the role of the stimulatory Gs alpha (GS-α) gene as a potential candidate oncogene in ODOMYX, Boson et al. (755) used polymerase chain reaction (PCR) to amplify the appropriate genomic fractions extracted from 23 biopsies followed by denaturing gradient gel electrophoresis (DGGE) analysis. Although Gs-α gene mutations have been demonstrated in other neoplasms, they could not be demonstrated in any of the tumors analyzed.

Myxomas of bones and other sites occur as part of the Carney complex (CNC), a multiple neoplasia syndrome caused by mutations in the *PRKAR1A* gene, which codes for the regulatory subunit of protein kinase A (PKA). Perdigão et al. (756) screened 17 ODOMYXs for *PRKAR1A* mutations by DNA analysis and for *PRKAR1A* protein expression by immunohistochemistry. Mutations of the coding region of the *PRKAR1A* gene were identified in two tumors; both these lesions showed no or significantly decreased immunostaining of *PRKAR1A* in the tumor compared with that in the surrounding normal tissue. Of the remaining tumors, 7 of the 15 without mutations showed almost no *PRKAR1A* in the tumor cells, whereas immunohistochemistry showed that the protein was abundant in nontumorous cells. The authors concluded that *PRKAR1A* may be involved in the pathogenesis of ODOMYX.

Differential Diagnosis. ODOMYXs may be confused microscopically with nonneoplastic normal tissue and with benign and malignant neoplasms (726). Most enlarged dental follicles are myxoid and may easily be misdiagnosed microscopically as ODOMYX (757). Accurate clinical and radiographic information should exclude this possibility. If the lesion submitted for diagnosis is radiologically confined to the crown of an unerupted tooth and a few millimeters around it, then an enlarged follicle is almost certainly the diagnosis (54). The appearance of such a follicle under a high-power objective may be identical to that of a myxoma. Kim et al. (758) found that among 847 dental follicles and/or dental papillae referred to the AFIP, Washington, DC, about 20% were misdiagnosed. The dental follicle is usually more collagenous than myxomas and may contain reduced enamel epithelium and numerous islands of odontogenic epithelium, some of which may be calcified. ODOMYX rarely contains islands of odontogenic epithelium, and if so usually few. The formative dental pulp, the dental papilla may be separated from a developing tooth during surgery and may be included within a surgical specimen separate from any formed tooth elements (381). Kim et al. (758) quote a 5.8% incidence of misinterpretation of dental follicles and/or papillas for ODOMYX. Macroscopically the dental papilla is a doughnut-shaped or flattened sphere of gelatinous tissue up to 12 mm in diameter. Usually a few odontoblasts remain in the tissue close to the surface and a narrow cell-free zone is seen below them and along the margin elsewhere (54), a histological feature that distinguishes it from ODOMYX. Among odontogenic neoplasms the odontogenic fibroma may cause differential diagnostic problems. Other myxoid neoplasms to consider are myxoid neurofibroma, myxoid lipoma, low-grade myxoid fibrosarcoma, and liposarcoma, mesenchymal chondrosarcoma, chondromyxoid fibroma, and in the maxilla, chordoma, and nasal polyps. These can usually be ruled out by good sampling, characteristic light microscopic features, and immunohistochemistry (54,726).

Treatment and Prognosis. Smaller ODOMYXs have been treated successfully with curettage, but in general, conservative treatment has resulted in unacceptable high recurrence rates. In the literature, recurrence rates range from 10% to 33%, with a reported average of 25% (721,746). Although a slow-growing neoplasm, it is never encapsulated, but infiltrative and may be aggressive. For larger lesions radical surgery in terms of resection is the treatment of choice, especially in maxillary lesions, and they require subsequent reconstruction of the jaw. Complete removal can be difficult. Among 25 cases Li et al. (738) reported 5 cases to be treated by enucleation followed by curettage. Four patients showed no signs of recurrence after being followed 7 to 11 years. One patient with a maxillary tumor exhibited recurrent tumor six months after surgery. The majority of the patients (17 cases) were treated by relatively radical procedures (segmental resection, partial, or complete maxillectomy); follow-up data ranging from 2 to 12 years (mean, 3.9 years) were available for 12 patients, and none of them developed recurrence. Although the majority of recurrences are diagnosed within two years after surgery, some tumors recur after many years. One case, followed for 35 years, recurred after prolonged remissions after 20, and then 10 years (759). MacDonald-Jankowski et al. (720) recommended lifelong or at least long-term follow-up.

Malignant transformation (odontogenic myxosarcoma) is extremely rare; only four cases have been reported (760–762).

3.4 Cementoblastoma

Introduction. The neoplasm (CEMBLA) is characterized by the formation of sheets of cementum-like tissue containing a large number of reversal lines developing on the surface of a root of a tooth, and being unmineralized at the periphery of the mass or in the more active growth areas (23,763). A simultaneous resorption of the root takes place.

ICD-O code 9273/0

Synonyms: Benign CEMBLA, true cementoma.

Clinical Features. The prevalence and incidence of the CEMBLA is unknown. The relative frequency of the tumor in material received for histological diagnosis in services of diagnostic pathology in various countries for various amounts of years ranges from 0.1% to 4.2% in studies comprising more than 300 samples of odontogenic tumors. The results are indicated as follows: number of odontogenic tumors/number of CEMBLAs/%. Regezzi et al., Michigan, U.S.A. (31): 706/1/0.1%, Daley et al., Canada (33): 392/7/1.8%, Mosqueda-Taylor et al., Mexico (34): 349/3/0.8%, Ochsenius et al., Chile (35): 362/6/1.7%, Fernandes et al., Brazil (37): 340/8/2.3%, Ladeinde et al., Nigeria (38): 319/2/0.6%, Buchner et al., California (30): 1088/10/0.9%, Jones et al., England (2006, pooled figures from two studies) (39,40): 523/22/4.2%, Olgac et al., Turkey (41): 527/10/1.9%, and Jing et al., China (42): 1642/33/2.0%. The data are skewed; however, the figures reflect regional differences in type of lesions sent for histopathological confirmation rather than effects of genetical or environmental factors.

Only about 120 cases have been published (764,765). In a review of 44 cases of CEMBLA from AFIP, Washington, DC, and 74 cases from the literature the gender distribution was: males: 58.1% and females: 41.9% (765). The ratio 1.4:1 may not be statistically significant since the material is likely to be biased. Caucasians made up 65.7% of the patients.

The tumor occurs primarily in teenagers and young adults, age range is 6 to 71 years, with a mean age of 21.3 years (764–766).

The lesion has a predilection for the mandible molars, particularly the mandibular first molar, 20.5% were located in the maxilla, and 79.5% in the mandible; in 47% of the cases the tumor was attached to the mandibular first permanent molar. Only two cases of incisor involvement have been reported (767,768). Involvement of deciduous teeth have been documented, but is an infrequent finding (769–773). A patient with bilateral mandibular CEMBLAs has been reported (774).

The growth rate is estimated to be 0.5 cm/yr (775,769). The average duration of clinical symptoms before treatment in 44 patients was found to be 12.4 months (765). The following symptoms were registered: 10 patients were symptom free; swelling accompanied by pain was seen in 17 patients, swelling alone in 8 patients, pain alone in 3 patients. The swelling may be considerable, and manifested as buccal and lingual/palatal expansion of the bony cortical plates. The pain in seven cases was described as severe or "worsening." It may simulate pulpitis making the diagnosis difficult without a radiogram in early cases. The tooth may be sensitive to percussion, and tooth mobility has been noted in some cases. Despite the root resorption the pulp is usually vital, unless it has been endodontically treated or died for other reasons.

Imaging. Radiographic examination is crucial in establishing the diagnosis. The typical finding is a well-defined, circumscribed, radiopaque mass fused to the root of a tooth and surrounded by a narrow radiolucent zone of uniform width (381,764,765). A variable degree of root resorption is present but may be obscured by the density of the tumor, and the periodontal ligament space may be obliterated. If the tumor is diagnosed in the initial phase, the lesion is radiolucent or has a mixed density; the radiographic appearance depends on the degree of mineralization. In such cases a vitality test of the pulp is particularly important for differential diagnostic reasons. Occlusal radiograph may be useful to evaluate the expansion of the tumor; CT or MRI is usually not indicated (766). The size of the lesion has ranged from 0.5 to 5.5 cm, with an average of 2 cm (765,774). Fusion to adjacent teeth, displacement of adjacent teeth, and external resorption of adjacent tooth roots may be seen in rare cases. Recurrent CEMBLAs consistently showed radiographic evidence of a locally destructive neoplasm characterized by somewhat irregular margins with radiopaque foci (698).

Pathology. The etiology of the CEMBLA is unknown and difficult to study, since the lesion is rare and experimental studies have been unfeasible. A further complication is that specific cementum markers are not yet available. In earlier classifications of odontogenic tumors (9,22,23) the lesions, which are now considered osseous dysplasias in the 2005 WHO classification (12), were included in the group of cementum producing tumors. They have been excluded as a consequence of the lack of a specific cementum marker and the unreliability of histomorphology as a mean of differentiating between pathological bone and cementum. There are conspicuous physiological differences between normal bone and cementum, however, the most important being a different reaction to physical pressure. Orthodontic treatment is based on the fact that mild physical pressure to a tooth causes resorption of the surrounding bone without resorption of the cementum of the root. The availability of a reliable specific cementum marker may well change our concept of cemento-osseous lesions.

The tumor is considered a neoplasm with unlimited growth potential. It is supposed to arise from the ectomesenchymal cells of the periodontium and is initially characterized by periapical osteolysis and beginning resorption of the surface of the root of the tooth. Eventually increasing formation of hard tissue takes place together with root resorption and later stages are dominated by calcified hard tissue (776).

Macroscopically, the CEMBLA appears as a hard, rounded, or nodular mass fused to the apical part of one or more teeth roots (Fig. 82) and surrounded by a grayish layer of irregular soft tissue. The lesion may be submitted in fragments. Tissue from recurrent tumors have been described as "poorly calcified chalklike tissue," "gritty," and "irregular-shaped calcifications" (765,777).

Histologically the tumor is composed of irregular cementum-like trabeculae with numerous basophilic reversal lines. The hard tissue is attached to the resorbed surface of the root of a tooth (Fig. 83), and this is the main feature that distinguishes the lesion from an osteoblastoma or osteoid osteoma, which may have a similar histomorphology. The root of the associated tooth is usually shortened by resorption, and the tumor may involve the pulp. In more mature parts the hard tissue contains entrapped cells. In numerous places the trabeculae are rimmed with large, plump cementoblasts, which may exhibit some

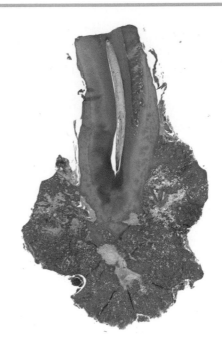

Figure 82 Cementoblastoma. The tumor developed around the mesial root of a left first mandibular molar of a 14-year-old boy. It is fused to the surface of the root and causes resorption of cementum and dentin. The pulp of the root was vital. The hard tissue shows varying degree of calcification and is mixed with areas composed of soft tissue. H&E stain.

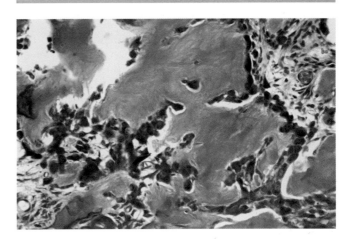

Figure 83 Cementoblastoma. High-power view of an area with cementogenesis, they are primarily found in the periphery of the tumor. Cementoid is seen lined by numerous large cementoblasts with darkly stained nuclei. H&E stain.

degree of pleomorphism (Fig. 84). At the periphery and in other areas of active growth, extensive sheets of unmineralized tissue may be seen, which show no remodeling (23). At the periphery radiating columns of unmineralized matrix is typically seen. There is no permeation of the surrounding bone; often a capsule-like layer of fibrous tissue is seen at the border of the

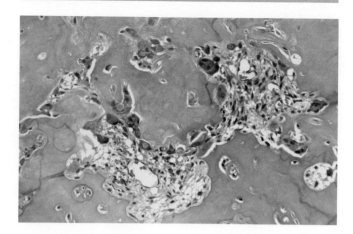

Figure 84 Cementoblastoma. High-power view of an area with resorption; cementoclasts are seen in the lacunae. Remodeling does not take place in normal cementum, but is a characteristic of the cementoblastoma and explains the basophilic reversal lines. H&E stain.

lesion. The soft tissue component consists of vascular, loose-textured fibrous tissue containing large, deeply staining cells with a single nucleus and multinucleated cells. Mitotic activity has not been reported (23,381,765,766). Recurrent lesions have shown multiple small foci of cementum between trabeculae of normal bone. The cemental foci frequently exhibit radiating columns of partly calcified matrix at their periphery (765).

Immunohistochemistry. A CEMBLA-conditioned medium-derived protein has been purified and corresponding antibody used in a study of human periodontal tissue with a positive reaction from cementoblasts, cementocytes, and acellular and cellular cementum throughout the cementoid phase (778). However, no immunohistochemical studies of CEMBLA with cementum markers have been published to date. Monoclonal antibody against bovine morphogenetic protein (BMPMcAb) has been used on sections from five cases of CEMBLA. Both cemento-blasts-like tumor cells and connective tissue matrix showed a positive reaction to BMPMcAb, but no staining was found in the calcified cementum-like tissue (168).

Electron Microscopy. No studies have been published.

Molecular-Genetic Data. No studies have been published.

Differential Diagnosis. The most obvious differential diagnosis is the osteoblastoma, which has a similar histomorphology. If sufficient clinical information including radiograms is available or the removed specimen is received with the tumor attached to the tooth, the diagnosis is uncomplicated. Osteoblastomas do not fuse with the surface of tooth roots and CEMBLAs remain separated from bone (765,779,780). The CEMBLA's fusion to the surface of a tooth root is not a fortuitous event; it is a morphological expression

of a specific property of the cells, which produce the neoplasm.

In some cases the lesion may show a slight pleomorphism of the cementoblasts, which make it resemble an atypical osteosarcoma, but malignancy has never been reported, and its distinctive relationship to the root of a tooth is unique. Diagnosis should not be made on the basis of biopsy material alone.

In case of a recurrent CEMBLA the pathologist may be dependent on sufficient clinical information.

Treatment and Prognosis. Until recently the CEMBLA has been considered a slowly growing neoplasm, which is readily enucleated and does not recur (766). Due to the capsule and the unmineralized margins the removal is usually uncomplicated. The studies of Brannon et al. (765) have shown, however, that recurrence of the tumor is more common than previously reported. The recurrence rate was 37.1% in 44 own cases, and 21.7% for 118 cases, which included 74 cases from the literature. The recurrence is primarily caused by incomplete removal of tumor tissue. Residual tumor cells will continue to grow (781); hence appropriate treatment should consist of removal of the lesion, including the affected tooth or teeth, followed by thorough curettage or peripheral ostectomy (782). If less than half of the root of the tooth is resorbed by the tumor, it is technically possible to remove the tumor and retain the tooth by amputation of the root in conjunction with endodontic therapy. However, most attempts to retain the tooth by means of this therapy have ultimately ended with subsequent extraction of the tooth (764). Malignant development of the neoplasm has not been reported.

II. MALIGNANT ODONTOGENIC TUMORS

1. Odontogenic Carcinomas

Odontogenic carcinomas include METAM, AMCA, PIOSCC, CCOC, and GCOC.

1.1 Metastasizing Ameloblastoma

Introduction. A METAM is an ameloblastoma that metastasizes in spite of a benign histological appearance (783).

ICD-O code 9310/3

Synonym: Metastasizing, malignant ameloblastoma

Per definition the histopathological features of the METAM do not differ from those of ameloblastomas that do not metastasize. An ameloblastoma with histological sign of malignancy should be classified as an AMCA. Therefore the diagnosis of a METAM can only be made in retrospect, after the occurrence of metastatic deposits (783). It is thus its clinical behavior and not the histopathology that justifies a diagnosis of METAM. Despite suggestions from Elzay (784), Slootweg et al. (785), and Waldron et al. (786) to change the classification of odontogenic carcinomas and separate the two entities, it was first done in the 2005 WHO classification (12). This lack of distinguishing between the two entities has caused much confusion; cases published as malignant ameloblastoma, METAM, or atypical ameloblastomas have been METAMs as well as AMCAs, resulting in a grouping of entities showing considerable differences in clinical course and histological appearance (785). Furthermore reviewing the literature on the subject is made complicated; reviews where the entities are not separated have become obsolete.

Clinical Features. METAM is a rare tumor; only about 70 cases have been reported. In a Chinese review (42) of cases received for diagnosis from 1952 to 2004 a total of 1642 odontogenic tumors were diagnosed; 50 cases were malignant (3.0%); none of these were METAM.

It has been estimated that approximately 2% of ameloblastomas do metastasize, but the estimate is probably too high (787). In a long-term follow-up on recurrence of 305 ameloblastoma cases, Hong et al. found one case (0.3%) with metastasis. Reviews of reported cases have been published by Slootweg et al. (785), Kunze et al. (788), Laughlin (789), Ueda et al. (790), Ameerally et al. (791), and Henderson et al. (792). Reichart and Philipsen (793) pooled the data from the 43 cases published by Laughlin , the 7 cases by Ueda , 11 cases by Ameerally, and single cases reported by Duffey et al. (794), Sugiyama et al. (795), Weir et al. (796), and Witterick et al. (797).

Among the 65 pooled patients 35 were males and 30 females, the male:female ratio was thus 1:0.86.

The data showed an age range of 5 to 74 years, and the mean age was 34.4 years. There was an age peak in the fifth decade, though.

The location of METAM does not differ significantly from that of non-METAM (789,792); about 80% of ameloblastomas, s/m type occur in the mandible, primarily in the posterior region.

A case of peripheral METAM was published by Lin et al. (798).

No differences in clinical signs between the primary tumor in METAM and non-METAM has been found, but multiple recurrences evidently increase the probability of malignant behavior (55,788).

The metastases seem to grow slowly in most cases. The time between operation of primary tumor and diagnosis of metastasis is long. The data differ somewhat in the reviews of published cases. On the basis of 31 cases Ueda et al. (790) found a range of time to be 0.25 to 31 years, with a mean time of 10.3 years. Eleven metastases (35.5%) were diagnosed within the first five years. Ameerally et al. (791) reviewed 28 cases and found a time range from seven weeks to 38 years between primary tumor and metastases; the mean time was 13.5 years. In five cases (17.9%) the metastasis was diagnosed within the first five years.

The most common site of metastases is the lung (785,788,789). Ameerally et al. (791) reviewed 28 cases from 1965 to 1995; 75% of the cases had lung metastases, including hilar lymph nodes; 25% involved bones, including skull, vertebrae, and femur; 18% cervical lymph nodes; 11% liver; 10% brain, and 3.5% other lymph nodes, spleen, and kidney. Pulmonary metastases are most commonly found bilaterally and with multiple nodes (792). Metastasis to cervical lymphn-

odes from METAM are usually diagnosed many years after first operation (799); Duffey et al. (794) analyzed published cases of METAMs with metastases to cervical lymphnodes and found nine cases to which they added their own case. The range of time from first presentation to the detection of metastases was 2 to 24 years (7 cases), with a mean of 11.7 years.

Several factors appear to contribute to the development of metastatic disease, inclusive the size and duration of the initial tumor, multiple local recurrences, inadequate surgical procedures, radiotherapy, or chemotherapy (792). The exact importance of each parameter has not been unraveled.

Ameerally et al. (791) put attentions to the fact that there has been a propensity to unrestrained soft tissue invasion in several cases of METAM. Ameloblastomas are usually confined to bone.

Imaging. The primary tumor of METAM presents as a typical ameloblastoma, and its radiological features do not differ from those of the non-metastasizing counterpart.

Pathology. The etiology of the tumor is unknown. It is suspected that the ameloblastoma possess an inherent low-grade malignancy, which is stimulated by multiple recurrences (788). It shares many features with the basal cell carcinoma of the skin, in terms of histopathology as well as behavior. Like ameloblastomas basal cell carcinomas usually do not metastasize; the frequency is less than 1% (800).

The histopathological features of the METAM are the same as those of the non-METAM. There is no cytonuclear atypia or other indication of ability to metastasize. Among the different cell types encountered in ameloblastomas, Hartman (59) found that the granular cell type of ameloblastoma demonstrated a marked tendency to recur following conservative therapy. This finding has been partly confirmed; in a long-term follow-up on recurrence of 305 ameloblastoma cases with statistical analysis (55) it was found that the histopathology of an ameloblastoma is significantly associated with a recurrence. The follicular growth pattern and the granular and acanthomatous cell types have a relatively high likelihood of recurrence. However, the recurrence of an ameloblastoma in large part reflects the inadequacy or failure of the primary surgical procedure. The majority of patients with METAMs have a history of multiple recurrences (788).

All METAMs have originated from solid/cystic ameloblastomas. Metastases from desmoplastic, peripheral, or UNAMs have not been reported.

The metastases of some METAMs show histomorphological signs of malignancy (785). Some authors require that both the primary and metastatic foci lack any features of malignancy (793,800). However, the primary tumor in such cases cannot be classified as AMCA; if it can be established that a metastasis with histomorphological sign of malignancy has derived from the benign looking ameloblastoma, it is meaningful to classify the lesion as METAM.

Immunohistochemistry. Kumamoto et al. (163) used antibodies against amelogenin and CK-19 on sections from a case of METAM. The immunoreactivity for amelogenin and CK-19 was similar to that of the non-METAMs, which showed expression of amelogenin in peripheral columnar or cuboidal epithelial cells and some central polyhedral cells. Immunoreactivity for CK-19 was diffusely present in neoplastic cells. There was no distinct difference in amelogenin or CK-19 expression between the primary and recurrent ameloblastomas.

Kumamoto et al. (178) investigated the immunoreaction of extracellular matrix-degrading serine proteinase in odontogenic tumors and detected expression of urokinase-type uPA, uPAR, PAI-1, and maspin in two cases of METAM.

To evaluate roles of the Akt-signaling pathway in oncogenesis and cytodifferentiation of odontogenic tumors, Kumamoto et al. (250) investigated the expression of phosphorylated Akt, P13K, and PTEN in two cases of METAM, which both reacted positive.

The roles of MAPKs in oncogenesis and cytodifferentiation of odontogenic tumors were investigated by Kumamoto et al. (78), who detected expression of p-p38 MAPK, and p-ERK5, but not p-JNK in two cases of METAM.

To clarify the roles of rat sarcoma (Ras)/MAPK-signaling pathway in oncogenesis and cytodifferentiation of odontogenic tumors, K-Ras status and expression of Ras, Raf1, MAPK/ERK, kinase (MEK), and ERK 1/2 proteins were analyzed in two cases of METAM together with other odontogenic tumors, and were compared with the reactivity in human tooth germs by Kumamoto et al. (801). The reactivity for K-Ras, Raf1, MEK1, and ERK 1/2 was detected chiefly within odontogenic epithelial cells neighboring the basement membrane. The reactivity was lower than that in dental lamina of tooth germs.

Miyake et al. (157) detected β-catenin (CTNNB1), but no mutation of the corresponding gene in a case of METAM. CTNNB1 is believed to play an important role in promoting tumor progression by stimulating tumor cell proliferation.

To clarify the roles of the p53–MDM2–p14^{arf} cell cycle regulation system in oncogenesis and cytodifferentiation of odontogenic tumors frozen sections from a case of METAM (and 10 benign ameloblastomas) were used for direct DNA sequencing by Kumamoto et al. (116). No alterations of the p53 gene exons 5–8 in METAM were found. Immunohistochemical reactivity of p53, MDM2, and p14(ARF) was increased in two METAS (and 1 AMCA) compared with normal tooth germs. Immunoreactivity for p63 and p73 was detected in epithelial cells adjacent to basement membrane in METAM by Kumamoto et al. (120); the p63 and p73 protein-producing genes are homolog to p53 tumor-suppressor genes and have been identified at loci 3q27–29 and 1p36, respectively.

Tissue from a case of METAM and 36 benign ameloblastomas was examined by RT-PCR and immunohistochemistry for the expression of SHH signaling molecules, *PTCH* protein, SMO protein, and GLI1 by Kumamoto et al. (155). The detected PCR products of SHH, *PTCH*, SMO, and GLI1 were 233, 144, 140, and 412 bp, respectively. There were no distinct differences in the expression between the malignant and the benign ameloblastomas.

Electron Microscopy. No data are published.
Molecular-Genetic Data. No data are published.

Differential Diagnosis. Since the histopathology of the primary tumor of a METAM is similar to that of a nonmetastasizing ameloblastoma the differential problems are the same.

Treatment and Prognosis. There is strong evidence that adequate surgical treatment of any ameloblastoma is of paramount importance to reduce the risk of recurrence and thereby reduce the risk of metastasizing (55,788). A resection with some safety margin is the best method for treating the majority of proven ameloblastomas.

Since the metastases in the majority of cases are diagnosed several years after the removal of the primary tumor, and the growth rate seems to be slow and constant during long periods (790), Goldenberg et al. (802) recommended that patients with ameloblastoma be followed serially and for a long time; they recommended annual chest radiographs to evaluate the most likely site for distant metastasis.

The metastases have been treated in various ways depending on their location and how advanced the disease is at the time of diagnosis. Regarding metastases to the lungs significant resection with preservation of as much viable lung tissue as possible has been the treatment of choice, as this is the only way to offer a significant disease-free survival (803).

Radiation therapy and chemotherapy is recommended as palliative care for inoperable cases only (792). The response to radiation therapy cannot be predicted (789) and the recurrence rate is high. Chemotherapy is not curative (804), but has been shown to have a palliative effect on patient's symptoms, and in a limited number of cases it has shown a reduction in the size of the metastasis (792).

The median survival time after treatment of the primary tumor has ranged from 11 to 14 years; however, the median survival time after the appearance of metastatic disease has ranged from three months to just five years (792). Nineteen (44.2%) of the forty-three patients reviewed by Laughlin (789) died of tumor and/or metastasis. The longest-reported survival time after the appearance of metastatic disease has been 25 years (787).

1.2 Ameloblastic Carcinoma

1.2.1 Primary.
Introduction. The term "primary type of ameloblastic carcinoma" covers a rare malignant odontogenic tumor that combines the histological features of ameloblastoma with cytological atypia. The diagnosis is used whether the tumor has metastasized or not (783).

ICD-O code 9270/3

Clinical Features. The incidence and prevalence of AMCA is unknown. In a Chinese review (42) of cases received for diagnosis from 1952 to 2004 a total of 1642 odontogenic tumors were diagnosed; 50 cases were malignant (3.0%); 27 (1.6%) of these were AMCA.

About 80 cases have been published, all subtypes (primary, secondary, peripheral) included. The relative frequency of AMCA in material received for histological diagnosis in services of diagnostic pathology for varies amount of time has been recorded in four studies, which comprise more than 300 cases of odontogenic tumors. The figures have varied from 0.3% to 2.2% in different countries; the numbers in square brackets are the total number of odontogenic tumors in the study. Brazil 0.3% [340] (37), Turkey 0.4% [527] (41), China 1.6% [1642] (42), and Nigeria 2.2% [319] (38).

Slootweg et al. (785) reviewed the cases published from 1927 to 1983. Akrish et al. (805) have reviewed the cases published from 1984 to 2004. Since then five reports of single cases have been published (806–810). Furthermore Hall et al. (811) have published 14 cases, among which 9 contained clear cells, and might be classified as CCOC by others, but 5 of the AMCAs did not contain clear cells. Slootweg et al. (785) reviewed 9 cases of AMCA with metastases and 14 cases without. Among these 23 patients 13 (56.5%) were males and 10 (43.5%) were females (ratio 1:0.8). The age range was 4 to 62 years, with a mean age of 34.4 years. Regarding location of the tumors 19 were diagnosed in the mandible and 4 in the maxilla, with a ratio of 4.8:1. Akrish et al. (805) reviewed 37 cases from the literature and added one case of their own. Four of them were secondary, dedifferentiated tumors, i.e., they developed in benign ameloblastomas. Their results differ from those of Slootweg et al. Among the 38 patients 25 (66%) were males, and 13 (34%) were females (ratio 1:0.5). The age range was 15 to 84 years, the mean age: 52 years, and median age 59 years. The mean age of males (54 years) was five years higher than that of females (49 years).

The locations of the tumors were as follows: 25 (66%) in the mandible, and 13 (34%) in the maxilla, the ratio was thus 2:1. The location within the jaws was reported in 29 cases. Among 17 tumors in the mandible, 3 were in the posterior region, 11 extended from the posterior region to the ramus, and 3 involved the anterior and posterior region extending to the ramus. Twelve of the lesions were located in the maxilla, eleven in the posterior, and one in the anterior and posterior region.

The most reported symptom ($N = 22$; 58%) was swelling ("expansion" or "hard mass"), followed by pain or discomfort ($N = 12$; 31%), and tooth ache or tooth mobility ($N = 7$; 18%). Other less commonly reported symptoms were a nonhealing extraction site, ulcer or fistula, facial asymmetry, and trismus. Perforation of the cortex is a very unusual symptom in benign ameloblastomas; it was reported in 12 (31%) cases. Paresthesia of the lower lip is an important symptom; it was reported in six cases (16%).

The growth rate was rapid in eight (21%) of the cases; the mean duration of symptoms to initial diagnosis was 11 months. For ameloblastomas the mean duration of symptoms has been calculated to be 27 months.

Imaging. Since many of the AMCAs have perforated the cortex, CT and MRI are important tools to establish the borders of the tumor. In the review by Akrish et al. (805) the locularity of the lesions on radiograms was described in 15 cases; 10 (76%) were multilocular, and 5 (33%) were unilocular. Border information could be obtained in 13 cases: six (46%) were well defined and seven (54%) were ill defined.

Pathology. The etiology of the AMCA is unknown. Per definition the tumor is a de novo neoplasm, if areas of ameloblastoma are present together with malignant features, the tumor is considered a secondary (dedifferentiated) type. Resemblance to an ameloblastic phenotype together with cytological features of malignancy is crucial to establishment of the diagnosis. The growth pattern may be follicular, or plexiform, or both. The cytology may vary, but peripheral palisading of tall columnar cells must be present in some areas, and inverted nuclear polarity may also be evident (224). A stellate reticulum-like structure in the epithelial islands and strands will usually be discernable, but may be absent, and basaloid cells may dominate in the centermost areas of the tumor islands (Fig. 85). Criteria for the malignant features have been suggested by Hall et al. (811) to include hypercellularity, hyperchromatism, loss of ameloblastic differentiation, spindling, more than two mitotic figures per high-power field, vascular invasion, and neural invasion. No single of these features is by itself a determinant of malignancy, and there is no single definitive microscopic criterion for AMCA. Pseudosarcomatous areas with a storiform pattern may be seen, which may require detection of CKs to disclose their epithelial origin. Areas may be encountered, which are undifferentiated to the extent that those areas alone are not recognizable as ameloblastic in origin. Necrosis may be seen as focal areas of

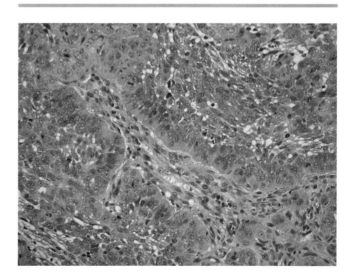

Figure 85 Ameloblastic carcinoma. Section of a peripheral primary AMCA which developed in the gingiva around the extraction wound of a newly extracted right third mandibular molar in a 60-year-old man. Numerous mitotic figures are seen and several were abnormal. Some central areas are stellate reticulum-like and the peripheral cells are columnar with distinct reverse polarity of the nuclei. H&E stain.

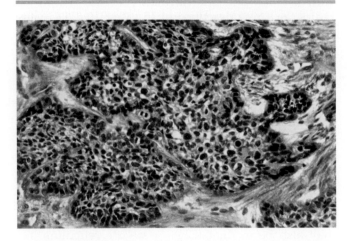

Figure 86 Ameloblastic carcinoma . Section of a primary AMCA with many clear cells, with pleomorphism and mitotic figures. If a major part of the tumor cells are clear cells, the tumor is better classified as a clear cell odontogenic carcinoma. There is substantial evidence that tumors with many clear cells have a worse prognosis than those without. H&E stain.

subtle necrosis to more obvious central, comedo necrosis-like areas (783). Hall et al. (811) have suggested the presence of clear cells (Fig. 86) as a criterion for AMCA if there are other features of malignant ameloblastoma in the tumor; such neoplasms have hitherto been classified as clear cell carcinomas (812). Keratin production and clusters of ghost cells may be seen (811).

The stroma is collagenous with a moderate cellularity. Focal areas of dense hyaline matrix was observed in five (35.7%) of the cases studies by Hall et al. (811); two cases showed dentinoid/osteoid formation, and small dystrophic calcifications was seen in one case, an unusual feature of an ameloblastoma.

Immunohistochemistry. Zarbo et al. (813) detected CK (CK types not specified) in the tumor cells of a spindle-cell variant of AMCA. Datta et al. (814) used antibodies against pancytokeratin (AE1/ AE3) and CK-8 and CK-18 (CAM 5.2) and found a strong immunoreactivity. Kumamoto et al. (163) used antibodies against CK-19, which was expressed diffusely in neoplastic cells of both well- and poorly differentiated cases. There was no distinct difference among the primary, recurrent, and metastatic lesions. Monoclonal antibodies against CK (33βE12), against EMA, and against vimentin were used by Kawauchi et al. (815) on sections from a spindle-cell AMCA. The epithelial carcinomatous cells were positive for CK and EMA, whereas few cells were positive for vimentin. Spindle-shaped sarcomatous cells were stained positively for vimentin, but only occasional cells were positive for CK; spindle-shaped cells were negative for EMA.

Basement membrane–related molecules were studied by Sauk (816) who used antibodies against type IV collagen and laminin. The AMCA and its metastases showed only scattered foci of extracellular staining of both these basement membrane proteins,

only in the most differentiated portions of the neoplasm could some focal linear staining be seen. These findings are in agreement with those of Nagatsuka et al. (75) who found that collagen IV α chain staining in the AMCA demonstrated an irregular and disrupted expression pattern with specific loss of α1(IV)/α2(IV) chains. Poorly differentiated tumor nests showed complete disappearance of αIV chain expression. In well-differentiated areas the basement membranes demonstrated a discontinuous and fragmented expression pattern for α5(IV)/α6(IV) chains.

Ito et al. (67) detected versican in two cases of AMCA. Versican is a large aggregating chondroitin sulfate proteoglycans, which might be involved in epithelial growth. The reaction was strong and located to the tumor nests.

Kumamoto et al. (178) investigated the immunoreaction of extracellular matrix-degrading serine proteinase in odontogenic tumors, and detected expression of urokinase-type uPA, uPAR, PAI-1, and maspin in three cases of AMCA.

To evaluate roles of the Akt-signaling pathway in oncogenesis and cytodifferentiation of odontogenic tumors Kumamoto et al. (250) investigated the expression of phosphorylated Akt, P13K, and PTEN in three cases of AMCA, which all reacted positive.

The roles of MAPKs in oncogenesis and cytodifferentiation of odontogenic tumors were investigated by Kumamoto et al. (78), who detected expression of p-p38 MAPK, and p-ERK5, but not p-JNK in three cases of AMCA.

The tumor cells do not react with S-100 protein antibodies (815).

Amelogenin expression in peripheral cuboidal cells in well-differentiated areas of AMCA was detected by Kumamoto et al. (163). Poorly differentiated areas reacted sporadically and faintly.

Lo Muzio et al. (121) studied expression of the TP63 gene (a member of the TP53 gene family) in odontogenic tumors. Reactivity for p63 was detected in the epithelial cells of all odontogenic tumors, and was only nuclear. In sections from three AMCAs p63 was found in more than 50% of the tumor cells. The expression was significantly higher than in benign nonaggressive odontogenic tumors, but did not differ significantly from the expression in benign, local aggressive tumors with high risk of recurrence.

Kim et al. (79) studied the occurrence of PCNA in sections from a case of AMCA. The reactivity showed a variable pattern, but the fraction of positive cells was remarkably high with a mean score of 379.1, compared with a mean score between 70 and 78 in benign ameloblastomas.

Electron Microscopy. Kawauchi et al. (815) studies the ultrastructure of a case of spindle-cell AMCA. The finding of desmosomes and perinuclear aggregates of tonofilaments confirmed the epithelial character of the spindle-shaped sarcomatous cells. The epithelial ultrastructural phenotype was compared with genomic analysis (*vide infra*).

Molecular-Genetic Data. DNA ploidy was studied by means of image and flow cytometry in 22 ameloblastomas and 5 AMCAs by Muller et al. (817).

Aneuploidy was found to be significantly more common in AMCAs than in primary and recurrent ameloblastomas and was considered a strong predictor for malignant potential.

Kawauchi et al. (815) used CGH to study the chromosomes of tumor cells from a spindle-cell AMCA. Gains of 5q and 6q and amplification of 5q13 were shown in the tumor as chromosomal imbalances. No loss of chromosomal fragments was detected.

DNA microarray technology was used by Carinci et al. (806) to detect possible upregulated or down-regulated genes in a case of AMCA. Several genes were found to be differently expressed, and they covered a broad range of functional activities: (*i*) transcription, (*ii*) translation, (*iii*) signaling transduction, (*iv*) cell-cycle regulation, and (*v*) differentiation.

Nodit et al. (110) used tissue from 12 ameloblastomas and 3 AMCAs to study for loss of heterozygosity of tumor-suppressor genes on chromosomes 1p, 3p, 9p, 10q, and 17p (L-*myc*, hOGG1, p 16, pten, and p53). The rate of allelic loss in the three AMCAs was similar to that seen in benign tumors. The authors concluded that since tumors that behaved aggressively did not harbor more allelic losses, it is likely that DNA damage in ameloblastomas and AMCAs is sporadic and cumulative; other genetic or epigenetic mechanisms may be responsible for malignant behavior in AMCAs.

Differential Diagnosis. The differential diagnosis includes other odontogenic carcinomas and ameloblastomas. Occasional mitoses, keratinization, and formation of hyaline material adjacent to the epithelium in ameloblastomas are not signs of malignancy (811). If areas of cytological benign ameloblastoma are present in a tumor, which otherwise shows signs of malignancy with ameloblastic feature, the tumor is an AMCA ex ameloblastoma, and should be diagnosed as a secondary type. If the malignant part is a squamous carcinoma, the diagnosis is intraosseous squamous carcinoma ex ameloblastoma, and not AMCA. Carcinomas metastatic to the jaws should also be considered, but they do not show ameloblastic features (783).

Some AMCAs have been reported to contain clear cells. If the presence of clear cells is conspicuous, most pathologists will classify the tumor as a clear cell carcinoma (812). Hall et al. (811) have suggested they should be regarded as clear cell type of AMCA and have demonstrated that those with a significant amount of clear cells have a worse prognosis, than those without.

AMCAs may be dominated by spindle cells and areas with sarcomatoid proliferation. Pancytokeratin and vimentin stainings are useful means to establish the epithelial quality of the tumor cells. Cases have been reported with such a histomorphology and been considered carcinonosarcomas or AMCA with development of sarcoma (818,819). No immunohistochemistry was done to clear up the origin of the tumor cells.

Treatment and Prognosis. Patients with AMCA have been treated with curettage, resection, irradiation, and chemotherapy (805,811). Patients treated with radical surgical removal early in the course of the disease had the fewest recurrences and were apparently cured (811). Resection in terms of complete removal of the tumor with a wide margin of clinically uninvolved tissue is the treatment of choice. The study of Hall et al. (811) comprising 14 cases from the Mayo Clinic, Rochester, 9 of which contained clear cells, showed that surgical resection was more successful in eradicating disease earlier in the course of the disease than later, and after multiple recurrences it was not successful. Eight patients were cured by surgical intervention. All tumors treated with irradiation or curettage recurred. Primary radiotherapy may be considered when an adequate surgical invention is impossible. It is doubtful whether chemotherapy has any effect on AMCA or metastases from AMCA.

In their review of 30 cases, mainly from the literature Akrish et al. (805) found a history of metastatic tumor in 8 (28%) patients, all with the primary tumor located in the mandible. All metastases were diagnosed within 1.5 years after the initial treatment. Follow-up information on recurrence was available for 29 patients. Seven (24%) of these had a history of recurrent tumor. The time span from initial surgery to recurrence was three years for one patient and within 1.5 years for six patients. Four of the patients were reported to have died from the disease, either because of uncontrollable local tumor or metastasis.

1.2.2 Secondary (Dedifferentiated), Intraosseous (Arising in a Preexisting Benign Ameloblastoma).

Introduction. AMCA may arise in a preexisting benign ameloblastom. The term "dedifferentiated ameloblastoma" has been applied when morphological features of typical ameloblastoma were noted (783).

ICD-O code 9270/3

Synonym: Carcinoma ex intraosseous ameloblastoma.

Clinical Features. Seven cases of secondary, intraosseous AMCA have been published (785,810,814,820–823). All cases have been located in the mandible. In two of these, areas of ameloblastoma and AMCA were found in the tumor at the first operation, one patient was a 22-year-old man (814), the other was a 74-year-old-man (810). In the remaining cases the AMCA occurred after one or more recurrences often after many years: 5 years (M 65 years at diagnosis of ameloblastoma/70 years at diagnosis of AMCA) (822), 12 years (F 32years/44years) (823), 18 years (M 25years/43years) (821), 19 years (F 33years/52years) (785), and 25 years (F 36years/64years) (820) after the diagnosis of the primary ameloblastoma. The patients' gender and age at diagnosis of the primary tumor and at the diagnosis of the AMCA is indicated in the parentheses.

The clinical symptoms of ameloblastomas, which dedifferentiate to AMCA over time do not differ from those of ameloblastomas. In most of the cases the tumor has been very large when it was diagnosed. The course of the disease has varied considerably in the reported cases; no general conclusions can be drawn.

Imaging. At the time of malignant transformation an increased growth rate can be expected with more rapid destruction of bone with ill-defined borders and cortical destruction with invasion into the soft tissue, a feature that is not typically found in an ameloblastoma.

Pathology. The etiology of the tumor is unknown, as is the reason for the malignant transformation, although previous radiotherapy has been suspected in some cases (814).

Macroscopically the tumor has been described as a firm, homogenous, ivory-colored mass with an ill-defined border with respect from the surrounding bone (814).

Per definition the primary tumor must contain at least some areas histologically compatible with a benign ameloblastoma. In the majority of cases the primary tumor and sometimes even the first recurrence (820) has shown ameloblastoma without signs of malignancy. The malignant features have appeared in the first, second, or third recurrence.

Immunohistochemistry. In a case of AMCA, which showed dominating cytological malignancy in the primary tumor with areas of ameloblastoma, Datta et al. (814) detected CKs (with AE1/AE3 and Cam 5.2) and vimentin. Epithelial cells do not usually react with antibodies against vimentin. The reaction to a number of other antibodies including muscle-specific actin, desmin, S-100, and neurofilament was negative. Glycogen was found in the tumor cells.

A histochemical study of tissue from the first, second, and third recurrence and the metastases of an AMCA was performed by Hayashi et al. (820). At first recurrence the tumor was an ameloblastoma, at second recurrence the tumor was partly ameloblastoma, partly AMCA. At third recurrence the tumor disclosed a poorly differentiated squamoid pattern. Tissue from first recurrence, second recurrence,benign as well as malignant areas, and the third recurrence all stained positively for a cocktail of antibodies against CK-1, CK-5, CK-10, and CK-11, but none of them reacted to CK-1 alone, nor to EMA or vimentin. CK-7 was detected exclusively in benign areas of the second metastasis and the squamoid areas of the third metastasis. CK-8 was detected in the first recurrence, the benign areas only in the second metastasis, and in the squamoid tumor epithelium of the third metastasis. A dedifferentiated metastasis to the orbital area without features of typical ameloblastoma was negative to all the antibodies used.

Kumamoto et al. (178) investigated the immunoreaction of extracellular matrix-degrading serine proteinase in odontogenic tumor, and detected expression of uPA, uPAR, PAI-1, and maspin in three cases of AMCA.

To evaluate roles of the Akt-signaling pathway in oncogenesis and cytodifferentiation of odontogenic tumors Kumamoto et al. (250) investigated the expression of phosphorylated Akt, P13K, and PTEN in three cases of AMCA, which all reacted positive.

The roles of MAPKs in oncogenesis and cytodifferentiation of odontogenic tumors were investigated by Kumamoto et al. (78), who detected expression of p-p38 MAPK, and p-ERK5, but not p-JNK in three cases of AMCA.

Abiko et al. (810) stained sections of an AMCA ex ameloblastoma using anti-p53 antibodies. No staining was observed neither in the benign nor in the malignant areas. The study was made in connection with a genetic analysis (*vide infra*).

Electron Microscopy. In a case of secondary AMCA Datta et al. (814) described rare tight cell junctions, well-defined basal lamina, numerous glycogen granules, and abundant mitochondriae in the tumor cells.

Molecular-Genetic Data. Abiko et al. (810) extracted DNA separately from cytological benign and malignant areas in an AMCA ex ameloblastoma. The isolated DNA was separately amplified for exons 5 to 8 for the p53 gene with PCR and sequenced in a genetic analyzer. Direct sequencing showed no genetic mutation of exons 5 to 8 of the p53 gene. Hypermethylation of CpG islands of the p16 gene was detected in the malignant parts of the tumor. It was concluded that hypermethylation of p16 may have been involved in the malignant transformation of the ameloblastoma.

Differential Diagnosis. To fulfill the requirements suggested in the definition by WHO 2005 (783) there must be evidence of a preexisting benign ameloblastoma. If the tumor is a recurrence, which does not show areas of ameloblastoma together with malignant ameloblastic tumor epithelium, there must be evidence that a previous metastasis or primary tumor was indeed an ameloblastoma. Otherwise the differential problems are similar to those of a primary AMCA.

Treatment and Prognosis. Radical surgical resection with clear margins of uninvolved surrounding tissue as early as possible is undoubtedly the treatment of choice. It appears from the case reports, however, that the tumor is likely to have eroded the cortical bone and invaded the surrounding soft tissue sometimes making a radical surgical removal technically impossible. In some of these cases and in cases that have been considered intractable, radiotherapy has been used postoperatively or alone. The course of the disease in the reported cases have differed considerably and the follow-up time after the last treatment been short. As with de novo AMCA, prognosis must remain guarded over an observation period of several years.

1.2.3   Secondary (Dedifferentiated) Peripheral (Arising in a Preexisting Benign Ameloblastoma).

Introduction. The term covers a preexisting peripheral (extraosseous) ameloblastoma with transformation to a malignant cellular phenotype. Prior cases of so-called intraoral basal cell carcinomas (gingiva) may, in retrospect be considered in this category as well (783). Basal cell carcinomas develop from the annexes of the skin and do not occur in the jaws or the oral mucosa.

ICD-O code 9270/3

Synonym: Carcinoma ex PERAM

Clinical Features. In a review of 160 published cases of PERAM Philipsen et al. (192) found six cases of malignant PERAM. Another three cases have been published (195,824,825). Six have occurred in men and three in women. Nearly all patients have been past 50 years. The age range is 40 to 83 years, the mean age 65.1 years, median age is 71 years. A possible case has been published by Dufau et al. (826) as a peripheral AFS, which developed in a recurrent PERAM in an 89-year-old man. No immunohistochemistry was done.

The gingival soft tissues are the sites of the transformed PERAM. The tumors may present with variable surface alterations including irregularity, concavity, sessile, and pedunculated features as well as resorption of the underlying bone (783). They are generally nontender. Four of the peripheral AMCAs occurred in the upper jaw, one in the left canine area (220), one in the left premolar area, and two in the left tuber area (219,827). Five tumors were diagnosed in the mandible, one in the left lateral incisor area (824), one in the right premolar area extending to the floor of the mouth (828), two in the left third molar or retromolar area (825,829), and one extending from the right third molar to the right canine area (798).

Imaging. Radiograms may disclose erosion of the underlying bone (195,219,824,829,827). In one case occurring in the maxillary premolar area all bone between the roots of the premolars was resorbed, but no resorption of the teeth was seen (195). In some cases the bone is not involved (220,798,825), even in a case that has metastasized (798).

A CT scanning is often more informative than radiograms in these cases (219,827).

Pathology. The etiology of the tumor is unknown. The origin of the tumor is believed to be from remnants of the dental lamina in the gingival submucosa. It has also been suggested that the tumor may develop from the basal cell layer of the surface epithelium, but the question is controversial. The amalgamation of the tumor with the surface layer, which is seen in some cases (195,219,825,827,829), may represent fusion of tumor from below with surface epithelium. In the majority of cases the primary tumor shows areas of PERAM together with cytological malignant areas. In two cases the AMCA did develop in a recurrence and was not present in the primary tumor (219,825). The tumor is usually characterized by an extensive network of strands and islands of recognizable ameloblastoma-type histology with peripherally located columnar cells and centrally located stellate reticulum-like areas, which may show variable degree of squamous differentiation. To fulfill the criteria for the diagnosis of AMCA some areas must show signs of cytological malignancy in terms of cellular and nuclear pleomorphism, abnormal mitotic figures, invasion of alveolar bone, or the sheets of peripheral nerves (783). Spindle-cell dedifferentiation may bee seen.

Immunohistochemistry. A case of peripheral AMCA was examined immunohistochemically for CKs, CK-10/13; CK-14; CK-18; CK-19, and pankeratin by Tajima et al. (195). There was a fusion between the tumor epithelium and the gingival surface epithelium. Stellate reticulum-like cells exclusively showed CK-18. CK-19 could be detected in peripheral columnar cells, stellate reticulum-like cells, cells with squamous metaplasia, and round and spindle neoplastic cells. Neither CK-18 nor CK-19 was present in the gingival epithelium. CK-19 is usually present in odontogenic epithelium.

Putzke (824) studied the proliferation activity in a case of peripheral AMCA by measuring the Ki-67 L. I. In the central areas of well-differentiated follicular ameloblastoma the index was 4.9% and in the peripheral cylindrical basal cells 10.4%. In contrast an index of 43.6% was found in the dedifferentiated areas. The tumor had metastasized to regional lymph nodes where indexes varying between 18.9% and 41.1% were found.

Electron Microscopy. Edmondson et al. (829) studied the ultrastructure of a peripheral AMCA, which they diagnosed as an intraoral basal cell carcinoma. Tumor cells contained scattered mitochondriae, tonofilaments, and free and polyribosomes. Occasionally endoplasmic reticulum was present. The nuclei contained one or two discrete nucleoli. The plasma membranes were generally smooth, containing few microvilli and scattered desmosomes. At the periphery of tumor islands there was a lamina-densa and -scattered hemidesmosomes.

Molecular-Genetic Data. No data published.

Differential Diagnosis. Proliferation of hyperplastic odontogenic epithelium in the gingival submucosa may be difficult to diagnose. To fulfill the criteria for the diagnosis of AMCA some areas must show signs of cytological malignancy in terms of cellular and nuclear pleomorphism, in combination with the histological patterns of an ameloblastoma. Lesions that, besides the odontogenic epithelium, show cell-rich embryonic pulp-like tissue can easily be excluded. The epithelial-rich type of the peripheral odontogenic fibroma (830) may be difficult to distinguish from a PERAM but not from an AMCA because of its lack of features of malignancy. Similar considerations are valid with regard to the rare peripheral variant of the SOT.

Treatment and Prognosis. Wide local excision with en bloc resection of the involved segment of the affected jawbone is the indicated treatment (783). None of the reported cases contain long-term follow-up. Experience from other types of AMCAs and from METAMs underlines the importance of long-term follow-up.

1.3 *Primary Intraosseous Squamous Cell Carcinoma*

PIOSCC is a central jaw carcinoma having no initial connection with the oral mucosa and is presumably originating from residual odontogenic epithelial elements. To fulfill the criteria for this lesion there must be no evidence to suggest metastatic tumor and tumors originating from salivary gland tissues are excluded (831,832). Invasion from an antral primary carcinoma must also be excluded.

ICD-O 9270/3

Synonym: Primary intra-alveolar epidermoid carcinoma of the jaw (833).

With regard to the pathogenesis three subcategories of PIOSCC are recognized (832): (*i*) a solid tumor that invades marrow spaces and induces osseous resorption, (*ii*) as SCC arising from the lining of an odontogenic cyst, and (*iii*) a SCC arising in association with a benign epithelial odontogenic tumor (832,834). When the tumor destroys the cortex and invades the surface mucosa it may be impossible to distinguish a PIOSCC and a carcinoma arising from the oral mucosa (832).

Other classifications have been suggested previously (784–786).

1.3.1 Solid Type (Arising De Novo).

Introduction. A primary intraosseous SCC arising from a noncystic source like remnants of odontogenic epithelium, reduced enamel epithelium (835) or from a benign odontogenic tumor (836,837).

Clinical Features. The prevalence and incidence of this rare tumor is unknown. The relative frequency was indicated in a Chinese review (42) of cases received for diagnosis from 1952 to 2004; a total of 1642 odontogenic tumors were diagnosed; 50 cases were malignant (3.0%), 14 of these (0.9%) were PIOSCC, subtypes were not specified.

About 51 cases of this rare lesion have been published. Reviews have been written by Elzay et al. (784): 12 cases, Ohtake et al. (838): 28 cases including cystogenic types, Suei et al. (839): 39 cases, Kaffe et al. (840): 24 cases, Thomas et al. (841): 35 cases. Eight cases have been published later or were not included (315,835,837,842–846).

There is a male predominance, with a male: female ratio higher than 2:1 (839,841). The age range is 4 to 81 year, and the mean age about 50 to 53 years (839,841), it is about three years higher for women than for men. More than 60% of the patients have been older than 50 years.

Only 10% of the lesions have been located in the maxilla, and all in the anterior part. The posterior mandible is the predominant site; 80% of all PIOSCC, solid type, have been located in that region.

Swelling of the mucosa at the affected site is a common symptom (81%), as well as pain (74%) (839). Sensory disturbances (numbness or paresthesia of the mandibular nerve), an important symptom, were found in 9 of 15 cases in which this data was available (839).

Many of the cases were diagnosed during the course of routine dental examination or in patients presenting with persistent symptoms from dental disorders (847). The diagnosis of PIOSCC was delayed in such patients, because the dental problem was given prior attention.

Metastases to regional lymph nodes were confirmed histologically in 13 of 33 cases (839).

Imaging. Radiograms have shown osteolytic bone changes in all cases, and only a few with mixed radiopaque areas. Among 22 cases (839) the margins were diffuse, irregular or ill defined in 16 cases, and well defined in 6. Among 23 cases 15 were unilocular, 1 multilocular, and 7 not loculated (840). The lesions extended into the alveolar bone and/or the body of the jaw and the mandibular ramus. Root resorption was

only reported in two cases (839). The supplementary use of CT examination has proved to increase the level of image information considerably (840).

Pathology. The etiology of the tumor is unknown. It is presumed to arise within the jawbones from periradicular rests of the epithelial root sheet (Malassez) or from the reduced enamel epithelium (835,843). A few cases have developed in benign ameloblastomas (837,848) or SOT (315).

The histomorphology of the PIOSCC is similar to the conventional SCC (849) with islands of neoplastic squamous epithelium in a fibrous connective tissue with varying degree of diffuse infiltration of lymphocytes (Figs. 87, 88). The extent of keratinization varies;

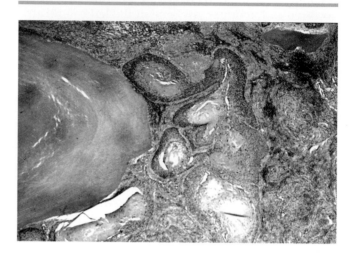

Figure 87 Primary intra-osseous squamous cell carcinoma, solid type. The root of a tooth is seen to the left, but there was no radicular cyst, the tumor arose de novo. H&E stain. *Source*: Image courtesy of Professor M. Shear, Cape Town, South Africa.

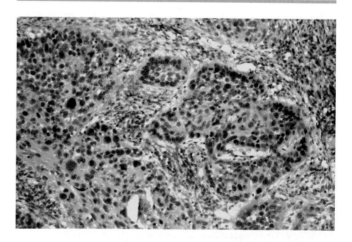

Figure 88 Primary intra-osseous squamous cell carcinoma, solid type. Higher magnification of the tumor seen in Figure 87. The islands of the neoplasm exhibit pleomorphism, abnormal mitoses, and loss of basal cell differentiation. H&E stain. *Source*: Image courtesy of Professor M. Shear, Cape Town, South Africa.

most tumors are moderately differentiated without prominent keratinization (832).

In a few cases the formation of hard tissue in the tumor has been observed (850), it has been interpreted as osseous metaplasia.

Immunohistochemistry. Abiko et al. (548) used antibodies against amelogenin on sections from a case of PIOSCC and found positive reactions in small foci of mineralized products in epithelial nests, but only in a few areas. Nagatsuka et al. (75) used antibodies against type IV collagen chains on a case of PIOSCC. Type IV collagen is the major component of basement membranes. Differential α(IV) chain staining revealed a disrupted immunolabelling profile. Coexpression of α1(IV)/α2(IV) chains occurred as thin linear discontinuous patterns around well-differentiated tumor clusters. An irregular staining reaction was observed for α5(IV)/α6(IV) chains as well, except that α5(IV) chain disposition appeared granular, with a tendency to enclose small nests of peripheral tumor cells in a cuff-like manner. No immunoreaction for α4 (IV) chains was observed. The authors suggested that the modification and remodeling of basement collagen is a process of crucial importance to tumor cell growth and progression.

Miyake et al. (157) detected β-catenin (CTNNB1), but no mutations of the corresponding gene in a case of solid PIOSCC. CTNNB1 can play important roles in promoting tumor progression by stimulating tumor cell proliferation.

Lo Mutio et al. (121) studied the expression of p63 protein, a member of the TP53 gene family in a case of PIOSCC. A strong overexpression of p63 was detected in all tumor cells and the positivity was only nuclear. The expression was significantly higher than in benign, nonaggressive odontogenic tumors, indicating an abnormal control of the cell cycle leading to increased growth potential.

Electron Microscopy. Ruskin et al. (851) studied the ultrastructure of two cases of PIOSCC. Their documentation shows groups of squamous epithelial cells with wide intercellular spaces, prominent desmosomal connections, and large, irregularly shaped nuclei with prominent nucleoli.

Molecular-Genetic Data. Alevizos et al. (852) performed a cytogenetic analysis on 120,000 keratinocytes harvested from 5 μmol cryosections of a moderately to poorly differentiated PIOSCC associated with a displaced mandibular third molar. There were no odontogenic cyst remnants in the area. Functional genomic analysis of about 6800 human sequences was performed, and the database generated was compared with the gene expression demonstrated in four oral mucosa SCC databases generated in a similar fashion. Comparison of the databases revealed numerous, verifiable upregulated ($N = 102$) and downregulated ($N = 99$) genetic events unique to PIOSCC. On the other hand 1340 genes appeared to be commonly expressed between all five tumors. There were eight PIOSCC genes, which had a more than threefold upregulated expression and 20 genes with a more than threefold downregulated gene expression, among these 10 ribosomal protein genes and 4 CK

type genes. Thus only a small subset of genes seemed to distinguish this PIOSCC from oral mucosal epidermoid carcinoma.

Differential Diagnosis. The diagnosis of PIOSCC is not possible without supporting clinical and radiographic information. A distant primary site can only be excluded about six months after treatment. To distinguish a solid PIOSCC from a PIOSCC derived from an odontogenic cyst may be impossible; a PIOSCC in an advanced stage may have obliterated any residual tissue of origin. Histologically differential diagnosis should include a central mucoepidermoid carcinoma in which epidermoid cells predominate (54) and an acanthomatous ameloblastoma and a SOT, which may be misdiagnosed as SCC (853).

Treatment and Prognosis. Patients with PIOSCC have been treated with radical surgery, radiotherapy and chemoradiation, and combinations of these treatment modalities (841,847). Partial to hemimaxillectomy is appropriate when the tumor is located in the maxilla depending of the size of the lesion with postoperative radiation as an elective option (849). Hemimandibulectomy may be required for extensive mandibular lesions; involved lymph nodes require block dissection. Postoperative radiation therapy is an elective option.

The prognosis is difficult to determine because of the paucity of cases reported and the very few cases with a follow-up period of five years or more, but it seems quite poor. Shear (833) estimated a five-year survival rate between 30% and 40%. This estimate was confirmed by To et al. (854); in a group of 29 patients 11 died within a year, 4 died within two years, 3 were alive and well for two to five years, and 11 survived more than five years.

Metastases at the time of presentation were seen in 31.4% of the cases analyzed by Thomas et al. (841), but they did not find any significant effect of lymph node involvement on survival time. In an analysis of 35 cases Thomas et al. found an overall survival rate at one year, two years, and three years to be 75.7%, 62.1%, and 37.8%. Only 29.8% were disease free after three years.

1.3.2 Cystogenic Type (Arising From Odontogenic Cyst or Keratocystic Odontogenic Tumor).

Introduction. The lesion is defined as a SCC arising within the jaws in the presence of an odontogenic cyst and without connection to the oral mucosa. Evidence of dysplastic or malignant transformation of the squamous epithelium in a cyst wall is essential for the diagnosis of PIOSCC ex odontogenic cyst (855).

Estimated about 75 cases of PIOSCC ex odontogenic cysts including keratinizing cystic odontogenic tumor (former odontogenic keratocyst) have been published. A few reviews have been published on various amounts of cases (786,856–859). PIOSCC has arisen in several types of cysts: radicular (apical and lateral), residual, dentigerous, lateral periodontal (1 dubious case reported), COC (1 case published), and keratinizing cystic odontogenic tumor.

Clinical Features. In three reviews (786,856,857) data from case reports have been listed; if the data are pooled together and PIOSCC derived from the COC and the KCOTs are excluded, data from a total of 43 cases of PIOSCC derived from radicular, residual, and dentigerous cysts give the following information about age at time of diagnosis and location. Among the 43 cases 30 were males, and 13 females; the male:female ratio is thus 2.3:1. The age range is 22 to 90 years (for males: 22–75 years, for females: 30–90 years), the mean age is 56.7 years (for males: 54.8 years, for females: 61 years); the median age is 57 years (for males: 57 years, for females: 67 years). Thirty of the forty-three patients (58.9%) were older than 50 years.

Like the solid type of PIOSCC the carcinomas derived from odontogenic cysts are more common in the mandible than in the maxilla. Among the 43 cases, 13 were located in the maxilla (10 males, 3 females) and 30 in the mandible (20 males, 10 females); the ratio maxilla:mandible being 1:2.3.

Regarding PIOSCC derived from the KCOT about 26 cases have been published, six of them in the Japanese or Korean language (860). Data from 20 cases published in English (861–879) show that 13 of the 20 patients were males and 7 were females, making the male:female ratio 1.9:1 The age range is 18 to 81 years (males: 25–79 years, females: 18–81 years). The mean age is 51.3 years (for males: 51 years, for females: 51.7 years). The median age is 54 years (for males: 46 years, for females: 54 years).

The tumor is more common in the mandible, where it was located in 14 cases (9 males and 5 females), than in the maxilla: 6 cases (3 males and 2 females). The ratio maxilla:mandible is 1:2.3. Among the six tumors in the maxilla, three were located in the anterior region and three in the posterior. None of the tumors in the mandible were located in the anterior region, apart from two cases where the tumor occupied the entire left or right side of the jaw. The remaining 12 cases were located in the posterior region.

There are no obvious differences in the data from patients with PIOSCC ex KCOT and PIOSCC from other types of odontogenic cysts except that the mean and median age in patients with PIOSCC ex KCOT is somewhat lower, but the number of patients is small, so the difference may not be significant.

Since more than 50% of the KCOT and more than 50% of the dentigerous cysts are diagnosed in the posterior part of the mandible, and the majority of the radicular and residual cysts occur in the anterior part of the maxilla (228), a difference in the prevailing locations between PIOSCCs derived from various types of cysts could be expected, but the study has not been done.

Irrespective of the source of the tumor there is an absence of any indication of malignancy in most cases, even at the time of biopsy or enucleation. The diagnosis of PIOSCC derived from a cyst is often made on the basis of a histological examination. When symptoms are present they are mainly nonspecific, including swelling and pain. In a review of 56 cases Schwimmer et al. (858) found enlargement in 58.9%, pain in 19.6%, and painful swelling in 21.5% of the patients. In a review of 39 cases Suei et al. (839) recorded swelling in 64.1%, pain in 64.1%, sensory disturbance in 23%, and

local lymph node metastasis in 33% of the cases. Significant symptoms apart from swelling of lymph nodes are paresthesia or anesthesia, rapid, firm non-tender enlargement of the jaw, and failure of an extraction alveolus to heal.

Imaging. In the majority of cases the lesion presents itself on the radiogram as a round to ovoid unilocular, sometimes multilocular radiolucency with well-defined, sometimes ill-defined margins. Early lesions are diagnosed as cysts; in more advanced stages at least some parts of the border is indistinct and may be jagged with indentations, thus distinguishing the cyst-derived PIOSCC from a benign odontogenic cyst (856). Thinning of the cortex of the jaw may be seen, and resorption of roots of teeth adjacent to the radiolucency has been observed.

Pathology. The etiology is unknown; there are no predisposing factors (832). It has been noted that a surprising amount of cysts in which PIOSCC developed, and which were not KCOT showed some keratinization (880,881,863), a feature that could be related to the carcinomatous potential.

Histopathologically, the tumor is characterized as a cyst in association with a SCC. The histomorphology of the lining of the cyst depends on its type, radicular/residual, dentigerous, COC, or keratinizing cystic odontogenic tumor. The latter is usually para-keratinized, but it may be orthokeratinized (870,875). The diagnosis requires documentation in the microscope of transition from a benign cyst with its characteristic epithelial lining to an invasive carcinoma (849). The transition may be abrupt or gradual in terms of various degrees of epithelial dysplasia in the epithelial lining (Fig. 89). The SCC extends from the epithelial lining of the cyst into the connective tissue wall accompanied by chronic inflammation. The carcinoma is well differentiated in most cases, but a case of spindle cell carcinoma arising in an odontogenic cyst has been published (882). Sawyer et al. (883) published a case in which they observed hard tissue

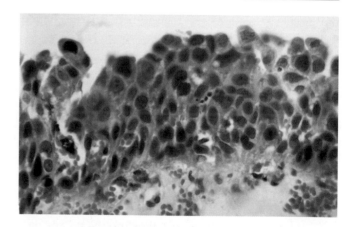

Figure 89 Primary intra-osseous squamous cell carcinoma, cystogenic type. Carcinoma in situ is seen in this part of the lining of a cyst, which in other areas showed invasive carcinoma. The tumor developed in a large cyst in the left mandible of a 76-year-old woman. H&E stain.

formation in the PIOSCC; it was interpreted as dysplastic dentin (dentinoid).

Immunohistochemistry. McDonald et al. (884) studied the expression of p53-protein with a monoclonal antibodies in a SCC derived from a cyst around the crown of a mesially impacted lower right molar. An overexpression of p53 was found in the nuclei of tumor cells, but not in the cystic epithelium.

Electron Microscopy. Herbener et al. (870) studied the ultrastructure of a SCC juxtaposed to a KCOT. Dysplasia in the cyst epithelium could not be found, the ultrastructure of the cystic lining was in accordance with other similar studies (228). The tumor cells were loosely bound to one another and had a tortuous outline. The nuclei had an irregular outline and contained multiple prominent nucleoli. The cytoplasm was rich in mitochondria, contained a dilated RER, and inclusions that resembled lysosomes. Occasionally Golgi apparatus, vacuoles, and glycogen were found. Some cells contained irregularly distributed bundles of tonofilaments throughout the cytoplasm. The authors stated that some of the cells had a remarkable resemblance to the ameloblasts of developing teeth and ameloblast-like cells in the ameloblastoma.

Molecular-Genetic Data. By means of flow cytometry, High et al. (864) studied the DNA of cells from a keratinizing cystic odontogenic tumor (odontogenic keratocyst) with epithelial dysplasia, which underwent subsequent malignant transformation. The cells from the cyst showed a type of DNA-aneuploidy, which was found in the subsequent SCC as well.

Differential Diagnosis. Any connection with a mucosal surface SCC as well as a metastatic must be excluded. The main differential diagnosis should include a central mucoepidermoid carcinoma dominated by epidermoid cells, and SOT-like proliferations in the cyst wall (315). In the latter case there will be no epithelial dysplasia in the cyst lining.

Treatment and Prognosis. In the few cases where the malignancy is detected before the initial treatment, aggressive resection like a bloc resection, hemimaxillectomy, and hemimandibulectomy have been performed (786,838,857). The recurrence rate is difficult to assess. In the review by Waldron et al. (786) recurrence was seen in 7 of 14 cases, in the review by Ohtake et al. (838) it was considerably lower. Relatively few patients have been reported dead of disease, but the follow-up period in most reported cases is short. Long-term follow-up is mandatory. The prognosis is thus difficult to estimate, in a review of 36 cases Eversole et al. (885) calculated the two-years survival to be 53%.

1.4   Clear Cell Odontogenic Carcinoma

Introduction. The WHO definition of the CCOC is as follows: CCOC is characterized by sheets and islands of vacuolated and clear cells (812).

ICD-O code 9341/3.

Synonym: None, but cases have been published with various diagnoses before 1985.

CCOC was described as a new entity by Hansen et al. in 1985, although the term "clear cell odontogenic tumor" was used (886) and by Waldron et al. who used the term "clear cell ameloblastoma" (887). It is a locally invasive neoplasm with potential for metastasizing and is considered malignant even in cases without cytological signs of malignancy. The entity CCOC as defined by WHO (812) embraces two somewhat different histomorphological patterns. One of them—being the most common—shows the histomorphology originally described by Hansen et al. (886). The tumor is composed of sheets, islands, and strands of epithelial clear cells surrounded by narrow or broader bands of fibrous connective tissue. Often the clear cells are intermixed with smaller islands of polygonal cells with an eosinophilic, slightly granular cytoplasm. The two cell types may coexist in the same tumor island (biphasic pattern). The tumor does not show areas of ameloblastoma pattern. The other histomorphological pattern embraced by the term "CCOC" was first described by Waldron et al. (887), who named the tumor "clear cell ameloblastoma" (CCAM). The histology resembles in many aspects a s/mAM with follicular growth pattern: epithelial islands with stellate reticulum-like cells, areas with peripheral, palisading, elongated cells with reverse polarization of nuclei together with a substantial amount of islands consisting of clear cells (biphasic pattern). According to the opinion of some authors (563,812,888–894), the two types represent variations along a single histopathological spectrum rather than separate entities. Others suggest that the latter variant (CCAM) should be separated from CCOC (890,895–898).

It is generally agreed upon that both variants should be considered as low-grade carcinomas.

Some authors (890,899) suggested the term "clear cell ameloblastic carcinoma" for this variant instead of the term "clear cell ameloblastoma," which falsely implies a benign tumor. However, the term *"ameloblastic carcinoma"* is used exclusively for tumors with the histological features of ameloblastoma in combination with cytological atypia (783).

Hall et al (811) have shown in a study of 14 cases of AMCAs that the presence of clear cells in more than 15% of an ameloblastoma strongly suggests an AMCA. They suggested that tumors, which contain ameloblastoma-like areas, areas with clear cells, and histomorphological signs of malignances should be classified as a subgroup (clear cell AMCA) of the AMCA.

If the presence of a substantial amount of clear cells in an odontogenic tumor is regarded as a histomorphological sign of malignancy in itself, then the entire entity CCOC should be classified as AMCAs.

Clinical Features. The prevalence and incidence of CCOC is unknown. The relative frequency was indicated in a Chinese review (42) of cases received for diagnosis from 1952 to 2004; a total of 1642 odontogenic tumors were diagnosed; 50 cases were malignant (3.0%), 2 of these (0.1%) were CCOC.

Only about 55 cases of this rare tumor (both variants) have been published, so no epidemiological data are available. Reviews of published cases with the two variants pooled together are found in three publications (900–902). Only in two reviews are the data separated for the variants CCOC and CCAM (898,899). The latter (899) in particular is detailed, and the authors use stringent criteria for separation of the two variants; the following description of clinical features is based on that review.

Among 27 cases of CCOC, 8 were males and 19 females, with a male-to-female ratio of 1:2.4. Among eight cases of CCAM there were five males and three females (ratio 1.7:1).

Age at the time of diagnosis ranged from 17 to 89 years in CCOC with a mean age of 59 years and a median age of 61 years. The mean age of females was eight year higher than that of men (61 and 53 years, respectively). Regarding the eight cases of CCAM, age ranged from 14 to 71 years, with a mean age of 44 and a median age of 46 years. The mean age of females was about the same as that of the males, 45 and 43 years, respectively.

CCOC and CCAM are primarily intraosseous neoplasms. A single case of PERAM with clear cells has been published (903); the amount of clear cells was very limited and it was apparently a benign lesion. No case of multiple lesions has been published. The CCOC is by far most often located in the mandible. Among 29 cases, 3 were in the maxilla (2 anterior, 1 posterior) and 24 in the mandible (12 anterior, 11 posterior, 1 unknown). The eight cases of CCAM were distributed with two in the maxilla (both posterior) and six in the mandible (4 anterior, 2 posterior).

The size of the neoplasm has varied considerably. A few were small, about 2 cm at longest diameter, many were about 5 cm, and some have been very large, about 10 cm. The growth rate seems to be fast; the time from first symptom to diagnosis is generally short, often between two and six months. In some cases it was two years or more, but in such cases the tumor has often developed in continuation of or as recurrence of another lesion. Very few, and they were all small tumors, were diagnosed during routine examination.

Swelling and expansion are the most common symptoms in CCOC as well as in CCAM. A few have complained of mild pain or a dull ache. Among 27 cases of CCOC tooth mobility was found in seven cases, and tooth displacement in six cases. Among eight cases of CCAM tooth mobility was found in one case, and tooth displacement in 2 cases (899).

Imaging. The information on radiographic characteristics have been incomplete in many reported cases (899). The lesions have been described as radiolucent; nine cases of CCOC as unilocular and four as multilocular. The lesions had well-defined borders in 5 cases and poorly defined borders in 9 cases; root resorption has been reported in 1 case and cortical destruction in 11 cases. Among the CCAM lesions all eight were radiolucent; five of them were unilocular and one multilocular. Well-defined borders were seen in two lesions, and one was poorly defined. Root resorption occurred in one case. Cortical destruction was seen in five of seven cases in which this data was available. CT scanning has proven to be very useful in tracing the extension of the lesion (888,904,895).

Pathology. The etiology and pathogenesis of the CCOC and the CCAM are unknown. Since they are both exclusively intraosseous, they arise most likely in residues of the dental lamina and proliferations of odontogenic epithelium adjacent to reduced enamel epithelium (448), although histological similarities to tissue in the developing tooth germ are lacking in the CCOC (800). Clear cells have been found in the wall of gingival cysts of the adult, in the wall of the lateral periodontal cyst, and in rests of dental lamina in the gingival, and in operculae, but not in radicular or dentigerous cysts (228,905,906). Some tumors seem to arise in preexisting recurring ameloblastomas (cases 2 and 3) (894,907) .

Macroscopically the tumor has been described as a white or pinkish-gray, solid mass with (908) and without (886) necrosis.

Histologically, the CCOC is composed of irregular bands and islands of relatively uniform, round to oval epithelial cells with abundant clear cytoplasm and round, lightly stained vesicular nuclei (Fig. 90). Other islands may consist of smaller polygonal cells with an eosinophilic, faintly fibrillar cytoplasm and monomorphic hyperchromatic nuclei. The two cell populations may exist in the same tumor island (biphasic pattern), and transition to clear cells may be observed (849,886,898,908). Strands of small eosinophilic cells may be present. Neither nuclear pleomorphism nor mitotic activity is necessarily present, but moderate nuclear pleomorphism is not uncommon (Fig. 91). Mitotic activity is usually rare (886), but in some cases mitoses are frequent (891) or numerous (909). No squamous, glandular, or ameloblastoma-like features are seen. The tumor islands are separated by narrow bands of mature, fibrous, sometimes hyalinized connective tissue with few cells. There is no encapsulation, and the tumor invades the surrounding medullary bone and sometimes even dental pulp (831). Cortical destruction with growth into the

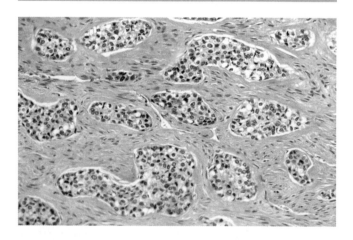

Figure 90 Clear cell odontogenic carcinoma. The tumor is composed of oblong, rounded epithelial islands with many clear cells and moderate pleomorphism. The histology shows no resemblance to an ameloblastoma, no palisading columnar cells are seen in the periphery, and no stellate reticulum-like epithelium is present in the islands. H&E stain. *Source*: Section by courtesy of Professor G. Bang, Bergen.

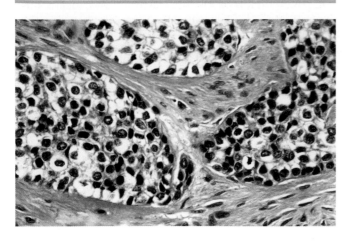

Figure 91 Clear cell odontogenic carcinoma. Higher magnification of another area of the tumor seen in Figure 90. The tumor islands show a moderate, but distinct pleomorphism in a mixed population of clear cells and eosinophilic polyhedral cells. The histology differs clearly from that of an ameloblastoma. H&E stain. *Source*: Section by courtesy of Prof. G. Bang, Bergen.

surrounding soft tissue is a common feature, and that is highly unusual for ameloblastomas (831,899).

The CCAM variant is characterized by a histomorphology, which is in some aspects similar to that of an ameloblastoma with follicular growth pattern, but often with cuboidal central cells with vesicular nuclei and abundant eosinophilic, slightly granular or fibrillar cytoplasm instead of a stellate reticular pattern. Together with this pattern a prominent clear cell component is present within the follicular nests with areas showing transition between the two patterns (biphasic pattern). Squamous cells may be seen, particularly in the central areas of the islands. A few mitoses may be observed. However, if signs of malignancy are present, like hypercellularity, hyperchromatism, loss of ameloblastic differentiation, spindling, more than two mitotic figures per high power field (40×), vascular invasion or neural invasion, the tumor should be classified as AMCA (811).

The stroma consists of dense fibrous, connective tissue with hyalinized areas. The stroma is often more abundant than in tumors with the CCOC pattern.

A few ghost cells may be seen, which is not unusual for many odontogenic tumors. In very few cases a formation of dentinoid or even canalicular dentin has been observed (891,910). Similar findings have been described in AMCAs (811). While the case reported by Ariyoshi et al. (910) is likely to be a DGCT with clear cells, other cases published by Miyauchi et al. (891) and Kumamoto et al. (911) are more difficult to explain, since no odontogenic ectomesenchyme was detected in the tumors. Small cystic spaces with amorphous, eosinophilic, Congo red negative content has been described (900,911,912).

Immunohistochemistry. A considerable amount of histochemical and immunohistochemical studies have been published; it remains unclear if differences exist between the CCOC and the CCAM.

Glycogen (diastase-digested, PAS-positive granules) in the cytoplasm of the clear cells is a common finding (891,900,913). The cells are consistently negative when stained with mucicarmine and alcian blue, thus excluding glandular activity (563,900,914,915).

Intracellular enzymes have been detected: acid phosphatase in lysosomes (909,913), nonspecific esterase and NADH diaphorase, while alkaline phosphatase, which is related to mineralization is absent (913).

Most investigators have found the tumor cells S-100 protein-negative (891,900,911,912,914,916,917). EMA has been detected (891,915,917,918), but the tumor cells do neither contain involucrin (563,911), smooth muscle actin (891,900,911,914,916,917) nor vimentin (891,900,914–918).

Filagrin has been detected (911), as well as various types of CK. Tumor cells have reacted positively to pankeratin antibodies (AE1/AE3, KL1) sporadically in clear cells, invariably in eosinophilic cells (563,891, 900,907,909,917). Reaction to CK-10, which is found in keratinized squamous epithelium has been negative (563). CK-5, CK-6, CK-13, and CK-14, which are usually found in lower or middle layers of squamous epithelium have been detected in tumor cells (889, 912,916). CK-14 is a common finding in ameloblastomas. Among the CKs usually found in simple epithelia, CK-8 has been found by some (891,900, 912,916,). Investigations of CK-18 have given contradicting results, some were negative (916), some found weak focal reactions (912,918). CK-19 is a constant finding in odontogenic epithelium and has been detected in the tumor cells repeatedly (163,891,900, 907,912,916,917). CK-20 could not be detected (563).

Amelogenin, an enamel protein has been disclosed in the tumor cells (163).

An overexpression of MDM2, an oncogene product has been detected in the tumor cells as well.

Electron Microscopy. Ultrastructural studies have shown nests of epithelial cells surrounded by a continuous basement membrane (909,914,915). The islands are surrounded by fibrous stroma of collagen and fibroblasts (913). No glandular or luminal structures are seen. The plasma membrane is often very convoluted (913) and the cells tightly interdigitated by microvillous projections (891,914). Desmosomes are small (891,915,914). Basal lamina-like deposits between the tumor cells have been observed (891,913). Palisading cubic or elongated basal cells are found in some places in the CCAM variant (914). The clear cells show an abundant clear cytoplasm with a paucity of cell organelles. Organelles are more numerous in the eosinophilic cells (914). Mitochondria that appear normal are sparsely dispersed or clustered in one end of the cell (913,914); some are swollen. Glycogen rosettes are commonly found, sometimes in accumulations (891,919). Lysosomes are present (913), and sometimes abundant (909). Short segments of RER have been detected and annulate lamellae are frequently seen in the cytoplasm, often adjacent to cell nucleus (913). No well-developed Golgi apparatus or secretory granules are found (913,914). A concentration of microfilaments may be seen, particularly in eosinophilic cells (915). Many cells have centrioles or microtubule organizing centers adjacent to the nuclei (913). Large empty or clear areas in the cytoplasm may be seen. The nuclei have complex invaginations and one or two nucleoli (891,914). Many nuclei look pycnotic.

The fibroblasts of the stroma are elongated, with a rough endoplasmatic reticulum, which appears swollen (913,914).

Molecular-Genetic Data. Flow cytometry DNA-analysis has disclosed a polyploid tumor cell population with DNA-index 1.93 and an S-phase of 10.2% (920).

CGH analysis of tumor cell chromosomes have disclosed aberrations in terms of gains for chromosomes 19 and 20, and the long arm of chromosome 14, as well as loss for chromosomes 6 and 9 (916).

DNA-microarray has been used to detect gene expression changes in CCOC compared with reference tissue (921). Several genes were found whose expression was definitely upregulated or downregulated. The genes were found to be differently expressed over a broad range of functional activity: transcription, signaling transduction, cell cycle regulation, apoptotic stimulation, and differentiation.

Tumor suppressor genes have been studied (5); a high expression of p63—a member of the TP53 gene family—was found in peripheral as well as in central epithelial cells (121).

The cell proliferation marker Ki-67 has been studied in sections of CCOC. The activity was conspicuously increased (40% positive nuclei) (909).

Differential Diagnosis. Differential diagnosis from other tumors of the jaws with a prominent clear cell component may be very difficult. They include primary odontogenic, primary intraosseous salivary gland, and metastatic neoplasms. A detailed setting up of differential diagnostic features of head and neck tumors with clear cells has been published by Eversole (677) and by Brandwein et al. (915).

CEOT with clear cells is a very rare tumor; about 15 cases have been published (332). Most CEOTs will show typical sheets of polygonal epithelial cells some of which are transformed into eosinophilic material that stains for amyloid and eventually calcifies. They should be easy to identify. Even in absence of these features the differential diagnosis should not be too difficult, since the clear cell nests are usually small and form clusters, and the cytomorphology of the CEOT cells differs conspicuously even from the eosinophilic polygonal cells of the CCOC.

S/mAMs may contain areas with clear cells. The only difference to the CCAM variant of the CCOC with absence of mitoses and cellular atypia may be the proportional amount of clear cells in the tumor. While the CCAM has been documented to be a malignant tumor, it is unknown whether a limited amount of clear cells in an s/mAM does influence its pathogenesis.

Salivary gland neoplasms arising within the jaws are extremely rare, but may cause differential diagnostic problems particularly if the CCOC is monophasic, consisting entirely of clear cells. Mucoepidermoid carcinomas are usually biphasic with a squamous cell and a mucous cell component. The latter is stainable with mucicarmine and alcian blue in contrast to CCOC clear cells. Sometimes the mucoepidermoid carcinoma may be composed almost exclusively of clear cell sheets, but this clear cell variant is distinctive (677).

About 6% of acinic cell carcinoma irrespective of location contain clear cells with a cytoplasm that is nonreactive with a PAS staining (922), but they usually contain some areas with serous acinar cells with zymogen-like granules, which are PAS-positive and resistant to diastase. Ultrastructural examination will demonstrate evidence of glandular differentiation, which is absent in CCOC.

The most difficult differential diagnosis is CCOC versus an intraosseous *hyalinizing clear cell carcinoma* (HCCC), a very rare salivary gland tumor (922). Histochemistry is not useful. Berho et al. (923) argue that the cells of the CCOC are S-100 protein-positive, and those of the HCCC are negative. However, later investigations have invariably shown the CCOC to be S-100 protein-negative (*vide supra*). The most conspicuous difference is the stromal component, which is less prominent and less hyalinized in CCOC than in HCCC, which may show a heavy hyalinized stroma almost completely obliterating the epithelial elements (915,923,924).

Metastases to the jaws with clear cell features are primarily of renal origin. Histomorphologically the differential diagnosis to CCOC may be difficult, but renal clear cell carcinoma tends to be composed of smaller islands of clear cells, and the capillary septa are more extensive. Furthermore the renal carcinoma cells are vimentin-positive; the CCOC cells are vimentin-negative. Careful physical examination of the patient and meticulous metastatic work-up should contribute to solve this issue (923).

Treatment and Prognosis. The treatment of choice for CCOC as well as the CCAM variant is resection with at least 1 cm tumor-free margins, and long-term follow-up (10–15 years or more). Adjuvant radiotherapy is a rational option in case of eroded cortical bone and invasion into soft tissue (915). Patients treated with local enucleation and curettage have eventually developed multiple recurrences, metastasis and died of the tumor (899–901,902,915). Recurrences and/or metastases may occur even despite aggressive surgery. There is no obvious difference in the prognosis of CCOC and CCAM, although the mean time between diagnosis and appearance of metastasis was three years for CCOC patients and 13 years for CCAM in the cases published. More CCAM patients (38%) than CCOC patients (13%) died of their tumor (899). It is worth noting in this context that in a study of 14 cases of AMCAs, with clear cells present in nine of the tumors, Hall et al. (811) observed that three of four patients who died of or with the tumor had a substantial amount of clear cells in the tumor.

1.5 Ghost Cell Odontogenic Carcinoma

Introduction. GCOC is the malignant counterpart of the calcifying odontogenic cyst COC, CCOT, and the DGCT. It is characterized by cell-rich usually large islands of various shapes consisting of small round epithelial cells with hyperchromatic nuclei and numerous mitoses admixed with ghost cells and sometimes calcification (597).

ICD-O code 9302/3

Synonyms: Odontogenic ghost cell carcinoma; calcifying GCOC; malignant epithelial odontogenic ghost cell tumor; malignant calcifying ghost cell odontogenic tumor.

Clinical Features. The prevalence and incidence of GCOC is unknown. The relative frequency was indicated in a Chinese review (42) of cases received for diagnosis from 1952 to 2004, a total of 1642 odontogenic tumors were diagnosed; 50 cases were malignant (3.0%), 5 of these (0.3%) were GCOC.

Only about 29 cases of this rare tumor has been reported in the English and Spanish language literature (142,578,579,581,626–631,925–935), some others have been published in Chinese and Japanese (657). The first case was published in Spanish in 1965 as "Tumor odontogenico epithelial calcificante" (578). On the basis of the reviewing of the 29 published cases the following data could be extracted. All cases have been intraosseous, but several have invaded the surrounding soft tissue. There is a male predominance; 24 males versus 5 females. The age range for both genders is 13 to 72 years, for males 17 to 57 years, for females 13 to 72 years. Mean age at time of operation is 37.7 years; for males 36.4 years, for females 44.0 years. The median age is 38 years; for males 38 years, for females 48 years. Nineteen patients (65.5%) have been between 30 and 48 years.

The tumor occurs primarily in the maxilla; 21 cases have been diagnosed in the maxilla (16 in males, and 5 in females), and 8 cases have been diagnosed in the mandible (all in males). The ratio maxilla:mandible is 2.6:1.

The tumors have been large, five of them involved the region of two to four teeth only, but eight of them have involved the entire left or right side of a jaw; four have crossed the midline, and one case (578) developed in the left mandible, but eventually invaded the left maxilla via the soft tissues after several recurrences. The size of the tumors has varied, but most have been larger than 5 cm at the longest diameter at the time of operation.

The growth rate is fast, but in several cases the tumor has arisen in, or in association with a COC, CCOT, or DGCT, which has been present as a painless swelling for years. Many patients have experienced even the malignant tumor as a painless swelling; pain has been reported in seven cases and paresthesia of the mandible in one case (628). Some patients have had symptoms related to the invasion of the tumor into the nasal cavities, maxillary sinuses, or the orbit.

Imaging. The typical radiographic picture shows a poorly demarcated osteolytic radiolucency with radiopaque foci (597); only five cases have been reported to be exclusively radiolucent (631). The lesion may be unilocular or multilocular. Supplementary CT and MRI scanning is recommended (936). Displacement of roots of teeth has been described in five cases and root resorption in six cases (631).

Although the specific diagnosis is difficult to make on the basis of the imaging, it does indicate a malignant tumor.

Pathology. The etiology of the tumor is unknown. It seems to arise either de novo or from, or at least in association with, a COC, CCOT, or the more rare DGCT, and sometimes in connection with recurrence of one of these entities. These benign lesions may be part of the operation specimen besides the malignant tumor mass; the malignant component may be separated from or admixed with the benign lesion. Some tumors are completely solid, but when it is associated with a COC or CCOT it consists macroscopically of a well-circumscribed cystic portion and a solid portion with gritty consistency on cut surface (597).

Histologically the tumor consists of rounded, irregularly shaped, varying-sized islands of closely packed, small epithelial cells with a sparse eosinophilic cytoplasm and with rounded, dark, moderately pleomorphic nucleoli (Fig. 92). Numerous mitoses are found. Admixed with the tumor cells varying-sized islands of ghost cells are seen; they present as large polygonal cells with a homogeneous pale eosinophilic cytoplasm (Fig. 93). The nuclei have disintegrated and left a rounded empty space, in some of these remnants of chromatin may be seen. Distinctly atypical ghost cells with retention of nuclei may also be seen as described by Ellis et al. (581) (case 1). Where ghost cell masses are in contact with the connective tissue stroma, a foreign body giant cell reaction is visible. There may be various amounts of calcification in the ghost cells. Clear cells or vacuolated cells may be admixed with the ghost cells. Necrosis within the central area of tumor islands is common and may be marked. Dysplastic dentin (dentinoid) has only been observed in cases admixed with an original COC,

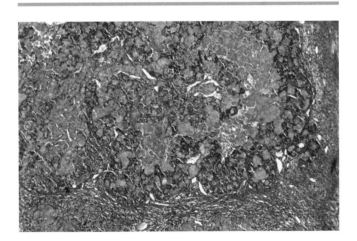

Figure 92 Ghost cell odontogenic carcinoma. The tumor developed in the posterior mandible of a 35-year-old man. It recurred several times and eventually invaded the maxilla. The case was published by Astacio et al. in 1965 (578). The large tumor islands are composed of numerous ghost cells and small closely packed epithelial cells with sparse cytoplasm and dark nuclei. H&E stain. *Source*: Section by courtesy of Dr. J.N. Astacio, San Salvador.

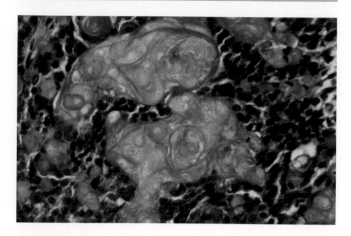

Figure 93 Ghost cell odontogenic carcinoma. Higher magnification of the tumor seen in Figure 92. Tumor cells are seen between clusters of ghost cells, they are small with sparse cytoplasm; the nuclei are rounded and hyperchromatic. Numerous mitoses are seen. H&E stain. *Source*: Section by courtesy of Dr. J.N. Astacio, San Salvador.

CCOT, or developed from a DGCT (930). The tumor invades surrounding bone and adjacent soft tissue.

Immunohistochemistry. Tumor cells have reacted positively to antibodies against high mw CKs (CK-1, KL-1, AE3, 34βE12) as well as low mw CKs (Cam 5.2, NCL-5D3, AE1). They have been strongly and uniformly positive for high mw CKs and more weakly and focally positive for low mw CKs (628,926,931). Kim et al. (142) used antibodies against low and high mw CKs (AE1/AE3) and against involucrin and found that the tumor cells were focally positive for both antibodies. Nucleated cells adjacent to the ghost cells were positive as well; ghost cells were not stained. The positivity for CKs and involucrin in the nucleated cells adjacent to the ghost cells appeared to disappear as the nuclei disappeared.

Results of reactions to antibodies against vimentin, CEA, S-100 protein, and p53 have been controversial (628,931,935).

Lu et al. (628) detected immunoreaction to NSE in tumor cells; these findings were confirmed by Sun et al. (935).

Takata et al. (615) assessed the proliferative activity of GCOC tumor cells by measuring the PCNA L.I. in four cases of GCOC and compare the results with the findings in 25 cases of COC. The PCNA L.I. of GCOC ($65.2 \pm 5.6\%$ and $65.9 \pm 7.3\%$) was significantly higher ($p = 0.002$) than that of the COC (29.3%) and the DGCT (45.8%). The authors concluded that the PCNA L.I. seems to be a possible parameter in differentiating the GCOC from its benign counterparts.

Overexpression of MIB-1, which detects the epitope of Ki-67 was found in three cases of GCOC by Lu et al. (628). In the same investigation an overexpression of p53 was found.

Electron Microscopy. Ultrastructural studies of a GCOC have been performed by Ikemura et al.

(626). The high nucleocytoplasmic ratio of the tumor cells, which is clearly seen in the light microscope, was confirmed. The cells have a prominent nucleolus in a polygonal nucleus and a well-developed RER with dilated cisternae, some free ribosomes, and numerous mitochondria. The cells have numerous microvilli on the surface; they are arranged in a pavement pattern and connected with a few desmosomes, which form poorly developed intercellular bridges. The loss of cohesion between many tumor cells was observed by Folpe et al. (931) who also described condensation of keratinfilaments around the nuclei.

Molecular-Genetic Data. Kim et al. (142) studied the possible involvement of apoptotic processes in the formation of ghost cells, which has been considered an abnormal from of keratinization. They performed immunohistochemical stains for Bcl-2 and Bcl-X_L, which prevent apoptotic cell death and for Bax, which induces apoptotic cell death. No cells had a positive response for Bcl-2, whereas Bcl-X_L was demonstrated in the pleomorphic tumor cells and in nucleated cells adjacent to the ghost cell areas. Some ghost cells were faintly positive for Bcl-X_L. Bax was expressed in ghost cells and in nucleated cells adjacent to ghost cells, but it was not found in the tumor cells, except for some nests of ameloblastoma-like cells, which were positive for Bax and Bcl-X_L. Furthermore a terminal deoxynucleotidyl transferase (Tdt)-mediated dUTP-nick-end-labeling (TUNEL) assay was used to detect cells undergoing apoptosis. On the basis of the results the authors suggested that the ghost cells might result from abnormal terminal differentiation toward keratinocytes or from the process of apoptosis of the poorly differentiated odontogenic cells.

Differential Diagnosis. The histological picture of the tumor is quite distinct with an admixture of small cells with hyperchromatic nuclei and many mitoses and with areas of necrosis and clusters of ghost cells. Since some of the neoplasms develop in association with a COC, it is important that representative areas of the often large operation specimen are examined. In almost all cases the clinical picture has clearly indicated a malignant tumor, but a preoperative biopsy may not necessarily produce tissue from the malignant part of such a process.

Treatment and Prognosis. Twelve of twenty-six patients from the published cases had recurrence after operation; most of them had multiple recurrences, and often despite aggressive surgery. Two had metastases and died because of the metastases. Four patients died from local tumor extension. Many cases have been reported with no or short-time follow-up, some were lost for follow-up, one refused treatment, and one died for other reason. Two patients have been reported to be tumor free after more than 5 years, one after 7 years (927), the patient was treated with hemimaxillectomy, and one after 10 years (627); this patient was treated with enucleation and postoperative irradiation. GCOC is obviously an aggressive tumor and radical surgery with clear margins is required. Postoperative irradiation may be indicated in some cases. It is unknown whether chemotherapy has any effect.

2. Odontogenic Sarcomas

This group of malignant ectomesenchymal odontogenic neoplasms comprises tumors named ameloblastic fibrosarcoma (AFS), ameloblastic fibrodentinosarcoma (AFDS), and ameloblastic fibro-odontosarcoma (AFOS). To this group belong as well two very rare malignant counterparts to the odontogenic fibroma and the ODOMYX or fibromyxoma called odontogenic fibrosarcoma and odontogenic myxo- (or fibromyxo-) sarcoma, respectively. None of the latter was included in the WHO classification 2005 of odontogenic sarcomas (937).

The term "ameloblastic sarcoma" is used as a collective name for AFS, AFDS, and AFOS (938); somewhat confusing it is also used as a synonym for AFS, mainly because some authors consider it unnecessary to subdifferentiate into variants without and with dental hard tissue. For therapeutic purposes there seems to be no reason for separating the three variants. Those containing hard dental tissue are extremely rare, and regarding clinical aspects, treatment, and prognosis they do not seem to differ significantly from the AFS. They do represent a higher level of histodifferentiation, though (937), which is the main reason for keeping the separate terms.

The ameloblastic sarcomas all contain benign odontogenic epithelium; they represent the malignant counterparts of the so-called mixed odontogenic tumors, which reflect the normal odontogenesis in the way that they contain odontogenic epithelium and odontogenic ectomesenchyme with mutual inductive effects similar to some of the interactions, which take place during normal odontogenesis. The AFS contains soft tissue exclusively; the ASDS contains additional hard tissue in terms of dentin or dentinoid, and the AFOS contains furthermore some enamel or enameloid.

A review of the literature of this group of tumors reveals a very inconsistent use of nomenclature; like lesions have been published under different terms.

2.1 Ameloblastic Fibrosarcoma

Introduction. AFS is an odontogenic tumor with a benign epithelial and a malignant ectomesenchymal component. The epithelial component is identical to that of the AMF, and the tumor is regarded as the malignant counterpart of the AMF (937,849). This malignant neoplasm may arise de novo or from a preexisting AMF.

ICD-O code 9330/3

Synonym: Ameloblastic sarcoma

Clinical Features. The tumor is rare; no data about prevalence and incidence are available. The relative frequency was indicated in a Chinese review (42) of cases received for diagnosis from 1952 to 2004; a total of 1642 odontogenic tumors were diagnosed; 50 cases were malignant (3.0%), 2 of these (0.1%) were AFS.

Detailed reviews of cases from the literature have been published by Leider et al. (939), Yamamoto et al. (940), Muller et al. (941), and Carlos-Bregni et al.

(942). The latter reviewed the literature and found 60 cases, including cases with formation of dentin/dentinoid and enamel/enameloid. They presented two cases, and since then three cases have been published (943–945). The total amount of published cases is thus about 66. In the review by Carlos-Bregni et al. (942) the gender was known in 60 cases, 37 (59.6%) were males and 23 (37.1%) were females, giving a male:female ratio of 1.6:1. The age range was 3 to 83 years for 62 cases, and the mean age at time of diagnosis was 27.3 years.

If the cases were divided in AFSs, which had arisen de novo (64.2%), and AFSs derived from malignant transformation of an AMF (35.8%), the mean age was 22.9 years for the former and 33.0 years for the latter group, this is a confirmation of the findings by Muller et al. (941).

The tumor was diagnosed in the mandible in 49 cases (79%) and in the maxilla in 13 cases (21%), with a ratio of about 5:1. The exact location was reported in 46 cases; the majority of the tumors were located in the posterior part of the mandible; 34 lesions were located in the mandible (32 posterior and 2 anterior), 9 were located in the maxilla, all in the posterior region.

A single case of peripheral AFS has been published (826). The diagnosis is controversial; the tumor was highly unusual; it developed in a recurrent PERAM in an 89-year-old man.

Various kinds of symptoms have been reported. Among the most constant findings are swelling and pain (938,939,941,946–949). Mobility of teeth was seen in some cases and paresthesia in a few cases (939,948). Growth may be rapid; some tumors have been more than 10 cm at longest diameter (942).

The potential for metastasis is low. It has been reported in one case (950) in which pleuropulmonary metastases and later hepatic metastases were diagnosed 10 years after the first symptoms of the tumor and without any local recurrence.

Imaging. Radiographically, a uni- or multilocular radiolucent area with indistinct margins is characteristic (Fig. 94). The margins may be partially distinct (951). Penetration of the cortex and extension into the surrounding soft tissue is not uncommon (467,939,952). Intralesional septa and periosteal new bone formation has been detected (951). Impaction of teeth has been described in several cases (942,951,953,954), and displacement of teeth is common (951,955–958); resorption of teeth has rarely been reported (959).

CT and MRI are important tools for evaluation of tumor extension and bone destruction (467,947,960).

Pathology. The etiology of the tumor is unknown. Pathogenetically it may develop de novo (958,961,962) or from malignant transformation of a preexisting AMF. About 36% of the reported AFSs developed from an AF, and the average age of these patients is higher (33.0 years) than that of patients with AFS, which arose de novo (22.9 years) (941,942).

Macroscopically, the tumor was described as tender but solid and whitish at the cut surface by Eda et al. (963), as tough and rubbery with some

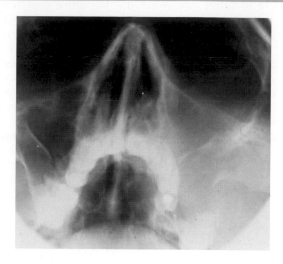

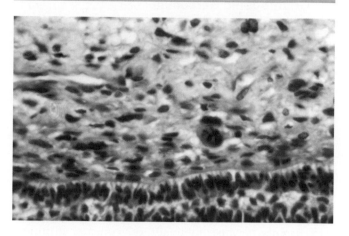

Figure 94 Ameloblastic fibrosarcoma in the maxilla of a 17-year-old man. The tumor involved the left maxillary sinus and the inferior part of the orbit. *Source*: From Ref. 955.

Figure 96 Ameloblastic fibrosarcoma. Higher magnification of the tumor seen in Figure 95. The highly differentiated odontogenic epithelium is seen below. The ectomesenchyme is the malignant component and exhibits pleomorphism and atypical mitosis. H&E stain.

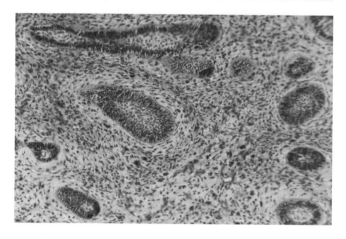

Figure 95 Ameloblastic fibrosarcoma. Section of the tumor shown in Figure 94. Islands of odontogenic epithelium without sign of malignancy are seen in a highly cellular ectomesenchyme with marked pleomorphism. H&E stain.

calcified spicules of bone by Dallera et al. (951), and as soft and pale with a few hemorrhagic areas by Yamamoto et al. (940).

The histomorphology of the AFS may resemble that of the AMF in many aspects (937,964,965). The tumor is composed by strands and slender branching cords of odontogenic epithelium with formation of buds imitating the formation of enamel organs from a dental lamina. No malignant features are detected in the epithelial component (Fig. 95). The basal cells are cubic or columnar with darkly stained nuclei, which are polarized away from the basement membrane when the basal cells are palisaded, columnar-shaped cells (Fig. 96). The epithelium also presents as small rounded or irregularly shaped islands with basal cells

of similar morphology and a central network of interconnected stellate-shaped cells with a clear or faintly stained, eosinophilic cytoplasm (Fig. 96). Mitoses are rare or nondetectable, the histomorphology of the epithelium may be indistinguishable from that of an AMF. The epithelium is growing in an abundant hypercellular ectomesenchymal tissue, which takes up about three-fourth of the tumor area (951). Cytological features of malignancy are found in this connective tissue, which shows a marked increase in cellularity. The cells are polygonal, rounded, or fusiform and closely packed. The cytoplasm is scanty, and the nuclei are hyperchromatic, and may show moderate variation in nuclear size and shape, but in some cases cellular and nuclear pleomorphism are prominent dominated by bizarre and hyperchromatic nuclei (Fig. 96). Mitoses are frequent and may be abnormal. In cases derived from AMFs (458,467,946,952,954, 957,966,967), areas without cytological features of malignancy may be found. Correct evaluation of the histology may require extensive sampling. Collagen may be seen in some areas, like in AMFs, but is usually only present in small amounts. The vascular component is inconspicuous. Variations in the cellularity may be seen. In some areas the greatest density of sarcomatous cells is seen in zones surrounding benign epithelial islands (964), but in other areas these zones may show conspicuously less cellular density than the main part of the tumor (937). AFS with areas with an Antoni A neurilemmoma-like pattern has been described (964), but the finding is quite unusual. Several authors have described a greater stromal cellularity and increased mitotic rate in recurrent tumors, and a decrease in the amount of the epithelial component, which after several recurrences may disappear completely (458,954,939,966).

Immunohistochemistry. Compared with other types of fibrosarcomas of the head and neck,

Chomette et al. (950) found a higher level of alkaline phosphatase and adenosinetriphosphatase (ATPase) in the ectomesenchymal tissue of three cases of AFS.

Several authors have detected CK in the epithelial component of the AFS (467,940,944,968). Yamamoto et al. (940) detected CK in the columnar and polyhedral cells of the ameloblastic epithelium. The intensity of the staining reaction was not uniform, and the polyhedral cells were more intensely stained. Lee et al. (944) found a positive immunoreactivity for pancytokeratin (AE1/AE3) in the ameloblastic epithelium, and Williams et al. (467) detected a uniformly positive reaction for pancytokeratin and CK-5 and CK-6 in the epithelial component in the benign areas of a recurrent AMF with malignant transformation. The reaction to CK-7, CK-19, and CAM 5.2 was negative.

Tajima et al. (968) found the epithelial cells of an AFS slightly positive to monoclonal EMA.

S-100 protein in AFS was investigated in two studies (944,968); both tumor component were negative.

Vimentin antibodies were used in two studies (940,944), the malignant fibroblastic spindle-shaped cells were positive in both investigations.

Fujita et al. (422) detected nestin in the ectomesenchymal tumor cells of two cases of AFS; the epithelium was negative. Nestin is an intermediate filament constituting the cytoskeleton, and is related to tooth development and repair of dentin; it is considered a useful marker for ectomesenchyme and odontoblasts in odontogenic tumors.

Lee et al. (944) detected CD34 in the malignant spindle-shaped cells in an AFS. The antigen is a transmembrane glycoprotein, which is considered a leukocyte antigen. It is usually found on the surface of some bone marrow and blood cells. They also used antibodies to CD117 and found all tumor cells to be negative in contrast to Williams et al. (467) who found that the sarcomatous component of a recurrent AMF with malignant transformation was strongly positive for c-KIT (CD117). No expression of the antigen was present in either the stroma or in the epithelial cells of the AMF areas. CD177 is a leukocyte differentiation antigen frequently found on early normal and leukemic hematopoietic cells.

The presence of p53 protein was investigated in three studies (943,467,969). They all detected the protein in the nuclei of the mesenchymal sarcomatous cells, but not in the epithelial cells and not in AMFs or the benign component of a recurrent AMF with malignant transformation (467). No overexpression of MDM2, a regulator of p53, was detected in either the benign or sarcomatous component.

Huguet et al. (969) used PCNA and Ki-67 in a study of AFS and AMF. The sarcomatous component of AFS was positive; AMFs were negative. Sano et al. (463) counted the L.I. of the monoclonal MIB-1 antibody in tissue from two AMFs, two AFODs, and one AFS. The antibody recognizes the epitope of Ki-67 antigen. Positive reaction for MIB-1 was observed in the nuclei of tumor cells in both the epithelial and mesenchymal components. The labeling indices were higher in the mesenchymal components than in epithelial ones in an AMF with late recurrence and in the

AFS. The highest label in the mesenchymal component was observed in the AFS. The authors concluded that the findings suggest that evaluation of the growth potential in AMFs and related lesions by means of proliferation-associated nuclear antigens could be of help in estimating the tumor's aggressiveness.

Electron Microscopy. The ultrastructure of the AFS have been described in several publications (940,946,949,950,963,970).

The epithelial nests were lined with columnar or more often cuboidal cells and had a core of stellate cells with large intercellular spaces; the cells were intermingled with epidermoid cells containing loosely arranged tonofilaments. On the whole these epithelial nests were poorly differentiated (950). Takeda et al. (946) found a stratum intermedium-like layer between the peripheral cells and the innermost cells. Various results have been reported from the study of the cytoplasm of the peripheral cells. According to Chomette et al. (950) the peripheral cells contained few organelles, they detected some mitochondriae, rare lysosomal bodies, poorly developed rough endoplasmatic reticulum and Golgi apparatus. Eda et al. (963) on the contrary found many organelles in the peripheral cells. Glycogen granules and tonofilaments were generally well preserved. A basal lamina around the peripheral cells was clearly seen. Their case contained minor areas of primitive dentin and enamel.

The malignant tumor cells of the ectomesenchymal connective tissue have been described by Chomette et al. (950) and Yamamota et al. (940). The latter described spindle-shaped fibroblasts with large irregularly shaped nuclei with one, two, or more nuclei and a variable amount of chromatin. Mitotic figures were present. In some cells bizarre mitochondria were observed and the Golgi fields were well preserved. A dilated smooth and rough endoplasmic reticulum could be detected, as well as glycogen granules. Polyribosomes were scattered throughout the cytoplasm. Collagen was relatively scarce in the matrix. Chomette et al. (950) detected various cell types in the connective tumor tissue. Closely packed clear round cells with numerous delicate, short filaments were detected, as well as more differentiated oval or spindle-shaped cells with well developed Golgi-apparatus and secretory vacuoles. Numerous microfilaments were present parallel to the plasmatic membrane. Other cells were of the granular type, they contained a vast number of osmiophilic heterophagosomes. Some well-differentiated fibroblasts and myofibroblastic cells with distinct myofilaments could also be identified.

Molecular-Genetic Data. Muller et al. (941) compared nuclear DNA content of five AFSs and three AMFs by image analysis of Feulgen stained nuclei by means of an image cytometer. A DNA index was generated for each tumor. The three AMFs were diploid, whereas 1 of 5 AFSs was aneuploid. There was no correlation between aneuploidy and the histological grade of malignancy. Williams et al. (467) analyzed an anaplastic AFS for genetic mutations in exons 9, 11, 13, and 17 of the c-KIT gene; a proto-oncogene located in chromosome 4, but found no mutations.

Differential Diagnosis.   The differentiation of an AFS from an AMF with high cellularity and presence of mitoses may be a difficult decision. Mitosis may occur in the epithelium and in the ectomesenchymal tissue of an AMF, but should be normal. More than a few mitoses and any atypia seen should provoke the suspicion of malignancy in the appropriate clinical setting (54). The patient's age may be taken in consideration as well, AMFs rarely occurs in patients older than 30 years. After recurrence, in particular multiple recurrences, the epithelial component of the tumor may decrease or disappear so traces of the odontogenic origin may eventually be lost (939,954,962); such cases risk to be diagnosed as conventional fibrosarcomas, unless the pathologist had access to sections of the tumor from earlier operations.

Treatment and Prognosis.   The AFS is a highly locally aggressive neoplasm with a very low potential for distant metastasis (937), only one of the published cases has been reported to metastasize (950). Lymph node metastases with histological documentation have not been reported (941), and are rare in any type of sarcoma of the head and neck (971). En bloc resection with wide margins and follow-up for at least 10 years is the recommended treatment. Postsurgical radiotherapy (952) or adjuvant chemotherapy has been used in some cases. Goldstein et al. (966) reported curative effects) from the use of Actinomycin D, Vincristine, and Cytoxane. Others have reported unsatisfactory results from the use of chemotherapy (947); chemotherapy may be indicated as an adjuvant with radiotherapy to surgical resection, where a wide margin of resection is difficult to achieve (971).

The prognosis for the AFS is apparently better than for other fibrosarcomas of the orofacial region, but recurrences are common. One, two, three, or multiple recurrences were reported in 20 of 49 cases reviewed by Muller et al. (941), and 20.4% of the patients with AFS died within 2 to 19 years. Takeda et al. (946) reviewed eight fatal cases, where the patients died from uncontrollable local infiltration.

2.2   *Ameloblastic Fibrodentino- and Fibro-Odontosarcoma*

Introduction.   The AFDS and the AFOS combine the histological features of AFS with dysplastic dentin (AFDS) and dentin or dentinoid together with enamel or enameloid (AFOS) (937).

ICD-O code 9290/3

Synonyms: Ameloblastic dentinosarcoma; ameloblastic odontosarcoma; ameloblastic sarcoma; odontogenic sarcoma.

Some have found the terms disturbing (964) since "ameloblastic odontosarcoma" evokes the notion of a "malignant tooth." The term is based on the knowledge that some of the tumors have developed from malignant transformation of an AFOD (950,480,501).

Clinical Features.   The tumors are exceedingly rare, and the exact amount of published cases is difficult to estimate because of inconsequent use of nomenclature. Some authors find it unnecessary to distinguish these tumors from the AFS (54,941,951,964,968,972). Cases of AFDS and AFOS (950,956) have thus been published under the term "AFS" or "ameloblastic sarcoma," and a case, which contained dentinoid, but no enamel, has been published as an ameloblastic odontosarcoma (973). According to Carlos et al., (937) 14 cases of these tumors were published before 2003; nine cases occurred in men and four in women. The age range was 12 to 83 years, with a peak in the third decade. Most of the cases have been found in the mandible. The clinical findings have been similar to those present in the AFS, swelling and pain being the most common symptoms, and sometimes mobility of teeth.

Imaging.   In the majority of cases the amount of dental hard tissue in the tumor is so limited that it does not show on a radiogram. In cases of AFOS developed in an AFOD (950,480,501), the dentin and enamel produced by the benign tumor before the malignant transformation will be detectable on the radiogram. The use of CT and MRI increases the information about the borders of the tumor considerably.

Pathology.   The etiology is unknown.

The resection specimens are usually large. Macroscopically, Forman et al. (956) described the tumor as fleshy and lobulated; the cut surface had a firm gelatinous appearance.

The major part of the tumor is histomorphologically indistinguishable from an AFS. In the AFDS scattered areas of dentinoid is found; such cases have been reported and well illustrated by Tahsinoglu et al. (974) [supplementary illustrated in *Thoma's Oral Pathology* (63)], Altini et al. (972), and Altini et al. (938). Eosinophilic hyalinized zones in the connective tissue without a cellular border, seen around the epithelial islands, are not regarded as dentinoid (938). Areas of benign ectomesenchymal tissue may be present (938,972), suggesting malignant development in an AMF or an AFD. The formation of dentinoid and dentin is dependent on complex interchange of signals and substances between the odontogenic epithelium and the odontogenic ectomesenchyme (975,976). The gene expressions necessary for this process seems conserved to some degree in these sarcomas, since the dentinoid can be found in areas with conspicuous polymorphism in the ectomesenchyme. Cases compatible with the definition of an AFOS have been reported by Chibret (977), the clinical features were described by Polaillon (978); and by Forman et al. (956), Eda et al. (963), Howell et al. (480), Chomette et al. (950), Takeda et al. (979), and Herzog et al. (501). In nearly all cases the amount of dentin and enamel has been very limited (963), and rather (Figs. 97, 98) dentinoid and enameloid (501,979,980). In Chibret's case though, formation of canalicular dentin was reported.

Immunohistochemistry.   Nagatsuka (75) included a case of AFOS in a study of differential expression of collagen IV α1 to α6 chains in basement membranes of benign and malignant odontogenic tumors. A moderate immunoreactivity of α1(IV)/α2 (IV) and α4(IV) chains was found along the basement membrane of ameloblastic epithelium. Chains of α5 (IV)/α6(IV) were strongly codistributed as continuous

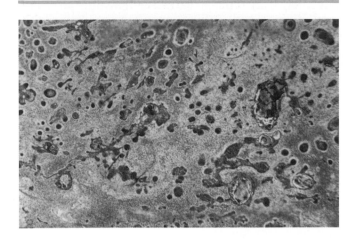

Figure 97 Ameloblastic fibro-odontosarcoma. The section is from the third recurrence of a tumor, which occupied the entire right mandible in a 21-year-old man. The histology in this area of the tumor is similar to that of an ameloblastic fibrosarcoma. H&E stain. *Source*: Section by courtesy of Dr. J. Payen, Paris.

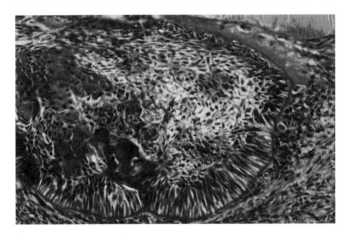

Figure 98 Ameloblastic fibro-odontosarcoma. Higher magnification of the tumor seen in Figure 97. Dentin and dentinoid is seen in the upper right corner, and dysplastic enamel is seen adjacent to the ameloblasts in the lower part of the epithelial island. H&E stain. *Source*: Section by courtesy of Dr. J. Payen, Paris.

linear patterns demarcating the benign epithelial tumor nests from the surrounding sarcomatous stroma. These α(IV) chains also randomly stained the tumoral and stromal cells. In the inductive dental hard tissue areas; no reactivity was found.

Electron Microscopy. Eda et al. published an ultrastructural study of a case of AFOS, but concentrated on the soft parts of the tumor, which showed changes similar to those described for the AFS apart from a higher concentration of organelles in the peripheral cells of the epithelial islands (950).

Molecular-Genetic Data. No data are published.

Differential Diagnosis. The amount of dental hard tissue in AFDS and AFOS is usually scarce, so its detection may depend on extensive sampling from a large tumor. It has no therapeutic consequences, however, to diagnose an AFDS or an AFOS as an AFS, which is the main argument for using the common diagnosis "ameloblastic sarcomas" for all three tumors. As it is the case with the AFS, the most difficult diagnostic problem is to decide if a large, fast-growing highly cellular AFDS or AFOS show histomorphological signs of malignancy. Any signs of pleomorphism and the presence of more than a limited amount of mitotic figures should be regarded as signs of malignant transformation in the appropriate clinical settings.

Treatment and Prognosis. The AFDS and the AFOS are highly locally aggressive neoplasms with a very low potential for distant metastases and should be treated with wide margin en bloc resections. In cases where complete surgical removal is impossible, adjuvant radiotherapy is indicated, but may not be curative as reported by Howell et al. (480) (case 1). In another case (case 2) reported by Howell et al. (480) an adjuvant-combined chemotherapeutic regimen of Cytoxan, Actinomycin, and Vincristine gave a favorable result.

The prognosis is difficult to assess. The two cases of AFDS reported by Altini et al. (1976 and 1985) (938,972) were cured after resection, but the follow-up time was short. In the case of AFOS (case 1) and in two other reported cases the patients were cured after hemimandibulectomy (956,963), but the follow-up time was relatively short.

A long-time follow-up is indicated, as clearly illustrated by the case of Herzog et al. (501). A 14-year-old girl had an AFOD removed from the angle of the left side of the mandible by means of curettage. The tumor recurred five years later, and was again treated by curettage. Twelve years after the first symptoms, the tumor recurred again and microscopy showed an AFDS. It had invaded the adjacent soft tissue, including the parotic gland. It was treated by extensive surgery and Cobalt 60. Two years later metastases to lymphnodes in the neck were diagnosed.

2.3 Odontogenic Fibrosarcoma

As pointed out by Slater (964) the cases reported as AFS by Tajima et al. (968) and by DeNittis et al. (960) contained slender cords of odontogenic epithelium more closely resembling those seen in odontogenic fibroma than those in AMF (454,687). Both tumors were fibrosarcoma de novo and both were characterized by short collagenous fibers and did not resemble the embryonic pulp-like tissue, which is typical for AMFs. They were both highly cellular with conspicuous pleomorphism and numerous mitoses. One of them contained some dentinoid or rather cementoid (968). Chan et al. (981) reported a case of COF in the premolar region of the mandible of a 34-year-old man. Radical resection was not possible for cardiac reasons, the tumor was enucleated and recurred 10 months later. It was now diagnosed as a low-grade odontogenic fibrosarcoma. A second recurrence was diagnosed 15 months later, and a hemimandibulectomy was performed. The mesenchyme was unchanged, the odontogenic epithelium had disappeared. There were no symptoms till eight years later when a lung metastasis measuring 60 mm was diagnosed. Chemotherapy was used without response. The patient died 20 months later from brain metastasis and hemoptysis. The authors recommended chest X rays every six months for prolonged periods of time after initial surgical resection.

The tumor reported by Tajima et al. (968) occurred in the right maxillary molar region of a 14-year-old male. Hemimaxillectomy was performed; the tumor recurred two months later with involvement of the maxillary sinus and with subsequent invasion of the orbital base. The patient died six months after the operation. Immunohistochemistry was done on sections from the operation specimen. The odontogenic epithelium reacted strongly to antibodies against wide spectrum CKs, and faintly to EMA. The sarcomatous cells reacted strongly to vimentin, but were negative to desmin, smooth muscle actin, neurofilament, and S-100 protein.

The case reported by DeNittis et al. (960) was a tumor in the molar area of the maxilla in a 32-year-old man; it had eroded the bone and infiltrated the adjacent soft tissues. An extended maxillectomy was done, which removed all tumor tissue except for a focus in the right nasopharynx penetrating bone. Adjuvant radiation therapy was given. The patient was tumor free at control six months later. No information was given about follow-up.

These tumors should be called odontogenic fibrosarcomas rather than AFSs. Although the number of cases is too limited for conclusions, they seem to be more aggressive than the AFSs.

The odontogenic fibrosarcomas were not classified in the 2005 WHO classification of tumors of the head and neck (982).

2.4 Odontogenic Myxosarcoma

Very few cases of odontogenic myxosarcomas have been published (760–762). Lamberg et al. (761) reported a maxillary myxoma in a 40-year-old man, which recurred three weeks after surgery. The tumor had infiltrated the adjacent soft tissues. Repeated biopsy as well as reassessment of the removed tumor lead to the diagnosis myxosarcoma. Microscopy showed a tumor composed of plump, pleomorphic, stellate cells with bizarre mitotic figures surrounded by an amorphic myxoid matrix. Electron microscopy showed that the tumor cells were similar to fibroblasts. Radiotherapy was unsuccessful, so the left part of the maxilla was removed with orbital excenteration. The patient died accidentally three years later. At autopsy no signs of recurrence or metastasis were found.

The tumor reported by Pahl et al. (762) was an ODOMYX with an aggressive clinical course, which developed in the maxilla of a 53-year-old man. Nuclear MRI was used to determine the extension of the tumor, which invaded the sinuses and the nasal cavity. The tumor recurred twice after extended maxillectomy and

ultimately caused the patient's death by uncontrollable local disease with infiltration of the cranial cavity. Microscopy showed a low grade myxosarcoma. A cytogenic analysis revealed an unexpectedly aberrant hypertetraploid chromosome complement, which was considered as incompatible with the usual karyotypic patterns of benign tumors.

Mlosek et al. (760) described sarcomatous changes in ODOMYX in two cases that resulted in death.

3. Odontogenic Carcinosarcoma

The odontogenic carcinosarcoma (ODCASA) was defined in the second edition of the WHO "Histological Typing of Odontogenic Tumours" (23) as "a very rare neoplasm, similar in pattern to AFS, but in which both the epithelial and the ectomesenchymal components show cytological features of malignancy." The entity was not included in the year 2005 edition of the WHO classification of head and neck tumors (12) because of the paucity of published cases and because of controversial opinions regarding the definition of the tumor (831,964,983).

Three acceptable cases have been published (964,980,984).

Phillips et al. (980) reported a case in a 29-year-old man. Ten months after the removal of an inflamed partly unerupted lower left third molar the patient presented with a fast growing, large, firm swelling extending from the lower left first molar to the coronoid process of the left mandible. The radiogram showed a radiolucency, which was scalloped and multilocular, relatively well circumscribed from the first molar and into the ramus. There was erosion of the base of the mandible and both the facial and the lingual plate. The left part of the mandible from the premolar area to the condyle was resected. The follow-up time was 13 months without sign of recurrence or metastasis. Microscopy showed a neoplasm with a histomorphology compatible with an AFOS, with small areas of dysplastic dentin and enamel. In some areas the odontogenic epithelium was pleomorphic, showed hyperchromatic nuclei, and mitotic figures.

The case reported by Slater (964) was a 55-year-old man with an $8 \times 6.2 \times 5$ cm large tumor in the right mandibular body and ramus. A hemimandibulectomy was done. There was no follow-up information. Microscopically, the tumor showed at low magnification architecture similar to a cell-rich AMF. At higher magnification the ectomesenchyme presented signs of sarcoma with closely packed mitotically active polygonal cells showing hyperchromatic nuclei and moderate nuclear polymorphism. The ameloblastic epithelial component showed epithelial dysplasia with peripheral large cells with crowded large hyperchromatic nuclei and mitotic figures. The central stellate reticulum showed high cellularity and plump cells.

Kunkel et al. (984) reported a tumor in the right posterior mandible of a 52-year-old man with a large swelling in the retromolar area and numbness of the right lower lip. There was no regional lymphadenopathy. Radiography showed an ill-defined radiolucency extending from the third molar to the coronoid process. A segmental resection of the mandible including adjacent soft tissue was performed. All margins were free of tumor. Two years later local recurrence occurred with infiltration of the condyle and the parotic gland. A second extensive resection was done. Three years later a second recurrence was diagnosed. The patient was treated with extended surgery, including exenteration of the infratemporal fossa and the pterigoid region, resection of the zygomatic arch, the lateral zygoma, and the infiltrated skin area. Twelve months later mediastinal and pulmonary metastases were diagnosed, but there was no local recurrence. Chemotherapy involving Adriamycin and Ifosmamid gave no response. Temporary reduction of pulmonary mass was recognized on administration of Etoposide and Cisplatin. After further spread of metastases to ribs and pelvis and development of an acute myelocytic leukemia the patient died 64 months after the initial surgical treatment. Sections from primary tumor and the first and second recurrence showed well-demarcated islands and cords of malignant epithelial cells embedded in hypercellular mesenchymal tissue with pleomorphic cells. Similar changes were found in the metastasis from the lung. The epithelium stained positively for CK-5, CK-6, CK-8, and CK-17 and the mesenchymal component reacted strongly to vimentin antibodies. A Ki-67 labeling indicated a high proportion of proliferating cells in both of the tumor components.

It is unknown if the primary tumor had an architecture similar to an AFS, it was neither described nor illustrated, but it seams reasonable to classify an odontogenic tumor consisting of malignant ameloblastic epithelium and malignant ectomesenchyme as an ODCASA.

Two cases have been published as ODCASA, which are better classified as biphasic AMCAs (985,986). None of these showed an AFS-like pattern, they consisted of an epithelial component resembling an AMCA and a sarcomatous component of spindle cells, which is sometimes seen in biphasic AMCAs. No immunohistochemical stainings for CK and vimentin to determine the nature of the tumor cells were done in the two cases. These stainings are mandatory for the differential diagnosis.

REFERENCES

1. Pflüger H, Schürmann P. Die Hypophysengangsgeschwülste und die Tumoren des zahnbildenden Gewebes, ihre Verwandtschaft im morphologischen Bild und ihrer Genese. In: Schürmann P, Pflüger H, Norrenbrock W, eds. Die Histogenese Ekto-Mesodermaler Mischgeschwülste der Mundhöhle. Ein Beitrag zur Frage der Organisatorenwirkung (Spemann) beim pathologischen Wachstum. Leipzig: Georg Thieme Verlag, 1931:1–62.
2. Kalnins V, Rossi E. Odontogenic craniopharyngioma: A case report. Cancer 1965; 18:899–906.
3. Bernstein ML, Buchino JJ. The histologic similarity between craniopharyngioma and odontogenic lesions: a reappraisal. Oral Surg Oral Med Oral Pathol 1983; 56(5):502–511.
4. Paulus W, Stöckel C, Krauss J, et al. Odontogenic classification of craniopharyngiomas: a clinicopathological study of 54 cases. Histopathology 1997; 30(2):172–176.
5. Kumamoto H. Molecular pathology of odontogenic tumors. J Oral Pathol Med 2006; 35(2):65–74.
6. Rivenson A, Mu B, Silverman J, et al. Chemically induced rat odontomas: morphogenetic considerations. Cancer Detect Prev 1984; 7(4):293–298.
7. Ida-Yonemochi H, Noda T, Shimokawa H, et al. Disturbed tooth eruption in osteopetrotic (op/op) mice: histopathogenesis of tooth malformation and odontomas. J Oral Pathol Med 2002, 31(6):361–373.
8. Gardner DG. Experimentally induced ameloblastomas: a critical review. J Oral Pathol Med 1992; 21(8):337–339.
9. Gorlin RJ, Chaudhry AP, Pindborg JJ. Odontogenic tumors. Classification, histopathology, and clinical behavior in man and domesticated animals. Cancer 1961; 14:73–101.
10. Baden E. Odontogenic tumors. Pathol Annu 1971; 6: 475–568.
11. Philipsen HP, Reichart PA. Classification of odontogenic tumours. A historical review. J Oral Pathol Med 2006; 35(9):525–529.
12. Barnes L, Eveson JW, Reichart P, et al. eds. World Health Organization Classification of Tumours. Pathology and Genetics of Head and Neck Tumours. Lyon: IARC Press, 2005:1–430.
13. Eversole LR, Tomich CE, Cherrick HM. Histogenesis of odontogenic tumors. Oral Surg Oral Med Oral Pathol 1971, 32(4):569–581.
14. Stoelinga PJ. Studies on the dental lamina as related to its role in the etiology of cysts and tumors. J Oral Pathol 1976, 5(2):65–73.
15. Gardner DG. The concept of hamartomas: its relevance to the pathogenesis of odontogenic lesions. Oral Surg Oral Med Oral Pathol 1978; 45(6):884–886.
16. Philipsen HP, Reichart PA. The development and fate of epithelial residues after completion of the human odontogenesis with special reference to the origins of epithelial odontogenic neoplasms, hamartomas and cysts. Oral Biosci Med 2004; 1(3):171–179.
17. Ide F, Obara K, Yamada H, et al. Hamartomatous proliferations of odontogenic epithelium within the jaws: a potential histogenetic source of intraosseous epithelial odontogenic tumors. J Oral Pathol Med 2007; 36(4): 229–235.
18. Garant PR. Early tooth development. Oral Cells and Tissues. Chicago: Quintessence Publishing Co, Inc, 2003: 1–23.
19. Thesleff I, Hurmerinta K. Tissue interactions in tooth development. Differentiation 1981; 18(2):75–88.
20. Peters H, Balling R. Teeth. Where and how to make them. Trends Genet 1999; 15(2):59–65.
21. Cobourne MT, Sharpe PT. Tooth and jaw: molecular mechanisms of patterning in the first branchial arch. Arch Oral Biol 2003; 48(1):1–14.
22. Pindborg JJ, Kramer IRH. Histological Typing of Odontogenic Tumours, Jaw Cysts, and Allied Lesions. Geneva: World Health Organization, 1971.
23. Kramer IRH, Pindborg JJ, Shear M. Histological Typing of Odontogenic Tumours. Second edition ed. Berlin: Springer-Verlag, 1992:1–118.
24. Sciubba JJ, Fantasia JE, Kahn LB. Tumors and Cysts of the Jaws. Third Series ed. Washington, D.C.: Armed Forces Institute of Pathology, 2001:1–275.
25. Reichart PA, Philipsen HP. Odontogenic Tumors and Allied Lesions. London: Quintessence Publishing Co Ltd, 2004:1–387.
26. Gardner DG, Heikinheimo K, Shear M, et al. Ameloblastomas. In: Barnes L, Eveson JW, Reichart P, et al. eds. World Health Organization Classification of Tumours. Pathology and Genetics of Head and Neck Tumours. Lyon: IARC Press, 2005:296–300.

27. Shear M, Singh S. Age-standardized incidence rates of ameloblastoma and dentigerous cyst on the Witwatersrand, South Africa. Community Dent Oral Epidemiol 1978; 6(4):195–199.

28. Gardner DG. Critique of the 1995 review by Reichart et al. of the biologic profile of 3677 ameloblastomas. Oral Oncol 1999; 35(4):443–449.

29. Larsson Å, Almeren H. Ameloblastoma of the jaws. An analysis of a consecutive series of all cases reported to the Swedish Cancer Registry during 1958–1971. Acta Pathol Microbiol Scand [A] 1978; 86A(5):337–349.

30. Buchner A, Merrell PW, Carpenter WM. Relative frequency of central odontogenic tumors: a study of 1,088 cases from Northern California and comparison to studies from other parts of the world. J Oral Maxillofac Surg 2006; 64(9): 1343–1352.

31. Regezi JA, Kerr DA, Courtney RM. Odontogenic tumors: analysis of 706 cases. J Oral Surg 1978; 36(10):771–778.

32. Günhan Ö, Erseven G, Ruacan S, et al. Odontogenic tumours. A series of 409 cases. Aust Dent J 1990; 35(6):518–522.

33. Daley TD, Wysocki GP, Pringle GA. Relative incidence of odontogenic tumors and oral and jaw cysts in a Canadian population. Oral Surg Oral Med Oral Pathol 1994; 77(3):276–280.

34. Mosqueda-Taylor A, Ledesma-Montes C, Caballero-Sandoval S, et al. Odontogenic tumors in Mexico: a collaborative retrospective study of 349 cases. Oral Surg Oral Med Oral Pathol Oral Radiol Endod 1997; 84(6): 672–675.

35. Ochsenius G, Ortega A, Godoy L, et al. Odontogenic tumors in Chile: a study of 362 cases. J Oral Pathol Med 2002; 31(7):415–420.

36. Adebayo ET, Ajike SO, Adekeye EO. A review of 318 odontogenic tumors in Kaduna, Nigeria. J Oral Maxillofac Surg 2005; 63(6):811–819.

37. Fernandes AM, Duarte EC, Pimenta FJ, et al. Odontogenic tumors: a study of 340 cases in a Brazilian population. J Oral Pathol Med 2005; 34(10):583–587.

38. Ladeinde AL, Ajayi OF, Ogunlewe MO, et al. Odontogenic tumors: a review of 319 cases in a Nigerian teaching hospital. Oral Surg Oral Med Oral Pathol Oral Radiol Endod 2005; 99(2):191–195.

39. Jones AV, Franklin CD. An analysis of oral and maxillofacial pathology found in children over a 30-year period. Int J Paediatr Dent 2006; 16(1):19–30.

40. Jones AV, Franklin CD. An analysis of oral and maxillofacial pathology found in adults over a 30-year period. J Oral Pathol Med 2006, 35(7):392–401.

41. Olgac V, Koseoglu BG, Aksakalli N. Odontogenic tumours in Istanbul: 527 cases. Br J Oral Maxillofac Surg 2006; 44(5):386–388.

42. Jing W, Xuan M, Lin Y, et al. Odontogenic tumours: a retrospective study of 1642 cases in a Chinese population. Int J Oral Maxillofac Surg 2007; 36(1):20–25.

43. Reichart PA, Philipsen HP, Sonner S. Ameloblastoma: biological profile of 3677 cases. Eur J Cancer B Oral Oncol 1995; 31B(2):86–99.

44. Ledesma-Montes C, Mosqueda-Taylor A, Carlos-Bregni R, et al. Ameloblastomas: a regional Latin-American multicentric study. Oral Dis 2007; 13:303–307.

45. Ord RA, Blanchaert RH Jr., Nikitakis NG, et al. Ameloblastoma in children. J Oral Maxillofac Surg 2002; 60(7):762–770.

46. Arotiba GT, Ladeinde AL, Arotiba JT, et al. Ameloblastoma in Nigerian children and adolescents: a review of 79 cases. J Oral Maxillofac Surg 2005; 63(6):747–751.

47. Carlson ER, Marx RE. The ameloblastoma: primary, curative surgical management. J Oral Maxillofac Surg 2006; 64(3):484–494.

48. Ueno S, Nakamura S, Mushimoto K, et al. A clinicopathologic study of ameloblastoma. J Oral Maxillofac Surg 1986; 44(5):361–365.

49. van Rensburg LJ, Thompson IO, Kruger HE, et al. Hemangiomatous ameloblastoma: Clinical, radiologic, and pathologic features. Oral Surg Oral Med Oral Pathol Oral Radiol Endod 2001; 91(3):374–380.

50. Asaumi J, Hisatomi M, Yanagi Y, et al. Assessment of ameloblastomas using MRI and dynamic contrast-enhanced MRI. Eur J Radiol 2005; 56(1):25–30.

51. Quinn JH, Fullmer HM. A small ameloblastoma of the mandible. Oral Surg Oral Med Oral Pathol 1953; 6(8): 949–952.

52. Motamedi MH. Periapical ameloblastoma–a case report. Br Dent J 2002; 193(8):443–445.

53. Heikinheimo K, Hormia M, Stenman G, et al. Patterns of expression of intermediate filaments in ameloblastoma and human fetal tooth germ. J Oral Pathol Med 1989; 18(5):264–273.

54. Odell EW, Morgan PR. Odontogenic tumours. In: Biopsy Pathology of the Oral Tissues. London: Chapman & Hall Medical, 1998:365–439.

55. Hong J, Yun PY, Chung IH, et al. Long-term follow up on recurrence of 305 ameloblastoma cases. Int J Oral Maxillofac Surg 2007; 36:283–288.

56. Pindborg JJ, Weinmann JP. Squamous cell metaplasia with calcification in ameloblastomas. Acta Pathol Microbiol Scand 1958; 44(3):247–252.

57. Altini M, Hille JJ, Buchner A. Plexiform granular cell odontogenic tumor. Oral Surg Oral Med Oral Pathol 1986; 61(2):163–167.

58. Siar CH, Ng KH. Unusual granular cell odontogenic tumor. Report of two undescribed cases with features of granular cell ameloblastoma and plexiform granular cell odontogenic tumor. J Nihon Univ Sch Dent 1993; 35(2): 134–138.

59. Hartman KS. Granular-cell ameloblastoma. Oral Surg Oral Med Oral Pathol 1974; 38(2):241–253.

60. Raubenheimer EJ, van Heerden WF, Noffke CE. Infrequent clinicopathological findings in 108 ameloblastomas. J Oral Pathol Med 1995; 24(5):227–232.

61. Wilson D, Walker M, Aurora N, et al. Ameloblastoma with mucous cell differentiation. Oral Surg Oral Med Oral Pathol Oral Radiol Endod 2001; 91(5):576–578.

62. Ide F, Tanaka A, Kitada M, et al. Histopathology of ameloblastomas with emphasis on infrequent features. Hospital Dentistry & Oral-Maxillofacial Surgery (Tokyo) 2001, 13(2):93–97.

63. Gorlin RJ. Odontogenic tumors. In: Gorlin RJ, Goldman HM, eds. Thoma's Oral pathology. St. Louis: The C. V. Mosby Company, 1970:481–515.

64. Müller H, Slootweg PJ. The growth characteristics of multilocular ameloblastomas. A histological investigation with some inferences with regard to operative procedures. J Maxillofac Surg 1985; 13(5):224–230.

65. Gortzak RA, Latief BS, Lekkas C, et al. Growth characteristics of large mandibular ameloblastomas: report of 5 cases with implications for the approach to surgery. Int J Oral Maxillofac Surg 2006; 35(8):691–695.

66. Crivelini MM, de Araujo V, de Sousa SO, et al. Cytokeratins in epithelia of odontogenic neoplasms. Oral Dis 2003; 9(1):1–6.

67. Ito Y, Abiko Y, Tanaka Y, et al. Immunohistochemical localization of large chondroitin sulfate proteoglycan in odontogenic tumor. Med Electron Microsc 2002; 35(3):173–177.

68. Heikinheimo K, Morgan PR, Happonen RP, et al. Distribution of extracellular matrix proteins in odontogenic tumours and developing teeth. Virchows Arch B Cell Pathol Incl Mol Pathol 1991; 61(2):101–109.

69. Nagai N, Yamachika E, Nishijima K, et al. Immunohistochemical demonstration of tenascin and fibronectin in odontogenic tumours and human fetal tooth germs. Eur J Cancer B Oral Oncol 1994; 30B(3):191–195.

70. Mori M, Yamada T, Doi T, et al. Expression of tenascin in odontogenic tumours. Eur J Cancer B Oral Oncol 1995; 31B(4):275–279.

71. Nadimi H, Toto PD. Product identification of ameloblastomas: an immunohistochemical study. J Oral Pathol 1986; 15(8):439–444.

72. Parikka M, Kainulainen T, Tasanen K, et al. Altered expression of collagen XVII in ameloblastomas and basal cell carcinomas. J Oral Pathol Med 2001; 30(10): 589–595.

73. Poomsawat S, Punyasingh J, Vejchapipat P. Expression of basement membrane components in odontogenic tumors. Oral Surg Oral Med Oral Pathol Oral Radiol Endod 2007; 104(5):666–675.

74. Nakano K, Siar CH, Nagai N, et al. Distribution of basement membrane type IV collagen alpha chains in ameloblastoma: an immunofluorescense study. J Oral Pathol Med 2002; 31(8):494–499.

75. Nagatsuka H, Siar CH, Nakano K, et al. Differential expression of collagen IV alpha1 to alpha6 chains in basement membranes of benign and malignant odontogenic tumors. Virchows Arch 2002; 441(4):392–399.

76. Souza Andrade ES, da Costa Miguel MC, Pinto LP, et al. Ameloblastoma and adenomatoid odontogenic tumor: the role of alpha2beta1, alpha3beta1, and alpha5beta1 integrins in local invasiveness and architectural characteristics. Ann Diagn Pathol 2007; 11(3):199–205.

77. Ida-Yonemochi H, Ikarashi T, Nagata M, et al. The basement membrane-type heparan sulfate proteoglycan (perlecan) in ameloblastomas: its intercellular localization in stellate reticulum-like foci and biosynthesis by tumor cells in culture. Virchows Arch 2002; 441(2):165–173.

78. Kumamoto H, Ooya K. Immunohistochemical detection of phosphorylated JNK, p38 MAPK, and ERK5 in ameloblastic tumors. J Oral Pathol Med 2007; 36(9):543–549.

79. Kim J, Yook JI. Immunohistochemical study on proliferating cell nuclear antigen expression in ameloblastomas. Eur J Cancer B Oral Oncol 1994; 30B(2):126–131.

80. Funaoka K, Arisue M, Kobayashi I, et al. Immunohistochemical detection of proliferating cell nuclear antigen (PCNA) in 23 cases of ameloblastoma. Eur J Cancer B Oral Oncol 1996; 32B(5):328–332.

81. Ong'uti MN, Cruchley AT, Howells GL, et al. Ki-67 antigen in ameloblastomas: correlation with clinical and histological parameters in 54 cases from Kenya. Int J Oral Maxillofac Surg 1997; 26(5):376–379.

82. Piattelli A, Fioroni M, Santinelli A, et al. Expression of proliferating cell nuclear antigen in ameloblastomas and odontogenic cysts. Oral Oncol 1998; 34(5):408–412.

83. Sandra F, Mitsuyasu T, Nakamura N, et al. Immunohistochemical evaluation of PCNA and Ki-67 in ameloblastoma. Oral Oncol 2001; 37(2):193–198.

84. Meer S, Galpin JS, Altini M, et al. Proliferating cell nuclear antigen and Ki67 immunoreactivity in ameloblastomas. Oral Surg Oral Med Oral Pathol Oral Radiol Endod 2003; 95(2):213–221.

85. Thosaporn W, Iamaroon A, Pongsiriwet S, et al. A comparative study of epithelial cell proliferation between the odontogenic keratocyst, orthokeratinized odontogenic cyst, dentigerous cyst, and ameloblastoma. Oral Dis 2004; 10(1):22–26.

86. Payeras MR, Sant'Ana Filho M, Lauxen IS, et al. Quantitative analysis of argyrophilic nucleolar organizer regions and epidermal growth factor receptor in ameloblastomas. J Oral Pathol Med 2007; 36:99–104.

87. Kumamoto H, Ooya K. Immunohistochemical and ultrastructural investigation of apoptotic cell death in granular cell ameloblastoma. J Oral Pathol Med 2001; 30(4): 245–250.

88. Moe H, Clausen F, Philipsen HP. The ultrastructure of the simple ameloblastoma. Acta Pathol Microbiol Scand 1961; 52:140–154.

89. Sujaku C, Oo T, Tokoshima A, et al. Electron microscopic observations on the ameloblastoma. Kurume Med J 1968; 15(3):127–136.

90. Csiba A, Okros I, Dzsinich C, et al. Virus-like particles in a human ameloblastoma. Arch Oral Biol 1970; 15(9):817–826.

91. Navarrette AR, Smith M. Ultrastructure of granular cell ameloblastoma. Cancer 1971; 27(4):948–955.

92. Lee KW, el-Labban NG, Kramer IR. Ultrastructure of a simple ameloblastoma. J Pathol 1972; 108(2):173–176.

93. Mincer HH, McGinnis JP. Ultrastructure of three histologic variants of the ameloblastoma. Cancer 1972; 30(4): 1036–1045.

94. Cutler LS. Intracytoplasmic desmosomes in human oral neoplasms. Arch Oral Biol 1976; 21(4):221–226.

95. Tandler B, Rossi EP. Granular cell ameloblastoma: electron microscopic observations. J Oral Pathol 1977; 6(6): 401–412.

96. Kim SK, Nasjleti CE, Weatherbee L. Fine structure of cell types in an ameloblastoma. J Oral Pathol 1979; 8(6): 319–332.

97. Matthiessen ME, Vedtofte P, Romert P. Morphology of a simple ameloblastoma related to the human enamel organ. Scand J Dent Res 1980; 88(3):181–186.

98. Rothouse LS, Majack RA, Fay JT. An ameloblastoma with myofibroblasts and intracellular septate junctions. Cancer 1980; 45(11):2858–2863.

99. Chomette G, Auriol M, Vaillant JM. Induction odontogène et améloblastome: données histoenzymologiques et ultrastructurale [Odontogenic induction and ameloblastoma. Histoenzymological and ultrastructural studies]. Ann Pathol 1981; 1(3):221–231.

100. Nasu M, Ishikawa G. Ameloblastoma. Light and electron microscopic study. Virchows Arch A Pathol Anat Histopathol 1983; 399(2):163–175.

101. Takeda Y, Kikuchi H, Suzuki A. Hyaline bodies in ameloblastoma: histological and ultrastructural observations. J Oral Pathol 1985; 14(8):639–643.

102. Smith SM, Bartov SA. Ameloblastoma with myofibroblasts: first report. J Oral Pathol 1986; 15(5):284–286.

103. Farman AG, Gould AR, Merrell E. Epithelium-connective tissue junction in follicular ameloblastoma and ameloblastic fibroma: an ultrastructural analysis. Int J Oral Maxillofac Surg 1986; 15(2):176–186.

104. Nasu M, Takagi M, Yamamoto H. Ultrastructural and histochemical studies of granular-cell ameloblastoma. J Oral Pathol 1984; 13(4):448–456.

105. Sandros J, Heikinheimo K, Happonen RP, et al. Expression of p21RAS in odontogenic tumors. APMIS 1991; 99(1):15–20.

106. Kumamoto H, Ooya K, Sasano H. Immunohistochemical localization of c-myc oncogene protein correlated with malignancy of oral epithelium. Jpn J Oral Biol 1991; 33:315–319.

107. Heikinheimo K, Jee KJ, Niini T, et al. Gene expression profiling of ameloblastoma and human tooth germ by means of a cDNA microarray. J Dent Res 2002; 81(8): 525–530.

108. Jääskeläinen K, Jee KJ, Leivo I, et al. Cell proliferation and chromosomal changes in human ameloblastoma. Cancer Genet Cytogenet 2002; 136(1):31–37.

109. Carinci F, Francioso F, Rubini C, et al. Genetic portrait of malignant granular cell odontogenic tumour. Oral Oncol 2003; 39(1):69–77.

110. Nodit L, Barnes L, Childers E, et al. Allelic loss of tumor suppressor genes in ameloblastic tumors. Mod Pathol 2004; 17(9):1062–1067.

111. Lim J, Ahn H, Min S, et al. Oligonucleotide microarray analysis of ameloblastoma compared with dentigerous cyst. J Oral Pathol Med 2006; 35(5):278–285.

112. Migaldi M, Sartori G, Rossi G, et al. Tumor cell proliferation and microsatellite alterations in human ameloblastoma. Oral Oncol 44(1):50–60. [Epub 2007, Feb 16].

113. Slootweg PJ. p53 protein and Ki-67 reactivity in epithelial odontogenic lesions. An immunohistochemical study. J Oral Pathol Med 1995; 24(9):393–397.

114. Kumamoto H. Detection of apoptosis-related factors and apoptotic cells in ameloblastomas: analysis by immunohistochemistry and an in situ DNA nick end-labeling method. J Oral Pathol Med 1997; 26(9):419–425.

115. Shibata T, Nakata D, Chiba I, et al. Detection of TP53 mutation in ameloblastoma by the use of a yeast functional assay. J Oral Pathol Med 2002; 31(9):534–538.

116. Kumamoto H, Izutsu T, Ohki K, et al. p53 gene status and expression of p53, MDM2, and p14 proteins in ameloblastomas. J Oral Pathol Med 2004; 33(5):292–299.

117. Appel T, Gath R, Wernert N, et al. Molekularbiologische und immunohistochemische Untersuchungen des tp53-Gens in menschlichen Ameloblastomen. Mund Kiefer Gesichtschir 2004; 8(3):167–172.

118. Sandra F, Nakamura N, Kanematsu T, et al. The role of MDM2 in the proliferative activity of ameloblastoma. Oral Oncol 2002; 38(2):153–157.

119. Carvalhais J, Aguiar M, Araujo V, et al. p53 and MDM2 expression in odontogenic cysts and tumours. Oral Dis 1999; 5(3):218–222.

120. Kumamoto H, Ohki K, Ooya K. Expression of p63 and p73 in ameloblastomas. J Oral Pathol Med 2005; 34(4):220–226.

121. Lo Muzio L, Santarelli A, Caltabiano R, et al. p63 expression correlates with pathological features and biological behavior of odontogenic tumours. Histopathology 2006; 49(2):211–214.

122. Kumamoto H, Ooya K. Immunohistochemical detection of beta-catenin and adenomatous polyposis coli (APC) in ameloblastomas. J Oral Pathol Med 2005; 34(7):401–406.

123. Kumamoto H, Ooya K. Immunohistochemical detection of retinoblastoma protein and E2 promoter-binding factor-1 in ameloblastomas. J Oral Pathol Med 2006; 35(3):183–189.

124. Castrilli G, Piantelli M, Artese L, et al. Expression of hMSH2 and hMLH1 proteins of the human DNA mismatch repair system in ameloblastoma. J Oral Pathol Med 2001; 30(5):305–308.

125. van Heerden WF, Van Rensburg EJ, Raubenheimer EJ, et al. Detection of human papillomavirus DNA in an ameloblastoma using the in situ hybridization technique. J Oral Pathol Med 1993; 22(3):109–112.

126. Sand L, Jalouli J, Larsson PA, et al. Presence of human papilloma viruses in intraosseous ameloblastoma. J Oral Maxillofac Surg 2000; 58(10):1129–1134.

127. Namin AK, Azad TM, Eslami B, et al. A study of the relationship between ameloblastoma and human papilloma virus. J Oral Maxillofac Surg 2003; 61(4):467–470.

128. Migaldi M, Pecorari M, Rossi G, et al. Does HPV play a role in the etiopathogenesis of ameloblastoma? An immunohistochemical, in situ hybridization and polymerase chain reaction study of 18 cases using laser capture microdissection. Mod Pathol 2005; 18(2):283–289.

129. Fujita S, Shibata Y, Takahashi H, et al. Latent infection with Epstein-Barr virus in odontogenic disorders: comparison among ameloblastoma, dentigerous cyst and odontogenic keratocyst. Pathol Int 1997; 47(7):449–453.

130. Heikinheimo K, Voutilainen R, Happonen RP, et al. EGF receptor and its ligands, EGF and TGF-alpha, in developing and neoplastic human odontogenic tissues. Int J Dev Biol 1993; 37(3):387–396.

131. Ueno S, Miyagawa T, Kaji R, et al. Immunohistochemical investigation of epidermal growth factor receptor expression in ameloblastomas. J Pathol 1994; 173(1):33–38.

132. Vered M, Shohat I, Buchner A. Epidermal growth factor receptor expression in ameloblastoma. Oral Oncol 2003; 39(2):138–143.

133. Heikinheimo K, Happonen RP, Miettinen PJ, et al. Transforming growth factor beta 2 in epithelial differentiation of developing teeth and odontogenic tumors. J Clin Invest 1993; 91(3):1019–1027.

134. Kumamoto H, Yoshida M, Ooya K. Immunohistochemical detection of hepatocyte growth factor, transforming growth factor-beta and their receptors in epithelial odontogenic tumors. J Oral Pathol Med 2002; 31(9):539–548.

135. Myoken Y, Myoken Y, Okamoto T, et al. Immunohistochemical localization of fibroblast growth factor-1 (FGF-1) and FGF-2 in cultured human ameloblastoma epithelial cells and ameloblastoma tissues. J Oral Pathol Med 1995; 24(9):387–392.

136. So F, Daley TD, Jackson L, et al. Immunohistochemical localization of fibroblast growth factors FGF-1 and FGF-2, and receptors FGFR2 and FGFR3 in the epithelium of human odontogenic cysts and tumors. J Oral Pathol Med 2001; 30(7):428–433.

137. Kumamoto H, Ooya K. Immunohistochemical detection of platelet-derived endothelial cell growth factor/thymidine phosphorylase and angiopoietins in ameloblastic tumors. J Oral Pathol Med 2006; 35(10):606–612.

138. Kumamoto H, Ooya K. Immunohistochemical detection of insulin-like growth factors, platelet-derived growth factor, and their receptors in ameloblastic tumors. J Oral Pathol Med 2007; 36(4):198–206.

139. Sumida T, Sogawa K, Hamakawa H, et al. Detection of telomerase activity in oral lesions. J Oral Pathol Med 1998; 27(3):111–115.

140. Kumamoto H, Kinouchi Y, Ooya K. Telomerase activity and telomerase reverse transcriptase (TERT) expression in ameloblastomas. J Oral Pathol Med 2001; 30(4):231–236.

141. Kumamoto H, Kimi K, Ooya K. Detection of cell cycle-related factors in ameloblastomas. J Oral Pathol Med 2001; 30(5):309–315.

142. Kim J, Lee EH, Yook JI, et al. Odontogenic ghost cell carcinoma: a case report with reference to the relation between apoptosis and ghost cells. Oral Surg Oral Med Oral Pathol Oral Radiol Endod 2000; 90(5):630–635.

143. Sandra F, Nakamura N, Mitsuyasu T, et al. Two relatively distinct patterns of ameloblastoma: an anti-apoptotic proliferating site in the outer layer (periphery) and a pro-apoptotic differentiating site in the inner layer (centre). Histopathology 2001; 39(1):93–98.

144. Kumamoto H, Kimi K, Ooya K. Immunohistochemical analysis of apoptosis-related factors (Fas, Fas ligand, caspase-3 and single-stranded DNA) in ameloblastomas. J Oral Pathol Med 2001; 30(10):596–602.

145. Luo HY, Yu SF, Li TJ. Differential expression of apoptosis-related proteins in various cellular components of ameloblastomas. Int J Oral Maxillofac Surg 2006; 35(8):750–755.

146. Kumamoto H, Ooya K. Expression of tumor necrosis factor alpha, TNF-related apoptosis-inducing ligand, and their associated molecules in ameloblastomas. J Oral Pathol Med 2005; 34(5):287–294.

147. Mitsuyasu T, Harada H, Higuchi Y, et al. Immunohistochemical demonstration of bcl-2 protein in ameloblastoma. J Oral Pathol Med 1997; 26(8):345–348.

148. Kumamoto H, Ooya K. Immunohistochemical analysis of bcl-2 family proteins in benign and malignant ameloblastomas. J Oral Pathol Med 1999; 28(8):343–349.

149. Kumamoto H, Ooya K. Expression of survivin and X chromosome-linked inhibitor of apoptosis protein in ameloblastomas. Virchows Arch 2004; 444(2):164–170.

150. Kumamoto H, Ooya K. Detection of mitochondria-mediated apoptosis signaling molecules in ameloblastomas. J Oral Pathol Med 2005; 34(9):565–572.

151. Sandra F, Hendarmin L, Nakao Y, et al. TRAIL cleaves caspase-8, -9 and -3 of AM-1 cells: a possible pathway for TRAIL to induce apoptosis in ameloblastoma. Tumour Biol 2005; 26(5):258–264.

152. Sandra F, Hendarmin L, Nakamura S. Osteoprotegerin (OPG) binds with tumor necrosis factor-related apoptosis-inducing ligand (TRAIL): suppression of TRAIL-induced apoptosis in ameloblastomas. Oral Oncol 2006; 42(4): 415–420.

153. Hendarmin L, Sandra F, Nakao Y, et al. TNFalpha played a role in induction of Akt and MAPK signals in ameloblastoma. Oral Oncol 2005; 41(4):375–382.

154. Sandra F, Hendarmin L, Nakao Y, et al. Inhibition of Akt and MAPK pathways elevated potential of TNFalpha in inducing apoptosis in ameloblastoma. Oral Oncol 2006; 42(1):39–45.

155. Kumamoto H, Ohki K, Ooya K. Expression of Sonic hedgehog (SHH) signaling molecules in ameloblastomas. J Oral Pathol Med 2004; 33(3):185–190.

156. Sekine S, Sato S, Takata T, et al. Beta-catenin mutations are frequent in calcifying odontogenic cysts, but rare in ameloblastomas. Am J Pathol 2003; 163(5):1707–1712.

157. Miyake T, Tanaka Y, Kato K, et al. Gene mutation analysis and immunohistochemical study of beta-catenin in odontogenic tumors. Pathol Int 2006; 56(12):732–737.

158. Leocata P, Villari D, Fazzari C, et al. Syndecan-1 and Wingless-type protein-1 in human ameloblastomas. J Oral Pathol Med 2007; 36(7):394–399.

159. Saku T, Okabe H, Shimokawa H. Immunohistochemical demonstration of enamel proteins in odontogenic tumors. J Oral Pathol Med 1992; 21(3):113–119.

160. Takata T, Zhao M, Uchida T, et al. Immunohistochemical detection and distribution of enamelysin (MMP-20) in human odontogenic tumors. J Dent Res 2000; 79(8): 1608–1613.

161. Takata T, Zhao M, Uchida T, et al. Immunohistochemical demonstration of an enamel sheath protein, sheathlin, in odontogenic tumors. Virchows Arch 2000; 436(4):324–329.

162. Mori M, Yamada K, Kasai T, et al. Immunohistochemical expression of amelogenins in odontogenic epithelial tumours and cysts. Virchows Arch A Pathol Anat Histopathol 1991; 418(4):319–325.

163. Kumamoto H, Yoshida M, Ooya K. Immunohistochemical detection of amelogenin and cytokeratin 19 in epithelial odontogenic tumors. Oral Dis 2001; 7(3):171–176.

164. Snead ML, Luo W, Hsu DD, et al. Human ameloblastoma tumors express the amelogenin gene. Oral Surg Oral Med Oral Pathol 1992; 74(1):64–72.

165. Perdigao PF, Gomez RS, Pimenta FJ, et al. Ameloblastin gene (AMBN) mutations associated with epithelial odontogenic tumors. Oral Oncol 2004; 40(8):841–846.

166. Tsujigiwa H, Nagatsuka H, Han PP, et al. Analysis of amelogenin gene (AMGX, AMGY) expression in ameloblastoma. Oral Oncol 2005; 41(8):843–850.

167. Chen J, Aufdemorte TB, Jiang H, et al. Neoplastic odontogenic epithelial cells express bone sialoprotein. Histochem J 1998; 30(1):1–6.

168. Gao YH, Yang LJ, Yamaguchi A. Immunohistochemical demonstration of bone morphogenetic protein in odontogenic tumors. J Oral Pathol Med 1997; 26(6):273–277.

169. Kumamoto H, Ooya K. Expression of bone morphogenetic proteins and their associated molecules in ameloblastomas and adenomatoid odontogenic tumors. Oral Dis 2006; 12(2):163–170.

170. Pripatnanont P, Song Y, Harris M, et al. In situ hybridisation and immunocytochemical localisation of osteolytic cytokines and adhesion molecules in ameloblastomas. J Oral Pathol Med 1998; 27(10):496–500.

171. Kumamoto H, Ooya K. Expression of E-cadherin and alpha-catenin in epithelial odontogenic tumors: an immunohistochemical study. J Oral Pathol Med 1999; 28(4):152–157.

172. Kumamoto H, Ohba S, Susuki T, et al. Immunohistochemical expression of integrins and CD44 in ameloblastomas. Oral Med Pathol 2001; 6:73–78.

173. Modolo F, Martins MT, Loducca SV, et al. Expression of integrin subunits alpha2, alpha3, alpha5, alphav, beta1, beta3 and beta4 in different histological types of ameloblastoma compared with dental germ, dental lamina and adult lining epithelium. Oral Dis 2004; 10(5):277–282.

174. Kumamoto H, Yamauchi K, Yoshida M, et al. Immunohistochemical detection of matrix metalloproteinases (MMPs) and tissue inhibitors of metalloproteinases (TIMPs) in ameloblastomas. J Oral Pathol Med 2003; 32(2):114–120.

175. Pinheiro JJ, Freitas VM, Moretti AI, et al. Local invasiveness of ameloblastoma. Role played by matrix metalloproteinases and proliferative activity. Histopathology 2004; 45(1):65–72.

176. Kumamoto H, Ooya K. Immunohistochemical detection of MT1-MMP, RECK, and EMMPRIN in ameloblastic tumors. J Oral Pathol Med 2006; 35(6):345–351.

177. Nagatsuka H, Han PP, Tsujigiwa H, et al. Heparanase gene and protein expression in ameloblastoma: possible role in local invasion of tumor cells. Oral Oncol 2005; 41(5):542–548.

178. Kumamoto H, Ooya K. Immunohistochemical detection of uPA, uPAR, PAI-1, and maspin in ameloblastic tumors. J Oral Pathol Med 2007; 36(8):88–494.

179. Kumamoto H, Ohki K, Ooya K. Association between vascular endothelial growth factor (VEGF) expression and tumor angiogenesis in ameloblastomas. J Oral Pathol Med 2002; 31(1):28–34.

180. MacPherson DW, Hopper C, Meghji S. Hypercalcaemia and the synthesis of interleukin-1 by an ameloblastoma. Br J Oral Maxillofac Surg 1991; 29(1):29–33.

181. Kubota Y, Nitta S, Oka S, et al. Discrimination of ameloblastomas from odontogenic keratocysts by cytokine levels and gelatinase species of the intracystic fluids. J Oral Pathol Med 2001; 30(7):421–427.

182. Kumamoto H, Ooya K. Expression of parathyroid hormone-related protein (PTHrP), osteoclast differentiation factor (ODF)/receptor activator of nuclear factor-kappaB ligand (RANKL) and osteoclastogenesis inhibitory factor (OCIF)/osteoprotegerin (OPG) in ameloblastomas. J Oral Pathol Med 2004; 33(1):46–52.

183. Tay JY, Bay BH, Yeo JF, et al. Identification of RANKL in osteolytic lesions of the facial skeleton. J Dent Res 2004; 83(4):349–353.

184. Sandra F, Hendarmin L, Kukita T, et al. Ameloblastoma induces osteoclastogenesis: a possible role of ameloblastoma in expanding the bone. Oral Oncol 2005; 41(6): 637–644.

185. Nakamura N, Higuchi Y, Mitsuyasu T, et al. Comparison of long-term results between different approaches to ameloblastoma. Oral Surg Oral Med Oral Pathol Oral Radiol Endod 2002; 93(1):13–20.

186. Huang IY, Lai ST, Chen CH, et al. Surgical management of ameloblastoma in children. Oral Surg Oral Med Oral Pathol Oral Radiol Endod 2007; 104(4):478–484.

187. Chala S, Nassih M, Rzin A, et al. Notre expérience des améloblastomes de la mandibule [Ameloblastoma of the mandible]. Rev Stomatol Chir Maxillofac 2002; 103(4):247–250.

188. Ghandhi D, Ayoub AF, Pogrel MA, et al. Ameloblastoma: a surgeon's dilemma. J Oral Maxillofac Surg 2006; 64(7): 1010–1014.

189. Demeulemeester LJ, Mommaerts MY, Fossion E, et al. Late loco-regional recurrences after radical resection for mandibular ameloblastoma. Int J Oral Maxillofac Surg 1988; 17(5):310–315.

190. Hayward JR. Recurrent ameloblastoma 30 years after surgical treatment. J Oral Surg 1973; 31(5):368–370.

191. Chapelle KA, Stoelinga PJ, de Wilde PC, et al. Rational approach to diagnosis and treatment of ameloblastomas and odontogenic keratocysts. Br J Oral Maxillofac Surg 2004; 42(5):381–390.

192. Philipsen HP, Reichart PA, Nikai H, et al. Peripheral ameloblastoma: biological profile based on 160 cases from the literature. Oral Oncol 2001; 37(1):17–27.

193. Orsini G, Fioroni M, Rubini C, et al. Peripheral ameloblastoma: a report of 2 cases. J Periodontol 2000; 71(7): 1174–1176.

194. Kelly JP, Said-Al-Naief N, Salehani D, et al. An exophytic submucosal mass overlying the ramus in a 79-year-old man. J Oral Maxillofac Surg 2001; 59(11):1345–1348.

195. Tajima Y, Kuroda-Kawasaki M, Ohno J, et al. Peripheral ameloblastoma with potentially malignant features: report of a case with special regard to its keratin profile. J Oral Pathol Med 2001; 30(8):494–498.

196. Ide F, Kusama K, Tanaka A et al. Peripheral ameloblastoma is not a hamartoma but rather more of a neoplasm. Oral Oncol 2002; 38(3):318–320.

197. Lentini M, Simone A, Carrozza G. Peripheral ameloblastoma: use of cytokeratin 19 and BER-EP4 to distinguish it from basal cell carcinoma. Oral Oncol 2004; 40:79–80.

198. Manor Y, Mardinger O, Katz J, et al. Peripheral odontogenic tumours–differential diagnosis in gingival lesions. Int J Oral Maxillofac Surg 2004; 33(3):268–273.

199. Gavaldá C. Ameloblastoma periférico [Peripheral ameloblastoma]. Med Oral Patol Oral Cir Bucal 2005; 10(2):187.

200. López-Jornet P, Bermejo-Fenoll A. Peripheral ameloblastoma of the gingiva: the importance of diagnosis. J Clin Periodontol 2005; 32(1):12–15.

201. Martelli-Júnior H, Souza LN, Santos LA, et al. Peripheral ameloblastoma: a case report. Oral Surg Oral Med Oral Pathol Oral Radiol Endod 2005; 99(5):E31–E33.

202. Shetty K. Peripheral ameloblastoma: An etiology from surface epithelium? Case report and review of literature. Oral Oncology EXTRA 2005; 41:211–215.

203. Hayes MI, Prince SE. Peripheral ameloblastoma: a case report. Dent Update 2006; 33(10):624–625.

204. LeCorn DW, Bhattacharyya I, Vertucci FJ. Peripheral ameloblastoma: a case report and review of the literature. J Endod 2006; 32(2):152–154.

205. Pekiner FN, Ozbayrak S, Sener BC, et al. Peripheral ameloblastoma: a case report. Dentomaxillofac Radiol 2007; 36(3):183–186.

206. Balfour RS, Loscalzo LJ, Sulka M. Multicentric peripheral ameloblastoma. J Oral Surg 1973; 31(7):535–538.

207. Hernandez G, Sanchez G, Caballero T, et al. A rare case of a multicentric peripheral ameloblastoma of the gingiva. A light and electron microscopic study. J Clin Periodontol 1992; 19(4):281–287.

208. Yamanishi T, Ando S, Aikawa T, et al. A case of extra-gingival peripheral ameloblastoma in the buccal mucosa. J Oral Pathol Med 2007; 36(3):184–186.

209. Wesley RK, Borninski ER, Mintz S. Peripheral ameloblastoma: report of case and review of the literature. J Oral Surg 1977; 35(8):670–672.

210. Moskow BS, Baden E. The peripheral ameloblastoma of the gingiva. Case report and literature review. J Periodontol 1982; 53(12):736–742.

211. Gardner DG. Peripheral ameloblastoma: a study of 21 cases, including 5 reported as basal cell carcinoma of the gingiva. Cancer 1977; 39(4):1625–1633.

212. Buchner A, Sciubba JJ. Peripheral epithelial odontogenic tumors: a review. Oral Surg Oral Med Oral Pathol 1987; 63(6):688–697.

213. Scheffer P, Attar A, Adouani A, et al. Améloblastome mandibulaire extra-osseux [Extra-osseous mandibular ameloblastoma]. Rev Stomatol Chir Maxillofac 1988; 89(3): 151–157.

214. Nauta JM, Panders AK, Schoots CJ, et al. Peripheral ameloblastoma. A case report and review of the literature. Int J Oral Maxillofac Surg 1992; 21(1):40–44.

215. Yamamoto T, Ueta E, Yoneda K, et al. Peripheral ameloblastoma: case report with immunohistochemical investigation. J Oral Maxillofac Surg 1990; 48(2):197–200.

216. Gould AR, Farman AG, DeJean EK, et al. Peripheral ameloblastoma: an ultrastructural analysis. J Oral Pathol 1982; 11(2):90–101.

217. Ficarra G, Hansen LS. Peripheral ameloblastoma. A case report. J Craniomaxillofac Surg 1987; 15(2):110–112.

218. Anneroth G, Johansson B. Peripheral ameloblastoma. Int J Oral Surg 1985; 14(3):295–299.

219. Baden E, Doyle JL, Petriella V. Malignant transformation of peripheral ameloblastoma. Oral Surg Oral Med Oral Pathol 1993; 75(2):214–219.

220. Califano L, Maremonti P, Boscaino A, et al. Peripheral ameloblastoma: report of a case with malignant aspect. Br J Oral Maxillofac Surg 1996; 34(3):240–242.

221. Takeda Y, Kuroda M, Suzuki A. Ameloblastoma of mucosal origin. Acta Pathol Jpn 1988; 38(8):1053–1060.

222. Greer RO Jr., Hammond WS. Extraosseous ameloblastoma: light microscopic and ultrastructural observations. J Oral Surg 1978; 36(7):553–556.

223. Ueda A, Kage T, Chino T, et al. A case report of peripheral ameloblastoma with unusual invasion. Oral Med Pathol 1998; 3:93–96.

224. Ward BB, Edlund S, Sciubba J, et al. Ameloblastic carcinoma (primary type) isolated to the anterior maxilla: case report with review of the literature. J Oral Maxillofac Surg 2007; 65(9):1800–1803.

225. Sciubba JJ, Zola MB. Odontogenic epithelial hamartoma. Oral Surg Oral Med Oral Pathol 1978; 45(2):261–265.

226. Baden E, Moskow BS, Moskow R. Odontogenic gingival epithelial hamartoma. J Oral Surg 1968; 26(11): 702–714.

227. Reichart PA, Philipsen HP. Peripheral Ameloblastoma. In: Odontogenic Tumors and Allied Lesions. London: Quintessence Publishing Co Ltd, 2004:59–67.

228. Shear M, Speight P. Cysts of the Oral and Maxillofacial Regions. Fourth edition ed. Oxford, United Kingdom: Blackwell Munksgaard, 2007:1–384.

229. Reichart PA, Philipsen HP. Desmoplastic Ameloblastoma. In: Odontogenic Tumors and Allied Lesions. London: Quintessence Publishing Co Ltd, 2004:69–76.

230. Eversole LR, Leider AS, Hansen LS. Ameloblastomas with pronounced desmoplasia. J Oral Maxillofac Surg 1984; 42(11):735–740.

231. Philipsen HP, Reichart PA, Takata T. Desmoplastic ameloblastoma (including "hybrid" lesion of ameloblastoma). Biological profile based on 100 cases from the literature and own files. Oral Oncol 2001; 37(5):455–460.

232. Waldron CA, El-Mofty SK. A histopathologic study of 116 ameloblastomas with special reference to the desmoplastic variant. Oral Surg Oral Med Oral Pathol 1987; 63(4): 441–451.

233. Keszler A, Paparella ML, Dominguez FV. Desmoplastic and non-desmoplastic ameloblastoma: a comparative clinicopathological analysis. Oral Dis 1996; 2(3):228–231.
234. Lam KY, Chan AC, Wu PC, et al. Desmoplastic variant of ameloblastoma in Chinese patients. Br J Oral Maxillofac Surg 1998; 36(2):129–134.
235. Takata T, Miyauchi M, Ito H, et al. Clinical and histopathological analyses of desmoplastic ameloblastoma. Pathol Res Pract 1999; 195(10):669–675.
236. Kishino M, Murakami S, Fukuda Y, et al. Pathology of the desmoplastic ameloblastoma. J Oral Pathol Med 2001; 30(1):35–40.
237. Ng KH, Siar CH. Desmoplastic variant of ameloblastoma in Malaysians. Br J Oral Maxillofac Surg 1993; 31(5):299–303.
238. Smullin SE, Faquin W, Susarla SM, et al. Peripheral desmoplastic ameloblastoma: report of a case and literature review. Oral Surg Oral Med Oral Pathol Oral Radiol Endod 2008; 105(1):37–40.
239. Philipsen HP, Ormiston IW, Reichart PA. The desmo- and osteoplastic ameloblastoma. Histologic variant or clinicopathologic entity? Case reports. Int J Oral Maxillofac Surg 1992; 21(6):352–357.
240. Kaffe I, Buchner A, Taicher S. Radiologic features of desmoplastic variant of ameloblastoma. Oral Surg Oral Med Oral Pathol 1993; 76(4):525–529.
241. Iida S, Kogo M, Kishino M, et al. Desmoplastic ameloblastoma with large cystic change in the maxillary sinus: report of a case. J Oral Maxillofac Surg 2002; 60(10):1195–1198.
242. Kawai T, Kishino M, Hiranuma H, et al. A unique case of desmoplastic ameloblastoma of the mandible: report of a case and brief review of the English language literature. Oral Surg Oral Med Oral Pathol Oral Radiol Endod 1999; 87(2):258–263.
243. Thompson IO, van Rensburg LJ, Phillips VM. Desmoplastic ameloblastoma: correlative histopathology, radiology and CT-MR imaging. J Oral Pathol Med 1996; 25(7):405–410.
244. Higuchi Y, Nakamura N, Ohishi M, et al. Unusual ameloblastoma with extensive stromal desmoplasia. J Craniomaxillofac Surg 1991; 19(7):323–327.
245. Takata T, Miyauchi M, Ogawa I, et al. So-called 'hybrid' lesion of desmoplastic and conventional ameloblastoma: report of a case and review of the literature. Pathol Int 1999; 49(11):1014–1018.
246. dos Santos JN, De Souza VF, Azevêdo RA, et al. "Hybrid" lesion of desmoplastic and conventional ameloblastoma: immunohistochemical aspects. Rev Bras Otorrinolaringol (Engl Ed) 2006; 72(5):709–713.
247. Hirota M, Aoki S, Kawabe R, et al. Desmoplastic ameloblastoma featuring basal cell ameloblastoma: a case report. Oral Surg Oral Med Oral Pathol Oral Radiol Endod 2005; 99(2):160–164.
248. Siar CH, Ng KH. Patterns of expression of intermediate filaments and S-100 protein in desmoplastic ameloblastoma. J Nihon Univ Sch Dent 1993; 35(2):104–108.
249. Takata T, Miyauchi M, Ogawa I, et al. Immunoexpression of transforming growth factor beta in desmoplastic ameloblastoma. Virchows Arch 2000; 436(4):319–323.
250. Kumamoto H, Ooya K. Immunohistochemical detection of phosphorylated Akt, PI3K, and PTEN in ameloblastic tumors. Oral Dis 2007; 13(5):461–467.
251. Tatemoto Y, Okada Y, Mori M. Squamous odontogenic tumor: immunohistochemical identification of keratins. Oral Surg Oral Med Oral Pathol 1989; 67(1):63–67.
252. Hietanen J, Lukinmaa PL, Ahonen P, et al. Peripheral squamous odontogenic tumour. Br J Oral Maxillofac Surg 1985; 23(5):362–365.
253. Favia GF, Di Alberti L, Scarano A, et al. Squamous odontogenic tumour: report of two cases. Oral Oncol 1997; 33(6):451–453.
254. Muller H, Slootweg PJ. The ameloblastoma, the controversial approach to therapy. J Maxillofac Surg 1985; 13(2):79–84.
255. Pillai RS, Ongole R, Ahsan A et al. Recurrent desmoplastic ameloblastoma of the maxilla: a case report. J Can Dent Assoc 2004; 70(2):100–104.
256. Robinson L, Martinez MG. Unicystic ameloblastoma: a prognostically distinct entity. Cancer 1977; 40(5):2278–2285.
257. Ackermann GL, Altini M, Shear M. The unicystic ameloblastoma: a clinicopathological study of 57 cases. J Oral Pathol 1988; 17(9–10):541–546.
258. Li T, Wu Y, Yu S, et al. Clinicopathological features of unicystic ameloblastoma with special reference to its recurrence. Zhonghua Kou Qiang Yi Xue Za Zhi 2002; 37(3):210–212.
259. Philipsen HP, Reichart PA. Unicystic ameloblastoma. A review of 193 cases from the literature. Oral Oncol 1998; 34(5):317–325.
260. Eversole LR, Leider AS, Strub D. Radiographic characteristics of cystogenic ameloblastoma. Oral Surg Oral Med Oral Pathol 1984; 57(5):572–577.
261. Keszler A, Dominguez FV. Ameloblastoma in childhood. J Oral Maxillofac Surg 1986; 44(8):609–613.
262. Li T-J, Wu Y-T, Yu S-F, et al. Unicystic ameloblastoma: a clinicopathologic study of 33 Chinese patients. Am J Surg Pathol 2000; 24(10):1385–1392.
263. Rosenstein T, Pogrel MA, Smith RA, et al. Cystic ameloblastoma–behavior and treatment of 21 cases. J Oral Maxillofac Surg 2001; 59(11):1311–1316.
264. Gardner DG. Plexiform unicystic ameloblastoma: a diagnostic problem in dentigerous cysts. Cancer 1981, 47(6), 1358–1363.
265. Leider AS, Eversole LR, Barkin ME. Cystic ameloblastoma. A clinicopathologic analysis. Oral Surg Oral Med Oral Pathol 1985; 60(6):624–630.
266. Lee PK, Samman N, Ng IO. Unicystic ameloblastoma–use of Carnoy's solution after enucleation. Int J Oral Maxillofac Surg 2004; 33(3):263–267.
267. Olaitan AA, Adekeye EO. Unicystic ameloblastoma of the mandible: a long-term follow-up. J Oral Maxillofac Surg 1997; 55(4):345–348.
268. Konouchi H, Asaumi J, Yanagi Y, et al. Usefulness of contrast enhanced-MRI in the diagnosis of unicystic ameloblastoma. Oral Oncol 2006; 42(5):481–486.
269. Melrose RJ. Benign epithelial odontogenic tumors. Semin Diagn Pathol 1999; 16(4):271–287.
270. Vickers RA, Gorlin RJ. Ameloblastoma: delineation of early histopathologic features of neoplasia. Cancer 1970; 26(3):699–710.
271. Gardner DG, Corio RL. Plexiform unicystic ameloblastoma. A variant of ameloblastoma with a low-recurrence rate after enucleation. Cancer 1984; 53(8):1730–1735.
272. Buchner A. Granular-cell odontogenic cyst. Oral Surg Oral Med Oral Pathol 1973; 36(5):707–712.
273. Siar CH, Ng KH, Jalil NA. Plexiform granular cell odontogenic tumor: unicystic variant. Oral Surg Oral Med Oral Pathol 1991; 72(1):82–85.
274. Dresser WJ, Segal E. Ameloblastoma associated with a dentigerous cyst in a 6-year-old child. Report of a case. Oral Surg Oral Med Oral Pathol 1967; 24(3):388–391.
275. Altini M, Coleman H, Doglioni C, et al. Calretinin expression in ameloblastomas. Histopathology 2000; 37(1):27–32.
276. Coleman H, Altini M, Ali H, et al. Use of calretinin in the differential diagnosis of unicystic ameloblastomas. Histopathology 2001; 38(4):312–317.

277. Piattelli A, Fioroni M, Iezzi G, et al. Calretinin expression in odontogenic cysts. J Endod 2003; 29(6):394–396.

278. Coleman HG, Altini M, Groeneveld HT. Nucleolar organizer regions (AgNORs) in odontogenic cysts and ameloblastomas. J Oral Pathol Med 1996; 25(8):436–440.

279. Eslami B, Yaghmaei M, Firoozi M, et al. Nucleolar organizer regions in selected odontogenic lesions. Oral Surg Oral Med Oral Pathol Oral Radiol Endod 2003; 95(2): 187–192.

280. Li TJ, Browne RM, Matthews JB. Expression of proliferating cell nuclear antigen (PCNA) and Ki-67 in unicystic ameloblastoma. Histopathology 1995; 26(3):219–228.

281. Piattelli A, Lezzi G, Fioroni M, et al. Ki-67 expression in dentigerous cysts, unicystic ameloblastomas, and ameloblastomas arising from dental cysts. J Endod 2002; 28(2): 55–58.

282. Lau SL, Samman N. Recurrence related to treatment modalities of unicystic ameloblastoma: a systematic review. Int J Oral Maxillofac Surg 2006; 35(8):681–690.

283. Nakamura N, Higuchi Y, Tashiro H, et al. Marsupialization of cystic ameloblastoma: a clinical and histopathologic study of the growth characteristics before and after marsupialization. J Oral Maxillofac Surg 1995; 53(7):748–754.

284. Siar CH, Ng KH. 'Combined ameloblastoma and odontogenic keratocyst' or 'keratinising ameloblastoma'. Br J Oral Maxillofac Surg 1993; 31(3):183–186.

285. Norval EJ, Thompson IO, Van Wyk CW. An unusual variant of keratoameloblastoma. J Oral Pathol Med 1994; 23(10):465–467.

286. Said-al-Naief NA, Lumerman H, Ramer M, et al. Keratoameloblastoma of the maxilla. A case report and review of the literature. Oral Surg Oral Med Oral Pathol Oral Radiol Endod 1997; 84(5):535–539.

287. Ide F, Mishima K, Saito I. Solid-cystic tumor variant of odontogenic keratocyst: an aggressive but benign lesion simulating keratoameloblastoma. Virchows Arch 2003; 442(5):501–503.

288. Whitt JC, Dunlap CL, Sheets JL, et al. Keratoameloblastoma: a tumor sui generis or a chimera? Oral Surg Oral Med Oral Pathol Oral Radiol Endod 2007; 104(3):368–376.

289. Lurie R, Altini M, Shear M. A case report of keratoameloblastoma. Int J Oral Surg 1976; 5(5):245–249.

290. Omura S, Kawabe R, Kobayashi S, et al. Odontogenic keratocyst appearing as a soap-bubble or honeycomb radiolucency: Report of a case. J Oral Maxillofac Surg 1997; 55:185–189.

291. Vered M, Buchner A, Dayan D, et al. Solid variant of odontogenic keratocyst. J Oral Pathol Med 2004; 33(2): 125–128.

292. Pindborg JJ. Odontogenic tumors. In: Pathology of the Dental Hard Tissue. Copenhagen: Munksgaard, 1970: 367–428.

293. Altini M, Slabbert HD, Johnston T. Papilliferous keratoameloblastoma. J Oral Pathol Med 1991; 20(1):46–48.

294. Takeda Y, Satoh M, Nakamura S, et al. Keratoameloblastoma with unique histological architecture: an undescribed variation of ameloblastoma. Virchows Arch 2001; 439(4):593–596.

295. Reichart PA. Squamous odontogenic tumour. In: Barnes L, Eveson JW, Reichart P, et al. eds. World Health Organization Classification of Tumours. Pathology and Genetics of Head and Neck Tumours. Lyon: IARC Press, 2005:301.

296. Pullon PA, Shafer WG, Elzay RP, et al. Squamous odontogenic tumor. Report of six cases of a previously undescribed lesion. Oral Surg Oral Med Oral Pathol 1975; 40(5):616–630.

297. Philipsen HP, Reichart PA. Squamous odontogenic tumor (SOT): a benign neoplasm of the periodontium. A review of 36 reported cases. J Clin Periodontol 1996; 23(10):922–926.

298. Doyle JL, Grodjesk JE, Dolinsky HB, et al. Squamous odontogenic tumor: report of three cases. J Oral Surg 1977; 35(12):994–996.

299. McNeill J, Price HM, Stoker NG. Squamous odontogenic tumor: report of case with long-term history. J Oral Surg 1980; 38(6):466–471.

300. Hopper TL, Sadeghi EM, Pricco DF. Squamous odontogenic tumor. Report of a case with multiple lesions. Oral Surg Oral Med Oral Pathol 1980; 50(5):404–410.

301. Carr RF, Carlton DM Jr., Marks RB. Squamous odontogenic tumor: report of case. J Oral Surg 1981; 39(4):297–298.

302. Leventon GS, Happonen RP, Newland JR. Squamous odontogenic tumor. Am J Surg Pathol 1981; 5(7):671–677.

303. Kangvonkit P, Sirichitra V, Hansasuta C. [Squamous odontogenic tumor (report of a case and review of the literature)]. J Dent Assoc Thai 1981; 31(1):25–33.

304. Goldblatt LI, Brannon RB, Ellis GL. Squamous odontogenic tumor. Report of five cases and review of the literature. Oral Surg Oral Med Oral Pathol 1982; 54(2): 187–196.

305. Cataldo E, Less WC, Giunta JL. Squamous odontogenic tumor. A lesion of the periodontium. J Periodontol 1983; 54(12):731–735.

306. Norris LH, Baghaei-Rad M, Maloney PL, et al. Bilateral maxillary squamous odontogenic tumors and the malignant transformation of a mandibular radiolucent lesion. J Oral Maxillofac Surg 1984; 42(12):827–834.

307. Kristensen S, Andersen J, Jacobsen P. Squamous odontogenic tumour: review of the literature and a new case. J Laryngol Otol 1985; 99(9):919–924.

308. Monteil RA, Terestri P. Squamous odontogenic tumor related to an unerupted lower canine. J Oral Maxillofac Surg 1985; 43(11):888–895.

309. Warnock GR, Pierce GL, Correll RW, et al. Triangular-shaped radiolucent area between roots of the mandibular right canine and first premolar. J Am Dent Assoc 1985; 110(6):945–946.

310. Mills WP, Davila MA, Beuttenmuller EA, et al. Squamous odontogenic tumor. Report of a case with lesions in three quadrants. Oral Surg Oral Med Oral Pathol 1986; 61(6): 557–563.

311. Leider AS, Jonker LA, Cook HE. Multicentric familial squamous odontogenic tumor. Oral Surg Oral Med Oral Pathol 1989; 68(2):175–181.

312. Yaacob HB. Squamous odontogenic tumor. J Nihon Univ Sch Dent 1990; 32(3):187–191.

313. Reichart PA, Philipsen HP. Squamous odontogenic tumor. J Oral Pathol Med 1990; 19(5):226–228.

314. Baden E, Doyle J, Mesa M, et al. Squamous odontogenic tumor. Report of three cases including the first extraosseous case. Oral Surg Oral Med Oral Pathol 1993; 75(6): 733–738.

315. Ide F, Shimoyama T, Horie N, et al. Intraosseous squamous cell carcinoma arising in association with a squamous odontogenic tumour of the mandible. Oral Oncol 1999; 35(4):431–434.

316. Haghighat K, Kalmar JR, Mariotti AJ. Squamous odontogenic tumor: diagnosis and management. J Periodontol 2002; 73(6):653–656.

317. Matras RC, Nattestad A, Reibel J. Squamous odontogenic tumour. En oversigt og præsentation af et tilfælde. Tandlaegebladet (Danish Dental Journal) 2002; 106(9):712–716.

318. Cillo JE Jr., Ellis E III, Kessler HP. Pericoronal squamous odontogenic tumor associated with an impacted mandibular third molar: a case report. J Oral Maxillofac Surg 2005; 63(3):413–416.

319. Gardner DG. Peripheral squamous odontogenic tumor. Oral Surg Oral Med Oral Pathol 1987; 64(5):609–610.

320. Kim K, Mintz SM, Stevens J. Squamous odontogenic tumor causing erosion of the lingual cortical plate in the mandible: a report of 2 cases. J Oral Maxillofac Surg 2007; 65(6):1227–1231.

321. Simon JH, Jensen JL. Squamous odontogenic tumor-like proliferations in periapical cysts. J Endod 1985; 11(10): 446–448.

322. Wright JM Jr. Squamous odontogenic tumor like proliferations in odontogenic cysts. Oral Surg Oral Med Oral Pathol 1979; 47(4):354–358.

323. Fay JT, Banner J, Rothouse L, et al. Squamous odontogenic tumors arising in odontogenic cysts. J Oral Med 1981; 36(2):35–38.

324. Unal T, Gomel M, Gunel O. Squamous odontogenic tumor-like islands in a radicular cyst: report of a case. J Oral Maxillofac Surg 1987; 45(4):346–349.

325. Olivera JA, Costa IM, Loyola AM. Squamous odontogenic tumor-like proliferation in residual cyst: case report. Braz Dent J 1995; 6(1):59–64.

326. Yamada K, Tatemoto Y, Okada Y, et al. Immunostaining of involucrin in odontogenic epithelial tumors and cysts. Oral Surg Oral Med Oral Pathol 1989; 67(5):564–568.

327. Pindborg JJ, Vedtofte P, Reibel J, et al. The calcifying epithelial odontogenic tumor. A review of recent literature and report of a case. APMIS Suppl 1991; 23: 152–157.

328. Takata T, Slootweg PJ. Calcifying epithelial odontogenic tumour. In: Barnes L, Eveson JW, Reichart P, et al. eds. Pathology and Genetics of Head and Neck Tumours. World Health Organization Classification of Tumours. Lyon: IARC Press, 2005:302–303.

329. Pindborg JJ. Calcifying epithelial odontogenic tumors. Acta Pathol Microbiol Scand Suppl 1955; 111:71.

330. Pindborg JJ. A calcifying epithelial odontogenic tumor. Cancer 1958; 11(4):838–843.

331. Franklin CD, Pindborg JJ. The calcifying epithelial odontogenic tumor. A review and analysis of 113 cases. Oral Surg Oral Med Oral Pathol 1976; 42(6):753–765.

332. Philipsen HP, Reichart PA. Calcifying epithelial odontogenic tumour: biological profile based on 181 cases from the literature. Oral Oncol 2000; 36(1):17–26.

333. Kaplan I, Buchner A, Calderon S, et al. Radiological and clinical features of calcifying epithelial odontogenic tumour. Dentomaxillofac Radiol 2001; 30(1):22–28.

334. Reichart PA, Philipsen HP. Adenomatoid odontogenic tumor. In: Odontogenic Tumors and Allied Lesions. London: Quintessence Publishing Co Ltd, 2004:105–115.

335. da Silveira EJ, Gordon-Nunez MA, Seabra FR, et al. Peripheral calcifying epithelial odontogenic tumor associated with generalized drug-induced gingival growth: A case report. J Oral Maxillofac Surg 2007; 65(2):341–345.

336. Chomette G, Auriol M, Guilbert F. Tumeur épithéliale odontogène calcifiée bifocale (tumeur de Pindborg). Etude morphologique et ultrastructurale [Bifocal odontogenic calcified epithelial tumor (Pindborg's tumor). A morphologic and ultrastructural study]. Rev Stomatol Chir Maxillofac 1984; 85(4):329–336.

337. Busch HP, Hoppe W. Multilokulärer kalzifizierender epithelialer odontogener Tumor (CEOT) [Multilocular calcifying epithelial odontogenic tumor (CEOT)]. Dtsch Z Mund-Kiefer-Gesichts-Chir 1988; 12(3):193–194.

338. Sedghizadeh PP, Wong D, Shuler CF, et al. Multifocal calcifying epithelial odontogenic tumor. Oral Surg Oral Med Oral Pathol Oral Radiol Endod 2007; 104(1):e30–e34.

339. Bridle C, Visram K, Piper K, et al. Maxillary calcifying epithelial odontogenic (Pindborg) tumor presenting with abnormal eye signs: case report and literature review. Oral Surg Oral Med Oral Pathol Oral Radiol Endod 2006; 102(4):e12–e15.

340. Anavi Y, Kaplan I, Citir M, et al. Clear-cell variant of calcifying epithelial odontogenic tumor: clinical and radiographic characteristics. Oral Surg Oral Med Oral Pathol Oral Radiol Endod 2003; 95(3):332–339.

341. Gon F. The calcifying epithelial odontogenic tumour: report of a case and a study of its histogenesis. Br J Cancer 1965; 19:39–50.

342. Takeda Y, Suzuki A, Sekiyama S. Peripheral calcifying epithelial odontogenic tumor. Oral Surg Oral Med Oral Pathol 1983; 56(1):71–75.

343. Blank DM, Solomon M, Berger J. A microscopic focus of calcifying epithelial odontogenic tumor arising in an operculum: an incidental finding. J Oral Surg 1981; 39(6): 454–456.

344. Gopalakrishnan R, Simonton S, Rohrer MD, et al. Cystic variant of calcifying epithelial odontogenic tumor. Oral Surg Oral Med Oral Pathol Oral Radiol Endod 2006; 102(6):773–777.

345. Basu MK, Matthews JB, Sear AJ et al. Calcifying epithelial odontogenic tumour: a case showing features of malignancy. J Oral Pathol 1984; 13(3):310–319.

346. Cheng YS, Wright JM, Walstad WR, et al. Calcifying epithelial odontogenic tumor showing microscopic features of potential malignant behavior. Oral Surg Oral Med Oral Pathol Oral Radiol Endod 2002; 93(3):287–295.

347. Veness MJ, Morgan G, Collins AP, et al. Calcifying epithelial odontogenic (Pindborg) tumor with malignant transformation and metastatic spread. Head Neck 2001; 23(8):692–696.

348. Pindborg JJ. The calcifying epithelial odontogenic tumor. Review of the literature and report of one extraosseous case. Acta Odontol Scand 1966; 24:419–430.

349. Gardner DG, Michaels L, Liepa E. Calcifying epithelial odontogenic tumor: an amyloid-producing neoplasm. Oral Surg Oral Med Oral Pathol 1968; 26(6):812–823.

350. Mainwaring AR, Ahmed A, Hopkinson JM, et al. A clinical and electron microscopic study of a calcifying epithelial odontogenic tumour. J Clin Pathol 1971; 24(2): 152–158.

351. Mori M, Makino M. Calcifying epithelial odontogenic tumor: histochemical properties of homogeneous acellular substances in the tumor. J Oral Surg 1977; 35(8): 631–639.

352. Aviel-Ronen S, Liokumovich P, Rahima D, et al. The amyloid deposit in calcifying epithelial odontogenic tumor is immunoreactive for cytokeratins. Arch Pathol Lab Med 2000; 124(6):872–876.

353. Vickers RA, Dahlin DC, Gorlin RJ. Amyloid-containing odontogenic tumors. Oral Surg Oral Med Oral Pathol 1965; 20(4):476–480.

354. Ranløv P, Pindborg JJ. The amyloid nature of the homogeneous substance in the calcifying epithelial odontogenic tumour. Acta Pathol Microbiol Scand 1966; 68(2):169–174.

355. Chaudhry AP, Hanks CT, Leifer C et al. Calcifying epithelial odontogenic tumor. A histochemical and ultrastructural study. Cancer 1972; 30(2):519–529.

356. Franklin CD, Martin MV, Clark A, et al. An investigation into the origin and nature of 'amyloid' in a calcifying epithelial odontogenic tumour. J Oral Pathol 1981; 10(6): 417–429.

357. Asano M, Takahashi T, Kusama K, et al. A variant of calcifying epithelial odontogenic tumor with Langerhans cells. J Oral Pathol Med 1990; 19(9):430–434.

358. Takata T, Ogawa I, Miyauchi M, et al. Non-calcifying Pindborg tumor with Langerhans cells. J Oral Pathol Med 1993; 22(8):378–383.

359. Krolls SO, Pindborg JJ. Calcifying epithelial odontogenic tumor. A survey of 23 cases and discussion of histomorphologic variations. Arch Pathol 1974; 98(3):206–210.

360. Mesquita RA, Lotufo MA, Sugaya NN, et al. Peripheral clear cell variant of calcifying epithelial odontogenic tumor: report of a case and immunohistochemical investigation. Oral Surg Oral Med Oral Pathol Oral Radiol Endod 2003; 95(2):198–204.

361. Germanier Y, Bornstein MM, Stauffer E, et al. Calcifying epithelial odontogenic (Pindborg) tumor of the mandible with clear cell component treated by conservative surgery: report of a case. J Oral Maxillofac Surg 2005; 63(9): 1377–1382.

362. Kumamoto H, Sato I, Tateno H, et al. Clear cell variant of calcifying epithelial odontogenic tumor (CEOT) in the maxilla: report of a case with immunohistochemical and ultrastructural investigations. J Oral Pathol Med 1999; 28(4):187–191.

363. Seim P, Regezi JA, O'Ryan F. Hybrid ameloblastoma and calcifying epithelial odontogenic tumor: case report. J Oral Maxillofac Surg 2005; 63(6):852–855.

364. Mori M, Tatemoto Y, Yamamoto N, et al. Immunohistochemical localization of intermediate filament proteins in calcifying epithelial odontogenic tumors. J Oral Pathol 1988; 17(5):236–240.

365. Maiorano E, Renne G, Tradati N, et al. Cytogical features of calcifying epithelial odontogenic tumor (Pindborg tumor) with abundant cementum-like material. Virchows Arch 2003; 442(2):107–110.

366. Poomsawat S, Punyasingh J. Calcifying epithelial odontogenic tumor: an immunohistochemical case study. J Mol Histol 2007; 38:103–109.

367. Sauk JJ, Cocking-Johnson D, Warings M. Identification of basement membrane components and intermediate filaments in calcifying epithelial odontogenic tumors. J Oral Pathol 1985; 14(2):133–140.

368. Matsumura T, Matsuura H, Hirose I, et al. Calcifying epithelial odontogenic tumor - enzyme histochemical and electronmicroscopic considerations. J Osaka Univ Dent Sch 1975; 15(1):25–36.

369. Morimoto C, Tsujimoto M, Shimaoka S, et al. Ultrastructural localization of alkaline phosphatase in the calcifying epithelial odontogenic tumor. Oral Surg Oral Med Oral Pathol 1983; 56(4):409–414.

370. Chomette G, Auriol M, Guilbert F. Histoenzymological and ultrastructural study of a bifocal calcifying epithelial odontogenic tumor. Characteristics of epithelial cells and histogenesis of amyloid-like material. Virchows Arch A Pathol Anat Histopathol 1984; 403(1):67–76.

371. Kawano K, Ono K, Yada N, et al. Malignant calcifying epithelial odontogenic tumor of the mandible: report of a case with pulmonary metastasis showing remarkable response to platinum derivatives. Oral Surg Oral Med Oral Pathol Oral Radiol Endod 2007; 104(1):76–81.

372. Page DL, Weiss SW, Eggleston JC. Ultrastructural study of amyloid material in the calcifying epithelial odontogenic tumor. Cancer 1975; 36(4):1426–1435.

373. el-Labban NG, Lee KW, Kramer IR. The duality of the cell population in a calcifying epithelial odontogenic tumour (CEOT). Histopathology 1984; 8(4):679–691.

374. el-Labban NG, Lee KW, Kramer IR, et al. The nature of the amyloid-like material in a calcifying epithelial odontogenic tumour: an ultrastructural study. J Oral Pathol 1983; 12(5):366–374.

375. Solomon A, Murphy CL, Weaver K, et al. Calcifying epithelial odontogenic (Pindborg) tumor-associated amyloid consists of a novel human protein. J Lab Clin Med 2003; 142(5):348–355.

376. Kestler DP, Foster JS, Macy SD, et al. Expression of odontogenic ameloblast-associated protein (ODAM) in dental and other epithelial neoplasms. Mol Med 2008; 14(5–6):318–326.

377. el-Labban NG. Cementum-like material in a case of Pindborg tumor. J Oral Pathol Med 1990; 19(4):166–169.

378. Slootweg PJ. Bone and cementum as stromal features in Pindborg tumor. J Oral Pathol Med 1991; 20(2):93–95.

379. Dunlap CL. Odontogenic fibroma. Semin Diagn Pathol 1999; 16(4):293–296.

380. Smith RA, Hansen LS, Decker D. Atypical calcifying epithelial odontogenic tumor of the maxilla. J Am Dent Assoc 1980; 100(5):706–709.

381. Sciubba JJ, Fantasia JE, Kahn LB. Benign odontogenic tumors. In: Tumors and Cysts of the Jaws. Washington, D.C.: Armed Forces Institute of Pathology, 2001:71–127.

382. Philipsen HP, Nikai H. Adenomatoid odontogenic tumour. In: Barnes L, Eveson JW, Reichart P, et al. eds. World Health Organization Classification of Tumours. Pathology and Genetics of Head and Neck Tumours. Lyon: IARC Press, 2005:304–305.

383. Philipsen HP, Reichart PA, Siar CH, et al. An updated clinical and epidemiological profile of the adenomatoid odontogenic tumour: a collaborative retrospective study. J Oral Pathol Med 2007; 36(7):383–393.

384. Philipsen HP, Reichart PA. Adenomatoid odontogenic tumour: facts and figures. Oral Oncol 1998; 35(2):125–131.

385. Swasdison S, Dhanuthai K, Jainkittivong A, et al. Adenomatoid odontogenic tumors: an analysis of 67 cases in a Thai population. Oral Surg Oral Med Oral Pathol Oral Radiol Endod 2008; 105(2):210–215.

386. Yazdi I, Nowparast B. Extraosseous adenomatoid odontogenic tumor with special reference to the probability of the basal-cell layer of oral epithelium as a potential source of origin. Report of a case. Oral Surg Oral Med Oral Pathol 1974; 37(2):249–256.

387. Kearns GJ, Smith R. Adenomatoid odontogenic tumour: an unusual cause of gingival swelling in a 3-year-old patient. Br Dent J 1996; 181(10):380–382.

388. Giansanti JS, Someren A, Waldron CA. Odontogenic adenomatoid tumor (adenoameloblastoma). Survey of 3 cases. Oral Surg Oral Med Oral Pathol 1970; 30(1):69–88.

389. Philipsen HP, Reichart PA, Zhang KH, et al. Adenomatoid odontogenic tumor: biologic profile based on 499 cases. J Oral Pathol Med 1991; 20(4):149–158.

390. Leon JE, Mata GM, Fregnani ER, et al. Clinicopathological and immunohistochemical study of 39 cases of Adenomatoid Odontogenic Tumour: a multicentric study. Oral Oncol 2005; 41(8):835–842.

391. Toida M, Hyodo I, Okuda T, et al. Adenomatoid odontogenic tumor: report of two cases and survey of 126 cases in Japan. J Oral Maxillofac Surg 1990; 48(4):404–408.

392. Nomura M, Tanimoto K, Takata T, et al. Mandibular adenomatoid odontogenic tumor with unusual clinicopathologic features. J Oral Maxillofac Surg 1992; 50(3): 282–285.

393. Dayi E, Gurbuz G, Bilge OM, et al. Adenomatoid odontogenic tumour (adenoameloblastoma). Case report and review of the literature. Aust Dent J 1997; 42(5):315–318.

394. Nigam S, Gupta SK, Chaturvedi KU. Adenomatoid odontogenic tumor - a rare cause of jaw swelling. Braz Dent J 2005; 16:251–253.

395. Chuan-Xiang Z, Yan G. Adenomatoid odontogenic tumor: a report of a rare case with recurrence. J Oral Pathol Med 2007; 36(7):440–443.

396. Takahashi K, Yoshino T, Hashimoto S. Unusually large cystic adenomatoid odontogenic tumour of the maxilla: case report. Int J Oral Maxillofac Surg 2001; 30(2):173–175.

397. Takeda Y, Kudo K. Adenomatoid odontogenic tumor associated with calcifying epithelial odontogenic tumor. Int J Oral Maxillofac Surg 1986; 15(4):469–473.

398. Philipsen HP, Birn H. The adenomatoid odontogenic tumour. Ameloblastic adenomatoid tumour or

adeno-ameloblastoma. Acta Pathol Microbiol Scand 1969; 75(3):375–398.

399. el-Labban NG, Lee KW. Vascular degeneration in adenomatoid odontogenic tumour: an ultrastructural study. J Oral Pathol 1988; 17(6):298–305.

400. Mori M, Makino M, Imai K. The histochemical nature of homogeneous amorphous materials in odontogenic epithelial tumors. J Oral Surg 1980; 38(2):96–102.

401. Moro I, Okamura N, Okuda S, et al. The eosinophilic and amyloid-like materials in adenomatoid odontogenic tumor. J Oral Pathol 1982; 11(2):138–150.

402. Murata M, Cheng J, Horino K, et al. Enamel proteins and extracellular matrix molecules are co-localized in the pseudocystic stromal space of adenomatoid odontogenic tumor. J Oral Pathol Med 2000; 29(10):483–490.

403. Evans BL, Carr RF, Phillipe LJ. Adenoid ameloblastoma with dentinoid: a case report. Oral Surg Oral Med Oral Pathol Oral Radiol Endod 2004; 98(5):583–588.

404. Takeda Y, Shimono M. Adenomatoid odontogenic tumor with extensive formation of tubular dentin. Bull Tokyo Dent Coll 1996; 37(4):189–193.

405. Philipsen HP, Reichart PA, Nikai H. The adenomatoid odontogenic tumor (AOT): an update. Oral Med Pathol 1998; 2:55–60.

406. Damm DD, White DK, Drummond JF, et al. Combined epithelial odontogenic tumor: adenomatoid odontogenic tumor and calcifying epithelial odontogenic tumor. Oral Surg Oral Med Oral Pathol 1983; 55(5):487–496.

407. Bingham RA, Adrian JC. Combined epithelial odontogenic tumor - adenomatoid odontogenic tumor and calcifying epithelial odontogenic tumor: report of a case. J Oral Maxillofac Surg 1986; 44(7):574–577.

408. Siar CH, Ng KH. Combined calcifying epithelial odontogenic tumor and adenomatoid odontogenic tumor. Int J Oral Maxillofac Surg 1987; 16(2):214–216.

409. Miyake M, Nagahata S, Nishihara J, et al. Combined adenomatoid odontogenic tumor and calcifying epithelial odontogenic tumor: report of case and ultrastructural study. J Oral Maxillofac Surg 1996; 54(6):788–793.

410. Ledesma-Montes C, Mosqueda Taylor A, Romero de Leon E, et al. Adenomatoid odontogenic tumour with features of calcifying epithelial odontogenic tumour. (The so-called combined epithelial odontogenic tumour.) Clinicopathological report of 12 cases. Eur J Cancer B Oral Oncol 1993; 29B(3):221–224.

411. Dunlap CL, Fritzlen TJ. Cystic odontoma with concomitant adenoameloblastoma (adenoameloblastic odontoma). Oral Surg Oral Med Oral Pathol 1972; 34(3):450–456.

412. Allen CM, Neville BW, Hammond HL. Adenomatoid dentinoma. Report of four cases of an unusual odontogenic lesion. Oral Surg Oral Med Oral Pathol Oral Radiol Endod 1998; 86(3):313–317.

413. Ide F, Kusama K. Adenomatoid odontoma. Oral Surg Oral Med Oral Pathol Oral Radiol Endod 2002; 94(2):149–150.

414. Vargas PA, Carlos-Bregni R, Mosqueda-Taylor A, et al. Adenomatoid dentinoma or adenomatoid odontogenic hamartoma: what is the better term to denominate this uncommon odontogenic lesion? Oral Dis 2006; 12(2):200–203.

415. Aldred MJ, Gray AR. A pigmented adenomatoid odontogenic tumor. Oral Surg Oral Med Oral Pathol 1990; 70(1):86–89.

416. Warter A, George-Diolombi G, Chazal M, et al. Melanin in a dentigerous cyst and associated adenomatoid odontogenic tumor. Cancer 1990; 66(4):786–788.

417. Yamamoto K, Yoneda K, Yamamoto T, et al. An immunohistochemical study of odontogenic mixed tumours. Eur J Cancer B Oral Oncol 1995; 31B(2):122–128.

418. Takahashi H, Fujita S, Shibata Y, et al. Adenomatoid odontogenic tumour: immunohistochemical demonstration of transferrin, ferritin and alpha-one-antitrypsin. J Oral Pathol Med 2001; 30(4):237–244.

419. Vera Sempere FJ, Artes Martinez MJ, Vera SB, et al. Follicular adenomatoid odontogenic tumor: immunohistochemical study. Med Oral Patol Oral Cir Bucal 2006; 11(4):E305–E308.

420. Crivelini MM, Soubhia AMP, Felipini RC. Study on the origin and nature of the adenomatoid odontogenic tumor by immunohistochemistry. Journal of Applied Oral Science 2005; 13(4):406–412.

421. Tatemoto Y, Tanaka T, Okada Y, et al. Adenomatoid odontogenic tumour: co-expression of keratin and vimentin. Virchows Arch A Pathol Anat Histopathol 1988; 413(4):341–347.

422. Fujita S, Hideshima K, Ikeda T. Nestin expression in odontoblasts and odontogenic ectomesenchymal tissue of odontogenic tumours. J Clin Pathol 2006; 59(3):240–245.

423. Philipsen HP, Reichart PA. The adenomatoid odontogenic tumour: ultrastructure of tumour cells and non-calcified amorphous masses. J Oral Pathol Med 1996; 25(9):491–496.

424. Smith RR, Olson JL, Hutchins GM, et al. Adenomatoid odontogenic tumor: ultrastructural demonstration of two cell types and amyloid. Cancer 1979; 43(2):505–511.

425. Poulson TC, Greer RO Jr. Adenomatoid odontogenic tumor: clinicopathologic and ultrastructural concepts. J Oral Maxillofac Surg 1983; 41(12):818–824.

426. Hatakeyama S, Suzuki A. Ultrastructural study of adenomatoid odontogenic tumor. J Oral Pathol 1978; 7(5):295–300.

427. Yamamoto H, Kozawa Y, Hirai G, et al. Adenomatoid odontogenic tumor: light and electron microscopic study. Int J Oral Surg 1981; 10(4):272–278.

428. Lee KW. A light and electron microscopic study of the adenomatoid odontogenic tumor. Int J Oral Surg 1974; 3(4):183–193.

429. el-Labban NG. The nature of the eosinophilic and laminated masses in the adenomatoid odontogenic tumor: a histochemical and ultrastructural study. J Oral Pathol Med 1992; 21(2):75–81.

430. Sato D, Matsuzaka K, Yama M, et al. Adenomatoid odontogenic tumor arising from the mandibular molar region: a case report and review of the literature. Bull Tokyo Dent Coll 2004; 45(4):223–227.

431. Geist SM, Mallon HL. Adenomatoid odontogenic tumor: report of an unusually large lesion in the mandible. J Oral Maxillofac Surg 1995; 53(6):714–717.

432. Motamedi MH, Shafeie HA, Azizi T. Salvage of an impacted canine associated with an adenomatoid odontogenic tumour: a case report. Br Dent J 2005; 199(2):89–90.

433. Tomich CE. Benign mixed odontogenic tumors. Semin Diagn Pathol 1999; 16(4):308–316.

434. Slavkin HC. Embryonic Tooth Formation. A Tool for Developmental Biology. In: Melcher AH, Zarb GA, eds. Oral Sciences Reviews. Copenhagen: Munksgaard, 1974; 4:1–136.

435. Tucker AS, Sharpe PT. Molecular genetics of tooth morphogenesis and patterning: the right shape in the right place. J Dent Res 1999; 78(4):826–834.

436. Sharpe PT. Neural crest and tooth morphogenesis. Adv Dent Res 2001; 15:4–7.

437. Slootweg PJ. An analysis of the interrelationship of the mixed odontogenic tumors–ameloblastic fibroma, ameloblastic fibro-odontoma, and the odontomas. Oral Surg Oral Med Oral Pathol 1981; 51(3):266–276.

438. Chen Y, Wang J-M, Li T-J. Ameloblastic fibroma: a review of published studies with special reference to its nature and biological behavior. Oral Oncol 2007; 43(10):960–969. [Epub 2007, Aug 3].

439. Trodahl JN. Ameloblastic fibroma. A survey of cases from the Armed Forces Institute of Pathology. Oral Surg Oral Med Oral Pathol 1972; 33(4):547–558.

440. Chen Y, Li TJ, Gao Y, et al. Ameloblastic fibroma and related lesions: a clinicopathologic study with reference to their nature and interrelationship. J Oral Pathol Med 2005; 34(10):588–595.

441. Philipsen HP, Reichart PA, Praetorius F. Mixed odontogenic tumours and odontomas. Considerations on interrelationship. Review of the literature and presentation of 134 new cases of odontomas. Oral Oncol 1997; 33(2):86–99.

442. Lu Y, Xuan M, Takata T, et al. Odontogenic tumors. A demographic study of 759 cases in a Chinese population. Oral Surg Oral Med Oral Pathol Oral Radiol Endod 1998; 86(6):707–714.

443. Kusama K, Miyake M, Moro I. Peripheral ameloblastic fibroma of the mandible: report of a case. J Oral Maxillofac Surg 1998; 56(3):399–401.

444. Daley TD, Wysocki GP. Peripheral odontogenic fibroma. Oral Surg Oral Med Oral Pathol 1994; 78(3):329–336.

445. Ide F, Kitada M, Tanaka A, et al. Ameloblastic fibroma and related lesions: histological variability and potentially diagnostic pitfall. Hospital Dentistry & Oral-Maxillofacial Surgery (Tokyo) 2002; 14(1):15–21.

446. Ide F, Shimoyama T, Horie N. Peripheral ameloblastic fibroma. Oral Oncol 2000; 36(3):308.

447. Schmidt-Westhausen A, Philipsen HP, Reichart PA. Das ameloblastische fibrom - ein odontogener Tumor im Wachstumsalter [The ameloblastic fibroma. An odontogenic tumor in the growth period]. Dtsch Zahnärztl Z 1991; 46(1):66–68.

448. Philipsen HP, Thosaporn W, Reichart P, et al. Odontogenic lesions in opercula of permanent molars delayed in eruption. J Oral Pathol Med 1992; 21(1):38–41.

449. Pflüger H. Über die vom Zahnbildenden Gewebe ausgehenden Geschwülste Adamantinom und Odontom. Dtsch Zahn Mund Kieferheilkd Zentralbl Gesamte 1956; 25(3–4): 97–121.

450. Nilsen R, Magnusson BC. Ameloblastic fibroma. Int J Oral Surg 1979; 8(5):370–374.

451. Edwards MB, Goubran GF. Cystic, melanotic ameloblastic fibroma with granulomatous inflammation. Oral Surg Oral Med Oral Pathol 1980; 49(4):333–336.

452. Trott JR. Ameloblastic fibroma–case report. Br J Oral Surg 1967; 5(1):11–15.

453. Becker J, Reichart PA, Schuppan D, et al. Ectomesenchyme of ameloblastic fibroma reveals a characteristic distribution of extracellular matrix proteins. J Oral Pathol Med 1992; 21(4):156–159.

454. Slootweg PJ. Ameloblastic fibroma/fibrodentinoma. In: Barnes L, Eveson JW, Reichart P, et al. eds. World Health Organization Classification of Tumours. Pathology and Genetics of Head and Neck Tumours. Lyon: IARC Press, 2005:308.

455. Couch RD, Morris EE, Vellios F. Granular cell ameloblastic fibroma. Am J Clin Pathol 1962; 27:398–404.

456. White DK, Chen SY, Hartman KS, et al. Central granular-cell tumor of the jaws (the so-called granular-cell ameloblastic fibroma). Oral Surg Oral Med Oral Pathol 1978; 45(3):396–405.

457. Takeda Y. Granular cell ameloblastic fibroma, ultrastructure and histogenesis. Int J Oral Maxillofac Surg 1986; 15(2):190–195.

458. Takeda Y. Ameloblastic fibroma and related lesions: current pathologic concept. Oral Oncol 1999; 35(6): 535–540.

459. Tatemoto Y, Yamamoto N, Onojima M, et al. Ameloblastic fibroma: growth potentiality of odontogenic epithelium and coexpression of intermediate filament proteins in fibromatous cells. J Oral Pathol 1988; 17(4):168–174.

460. Heikinheimo K, Sandberg M, Happonen RP, et al. Cytoskeletal gene expression in normal and neoplastic human odontogenic epithelia. Lab Invest 1991; 65(6):688–701.

461. Papagerakis P, Peuchmaur M, Hotton D, et al. Aberrant gene expression in epithelial cells of mixed odontogenic tumors. J Dent Res 1999; 78(1):20–30.

462. Takeda Y, Sato H, Satoh M, et al. Immunohistochemical expression of neural tissue markers (neuron-specific enolase, glial fibrillary acidic protein, S100 protein) in ameloblastic fibrodentinoma: a comparative study with ameloblastic fibroma. Pathol Int 2000; 50(8):610–615.

463. Sano K, Yoshida S, Ninomiya H, et al. Assessment of growth potential by MIB-1 immunohistochemistry in ameloblastic fibroma and related lesions of the jaws compared with ameloblastic fibrosarcoma. J Oral Pathol Med 1998; 27(2):59–63.

464. Csiba A, Lapis K. Ultrastructure de l'améloblastome fibromateux [The ultrastructure of ameloblastic fibroma]. Bull Group Int Rech Sci Stomatol 1972; 15(3):233–250.

465. Ide F, Sakashita H, Kusama K. Ameloblastomatoid, central odontogenic fibroma: an epithelium-rich variant. J Oral Pathol Med 2002; 31(10):612–614.

466. Monteil RA, Le Bas V, Favot C, et al. Stereologic analysis of histologic parameters of a twice-recurrent ameloblastic fibroma. Oral Surg Oral Med Oral Pathol 1986; 61(2):168–172.

467. Williams MD, Hanna EY, El-Naggar AK. Anaplastic ameloblastic fibrosarcoma arising from recurrent ameloblastic fibroma: restricted molecular abnormalities of certain genes to the malignant transformation. Oral Surg Oral Med Oral Pathol Oral Radiol Endod 2007; 104(1): 72–75.

468. Hietanen J, Calonius PE, Collan Y, et al. Histology and ultrastructure of an ameloblastic fibroma. A case report. Proc Finn Dent Soc 1973; 69(4):129–140.

469. Van Wyk CW, van der Vyver PC. Ameloblastic fibroma with dentinoid formation/immature dentinoma. A microscopic and ultrastructural study of the epithelial-connective tissue interface. J Oral Pathol 1983; 12(1):37–46.

470. Baker WR, Swift JQ. Ameloblastic fibro-odontoma of the anterior maxilla. Report of a case. Oral Surg Oral Med Oral Pathol 1993; 76(3):294–297.

471. Gardner DG. The mixed odontogenic tumors. Oral Surg Oral Med Oral Pathol 1984; 58(2):166–168.

472. Takeda Y. So-called "immature dentinoma": a case presentation and histological comparison with ameloblastic fibrodentinoma. J Oral Pathol Med 1994; 23(2):92–96.

473. Lukinmaa PL, Hietanen J, Laitinen JM, et al. Mandibular dentinoma. J Oral Maxillofac Surg 1987; 45(1):60–64.

474. Ulmansky M, Bodner L, Praetorius F, et al. Ameloblastic fibrodentinoma: report on two new cases. J Oral Maxillofac Surg 1994; 52(9):980–984.

475. Husted E, Pindborg JJ. Odontogenic tumours; clinical and roentgenological aspects, treatment and pathology. Odontol Tidskr 1953; 61(5):275–292.

476. McKelvy BD, Cherrick HM. Peripheral ameloblastic fibrodentinoma. J Oral Surg 1976; 34(9):826–829.

477. Grodjesk JE, Doblinsky HB, Schneider LC, et al. Ameloblastic fibrodentinoma in the gingiva: Report of a case. J Oral Med 1980; 35(3):59–61.

478. Reichart PA, Philipsen HP. Ameloblastic Fibrodentinoma. In: Odontogenic Tumors and Allied Lesions. London: Quintessence Publishing Co Ltd, 2004:129–132.

479. Pindborg JJ. On dentinomas; with report of a case. Acta Pathol Microbiol Scand Suppl 1955; 105:135–144.

480. Howell RM, Burkes EJ Jr. Malignant transformation of ameloblastic fibro-odontoma to ameloblastic fibrosarcoma. Oral Surg Oral Med Oral Pathol 1977; 43(3):391–401.

481. Sekine J, Kitamura A, Ueno K, et al. Cell kinetics in mandibular ameloblastic fibro-odontoma evaluated by bromodeoxyuridine and proliferating cell nuclear antigen immunohistochemistry: case report. Br J Oral Maxillofac Surg 1996; 34(5):450–453.

482. Favia GF, Di AL, Scarano A, et al. Ameloblastic fibro-odontoma: report of two cases. Oral Oncol 1997; 33(6):444–446.

483. Ozer E, Pabuccuoglu U, Gunbay U, et al. Ameloblastic fibro-odontoma of the maxilla: case report. J Clin Pediatr Dent 1997; 21(4):329–331.

484. Yagishita H, Taya Y, Kanri Y, et al. The secretion of amelogenins is associated with the induction of enamel and dentinoid in an ameloblastic fibro-odontoma. J Oral Pathol Med 2001; 30(8):499–503.

485. Chang H, Precious DS, Shimizu MS. Ameloblastic fibro-odontoma: a case report. J Can Dent Assoc 2002; 68(4):243–246.

486. Fantasia JE, Damm DD. Mandibular radiolucency. Ameloblastic fibro-odontoma. Gen Dent 2002; 50(2):202,204.

487. Reichart PA, Philipsen HP, Gelderblom HR, et al. Ameloblastic fibro-odontoma - report of two cases with ultrastructural study of tumour dental hard structures. Oral Oncology EXTRA 2004; 40:8–12.

488. Oghli AA, Scuto I, Ziegler C, et al. A large ameloblastic fibro-odontoma of the right mandible. Med Oral Patol Oral Cir Bucal 2007; 12(1):E34–E37.

489. Hawkins PL, Sadeghi EM. Ameloblastic fibro-odontoma: report of case. J Oral Maxillofac Surg 1986; 44(12):1014–1019.

490. Savage MG, Heldt L, Dann JJ, et al. Encephalocraniocutaneous lipomatosis and mixed odontogenic tumors. J Oral Maxillofac Surg 1985; 43(8):617–620.

491. Herrmann M. Über vom Zahnsystem ausgehenden Tumoren bei Kindern. Fortschr Kiefer Gesichtschir 1957; 3:257–264.

492. Herrmann M. Über vom Zahnsystem audgehende Tumoren bei Kindern. (Ergänzungen zu dem 1956 gegebenen Bericht). Fortschr Kiefer Gesichtschir 1958; 4:226–229.

493. Schmidseder R, Hausamen JE. Multiple odontogenic tumors and other anomalies. An autosomal dominantly inherited syndrome. Oral Surg Oral Med Oral Pathol 1975; 39(2):249–258.

494. Kitano M, Tsuda-Yamada S, Semba I, et al. Pigmented ameloblastic fibro-odontoma with melanophages. Oral Surg Oral Med Oral Pathol 1994; 77(3):271–275.

495. Matsuzaka K, Inoue T, Nashimoto M, et al. A case of an ameloblastic fibro-odontoma arising from a calcifying odontogenic cyst. Bull Tokyo Dent Coll 2001; 42(1):51–55.

496. Miyauchi M, Takata T, Ogawa I, et al. Immunohistochemical observations on a possible ameloblastic fibro-odontoma. J Oral Pathol Med 1996; 25(2):93–96.

497. Hanna RJ, Regezi JA, Hayward JR. Ameloblastic fibro-odontoma: report of case with light and electron microscopic observations. J Oral Surg 1976; 34(9):820–825.

498. Josephsen K, Larsson A, Fejerskov O. Ultrastructural features of the epithelial-mesenchymal interface in an ameloblastic fibro-odontoma. Scand J Dent Res 1980; 88(2):79–95.

499. Slootweg PJ. Epithelio-mesenchymal morphology in ameloblastic fibro-odontoma: a light and electron microscopic study. J Oral Pathol 1980; 9(1):29–40.

500. Reich RH, Reichart PA, Ostertag H. Ameloblastic fibro-odontome. Report of a case, with ultrastructural study. J Maxillofac Surg 1984; 12(5):230–234.

501. Herzog U, Putzke HP, Bienengraber V, et al. Das ameloblastische Fibroodontom - ein odontogener Mischtumor mit Übergang in ein odontogenes Sarkom [The amelo-blastic fibro-odontoma–an odontogenic mixed tumor progressing into an odontogenic sarcoma]. Dtsch Z Mund-Kiefer-Gesichts-Chir 1991; 15(2):90–93.

502. Prætorius F, Piatelli A. Odontoma, complex type. In: Barnes L, Eveson JW, Reichart P, et al. eds. World Health Organization Classification of Tumours. Pathology and Genetics of Head and Neck Tumours. Lyon: IARC Press, 2005:310.

503. Hisatomi M, Asaumi JI, Konouchi H, et al. A case of complex odontoma associated with an impacted lower deciduous second molar and analysis of the 107 odontomas. Oral Dis 2002; 8(2):100–105.

504. O'Grady JF, Radden BG, Reade PC. Odontomes in an Australian population. Aust Dent J 1987; 32(3):196–199.

505. Budnick SD. Compound and complex odontomas. Oral Surg Oral Med Oral Pathol 1976; 42(4):501–506.

506. Zachariades N, Koundouris J, Angelopoulous AP. Odontoma of the maxillary sinus: report of case. J Oral Surg 1981; 39(9):697–698.

507. McClure G. Odontoma of the nasopharynx. Arch Otolaryngol Head Neck Surg 1946; 44:51–60.

508. McClatchey KD, Hakimi M, Batsakis JG. Retrotympanic odontoma. Am J Surg Pathol 1981; 5(4):401–404.

509. Bellucci RJ, Zizmor J, Goodwin RE. Odontoma of the middle ear. A case presentation. Arch Otolaryngol Head Neck Surg 1975; 101(9):571–573.

510. Mani NJ. Odontoma syndrome: report of an unusual case with multiple multiform odontomas of both jaws. J Dent 1974; 2(4):149–152.

511. Bader G. Odontomatosis (multiple odontomas). Oral Surg Oral Med Oral Pathol 1967; 23(6):770–773.

512. Bodin I, Julin P, Thomsson M. Odontomas and their pathological sequels. Dentomaxillofac Radiol 1983; 12(2):109–114.

513. Amado-Cuesta S, Gargallo-Albiol J, Berini-Aytés L, et al. Review of 61 cases of odontoma. Presentation of an erupted complex odontoma. Med Oral 2003; 8(5):366–373.

514. Riddet SA. A composite odontoma at a very early age. Br Dent J 1944; 77:129–131.

515. Clausen F. Les odontômes améloblastiques. Revue de Stomatologie 1959; 60:590–609.

516. Pantoja E, Wendth AJ, Luther PM. Ameloblastic odontoma. Clinicopathologic study. N Y State J Med 1976; 76(2):224–227.

517. Morning P. Impacted teeth in relation to odontomas. Int J Oral Surg 1980; 9(2):81–91.

518. Or S, Yucetas S. Compound and complex odontomas. Int J Oral Maxillofac Surg 1987; 16(5):596–599.

519. Yonemochi H, Noda T, Saku T. Pericoronal hamartomatous lesions in the opercula of teeth delayed in eruption: an immunohistochemical study of the extracellular matrix. J Oral Pathol Med 1998; 27(9):441–452.

520. Goldberg H, Schofield ID, Popowich LD, et al. Cystic complex composite odontoma. Report of two cases. Oral Surg Oral Med Oral Pathol 1981; 51(1):16–20.

521. De Visscher JG, Guven O, Elias AG. Complex odontoma in the maxillary sinus. Report of 2 cases. Int J Oral Surg 1982; 11(4):276–280.

522. Salama N, Hilmy A. Extensive complex composite odontome occupying the whole of the left maxilla. Br Dent J 1950; 89:68–70.

523. Wainwright WW. Complex odontoma. Report of a case. Am J Orthod Oral Surg section 1945; 31:447–454.

524. Kristen K, Singer R. Über Odontome unter besonderer Berüchsichtigung des Gardner-Syndroms [Odontomas with special reference to Gardner's syndrome]. Dtsch Zahnärztl Z 1977; 32(10):785–787.

525. Schalow W, Bader G. Das angeborene systematisierte Odontom. Dtsch Zahnärztl Z 1967; 22:1514.

526. Yoda T, Ishii Y, Honma Y, et al. Multiple macrodonts with odontoma in a mother and son–a variant of Ekman-Westborg-Julin syndrome. Report of a case. Oral Surg Oral Med Oral Pathol Oral Radiol Endod 1998; 85(3):301–303.

527. Carol-Montfort J. Significacion e histogenesis de los odontomas. Revista Española d'Estomatologia 1957; 5(5):433–442.

528. Gardner DG, Farquhar DA. A classification of dysplastic forms of dentin. J Oral Pathol 1979; 8(1):28–46.

529. Marchetti C. Some information on dental tissues obtained from observations on a complex odontoma. Acta Anat (Basel) 1993; 147(1):40–44.

530. Gardner DG, Dort LC. Dysplastic enamel in odontomas. Oral Surg Oral Med Oral Pathol 1979; 47(3):238–246.

531. Marchetti C, Piacentini C, Menghini P, et al. Observations on the enamel of odontomas. Scanning Microsc 1993; 7(3):999–1006.

532. Kerebel B, Kerebel LM. Ghost cells in complex odontoma: a light microscopic and SEM study. Oral Surg Oral Med Oral Pathol 1985; 59(4):371–378.

533. Piattelli A, Trisi P. Ghost cells in compound odontoma: a study of undemineralized material. Bull Group Int Rech Sci Stomatol Odontol 1991; 34(3–4):145–149.

534. Sedano HO, Pindborg JJ. Ghost cell epithelium in odontomas. J Oral Pathol 1975; 4(1):27–30.

535. Tanaka A, Okamoto M, Yoshizawa D, et al. Presence of ghost cells and the Wnt signaling pathway in odontomas. J Oral Pathol Med 2007; 36(7):400–404.

536. Sapp JP, Jensvold J. The distribution and morphologic variation of hyaline deposits in odontogenic lesions. Oral Surg Oral Med Oral Pathol 1983; 55(2):151–161.

537. Prætorius F, Piatelli A. Odontoma, compound type. In: Barnes L, Eveson JW, Reichart P, et al. eds. World Health Organization Classification of Tumours. Pathology and Genetics of Head and Neck Tumours. Lyon: IARC Press, 2005:311.

538. Castro GW, Houston G, Weyrauch C. Peripheral odontoma: report of case and review of literature. ASDC J Dent Child 1994; 61(3):209–213.

539. Ledesma-Montes C, Perez-Bache A, Garces-Ortiz M. Gingival compound odontoma. Int J Oral Maxillofac Surg 1996; 25(4):296–297.

540. Schreiber LK. Bilateral odontomas preventing eruption of maxillary central incisors. Report of a case. Oral Surg Oral Med Oral Pathol 1963; 16:503–507.

541. Thompson RD, Hale ML, McLeran JH. Multiple compound composite odontomas of maxilla and mandible: report of case. J Oral Surg 1968; 26(7):478–480.

542. Melnick M. Odontomatosis. Oral Surg Oral Med Oral Pathol 1975; 40(1):163.

543. Ajike SO, Adekeye EO. Multiple odontomas in the facial bones. A case report. Int J Oral Maxillofac Surg 2000; 29(6):443–444.

544. Jacobs HG. Der Zeitraum der Hartsubstanzbildung von zusammengesetzten Odontomen. Ein klinisch-röntgenologischer Beitrag [The period of hard substance formation in compound composite odontomas. A clinical/radiographic documentation]. Dtsch Z Mund-Kiefer-Gesichts-Chir 1988; 12(3):201–204.

545. Lopez-Areal L, Silvestre Donat F, Gil Lozano J. Compound odontoma erupting in the mouth: 4-year follow-up of a clinical case. J Oral Pathol Med 1992; 21(6):285–288.

546. De Visscher JG. Compound odontoma with displaced toothbuds: report of case with four-year follow-up. J Oral Surg 1981; 39(5):359–361.

547. Piattelli A, Trisi P. Morphodifferentiation and histodifferentiation of the dental hard tissues in compound odontoma: a study of undemineralized material. J Oral Pathol Med 1992; 21(8):340–342.

548. Abiko Y, Murata M, Ito Y, et al. Immunohistochemical localization of amelogenin in human odontogenic tumors, using a polyclonal antibody against bovine amelogenin. Med Electron Microsc 2001; 34(3):185–189.

549. Sapp JP, Gardner DG. An ultrastructural study of the calcifications in calcifying odontogenic cysts and odontomas. Oral Surg Oral Med Oral Pathol 1977; 44(5):754–766.

550. Blinder D, Peleg M, Taicher S. Surgical considerations in cases of large mandibular odontomas located in the mandibular angle. Int J Oral Maxillofac Surg 1993; 22(3):163–165.

551. Kamakura S, Matsui K, Katou F, et al. Surgical and orthodontic management of compound odontoma without removal of the impacted permanent tooth. Oral Surg Oral Med Oral Pathol Oral Radiol Endod 2002; 94(5):540–542.

552. Friedrich RE, Siegert J, Donath K, et al. Recurrent ameloblastic fibro-odontoma in a 10-year-old boy. J Oral Maxillofac Surg 2001; 59(11):1362–1366.

553. Tomizawa M, Otsuka Y, Noda T. Clinical observations of odontomas in Japanese children: 39 cases including one recurrent case. Int J Paediatr Dent 2005; 15(1):37–43.

554. Mosqueda-Taylor A. Odontoameloblastoma. In: Barnes L, Eveson JW, Reichart P, et al. eds. World Health Organization Classification of Tumours. Pathology and Genetics of Head and Neck Tumours. Lyon: IARC Press, 2005:312.

555. Frissell CT, Shafer WG. Ameloblastic odontoma: report of a case. Oral Surg Oral Med Oral Pathol 1953; 6:1129–1133.

556. Silva CA. Odontoameloblastoma. Oral Surg Oral Med Oral Pathol 1956; 9(5):545–552.

557. Jacobsohn PH, Quinn JH. Ameloblastic odontomas. Report of three cases. Oral Surg Oral Med Oral Pathol 1968; 26(6):829–836.

558. LaBriola JD, Steiner M, Bernstein ML, et al. Odontoameloblastoma. J Oral Surg 1980; 38(2):139–143.

559. Kaugars GE, Zussmann HW. Ameloblastic odontoma (odonto-ameloblastoma). Oral Surg Oral Med Oral Pathol 1991; 71(3):371–373.

560. Orlowski WA, Doyle JL, Salb R. Unique odontogenic tumor with dentinogenesis and features of unicystic plexiform ameloblastoma. Oral Surg Oral Med Oral Pathol 1991; 72(1):91–94.

561. Matsumoto Y, Mizoue K, Seto K. Atypical plexiform ameloblastoma with dentinoid: adenoid ameloblastoma with dentinoid. J Oral Pathol Med 2001; 30(4):251–254.

562. Mosqueda-Taylor A, Carlos-Bregni R, Ramirez-Amador V, et al. Odontoameloblastoma. Clinico-pathologic study of three cases and critical review of the literature. Oral Oncol 2002; 38(8):800–805.

563. Kumamoto H, Kawamura H, Ooya K. Clear cell odontogenic tumor in the mandible: report of a case with an immunohistochemical study of epithelial cell markers. Pathol Int 1998; 48(8):618–622.

564. Wächter R, Remagen W, Stoll P. Kann man zwischen Odonto-Ameloblastom und ameloblastischem Fibro-Odontom unterscheiden? Kritische Stellungnahme auf der Basis von 18 Fallen im DÖSAK-Register [Is it possible to differentiate between odontoameloblastoma and fibro-odontoma? Critical position on basis of 18 cases in DOSAK list]. Dtsch Zahnärztl Z 1991; 46(1):74–77.

565. Thoma KH, Goldman HM. Odontogenic tumors, a classification based on observation of the epithelial, mesenchymal, and mixed varieties. Am J Pathol 1946; 22:433–471.

566. Rywkin AW. Beitrag zur pathologie der cholesteatome. Virchows Arch A Pathol Anat Histol 1932; 283:13–28.

567. Boss JH. A rare variant of ameloblastoma. Arch Pathol 1959; 68:299–305.

568. Spirgi M. Un cas d'épithélioma adamantin calcifié au niveau de la muqueuse buccale. Schweizerische Monatsschrift für Zahnheilkunde 1960; 70:1077–1090.

569. Lurie HI. Congenital melanocarcinoma, melanotic adamantinoma, retinal anlage tumor, progonoma, and pigmented epulis of infancy; summary and review of literature and report of first case in adult. Cancer 1961; 14:1090–1108.

570. Gorlin RJ, Pindborg JJ, Clausen FP, et al. The calcifying odontogenic cyst–a possible analogue of the cutaneous calcifying epithelioma of Malherbe. An analysis of fifteen cases. Oral Surg Oral Med Oral Pathol 1962; 15:1235–1243.

571. Gold L. The keratinizing and calcifying odontogenic cyst. Oral Surg Oral Med Oral Pathol 1963; 16:1414–1424.

572. Gorlin RJ, Pindborg JJ, Redman RS, et al. The calcifying odontogenic cyst. A new entity and possible analogue of the cutaneous calcifying epithelioma of Malherbe. Cancer 1964; 17:723–729.

573. Abrams AM, Howell FV. Calcifying epithelial odontogenic tumors: report of four cases. J Am Dent Assoc 1967; 74(6):1231–1240.

574. Chaves E. The calcifying odontogenic cyst. Report of two cases. Oral Surg Oral Med Oral Pathol 1968; 25(6):849–855.

575. Jones JH, McGowan DA, Gorman JM. Calcifying epithelial odontogenic and keratinizing odontogenic tumors. Oral Surg Oral Med Oral Pathol 1968; 25(3):465–469.

576. Ulmansky M, Azaz B, Sela J. Calcifying odontogenic cyst: report of cases. J Oral Surg 1969; 27:415–419.

577. Fejerskov O, Krogh J. The calcifying ghost cell odontogenic tumor - or the calcifying odontogenic cyst. J Oral Pathol 1972; 1(6):273–287.

578. Astacio JN, Pineda Martinez A. Tumor odontogenico epitelial calcificante. Reporte de un caso [Calcifying epithelial odontogenic tumor. Report of a case]. Archivos del Colegio Médico de El Salvador 1965; 18(4):283–290.

579. Li TJ, Yu SF. Clinicopathologic spectrum of the so-called calcifying odontogenic cysts: a study of 21 intraosseous cases with reconsideration of the terminology and classification. Am J Surg Pathol 2003; 27(3):372–384.

580. Prætorius F, Hjørting-Hansen E, Gorlin RJ, et al. Calcifying odontogenic cyst. Range, variations and neoplastic potential. Acta Odontol Scand 1981; 39(4):227–240.

581. Ellis GL, Shmookler BM. Aggressive (malignant?) epithelial odontogenic ghost cell tumor. Oral Surg Oral Med Oral Pathol 1986; 61(5):471–478.

582. Hong SP, Ellis GL, Hartman KS. Calcifying odontogenic cyst. A review of ninety-two cases with reevaluation of their nature as cysts or neoplasms, the nature of ghost cells, and subclassification. Oral Surg Oral Med Oral Pathol 1991; 72(1):56–64.

583. Altini M, Farman AG. The calcifying odontogenic cyst. Eight new cases and a review of the literature. Oral Surg Oral Med Oral Pathol 1975; 40(6):751–759.

584. Freedman PD, Lumerman H, Gee JK. Calcifying odontogenic cyst. A review and analysis of seventy cases. Oral Surg Oral Med Oral Pathol 1975; 40(1):93–106.

585. McGowan RH, Browne RM. The calcifying odontogenic cyst: a problem of preoperative diagnosis. Br J Oral Surg 1982; 20(3):203–212.

586. Shamaskin RG, Svirsky JA, Kaugars GE. Intraosseous and extraosseous calcifying odontogenic cyst (Gorlin cyst). J Oral Maxillofac Surg 1989; 47(6):562–565.

587. Buchner A, Merrell PW, Carpenter WM, et al. Central (intraosseous) calcifying odontogenic cyst. Int J Oral Maxillofac Surg 1990; 19(5):260–262.

588. Mascrès C, Donohue WB, Vauclair R. The calcifying odontogenic cyst: report of a case. J Oral Maxillofac Surg 1990; 48(3):319–322.

589. Johnson A III, Fletcher M, Gold L, et al. Calcifying odontogenic cyst: a clinicopathologic study of 57 cases with immunohistochemical evaluation for cytokeratin. J Oral Maxillofac Surg 1997; 55(7):679–683.

590. Moleri AB, Moreira LC, Carvalho JJ. Comparative morphology of 7 new cases of calcifying odontogenic cysts. J Oral Maxillofac Surg 2002; 60:689–696.

591. Orsini G, Fioroni M, Rubini C, et al. Peripheral calcifying odontogenic cyst. J Clin Periodontol 2002; 29(1):83–86.

592. Iida S, Ueda T, Aikawa T, et al. Ameloblastomatous calcifying odontogenic cyst in the mandible. Dentomaxillofac Radiol 2004; 33(6):409–412.

593. Buchner A, Merrell PW, Hansen LS, et al. Peripheral (extraosseous) calcifying odontogenic cyst. A review of forty-five cases. Oral Surg Oral Med Oral Pathol 1991; 72(1):65–70.

594. Buchner A. The central (intraosseous) calcifying odontogenic cyst: an analysis of 215 cases. J Oral Maxillofac Surg 1991; 49(4):330–339.

595. Toida M. So-called calcifying odontogenic cyst: review and discussion on the terminology and classification. J Oral Pathol Med 1998; 27(2):49–52.

596. Prætorius F, Ledesma-Montes C. Dentinogenic ghost cell tumour. In: Barnes L, Eveson JW, Reichart P, et al. eds. World Health Organization Classification of Tumours. Pathology and Genetics of Head and Neck Tumours. Lyon: IARC Press, 2005:314.

597. Takata T, Lu Y. Ghost cell odontogenic carcinoma. In: Barnes L, Eveson JW, Reichart P, et al. eds. World Health Organization Classification of Tumours. Pathology and Genetics of Head and Neck Tumours. Lyon: IARC Press, 2005:293.

598. Prætorius F, Ledesma-Montes C. Calcifying cystic odontogenic tumour. In: Barnes L, Eveson JW, Reichart P, et al. eds. World Health Organization Classification of Tumours. Pathology and Genetics of Head and Neck Tumours. Lyon: IARC Press, 2005:313.

599. Tanimoto K, Tomita S, Aoyama M, et al. Radiographic characteristics of the calcifying odontogenic cyst. Int J Oral Maxillofac Surg 1988; 17(1):29–32.

600. Yoshiura K, Tabata O, Miwa K, et al. Computed tomographic features of calcifying odontogenic cysts. Dentomaxillofac Radiol 1998; 27(1):12–16.

601. Wang YP, Chang YF, Wang JT, et al. Characteristics of calcifying odontogenic cyst in Taiwanese. J Formos Med Assoc 2003; 102(10):715–721.

602. Soames JV. A pigmented calcifying odontogenic cyst. Oral Surg Oral Med Oral Pathol 1982; 53(4):395–400.

603. Clausen FP, Dabelsteen E. Increase in sensitivity of the rhodamine B method for keratinisation by use of fluorescent light. Acta Pathol Microbiol Scand (A) 1969; 77:169–171.

604. Monteil RA, Bauduin D, Marcelet B. Étude signalétique et immunohistochimique de la kératinisation des cellules fantômes du kyste odontogène calcifié [Descriptive and immunohistochemical study of ghost cell keratinization in the calcifying odontogenic cyst]. J Biol Buccale 1986; 14(2):147–153.

605. Takeda Y, Suzuki A, Yamamoto H. Histopathologic study of epithelial components in the connective tissue wall of unilocular type of calcifying odontogenic cyst. J Oral Pathol Med 1990; 19(3):108–113.

606. Yoshida M, Kumamoto H, Ooya K, et al. Histopathological and immunohistochemical analysis of calcifying odontogenic cysts. J Oral Pathol Med 2001; 30(10):582–588.

607. Fregnani ER, Pires FR, Quezada RD, et al. Calcifying odontogenic cyst: clinicopathological features and immunohistochemical profile of 10 cases. J Oral Pathol Med 2003; 32(3):163–170.

608. Ng KH, Siar CH. Clear cell change in a calcifying odontogenic cyst. Oral Surg Oral Med Oral Pathol 1985; 60(4): 417–419.

609. Yamamoto Y, Hiranuma Y, Eba M, et al. Calcifying odontogenic cyst immunohistochemical detection of keratin and involucrin in cyst wall. Virchows Arch A Pathol Anat Histopathol 1988; 412(3):189–196.

610. Kakudo K, Mushimoto K, Shirasu R, et al. Calcifying odontogenic cysts: co-expression of intermediate filament proteins, and immunohistochemical distribution of keratins, involucrin, and filaggrin. Pathol Res Pract 1989; 185(6):891–899.

611. Gordeeff M, Clergeau-Guerithault S. L'expression de certaines cytokératines par les cellules epithéliales d'un kyste odontogène calcifié [The expression of various cytokeratins by epithelial cells of calcified odontogenic cysts]. J Biol Buccale 1991; 19(4):319–328.

612. Murakami S, Koike Y, Matsuzaka K, et al. A case of calcifying odontogenic cyst with numerous calcifications: Immunohistochemical analysis. Bull Tokyo Dent Coll 2003; 44(2):61–66.

613. Kusama K, Katayama Y, Oba K, et al. Expression of hard alfa-keratins in pilomatrixoma, craniopharyngeoma, and calcifying odontogenic cyst. Am J Clin Pathol 2005; 123:376–381.

614. Takata T, Zhao M, Nikai H, et al. Ghost cells in calcifying odontogenic cyst express enamel-related proteins. Histochem J 2000; 32(4):223–229.

615. Takata T, Lu Y, Ogawa I, et al. Proliferative activity of calcifying odontogenic cysts as evaluated by proliferating cell nuclear antigen labeling index. Pathol Int 1998; 48(11): 877–881.

616. Hassanein AM, Glanz SM, Kessler HP, et al. Beta-Catenin is expressed aberrantly in tumors expressing shadow cells. Pilomatricoma, craniopharyngioma, and calcifying odontogenic cyst. Am J Clin Pathol 2003; 120 (5):732–736.

617. Donath K, Kleinhans V, Gundlach KK. Zur Pathogenese der calcifizierenden odontogenen Cyste (Gorlin-Cyste) [The pathogenesis of the calcifying odontogenic cyst (Gorlin-cyst) (author's transl)]. Virchows Arch A Pathol Anat Histol 1979; 384(3):307–324.

618. Abaza NA. Ultrastructural features and biologic aspects of odontogenic cysts and tumors. Oral Maxillofac Surg Clin North Am 1994; 6:523–576.

619. Chen SY, Miller AS. Ultrastructure of the keratinizing and calcifying odontogenic cyst. Oral Surg Oral Med Oral Pathol 1975; 39(5):769–780.

620. Mimura M, Tanaka N, Kimijima Y, et al. An ultrastructural study of calcifying odontogenic cyst, especially calcified material. Med Electron Microsc 2002; 35:109–116.

621. Swinson TW. A clinico-pathological comparison of the ameloblastoma with the calcifying odontogenic cyst. Br J Oral Surg 1976; 13(3):217–229.

622. Slootweg PJ, Koole R. Recurrent calcifying odontogenic cyst (case report). J Maxillofac Surg 1980; 8(2):143–145.

623. Dominguez FV, Espinal EG. The calcifying odontogenic cyst. Clinical and histological analysis of 10 cases. Acta Odontol Latinoam 1984; 1(2):77–83.

624. Stoelinga PJ, Bronkhorst FB. The incidence, multiple presentation and recurrence of aggressive cysts of the jaws. J Craniomaxillofac Surg 1988; 16(4):184–195.

625. Daniels JS. Central odontogenic fibroma of mandible: a case report and review of the literature. Oral Surg Oral Med Oral Pathol Oral Radiol Endod 2004; 98 (3):295–300.

626. Ikemura K, Horie A, Tashiro H, et al. Simultaneous occurrence of a calcifying odontogenic cyst and its malignant transformation. Cancer 1985; 56(12):2861–2864.

627. Alcalde RE, Sasaki A, Misaki M, et al. Odontogenic ghost cell carcinoma: report of a case and review of the literature. J Oral Maxillofac Surg 1996; 54(1):108–111.

628. Lu Y, Mock D, Takata T, et al. Odontogenic ghost cell carcinoma: report of four new cases and review of the literature. J Oral Pathol Med 1999; 28(7):323–329.

629. Kamijo R, Miyaoka K, Tachikawa T, et al. Odontogenic ghost cell carcinoma: report of a case. J Oral Maxillofac Surg 1999; 57(10):1266–1270.

630. Goldenberg D, Sciubba J, Tufano RP. Odontogenic ghost cell carcinoma. Head Neck 2004; 26(4):378–381.

631. Cheng Y, Long X, Li X, et al. Clinical and radiological features of odontogenic ghost cell carcinoma: review of the literature and report of four new cases. Dentomaxillofac Radiol 2004; 33(3):152–157.

632. Tajima Y, Yokose S, Sakamoto E, et al. Ameloblastoma arising in calcifying odontogenic cyst. Report of a case. Oral Surg Oral Med Oral Pathol 1992; 74 (6):776–779.

633. Aithal D, Reddy BS, Mahajan S, et al. Ameloblastomatous calcifying odontogenic cyst: a rare histologic variant. J Oral Pathol Med 2003; 32(6):376–378.

634. Ide F, Obara K, Mishima K, et al. Ameloblastoma ex calcifying odontogenic cyst (dentinogenic ghost cell tumor). J Oral Pathol Med 2005; 34(8):511–512.

635. Zeitoun IM, Dhanrajani PJ, Mosadomi HA. Adenomatoid odontogenic tumor arising in a calcifying odontogenic cyst. J Oral Maxillofac Surg 1996; 54(5):634–637.

636. Lukinmaa PL, Leppaniemi A, Hietanen J, et al. Features of odontogenesis and expression of cytokeratins and tenascin-C in three cases of extraosseous and intraosseous calcifying odontogenic cyst. J Oral Pathol Med 1997; 26(6): 265–272.

637. Buch RS, Coerdt W, Wahlmann U. Adenomatoider odontogener Tumor in kalzifizierender odontogener Zyste [Adenomatoid odontogenic tumor in calcifying odontogenic cyst]. Mund Kiefer Gesichtschir 2003; 7(5): 301–305.

638. Lin CC, Chen CH, Lin LM, et al. Calcifying odontogenic cyst with ameloblastic fibroma: report of three cases. Oral Surg Oral Med Oral Pathol Oral Radiol Endod 2004; 98(4):451–460.

639. Yoon JH, Kim HJ, Yook JI, et al. Hybrid odontogenic tumor of calcifying odontogenic cyst and ameloblastic fibroma. Oral Surg Oral Med Oral Pathol Oral Radiol Endod 2004; 98(1):80–84.

640. Farman AG, Smith SN, Nortje CJ, et al. Calcifying odontogenic cyst with ameloblastic fibro-odontome: one lesion or two? J Oral Pathol 1978; 7(1):19–27.

641. Ledesma-Montes C, Gorlin RJ, Shear M, et al. International collaborative study on ghost cell odontogenic tumours: calcifying cystic odontogenic tumour, dentinogenic ghost cell tumour and ghost cell odontogenic carcinoma. J Oral Pathol Med 2008; 37(5):302–308.

642. Nagao T, Nakajima T, Fukushima M, et al. Calcifying odontogenic cyst: a survey of 23 cases in the Japanese literature. J Maxillofac Surg 1983; 11(4):174–179.

643. Hirshberg A, Kaplan I, Buchner A. Calcifying odontogenic cyst associated with odontoma: a possible separate entity (odontocalcifying odontogenic cyst). J Oral Maxillofac Surg 1994; 52(6):555–558.

644. Duckworth R, Seward GR. A melanotic ameloblastic odontoma. Oral Surg Oral Med Oral Pathol 1965; 19:73–85.

645. Nagao T, Nakajima T, Fukushima M, et al. Calcifying odontogenic cyst with complex odontoma. J Oral Maxillofac Surg 1982; 40(12):810–813.

646. Satomura K, Nakanishi H, Fujisawa K, et al. Initiation of ectopic epithelial calcification in a calcifying odontogenic cyst. J Oral Pathol Med 1999; 28(7):330–335.

647. Pistóia GD, Gerlach RF, dos Santos JCB, et al. Odontoma-producing intraosseous calcifying odontogenic cyst: Case report. Braz Dent J 2001; 12(1):67–70.

648. Martin-Duverneuil N, Roisin-Chausson MH, Behin A, et al. Combined benign odontogenic tumors: CT and MR findings and histomorphologic evaluation. AJNR Am J Neuroradiol 2001; 22(5):867–872.

649. Saito I, Suzuki T, Yamamura J, et al. Calcifying odontogenic cyst. Case reports, variations, and tumorous potential. J Nihon Univ Sch Dent 1982; 24(2):69–78.

650. Gallana-Alvarez S, Mayorga-Jimenez F, Torres-Gomez FJ, et al. Calcifying odontogenic cyst associated with complex odontoma: case report and review of the literature. Med Oral Patol Oral Cir Bucal 2005; 10(3): 243–247.

651. Toida M, Ishimaru J, Tatematsu N. Calcifying odontogenic cyst associated with compound odontoma: report of a case. J Oral Maxillofac Surg 1990; 48(1):77–81.

652. Oliveira JA, da Silva CJ, Costa IM, et al. Calcifying odontogenic cyst in infancy: report of case associated with compound odontoma. ASDC J Dent Child 1995; 62(1):70–73.

653. Piattelli A, Scarano A, Piatteli M. Calcifying odontogenic cyst associated with compound odontoma: A study on undemineralized material. Bull Group Int Rech Sci Stomatol Odontol 1995; 38(3–4):105–109.

654. Eda S, Uanagisawa Y, Koike H, et al. Two cases of calcifying odontogenic cyst associated with odontoma, with an electron-microscopic observation. Bull Tokyo Dent Coll 1974; 15(2):77–90.

655. Wright BA, Bhardwaj AK, Murphy D. Recurrent calcifying odontogenic cyst. Oral Surg Oral Med Oral Pathol 1984; 58(5):579–583.

656. Ellis GL. Odontogenic ghost cell tumor. Semin Diagn Pathol 1999; 16(4):288–292.

657. Reichart PA, Philipsen HP. Calcifying Ghost Cell Odontogenic Cysts/Tumors (Odontogenic Ghost Cell Lesions). In: Odontogenic Tumors and Allied Lesions. London: Quintessence Publishing Co Ltd, 2004:155–170.

658. Bhaskar SN. Oral Surgery–Oral Pathology Conference NO. 13, Walter Reed Army Medical Center. Oral Surg Oral Med Oral Pathol 1965; 19:796–807.

659. Sauk JJ Jr. Calcifying and keratinizing odontogenic cyst. J Oral Surg 1972; 30(12):893–897.

660. Winter WA. Kalzifizierende odontogene Zyste und fibromatöser Tumor. Dtsch Z Mund-Kiefer-Gesichts-Chir 1980; 4:225–227.

661. Hirshberg A, Dayan D, Horowitz I. Dentinogenic ghost cell tumor. Int J Oral Maxillofac Surg 1987; 16(5): 620–625.

662. McClatchey KD, Stewart JC, Patterson BD. Dentinogenic ghost cell tumor presenting as a gingival mass. Ann Dent 1988; 47(1):31–32.

663. Günhan Ö, Mocan A, Can C, et al. Epithelial odontogenic ghost cell tumor: report of a peripheral solid variant and review of the literature. Ann Dent 1991; 50(2):8–11, 48.

664. Raubenheimer EJ, van Heerden WF, Sitzmann F, et al. Peripheral dentinogenic ghost cell tumor. J Oral Pathol Med 1992; 21(2):93–95.

665. Castro WH, de Aguiar MC, Gomez RS. Peripheral dentinogenic ghost-cell tumor: a case report. Quintessence Int 1997; 28(1):45–47.

666. Piattelli A, Fioroni M, Di Alberti L, et al. Immunohistochemical analysis of a dentinogenic ghost cell tumour. Oral Oncol 1998; 34(6):502–507.

667. Lombardi T, Kuffer R, Di Felice R, et al. Epithelial odontogenic ghost cell tumour of the mandibular gingiva. Oral Oncol 1999; 35(4):439–442.

668. Iezzi G, Rubini C, Fioroni M, et al. Peripheral dentinogenic ghost cell tumor of the gingiva: case report. J Periodontol 2007; 78:1635–1638.

669. Tajima Y, Ohno J, Utsumi N. The dentinogenic ghost cell tumor. J Oral Pathol 1986; 15(6):359–362.

670. Günhan Ö, Sengun O, Celasun B. Epithelial odontogenic ghost cell tumor: report of a case. J Oral Maxillofac Surg 1989; 47(8):864–867.

671. Colmenero C, Patron M, Colmenero B. Odontogenic ghost cell tumours. The neoplastic form of calcifying odontogenic cyst. J Craniomaxillofac Surg 1990; 18(5): 215–218.

672. Limongelli WA, Anilesh K, Pulse CL, et al. Surgical treatment of central epithelial ghost cell tumor. N Y State Dent J 1997; 63(7):42–46.

673. López-Tarruella VC, Knezevic MR, Vincente-Barrero M, et al. The central (intraosseous) epithelial odontogenic ghost cell tumor: report of a case. Med Oral 1998; 3: 101–106.

674. Kasahara K, Iizuka T, Kobayashi I, et al. A recurrent case of odontogenic ghost cell tumour of the mandible. Int J Oral Maxillofac Surg 2002; 31(6):684–687.

675. Yoon JH, Ahn SG, Kim SG, et al. Odontogenic ghost cell tumour with clear cell components: clear cell odontogenic ghost cell tumour? J Oral Pathol Med 2004; 33(6): 376–379.

676. Kim S-A, Ahn S-G, Kim S-G, et al. Investigation of the beta-catenin gene in a case of dentinogenic ghost cell tumor. Oral Surg Oral Med Oral Pathol Oral Radiol Endod 2007; 103(1):97–101.

677. Eversole LR. On the differential diagnosis of clear cell tumours of the head and neck. Eur J Cancer B Oral Oncol 1993; 29B(3):173–179.

678. Günhan Ö, Celasun B, Can C, et al. The nature of ghost cells in calcifying odontogenic cyst: an immunohistochemical study. Ann Dent 1993; 52(1):30–33.

679. Handlers JP, Abrams AM, Melrose RJ, et al. Central odontogenic fibroma: clinicopathologic features of 19 cases and review of the literature. J Oral Maxillofac Surg 1991; 49(1):46–54.

680. Kaffe I, Buchner A. Radiologic features of central odontogenic fibroma. Oral Surg Oral Med Oral Pathol 1994; 78(6):811–818.

681. Heimdal A, Isacsson G, Nilsson L. Recurrent central odontogenic fibroma. Oral Surg Oral Med Oral Pathol 1980; 50(2):140–145.

682. Raubenheimer EJ, Noffke CE. Central odontogenic fibroma-like tumors, hypodontia, and enamel dysplasia: review of the literature and report of a case. Oral Surg Oral Med Oral Pathol Oral Radiol Endod 2002; 94(1):74–77.

683. Dahl EC, Wolfson SH, Haugen JC. Central odontogenic fibroma: review of literature and report of cases. J Oral Surg 1981; 39(2):120–124.

684. Wright BA, Jennings EH. Oxytalan fibers in peripheral odontogenic fibromas. A histochemical study of eighteen cases. Oral Surg Oral Med Oral Pathol 1979; 48 (5):451–453.

685. Kinney LA, Bradford J, Cohen M, et al. The aggressive odontogenic fibroma: report of a case. J Oral Maxillofac Surg 1993; 51(3):321–324.

686. Wesley RK, Wysocki GP, Mintz SM. The central odontogenic fibroma. Clinical and morphologic studies. Oral Surg Oral Med Oral Pathol 1975; 40(2):235–245.

687. Philipsen HP, Reichart PA, Sciubba JJ, et al. Odontogenic fibroma. In: Barnes L, Eveson JW, Reichart P, et al. eds. World Health Organization Classification of Tumours. Pathology and Genetics of Head and Neck Tumours. Lyon: IARC Press, 2005:315.

688. de Villiers Slabbert H, Altini M. Peripheral odontogenic fibroma: a clinicopathologic study. Oral Surg Oral Med Oral Pathol 1991; 72(1):86–90.

689. Allen CM, Hammond HL, Stimson PG. Central odontogenic fibroma, WHO type. A report of three cases with an unusual associated giant cell reaction. Oral Surg Oral Med Oral Pathol 1992; 73(1):62–66.

690. Fowler C, Tomich C, Brannon R, et al. Central odontogenic fibroma: clinicopathologic features of 24 cases and review of the literature. Oral Surg Oral Med Oral Pathol 1993; 76(5):587.

691. Odell EW, Lombardi T, Barrett AW, et al. Hybrid central giant cell granuloma and central odontogenic fibroma-like lesions of the jaws. Histopathology 1997; 30(2):165–171.

692. Watt-Smith SR, Ell-Labban NG, Tinkler SM. Central odontogenic fibroma. Int J Oral Maxillofac Surg 1988; 17(2):87–91.

693. Dunlap CL, Barker BF. Central odontogenic fibroma of the WHO type. Oral Surg Oral Med Oral Pathol 1984; 57(4):390–394.

694. Jones GM, Eveson JW, Shepherd JP. Central odontogenic fibroma. A report of two controversial cases illustrating diagnostic dilemmas. Br J Oral Maxillofac Surg 1989; 27(5):406–411.

695. Buchner A. Peripheral odontogenic fibroma. Report of 5 cases. J Craniomaxillofac Surg 1989; 17(3):134–138.

696. Siar CH, Ng KH. Clinicopathological study of peripheral odontogenic fibromas (WHO-type) in Malaysians (1967–95). Br J Oral Maxillofac Surg 2000; 38(1):19–22.

697. Garcia BG, Johann AC, da Silveira-Junior JB, et al. Retrospective analysis of peripheral odontogenic fibroma (WHO-type) in Brazilians. Minerva Stomatol 2007; 56(3): 115–119.

698. Brannon RB, Goode RK, Eversole LR, et al. The central granular cell odontogenic tumor: report of 5 new cases. Oral Surg Oral Med Oral Pathol Oral Radiol Endod 2002; 94(5):614–621.

699. Calvo N, Alonso D, Prieto M, et al. Central odontogenic fibroma granular cell variant: a case report and review of the literature. J Oral Maxillofac Surg 2002; 60(10): 1192–1194.

700. Meer S, Altini M, Coleman H, et al. Central granular cell odontogenic tumor: immunohistochemistry and ultrastructure. Am J Otolaryngol 2004; 25(1):73–78.

701. Rinaggio J, Cleveland D, Koshy R, et al. Peripheral granular cell odontogenic fibroma. Oral Surg Oral Med Oral Pathol Oral Radiol Endod 2007; 104(5):676–679.

702. Lownie JF, Altini M, Shear M. Granular cell peripheral odontogenic fibroma. J Oral Pathol 1976; 5(5):295–304.

703. Piattelli A, Rubini C, Goteri G, et al. Central granular cell odontogenic tumour: report of the first malignant case and review of the literature. Oral Oncol 2003; 39(1):78–82.

704. Vincent SD, Hammond HL, Ellis GL, et al. Central granular cell odontogenic fibroma. Oral Surg Oral Med Oral Pathol 1987; 63(6):715–721.

705. Rühl GH, Akuamoa-Boateng E. Granular cells in odontogenic and non-odontogenic tumours. Virchows Arch A Pathol Anat Histopathol 1989; 415(5):403–409.

706. Mirchandani R, Sciubba JJ, Mir R. Granular cell lesions of the jaws and oral cavity: a clinicopathologic, immunohistochemical, and ultrastructural study. J Oral Maxillofac Surg 1989; 47(12):1248–1255.

707. Shiro BC, Jacoway JR, Mirmiran SA, et al. Central odontogenic fibroma, granular cell variant. A case report with S-100 immunohistochemistry and a review of the literature. Oral Surg Oral Med Oral Pathol 1989; 67(6):725–730.

708. Chen SY. Central granular cell tumor of the jaw. An electron microscopic and immunohistochemical study. Oral Surg Oral Med Oral Pathol 1991; 72(1):75–81.

709. Gesek DJ Jr., Adrian JC, Reid EN. Central granular cell odontogenic tumor: a case report including light microscopy, immunohistochemistry, and literature review. J Oral Maxillofac Surg 1995; 53(8):945–949.

710. Yih WY, Thompson C, Meshul CK, et al. Central odontogenic granular cell tumor of the jaw: report of case and immunohistochemical and electron microscopic study. J Oral Maxillofac Surg 1995; 53(4):453–459.

711. Machado de Sousa SO, de Araujo NS, Melhado RM, et al. Central odontogenic granular cell tumor: immunohistochemical study of two cases. J Oral Maxillofac Surg 1998; 56(6):787–791.

712. Buchner A, Odell EW. Odontogenic myxoma/myxofibroma. In: Barnes L, Eveson JW, Reichart P, et al. eds. World Health Organization Classification of Tumours. Pathology and Genetics of Head and Neck Tumours. Lyon: IARC Press, 2005:316–317.

713. Simon EN, Merkx MA, Vuhahula E, et al. Odontogenic myxoma: a clinicopathological study of 33 cases. Int J Oral Maxillofac Surg 2004; 33(4):333–337.

714. Slater LJ. Infantile lateral nasal myxoma: is it odontogenic? J Oral Maxillofac Surg 2004; 62(3):391.

715. James DR, Lucas VS. Maxillary myxoma in a child of 11 months. A case report. J Craniomaxillofac Surg 1987; 15(1):42–44.

716. Leiberman A, Forte V, Thorner P, et al. Maxillary myxoma in children. Int J Pediatr Otorhinolaryngol 1990; 18(3): 277–284.

717. Wachter BG, Steinberg MJ, Darrow DH, et al. Odontogenic myxoma of the maxilla: a report of two pediatric cases. Int J Pediatr Otorhinolaryngol 2003; 67(4):389–393.

718. Fenton S, Slootweg PJ, Dunnebier EA, et al. Odontogenic myxoma in a 17-month-old child: a case report. J Oral Maxillofac Surg 2003; 61(6):734–736.

719. Boussault P, Boralevi F, Raux-Rakotomalala F, et al. Odontogenic myxoma: a diagnosis to add to the list of facial tumours in infants. J Eur Acad Dermatol Venereol 2006; 20(7), 864–867.

720. MacDonald-Jankowski DS, Yeung R, Lee KM, et al. Odontogenic myxomas in the Hong Kong Chinese: clinicoradiological presentation and systematic review. Dentomaxillofac Radiol 2002; 31(2):71–83.

721. Kaffe I, Naor H, Buchner A. Clinical and radiological features of odontogenic myxoma of the jaws. Dentomaxillofac Radiol 1997; 26(5):299–303.

722. Farman AG, Nortje CJ, Grotepass FW, et al. Myxofibroma of the jaws. Br J Oral Surg 1977; 15(1):3–18.

723. Tahsinoglu M, Cöloglu AS, Kuralay T. Myxoma of the gingiva: a case report. Br J Oral Surg 1975; 13(1):95–97.

724. Tomich CE. Oral focal mucinosis. A clinicopathologic and histochemical study of eight cases. Oral Surg Oral Med Oral Pathol 1974; 38(5):714–724.

725. Schmidseder R, Groddeck A, Scheunemann H. Diagnostic and therapeutic problems of myxomas (myxofibromas) of the jaws. J Maxillofac Surg 1978; 6(4):281–286.

726. Barker BF. Odontogenic myxoma. Semin Diagn Pathol 1999; 16(4):297–301.

727. Noffke CE, Raubenheimer EJ, Chabikuli NJ, et al. Odontogenic myxoma: review of the literature and report of 30 cases from South Africa. Oral Surg Oral Med Oral Pathol Oral Radiol Endod 2007; 104(1):101–109.

728. Large ND, Niebel HH, Fredricks WH. Myxoma of the jaws. Report of two cases. Oral Surg Oral Med Oral Pathol 1960; 13(12):1462–1468.

729. Peltola J, Magnusson B, Happonen RP, et al. Odontogenic myxoma–a radiographic study of 21 tumours. Br J Oral Maxillofac Surg 1994; 32(5):298–302.

730. Kawai T, Murakami S, Nishiyama H, et al. Diagnostic imaging for a case of maxillary myxoma with a review of

the magnetic resonance images of myxoid lesions. Oral Surg Oral Med Oral Pathol Oral Radiol Endod 1997; 84(4):449–454.

731. Sumi Y, Miyaishi O, Ito K, et al. Magnetic resonance imaging of myxoma in the mandible: a case report. Oral Surg Oral Med Oral Pathol Oral Radiol Endod 2000; 90(5):671–676.

732. Hisatomi M, Asaumi J, Konouchi H, et al. Comparison of radiographic and MRI features of a root-diverging odontogenic myxoma, with discussion of the differential diagnosis of lesions likely to move roots. Oral Dis 2003; 9(3):152–157.

733. Koseki T, Kobayashi K, Hashimoto K, et al. Computed tomography of odontogenic myxoma. Dentomaxillofac Radiol 2003; 32(3):160–165.

734. Goldblatt LI. Ultrastructural study of an odontogenic myxoma. Oral Surg Oral Med Oral Pathol 1976; 42(2):206–220.

735. Happonen RP, Peltola J, Ylipaavalniemi P, et al. Myxoma of the jaw bones. An analysis of 13 cases. Proc Finn Dent Soc 1988; 84(1):45–52.

736. Martins C, Carvalho YR, do Carmo MA. Argyrophilic nucleolar organizer regions (AgNORs) in odontogenic myxoma (OM) and ameloblastic fibroma (AF). J Oral Pathol Med 2001; 30(8):489–493.

737. Harder F. Myxomas of the jaws. Int J Oral Surg 1978; 7(3):48–155.

738. Li TJ, Sun LS, Luo HY. Odontogenic myxoma: a clinicopathologic study of 25 cases. Arch Pathol Lab Med 2006; 130(12):1799–1806.

739. Hodson JJ, Prout RE. Chemical and histochemical characterization of mucopolysaccharides in a jaw myxoma. J Clin Pathol 1968; 21(5):582–589.

740. Sedano HO, Gorlin RJ. Odontogenic myxoma: some histochemical considerations. Arch Oral Biol 1965; 10(4):727–729.

741. Mori M, Murakami M, Hirose I, et al. Histochemical studies of myxoma of the jaws. J Oral Surg 1975; 33:529–536.

742. Lombardi T, Kuffer R, Bernard JP, et al. Immunohistochemical staining for vimentin filaments and S-100 protein in myxoma of the jaws. J Oral Pathol 1988; 17(4):175–177.

743. Takahashi H, Fujita S, Okabe H. Immunohistochemical investigation in odontogenic myxoma. J Oral Pathol Med 1991; 20(3):114–119.

744. Green TL, Leighty SM, Walters R. Immunohistochemical evaluation of oral myxoid lesions. Oral Surg Oral Med Oral Pathol 1992; 73(4):469–471.

745. Moshiri S, Oda D, Worthington P, et al. Odontogenic myxoma: histochemical and ultrastructural study. J Oral Pathol Med 1992; 21(9):401–403.

746. Lo Muzio L, Nocini P, Favia G, et al. Odontogenic myxoma of the jaws: a clinical, radiologic, immunohistochemical, and ultrastructural study. Oral Surg Oral Med Oral Pathol Oral Radiol Endod 1996; 82(4):426–433.

747. Schmidt-Westhausen A, Becker J, Schuppan D, et al. Odontogenic myxoma–characterisation of the extracellular matrix (ECM) of the tumour stroma. Eur J Cancer B Oral Oncol 1994; 30B(6):377–380.

748. Slootweg PJ, van den BT, Straks W. Glycosaminoglycans in myxoma of the jaw: a biochemical study. J Oral Pathol 1985; 14(4):299–306.

749. Bast BT, Pogrel MA, Regezi JA. The expression of apoptotic proteins and matrix metalloproteinases in odontogenic myxomas. J Oral Maxillofac Surg 2003; 61(12):1463–1466.

750. Harrison JD. Odontogenic myxoma: ultrastructural and histochemical studies. J Clin Pathol 1973; 26(8):570–582.

751. Westwood RM, Alexander RW, Bennett DE. Giant odontogenic myxofibroma. Report of a case with histochemical and ultrastructural studies and a review of the literature. Oral Surg Oral Med Oral Pathol 1974; 37(1):83–92.

752. White DK, Chen S, Mohnac AM, et al. Odontogenic myxoma. A clinical and ultrastructural study. Oral Surg Oral Med Oral Pathol 1975; 39(6):901–917.

753. Simes RJ, Barros RE, Klein-Szanto AJ, et al. Ultrastructure of an odontogenic myxoma. Oral Surg Oral Med Oral Pathol 1975; 39(4):640–646.

754. Jaeger M, Santos J, Domingues M, et al. A novel cell line that retains the morphological characteristics of the cells and matrix of odontogenic myxoma. J Oral Pathol Med 2000; 29(3):129–138.

755. Boson WL, Gomez RS, Araujo L, et al. Odontogenic myxomas are not associated with activating mutations of the Gs alpha gene. Anticancer Res 1998; 18(6A):4415–4417.

756. Perdigao PF, Stergiopoulos SG, De Marco L, et al. Molecular and immunohistochemical investigation of protein kinase a regulatory subunit type 1A (PRKAR1A) in odontogenic myxomas. Genes Chromosomes Cancer 2005; 44(2):204–211.

757. Shear M, Copelyn M. Myxofibroma of the jaws. Proc Int Acad Oral Pathol 1969; 195–201.

758. Kim J, Ellis GL. Dental follicular tissue: misinterpretation as odontogenic tumors. J Oral Maxillofac Surg 1993; 51(7):762–767.

759. Cawson RA. Myxoma of the mandible with a 35 year follow-up. Br J Oral Surg 1972; 10(1):59–63.

760. Mlosek K, Kryst L, Piekarczyk J. [Odontogenic myxomas] In Polish. Pol Przegl Radiol Med Nukl 1982; 46(1–3):21–26.

761. Lamberg MA, Calonius BP, Makinen JE, et al. A case of malignant myxoma (myxosarcoma) of the maxilla. Scand J Dent Res 1984; 92(4):352–357.

762. Pahl S, Henn W, Binger T, et al. Malignant odontogenic myxoma of the maxilla: case with cytogenetic confirmation. J Laryngol Otol 2000; 114(7):533–535.

763. van der Waal I. Cementoblastoma. In: Barnes L, Eveson JW, Reichart P, et al, eds. Pathology and Genetics of Head and Neck Tumours. World Health Organization Classification of Tumours. Lyon: IARC Press, 2005:318.

764. Ulmansky M, Hjørting-Hansen E, Praetorius F, et al. Benign cementoblastoma. A review and five new cases. Oral Surg Oral Med Oral Pathol 1994; 77(1):48–55.

765. Brannon RB, Fowler CB, Carpenter WM, et al. Cementoblastoma: an innocuous neoplasm? A clinicopathologic study of 44 cases and review of the literature with special emphasis on recurrence. Oral Surg Oral Med Oral Pathol Oral Radiol Endod 2002; 93(3):311–320.

766. Reichart PA, Philipsen HP. Benign Cemetoblastoma. Odontogenic Tumors and Allied Lesions. London: Quintessence Publishing Co Ltd, 2004:199–203.

767. Papageorge MB, Cataldo E, Nghiem FT. Cementoblastoma involving multiple deciduous teeth. Oral Surg Oral Med Oral Pathol 1987; 63(5):602–605.

768. Keyes G, Hilderbrand K. Successful surgical endodontics for benign cementoblastoma. J Endod 1987; 13(12):566–569.

769. Vindenes H, Nilsen R, Gilhuus-Moe O. Benign cementoblastoma. Int J Oral Surg 1979; 8(4):318–324.

770. Zachariades N, Skordalaki A, Papanicolaou S, et al. Cementoblastoma: review of the literature and report of a case in a 7 year-old girl. Br J Oral Maxillofac Surg 1985; 23(6):456–461.

771. Herzog S. Benign cementoblastoma associated with the primary dentition. J Oral Med 1987; 42:106–108.

772. Chaput A, Marc A. Un cas de cémentome localisé sur une molaire temporaire [A case of cementoma localised on a temporary molar]. SSO Schweiz Monatsschr Zahnheilkd 1965; 75:48–52.

773. Vilasco J, Mazere J, Douesnard JC, et al. Un cas de cémentoblastome [A case of cementoblastoma]. Rev Stomatol Chir Maxillofac 1969; 70(5):329–332.

774. Jelic JS, Loftus MJ, Miller AS, et al. Benign cementoblastoma: report of an unusual case and analysis of 14 additional cases. J Oral Maxillofac Surg 1993; 51 (9):1033–1037.

775. Anneroth G, Isacssom G, Sigurdsson A. Benign cementoblastoma (true cementoma). Oral Surg Oral Med Oral Pathol 1975; 40(1):141–146.

776. Cundiff EJ. Developing cementoblastoma: case report and update of differential diagnosis. Quintessence Int 2000, 31(3), 191–195.

777. Esguep A, Belvederessi M, Alfaro C. Benign cementoblastoma. (Report of an atypical case). J Oral Med 1983; 38(3):99–102.

778. Arzate H, Jimenez-Garcia LF, Alvarez-Perez MA, et al. Immunolocalization of a human cementoblastoma-conditioned medium-derived protein. J Dent Res 2002; 81(8):541–546.

779. Smith RA, Hansen LS, Resnick D, et al. Comparison of the osteoblastoma in gnathic and extragnathic sites. Oral Surg Oral Med Oral Pathol 1982; 54(3):285–298.

780. Slootweg PJ. Cementoblastoma and osteoblastoma: a comparison of histologic features. J Oral Pathol Med 1992; 21(9):385–389.

781. Zaitoun H, Kujan O, Sloan P. An unusual recurrent cementoblastoma associated with a developing lower second molar tooth: a case report. J Oral Maxillofac Surg 2007; 65(10):2080–2082.

782. Williams TP. Aggressive odontogenic cysts and tumors. Atlas Oral Maxillofac Surg Clin North Am 1997; 9: 329–338.

783. Sciubba JJ, Eversole LR, Slootweg PJ. Odontogenic/ameloblastic carcinomas. In: Barnes L, Eveson JW, Reichart P, et al, eds. Pathology and Genetics of Head and Neck Tumours. World Health Organization Classification of Tumours. Lyon: IARC Press, 2005:287–289.

784. Elzay RP. Primary intraosseous carcinoma of the jaws. Review and update of odontogenic carcinomas. Oral Surg Oral Med Oral Pathol 1982; 54(3):299–303.

785. Slootweg PJ, Müller H. Malignant ameloblastoma or ameloblastic carcinoma. Oral Surg Oral Med Oral Pathol 1984; 57(2):168–176.

786. Waldron CA, Mustoe TA. Primary intraosseous carcinoma of the mandible with probable origin in an odontogenic cyst. Oral Surg Oral Med Oral Pathol 1989; 67(6):716–724.

787. Houston G, Davenport W, Keaton W, et al. Malignant (metastatic) ameloblastoma: report of a case. J Oral Maxillofac Surg 1993; 51(10):1152–1155.

788. Kunze E, Donath K, Luhr HG, et al. Biology of metastasizing ameloblastoma. Pathol Res Pract 1985; 180(5): 526–535.

789. Laughlin EH. Metastasizing ameloblastoma. Cancer 1989; 64(3):776–780.

790. Ueda M, Kaneda T, Imaizumi M, et al. Mandibular ameloblastoma with metastasis to the lungs and lymph nodes: a case report and review of the literature. J Oral Maxillofac Surg 1989; 47(6):623–628.

791. Ameerally P, McGurk M, Shaheen O. Atypical ameloblastoma: report of 3 cases and a review of the literature. Br J Oral Maxillofac Surg 1996; 34(3):235–239.

792. Henderson JM, Sonnet JR, Schlesinger C, et al. Pulmonary metastasis of ameloblastoma: case report and review of the literature. Oral Surg Oral Med Oral Pathol Oral Radiol Endod 1999; 88(2):170–176.

793. Reichart PA, Philipsen HP. Metastasizing, Malignant Ameloblastoma. Odontogenic Tumors and Allied Lesions. London: Quintessence Publishing Co Ltd, 2004: 207–213.

794. Duffey DC, Bailet JW, Newman A. Ameloblastoma of the mandible with cervical lymph node metastasis. Am J Otolaryngol 1995; 16(1):66–73.

795. Sugiyama M, Ogawa I, Katayama K, et al. Simultaneous metastatic ameloblastoma and thyroid carcinoma in the cervical region: report of a case. J Oral Maxillofac Surg 1999; 57(10):1255–1258.

796. Weir MM, Centeno BA, Szyfelbein WM. Cytological features of malignant metastatic ameloblastoma: a case report and differential diagnosis. Diagn Cytopathol 1998; 18(2):125–130.

797. Witterick IJ, Parikh S, Mancer K, et al. Malignant ameloblastoma. Am J Otolaryngol 1996; 17(2): 122–126.

798. Lin SC, Lieu CM, Hahn LJ, et al. Peripheral ameloblastoma with metastasis. Int J Oral Maxillofac Surg 1987; 16(2):202–204.

799. Gilijamse M, Leemans CR, Winters HAH, et al. Metastasizing ameloblastoma. Int J Oral Maxillofac Surg 2007; 36:462–464.

800. Eversole LR. Malignant epithelial odontogenic tumors. Semin Diagn Pathol 1999; 16(4):317–324.

801. Kumamoto H, Takahashi N, Ooya K. K-Ras gene status and expression of Ras/mitogen-activated protein kinase (MAPK) signaling molecules in ameloblastomas. J Oral Pathol Med 2004; 33(6):360–367.

802. Goldenberg D, Sciubba J, Koch W, et al. Malignant odontogenic tumors: a 22-year experience. Laryngoscope 2004; 114(10):1770–1774.

803. Ciment LM, Ciment AJ. Malignant ameloblastoma metastatic to the lungs 29 years after primary resection: a case report. Chest 2002; 121(4):1359–1361.

804. Eliasson AH, Moser RJ III, Tenholder MF. Diagnosis and treatment of metastatic ameloblastoma. South Med J 1989; 82(9):1165–1168.

805. Akrish S, Buchner A, Shoshani Y, et al. Ameloblastic carcinoma: report of a new case, literature review, and comparison to ameloblastoma. J Oral Maxillofac Surg 2007; 65(4):777–783.

806. Carinci F, Palmieri A, Delaiti G, et al. Expression profiling of ameloblastic carcinoma. J Craniofac Surg 2004; 15(2): 264–269.

807. Üzüm N, Akyol G, Asal K, et al. Ameloblastic carcinoma containing melanocyte and melanin pigment in the mandible: a case report and review of the literature. J Oral Pathol Med 2005; 34(10):618–620.

808. Khalbuss WE, Loya A, Bazooband A. Fine-needle aspiration cytology of pulmonary ameloblastic carcinoma of mandibular origin. Diagn Cytopathol 2006; 34(3): 208–209.

809. Yazici N, Karagoz B, Varan A, et al. Maxillary ameloblastic carcinoma in a child. Pediatr Blood Cancer 2008; 50(1): 175–176.

810. Abiko Y, Nagayasu H, Takeshima M, et al. Ameloblastic carcinoma ex ameloblastoma: report of a case-possible involvement of CpG island hypermethylation of the p16 gene in malignant transformation. Oral Surg Oral Med Oral Pathol Oral Radiol Endod 2007; 103(1):72–76.

811. Hall JM, Weathers DR, Unni KK. Ameloblastic carcinoma: an analysis of 14 cases. Oral Surg Oral Med Oral Pathol Oral Radiol Endod 2007; 103(6):799–807.

812. Bang G, Koppang H. Clear cell odontogenic carcinoma. In: Barnes L, Eveson JW, Reichart P, et al. , eds. Pathology and Genetics of Head and Neck Tumours. World Health Organization Classification of Tumours. Lyon: IARC Press, 2005:292.

813. Zarbo RJ, Marunick MT, Johns R. Malignant ameloblastoma, spindle cell variant. Arch Pathol Lab Med 2003; 127(3):352–355.

814. Datta R, Winston JS, az-Reyes G, et al. Ameloblastic carcinoma: report of an aggressive case with multiple bony metastases. Am J Otolaryngol 2003; 24(1):64–69.

815. Kawauchi S, Hayatsu Y, Takahashi M, et al. Spindle-cell ameloblastic carcinoma: a case report with immunohistochemical, ultrastructural, and comparative genomic hybridization analyses. Oncol Rep 2003; 10(1):31–34.

816. Sauk JJ. Basement membrane confinement of epithelial tumor islands in benign and malignant ameloblastomas. J Oral Pathol 1985; 14(4):307–314.

817. Muller S, DeRose PB, Cohen C. DNA ploidy of ameloblastoma and ameloblastic carcinoma of the jaws. Analysis by image and flow cytometry. Arch Pathol Lab Med 1993; 117(11):1126–1131.

818. Yoshida T, Shingaki S, Nakajima T, et al. Odontogenic carcinoma with sarcomatous proliferation. A case report. J Craniomaxillofac Surg 1989; 17(3):139–142.

819. Tanaka T, Ohkubo T, Fujitsuka H, et al. Malignant mixed tumor (malignant ameloblastoma and fibrosarcoma) of the maxilla. Arch Pathol Lab Med 1991; 115(1):84–87.

820. Hayashi N, Iwata J, Masaoka N, et al. Ameloblastoma of the mandible metastasizing to the orbit with malignant transformation. A histopathological and immunohistochemical study. Virchows Arch 1997; 430(6):501–507.

821. Cox DP, Muller S, Carlson GW, et al. Ameloblastic carcinoma ex ameloblastoma of the mandible with malignancy-associated hypercalcemia. Oral Surg Oral Med Oral Pathol Oral Radiol Endod 2000; 90(6):716–722.

822. Oginni FO, Ugboko VI, Owotade JF, et al. Ameloblastic carcinoma of the jaws. A report of three Nigerian cases. Odontostomatol Trop 2003; 26(104):19–22.

823. Cizmecy O, Aslan A, Onel D, et al. Ameloblastic carcinoma ex ameloblastoma of the mandible: case report. Otolaryngol Head Neck Surg 2004; 130(5):633–634.

824. Putzke H-P. Histopathologie eines peripheren malignen Ameloblastoms der Gingiva. Dtsch Z Mund-Kiefer-Gesichts-Chir 1994; 18:204–206.

825. Wettan HL, Patella PA, Freedman PD. Peripheral ameloblastoma: review of the literature and report of recurrence as severe dysplasia. J Oral Maxillofac Surg 2001; 59(7):811–815.

826. Dufau JP, Paume P, Soulard R, et al. Fibrosarcome améloblastique périphérique [Peripheral ameloblastic fibrosarcoma]. Ann Pathol 2002; 22(4):310–313.

827. McClatchey KD, Sullivan MJ, Paugh DR. Peripheral ameloblastic carcinoma: a case report of a rare neoplasm. J Otolaryngol 1989; 18(3):109–111.

828. Bucci E, Lo Muzio L, Mignogna MD, et al. Peripheral ameloblastoma: case report. Acta Stomatol Belg 1992; 89(4):267–269.

829. Edmondson HD, Browne RM, Potts AJ. Intra-oral basal cell carcinoma. Br J Oral Surg 1982; 20(4):239–247.

830. Gardner DG. The peripheral odontogenic fibroma: an attempt at clarification. Oral Surg Oral Med Oral Pathol 1982; 54(1):40–48.

831. Slootweg PJ. Malignant odontogenic tumors: an overview. Mund Kiefer Gesichtschir 2002; 6(5):295–302.

832. Eversole LR, Siar CH, van der Waal I. Primary intraosseous squamous cell carcinomas. In: Barnes L, Eveson JW, Reichart P, et al, eds. Pathology and Genetics of Head and Neck Tumours. World Health Organization Classification of Tumours. Lyon: IARC Press, 2005:290–291.

833. Shear M. Primary intra-alveolar epidermoid carcinoma of the jaw. J Pathol 1969; 97(4):645–651.

834. González-García R, Sastre-Peréz J, Nam-Cha SH, et al. Primary intraosseous carcinomas of the jaws arising within an odontogenic cyst, ameloblastoma, and de novo: report of new cases with reconstruction considerations. Oral Surg Oral Med Oral Pathol Oral Radiol Endod 2007; 103(2):e29–e33.

835. Slootweg PJ. Carcinoma arising from reduced enamel epithelium. J Oral Pathol 1987; 16:479–482.

836. Tucker MR, Dechamplain RW, Jarrett JH. Simultaneous occurrence of an ameloblastoma and a squamous cell carcinoma of the mandible. J Oral Maxillofac Surg 1984; 42(2):127–130.

837. Ueta E, Yoneda K, Ohno A, et al. Intraosseous carcinoma arising from mandibular ameloblastoma with progressive invasion and pulmonary metastasis. Int J Oral Maxillofac Surg 1996; 25(5):370–372.

838. Ohtake K, Yokobayashi Y, Shingaki S, et al. Central carcinoma of the jaw. A survey of 28 cases in the Japanese literature. J Craniomaxillofac Surg 1989; 17(4):155–161.

839. Suei Y, Tanimoto K, Taguchi A, et al. Primary intraosseous carcinoma: review of the literature and diagnostic criteria. J Oral Maxillofac Surg 1994; 52(6):580–583.

840. Kaffe I, Ardekian L, Peled M, et al. Radiological features of primary intra-osseous carcinoma of the jaws. Analysis of the literature and report of a new case. Dentomaxillofac Radiol 1998; 27(4):209–214.

841. Thomas G, Pandey M, Mathew A, et al. Primary intraosseous carcinoma of the jaw: pooled analysis of world literature and report of two new cases. Int J Oral Maxillofac Surg 2001; 30(4):349–355.

842. Bridgeman A, Wiesenfeld D, Buchanan M, et al. A primary intraosseous carcinoma of the anterior maxilla. Report of a new case. Int J Oral Maxillofac Surg 1996; 25(4):279–281.

843. Ide F, Shimoyama T, Horie N, et al. Primary intraosseous carcinoma of the mandible with probable origin from reduced enamel epithelium. J Oral Pathol Med 1999; 28(9):420–422.

844. Zwetyenga N, Majoufre-Lefebvre C, Pinsolle V, et al. [Primary intraosseous carcinoma of the jaws: results of treatment of 9 cases and proposed classification]. Rev Stomatol Chir Maxillofac 2003; 104(5):265–273.

845. el-Naaj IA, Krausz AA, Ardekian L, et al. Primary intraosseous carcinoma of the anterior maxilla: report of a new case. J Oral Maxillofac Surg 2005; 63(3):405–409.

846. Hayashido Y, Yoshioka Y, Shintani T, et al. Primary intraosseous carcinoma of mandible associated with elevation of serum carcinoembryonic antigen level. Oral Oncology EXTRA 2005; 41:267–271.

847. Thomas G, Sreelatha KT, Balan A, et al. Primary intraosseous carcinoma of the mandible–a case report and review of the literature. Eur J Surg Oncol 2000; 26(1):82–86.

848. Suomalainen A, Hietanen J, Robinson S, et al. Ameloblastic carcinoma of the mandible resembling odontogenic cyst in a panoramic radiograph. Oral Surg Oral Med Oral Pathol Oral Radiol Endod 2006; 101(5):638–642.

849. Sciubba JJ, Fantasia JE, Kahn LB. Malignant odontogenic tumors. Tumors and Cysts of the Jaw. Washington, D.C.: Armed Forces Institute of Pathology, 2001:129–139.

850. Bennett JH, Jones J, Speight PM. Odontogenic squamous cell carcinoma with osseous metaplasia. J Oral Pathol Med 1993; 22(6):286–288.

851. Ruskin JD, Cohen DM, Davis LF. Primary intraosseous carcinoma: report of two cases. J Oral Maxillofac Surg 1988; 46(5):425–432.

852. Alevizos I, Blaeser B, Gallagher G, et al. Odontogenic carcinoma: a functional genomic comparison with oral mucosal squamous cell carcinoma. Oral Oncol 2002; 38(5):504–507.

853. Anneroth G, Hansen LS. Variations in keratinizing odontogenic cysts and tumors. Oral Surg Oral Med Oral Pathol 1982; 54(5):530–546.

854. To EH, Brown JS, Avery BS, et al. Primary intraosseous carcinoma of the jaws. Three new cases and a review of the literature. Br J Oral Maxillofac Surg 1991; 29(1):19–25.

855. Sciubba JJ, Fantasia JE, Kahn LB. Fibro-osseous lesions. Tumors and Cysts of the Jaw. Washington, D.C.: Armed Forces Institute of Pathology, 2001:141–160.

856. Gardner AF. The odontogenic cyst as a potential carcinoma: a clinicopathologic appraisal. J Am Dent Assoc 1969; 78 (4):746–755.

857. Maxymiw WG, Wood RE. Carcinoma arising in a dentigerous cyst: a case report and review of the literature. J Oral Maxillofac Surg 1991; 49(6):639–643.

858. Schwimmer AM, Aydin F, Morrison SN. Squamous cell carcinoma arising in residual odontogenic cyst. Report of a case and review of literature. Oral Surg Oral Med Oral Pathol 1991; 72(2):218–221.

859. Berens A, Kramer FJ, Kuettner C, et al. Entstehung eines plattenepithelkarzinoms auf dem boden einer odontogenen Zyste [Growth of a squamous epithelial carcinoma in an odontogenic cyst]. Mund Kiefer Gesichtschir 2000; 4(5):330–334.

860. Saito T, Okada H, Akimoto Y, et al. Primary intraosseous carcinoma arising from an odontogenic cyst: a case report and review of the Japanese cases. J Oral Sci 2002; 44(1): 49–53.

861. Ramsden RT, Barrett A. Gorlin's syndrome. J Laryngol Otol 1975; 89(6):615–629.

862. Areen RG, McClatchey KD, Baker HL. Squamous cell carcinoma developing in an odontogenic keratocyst. Report of a case. Arch Otolaryngol 1981; 107(9):568–569.

863. van der Waal I, Rauhamaa R, van der Kwast WA, et al. Squamous cell carcinoma arising in the lining of odontogenic cysts. Report of 5 cases. Int J Oral Surg 1985; 14(2):146–152.

864. High AS, Quirke P, Hume WJ. DNA-ploidy studies in a keratocyst undergoing subsequent malignant transformation. J Oral Pathol 1987; 16(3):135–138.

865. Moos KF, Rennie JS. Squamous cell carcinoma arising in a mandibular keratocyst in a patient with Gorlin's syndrome. Br J Oral Maxillofac Surg 1987; 25(4):280–284.

866. Siar CH, Ng KH. Squamous cell carcinoma in an orthokeratinised odontogenic keratocyst. Int J Oral Maxillofac Surg 1987; 16(1):95–98.

867. Macleod RI, Soames JV. Squamous cell carcinoma arising in an odontogenic keratocyst. Br J Oral Maxillofac Surg 1988; 26(1):52–57.

868. Foley WL, Terry BC, Jacoway JR. Malignant transformation of an odontogenic keratocyst: report of a case. J Oral Maxillofac Surg 1991; 49(7):768–771.

869. Hennis HL III, Stewart WC, Neville B, et al. Carcinoma arising in an odontogenic keratocyst with orbital invasion. Doc Ophthalmol 1991; 77(1):73–79.

870. Herbener GH, Gould AR, Neal DC, et al. An electron and optical microscopic study of juxtaposed odontogenic keratocyst and carcinoma. Oral Surg Oral Med Oral Pathol 1991; 71(3):322–328.

871. Minic AJ. Primary intraosseous squamous cell carcinoma arising in a mandibular keratocyst. Int J Oral Maxillofac Surg 1992; 21(3):163–165.

872. Anand VK, Arrowood JP Jr., Krolls SO. Malignant potential of the odontogenic keratocyst. Otolaryngol Head Neck Surg 1994; 111(1):124–129.

873. Dabbs DJ, Schweitzer RJ, Schweitzer LE, et al. Squamous cell carcinoma arising in recurrent odontogenic keratocyst: case report and literature review. Head Neck 1994; 16(4):375–378.

874. Zachariades N, Markaki S, Karabela-Bouropoulou V. Squamous cell carcinoma developing in an odontogenic keratocyst. Arch Anat Cytol Pathol 1995; 43(5–6): 350–353.

875. Yoshida H, Onizawa K, Yusa H. Squamous cell carcinoma arising in association with an orthokeratinized odontogenic keratocyst. Report of a case. J Oral Maxillofac Surg 1996; 54(5):647–651.

876. Ota Y, Karakida K, Watanabe D, et al. A case of central carcinoma of the mandible arising from a recurrent odontogenic keratocyst: delineation of surgical margins and reconstruction with bilateral rectus abdominis myocutaneous free flaps. Tokai J Exp Clin Med 1998; 23(4): 157–165.

877. Makowski GJ, McGuff S, Van Sickels JE. Squamous cell carcinoma in a maxillary odontogenic keratocyst. J Oral Maxillofac Surg 2001; 59(1):76–80.

878. Keszler A, Piloni MJ. Malignant transformation in odontogenic keratocysts. Case report. Med Oral 2002; 7(5): 331–335.

879. Chaisuparat R, Coletti D, Kolokythas A, et al. Primary intraosseous odontogenic carcinoma arising in an odontogenic cyst or de novo: a clinicopathologic study of six new cases. Oral Surg Oral Med Oral Pathol Oral Radiol Endod 2006; 101(2):194–200.

880. Browne RM, Gough NG. Malignant change in the epithelium lining odontogenic cysts. Cancer 1972; 29(5): 1199–1207.

881. Enriquez RE, Ciola B, Bahn SL. Verrucous carcinoma arising in an odontogenic cyst. Report of a case. Oral Surg Oral Med Oral Pathol 1980; 49(2):151–156.

882. El-Mofty SK, Shannon MT, Mustoe TA. Lymph node metastasis in spindle cell carcinoma arising in odontogenic cyst. Report of a case. Oral Surg Oral Med Oral Pathol 1991; 71(2):209–213.

883. Sawyer DR, Nwoku AL, Mosadomi A, et al. Odontogenic carcinoma with dentinoid. Int J Oral Maxillofac Surg 1986; 15(1):105–107.

884. McDonald AR, Pogrel MA, Carson J, et al. p53-positive squamous cell carcinoma originating from an odontogenic cyst. J Oral Maxillofac Surg 1996; 54(2):216–218.

885. Eversole LR, Sabes WR, Rovin S. Aggressive growth and neoplastic potential of odontogenic cysts: with special reference to central epidermoid and mucoepidermoid carcinomas. Cancer 1975; 35(1):270–282.

886. Hansen LS, Eversole LR, Green TL, et al. Clear cell odontogenic tumor–a new histologic variant with aggressive potential. Head Neck Surg 1985; 8(2):115–123.

887. Waldron CA, Small IA, Silverman H. Clear cell ameloblastoma–an odontogenic carcinoma. J Oral Maxillofac Surg 1985; 43(9):707–717.

888. Milles M, Doyle JL, Mesa M, et al. Clear cell odontogenic carcinoma with lymph node metastasis. Oral Surg Oral Med Oral Pathol 1993; 76(1):82–89.

889. de Aguiar MC, Gomez RS, Silva EC, et al. Clear-cell ameloblastoma (clear-cell odontogenic carcinoma): report of a case. Oral Surg Oral Med Oral Pathol Oral Radiol Endod 1996; 81(1):79–83.

890. Gardner DG. Some current concepts on the pathology of ameloblastomas. Oral Surg Oral Med Oral Pathol Oral Radiol Endod 1996; 82(6):660–669.

891. Miyauchi M, Ogawa I, Takata T, et al. Clear cell odontogenic tumour: a case with induction of dentin-like structures? J Oral Pathol Med 1998; 27(5):220–224.

892. Yamamoto H, Inui M, Mori A, et al. Clear cell odontogenic carcinoma: a case report and literature review of odontogenic tumors with clear cells. Oral Surg Oral Med Oral Pathol Oral Radiol Endod 1998; 86 (1):86–89.

893. Nair MK, Burkes EJ, Chai UD. Radiographic manifestation of clear cell odontogenic tumor. Oral Surg Oral Med Oral Pathol Oral Radiol Endod 2000; 89(2):250–254.

894. Benton DC, Eisenberg E. Clear cell odontogenic carcinoma: report of a case. J Oral Maxillofac Surg 2001; 59(1): 83–88.

895. Mari A, Escutia E, Carrera M, et al. Clear cell ameloblastoma or odontogenic carcinoma. A case report. J Craniomaxillofac Surg 1995; 23(6):387–390.

896. Maiorano E, Altini M, Favia G. Clear cell tumors of the salivary glands, jaws, and oral mucosa. Semin Diagn Pathol 1997; 14(3):203–212.

897. Sadeghi EM, Levin S. Clear cell odontogenic carcinoma of the mandible: report of a case. J Oral Maxillofac Surg 1995; 53(5):613–616.

898. Reichart PA, Philipsen HP. Clear Cell Odontogenic Carcinoma. Odontogenic Tumors and Allied Lesions. London: Quintessence Publishing Co Ltd, 2004:239–247.

899. Braunshtein E, Vered M, Taicher S, et al. Clear cell odontogenic carcinoma and clear cell ameloblastoma: a single clinicopathologic entity? A new case and comparative analysis of the literature. J Oral Maxillofac Surg 2003; 61(9):1004–1010.

900. Maiorano E, Altini M, Viale G, et al. Clear cell odontogenic carcinoma. Report of two cases and review of the literature. Am J Clin Pathol 2001; 116(1):107–114.

901. Adamo AK, Boguslaw B, Coomaraswarmy MA, et al. Clear cell odontogenic carcinoma of the mandible: case report. J Oral Maxillofac Surg 2002; 60(1):121–126.

902. August M, Faquin W, Troulis M, et al. Clear cell odontogenic carcinoma: evaluation of reported cases. J Oral Maxillofac Surg 2003; 61(5):580–586.

903. Ng KH, Siar CH. Peripheral ameloblastoma with clear cell differentiation. Oral Surg Oral Med Oral Pathol 1990; 70(2):210–213.

904. Mosqueda-Taylor A, Meneses-Garcia A, Ruiz-Godoy Rivera LM, et al. Clear cell odontogenic carcinoma of the mandible. J Oral Pathol Med 2002; 31(7):439–441.

905. Cutright DE. Histopathologic findings in third molar opercula. Oral Surg Oral Med Oral Pathol 1976; 41(2): 215–224.

906. Wysocki GP, Brannon RB, Gardner DG, et al. Histogenesis of the lateral periodontal cyst and the gingival cyst of the adult. Oral Surg Oral Med Oral Pathol 1980; 50(4):327–334.

907. Li TJ, Yu SF, Gao Y, et al. Clear cell odontogenic carcinoma: a clinicopathologic and immunocytochemical study of 5 cases. Arch Pathol Lab Med 2001; 125(12):1566–1571.

908. Muramatsu T, Hashimoto S, Inoue T, et al. Clear cell odontogenic carcinoma in the mandible: histochemical and immunohistochemical observations with a review of the literature. J Oral Pathol Med 1996; 25(9):516–521.

909. Guilbert F, Auriol M, Chomette G. Une forme rare d'épithelioma primitif de la mandibule: Le carcinome odontogénique à cellules claires. Etude clinique et morphologique [An unusual form of primary epithelioma of the mandible: odontogenic clear cell carcinoma. Clinical and morphologic study]. Rev Stomatol Chir Maxillofac 1991; 92(4):277–280.

910. Ariyoshi Y, Shimahara M, Miyauchi M, et al. Clear cell odontogenic carcinoma with ghost cells and inductive dentin formation–report of a case in the mandible. J Oral Pathol Med 2002; 31(3):181–183.

911. Kumamoto H, Yamazaki S, Sato A, et al. Clear cell odontogenic tumor in the mandible: report of a case with duct-like appearances and dentinoid induction. J Oral Pathol Med 2000; 29(1):43–47.

912. Kumar M, Fasanmade A, Barrett AW, et al. Metastasising clear cell odontogenic carcinoma: a case report and review of the literature. Oral Oncol 2003; 39(2):190–194.

913. Eversole LR, Belton CM, Hansen LS. Clear cell odontogenic tumor: histochemical and ultrastructural features. J Oral Pathol 1985; 14(8):603–614.

914. Fan J, Kubota E, Imamura H, et al. Clear cell odontogenic carcinoma. A case report with massive invasion of neighboring organs and lymph node metastasis. Oral Surg Oral Med Oral Pathol 1992; 74(6):768–775.

915. Brandwein M, Said-Al-Naief N, Gordon R, et al. Clear cell odontogenic carcinoma: report of a case and analysis of the literature. Arch Otolaryngol Head Neck Surg 2002; 128(9):1089–1095.

916. Brinck U, Gunawan B, Schulten HJ, et al. Clear-cell odontogenic carcinoma with pulmonary metastases resembling pulmonary meningothelial-like nodules. Virchows Arch 2001; 438(4):412–417.

917. Iezzi G, Rubini C, Fioroni M, et al. Clear cell odontogenic carcinoma. Oral Oncol 2002; 38(2):209–213.

918. Dahiya S, Kumar R, Sarkar C, et al. Clear cell odontogenic carcinoma: a diagnostic dilemma. Pathol Oncol Res 2002; 8(4):283–285.

919. Eversole LR, Duffey DC, Powell NB. Clear cell odontogenic carcinoma. A clinicopathologic analysis. Arch Otolaryngol Head Neck Surg 1995; 121(6):685–689.

920. Bang G, Koppang HS, Hansen LS, et al. Clear cell odontogenic carcinoma: report of three cases with pulmonary and lymph node metastases. J Oral Pathol Med 1989; 18(2):113–118.

921. Carinci F, Volinia S, Rubini C, et al. Genetic profile of clear cell odontogenic carcinoma. J Craniofac Surg 2003; 14(3): 356–362.

922. WHO Working group on classification of head and neck tumours. Tumours of the Salivary Glands. In: Barnes L, Eveson JW, Reichart P, et al, eds. Pathology and Genetics of Head and Neck Tumours. World Health Organization Classification of Tumours. Lyon: IARC Press, 2005: 209–281.

923. Berho M, Huvos AG. Central hyalinizing clear cell carcinoma of the mandible and the maxilla a clinicopathologic study of two cases with an analysis of the literature. Hum Pathol 1999; 30(1):101–105.

924. Urban SD, Keith DA, Goodman M. Hyalinizing clear cell carcinoma: report of a case. J Oral Pathol Med 1996; 25(10):562–564.

925. Grodjesk JE, Dolinsky HB, Schneider LC, et al. Odontogenic ghost cell carcinoma. Oral Surg Oral Med Oral Pathol 1987; 63(5):576–581.

926. Scott J, Wood GD. Aggressive calcifying odontogenic cyst–a possible variant of ameloblastoma. Br J Oral Maxillofac Surg 1989; 27(1):53–59.

927. McCoy BP, Carroll MKO, Hall JM. Carcinoma arising in a dentinogenic ghost cell tumor. Oral Surg Oral Med Oral Pathol 1992; 74(3):371–378.

928. Dubiel-Bigaj M, Olszewski E, Stachura J. The malignant form of calcifying odontogenic cyst. A case report. Patol Pol 1993; 44(1):39–41.

929. Siar CH, Ng KH. Aggressive (malignant?) epithelial odontogenic ghost cell tumour of the maxilla. J Laryngol Otol 1994; 108(3):269–271.

930. Kao SY, Pong BY, Li WY, et al. Maxillary odontogenic carcinoma with distant metastasis to axillary skin, brain, and lung: case report. Int J Oral Maxillofac Surg 1995; 24(3):229–232.

931. Folpe AL, Tsue T, Rogerson L, et al. Odontogenic ghost cell carcinoma: a case report with immunohistochemical and ultrastructural characterization. J Oral Pathol Med 1998; 27(4):185–189.

932. Castle JT, Arendt DM. Aggressive (malignant) epithelial odontogenic ghost cell tumor. Ann Diagn Pathol 1999; 3(4):243–248.

933. Zadeh AH, Deihimy P. Aggressive recurrent odontogenic ghost tumor with cranial invasion. Iran Journal Medical Science 2002; 27(4):196–198.

934. Nazaretian SP, Schenberg ME, Simpson I, et al. Ghost cell odontogenic carcinoma. Int J Oral Maxillofac Surg 2007; 36(5):455–458.

935. Sun ZJ, Zhao YF, Zhang L, et al. Odontogenic ghost cell carcinoma in the maxilla: a case report and literature review. J Oral Maxillofac Surg 2007; 65(9):1820–1824.

936. Kim HJ, Choi SK, Lee CJ, et al. Aggressive epithelial odontogenic ghost cell tumor in the mandible: CT and MR imaging findings. AJNR Am J Neuroradiol 2001; 22(1):175–179.

937. Carlos R, Altini M, Takeda Y. Odontogenic sarcomas. In: Barnes L, Eveson JW, Reichart P, et al, eds. Pathology and Genetics of Head and Neck Tumours. World Health Organization Classification of Tumours. Lyon: IARC Press, 2005:294–295.

938. Altini M, Thompson SH, Lownie JF, et al. Ameloblastic sarcoma of the mandible. J Oral Maxillofac Surg 1985; 43(10):789–794.

939. Leider AS, Nelson JF, Trodahl JN. Ameloblastic fibrosarcoma of the jaws. Oral Surg Oral Med Oral Pathol 1972; 33(4):559–569.

940. Yamamoto H, Caselitz J, Kozawa Y. Ameloblastic fibrosarcoma of the right mandible: immunohistochemical and electron microscopical investigations on one case, and a review of the literature. J Oral Pathol 1987; 16(9):450–455.

941. Muller S, Parker DC, Kapadia SB, et al. Ameloblastic fibrosarcoma of the jaws. A clinicopathologic and DNA analysis of five cases and review of the literature with discussion of its relationship to ameloblastic fibroma. Oral Surg Oral Med Oral Pathol Oral Radiol Endod 1995; 79(4):469–477.

942. Carlos-Bregni R, Taylor AM, Garcia AM. Ameloblastic fibrosarcoma of the mandible: report of two cases and review of the literature. J Oral Pathol Med 2001; 30(5):316–320.

943. Batista de Paula AM, da Costa Neto JQ, da Silva GE, et al. Immunolocalization of the p53 protein in a case of ameloblastic fibrosarcoma. J Oral Maxillofac Surg 2003; 61(2):256–258.

944. Lee OJ, Kim HJ, Lee BK, et al. CD34 expressing ameloblastic fibrosarcoma arising in the maxilla: a new finding. J Oral Pathol Med 2005; 34(5):318–320.

945. Kobayashi K, Murakami R, Fujii T, et al. Malignant transformation of ameloblastic fibroma to ameloblastic fibrosarcoma: case report and review of the literature. J Craniomaxillofac Surg 2005; 33(5):352–355.

946. Takeda Y, Kaneko R, Suzuki A. Ameloblastic fibrosarcoma in the maxilla, malignant transformation of ameloblastic fibroma. Virchows Arch A Pathol Anat Histopathol 1984; 404(3), 253–263.

947. Park HR, Shin KB, Sol MY, et al. A highly malignant ameloblastic fibrosarcoma. Report of a case. Oral Surg Oral Med Oral Pathol Oral Radiol Endod 1995; 79(4): 478–481.

948. Wood RM, Markle TL, Barker BF, et al. Ameloblastic fibrosarcoma. Oral Surg Oral Med Oral Pathol 1988; 66(1):74–77.

949. Nasu M, Matsubara O, Yamamoto H. Ameloblastic fibrosarcoma: an ultrastructural study of the mesenchymal component. J Oral Pathol 1984; 13(2):178–187.

950. Chomette G, Auriol M, Guilbert F, et al. Ameloblastic fibrosarcoma of the jaws–report of three cases. Clinicopathologic, histoenzymological and ultrastructural study. Pathol Res Pract 1983; 178(1):40–47.

951. Dallera P, Bertoni F, Marchetti C, et al. Ameloblastic fibrosarcoma of the jaw: report of five cases. J Craniomaxillofac Surg 1994; 22(6):349–354.

952. De Oliveira Nogueira T, Carvalho YR, Rosa LE, et al. Possible malignant transformation of an ameloblastic fibroma to ameloblastic fibrosarcoma: a case report. J Oral Maxillofac Surg 1997; 55(2):180–182.

953. Cina MT, Dahlin DC, Gores RJ. Ameloblastic sarcoma. Report of two cases. Oral Surg Oral Med Oral Pathol 1962; 15:696–700.

954. Reichart PA, Zobl H. Transformation of ameloblastic fibroma to fibrosarcoma. Int J Oral Surg 1978; 7(5):503–507.

955. Pindborg JJ. Ameloblastic sarcoma in the maxilla. Report of a case. Cancer 1960; 13:917–920.

956. Forman G, Garrett J. Ameloblastic sarcoma: report of case. J Oral Surg 1972; 30(1):50–54.

957. Prein J, Remagen W, Spiessl B, et al. Ameloblastic fibroma and its sarcomatous transformation. Pathol Res Pract 1979; 166(1):123–130.

958. Daramola JO, Ajagbe HA, Oluwasanmi JO, et al. Ameloblastic sarcoma of the mandible: report of case. J Oral Surg 1979; 37(6):432–435.

959. Dallera P, Bertoni F, Marchetti C, et al. Ameloblastic fibroma: a follow-up of six cases. Int J Oral Maxillofac Surg 1996; 25(3):199–202.

960. DeNittis AS, Stambaugh MD, Looby C. Ameloblastic fibrosarcoma of the maxilla: report of a case. J Oral Maxillofac Surg 1998; 56(5):672–675.

961. Cataldo E, Nathanson N, Shklar G. Ameloblastic sarcoma of the mandible. Oral Surg Oral Med Oral Pathol 1963; 16:953–957.

962. Hatzifotiadis D, Economou A. Ameloblastic sarcoma in the maxilla–a case report. J Maxillofac Surg 1973; 1(1):62–64.

963. Eda S, Saito T, Morimura G, et al. A case of ameloblastic fibrosarcoma, with an electron-microscopic observation. Bull Tokyo Dent Coll 1976; 17(1):11–25.

964. Slater LJ. Odontogenic sarcoma and carcinosarcoma. Semin Diagn Pathol 1999; 16(4):325–332.

965. Reichart PA, Philipsen HP. Ameloblastic Fibrosarcoma. Odontogenic Tumors and Allied Lesions. London: Quintessence Publishing Co Ltd, 2004:255–262.

966. Goldstein G, Parker FP, Hugh GS. Ameloblastic sarcoma: pathogenesis and treatment with chemotherapy. Cancer 1976; 37(4):1673–1678.

967. Navone R, Mela F, Romagnoli R, et al. Studio clinico-patologico di un caso di evoluzione sarcomatosa di fibroma amloblastico [Clinico-pathological study of a case of sarcomatous evolution of an ameloblastic fibroma]. Minerva Stomatol 1982; 31(6):673–678.

968. Tajima Y, Utsumi N, Suzuki S, et al. Ameloblastic fibrosarcoma arising de novo in the maxilla. Pathol Int 1997; 47(8):564–568.

969. Huguet P, Castellvi J, Avila M, et al. Ameloblastic fibrosarcoma: report of a case. Immunohistochemical study and review of the literature. Med Oral 2001; 6(3):173–179.

970. Chomette G, Auriol M, Guilbert F, et al. Fibrosarcome améloblastique. Etude clinique et anatomopathologique de trois observations données histo-enzymologiques et ultrastucturales [Ameloblastic fibrosarcoma. A clinical and anatomopathological study of three cases. Histoenzymological and ultrastructural data]. Arch Anat Cytol Pathol 1982; 30(3):172–178.

971. Pellitteri PK, Ferlito A, Bradley PJ, et al. Management of sarcomas of the head and neck in adults. Oral Oncol 2003; 39(1):2–12.

972. Altini M, Smith I. Ameloblastic dentinosarcoma–a case report. Int J Oral Surg 1976; 5(3):142–147.

973. Corominas-Villafane O, Cuestas-Carnero R, Corominas O Jr. et al. Ameloblastic odontosarcoma: report of a case. Acta Stomatol Belg 1993; 90(3):149–156.

974. Tahsinoglu M, Ozmerzifonlu S. Ameloblastik odontosarkom. Odonto-Stomat (Istanbul) 1964; 3:14–22.

975. Zhang YD, Chen Z, Song YQ, et al. Making a tooth: growth factors, transcription factors, and stem cells. Cell Res 2005; 15(5):301–316.

976. Tompkins K. Molecular mechanisms of cytodifferentiation in mammalian tooth development. Connect Tissue Res 2006; 47(3):111–118.

977. Chibret MA. Étude anatomo-pathologique d'un cas d'épithélioma adamantin. Archives de Médicine expérimentale et d'Anatomie pathologique 1894; 6(1 série):278–302.

978. Polaillon. Epithéliome paradentaire présentant tous les signes d'un sarcome du maxillaire inférieur. Résection du maxillaire. Guérison. Union Médicale 1889; 47–48(3. série), 474–476.

979. Takeda Y, Kuroda M, Suzuki A. Ameloblastic odontosarcoma (ameloblastic fibro-odontosarcoma) in the mandible. Acta Pathol Jpn 1990; 40(11):832–837.

980. Phillips VM, Grotepass FW, Hendricks R. Ameloblastic odontosarcoma with epithelial atypia: a case report. Br J Oral Maxillofac Surg 1988; 26(1):45–51.

981. Chan WK, Li CP, Liu JM, et al. Mandibular odontogenic fibrosarcoma. Case report. Aust Dent J 1997; 42(6):409–412.

982. WHO Working group on classification of head and neck tumours. Odontogenic Tumours. In: Barnes L, Eveson JW, Reichart P, et al, eds. Pathology and Genetics of Head and Neck Tumours. World Health Organization Classification of Tumours. Lyon: IARC Press, 2005:283–327.

983. Reichart PA, Philipsen HP. Odontogenic Carcinosarcoma. Odontogenic Tumors and Allied Lesions. London: Quintessence Publishing Co Ltd, 2004:269–270.

984. Kunkel M, Ghalibafian M, Radner H, et al. Ameloblastic fibrosarcoma or odontogenic carcinosarcoma: a matter of classification? Oral Oncol 2004; 40(4):444–449.

985. Shinoda T, Iwata H, Nakamura A, et al. Cytologic appearance of carcinosarcoma (malignant ameloblastoma and fibrosarcoma) of the maxilla. A case report. Acta Cytol 1992; 36(2):132–136.

986. Slama A, Yacoubi T, Khochtali H, et al. Carcinosarcome odontogène mandibulaire. A propos d'un cas [Mandibular odontogenic carcinosarcoma: a case report]. Rev Stomatol Chir Maxillofac 2002; 103(2):124–127.

ABBREVIATIONS

AFD	Ameloblastic fibrodentinoma
AFDS	Ameloblastic fibrodentinosarcoma
AFOD	Ameloblastic fibro-odontoma
AFOS	Ameloblastic fibro-odontosarcoma
AFS	Ameloblastic fibrosarcoma
AMCA	Ameloblastic carcinoma
AMF	Ameloblastic fibroma
AOT	Adenomatoid odontogenic tumor
CCAM	Clear cell ameloblastoma
CCOC	Clear cell odontogenic carcinoma
CCOT	Calcifying cystic odontogenic tumor
CEMBLA	Cementoblastoma
CEOT	Calcifying epithelial odontogenic tumor
COC	Calcifying odontogenic cyst
COF	Central odontogenic fibroma
DESAM	Desmoplastic ameloblastoma
DGCT	Dentinogenic ghost cell tumor
GCOC	Ghost cell odontogenic carcinoma
GCOT	Granular cell odontogenic tumor
HCCC	Hyalinizing clear cell carcinoma
KCOT	Keratocystic odontogenic tumor
METAM	Metastasizing ameloblastoma
O-A	Odontoameloblastoma
OaCCOT	Odontoma-associated calcifying cystic odontogenic tumor
ODCASA	Odontogenic carcinosarcoma
ODOMYX	Odontogenic myxoma/myxofibroma
ODTp	Compound odontoma
ODTx	Complex odontoma
PERAM	Solid/multicystic ameloblastoma - peripheral
PIOSCC	Primary intraosseous squamous cell carcinoma
POF	Peripheral odontogenic fibroma
s/mAM	Solid/multicystic ameloblastoma - central
SCC	Squamous cell carcinoma
SOHL	Squamous odontogenic hamartoid lesion
SOT	Squamous odontogenic tumor
UNAM	Unicystic ameloblastoma

20

Maldevelopmental, Inflammatory, and Neoplastic Pathology in Children

Louis P. Dehner and Samir K. El-Mofty

Lauren V. Ackerman Laboratory of Surgical Pathology, Barnes-Jewish and St. Louis Children's Hospitals, Washington University Medical Center, Department of Pathology and Immunology, St. Louis, Missouri, U.S.A.

I. INTRODUCTION

Whether one's surgical pathology practice is in the setting of a general or children's hospital, the perspective on head and neck pathology in children is limited or dominated by small scraps of keratotic tissue from a middle ear cholesteatoma or paranasal sinus contents in a child with chronic or allergic sinusitis, an important distinction to be made pathologically for purposes of clinical management. Most masses in the head and neck region of children are one or other congenital lesion, often cystic, or an inflammatory process presenting with enlarged lymph nodes (1–9). Approximately 50% to 60% of neck masses in children are congenital cystic lesions such as the dermoid cyst, branchial cleft cyst, or thyroglossal duct cyst (TGDC); 25% to 30% are inflammatory and reactive lymphadenitis in most cases; 5% are benign neoplasms represented mainly by melanocytic nevi, hemangiomas, and lymphangiomas or cystic hygromas; and 5% to 10% are malignancies especially in pediatric referral institutions with lymphoma and rhabdomyosarcoma (RMS) as the most common tumor types (8,10,11). One of the variables in the proportion of malignant tumors in the head and neck of children is the inclusion or exclusion of lymphomas (1).

Unlike most of the other chapters in this reference, which are mainly concerned with a specific organ such as the thyroid or salivary glands or anatomic sites such as the oral cavity, this chapter takes a more regional anatomic approach to include a large portion of the head and neck region and the several unique expressions of pathology that are seen mainly in patients younger than 20 years at diagnosis and may be present in some cases at birth or even detected in utero. Other types of pathology to be considered briefly in this chapter are found more often in adults but are discussed for the sake of completeness.

We acknowledge that some topics in this chapter may overlap with those in other chapters, but the emphasis is upon those lesions in children that reflect active pediatric surgical and otolaryngological services at the St. Louis Children's Hospital at the Washington University Medical Center, St. Louis, Missouri.

II. SKIN

A review of our surgical pathology files shows that the skin, soft tissue, and lymph node specimens have accounted for a substantial proportion of our cases from the head and neck region of children with the exclusion of the tonsils and adenoids.

A. Pigmented Lesions

Melanocytic nevi are the most common cutaneous tumefactions from children, and the vast majority are uncomplicated acquired compound melanocytic nevi, but a disproportionate number of these are congenital and arise in the head and neck region (12,13). Most congenital melanocytic nevi (CMN) offer few difficulties in diagnosis, since maturation is clearly present with depth, though the pattern is that of individual melanocytes sweeping through the dermis (14,15). Some lesions, usually less than 2 cm, may be evident at birth. Large CMN, in excess of 2 cm in diameter, in the head and neck, can involve the face and the contiguous neck and upper trunk, in which case they often exceed 20 cm and are regarded as "giant CMNs." Approximately 2% of large CMNs present on the face (16). One of the microscopic hallmarks of a CMN is the diffuse involvement of the dermis by a uniform infiltrate of small, individual melanocytes with the maintenance of existing dermal adnexa (15–17) (Fig. 1). These cells may infiltrate along the fibrous septa in the subcutis and even into the skeletal muscle (Fig. 2A, B). Lymphatic space involvement and perineural growth may be present as well. "Proliferative" nodules composed of "ballooned" darker-pigmented epithelioid melanocytes with a clonal appearance may cause concern about melanoma in the presence of some mitotic activity, but high-grade atypia and atypical mitoses are absent (18).

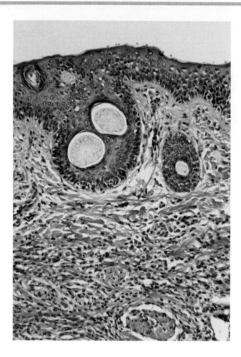

Figure 1 Congenital melanocytic nevus has a nested and lentiginous junctional component, like an acquired nevus, but even in the superficial dermis, the pattern of individual melanocytes streaming through the interstitial collagen is appreciated rather than the formation of discrete nests.

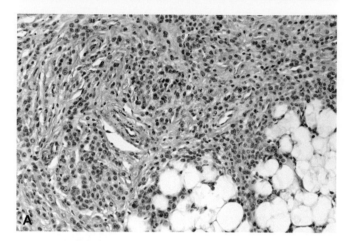

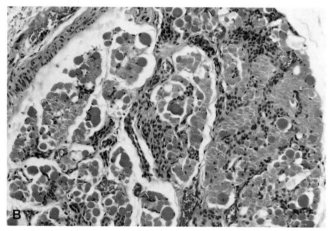

Figure 2 (**A**) Congenital melanocytic nevus is demonstrating the characteristic single cell pattern of growth into the deep reticular dermis and subcutaneous fat. (**B**) The nevus cells are shown here as they infiltrate into the temporalis muscle of an infant with a large congenital nevus involving one-half of the face and scalp.

Benign-appearing melanocytes may be found in regional lymph nodes. Multiple specimens from a single patient are not unusual, as these lesions are excised in stages. The risk of a malignancy in CMN, usually confined to the large lesions, is well below 5% (17,19).

Spitz nevus or, as Spitz herself referred to this problematic melanocytic proliferation, "juvenile melanoma," presents in the head and neck region in approximately 25% to 30% of cases in childhood, especially the cheek (20,21). A dome-shaped lesion is more often than not amelanotic so that the clinical impression is often that of a lobular capillary hemangioma (LCH) or "pyogenic granuloma." Most Spitz nevi are compound nevi with a prominent symmetric junctional population of epithelioid and/or spindled nevus cells with uniform eosinophilic cytoplasm with minimal melanin pigment (Fig. 3A) (20,22). The epidermis is often acanthotic, and the suprapapillary dermis contains ectatic thin-walled vascular spaces to account for the hemangioma-like clinical appearance. An enlarged nucleus with a prominent nucleolus but not out of proportion to the cell itself is a hallmark of the epithelioid and spindled melanocytes (23) (Fig. 3B). Large, hyperchromatic, and pleomorphic nuclei and deep mitotic figures, especially if atypical, should alert to the distinct possibility of a malignant melanoma with Spitz-like features (spitzoid melanoma) even in a young child. However, individual pleomorphic cells and nuclear pseudoinclusions are found in some Spitz nevi, and their presence is not indicative of a spitzoid or Spitz-like melanoma. Note

also the ectatic vessels. There is still no resolution about the significance of mitotic activity in the Spitz nevus, but if the mitotic figures are deep and atypical, then an interpretation of spitzoid melanoma would seem appropriate. It is generally recognized that some of these spitzoid lesions do not acquire a consensus diagnosis even among "experts" (23,24). All can agree to the management with complete excision and consideration of a sentinel lymph node biopsy. Both CMN at birth and the Spitz nevus can have a pagetoid pattern of individual melanocytes migrating through the epidermis (21). Rarely a CMN may have Spitz-like features.

Other melanocytic lesions found in the head and neck of children include the cellular blue nevus, which is a dermal and subcutaneous proliferation of relatively uniform spindle cells (25). The scalp is one of the favored sites, and these lesions may be locally aggressive in some cases. Some melanocytic nevi may have so-called combined features with the usual compound pattern and spitz-like, deep penetrating, or blue nevus-like features (26). The so-called neurocytic

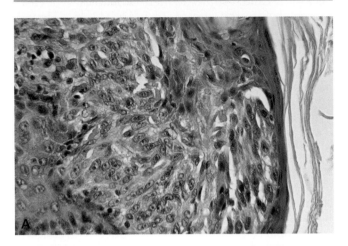

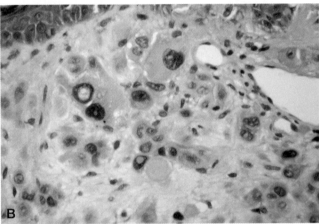

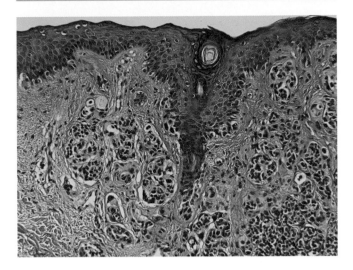

Figure 4 Compound melanocytic nevus from the scalp of a 15-year-old female shows an atypical pattern of lentiginous proliferation with extension down a hair follicle, but otherwise orderly maturation of dermal component. These atypical features in a nevus on the scalp of adolescents are similar to those seen in other "special sites including the axilla, umbilicus, perineum and acral region."

Figure 3 **(A)** Spitz nevus arising on the cheek of a 12-year-old male is showing an intermixture of epithelioid and spindle melanocytes at the epidermal junction. Note the vesicular nuclei and prominent nucleoli of these cells but an absence of overt pleomorphism. Mitotic figures (not shown) are not unusual at the junction. **(B)** The presence of individual, enlarged pleomorphic cells with abundant eosinophilic cytoplasm and nuclear pseudoinclusions without the presence of atypical mitotic figures in the superficial dermis is worrisome, but insufficient for a diagnosis of a spitzoid melanoma in most cases.

hamartoma is a complex lesion, with elements of a CMN and a nerve sheath neoplasm typically arising in the scalp (27,28).

Malignant melanoma occurs rarely in children where we have seen individual examples on the ear and face. Most cases are sporadic and, in our experience, are not associated with a preexisting syndrome such as xeroderma pigmentosa or giant CMN (19,22,24,29–32). The most common histologic patterns are those of a superficial spreading and spitzoid melanoma. One cautionary note is that acquired nevi on the scalp of adolescents can have atypical features with irregular junctional nests and pagetoid spread; this pattern is like the other "special site" nevi. The scalp in the adolescent is another site for an "atypical" nevus with lentiginous and even pagetoid features, yet appears entirely benign (35) (Fig. 4).

B. Epidermal and Cutaneous Adnexal Lesions

These include a variety of congenital and acquired lesions from the epidermal nevus, nevus sebaceous of Jadassohn (NSJ), and subepidermal cysts to neoplasms (33). The *epidermal nevus* involves the scalp as a variably sized lesion with a yellowish, verrucous or papillomatous appearance clinically (34,35). There are any number of histologic patterns of epidermal proliferation, resembling in some respects a common verruca vulgaris or seborrheic keratosis. Some of these lesions have a pattern of epidermolytic hyperkeratosis. There are a number of associated syndromes, several with other manifestations in the head and neck. NSJ has a predilection for the head and neck region and is noted at birth, and unlike the epidermal nevus does not spread but rather involutes during childhood until adolescence with the hormonal stimulation of sebaceous glands. At birth, there is a raised yellowish-orange lesion on the scalp, which is devoid of hair. As infancy gives way to early childhood, the lesion tends to flatten out with associated alopecia. Infrequently, NSJ can be multifocal in the head and neck or even more generalized. Unlike the epidermal nevus, there are numerous pilosebaceous units with immature-appearing hair follicles and hyperplastic sebaceous glands, which account for the clinical appearance (36) (Fig. 5A). The stroma around the pilar units has a hypercellular quality. Follicular plugs may be present but are more prominent in later childhood. In addition to the cosmetic indication for resection, there is also the risk for the development of a variety of cutaneous and adnexal neoplasms, which are not seen until puberty or later (37). It is estimated

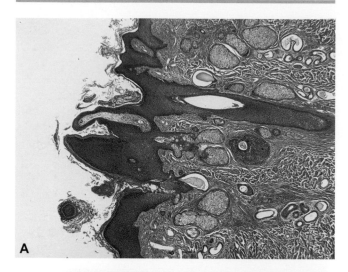

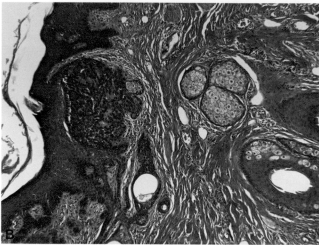

Figure 5 (**A**) Nevus sebaceous of Jahassohn presenting on the scalp of a child shows epidermal papillomatosis, but in addition numerous, enlarged sebaceous glands for age and sweat ducts, some lined by apocrine cells. (**B**) Elsewhere in the same excision, a basaloid proliferation with features of a trichoblastoma is present. Note that there is a contiguous abnormally formed pilosebaceous unit.

that one-fourth of NSJs harbor an adnexal tumor, most commonly the trichoblastoma, the revised interpretation of a basaloid neoplasm formerly diagnosed as basal cell carcinoma (BCC) (Fig. 5B). The rare squamous cell carcinoma has been reported in a child with NSJ (38).

BCC is reported in childhood and typically in the head and neck region (90% of cases) (39). An inquiry about the basal cell nevus syndrome (chromosome q22.3 deletion) or xeroderma pigmentosa is appropriate when a BCC is encountered in a child (40–42). The histopathologic differential diagnosis includes trichoblastoma and trichoepithelioma.

Pilomatrixoma is the most common of the pilar neoplasms as well as the most common cutaneous adnexal neoplasm in childhood and is one of the more common causes of a "lump or bump" in the head and neck of a child. Approximately 40% to 50% of cases present before the age of 18 years (43–45). Though reported in a variety of anatomic sites, there is a predilection for the periorbital region, scalp, cheek, and neck (in aggregate 50–70% of cases), where it is a mobile, firm nodule in the skin or subcutis (46,47). Multiple lesions are seen in 5% or so of cases. The age range at diagnosis is 6 months to 15 years (average 6–10 years). The diagnosis can be anticipated at times if the "cyst" is grossly solid, has circumscribed, contoured margins, and has a yellowish, gritty appearance representing dystrophic calcifications and metaplastic bone as features of regression. Sheets of uniform basaloid cells are accompanied by pale, eosinophilic ghost cells with abundant cytoplasm (Fig. 6A). Numerous mitotic figures in the basaloid or germinal cells should not be regarded with concern. A foreign body giant cell reaction, dystrophic calcifications, and metaplastic bone are other histologic features (Fig. 6B).

Syringoma presents as a solitary or multiple papules on the lower eyelid and cheek, which are seen around puberty and more commonly in females (48). Multiple syringomas can be associated with trisomy 21 (Down syndrome) (49). Lesions on the neck are also seen in a minority of cases. Histologically, a cluster of small, duct-like structures lined by cuboidal epithelial cells with or without clear cell features are present in the superficial dermis.

Epithelial-lined cysts arising in the head and neck constitute a varied histogenetic and pathogenetic category of lesions, which are clinically recognized as a cyst or as a "tumor." The most common acquired cysts are the *keratinous cysts* of the infundibular type, which are lined by epidermal or infundibular squamous epithelium and desquamated cyst contents, and of the pilar or tricholemmal type, which are lined by plump eosinophilic squamous cells and contents of acellular pilar-type keratin with or without dystrophic calcifications. Rupture of these cysts, especially the infundibular cyst, is associated with an intense, mixed inflammatory reaction and foreign body giant cells with ingested squamous debris. Pilar cysts have a predilection for the scalp and posterior neck and may be multiple, whereas the infundibular cyst has a wider anatomic distribution and is usually solitary. Both types of cysts are generally not seen until later childhood or adolescence. Severe acne keloidolis may be accompanied by deep infundibular cysts. Milial cysts are more superficial and commonly multiple. Severe scarring epidermolysis bullosa is complicated by milial cysts.

Dermoid cyst, unlike the keratinous cysts, is considered a maldevelopment of the embryo-fetal ectoderm, which invaginates or is otherwise displaced into the underlying tissues along sites of embryonic suture closure in the periorbital and nasal region (3,50–52). A firm nodule is the clinical presentation. The essential distinction between the keratinous cyst and the dermoid cyst is the presence of adnexal structures found along the periphery of the cyst wall as a manifestation of the embryo-fetal epidermis as the source of supporting adnexal structures as small attached or contiguous infundibular structures with

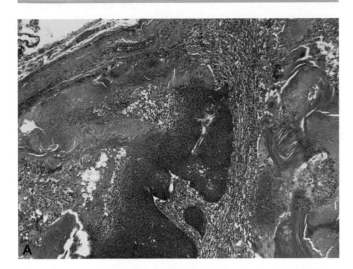

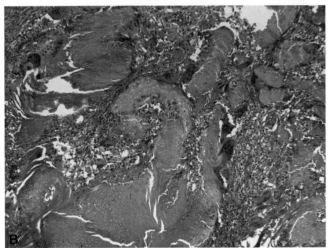

Figure 6 Pilomatrixoma from the neck of an eight-year-old male presented as a "cyst." (**A**) These well-circumscribed, noncystic lesions are composed in part of basaloid cells in sheets and nests and the paler-staining ghost cells with the associated giant cell reaction. A mixed inflammatory infiltrate is found in the interstitium. (**B**) Entire tumors may be devoid of germinal or basaloid cells, but only of islands and sheets of ghost cells with a foreign body granulomatous reaction. Dystrophic calcifications and metaplastic bone formation (not illustrated) are other microscopic features.

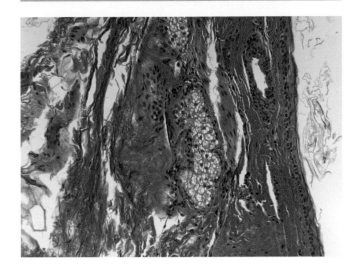

Figure 7 Dermoid cyst presented as a periorbital nodule in an infant. The microscopic appearance is a cyst lined by keratinizing squamous epithelium or epidermis and with cutaneous adnexal structures in the wall, most commonly sebaceous glands (as illustrated) and/or small duct-like structures. These cysts are rarely pigmented.

sebaceous glands (Fig. 7). If the dermoid cyst is in the midline and associated with the nose, it may have a posterior tract into the central nervous system (53,54). Other sites for the dermoid cyst include the orbit, floor of the mouth, and neck, where it can be coincidental with a TGDC. So-called congenital teratoid cyst in the floor of the mouth has the microscopic features of a dermoid cyst, but mesodermal derivatives like smooth and striated muscle and enteric and respiratory-lined cysts are present as well.

Eruptive vellus hair cyst is another developmental cyst, which occurs infrequently in the head and neck region and is not restricted to children, but is seen in association with steatocystoma multiplex and milia

cysts (55). Vellus hairs are a component of the cyst contents.

III. UPPER AERODIGESTIVE TRACT

A. Oral cavity, Oropharynx, Nasal Cavity, and Nasopharynx

Oral Cavity and Oropharynx

Developmental and/or congenital lesions in and around the oral cavity include a variety of common and not so common cystic and tumefactive entities. *Palatal* and *alveolar cysts*, lined by a stratified squamous epithelium and filled with keratin with or without a communication with the surface mucosa, are seen in 50% or more of term neonates, but are less common in preterm infants (56–58). These cysts are eponymically known as Epstein's pearls and Bohn's nodules, which are present along the median palatine raphe and the junction of the hard and soft palate, respectively. These cysts undergo spontaneous involution. Another type of cyst, dental lamina cyst, is found along the crests of the edentulous mandibular and maxillary alveolar ridge and is thought to be derived from remnants of the dental lamina. These lesions present as 1 to 3 mm whitish to whitish-yellow papules.

Other lesions in and around the oral cavity and underlying bony structures in children include a diverse number of entities (59–65). One of the more common lesions is the *mucocele* of the lip, which is characterized by a cystic space(s) occupied by extravasated mucin with accompanying neutrophils and histiocytes (66). Similar lesions in the floor of the mouth are known as ranulas (67,68). Injury to the duct of a minor salivary gland is the favored

Table 1 Hereditary Gingival Overgrowth and Infiltrative Fibroblastic Disorders

Syndrome	Phenotype	Mode of inheritance and genetic foci
GF, hypertrichosis and epilepsy syndrome	—	AD, 2p21-22, 2p 22.3–23.3, 5q13–q22
Zimmermann–Laband syndrome	GF, ear, nose, bone and nail defects, hepatosplenomegaly, hypertrichosis	AD, 3p21. 2, 8q24.3,mutant 3p14-p21 (AR deafness gene)
Cross syndrome	GF, microphthalimia, mental retardation, hypopigmentation, athetosis	AR
Winchester syndrome[a]	GF, progressive coarening of focal features, multicenteric osteolysis (hands and feet)	AR MMP2 mutation, 16q13
Jones syndrome	GF, progressive sensorineural deafness, odontogenic cyst	—
Rutherford syndrome	GF, corneal dystrophy	—
Juvenile hyaline fibromatosis and infantile systemic hyalinosis (allelic disease)	Oral, cutaneous and subcutaneous deposits and visceral involvement	AR, CMG 2 mutation, 4q21

[a]Other hereditary hands and feet osteolysis syndromes: Torg syndrome and nodulosis—arthropathy—osteolysis syndrome. *Abbreviations*: GF, gingival fibromatosis; AD, autosomal dominant; AR, autosmal recessive.

pathogenesis. Cysts of various types related to an erupted or unerupted tooth include the dentigerous, periapical, and odontogenic keratocyst and paradental and radicular cysts (69).

Odontogenic keratocysts are found in 60% to 80% of those with nevoid BCC syndrome (NBCCS, Gorlin–Goltz syndrome); these are seen in children, usually in early to mid-adolescence (40,70). A recurrence or the development of a second cyst is a reliable indication of NBCCS. These cysts have undulating parakeratosis on the surface, some basal nuclear hyperchromatism, six to eight epithelial layers, and a linear basement membrane zone (71). Differential cytokeratin expression (CK17 vs. CK19) is useful in the diagnosis (72). Odontogenic neoplasms are rare in children, but the odontoma is one of the more common, followed by the ameloblastoma, in particular the cystic type, and odontogenic myxoma. Less than 10% of all odontogenic neoplasms present in the first two decades of life (73,74).

Gingival fibrous overgrowth or infiltrative disorders of a hereditary nature include several syndromes and the entity of isolated hereditary gingival fibromatosis, which is the most common clinical type (75–77) (Table 1). The overgrowth syndromes are characterized by progressive enlargement of the gingival tissues at the time of eruption of the permanent teeth or less often with eruption of deciduous teeth. Dense collagenous bundles without any particular orientation replace the normal gingival stroma. Unlike desmoid fibromatosis or one of the other fibrous tumors of childhood, a cellular fibroblastic or myofibroblastic component is inconspicuous in the hypocellular homogeneous collagenous deposition. Dystrophic calcifications are seen infrequently. Juvenile hyaline fibromatosis (JHF) and the apparently related infantile systemic hyalinosis are characterized by the deposition of amorphous material of an uncertain nature within the normal interstitial tissues, which are largely replaced or displaced (Fig. 8) (73,75,78). These are regarded as an allelic disorder involving different point mutations in the capillary morphogenesis gene-2 (CMG-2) (74,79,80). Gingival overgrowth has other etiologies in children, including several therapeutic agents (phenytoin, cyclosporine) and neurofibromatosis.

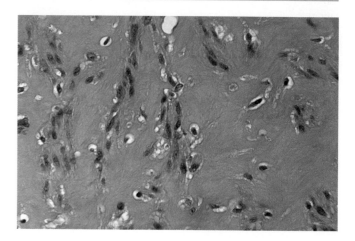

Figure 8 Juvenile hyaline fibromatosis and hereditary gingival fibromatosis have similar histological features of dense, hypocellular hyalinzed stroma.

Lipoid proteinosis (Urbach–Wiethe syndrome) is an autosomal recessive disorder (1q21, extracellular matrix protein 1 gene), which is characterized by an extracellular PAS-positive hyaline material in the head and neck (skin, pharynx, larynx) of infants as early as the neonatal period (81–83). The material resembles amyloid, but is Congo red–negative. However, amyloidosis is seen in the upper airway in children (84,85).

Granular cell tumor (GCT) has a predilection for the aerodigestive tract as well as the skin and soft tissues. Approximately 40% to 50% of GCTs in children usually older than three to four years present in the head and neck region, where they are seen on the lip, tongue, larynx, and orbit (86–88). These tumors are regarded as "neural"-type GCTs since the granular cells are immunopositive for S-100 protein.

Gingival GCT of the newborn (congenital epulis) is a unique clinicopathologic entity that presents as a pedunculated, erythematous mass, most often on the anterior alveolar ridge just lateral to the midline, with a preference for the maxillary over the mandibular ridge (2–3:1) (89,90). These lesions measure 2 cm or less, but rarely can exceed 5 cm in diameter. In 10% of

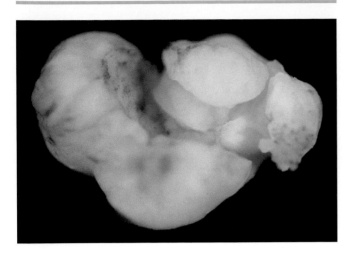

Figure 9 Congenital granular cell tumor in this 11-day-old female presented as a polypoid and multilobulated mass measuring 2.7 cm in great dimension. The grayish-white surface of the mass is appreciated on the partially sectioned surface.

cases, the tumors are multifocal on the maxillary and mandibular ridge and, rarer yet, with sites of involvement elsewhere in the oral cavity, including the tongue (91,92). Spontaneous regression is reported (93). There is an inexplicable female predilection (F:M, 8:1). These lesions have been detected by ultrasonography in utero (94).

An intact, glistening or occasionally ulcerated mucosa covers the polyp whose cut surface has a uniform white to grayish-white appearance (Fig. 9). The stroma is occupied by a monotonous, formless sheet of large polygonal cells with abundant granular cytoplasm and small, round to oval central or eccentric nuclei (Fig. 10A). Odontogenic epithelial islands may be seen among the granular cells. Pseudoepitheliomatous hyperplasia does not accompany the gingival GCT, unlike the more common cutaneous and mucous membrane-associated GCTs. It is thought that the gingival GCT is nonneural in derivation, since the cells, unlike most GCTs, are nonreactive for S-100 protein (Fig. 10D) but are positive for vimentin and CD68 (Fig. 10B, C). Smooth muscle differentiation

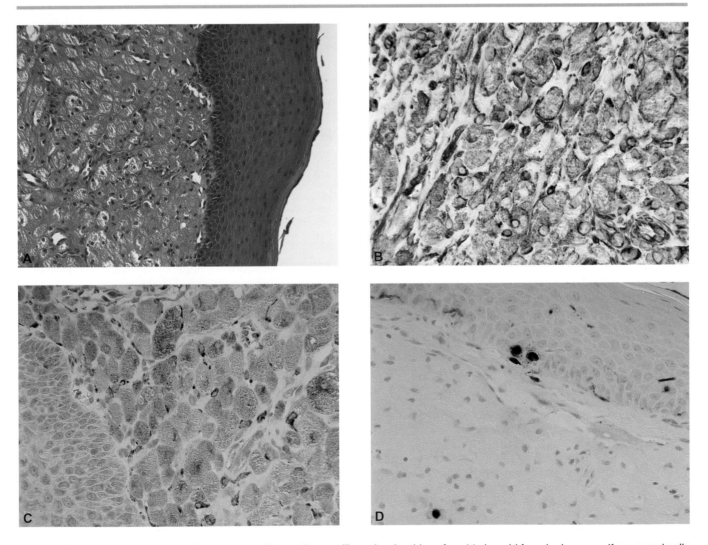

Figure 10 Congenital granular cell tumor presenting on the maxillary alveolar ridge of an 11-day-old female. Large, uniform round cells with abundant granular eosinophilic cytoplasm occupy the submucosa as a formless sheet of cells. (**B**) These cells are immunoreactive for vimentin. (**C**) The granular cells are diffusely positive for CD68. (**D**) There is lack of reactivity for S-100 protein.

has been reported (95). These lesions usually require resection, since they are known to interfere with feeding and/or to cause respiratory obstruction (96). Some are of the opinion that the gingival GCT should be regarded as a hamartoma rather than a true neoplasm.

Lingual thyroid is a rare anomaly and the arrested primordium of the thyroid, which, as a diverticulum of the foramen cecum, normally passes anterior to the hyoid bone. The ultimate destination of the thyroid is anterior to the trachea and occurs by the seventh embryonic week. A mass between the anterior two-thirds and the posterior one-third of the tongue is the typical location of the lingual thyroid (97). One estimate is that the lingual thyroid is seen as an incidental finding at autopsy in 10% of recognized cases, but during life is discovered in 1 per 10,000 individuals (98). For most individuals (70%), the lingual thyroid is the only functioning thyroid parenchyma (99). A lingual thyroid is a cause of congenital hypothyroidism (100,101). A biopsy of the mass without considering a lingual thyroid can result in hemorrhage with potential compromise in the functioning of the residual thyroid. Cellular microfollicles may be recognizable as thyroid tissue, but may require confirmation by immunohistochemistry for thyroglobulin and TTF-1. The base of the tongue is also the site for alveolar soft part sarcoma (ASPS) in children, which can be mistaken clinically for a lingual thyroid (102). Malignant transformation of lingual thyroid is rare at any age, but is mainly recorded in adults (103).

Melanotic neuroectodermal tumor of infancy (MNTI, retinal anlage tumor, melanotic progonoma) is a distinctive variably pigmented neoplasm generally diagnosed before the age of one year, but can be seen in somewhat older children. More than 90% of the cases present in the head and neck region with a predilection for the maxilla, where it accounts for 80% of all such cases (104,105). Other sites include the skull, mandible, orbit, and brain (106). These tumors can present as a rapidly growing expansile mass in the anterior maxilla or mandible. The surface mucosa may have a deep bluish or bluish-black coloration (Fig. 11). Not all MNTIs are deeply pigmented on gross examination, since the number of pigmented cells and the intensity of pigmentation can vary from case to case. Radiographically, developing teeth are displaced by an osteolytic lesion, which can have a multilocular appearance or may demonstrate a homogeneous lesion with a developing tooth. The tumors vary in size from 1 to 10 cm, and the larger ones may involve the entire maxilla. A small biopsy can be problematic if the pigmented cells are not prominent, and crush or compression artifact with multiple basophilic foci with poor preservation of cellular detail is present in a background of dense fibrous stroma. The resected tumor is well circumscribed, measuring 1 to 3 cm in greatest dimension, and has a firm fibrous appearance with or without obvious pigmentation. A fibrous stroma separates the many small nests of tumor cells (Fig. 12). Some nests are seemingly composed only of the small dark cells representing the neuroblasts with or without an apparent network of delicate

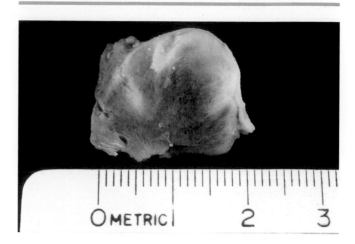

Figure 11 Melanotic neuroectodermal tumor of infancy presented as a mass in the mandible and soft tissues of a 10-month-old female. Abundant melaninin in this tumor accounted for bluish-black coloration.

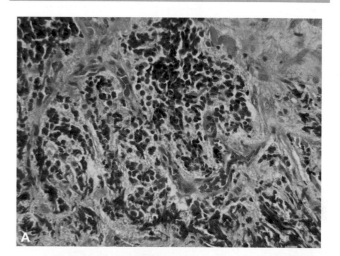

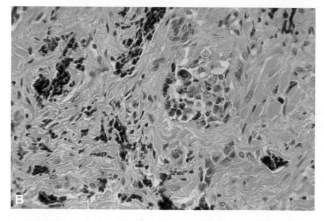

Figure 12 Melanotic neuroectodermal tumor of infancy is associated with a dense fibrous stroma in the background, but the prominence of the pigmented cells can vary from one tumor to another. (**A**) This microscopic field shows many nests of neuroblasts with crush artifact. (**B**) Another tumor is shown with a more prominent population of large pigment-containing cells.

eosinophilic fibrils or neuropil (Fig. 12A). The second cell type is a larger polygonal cell with finely pigmented granules in the cytoplasm, representing melanosomes, but these same cells may lack apparent melanin altogether (Fig. 12B). The two cell population has the ultrastructural and immunophenotypic attributes of neuroblasts and melanocytes. However, the immunophenotype is an idiosyncratic one, since the large cells, presumably melanocytes, express cytokeratin in addition to vimentin and HMB45 (107–109) (Fig. 13A–C). The neuroblasts are immunoreactive for neuron-specific enolase, synaptophysin, and chromogranin (Fig. 13D). Ganglion cells and myogenic elements have been observed infrequently in these tumors (110,111). The presence of melanocytes differentiates the MNTI from classic neuroblastoma (NB), retinoblastoma, and medulloblastoma, which can metastasize to the mandible or maxilla. Metastatic NB is generally not accompanied by a prominent fibrous stroma. The MNTI does not have any of the cytogenetic markers of classic NB (N-myc amplification or 1p deletion) or Ewing sarcoma–primitive neuroectodermal tumor (EWS-PNET) [t(11;22) (q24; q12)].

There is an element of unpredictability in the behavior of MNTI, but the majority of cases are managed successfully by surgical resection. The overall local recurrence rate is approximately 20% (105). However, 6% to 7% of tumors pursue a malignant course, and usually, these are the ones that have recurred on multiple occasions, with the eventual development of metastasis to regional lymph nodes and beyond. One well-studied case in the maxilla evolved into a purely neuroblastic neoplasm after multiple local recurrences and eventual widespread metastases as a classic NB (112). The recurrent MNTI of the maxilla may be more prone to malignant progression than in other primary sites.

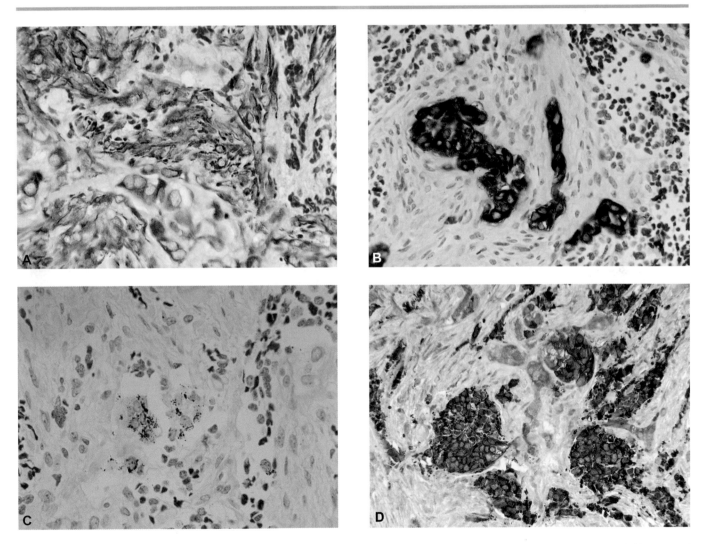

Figure 13 Melanotic neuroectodermal tumor presented on the forehead of a 12-week-old female involving the soft tissue and underlying bone. The immunophenotypical profile reflects the bilineal differentiation of these neoplasms. (**A**) Both the stroma and the larger pale cells are positive for vimentin. (**B**) The strong cytokeratin expression is one of the unique, inexplicable aspects of this tumor. (**C**) HMB-45 is positively expressed in the larger melanocytes. (**D**) Neuron-specific enolase is intensely positive in the individual nests of tumor.

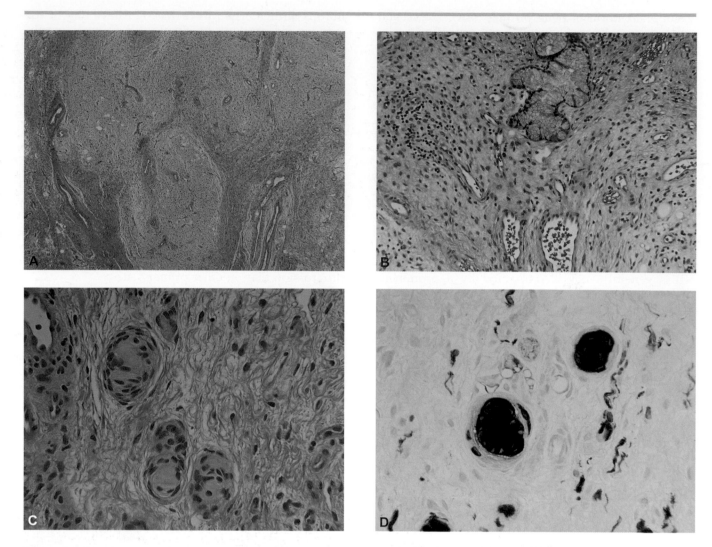

Figure 14 Mixed mesoneuroectodermal hamartoma presented as a soft tissue mass from the base of the skull to the neck in a four-month-old male. (**A**) Multiple pale-staining myxoid cellular nodules blend into each other or are partially surrounded by a dense fibrous stroma. (**B**) The immature mesenchymal cells are evenly spaced and lack any atypical features to suggest malignant rhabdomyoblasts. Isolated seromucinous glands are present in the background. (**C**) Small neuroid-tactoid bodies are present focally. (**D**) Those neuroid structures and surrounding individual spindle cells are strongly immunopositive for S-100 protein.

Hamartomas and other developmental tumefactive lesions present as cysts, polyps, and masses whose exact histogenesis and lines of differentiation are not obvious in all cases (Fig. 14A–D). Some of these cases have been interpreted as teratomas with some rationale. Striated and smooth muscle collections in the tongue, gingival and hard palate, (113–116) mature neuroglia, ganglioneuroma-like nodules, a mixture of differentiated mesenchymal tissue (bone, cartilage), and salivary gland are other tissue types that have been noted in these hamartomas (117). Those arising in the posterior oropharynx can lead to respiratory obstruction (118). Fibrous nodules of a presumed hamartomatous type are present in Cowden syndrome and tuberous sclerosis (119,120). Mucosal neuromas of multiple endocrine neoplasia (MEN) type 2B are considered as hamartomas in and around the oral cavity (121). Developmental cysts with a gastroenteric or

respiratory epithelial lining in and around the oral cavity have been interpreted as bronchoenteric duplications, but it is unlikely that their histogenesis is similar to the more distal duplications of endodermal-enteric origin. So-called foregut duplication cyst, typically found in the esophagus, is reported in the floor of the mouth or tongue. Another type of developmental cyst in the floor of the mouth is the dermoid cyst, with similar microscopic features to those found in the nasal and periorbital sites. Some midline or even lateral cysts in and around the oral cavity are difficult to classify (122–125).

B. Nasal Cavity and Nasopharynx

Polypoid or mass-like lesions of suspected developmental origin include the so-called hairy polyp, nasal glioma or nasal cerebral heterotopia, salivary gland anlage tumor, and nasal chondromesenchymal hamartoma.

Hairy, (teratoid, dermoid, or choristomatous) polyp presents as a pedunculated mass in the pharynx of a neonate, but similar lesions have been seen in the middle ear, tonsil, and eustachian tube or arising from the tongue (126–129). The polyp can have a smooth or lobulated contour and measures 1 to 2 cm in maximum dimension with an attachment to the lateral wall of the nasopharynx. Pilosebaceous units with supporting adnexa in a dense fibrous stroma are the microscopic features with a resemblance to the wall of a dermoid cyst. Meningothelial remnants have also been identified within the stroma, and skeletal muscle is present in the stalk where it is attached to the pharynx (130).

Nasal cerebral heterotopia (nasal glioma, sequestered encephalocele) is a tumefactive process of extracranial brain tissue without a direct connection to the brain or an encephalocele when there is continuity with the brain (3,131–133). An intranasal mass may be detected prenatally or within the first few years of life because of difficulty in breathing and feeding (134–136). The bridge of the nose, orbit, oral cavity, and oropharynx are other sites of glial heterotopia (137). A mass filling the nasal cavity with septal displacement is usually attached high on the lateral wall of the nose. It is important to exclude a true nasal encephalocele, which is usually soft and pulsatile, unlike the firmer nasal glioma, since surgical intervention in the former can have serious consequences.

Microscopically, nodules, small islands, or a diffuse pattern of mature neuroglia are embedded in a dense fibrovascular stroma (Fig. 15A, B). Glial fibrillary acidic protein immunostaining confirms the presence of the neuroglia (Fig. 15C) (3,138). When neuroglia extends to the mucosal surface, it may be intermingled with mucoserous glands. Multinucleated astrocytes and gemistocytic astrocytes, some with stellate cytoplasmic projections, may be present. Rarely, oliogodendrocytes, ependyma, and neurons may be found. Dystrophic calcifications with psammomatous features are present in some cases. An encephalocele generally lacks any nasal tissue elements but rather consists only of neuroglial tissue with some degree of organization and has the presence of leptomeninges and dura in some cases. It is not always possible to differentiate an encephalocele from a heterotopia simply on microscopic examination. The differential diagnosis also includes an intranasal teratoma. There is one report of a ganglioglioma presenting in the nose (139).

Rudimentary meningocele or ectopic meningothelial hamartoma presents as a nodule or plaque on the scalp and elsewhere as a soft tissue lesion that is composed of delicate, clefted spaces with a dense stroma in which the spaces encircle bundles of collagen (44,140,141) (Fig. 16A). Though resembling vascular structures, these spaces are immunoreactive for vimentin and epithelial membrane antigen in keeping with the presumed meningeal histogenesis (Fig. 16B). CD31 and CD34 are not expressed by the lining cells. The overlying skin may be alopecic, and the underlying bone may have a defect. This lesion may have mixed hamartomatous features with a resemblance to

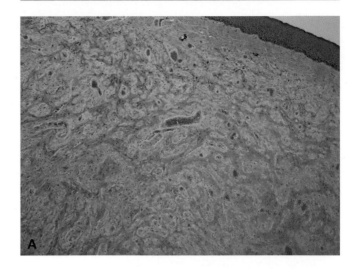

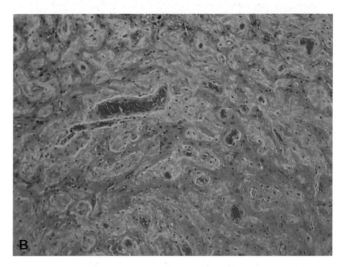

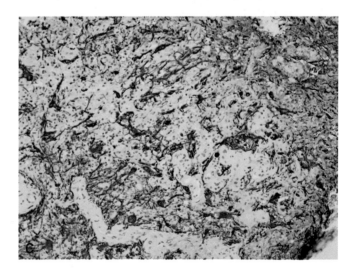

Figure 15 (**A** and **B**) Nasal cerebral heterotopia or nasal glioma is characterized by discrete islands or nodules of differentiated or mature neuroglia within a fibrous background or with a more diffuse pattern which is less apparent for neuroglia. (**C**) Glial fibrillary acidic protein immunostaining demonstrates and highlights the meshwork of astrocytes.

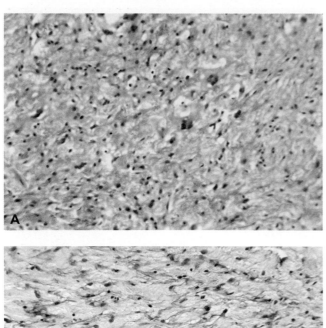

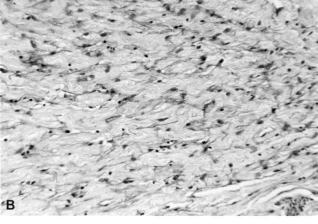

Figure 16 Rudimentary meningocele is usually discovered in an infant as a deep dermal and/or subcutandous mass in the occipital region or as part of a neuroglial heterotopia in the head and neck region. (**A**) A sieve-like or lattice network of apparent fibrous tissue has a vasoformative-like appearance with scattered, somewhat enlarged stromal cells. (**B**) These spaces display vimentin and epithelial membrane antigen (*shown*) immunopositivity in keeping with their meningothelial origin.

a NSJ (142). We have seen a case in an infant whose occipital lesion also had a glial heterotopia.

Salivary gland anlage tumor or so-called congenital pleomorphic adenoma, like the hairy polyp, presents as a pedunculated polyp at or near the midline of the nasopharynx in early infancy (3,143–145). There is a male predilection. Respiratory distress and/or feeding difficulties, as with the hairy or teratoid polyp and the congenital gingival GCT, is the usual clinical presentation. These lesions may be ulcerated with hemorrhage and necrosis (146). A simple excision or polypectomy is curative in virtually all cases reported to date. The polyp measures from 1.5 to 4 cm in diameter. Microscopically, the surface squamous mucosa is associated with focal projections of squamous nests and duct-like structures into and between spindle cell stromal nodules (Fig. 17A–C). The stroma between the nodules is less cellular than the more densely cellular pattern centrally.

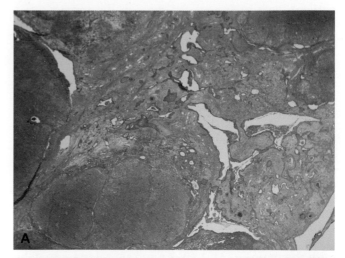

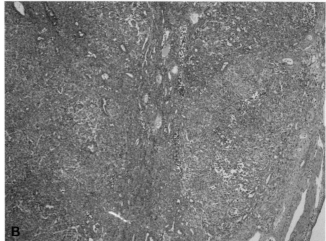

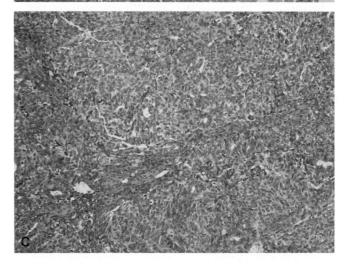

Figure 17 Salivary gland anlage tumor presents as a solitary, midline polyp of the nasaopharynx in a neonate with respiratory distress. (**A**) The low magnification appearance is that of a multiple solid nodules separated by a less-cellular stroma with a network of branching ducts and cysts. (**B**) The nodules are composed predominately of uncommitted mesenchyme and scattered small duct-like or glandular structures. (**C**) Despite the hypercellular appearance of the nodules, the spindled to ovoid cells have uniform nuclei and only occasional mitotic figures. These stromal cells are immunopositive for smooth muscle actin.

Duct-like structures and squamous nests with or without keratinization are more prominent toward the periphery of the more cellular stroma nodules. These lesions can undergo extensive hemorrhagic necrosis likely on the basis of torsion. The stromal cells have ultrastructural and immunophenotypic features of myoepithelial cells (143). Given the midline location, we favor a hamartoma of minor salivary gland tissue.

Nasal chondromesenchymal hamartoma (NCMH) is a tumefactive, presumably hamartomatous, mesenchymal lesion of the nasal cavity that presents predominantly in the first year of life but with several examples in older children and even the rare adult (147–150). An expansile inhomogeneous mass fills the nasal cavity, deviates the nasal septum, and displaces surrounding bony structures, including the orbit (151,152). These lesions are often excised in a piecemeal fashion, but if there is a substantial chondroid component, the tissue fragments have a glistening myxoid quality. A mixture of mesenchymal elements, including islands of hyaline cartilage and immature bony trabecula in a fibroblastic and histiocytic stroma is present in most cases (148). The cartilage nodules are hypercellular and usually well demarcated from the surrounding stroma (Fig. 18A). The bony trabeculae are irregular in shape and are reminiscent of the islands of woven bone in fibrous dysplasia. The cellularity of the stroma varies from loose myxoid areas to dense fascicles of spindle cells and the formation of storiform profiles (Fig. 18B). The spindle cells may merge with areas of polygonal histiocytic aggregates and osteoclast-like cells. Areas rich in thick-walled vessels are also seen. Cystic degeneration and aneurysmal bone cyst-like foci with blood-filled cysts are other features (153). Mitotic activity may be observed, but no atypical mitoses are found. The NCMH has been so designated because of its resemblance to the chest wall hamartoma, also presenting in infancy. We have seen two cases of NCMH in children with pleuropulmonary blastoma. Complete resection is the treatment of choice, but the NCMH can be a surgical challenge. Most NCMHs do not recur even though the resection is incomplete, but we have seen exceptions.

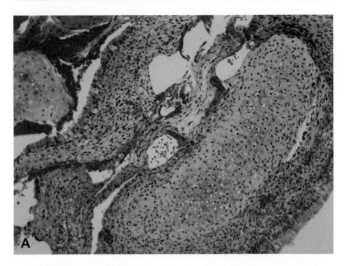

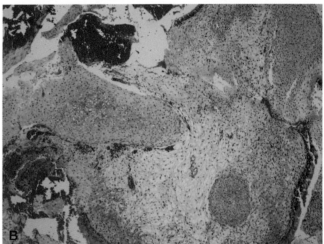

Figure 18 Nasal chondromesenchymal hamartoma presented as an expansile intranasal mass in an infant younger than one year. (**A**) The nodules of cartilage have an immature appearance in the infants, whereas the cartilage acquires a more mature character in somewhat older children. Note the spindle cell stroma around the nodule in the foreground. (**B**) A loose, spongy stroma is seen in the background. Blood-filled spaces may be lined by osteoclast-like giant cells resembling an aneurysmal bone cyst.

IV. SOFT TISSUES

Soft tissues are not precisely defined, but in terms of tissue types include the supporting, mainly mesenchymal tissues such as fibrous connective tissue, vascular structures, nerves, and adipose tissue. On the other hand, a "soft tissue" tumor in the head and neck of a child may not represent a conventional soft tissue neoplasm, and if so, it may involve one of the several organs in this anatomic region. In some cases, the soft tissue mass is a lymph node or a dense fibroinflammatory tumefactive process. When the pathologist receives a specimen from the head and neck region of a child that is "labeled as a soft tissue tumor or rule out as a soft tissue tumor," there are numerous diagnostic possibilities. The more superficial lesions arising in the skin and subcutaneous tissues are more likely to be benign, whereas the deeper "tumors" are usually more worrisome for a malignant neoplasm. Because of the intimacy of the soft tissue to the osseous anatomy in the head and neck region, the particular tumor may have its origin in the underlying bone as in the case of the melanotic neuroectodermal tumor of infancy or Langerhans cell histiocytosis (LCH).

A. Developmental Cysts of the Neck

Branchial cleft cyst and sinus and thyroglossal duct cyst (TGDC) are the two most common maldevelopmental entities presenting as a lateral or midline soft tissue mass in the neck of a child (3,154–156). Both

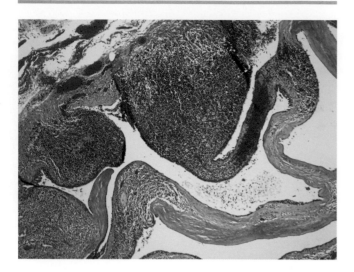

Figure 19 Branchial cleft cyst is typically lined by a squamous mucosa more often than respiratory epithelium. Subepithelial lymphoid aggregates are not present in all cases.

lesions share a common pathogenesis in that they represent the persistence of an embryonic remnant but differ in their respective histogenesis. Both types of cysts occur with an equal frequency in childhood, whereas a branchial cleft cyst is more likely to be seen in an adult.

Branchial cleft cyst is thought to be derived from the second branchial apparatus in the region of the bifurcation of the carotid artery; the second branchial apparatus accounts for 75% or more of all branchial anomalies (3,157–159) The cyst may measure up to 10 cm in greatest dimension, but most are smaller. If the cyst has ruptured or is infected, the surrounding soft tissues may be densely fibrotic, and the cyst itself may be obscured or obliterated by the fibroinflammatory reaction. A smooth-walled cyst with mucoid or watery contents is the appearance of an uncomplicated cyst. Either a nonkeratinizing squamous or a ciliated columnar respiratory-type epithelium lines the cyst. Scattered lymphoid aggregates are typically located immediately beneath the epithelium, but the lymphoid aggregates may vary from a few to many (Fig. 19). The germinal centers may be quite prominent. If the cyst is or has been infected in the past, the surrounding soft tissues may be inflamed with a prominent fibrohistiocytic reaction to raise concern about a neoplastic process. The inflammation and fibrosis may reposition the cyst more toward the midline with the clinical impression of a TGDC. If a mucinous type epithelium is encountered in a cystic lesion from the neck, which also has a bland squamous component, it is necessary to consider the possibility of a low-grade mucoepidermoid carcinoma (MEC). The less common first branchial cleft anomaly presents around the ear as a "skin tag," cyst or sinus and is lined by squamous epithelium without supporting adnexal structures, unlike the dermoid cyst (160,161). A nodule of cartilage in a presumed skin tag

in the preauricular region is the characteristic microscopic feature of the accessory tragus, a first branchial arch anomaly. The latter anomaly is seen in 2 per 1000 individuals and is bilateral in 5% to 6% of cases. A nodule of elastic cartilage is situated beneath immature vellus hair follicles. Anomalies of the third and fourth branchial clefts are rare but, importantly, may have remnants of parathyroid or thymus since these tissues are derived from the third and fourth branchial pouches. Heterotopic thymus in the neck of a child is often mistaken for an enlarged lymph node. The histologic features of normal thymus are seen. Fistula and sinus tracts in the neck are other manifestations of branchial anomalies, which are important from the surgical perspective. Other lymphoid associated epithelial cysts are the lymphoepithelial cyst and thymic cyst (162–164).

Thyroglossal duct cyst (TGDC) is a midline anomaly representing remnants of the diverticulum that forms from the embryonic foramen cecum. The embryonic tract is characterized by the presence of cystic epithelial-lined remnants and heterotopic thyroid tissue (165,166). Some surveys of head and neck surgery in children have reported that the Sistrunk and other like surgical procedures for branchial cleft cysts are the most common surgical procedures performed in children (167). Approximately 60% to 70% of congenital cysts of the neck are TGDCs (168,169). It has been estimated that 5% to 7% of the population have a TGDC. In addition to an anterior neck mass, signs of an infection or an inflammatory process may present as well (170). With inflammation and its attendant fibrosis, it can be difficult to document a TGDC pathologically as such in some cases. The TGDC is rarely a continuous tract from the base of the tongue with occasional exception, but is more often a dominant cyst with or without smaller cysts that are identified microscopically. The hyoid bone is part of the surgical specimen and should be examined for microscopic remnants of the cyst within the bone or immediately adjacent to it (171). Most cysts are positioned inferiorly to the hyoid bone. A dominant cyst can measure up to 4 cm in diameter, and the contents are either mucoid or mucopurulent. Grossly visible thyroid tissue is infrequently identified. If the lining of the cyst(s) has an irregular appearance and small excrescences, this finding may represent the effects of inflammation or, rarely, (1% of cases) a papillary thyroid carcinoma (PTC) (172). Columnar to stratified cuboidal epithelium with or without ciliated borders or squamous mucosa is present microscopically (Fig. 20). Subepithelial lymphocytes in some cases resemble the branchial cleft cyst. Individual thyroid follicles or small groups of follicles are found in up to 20% to 25% of cases, and if not found, there is always the alternative to return to the gross room for more sections (Fig. 21A, B). In some cases, it may be difficult to determine pathologically whether a particular cyst is TGDC or branchial cleft cyst, in which case, we will approach it as a "developmental cyst" with a comment.

Salivary gland heterotopias are found in the soft tissues at the base of the neck, in the tonsil, parathyroid,

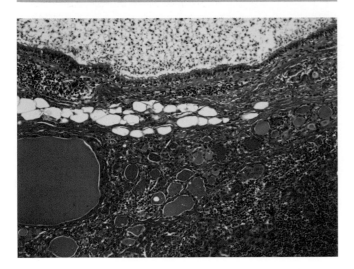

Figure 20 Thyroglossal duct cyst is shown here with a ciliated columnar-lined cyst and thyroid follicles in the wall with focal chronic inflammation.

and middle ear and in an association with thymic cysts (173–178) (Fig. 22).

B. Lymph Nodes

Inflammatory and Infectious Diseases

Lymph node(s) is a relatively common specimen from a child presenting as a "lump and bump" in the neck, usually in the anterior cervical chain. The lymph node enlargement has either developed over a relatively brief period of time or has persisted beyond the period of anticipated resolution (179). Srouji and associates (180) have discussed an approach to the child with cervical lymphadenopathy, as defined as a lymph node(s) in excess of 1 cm in diameter, in order to avoid unnecessary biopsies. In selected cases, there is the option of fine needle aspiration biopsy.

The overwhelming majority of lymph node biopsies show follicular hyperplasia of primary and secondary follicles whose features do not suggest a specific etiology, although a substantial proportion of these cases are thought to have a viral etiology (181–183). If there is evidence of acute inflammation or suppuration, then *Staphylococcus aureus* should be suspected. Suppurative granulomas with a pigmented histiocyic infiltrate are features of chronic granulomatous disease (CGD) of childhood (184,185). Chronic draining abscesses in and around the head and neck region in a child should suggest CGD or one of the other primary phagocytic disorders.

Necrotizing or nonnecrotizing granulomas may indicate the presence of a mycobacterial or Bartonella (cat scratch disease) infection, both of which are seen with some frequency in children. Unlike the transient lymphadenopathy of a self-limited infection, nontuberculous mycobacteriosis and bartonellosis tend to persist rather than to undergo resolution (186,187).

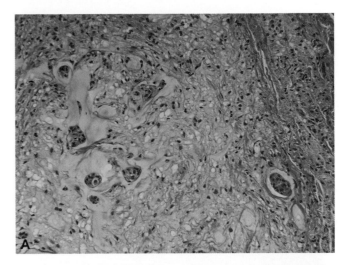

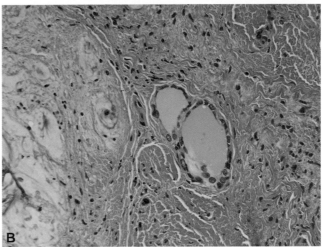

Figure 21 Thyroglossal duct cyst can be a difficult diagnosis to establish pathologically because of secondary changes related to disruption of small cysts and the focality and paucity of thyroid remnants. (**A**) The mucoid contents of the cysts can dissect into the surrounding soft tissues with small epithelial remnants whose features are similar to a ranula. (**B**) A thorough microscopic examination of the tissues may be rewarded with identification of isolated thyroid follicles.

Children aged between two and five years with chronic lymphadenitis in the cervicofacial region may have associated inflammatory changes in the overlying skin with breakdown of the skin. Microscopically, well-formed granulomas or a more diffuse granulomatous inflammatory reaction are the expected microscopic findings. Classic caseous necrosis should cause concern about *Mycobacteria tuberculosis* (188). Acid-fast bacilli (AFB) are difficult to identify in most cases of *Mycobacterium avium, scrofulaceum,* and *intracellulare* in our experience as well as that of Panesar and associates (189). Only 25% to 30% of cases have positive AFB stains. Unlike atypical mycobacteriosis, the granulomatous lymphadenitis in bartonellosis is characterized by microabscesses as early nodal

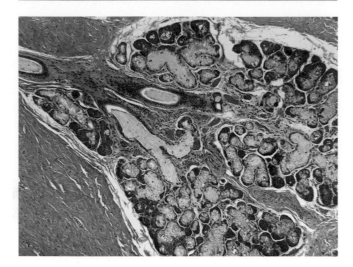

Figure 22 Salivary gland heterotopia shows the formation of diminutive lobulated seromucinous glands with mucin-filled ducts, which are surrounded by dense fibrous tissue from the base of the neck.

changes followed by a coalescence of the abscesses to form necrotizing or suppurative, palisading granulomas surrounded by a mantle of histiocytes and only a few multinucleated giant cells if any. The granulomas also have a gyriform geographic border. Other features include reactive follicular hyperplasia and expansion of the monocytoid B-cell population as sinusoidal collections of pale-staining intermediate-sized lymphocytes. The causative organism in the majority of cases is a diminutive gram-negative bacillus, *Bartonella henselae*, which is transmitted via kittens through a skin scratch or incidental handling, with the development of an erythematous papule or nodule followed by regional lymphadenopathy two to three weeks after the appearance of the cutaneous lesion (190) (Fig. 23A, B). We have found silver stains for the identification of organisms problematic, but Cheuk and associates (191) have successfully identified organisms by immunohistochemistry in the necrotic areas where they are often clumped. Nonnecrotizing or "naked" granulomas are the hallmark of *sarcoidosis*, which is relatively uncommon in childhood, but mediastinal and peripheral lymphadenopathy including cervical lymph node enlargement is seen in 30% to 40% of children older than 10 years (192,193). *Toxoplasma* lymphadenitis presents as cervical lymphadenopathy in adolescence and into early adulthood. The microscopic triad in the lymph node is follicular hyperplasia, sinusoidal monocytoid B-cell proliferation, and small parafollicular epithelioid granulomas (194). Necrotizing changes in a lymph node with neutrophilia and leukocytoclasis should suggest an infectious process or, in the presence of a histiocytic reaction and fibrinoid necrosis, should raise the possibility of *Kikuchi histiocytic necrotizing lymphadenitis* (195). The latter disorder presents in late adolescence or early adulthood with cervical lymphadenopathy

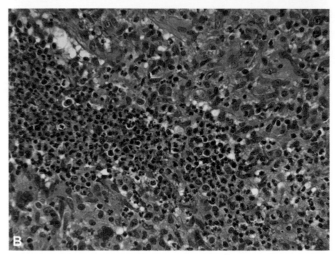

Figure 23 Necrotizing granulomatous lymphadenitis is present in this cervical lymph node of a five-year-old male with a suspected abscess in the neck. Molecular studies demonstrated the presence of *Bartonella henselae*, a gram-negative coccobacillus. (**A**) A low-magnification view demonstrates one of multiple pyogranulomas or septic granulomas with the characteristic stellate configuration. (**B**) The granuloma is characterized by the presence of neutrophils forming a central microabscess, which is surrounded by a palisaded array of histiocytes. Before the formation of the stellate pyogranulomas, a multifocal neutrophilic lymphadenitis is present, which should suggest the diagnosis.

(Fig. 24A, B). Similar reaction in the lymph node is seen in the setting of lupus erythematosus.

Neoplastic Diseases

As many as 10% or less in the more general experience of cervical lymph node biopsies in children harbor a malignant process, and the majority of these cases are non-Hodgkin lymphoma (NHL) or Hodgkin lymphoma (HL), accounting for 70% to 90% of all malignant diagnoses. There is some geographic and institutional variation in the distribution of lymphomatous

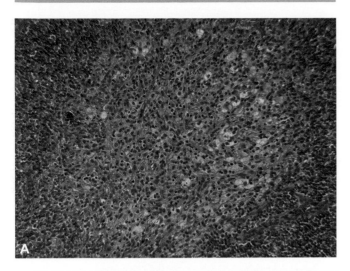

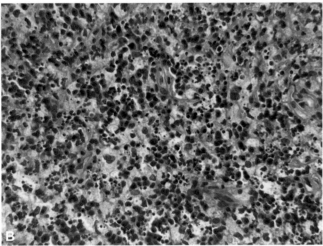

Figure 24 Histiocytic necrotizing lymphadenitis (Kikuchi-Fujimoto disease) presented with cervical lymphadenopathy in a 13-year-old female with neutropenia. (**A**) Multiple foci of histiocytes are scattered throughout the lymph node with a paracortical-interfollicular pattern of distribution. (**B**) The individual focus is characterized by larger, pale staining histiocytes in a background of karyorrhectic debris.

subtypes in cervical lymph node biopsies. The three principal subtypes in our experience are HL of the nodular sclerosis type, Burkitt lymphoma, and anaplastic large cell lymphoma (ALCL). One of the more common presentations of HL is cervical adenopathy, whereas NHL is as likely to appear in an extranodal site in the head and neck region in childhood (188,196,197). Burkitt lymphoma has a predilection for the mandible and maxilla (188,196,197). Precursor B-cell lymphoma and ALCL are known to occur in both nodal and extranodal sites (196). Nested and/or syncytial patterns in ALCL may suggest an epithelial malignancy. Extranodal marginal zone lymphoma is rare in children, but is reported in the parotid, or minor salivary gland tissue (198–200). The latter B-cell lymphoma is recognized in HIV/AIDS-infected children (201). Other detected malignancies are mainly

metastatic in nature with PTC, medullary thyroid carcinoma (MTC), and nasopharyngeal carcinoma (NPC) in descending order of frequency. Our institutional bias accounts for a number of cases of MTC in children with MEN types 2A and 2B. When nodal metastasis is found in a child who has undergone a prophylactic thyroidectomy for MTC, the disease is commonly microscopic and confined to the subcapsular sinuses. An undetected case of MTC in an older child may initially present with cervical lymph node metastasis (Fig. 25A–D). Cervical lymph node enlargement with bulky metastatic carcinoma is the most common clinical presentation of undifferentiated nasopharyngeal, nonkeratinizing carcinoma (so-called lymphoepithelioma) in children who are adolescents in most cases (202,203). A diffuse pattern (so-called Schmincke type) of nodal involvement with a background of lymphocytes and eosinophils may simulate Hodgkin or large cell lymphoma, whereas the more common nested or sheetlike pattern (so-called Regaud type) has the unmistakable features of a poorly differentiated carcinoma (Fig. 26A–C). Epstein–Barr virus (EBV) genome is detectable by in situ hybridization in a substantial proportion of pediatric NPCs, which vary from 80% to 100% (Fig. 26D). In fact, EBV is involved in the etiology of several lymphoid processes with head and neck manifestations in children, including Burkitt lymphoma, HL, and infectious mononucleosis. Florid interfollicular immunoblastic proliferation, follicular hyperplasia, and progressive transformation of germinal centers can simulate a malignant lymphoproliferative process (204–206). Neuroblastoma, embryonal and alveolar RMS, and granulocytic sarcoma (acute myeloid leukemia, M1, M5, and M7) are other malignancies that can present with nodal involvement in the neck as an initial manifestation of disease.

C. Soft Tissue Tumors

Soft tissue neoplasms and other nonneoplastic tumors of virtually all types are known to occur in the head and neck region of children and adolescents, but our attention is directed to those more common tumors, including vascular, fibroblastic-myofibroblastic, and myogenic neoplasms that in aggregate account for over 50% of all soft tissue tumors in children, and in each of these pathologic types, there is a predilection for the head and neck region.

Vascular neoplasms and other vascular tumefactions alone constitute 30% of all soft tumors in children where the skin, subcutis, deep soft tissues, including the orbit, sinonasal tract, and salivary gland, as in the case of infantile hemangioma-hemangioendothelioma of the parotid gland in the infant (see section "Salivary Gland"), are the various sites of presentation (207–214). There is a great deal of interest in the vascular biology as it relates to vasoproliferative lesions in children, since it is not always clear morphologically whether a particular vascular lesion is a neoplasm or a malformation (207–209,215–219). *Hemangiomas* are the most common type of soft tissue tumor of infancy, and over 50% of all cases present in the head and neck or cervicofacial region. These tumors are known for their rapid

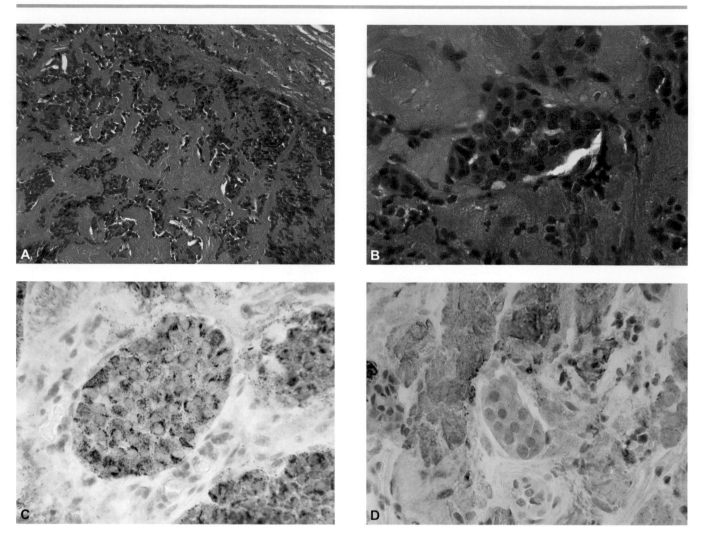

Figure 25 Medullary thyroid carcinoma in a nine-year-old female presented with cervical lymphadenopathy. (**A**) The entire lymph node is replaced by small rounded nests and elongated trabecular profiles of uniform, cohesive tumor cells. The amyloid stroma is prominent throughout the lymph node. (**B**) The individual nests are composed of uniform tumor cells with finely granular cytoplasm. (**C**) The tumor cells show finely granular cytoplasmic immunopositivity for chromogranin. (**D**) The immunostain for calcitonin is also positive.

proliferative phase followed by a longer period of resolution. The gross dimensions vary considerably from a few millimeters to several centimeters, and in the latter case, the clinical features are disconcerting at the least and alarming in the extreme. The tumors can involve all tissue layers from the dermis into the deep soft tissues. Some tumors have a less-obvious dermal component but are mainly in the deep tissues of the tongue or within the skeletal muscle (so-called skeletal muscle hemangioma). The pattern of growth may be exquisitely lobular or more often multilobular; the cellular lobules are composed of barely perceptible vascular spaces with interposed stromal cells giving these lesions a hypercellular appearance (Fig. 27). Mitotic figures are found without difficulty in these lesions during the proliferative phase whose presence should not be viewed with concern. Other capillary-sized vascular spaces may trail off into the surrounding soft tissues with the loss of apparent circumscription.

Extension into and around small nerves, replacement of subcutaneous fat, and involvement of small lymph nodes are some of the other microscopic findings. It is the nature of the capillary hemangioma to superimpose its growth on existing microanatomy such as the lobules of subcutaneous fat or the acinar-lobular architecture of the parotid gland. Growth on existing anatomy by a capillary hemangioma is seen also in the orbit, where the latter is the most common tumor of the orbit in childhood, usually presenting in the first three years of life (220,221). Lobular capillary hemangioma (so-called pyogenic granuloma) is a common vascular neoplasm presenting as a raised, erythematous cutaneous nodule with or without surface ulceration. This lesion may evolve over a period of a few weeks and, in a minority of cases, may present as multiple lesions. Periorbital skin, anterior nasal cavity, and oral mucous membranes are other sites of predilection for the LCH in the head and neck region. These

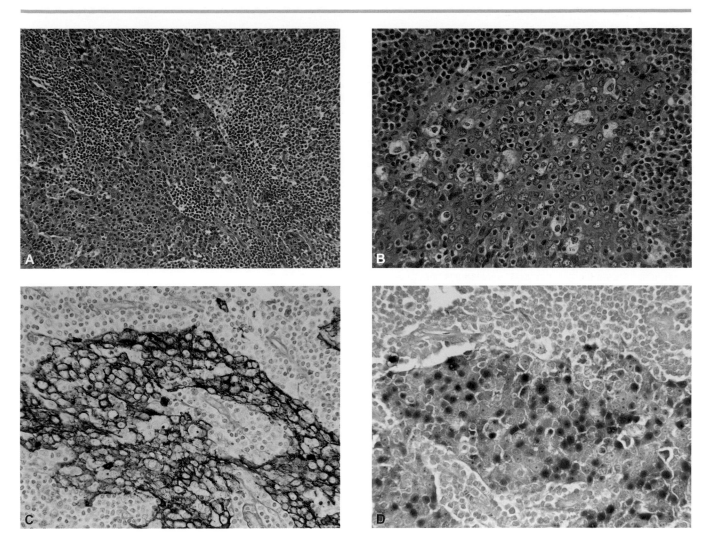

Figure 26 Undifferentiated nasopharyngeal nonkeratinizing carcinoma presented as a right neck mass in a 14-year-old male. **(A)** Irregular profiles of poorly differentiated carcinoma have replaced a substantial portion of the cervical lymph node. **(B)** The tumor cells have a syncytial-like growth pattern with poorly defined cell borders. Large, vesicular nuclei with a prominent central nucleolus are distinctive cytomorphological features. Note the intermingling of small lymphocytes within the nests of tumor. **(C)** Cytokeratin immunostain shows strong cytoplasmic positivity. **(D)** In situ hybridization for EBER demonstrates strong nuclear reactivity. *Abbreviation*: EBER, Epstein–Barr virus–encoded RNA

lesions measure less than 1 cm in most cases and have a characteristic multilobular pattern consisting of capillary-sized vessels with a large "feeder" vessel at the base of the polyp. When the epidermis is ulcerated, the surface has the features of granulation tissue with an inflammatory response. There is some microscopic resemblance between the LCH and bacillary angiomatosis, which is another manifestation of *B. henselae* in an immunocompromised patient, including children (222). *Kaposiform hemangioendothelioma* and the somewhat similar-appearing tufted angioma can present in the head and neck region (223) (Fig. 28A, B). These tumors, regardless of the presenting site, may be responsible for the Kasabach–Merritt syndrome (224–228). *Epithelioid hemangioma* also occurs in the head and neck region of children with a predilection for the lip, tongue, and nasal cavity (229) (Fig. 29). *Papillary endothelial hyperplasia* (Masson vegetant

hemangioma) is a well-described endothelial proliferation, which is either intra- or extravascular in location and represents the formation of endothelial papillary fronds in a thrombohematoma, which can simulate angiosarcoma. The lip, oral mucous membranes, and paranasal sinuses are some of the more common sites in the head and neck in children as well as adults (230–234).

Cystic hygroma-lymphangioma and cystic hygroma colli are distinct clinical and possibly pathologic entities. Despite their differences, both lesions are more likely malformations than true neoplasms. Cystic hygroma colli is congenital in its presentation as an abnormality that is most commonly detected on fetal ultrasonography and may indicate the presence of one of several chromosomal anomalies with the monosomy X or Turner syndrome as the archetype (235,236). Hydrops fetalis may be present as well

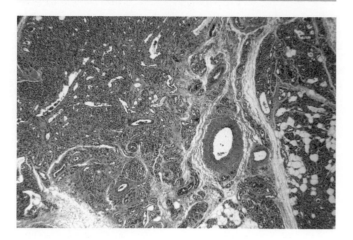

Figure 27 Capillary hemangioma in the soft tissues of the neck of an infant shows the characteristic multilobular pattern, which should suggest the diagnosis on low magnification.

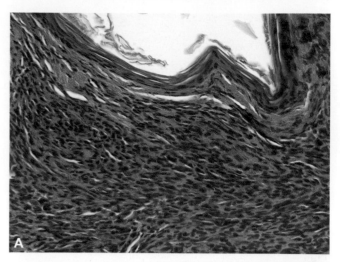

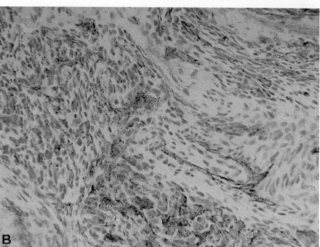

Figure 28 Kaposiform hemangioendothelioma presented as a locally destructive lesion in the middle ear of a one-year-old male. (**A**) Lobules of densely arranged spindle cells with slit-like spaces are present in association with keratinizing squamous epithelium of a secondary cholesteatoma. (**B**) Immunohisto-chemical staining for CD34 shows a diffuse, irregular pattern of positivity associated with the slit-like vascular spaces.

(237–239). The other cystic hygroma or true lymphangioma presents in the cervicofacial region as a unilateral mass (2,8,155). Most lesions present in infancy or early childhood and represent the most common or one of the most common soft tissue tumors in this anatomic region (240,241). Extensive regional involvement occurs in a minority of cases by a network of collapsible, thin-walled vascular channels throughout the soft tissues and even dissecting into and around the parotid and submandibular glands. The vascular spaces extend through tissue planes and along the stromal septa separating the lobules of fat. The multicystic spaces are either empty of contents or contain a watery, eosinophilic coagulum with or without accompanying lymphocytes. Occasional nodules of lymphocytes may be located beneath the endothelial lining in some but not all cases. Those cystic hygromas located above the hyoid bone have a local recurrence rate of 50% or greater (242). The histologic features of the recurrence often bear little resemblance to the original cystic hygroma because of the marked fibroblastic and myofibroblastic reaction that can impart a fibromatosis or myofibromatosis-like appearance except for the irregular empty vascular spaces in the background. More limited lymphangiomas may occur in the skin or the oral cavity.

Fibroblastic-myofibroblastic tumors with a predilection to the head and neck in children are the infantile myofibromatosis-myofibroma and nodular fasciitis to include the related cranial fasciitis and fibromatosis colli (243–246). Approximately 25% of fibrous tumors in children present in this anatomic region. Myofibromatosis-myofibroma occurs in a multiplicity of sites, including the scalp, face, oral cavity, and within the bone of the skull, nasal cavity, and orbit (51,247–253). The affected child is typically younger than two years, but may be older. Multifocal lesions are seen in a minority of infants with dermal and/or subcutaneous nodules as well as

circumscribed, osteolytic defects in the skull or elsewhere (254,255). Microscopically, the dermal component consists of multiple fibrohyaline or fibromyxoid nodules of plump fibroblasts separated to some extent by the stroma (Fig. 30). Small peripheral nodules with compressed, lunate vascular spaces are a useful finding in the diagnosis and reflect the suspected angiocentric origin of the myofibroma. Degenerative changes with apoptotic bodies, necrosis, and dystrophic calcifications are other changes that may be seen in one or more nodules. Another pattern is composed of spindle cells with or without a resemblance to a hemangiopericytoma; these combined patterns have resulted in the diagnostic designation of myopericytoma. So-called congenital hemangiopericytoma is considered part of the morphologic and biologic

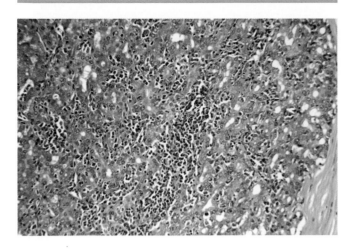

Figure 29 Epithelioid hemangioma presented in the dermis and soft tissues of the temporal region in a 12-year-old female. The multinodular neoplasm is composed of compactly arranged vessels formed by plump epithelioid-appearing endothelial cells. Eosinophils and lymphocytes are present in the background.

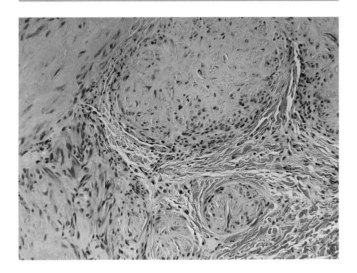

Figure 30 Infantile myofibroma (myofibromatosis) presented as a dermal-subcutaneous mass in the temporal region of a six-month-old male. Multiple circumscribed fibromyxoid nodules are separated by dermal collagen. The periphery of the individual nodules are often more cellular and are associated with a clefted vascular space.

spectrum of infantile myofibromatosis and has a preference for the head and neck region. Immunohistochemically, myofibromatosis is diffusely reactive for smooth muscle actin and vimentin but stains poorly for desmin and muscle-specific actin (HHF-35). Hemangiopericytoma-like foci are usually reactive for CD34, but less so for smooth muscle actin. *Nodular fasciitis* in children presents most often in the head and neck region, representing almost 40% to 60% of cases in our experience and others (245,256). The periorbital soft

tissues, orbit, periauricular region, oral cavity, and nose are the various reported sites in children (257–261). The microscopic features are similar regardless of age, but that does not diminish concern about a possible sarcoma in the presence of mitotic activity that is not subtle and a population of spindle cells in a loosely textured, myxoid background. The presence of scattered inflammatory cells, mucoid-filled microcysts and extravasated red cells are the critical features in the recognition of nodular fasciitis and the related cranial fasciitis. *Cranial fasciitis* occurs in infants and young children as a rapid-enlarging mass that can compress and erode the underlying calvarial bone and may have a predominant intracranial component (262–267) (Fig. 31A). These lesions are more uniformly myxoid than nodular fasciitis (Fig. 31B). *Fibromatosis colli* (sternomastoid tumor) presents in the lower

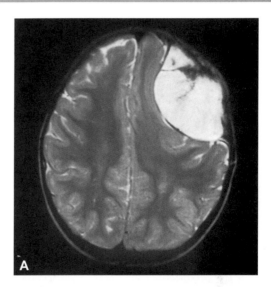

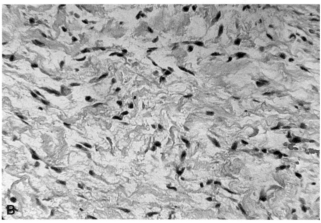

Figure 31 Cranial fasciitis is thought to be a reactive rather than a neoplastic proliferation of myofibroblasts typically presenting in early childhood as in this case. (**A**) The CT scan shows a large soft tissue mass pushing into the brain through a defect in the skull. (**B**) A bland proliferation of fibroblasts and/or myofibroblasts has a pale-staining myxofibrous appearance that seems to belie the gross characteristics of this mass.

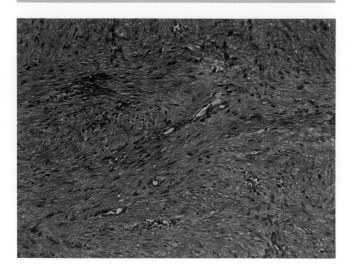

Figure 32 Infantile fibromatosis of the desmoid type presented as a soft tissue mass in the mandibular region of a two-year-old male. A uniformly dispersed proliferation of bland fibroblasts are arranged in short fascicles.

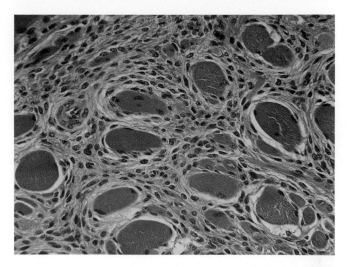

Figure 33 Infantile fibromatosis of the diffuse type presented in the tongue of a one-year-old female. Uniform spindle cells infiltrate into and through the normal skeletal muscle. These cells have somewhat immature features but are quite innocuous and generally lack mitotic activity. The characterization of "diffuse" is apparent from the growth pattern.

one-third of the sternocleidomastosid muscle in an infant who is six months or younger (268–270). Most of these lesions undergo spontaneous regression. When biopsied or excised, the fibrous nodule has largely replaced the skeletal muscle with isolated bundles of muscle separated by a variably cellular and collagenized process with features most like a desmoid fibromatosis when the histology is dominated by dense fibrous tissue. The earlier stage is considerably more cellular and vascularized and can resemble nodular fasciitis. If a presumed fibromatosis colli does not undergo spontaneous remission or recurs after resection, then an *infantile fibromatosis* with desmoid features becomes the more plausible diagnosis (Fig. 32). Another type of infantile fibromatosis is the so-called diffuse type, which is considerably more cellular and infiltrative. One of its favored sites is the head and neck and in particular the tongue (Fig. 33). JHF, an autosomal recessive disorder, is characterized by the development of firm, pearly papulonodular lesions in the skinand the head and neck region, including the scalp and gingival (75). Osteolytic lesions in the calvarium resemble those that are seen in infantile myofibromatosis. Both JHF and infantile systemic hyalinosis have mutations of the CMG-2 on chromosome 4q12 (Table 1). The histologic hallmark is the dense, hypocellular collagen with scattered rounded stromal cells in lacunar-like spaces and more spindled fibroblasts. These round cells have the phenotype of histiocytes. It is the hyalinized collagen that distinguishes JHF from the other fibrous tumors of childhood (Fig. 8). Infantile systemic hyalinosis has a microscopic resemblance of infantile myofibromatosis with its myxohyaline stroma. *Juvenile nasopharyngeal angiofibroma* (JNA) is classified with the fibrous tumors, but is unique in several respects from the other tumor types in this category in terms of specific localization, overwhelming male predilection, and age at presentation between 7 and 20 years, but mostly between 14 and 18 years (271). Like the desmoid fibromatosis, these tumors are highly aggressive locally (272). The tumor may arise in the region of the pterygopalatine fossa but presents in the nasopharynx on the posterior lateral wall. Pushing margins characterize the JNA (Fig. 34A). A bland fibrous stroma with uniformly distributed fibroblasts contain thin-walled vascular spaces that vary in shape and size and are more or less uniformly distributed throughout the stroma (273) (Fig. 34B). Malignant transformation is rare. Mutations in the β-catenin gene have been detected in JNAs, which is the molecular linkage between these tumors and desmoids and familial adenomatous polyposis (274–278). *Desmoid fibromatosis* is uncommon in the head and neck, but is well documented in the lower neck and supraclavicular region (279,280). Adolescents and young adults are affected more often than young children. These highly infiltrative neoplasms are composed of benign-appearing fibroblasts. The osseous counterpart is the desmoplastic fibroma with its predilection for the mandible.

Synovial sarcoma presents in the head, mainly in the neck in 5% of all cases, and is well documented in pediatric series (281–284). Both monophasic and biphasic patterns are recognized so that the differential diagnosis must include spindle cell RMS, leiomyosarcoma, malignant peripheral nerve sheath tumor, and the spindle epithelial tumor with thymus-like differentiation (285–290). A combination of immunohistochemistry and molecular genetic analysis may be necessary in some cases to establish the specific tumor type.

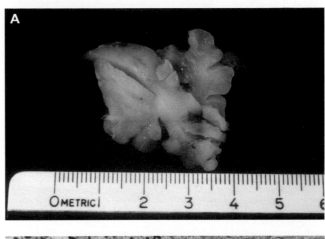

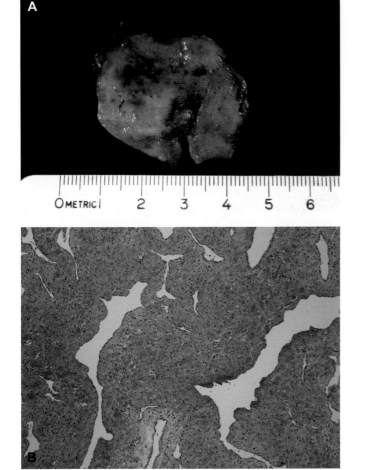

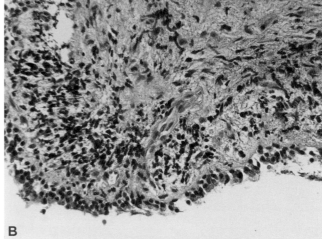

Figure 34 Juvenile nasopharyngeal angiofibroma presents in adolescent males with potentially life-threatening epistaxis. (**A**) A firm fibrous mass has a more homogenous cut surface than the usually trabeculated appearance of the desmoid fibromatosis. Vascular spaces can be identified on gross examination. The pushing margins are appreciated at the periphery. (**B**) The pattern of fibroblastic proliferation has a uniformly diffuse appearance with circular and branching thin-walled vascular spaces of varying sizes throughout.

Figure 35 Embryonal rhabdomyosarcoma is a neoplasm with a diversity of gross and microscopic features in terms of pattern and rhabdomyoblastic differentiation. (**A**) The polypoid mass presented in the nasal cavity of a one-year-old male and is an example of the sarcoma botryoides subtype of embryonal rhabdomyosarcoma. (**B**) A cambium layer of primitive small cells beneath a ciliated surface epithelium is seen in this sarcoma botryoides in the middle ear of an infant. There are also interspersed larger tumor cells with bright eosinophilic cytoplasm. When there is necrosis and inflammation, a biopsy of embryonal rhabdomyosarcoma from this site may be a diagnostic challenge.

Congenital-infantile fibrosarcoma with spindle cell features resembling the monophasic synovial sarcoma may rarely occur in the head and neck in children considerable younger than those with synovial sarcoma. A rare tumor presenting in the neck of infants has been reported as a "primitive myxoid mesenchymal tumor" by Alaggio and associates (291).

Myogenic neoplasms of the head and neck are dominated by RMS, which accounts for approximately 20% of all malignancies in this region in children and is only exceeded by HL and non-HL, which together constitute 50% to 55% of all head and neck malignancies in children (2,11,292). Approximately 35% of all RMSs in children present in the head and neck region with the orbit, nasal cavity middle ear/mastoid (Fig. 35A, B), pterogopalatine/infratemporal fossa (Fig. 36A–C), paranasal sinuses, salivary gland, and nasopharynx as the several specific anatomic primary sites (293–298). Embryonal RMS of the favorable sarcoma botryoides and spindle cell types and the intermediate prognosis "not otherwise specified'" type comprises 85% to 90% of all cases of RMS in the head and neck. Alveolar RMS is seen infrequently in the head and neck, and those that we have personally encountered have presented in young children in sites such as the periorbital soft tissues and in and around the paranasal sinuses. Cervical lymph node metastasis of alveolar RMS is found in those children with widespread disease (stage IV) at presentation. *Fetal rhabdomyoma*, arguably

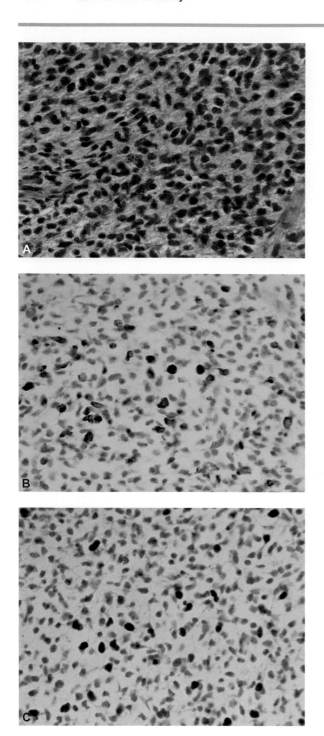

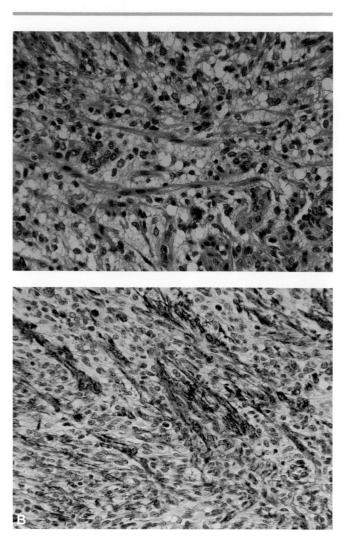

Figure 37 Fetal rhabdomyoma presented in the postauricular region of a two-year-old male. (**A**) The myxoid subtype is characterized by immature myotubes interspersed in a more or less regular pattern among immmature myoblasts, which themselves lack nuclear hyperchromatism, cellular pleomorphism, and mitotic figures to be found in an embryonal rhabdomyosarcoma. (**B**) The muscle-specific actin (HHF-35) immunostain demonstrates the histological pattern to better advantage than routine histology.

Figure 36 Embryonal rhabdomyosarcoma presented in the pterygoid fossa-base of skull in a three-year-old male. (**A**) The biopsy shows a primitive-appearing small cell neoplasm with considerable variation in cellular contours with a mixture of rounded to ovoid to spindle-shaped cells. Some of the latter cells have delicate threads of eosinophilic cytoplasm. The pale-staining myxoid to mucoid background is a feature of many embryonal rhabdomyosarcomas whose presence is helpful when one is considering the diagnosis. (**B**) Immunohistochemical staining for muscle-specific actin (HHF-35) shows that only scattered tumor cells are positive, which is often the case in a primitive embryonal rhabdomyosarcoma. (**C**) Only a minority of tumor cells have nuclear immunopositivity for myogenin.

a hamartomatous lesion, is seen in the pre-and post-auricular region in children younger than five years (299). These tumors are located in the superficial soft tissues and are composed of bundles of small immature mesenchymal cells layered between fetal myotubes in the so-called myxoid subtype (Fig. 37). Any mitotic activity should be viewed with concern about the possibility of a well-differentiated embryonal RMS. The cellular subtype has a uniform spindle cell pattern of more mature-appearing myotubes. *Rhabdomyomatous mesenchymal hamartoma* is a dermal and soft tissue lesion, typically presenting in neonates and older children through 15 years of age, as a peduncu-lated or sessile nodule on the nose, chin, eyelid, oral cavity, and neck (300). Bundles of striated skeletal muscle are present among adnexal structures and the subcutis. In several sites in the head and neck, skeletal muscle may be seen normally in the subcutis in a skin biopsy.

Malignant Round Cell Neoplasms

Other soft tissue neoplasms documented in the head and neck of children include a catalog of virtually every known pathologic type and on occasion those individual cases that seemingly defy classification into an established entity and are designated as a "malignant round cell neoplasm" or "undifferentiated sarcoma" (301). Two examples in the latter category in the head and neck of children are now recognized as the malignant rhabdoid tumor (MRT) and Ewing sarcoma–primitive neuroectodermal tumor (EWS-PNET). Desmoplastic small round cell tumor with its own distinctive EWS break apart from EWS-PNET is rarely seen in the head and neck of children (292). Classic NB is more common than EWS-PNET with a primary presentation in the cervical sympathetic chain, comprising 5% of all primary NBs in children, but metastatic NB is seen more commonly with bony lesions in the calvarium and/or mandible-maxilla, orbit, and cervical lymph nodes (302–305) (Fig. 38). Primary NB in the neck occurs in the first year of life for the most part, and the disease is usually localized to the neck. The histology is commonly that of a poorly differentiated NB without stroma and a low mitotic-karyorrhectic index. *Olfactory* NB (esthesioneuroblastoma) has microscopic similarities to the NB of childhood but is a different disease with its predominantly adult presentation, but there is a small age peak in the second decade of life. Overall, only 1% to 5% of cases are diagnosed before the age of 20 years (306,307).

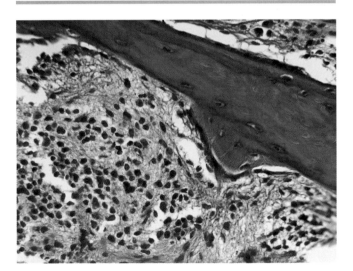

Figure 38 Metastatic neuroblastoma to the skull in a three-year-old male demonstrates a malignant small cell neoplasm, though poorly differentiated in a sense, has a prominent fibrillary network of cytoplasmic processes representing neurite differentiation.

These tumors do not have the molecular or metabolic (elevated urinary catecholamines) markers of childhood NB. Like the classic NB, there is a range in differentiation in terms of rosette formation and neurofibrillary formation. *Malignant ectomesenchymoma* is a rare malignant round cell neoplasm of childhood, which has been reported in the orbit and whose histologic and immunophenotypic features are chimeric with both rhabdomyoblastic and PNET-like features (301). EWS-PNET has been reported in soft tissue, but mainly in bony sites in the cranium and facial bones as young as the neonatal period (308–310). MRT as a primary neoplasm is well established in a number of extrarenal sites, including the head and neck, where it is seen as a soft tissue mass in infancy and even as a congenital neoplasm with widespread disease somewhat reminiscent of stage IV or IVs NB (311–313). The posterior fossa is another well-recognized primary site, where it is known as an *atypical teratoid/rhabdoid tumor*. The possibility of an MRT should be considered in the presence of a highly atypical malignant round cell neoplasm with prominent nucleoli (Fig. 39A–C). Actual rhabdoid cells with eosinophilic filamentous inclusions may not be readily apparent since their numbers seemingly vary in number and prominence from one case to another. However, the vimentin and/or cytokeratin immunostains are often impressive as well as the CD99 positivity and the lack of BAF nuclear-staining reflecting mutations or deletions that inactivate the hSNF5/INI1 gene on chromosome 22q11 (314,315) (Fig. 39D). In addition to the spindle cell RMS, other similar-appearing sarcomas include fibrosarcoma of the adult and congenital-infantile types, synovial sarcoma of the monophasic and poorly differentiated types, and malignant peripheral nerve sheath tumor.

Alveolar soft part sarcoma

This has two sites of predilection in the head and neck of children, the base of the tongue, and orbit (102,316–318). The youngest examples of alveolar soft part sarcoma (ASPS) are those cases in infants with a lingual mass thought to represent a lingual thyroid.

Peripheral Nerve Sheath Tumors

Schwannoma and *plexiform neurofibroma* are seen in children, and as anticipated, the plexiform neurofibroma may be the first clinical sign of neurofibromatosis in an infant with one or more superficial tumors in the neck, eyelid, oral cavity, and salivary gland as examples of the various sites of involvement (319–321) (Fig. 40). The schwannoma is the most common neurogenic neoplasm of childhood, usually occurring in older children or adolescents (322). Sporadic examples of schwannomas have been reported on an individual case basis in a number of sites in the head and neck (323–326) (Fig. 41). When these tumors arise from a peripheral nerve in the neck, the anatomic localization is straightforward, but a schwannoma in the retropharyngeal space or in and around the deeper air passages and spaces can be challenging with the differential diagnosis of the generic spindle cell neoplasm (322). Another important consideration is the

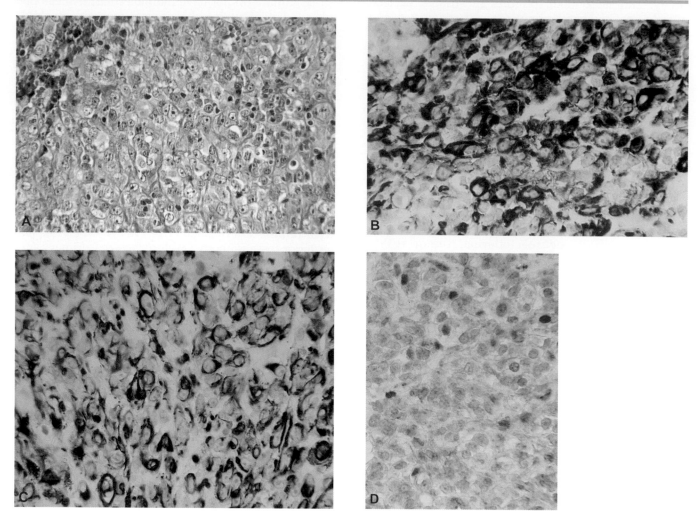

Figure 39 Malignant rhabdoid tumor presented in the floor of the mouth in a two-month-old female. This highly malignant neoplasm of infancy and early childhood occurs most often in the kidney, but is also recognized in a number of extrarenal primary sites including the soft tissues of the head and neck and brain (atypical teratoid/rhabdoid tumor). (**A**) Relative monotonous and cohesive malignant round cells have vesicular nuclei with a prominent central nucleolus. Filamentous inclusions in the cytoplasm may be inconspicuous on routine histology, but immunohistochemical staining for the intermediate filaments, vimentin and cytokeratin, consistently demonstrates their presence. (**B**) Vimentin immunostaining demonstrates numerous intensely positive inclusions. (**C**) Cytokeratin immunostaining also shows the inclusions, but fewer in number than the vimentin in this case (**B**). (**D**) Deletion of the INI1 gene on chromosome 22q11.2 results in the loss of nuclear staining for BAF47, as seen in this case. Positive nuclear staining for BAF47 is present in scattered nonneoplastic cells in the background.

possibility of neurofibromatosis type 2 if there are multiple schwannomas, especially of the VIII cranial nerve (327,328).

Lipomatous Tumors

Lipoblastoma, a lipomatous tumor almost exclusive seen in young children, is uncommon, but observed in the cervical region, parotid gland, as well as the parapharyngeal space (329,330). In a series of 16 cases, 5 (30%) arose in the neck where it can be mistaken clinically for a cystic hygroma (331). Immature multi-vacuolated lipoblasts and myxoid foci have a resemblance to myxoid liposarcoma. Unlike the latter with its

signature t(12;16) (q13;p11) translocation, lipoblastoma has the PLAG1-HAS2 fusion, which involves the chromosomal region 8q11-13 (332).

Germ Cell Neoplasms

Germ cell neoplasms, mainly with the microscopic features of an immature teratoma, are described in a number of sites in the head and neck region and are usually seen in neonates or within the first year of life. Polyhydraminios, fetal hydrops, and discovery of a mass prenatally by fetal ultrasonography are other aspects of these tumors. Approximately 2% to 4% of all germ cell neoplasms in the first two decades of life

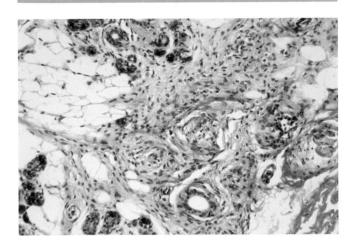

Figure 40 Plexiform neurofibroma with involvement of the parotid gland is seen in a six-year-old female as the presenting manifestation of neurofibromatosis type 1. Neuromatous nodules and spindle cells partially replace the glandular parenchyma and occupy the interstitium.

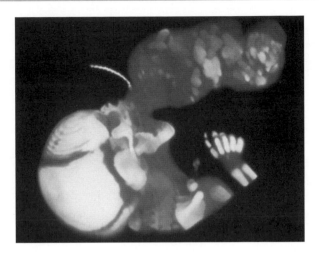

Figure 42 Immature teratoma presented as a mass projecting from the oral cavity of this neonate. The tumor was attached to the posterior nasopharynx.

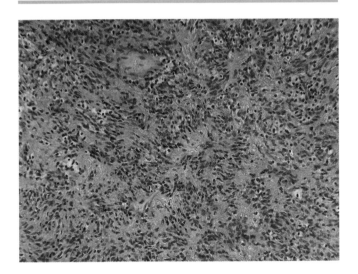

Figure 41 Schwannoma presented in the parapharyngeal space of a 12-year-old male. Numerous palisades of spindle cells are forming Verocay bodies. This tumor was apparently a sporadic occurrence.

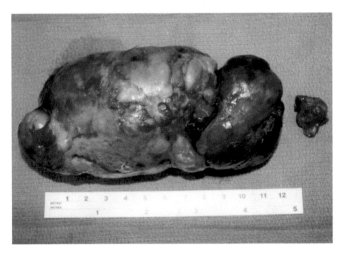

Figure 43 Immature teratoma in this resected specimen measured approximately 13 cm in greatest dimension. The external surface of this mass has a variegated appearance.

present in the head and neck with the exclusion of intracranial germ cell tumors from the latter figure (333–335). The various sites of presentation include the cervical thyroid, orbit, nasopharynx, nasal cavity, and oral cavity (336–343) (Fig. 42). Respiratory distress as a result of airway obstruction is one of the immediate clinical problems. A friable, soft and gelatinous mass measuring 5 to an excess of 10 cm is a typical gross appearance of these neoplasms (Fig. 43). Another relatively constant microscopic finding is the presence of immature somatic tissues, in particular immature neural tubes and sheets of neuroblasts often accompanied by a neuropil in the background (Fig. 44A, B). Cysts are usually lined by immature squamous or enteric-type epithelium. Nodules of immature cartilage, small islands of glandular or acinar tissue of an indeterminant type, and uncommitted mesenchyme complete the varied histologic appearance. Neuroglia and choroid plexus comprise some of the more mature tissue elements. *Endodermal sinus tumor or yolk sac carcinoma* can occur in the setting of immature teratoma or as an exclusive pathologic element (344–346). If small tubular-like profiles in a myxoid or reticulated background are found, these are the features of endodermal sinus tumor (Fig. 45). Thyroid parenchyma is found in a minority

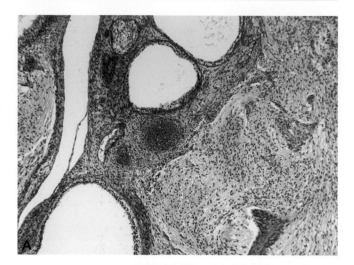

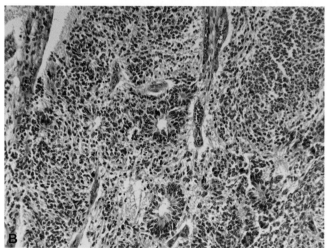

Figure 44 Immature teratoma is characterized by a spectrum of fetal-appearing somatic tissue elements with cystic and solid features. (**A**) Immature neuroglial tissue, cysts lined by bronchoenteric epithelium, nodules of immature cartilage, and a background of spindled mesenchyme represent one of many combinations of fetal-like tissues in these extranodal neoplasms in infants. (**B**) Embryonic neural tubules are often accompanied by neuroblasts. A large portion of an immature teratoma in an infant, whether in the head and neck region as in this case, is often composed of immature somatic tissues, especially neuroepithelial elements, whose presence is not an indication of malignancy. Pathological grading of these neoplasms in infancy is not predictive of outcome.

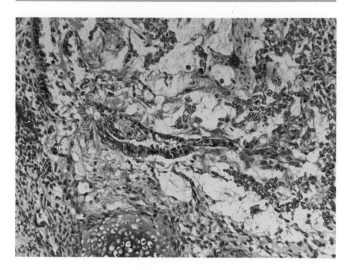

Figure 45 Endodermal sinus tumor (yolk sac carcinoma) is shown in an immature teratoma, which presented as an intranasal mass in a six-month-old male. Tubular profiles and irregular strands of tumor cells are contained within a mucoid background. Teratomatous elements are present at the periphery. The presence of endodermal sinus tumor in a teratoma defines it as a malignant germ cell neoplasm.

of cervical teratomas (347). We have seen several examples of immature and mature teratoma in cervical lymph nodes, which does not appear to alter an otherwise favorable prognosis upon successful surgical resection. The differential diagnosis of teratomas in the head and neck region is complicated by the presence of such lesions as heterotopic brain and developmental cysts with accompanying cartilage or salivary gland tissue. The dilemma is the pathogenetic boundary between a true teratoma and a heterotopia or

choristoma. One example is the case in an infant with an apparent "recurrent nasal glioma," which was reexcised and showed the presence of endodermal sinus tumor, which was inapparent in the original excision. When an immature teratoma recurs locally, mature neuroglia may be the only teratomatous remant (Fig. 46). *Teratocarcinosarcoma* is a rare and unique sinonasal neoplasm with a complex histologic pattern whose varied differentiation of epithelial and mesenchymal

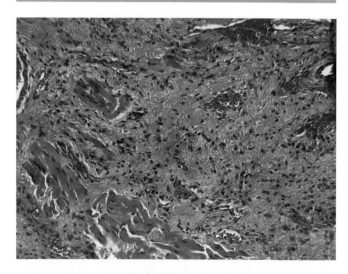

Figure 46 Recurrent teratoma of the neck presented two years after the initial resection. Mature neuroglial tissue is present within sternocleidomastoid muscle.

elements has features resembling a malignant teratoma. Although a neoplasm more common in adult males, it has been reported in childhood (348–350).

D. Tumorlike Lesions of Soft Tissue

Two nonneoplastic processes in the head and neck of children presenting as a soft tissue tumor are the tumefactive fibroinflammatory pseudotumor and deep granuloma annulare.

Tumefactive fibroinflammatory pseudotumor occurs in several extraorbital sites, including the neck, infratemporal or pterygopalatine fossa, buccal soft tissues, and the submandibular gland (351,352). These lesions are differentiated from the inflammatory myofibroblastic tumor and calcifying fibrous pseudotumor. We have seen several examples occurring throughout childhood to include infants younger than one year. In most cases, there is no clear etiology, although those in the neck are preceded by regional lymph node enlargement. Because of concern about a neoplastic process, a biopsy is performed and shows an infiltrate of small lymphocytes, plasma cells, and occasional eosinophils, but acute inflammation is inconspicuous in most cases. Fibrosis varies from case to case as does the intensity of the inflammatory reaction. Cultures are negative for microorganisms.

Deep or subcutaneous granuloma annulare (DSGA, pseudorheumatoid nodule) is an idiopathic process that presents as a solitary or multiple firm subcutaneous nodules with a predilection for the occipital scalp and periorbital region or more frequently on the lower anterior tibia. Infants may be affected, but most lesions develop before the age of 10 years (353–355). There is no consistent male to female preference. A nodule measuring less than 1 cm may or may not be mobile and is not associated with any skin discoloration. Necrobiosis with a palisading mantle of histiocytes is the basic histologic finding, but the latter is not always apparent or recognized upon initial examination. The overall architecture of the DSGA is optimally appreciated at low-power magnification. Several foci of necrobiosis comprise a single nodule, which is centered in the subcutis, and the dermis is usually free of involvement unlike most cases of granuloma annulare with a dermocentric localization (353). As the necrosis undergoes resolution, there is fibrosis surrounded by arcades of small vessels to suggest the possibility of a capillary hemangioma. It is important to include in the report that additional lesions may develop in the same site or elsewhere and are not associated with anything less than a favorable outcome. These children are not at risk by virtue of these lesions for any autoimmune-collagen vascular disease. Another important consideration in the differential diagnosis is epithelioid sarcoma (356,357).

Phakomatous choristoma (Zimmerman tumor) presents as a firm mass, measuring 1 to 1.5 cm in greatest dimension, in the inferonasal aspect of the lower eyelid or anterior orbit in early infancy (358–360). Cords and nests of epithelial cells are embedded in a dense fibrous stroma (Fig. 47A, B). The larger nests are lined by epithelial cells with prominent

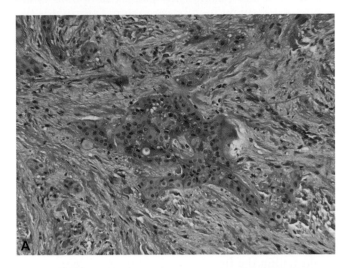

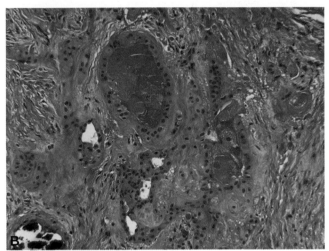

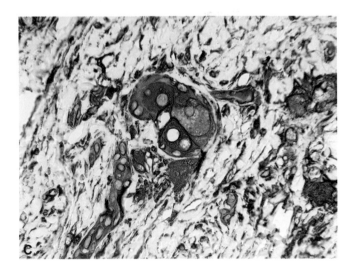

Figure 47 Phakomatous choristoma occurring in a four-month-old male presented with proptosis. (**A**) Irregular nests and strands of epithelioid cells are found in a dense fibrous stroma. (**B**) Gland-like structures are composed of rounded to ovoid epithelioid cells. Dystrophic calcifications are present in some areas. (**C**) The epithelioid nests as well as the surrounding stroma are strongly immunoreactive for vimentin.

eosinophilic cytoplasm with pale eosinophilic cystic contents. Basement membrane material surrounds the nests. The "epithelial" cells are immunoreactive for vimentin and S-100 protein (weak) and nonreactive for cytokeratin and epithelial membrane antigen (Fig. 47C). In addition, the cells express several lens-specific proteins (crystallins) to support the ectopic lenticular nature of this lesion (361).

V. SALIVARY GLANDS

For the most part, the spectrum of pathology seen in the salivary gland of a child is similar to the adult experience with some exceptions; these exceptions include the various nonepithelial neoplasms, including the hemangioma, lymphangioma, lipoma-lipomatosis, and RMS, which usually arise in or around the parotid gland within the first six years of life (362,363).

A. Nonepithelial Salivary Neoplasms

A review of 344 cases presenting in the region of the salivary gland in individuals younger than 18 years noted that the hemangioma accounted for almost 60% of tumors, followed by the lymphangioma in slightly over 25% of cases (364). *Hemangioma* of the salivary gland occurs almost exclusively in the parotid gland and is usually diagnosed before the age of one year. There is a female predilection, and as many as 25% of cases have bilateral involvement (211). These tumors often involve a substantial portion of the gland and may also extend into surrounding soft tissues. The microscopic findings are those of densely cellular, capillary-sized vascular spaces, which are more or less superimposed upon the lobular architecture of the gland to the point that the parenchyma is largely replaced (365) (Fig. 48). Virtually all of these tumors are capillary hemangiomas whose cellularlity and mitotic activity may be misjudged for a soft tissue malignancy like an embryonal RMS. Less often, the hemangioma has the spindle cell morphology of a kaposiform hemangioendothelioma, which is seen more commonly in the peripheral and retroperitoneal soft tissues.

Lymphangioma involving one or more salivary glands is often not restricted to the gland but is a component of a more diffuse process in the neck. In contrast to the growth pattern and cellularity of a hemangioma, the lymphangioma is composed of dilated lymphatic-like spaces that dissect through the interstitium of the salivary gland whose consequence is the separation of the acinar lobules from each other without replacing or overgrowing the lobules of salivary gland tissue. Plexiform neurofibroma in a child with neurofibromatosis 1 infiltrates within and around the salivary gland as myxoid neuromatous bundles (366).

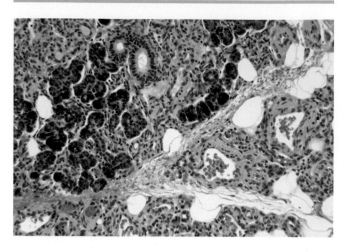

Figure 48 Hemangioma of the parotid gland in an infant shows partial replacement of the acinar parenchyma by small capillary-sized vascular spaces. Both, the gland itself and the surrounding soft tissues, are occupied by diffuse and lobular profiles of capillaries.

Embryonal RMS is the most common sarcoma involving the salivary gland(s) in childhood. These tumors are rarely restricted to the gland, which is often the parotid gland. A substantial portion of the tumor is in the soft tissues around the gland so that it is difficult to be certain about the exact primary site. The pattern of infiltration by the malignant small cells is generally along the interstitial planes of the gland and diffuse infiltration into the surrounding tissues. *Lipoma-Lipomatosis* has also been reported in the parotid gland of infants (367,368). Myeloid-monocytic leukemia presenting as a mass (granulocytic sarcoma), metastatic NB or retinoblastoma, EWS-PNETs, and non-HL (Burkitt or extranodal marginal zone lymphoma) are other neoplastic processes that involve the parotid and/or submandibular gland (369–373).

B. Epithelial Neoplasms of Salivary Glands

Epithelial neoplasms of the salivary glands in children account for only 1% to 3% of all such neoplasms in all age categories (363,374,375). Most of these tumors are sporadic occurrences, but it is known that MEC has a higher frequency than expected in older children and young adults who have received prior irradiation therapy in the management of an earlier, unrelated malignancy in the head and neck region (376,377). PA and MEC together account for 75% to 80% of all epithelial neoplasms in children with 70% to 80% of tumors arising in the parotid gland, but PAs have been reported in sites of minor salivary gland tissue (378,379). Most MECs are low to intermediate grade and often cystic, which accounts for the misdiagnosis

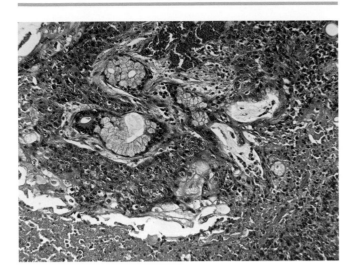

Figure 49 Mucoepidermoid carcinoma of the parotid gland in a 12-year-old male is composed in part of small mucinous gland and more solid squamous nests without keratinization.

of mucocele with secondary chronic inflammation and fibrosis in some cases (Fig. 49). Pathologic features and prognosis are the same as for adults (377). Acinic cell carcinoma, polymorphous low-grade adenocarcinoma, and adenoid cystic carcinoma are also reported in children (380–382).

Sialoblastoma (embryoma, congenital basal cell adenoma, low-grade basaloid adenocarcinoma) is the salivary gland analog of the other organ-based dysontogenetic neoplasms of childhood (383). The clinical presentation is a mass noted at birth or discovered shortly thereafter, but this tumor is known to occur later in childhood. There is a male predilection (M:F, 2:1), and the parotid gland is the preferred primary site and, less often, the submandibular gland (3:1) (384). These tumors vary remarkably in size from 1.3 to 15 cm and are lobulated and well circumscribed. The cut surface is gray-tan or tan-yellowish glistening in appearance. Solid islands and less well-delineated profiles of uniform, more or less primitive basaloid cells are contained within a fibrous or fibromyxomatous stroma (385,386) (Fig. 50A). The individual primitive-appearing tumor cells have indistinct cell borders, round to oval vesicular nuclei with one or more nucleoli, and scanty cytoplasm (Fig. 50B). Cells at the periphery of the nests have a vaguely palisaded appearance. More mature cuboidal cells with eosinophilic cytoplasm may be seen as well. Myoepithelial cells are found at the periphery. Small duct-like structures with luminal secretions when present are found at the periphery of the nests and islands (Fig. 50B). Less often, cribriform profiles are seen and may raise the possibility of another tumor type, adenoid cystic carcinoma, which is uncommon even in older children.

Mitotic activity is variable and is said to increase with subsequent recurrences. Necrosis and perineural invasion are the overt malignant features. Immunohistochemically, the tumor cells are positive for cytokeratin, vimentin, and S-100 protein, and the duct-like structures are more intensely positive for cytokeratin than the individual primitive small cells (Fig. 50C). Smooth muscle actin reactivity is seen in the peripheral cells, reflecting their myoepithelal phenotype (386) (Fig. 50D). The immunophenotype of the sialoblastoma is similar to the basal cell adenoma and adenocarcinoma. There is one case of a sialoblastoma that was accompanied by a marked elevation in serum α-fetoprotein, which was expressed by the tumor cells (387). It should be pointed out that there is at least one case of a concurrent sialoblatoma and hepatoblastoma (388).

The World Health Organization classification of salivary gland neoplasms includes the sialoblastoma among the malignant tumors (389). Since there have been so few cases with well-documented clinical follow-up, some uncertainty has been expressed in the past about the anticipated behavior of these tumors on the basis of the histologic features. If incompletely resected, the sialoblastoma recurs locally, and can do so on multiple occasions. Metastatic behavior has been reported in support of the malignant potential of this primitive epithelial neoplasm (390); widespread skeletal metastases were present in our illustrated case. Regional lymph node metastasis has been reported, and we have seen a case with widespread skeletal metastasis. A tumor resembling a sialoblastoma has been reported on the eyelid of an infant (391).

VI. THYROID GLAND

The thyroid is a relatively common site of pathology in children, more often in older children and adolescents. An exception to the latter statement is *cervicothyroidal teratoma*, which presents in the neonatal-infancy period. These neoplasms fill the anterior neck and involve the thyroid, which is not always apparent in the pathologic examination (see section "Germ Cell Neoplasms"). *Nodular hyperplasia* with a *dominant nodule* is the most common pathology in thyroid lobectomies in females aged between 10 and 12 years (392,393).

PTC is the most common adult carcinoma occurring in the first two decades of life (394–396) (Fig. 51A, B). RET/PTC rearrangements are commonly identified, either RET/PTC1 or RET/PTC3, in PTC in children and young adults (397–400). Follicular and sclerosing variants as well as the classic type are the two most common subtypes of PTC in children and adolescents. The prognosis is excellent for PTC in childhood even in the presence of bulky lymph node metastasis (401).

MTC is second to PTC in our institutional experience. These children have genetically proven MEN,

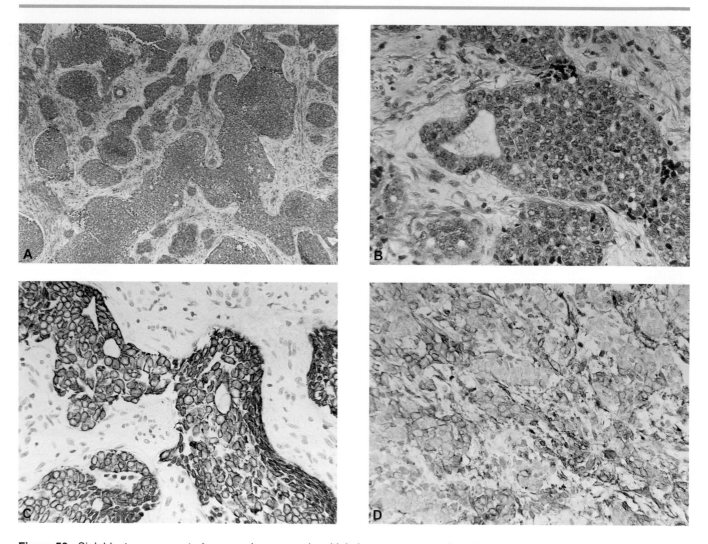

Figure 50 Sialoblastoma presented as a neck mass and multiple bony metastases in a 15-year-old male. (**A**) Circumscribed nests of relatively uniform immature basaloid cells have a variety of shapes and sizes. (**B**) Primitive-appearing basaloid tumor cells show focal gland-like or tubular formations toward the periphery of the solid nests. (**C**). The tumor cells are immunopositive for cytokeratin AE1/AE3. (**D**) Individual tumor cells are immunoreactive for smooth muscle actin with more diffuse positivity in the background stroma.

type 2A or 2B and are referred for prophylactic thyroidectomies (402–404). Because of the more aggressive behavior of MTC in the setting of MEN type 2B, it is recommended that these individuals should have a thyroidectomy as early as the infancy period. Most children with MEN have type 2A (60–90%) of cases (405). Virtually all of the resected thyroids are grossly unremarkable, but all have C-cell hyperplasia with diffuse or nodular patterns and about 25% have microscopic MTCs, mainly in the upper lobes (Fig. 52) (406). None of these thyroids have had grossly visible disease. The entire thyroid gland should be submitted for pathologic examination and labeled for purposes of localization of C-cell hyperplasia, which is multifocal and can be recognized by routine microscopy, but chromogranin and calcitonin immunostaining generally highlights more hyperplasia then is suspected

histologically. Small aggregates of larger, more atypical-appearing C-cells with nucleoli are the features of microscopic MTC (Fig. 53A, B). Both PTC and MTC are characterized by RET mutations (398,407).

VII. HISTIOCYTIC DISORDERS

LCH and juvenile xanthogranuloma (JXG) are the two histiocytic disorders of childhood that commonly have extranodal manifestations in the head and neck (408–411).

A. Langerhans Cell Histiocytosis

It has been variably reported that 30% to 45% of cases of LCH have head and neck involvement with the

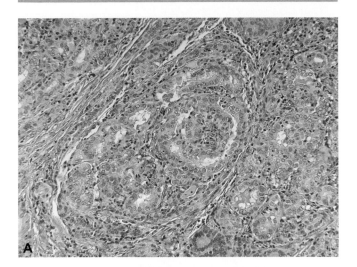

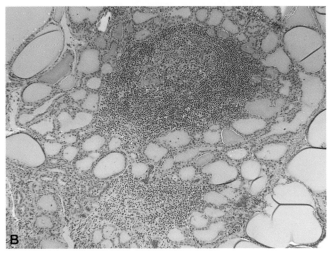

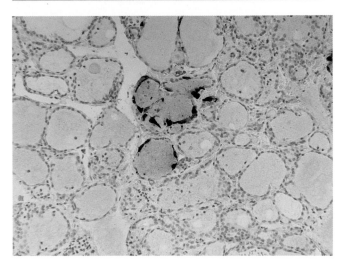

Figure 52 Medullary thyroid carcinoma in the setting of MEN types 2A or 2B is preceded and accompanied by C-cell hyperplasia. Some cases may require immunohistochemistry for calcitonin as in this case of a prophylactic thyroidectomy in an affected three-year-old male with the RET mutation from a kindred with MEN type 2B. *Abbreviation*: MEN, multiple endocrine neoplasia.

Figure 51 PTC is the most common "adult-type" carcinoma occurring in the first two decades of life, typically in older children and adolescents. (**A**) Regardless of the architectural pattern, the pathological diagnosis of PTC in the thyroid of this 15-year-old female is established on the basis of nuclear features. Even the follicular variant of PTC often has intrafollicular papillae. (**B**) A common accompanying feature is the presence of lymphocytic thyroiditis in over 50% of thyroids with PTC in young patients. *Abbreviation*: PTC, papillary thyroid carcinoma.

skull, orbit, and mandible as the sites of predilection. Otologic involvement is found in 10% to 20% of children, and greater than 80% to 90% of these have multisystem disease (412–416). Cutaneous and oral cavity lesions are other findings. In the oral cavity and ear, ulceration and secondary inflammation can obscure the underlying pathology of clusters of Langerhans cells with the characteristic reniform nucleus with a groove and pale-staining cytoplasm; the aggregation of Langerhans cells is often seen to better advantage in the S-100 protein and CD1a immunostains (Fig. 54A, B). Multinucleated, osteoclast-like

giant cells are found more often in those lesions involving bone. Eosinophils are variable in numbers, and plasma cells are present in those lesions with an element of chronicity.

B.   Juvenile Xanthogranuloma

This is a related dendritic cell proliferation to LCH, which is not only most commonly encountered in the head and neck as a solitary cutaneous lesion but also presents in the nasal cavity, temporal bone, paranasal sinus, upper and lower airway, eye, and soft tissues of the cervical region (410,411). A dense, transdermal infiltrate of nonlipidized and lipidized mononuclear cells with or without Touton giant cells and a variable number of eosinophils are the characteristic microscopic features of a cutaneous lesion.

C.   Rosai–Dorfman Disease

Rosai–Dorfman disease (sinus histiocytosis with massive lymphadenopathy) is one of the uncommon causes of cervical lymphadenopathy in a child, but the latter is the most common presentation, usually in individuals between 5 and 20 years. However, nasal cavity, paranasal sinuses, and salivary glands are relatively common extranodal sites of involvement (417–421) (Fig. 55). The skull and mandible are bony sites of disease as part of multifocal osteolytic lesions.

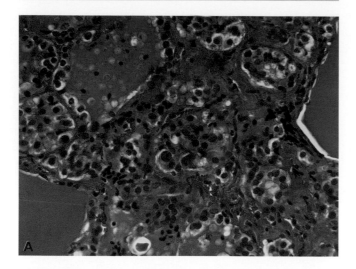

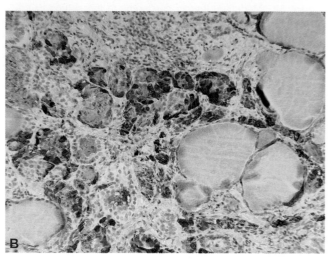

Figure 53 Medullary thyroid carcinoma if present is often microscopic in these prophylactic thyroidectomies from children with MEN type 2, as in this resected thyroid from a 10-year-old male with MEN type 2B. (**A**) One or more foci of small solid nests of tumor are budding from follicles and invading into the interstitium as follicles are displaced and overgrown. The individual malignant cells are larger than the hyperplastic C-cells and have prominent nucleoli. (**B**) Immunohistochemistry for calcitonin demonstrates the numerous small infiltrating nests of tumor. *Abbreviation*: MEN, multiple endocrine neoplasia.

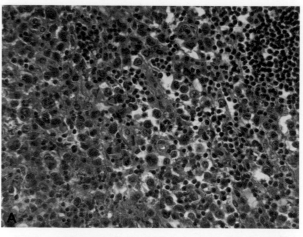

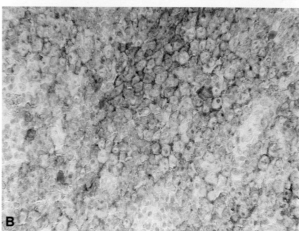

Figure 54 Langerhans cell histiocytosis presents in a number of sites in the head and neck region with osseous or extraosseous involvement or both. (**A**) This field shows an almost exclusive population of Langerhans cells with relatively few eosinophils. (**B**) Diffuse membrane immunopositivity for CD1a confirms the diagnosis.

Subcapsular and interfollicular sinusoids of an involved lymph node are expanded by large, pale-staining histiocytes with abundant pale cytoplasm with variably prominent emperipolesis (Fig. 56). Mature plasma cells are present among the histiocytes. In extranodal sinuses, the sinusoidal pattern is not present, but rather a mixed infiltrate of histiocytes and plasma cells with a variable degree of fibrosis (Fig. 57A). Emperipolesis if present is best identified in aggregates of S-100 protein (Fig. 57B) immunopositive histiocytes, which are CD1a-negative (422).

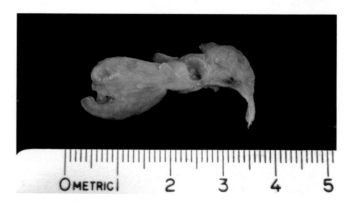

Figure 55 Rosai–Dorfman disease presents in several extranodal sites in the head and neck region. This nasal polypoid mass was thought to be an inflammatory polyp in a 16-year-old male without cervical lymphadenopathy.

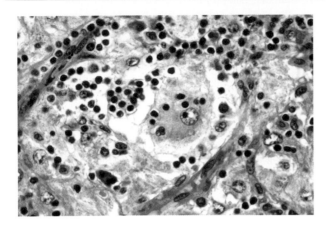

Figure 56 Rosai–Dorfman disease presenting as cervical lymphadenopathy in a five-year-old female shows emperipolesis with numerous lymphocytes in the cytoplasm of a large, pale-staining histiocyte. Plasma cells and lymphocytes are present within the surrounding tissues.

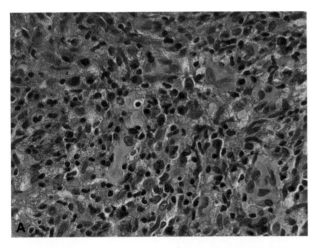

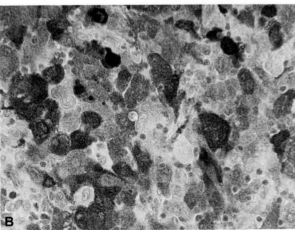

Figure 57 Rosai–Dorfman disease presented as several osteolytic lesions without other sites of involvement in a 10-year-old male. (**A**) A lesion of the frontal skull bone consists of a mixed cellular infiltrate, including large, pale histiocytes with isolated emperipolesis, lymphocytes and plasma cells. (**B**) The histiocytes are strongly and diffusely immunopositive for S-100 protein, but are nonreactive for CD1a.

REFERENCES

1. Biswas D, Saha S, Bera SP. Relative distribution of the tumours of ear, nose and throat in the paediatric patients. Int J Pediatr Otorhinolaryngol 2007; 71(5):801–805.
2. Brown RL, Azizkhan RG. Pediatric head and neck lesions. Pediatr Clin North Am 1998; 45(4):889–905.
3. Dehner LP. Congenital anomalies of the head and neck. In: Pilch B, ed. Head and Neck Surgical Pathology. Philadelphia, PA: Lippincott Williams & Wilkins, 2001:1–33.
4. Guarisco JL. Congenital head and neck masses in infants and children. Part II. Ear Nose Throat J 1991; 70(2):75–82.
5. Guarisco JL. Congenital head and neck masses in infants and children. Part I. Ear Nose Throat J 1991; 70(1):40–47.
6. Price HN, Zaenglein AI. Diagnosis and management of benign lumps and bumps in childhood. Curr Opin Pediatr 2007; 19(4):420–424.
7. Spinelli C, Ricci E, Berti P, et al. [Neck masses in childhood. Surgical experience in 154 cases]. Minerva Pediatr 1990; 42(5):169–172.
8. Torsiglieri AJ Jr., Tom LW, Ross AJ III, et al. Pediatric neck masses: guidelines for evaluation. Int J Pediatr Otorhinolaryngol 1988; 16(3):199–210.
9. Tracy TF Jr., Muratore CS. Management of common head and neck masses. Semin Pediatr Surg 2007; 16(1):3–13.
10. Ajayi OF, Adeyemo WL, Ladeinde AL, et al. Malignant orofacial neoplasms in children and adolescents: a clinicopathologic review of cases in a Nigerian tertiary hospital. Int J Pediatr Otorhinolaryngol 2007; 71(6):959–963.
11. Dickson PV, Davidoff AM. Malignant neoplasms of the head and neck. Semin Pediatr Surg 2006; 15(2):92–98.
12. English DR, Armstrong BK. Melanocytic nevi in children. I. Anatomic sites and demographic and host factors. Am J Epidemiol 1994; 139(4):390–401.
13. Changchien L, Dusza SW, Agero AL, et al. Age—and site-specific variation in the dermoscopic patterns of congenital melanocytic nevi: an aid to accurate classification and assessment of melanocytic nevi. Arch Dermatol 2007; 143(8):1007–1014.
14. Crowson AN, Megro MC, Mihm MC. The Melanocytic Proliferations. A Comprehensive Textbook of Pigmented Lesions. New York, NY: Wiley-Liss, 2001:209–223.
15. Massi G, LeBoit PE. Histological Diagnosis of Nevi and Melanoma. Darmstadt, Germany: Steinkopff-Verlag, 2004:71–120.
16. Barnhill RL, Fleischli M. Histologic features of congenital melanocytic nevi in infants 1 year of age or younger. J Am Acad Dermatol 1995; 33(5 pt 1):780–785.
17. Tannous ZS, Mihm MC Jr., Sober AJ, et al. Congenital melanocytic nevi: clinical and histopathologic features, risk of melanoma, and clinical management. J Am Acad Dermatol 2005; 52(2):197–203.
18. Herron MD, Vanderhooft SL, Smock K, et al. Proliferative nodules in congenital melanocytic nevi: a clinicopathologic and immunohistochemical analysis. Am J Surg Pathol 2004; (8):1017–1025.
19. Krengel S, Hauschild A, Schafer T. Melanoma risk in congenital melanocytic naevi: a systematic review. Br J Dermatol 2006; 155(1):1–8.
20. Ferrara G, Argenziano G, Soyer HP, et al. The spectrum of Spitz nevi: a clinicopathologic study of 83 cases. Arch Dermatol 2005; 141(11):1381–1387.
21. Massi G, LeBoit PE. Histological Diagnosis of Nevi and Melanoma. Darmstadt, Germany: Steinkopff-Verlag, 2004:169–234.
22. French JC, Rowe MR, Lee TJ, et al. Pediatric melanoma of the head and neck: a single institutions experience. Laryngoscope 2006; 116(12):2216–2222.
23. Yan AC, Smolinski KN. Melanocytic nevi: challenging clinical situations in pediatric dermatology. Adv Dermatol 2005; 21:65–80.

24. Barnhill RL, Argenyi ZB, From L, et al. Atypical Spitz nevi/tumors: lack of consensus for diagnosis, discrimination from melanoma, and prediction of outcome. Hum Pathol 1999; 30(5):513–520.

25. Temple-Camp CR, Saxe N, King H. Benign and malignant cellular blue nevus. A clinicopathological study of 30 cases. Am J Dermatopathol 1988; 10(4):289–296.

26. Scolyer RA, Zhuang L, Palmer AA, et al. Combined naevus: a benign lesion frequently misdiagnosed both clinically and pathologically as melanoma. Pathology 2004; 36(5):419–427.

27. Pearson JP, Weiss SW, Headington JT. Cutaneous malignant melanotic neurocristic tumors arising in neurocristic hamartomas. A melanocytic tumor morphologically and biologically distinct from common melanoma. Am J Surg Pathol 1996; 20(6):665–677.

28. Smith KJ, Mezebish D, Williams J, et al. The spectrum of neurocristic cutaneous hamartoma: clinicopathologic and immunohistochemical study of three cases. Ann Diagn Pathol 1998; 2(4):213–223.

29. Huynh PM, Grant-Kels JM, Grin CM. Childhood melanoma: update and treatment. Int J Dermatol 2005; 44(9): 715–723.

30. Leman JA, Evans A, Mooi W, et al. Outcomes and pathological review of a cohort of children with melanoma. Br J Dermatol 2005; 152(6):1321–1323.

31. Massi G. Melanocytic nevi simulant of melanoma with medicolegal relevance. Virchows Arch 2007; 451(3):623–647.

32. Schaffer JV. Pigmented lesions in children: when to worry. Curr Opin Pediatr 2007; 19(4):430–440.

33. Sugarman JL. Epidermal nevus syndromes. Semin Cutan Med Surg 2004; 23(2):145–157.

34. Happle R. How many epidermal nevus syndromes exist? A clinicogenetic classification. J Am Acad Dermatol 1991; 25(3):550–556.

35. Rogers M, McCrossin I, Commens C. Epidermal nevi and the epidermal nevus syndrome. A review of 131 cases. J Am Acad Dermatol 1989; 20(3):476–488.

36. Munoz-Perez MA, Garcia-Hernandez MJ, Rios JJ, et al. Sebaceus naevi: a clinicopathologic study. J Eur Acad Dermatol Venereol 2002; 16(4):319–324.

37. Santibanez-Gallerani A, Marshall D, Duarte AM, et al. Should nevus sebaceus of Jadassohn in children be excised? A study of 757 cases and literature review. J Craniofac Surg 2003; 14(5):658–660.

38. Hidvegi NC, Kangesu L, Wolfe KQ. Squamous cell carcinoma complicating naevus sebaceous of Jadassohn in a child. Br J Plast Surg 2003; 56(1):50–52.

39. Griffin JR, Cohen PR, Tschen JA, et al. Basal cell carcinoma in childhood: case report and literature review. J Am Acad Dermatol 2007; 57(5 suppl):S97–S102.

40. Gorlin RJ. Nevoid basal cell carcinoma (Gorlin) syndrome. Genet Med 2004; 6(6):530–539.

41. High Z, Zedan W. Basal cell nevus syndrome. Curr Opin Oncol 2005; 17(2):160–166.

42. Wicking C, Bale AE. Molecular basis of the nevoid basal cell carcinoma syndrome. Curr Opin Pediatr 1997; 9(6): 630–635.

43. Agarwal RP, Handler SD, Matthews MR, et al. Pilomatrixoma of the head and neck in children. Otolaryngol Head Neck Surg 2001; 125(5):510–515.

44. Marrogi AJ, Swanson PE, Kyriakos, M, et al. Rudimentary meningocele of the skin. Clinicopathologic features and differential diagnosis. J Cutan Pathol 1991; 18(3):178–188.

45. Marrogi AJ, Wick MR, Dehner LP. Pilomatrical neoplasms in children and young adults. Am J Dermatopathol 1992; 14(2):87–94.

46. Lan MY, Lan MC, Ho CY, et al. Pilomatricoma of the head and neck: a retrospective review of 179 cases. Arch Otolaryngol Head Neck Surg 2003; 129(12):1327–1330.

47. Yencha MW. Head and neck pilomatricoma in the pediatric age group: a retrospective study and literature review. Int J Pediatr Otorhinolaryngol 2001; 57(2):123–128.

48. Patrizi A, Neri I, Marzaduri S, et al. Syringoma: a review of twenty-nine cases. Acta Derm Venereol 1998; 78(6): 460–462.

49. Daneshpazhooh M, Nazemi TM, Bigdeloo L, et al. Mucocutaneous findings in 100 children with Down syndrome. Pediatr Dermatol 2007; 24(3):317–320.

50. Ahuja R, Azar NF. Orbital dermoids in children. Semin Ophthalmol 2006; 21(3):207–211.

51. Cummings TJ, George TM, Fuchs HE, et al. The pathology of extracranial scalp and skull masses in young children. Clin Neuropathol 2004; 23(1):34–43.

52. Pryor SG, Lewis JE, Weaver AL, et al. Pediatric dermoid cysts of the head and neck. Otolaryngol Head Neck Surg 2005; 132(6):938–942.

53. Blake WE, Chow CW, Holmes AD, et al. Nasal dermoid sinus cysts: a retrospective review and discussion of investigation and management. Ann Plast Surg 2006; 57(5):535–540.

54. Heywood RL, Lyons MJ, Cochrane LA, et al. Excision of nasal dermoids with intracranial extension—anterior small window craniotomy approach. Int J Pediatr Otorhinolaryngol 2007; 71(8):1193–1196.

55. Sexton M, Murdock DK. Eruptive vellus hair cysts. A follicular cyst of the sebaceous duct (sometimes). Am J Dermatopathol 1989; 11(4):364–368.

56. Donley CL, Nelson LP. Comparison of palatal and alveolar cysts of the newborn in premature and full-term infants. Pediatr Dent 2000; 22(4):321–324.

57. Flinck A, Paludan A, Matsson L, et al. Oral findings in a group of newborn Swedish children. Int J Paediatr Dent 1994; 4(2):67–73.

58. Paula JD, Dezan CC, Frossard WT, et al. Oral and facial inclusion cysts in newborns. J Clin Pediatr Dent 2006; 31(2):127–129.

59. Das S, Das AK. A review of pediatric oral biopsies from a surgical pathology service in a dental school. Pediatr Dent 1993; 15(3):208–211.

60. Dhanuthai K, Banrai M, Limpanaputtajak S. A retrospective study of paediatric oral lesions from Thailand. Int J Paediatr Dent 2007; 17(4):248–253.

61. Jones AV, Franklin CD. An analysis of oral and maxillofacial pathology found in adults over a 30-year period. J Oral Pathol Med 2006; 35(7):392–401.

62. Maia DM, Merly F, Castro WH, et al. A survey of oral biopsies in Brazilian pediatric patients. ASDC J Dent Child 2000; 67(2):128–131, 128–183.

63. Skiavounou A, Iakovou M, Kontos-Toutouzas J, et al. Intra-osseous lesions in Greek children and adolescents. A study based on biopsy material over a 26-year period. J Clin Pediatr Dent 2005; 30(2):153–156.

64. Sousa FB, Etges A, Correa L, et al. Pediatric oral lesions: a 15-year review from Sao Paulo, Brazil. J Clin Pediatr Dent 2002; 26(4):413–418.

65. Tanrikulu R, Erol B, Haspolat K. Tumors of the maxillofacial region in children: retrospective analysis and long-term follow-up outcomes of 90 patients. Turk J Pediatr 2004; 46(1):60–66.

66. Cohen L. Mucoceles of the oral cavity. Oral Surg Oral Med Oral Pathol 1965; 19:365–372.

67. Crysdale WS, Mendelsohn JD, Conley S. Ranulas—mucoceles of the oral cavity: experience in 26 children. Laryngoscope 1988; 98:296–298.

68. Pandit RT, Park AH. Management of pediatric ranula. Otolaryngol Head Neck Surg 2002; 127(1):115–118.
69. Bodner L, Goldstein J, Sarnat H. Eruption cysts: a clinical report of 24 new cases. J Clin Pediatr Dent 2004; 28(2): 183–186.
70. Meara JG, Li KK, Shah SS, et al. Odontogenic keratocysts in the pediatric population. Arch Otolaryngol Head Neck Surg 1996; 122(7):725–728.
71. Meara JG, Shah S, Li KK, et al. The odontogenic keratocyst: a 20-year clinicopathologic review. Laryngoscope 1998; 108(2):280–283.
72. Stoll C, Stollenwerk C, Riedliger D, et al. Cytokeratin expression patterns for distinction of odontogenic keratocysts from dentigerous and radicular cysts. J Oral Pathol Med 2005; 34:558–564.
73. Urbina F, Sazunic I, Murray G. Infantile systemic hyalinosis or juvenile hyaline fibromatosis? Pediatr Dermatol 2004; 21(2):154–159.
74. Antaya RJ, Cajaiba MM, Madri J, et al. Juvenile hyaline fibromatosis and infantile systemic hyalinosis overlap associated with a novel mutation in capillary morphogenesis protein-2 gene. Am J Dermatopathol 2007; 29(1): 99–103.
75. Al-Khateeb T, Al-Hadi Hamasha A, Almasri NM. Oral and maxillofacial tumours in north Jordanian children and adolescents: a retrospective analysis over 10 years. Int J Oral Maxillofac Surg 2003; 32(1):78–83.
76. Doufexi A, Mina M, Ioannidou E. Gingival overgrowth in children: epidemiology, pathogenesis, and complications. A literature review. J Periodontol 2005; 76(1):3–10.
77. Haytac MC, Ozcelik O. The phenotypic overlap of syndromes associated with hereditary gingival fibromatosis: follow-up of a family for five years. Oral Surg Oral Med Oral Pathol Oral Radiol Endod 2007; 103(4):521–527.
78. Barros SP, Merzel J, de Araujo VC, et al. Ultrastructural aspects of connective tissue in hereditary gingival fibromatosis. Oral Surg Oral Med Oral Pathol Oral Radiol Endod 2001; 92(1):78–82.
79. Rouzier C, Vanatka R, Bannwarth S, et al. A novel homozygous MMP2 mutation in a family with Winchester syndrome. Clin Genet 2006; 69(3):271–276.
80. Zankl A, Pachman L, Poznanski A, et al. Torg syndrome is caused by inactivating mutations in MMP2 and is allelic to NAO and Winchester syndrome. J Bone Miner Res 2007; 22(2):329–333.
81. Di Giandomenico S, Masi R, Cassandrini D, et al. Lipoid proteinosis: case report and review of the literature. Acta Otorhinolaryngol Ital 2006; 26(3):162–167.
82. Hamada T. Lipoid proteinosis. Clin Exp Dermatol 2002; 27(8):624–629.
83. Mirancea N, Hausser I, Metze D, et al. Junctional basement membrane anomalies of skin and mucosa in lipoid proteinosis (hyalinosis cutis et mucosae). J Dermatol Sci 2007; 45(3):175–185.
84. O'Halloran LR, Lusk RP. Amyloidosis of the larynx in a child. Ann Otol Rhinol Laryngol 1994; 103(8 pt 1): 590–594.
85. Woo P. Amyloidosis in children. Baillieres Clin Rheumatol 1994; 8(3):691–697.
86. Alessi DM, Zimmerman MC. Granular cell tumors of the head and neck. Laryngoscope 1988; 98(8 pt 1):810–814.
87. Brannon RB, Anand PM. Oral granular cell tumors: an analysis of 10 new pediatric and adolescent cases and a review of the literature. J Clin Pediatr Dent 2004; 29(1): 69–74.
88. Torsiglieri AJ Jr., Handler SD, Uri AK. Granular cell tumors of the head and neck in children: the experience at the Children's Hospital of Philadelphia. Int J Pediatr Otorhinolaryngol 1991; 21(3):249–258.
89. Lack EE, Perez-Atayde AR, McGill TJ, et al. Gingival granular cell tumor of the newborn (congenital "epulis"): ultrastructural observations relating to histogenesis. Hum Pathol 1982; 13(7):686–689.
90. Lack EE, Worsham GF, Callihan MD, et al. Gingival granula cell tumors of the newborn (congenital "epulis"): a clinical and pathologic study of 21 patients. Am J Surg Pathol 1981; 5(1):37–46.
91. Senoo H, Iida S, Kishino M, et al. Solitary congenital granular cell lesion of the tongue. Oral Surg Oral Med Oral Pathol Oral Radiol Endod 2007; 104(1):e45–e48.
92. Yavuzer R, Ataoglu O, Sari A. Multiple congenital epulis of the alveolar ridge and tongue. Ann Plast Surg 2001; 47(2): 199–202.
93. Sakai VT, Oliveira TM, Silva TC, et al. Complete spontaneous regression of congenital epulis in a baby by 8 months of age. Int J Paediatr Dent 2007; 17(4):309–312.
94. Messina M, Severi FM, Buonocore G, et al. Prenatal diagnosis and multidisciplinary approach to the congenital gingival granular cell tumor. J Pediatr Surg 2006; 41 (10):E35–E38.
95. Zarbo RJ, Lloyd RV, Beals TF, et al. Congenital gingival granular cell tumor with smooth muscle cytodifferentiation. Oral Surg Oral Med Oral Pathol 1983; 56(5):512–520.
96. Bilen BT, Alaybeyoglu N, Arslan A, et al. Obstructive congenital gingival granular cell tumour. Int J Pediatr Otorhinolaryngol 2004; 68(12):1567–1571.
97. Heitink-Polle KM, Ultee CA, van der Deure J, et al. A hypothyroid neonate with a lingual tumour. Arch Dis Child Fetal Neonatal Ed 2007; 92(2):F142.
98. Gillis D, Brnjac L, Perlman K, et al. Frequency and characteristics of lingual thyroid not detected by screening. J Pediatr Endocrinol Metab 1998; 11(2):229–233.
99. Benhammou A, Bencheikh R, Benbouzid MA, et al. Ectopic lingual thyroid. B-ENT 2006; 2(3):121–122.
100. Abdallah-Matta MP, Dubarry PH, Pessey JJ, et al. Lingual thyroid and hyperthyroidism: a new case and review of the literature. J Endocrinol Invest 2002; 25(3):264–267.
101. El-Desouki MI, Al-Herbish AS, Al-Jurayyan NA. Familial occurrence of congenital hypothyroidism due to lingual thyroid gland. Clin Nucl Med 1999; 24(6):421–423.
102. Fanburg-Smith JC, Miettinen M, Folpe AL, et al. Lingual alveolar soft part sarcoma; 14 cases: novel clinical and morphological observations. Histopathology 2004; 45(5): 526–537.
103. Winslow CP, Weisberger EC. Lingual thyroid and neoplastic change: a review of the literature and description of a case. Otolaryngol Head Neck Surg 1997; 117(6): S100–S102.
104. Fowler DJ, Chisholm J, Roebuck D, et al. Melanotic neuroectodermal tumor of infancy: clinical, radiological, and pathological features. Fetal Pediatr Pathol 2006; 25(2): 59–72.
105. Kruse-Losler B, Gaertner C, Burger H, et al. Melanotic neuroectodermal tumor of infancy: systematic review of the literature and presentation of a case. Oral Surg Oral Med Oral Pathol Oral Radiol Endod 2006; 102(2):204–216.
106. Hered RW, Smithwick W 4th, Sandler E, et al. Orbital melanotic neuroectodermal tumor of infancy successfully treated with chemotherapy and subtotal excision. J Aapos 2007; 11(5):504–505.
107. Barrett AW, Morgan M, Ramsay AD, et al. A clinicopathologic and immunohistochemical analysis of melanotic neuroectodermal tumor of infancy. Oral Surg Oral Med Oral Pathol Oral Radiol Endod 2002; 93(6):688–698.
108. Kapadia SB, Frisman DM, Hitchcock CL, et al. Melanotic neuroectodermal tumor of infancy. Clinicopathological, immunohistochemical, and flow cytometric study. Am J Surg Pathol 1993; 17(6):566–573.

109. Pettinato G, Manivel JC, d'Amore ES, et al. Melanotic neuroectodermal tumor of infancy. A reexamination of a histogenetic problem based on immunohistochemical, flow cytometric, and ultrastructural study of 10 cases. Am J Surg Pathol 1991; 15(3):233–245.

110. Ellison DA, Adada B, Qualman SJ, et al. Melanotic neuroectodermal tumor of infancy: report of a case with myogenic differentiation. Pediatr Dev Pathol 2007; 10(2): 157–160.

111. Shah RV, Jambhekar NA, Rana DN, et al. Melanotic neuroectodermal tumor of infancy: report of a case with ganglionic differentiation. J Surg Oncol 1994; 55(1):65–68.

112. Dehner LP, Sibley RK, Sauk JJ, et al. Malignant melanotic neuroectodermal tumor of infancy: a clinical, pathologic, ultrastructural and tissue culture study. Cancer 1979; 43(4):1389–1410.

113. de la Rosa-Garcia E, Mosqueda-Taylor A. Leiomyomatous hamartoma of the anterior tongue: report of a case and review of the literature. Int J Paediatr Dent 1999; 9(2): 129–132.

114. De la Sotta P, Salomone C, Gonzalez S. Rhabdomyomatous (mesenchymal) hamartoma of the tongue: report of a case. J Oral Pathol Med 2007; 36(1):58–59.

115. Kreiger PA, Ernst LM, Elden LM, et al. Hamartomatous tongue lesions in children. Am J Surg Pathol 2007; 31(8): 1186–1190.

116. Zaitoun H, Triantfyllou A. Smooth muscle hamartoma of the hard palate. J Oral Pathol Med 2007; 36(4):245–249.

117. Abdelsayed RA, Wetherington RW, Bent JP III, et al. Glial choristoma of the tongue: a case report and review of the literature. Oral Surg Oral Med Oral Pathol Oral Radiol Endod 1999; 87(2):215–222.

118. Alborno T, Hofmann T, Beham A, et al. Giant hamartoma of the retro- and parapharyngeal region. Case report and review of literature. Int J Pediatr Otorhinolaryngol 2004; 68(4):511–515.

119. Scheper MA, Nikitakis NG, Sarlani E, et al. Cowden syndrome: report of a case with immunohistochemical analysis and review of the literature. Oral Surg Oral Med Oral Pathol Oral Radiol Endod 2006; 101(5):625–631.

120. Sparling JD, Hong CH, Brahim JS, et al. Oral findings in 58 adults with tuberous sclerosis complex. J Am Acad Dermatol 2007; 56(5):786–790.

121. Pujol RM, Matias-Guiu X, Mirrales J, et al. Multiple idiopathic mucosal neuromas: a minor form of multiple endocrine neoplasia type 2B or a new entity? J Am Acad Dermatol 1997; 37(2 Pt 2):349–352.

122. Lipsett J, Sparnon AL, Byard RW. Embryogenesis of enterocystomas-enteric duplication cysts of the tongue. Oral Surg Oral Med Oral Pathol 1993; 75(5):626–630.

123. Manor Y, Buchner A, Peleg M, et al. Lingual cyst with respiratory epithelium: an entity of debatable histogenesis. J Oral Maxillofac Surg 1999; 57(2):124–127; discussion 128–129.

124. Said-Al-Naief N, Fantasia JE, Sciubba JJ, et al. Heterotopic oral gastrointestinal cyst: report of 2 cases and review of the literature. Oral Surg Oral Med Oral Pathol Oral Radiol Endod 1999; 88(1):80–86.

125. Willner A, Feghali J, Bassila M. An enteric duplication cyst occurring in the anterior two-thirds of the tongue. Int J Pediatr Otorhinolaryngol 1991; 21(2):169–177.

126. Aughton DJ, Sloan CT, Milad MP, et al. Nasopharyngeal teratoma ('hairy polyp'), Dandy-Walker malformation, diaphragmatic hernia, and other anomalies in a female infant. J Med Genet 1990; 27(12):788–790.

127. Erdogan S, Tunali N, Canpolat T, et al. Hairy polyp of the tongue: a case report. Pediatr Surg Int 2004; 20(11–12): 881–882.

128. Kelly A, Bough ID Jr., Luft JD, et al. Hairy polyp of the oropharynx: case report and literature review. J Pediatr Surg 1996; 31(5):704–706.

129. Simoni P, Wiatrak BJ, Kelly DR. Choristomatous polyps of the aural and pharyngeal regions: first simultaneous case. Int J Pediatr Otorhinolaryngol 2003; 67(2):195–199.

130. Olivares-Pakzad BA, Tazelaar HD, Dehner LP, et al. Oropharyngeal hairy polyp with meningothelial elements. Oral Surg Oral Med Oral Pathol Oral Radiol Endod 1995; 79(4):462–468.

131. Hoving EW. Nasal encephaloceles. Childs Nerv Syst 2000; 16(10–11):702–706.

132. Patterson K, Kapur S, Chandra RS. "Nasal gliomas" and related brain heterotopias: a pathologist's perspective. Pediatr Pathol 1986; 5(3–4):353–362.

133. Yeoh GP, Bale PM, de Silva M. Nasal cerebral heterotopia: the so-called nasal glioma or sequestered encephalocele and its variants. Pediatr Pathol 1989; 9(5):531–549.

134. De Biasio P, Scarso E, Prefumo F, et al. Prenatal diagnosis of a nasal glioma in the mid trimester. Ultrasound Obstet Gynecol 2006; 27(5):571–573.

135. Huisman TA, Schneider JF, Kellenberger CJ, et al. Developmental nasal midline masses in children: neuroradiological evaluation. Eur Radiol 2004; 14(2):243–249.

136. Rahbar R, Resto VA, Robson CD, et al. Nasal glioma and encephalocele: diagnosis and management. Laryngoscope 2003; 113(12):2069–2077.

137. Bajaj MS, Kashyap S, Wagh VB, et al. Glial heterotopia of the orbit and extranasal region: an unusual entity. Clin Experiment Ophthalmol 2005; 33(5):513–515.

138. Penner CR, Thompson L. Nasal glial heterotopia: a clinicopathologic and immunophenotypic analysis of 10 cases with a review of the literature. Ann Diagn Pathol 2003; 7(6):354–359.

139. Niedzielska G, Niedzielski A, Kotowski M. Nasal ganglioglioma—difficulties in radiological imaging. Int J Pediatr Otorhinolaryngol 2008; 72(2):285–287.

140. Sibley DA, Cooper PH. Rudimentary meningocele: a variant of "primary cutaneous meningioma". J Cutan Pathol 1989; 16(2):72–80.

141. Suster S, Rosai J. Hamartoma of the scalp with ectopic meningothelial elements. A distinctive benign soft tissue lesion that may simulate angiosarcoma. Am J Surg Pathol 1990; 14(1):1–11.

142. Ferran M, Tribo MJ, Gonzalez-Rivero MA, et al. Congenital hamartoma of the scalp with meningothelial, sebaceus, muscular, and immature glandular components. Am J Dermatopathol 2007; 29(6):568–572.

143. Dehner LP, Valbuena L, Perez-Atayde A, et al. Salivary gland anlage tumor ("congenital pleomorphic adenoma"). A clinicopathologic, immunohistochemical and ultrastructural study of nine cases. Am J Surg Pathol 1994; 18(1):25–36.

144. Har-El G, Zirkin HY, Tovi F, et al. Congenital pleomorphic adenoma of the nasopharynx (report of a case). J Laryngol Otol 1985; 99(12):1281–1287.

145. Hermann BW, Dehner LP, Lieu JE. Congenital salivary gland anlage tumor: a case series and review of the literature. Int J Pediatr Otorhinolaryngol 2005; 69(2): 149–156.

146. Michal M, Sokol L, Mukensnabl P. Salivary gland anlage tumor. A case with widespread necrosis and large cyst formation. Pathology 1996; 28(2):128–130.

147. Alrawi M, McDermott M, Orr D, et al. Nasal chondromesynchymal hamartoma presenting in an adolescent. Int J Pediatr Otorhinolaryngol 2003; 67(6):669–672.

148. McDermott MB, Ponder TB, Dehner LP. Nasal chondromesenchymal hamartoma: an upper respiratory tract

analogue of the chest wall mesenchymal hamartoma. Am J Surg Pathol 1998; 22(4):425–433.

149. Norman ES, Bergman S, Trupiano JK. Nasal chondromesenchymal hamartoma: report of a case and review of the literature. Pediatr Dev Pathol 2004; 7(5):517–520.

150. Ozolek JA, Carrau R, Barnes EL, et al. Nasal chondromesenchymal hamartoma in older children and adults: series and immunohistochemical analysis. Arch Pathol Lab Med 2005; 129(11):1444–1450.

151. Johnson C, Nagaraj U, Esguerra J, et al. Nasal chondromesenchymal hamartoma: radiographic and histopathologic analysis of a rare pediatric tumor. Pediatr Radiol 2007; 37(1):101–104.

152. Silkiss RZ, Mudvari SS, Shetlar D. Ophthalmologic presentation of nasal chondromesenchymal hamartoma in an infant. Ophthal Plast Reconstr Surg 2007; 23(3):243–244.

153. Shet T, Borges N, Nair C, et al. Two unusual lesions in the nasal cavity of infants—a nasal chondromesenchymal hamartoma and an aneurysmal bone cyst like lesion. More closely related than we think? Int J Pediatr Otorhinolaryngol 2004; 68(3):359–364.

154. Aclerno SP, Waldhausen JH. Congenital cervical cysts, sinuses and fistulae. Otolaryngol Clin North Am 2007; 40 (1):161–176, vii–viii.

155. Koch BL. Cystic malformations of the neck in children. Pediatr Radiol 2005; 35(5):463–477.

156. Koeller KK, Alamo L, Adair CF, et al. Congenital cystic masses of the neck: radiologic-pathologic correlation. Radiographics 1999; 19(1):121–146; quiz 152–153.

157. Kenealy JF, Torsiglieri AJ Jr., Tom LW. Branchial cleft anomalies: a five-year retrospective review. Trans Pa Acad Ophthalmol Otolaryngol 1990; 42:1022–1025.

158. Schroeder JW Jr., Mohyuddin N, Maddalozzo J. Branchial anomalies in the pediatric population. Otolaryngol Head Neck Surg 2007; 137(2):289–295.

159. Waldhausen JH. Branchial cleft and arch anomalies in children. Semin Pediatr Surg 2006; 15(2):64–69.

160. Jansen T, Romiti R, Altmeyer P. Accessory tragus: report of two cases and review of the literature. Pediatr Dermatol 2000; 17(5):391–394.

161. Triglia JM, Nicollas R, Ducroz V, et al. First branchial cleft anomalies: a study of 39 cases and a review of the literature. Arch Otolaryngol Head Neck Surg 1998; 124(3):291–295.

162. Mehta RP, Faquin WC, Cunningham MJ. Cervical bronchogenic cysts: a consideration in the differential diagnosis of pediatric cervical cystic masses. Int J Pediatr Otorhinolaryngol 2004; 68(5):563–568.

163. Millman B, Pransky S, Castillo J III, et al. Cervical thymic anomalies. Int J Pediatr Otorhinolaryngol 1999; 47(1):29–39.

164. Petropoulos I, Konstantinidis I, Joussios G, et al. Thymic cyst in the differential diagnosis of paediatric cervical masses. B-ENT 2006; 2(1):35–37.

165. Foley DS, Fallat ME. Thyroglossal duct and other congenital midline cervical anomalies. Semin Pediatr Surg 2006; 15(2):70–75.

166. Organ GM, Organ CH Jr. Thyroid gland and surgery of the thyroglossal duct: exercise in applied embryology. World J Surg 2000; 24(8):886–890.

167. Marianowski R, Ait Amer JL, Morisseau-Durand MP, et al. Risk factors for thyroglossal duct remnants after Sistrunk procedure in a pediatric population. Int J Pediatr Otorhinolaryngol 2003; 67(1):19–23.

168. Mondin V, Ferlito A, Muzzi E, et al. Thyroglossal duct cyst: personal experience and literature review. Auris Nasus Larynx 2008; 35(1):11–25.

169. Shah R, Gow K, Sobol SE. Outcome of thyroglossal duct cyst excision is independent of presenting age or symptomatology. Int J Pediatr Otorhinolaryngol 2007; 71(11): 1731–1735.

170. Ostlie DJ, Burjonrappa SC, Snyder CL, et al. Thyroglossal duct infections and surgical outcomes. J Pediatr Surg 2004; 39(3):396–399; discussion 396–369.

171. Ducic Y, Chou S, Drkulec J, et al. Recurrent thyroglossal duct cysts: a clinical and pathologic analysis. Int J Pediatr Otorhinolaryngol 1998; 44(1):47–50.

172. Peretz A, Leiberman E, Kapelushnik J, et al. Thyroglossal duct carcinoma in children: case presentation and review of the literature. Thyroid 2004; 14(9):777–785.

173. Carney JA. Salivary heterotopia, cysts, and the parathyroid gland: branchial pouch derivatives and remnants. Am J Surg Pathol 2000; 24(6):837–845.

174. Daniel E, McGuirt WF Sr. Neck masses secondary to heterotopic salivary gland tissue: a 25-year experience. Am J Otolaryngol 2005; 26(2):96–100.

175. Edwards PC, Bhuiya T, Kahn LB, et al. Salivary heterotopia of the parathyroid gland: a report of two cases and review of the literature. Oral Surg Oral Med Oral Pathol Oral Radiol Endod 2005; 99(5):590–593.

176. Haemel A, Gnepp DR, Carlsten J, et al. Heterotopic salivary gland tissue in the neck. J Am Acad Dermatol 2008; 58(2):251–256.

177. Park JY, Kim GY, Suh YL. Intrathyroidal branchial cleft-like cyst with heterotopic salivary gland-type tissue. Pediatr Dev Pathol 2004; 7(3):262–267.

178. Yazici D, Cetik F. An infrequent mass of the middle ear: salivary gland choristoma. Arch Otolaryngol Head Neck Surg 2006; 132(11):1260–1262.

179. Oguz A, Karadeniz C, Temel EA, et al. Evaluation of peripheral lymphadenopathy in children. Pediatr Hematol Oncol 2006; 23(7):549–561.

180. Srouji IA, Okpala N, Nilssen E, et al. Diagnostic cervical lymphadenectomy in children: a case for multidisciplinary assessment and formal management guidelines. Int J Pediatr Otorhinolaryngol 2004; 68(5):551–556.

181. Karadeniz C, Oguz A, Ezer U, et al. The etiology of peripheral lymphadenopathy in children. Pediatr Hematol Oncol 1999; 16(6):525–531.

182. Leung AK, Robson WL. Childhood cervical lymphadenopathy. J Pediatr Health Care 2004; 18(1):3–7.

183. Yaris N. Analysis of children with peripheral lymphadenopathy. Clin Pediatr (Phila) 2006; 45(6):544–549.

184. O'Shea PA. Chronic granulomatous disease of childhood. Perspect Pediatr Pathol 1982; 7:237–258.

185. Soler-Palacin P, Margareto C, Llobet P, et al. Chronic granulomatous disease in pediatric patients: 25 years of experience. Allergol Immunopathol (Madr) 2007; 35(3): 83–89.

186. Gosche JR, Vick L. Acute, subacute, and chronic cervical lymphadenitis in children. Semin Pediatr Surg 2006; 15(2): 99–106.

187. Rahal A, Abela A, Arcand PH, et al. Nontuberculous mycobacterial adenitis of the head and neck in children: experience from a tertiary care pediatric center. Laryngoscope 2001; 111(10):1791–1796.

188. Urquhart A, Berg R. Hodgkin's and non-Hodgkin's lymphoma of the head and neck. Laryngoscope 2001; 111 (9):1565–1569.

189. Marais BJ, Wright CA, Schaaf HS, et al. Tuberculous lymphadenitis as a cause of persistent cervical lymphadenopathy in children from a tuberculosis-endemic area. Pediatr Infect Dis J 2006; 25(2):142–146.

190. Cockerell CJ, Connor DH. Cat scratch disease. In: Connor DH, ed. Cat scratch disease. Pathology of Infectious Diseases. Stamford, CT: Appleton & Lange, 1997: 461–468.

191. Cheuk W, Chan AK, Wong MC, et al. Confirmation of diagnosis of cat scratch disease by immunohistochemistry. Am J Surg Pathol 2006; 30(2):274–275.

192. Fauroux B, Clement A. Paediatric sarcoidosis. Paediatr Respir Rev 2005; 6(2):128–133.

193. Iannuzzi MC, Rybicki BA, Teirstein AS. Aravindan, evidence based criteria for the histopathological diagnosis of toxoplasmic lymphadenopathy. J Clin Pathol 2005; 58 (11):1143–1146.

194. Eapen M, Mathew CF, Aravindan KP. Kikuchi-Fujimoto disease is a rare cause of lymphadenopathy and fever of unknown origin in children: report of two cases and review of the literature. J Pediatr Hematol Oncol 2005; 27(6):337–340.

195. Scagni P, Peisino MG, Bianchi M, et al. Childhood and adolescent non-Hodgkin lymphoma: new insights in biology and critical challenges for the future. Pediatr Blood Cancer 2005; 45(6):753–769.

196. Cairo MS, Raetz E, Lim MS, et al. Childhood and adolescent non-Hodgkin lymphoma: new insights in biology and critical challenges for the future. Pediatr Blood Cancer 2005; 45(6):753–769.

197. Roh JL, Huh J, Moon HN. Lymphomas of the head and neck in the pediatric population. Int J Pediatr Otorhinolaryngol 2007; 71(9):1471–1477.

198. Mo JQ, Dimashkieh H, Mallery SR, et al. MALT lymphoma in children: case report and review of the literature. Pediatr Dev Pathol 2004; 7(4):407–413.

199. Swerdlow SH. Pediatric follicular lymphomas, marginal zone lymphomas, and marginal zone hyperplasia. Am J Clin Pathol 2004; 122(suppl):S98–S109.

200. Zambrano E, Mejia-Mejia O, Bifulco C, et al. Extranodal marginal zone B-cell lymphoma/maltoma of the lip in a child: case report and review of cutaneous lymphoid proliferations in childhood. Int J Surg Pathol 2006; 14 (2):163–169.

201. Joshi VV, Gagnon GA, Chadwick EG, et al. The spectrum of mucosa-associated lymphoid tissue lesions in pediatric patients infected with HIV: a clinicopathologic study of six cases. Am J Clin Pathol 1997; 107(5):592–600.

202. Ayan I, Kaytan E, Ayan N. Childhood nasopharyngeal carcinoma: from biology to treatment. Lancet Oncol 2003; 4(1):13–21.

203. Laskar S, Sanghavi V, Muckaden MA, et al. Nasopharyngeal carcinoma in children: ten years' experience at the Tata Memorial Hospital, Mumbai. Int J Radiat Oncol Biol Phys 2004; 58(1):189–195.

204. Cohen JI. Benign and malignant Epstein-Barr virus-associated B-cell lymphoproliferative diseases. Semin Hematol 2003; 40(2):116–123.

205. Hicks J, Flaitz C. Progressive transformation of germinal centers: review of histopathologic and clinical features. Int J Pediatr Otorhinolaryngol 2002; 65(3):195–202.

206. Ramsay AD. Reactive lymph nodes in pediatric practice. Am J Clin Pathol 2004; 122(suppl):S87–S97.

207. Adams DM, Lucky AW. Cervicofacial vascular anomalies. I. Hemangiomas and other benign vascular tumors. Semin Pediatr Surg 2006; 15(2):124–132.

208. Elluru RG, Azizkhan RG. Cervicofacial vascular anomalies. II. Vascular malformations. Semin Pediatr Surg 2006; 15(2):133–139.

209. Fishman SJ, Mulliken JB. Hemangiomas and vascular malformations of infancy and childhood. Pediatr Clin North Am 1993; 40(6):1177–1200.

210. Garzon M. Hemangiomas: update on classification, clinical presentation, and associated anomalies. Cutis 2000; 66 (5):325–328.

211. Greene AK, Rogers GF, Mulliken JB. Management of parotid hemangioma in 100 children. Plast Reconstr Surg 2004; 113(1):53–60.

212. Heffner DK. Problems in pediatric otorhinolaryngic pathology. II. Vascular tumors and lesions of the sinonasal tract and nasopharynx. Int J Pediatr Otorhinolaryngol 1983; 5(2):125–138.

213. Requena L, Sangueza OP. Cutaneous vascular proliferation. Part II. Hyperplasias and benign neoplasms. J Am Acad Dermatol 1997; 37(6):887–919; quiz 920–922.

214. Rquena L, Sangueza OP. Cutaneous vascular anomalies. Part I. Hamartomas, malformations, and dilation of preexisting vessels. J Am Acad Dermatol 1997; 37(4):523–549; quiz 549–552.

215. Bruckner AL, Frieden IJ. Hemangiomas of infancy. J Am Acad Dermatol 2003; 48(4):477–493; quiz 494–496.

216. Dadras SS, North PE, Bertoncini J, et al. Infantile hemangiomas are arrested in an early developmental vascular differentiation state. Mod Pathol 2004; 17(9): 1068–1079.

217. Gampper TJ, Morgan RF. Vascular anomalies: hemangiomas. Plast Reconstr Surg 2002; 110(2):572–585; quiz 586; discussion 587–588.

218. Miller T, Frieden IJ, Hemangiomas: new insights and classification. Pediatr Ann 2005; 34(3):179–187.

219. North PE, Waner M, buckmiller L, et al. Vascular tumors of infancy and childhood: beyond capillary hemangioma. Cardiovasc Pathol 2006; 15(6):303–317.

220. Chung EM, Smirniotopoulos JG, Specht CS, et al. From the archives of the AFIP: pediatric orbit tumors and tumorlike lesions: nonosseous lesions of the extraocular orbit. Radiographics 2007; 27(6):1777–1799.

221. Shields JA, Shields CL, Scartozzi R. Survey of 1264 patients with orbital tumors and simulating lesions: the 2002 Montgomery Lecture, part 1. Ophthalmology 2004; 111(5):997–1008.

222. Turgut M, Alabaz D, Karakas M, et al. Bacillary angiomatosis in an immunocompetent child with a grafted traumatic wound. J Dermatol 2004; 31(10):844–847.

223. Birchler MT, Schmid S, Holzmann D, et al. Kaposiform hemangioendothelioma arising in the ethmoid sinus of an 8-year-old girl with severe epistaxis. Head Neck 2006; 28(8):761–764.

224. Alvarez-Mendoza A, Lourdes TS, Ridaura-Sanz C, et al. Histopathology of vascular lesions found in Kasabach-Merritt syndrome: review based on 13 cases. Pediatr Dev Pathol 2000; 3(6):556–560.

225. Enjolras O, Wassef M, Kazoyer E, et al. Infants with Kasabach-Merritt syndrome do not have "true" hemangiomas. J Pediatr 1997; 130(4):631–640.

226. Hall GW. Kasabach-Merritt syndrome: pathogenesis and management. Br J Haematol 2001; 112(4):851–862.

227. Lyons LL, North PE, Mac-Moune Lai F, et al. Kaposiform hemangioendothelioma: a study of 33 cases emphasizing its pathologic, immunophenotypic, and biologic uniqueness from juvenile hemangioma. Am J Surg Pathol 2004; 28(5):559–568.

228. Vin-Christian K, McCalmont TH, Frieden IJ. Kaposiform hemangioendothelioma. An aggressive, locally invasive vascular tumor that can mimic hemangioma of infancy. Arch Dermatol 1997; 133(12):1573–1578.

229. Sun ZJ, Zhang L, Zhang WF, et al. Epithelioid hemangioendothelioma of the oral cavity. Oral Dis 2007; 13(2): 244–250.

230. Cozzutto C, Guarino M, Dodero P, et al. Intravascular endothelial proliferations in children. Am J Clin Pathol 1979; 71(3):247–252.

231. Hashimoto H, Daimaru Y, Enjoji M. Intravascular papillary endothelial hyperplasia. A clinicopathologic study of 91 cases. Am J Dermatopathol 1983; 5(6):539–546.

232. Raghu AR, Tandon S, Rao NN, et al. Intraoral papillary endothelial hyperplasia: case discussion with supportive histochemistry and immunohistochemistry. J Clin Pediatr Dent 2005; 29(3):253–257.

233. Renshaw AA, Rosai J. Benign atypical vascular lesions of the lip. A study of 12 cases. Am J Surg Pathol 1993; 17(6): 557–565.

234. Tosios K, Koutlas IG, Papanicolaou SI. Intravascular papillary endothelial hyperplasia of the oral soft tissues: report of 18 cases and review of the literature. J Oral Maxillofac Surg 1994; 52(12):1263–1268.

235. Edwards MJ, Graham JM Jr. Posterior nuchal cystic hygroma. Clin Perinatol 1990; 17(3):611–640.

236. Ismail KM, Martin WL, Ghosh S, et al. Etiology and outcome of hydrops fetalis. J Matern Fetal Med 2001; 10 (3):175–181.

237. Abrams ME, Meredith KS, Kinnard P, et al. Hydrops fetalis: a retrospective review of cases reported to a large national database and identification of risk factors associated with death. Pediatrics 2007; 120(1):84–89.

238. Lallemand AV, Doco-Fenzy M, Gaillard DA. Investigation of nonimmune hydrops fetalis: multidisciplinary studies are necessary for diagnosis—review of 94 cases. Pediatr Dev Pathol 1999; 2(5):432–439.

239. Rodriguez MM, Chaves F, Romaguera RL, et al. Value of autopsy in nonimmune hydrops fetalis: series of 51 still-born fetuses. Pediatr Dev Pathol 2002; 5(4):365–374.

240. Alquhtani A, Nguyen LT, Flageole H, et al. 25 years' experience with lymphangiomas in children. J Pediatr Surg 1999; 34(7):1164–1168.

241. Orvidas LJ, Kasperauer JL. Pediatric lymphangiomas of the head and neck. Ann Otol Rhinol Laryngol 2000; 109 (4):411–421.

242. Okazaki T, Iwatani S, Yanai T, et al. Treatment of lymphangioma in children: our experience of 128 cases. J Pediatr Surg 2007; 42(2):386–389.

243. Beck JC, Devaney KO, Weatherly RA, et al. Pediatric myofibromatosis of the head and neck. Arch Otolaryngol Head Neck Surg 1999; 125(1):39–44.

244. Coffin CM, Dehner LP. Fibroblastic-myofibroblastic tumors in children and adolescents: a clinicopathologic study of 108 examples in 103 patients. Pediatr Pathol 1991; 11(4):569–588.

245. Dayan D, Nasrallah V, Vered M. Clinico-pathologic correlations of myofibroblastic tumors of the oral cavity: 1. Nodular fasciitis. J Oral Pathol Med 2005; 34(7):426–435.

246. Vered M, Allon I, Buchner A, et al. Clinico-pathologic correlations of myofibroblastic tumors of the oral cavity. II. Myofibroma and myofibromatosis of the oral soft tissues. J Oral Pathol Med 2007; 36(5):304–314.

247. Duffy MT, Harris M, Hornblass A. Infantile myofibromatosis of orbital bone. A case report with computed tomography, magnetic resonance imaging and histologic findings. Ophthalmology 1997; 104(9):1471–1474.

248. Foss RD, Ellis GL. Myofibromas and myofibromatosis of the oral region: a clinicopathologic analysis of 79 cases. Oral Surg Oral Med Oral Pathol Oral Radiol Endod 2000; 89(1):57–65.

249. Lingen MW, Mostofi RS, Solt DB. Myofibromas of the oral cavity. Oral Surg Oral Med Oral Pathol Oral Radiol Endod 1995; 80(3):297–302.

250. Rodrigues EB, Shields CL, Eagle RC Jr., et al. Solitary intraosseous orbital myofibroma in four cases. Ophthal Plast Reconstr Surg 2006; 22(4):292–295.

251. Soylemezoglu F, Tezel GG, Koybasoglu F, et al. Cranial infantile myofibromatosis: report of three cases. Childs Nerv Syst 2001; 17(9):524–527.

252. Tsuji M, Inagaki T, Kasai H, et al. Solitary myofibromatosis of the skull: a case report and review of literature. Childs Nerv Syst 2004; 20(5):366–369.

253. Walsh RM, Leen EJ, Gleeson MJ. Solitary infantile and adult myofibromatosis of the nasal cavity: a report of two cases. J Laryngol Otol 1996; 110(6):574–577.

254. Behar PM, Albritton FD, Muller S, et al. Multicentric infantile myofibromatosis. Int J Pediatr Otorhinolaryngol 1998; 45(3):249–254.

255. Vigneswaran N, Boyd DL, Waldron CA. Solitary infantile myofibromatosis of the mandible. Report of three cases. Oral Surg Oral Med Oral Pathol 1992; 73(1):84–88.

256. Carr MM, Fraser RB, Clarke KD. Nodular fasciitis in the parotid region of a child. Head Neck 1998; 20(7):645–648.

257. DiNardo LJ, Wetmore RF, Potsic WP. Nodular fasciitis of the head and neck in children. A deceptive lesion. Arch Otolaryngol Head Neck Surg 1991; 117(9):1001–1002.

258. Harrison HC, Motbey J, Kan AE, et al. Nodular fasciitis of the nose in a child. Int J Pediatr Otorhinolaryngol 1995; 33 (3):257–264.

259. Hymas DC, Mamalis N, Pratt DV, et al. Nodular fasciitis of the lower eyelid in a pediatric patient. Ophthal Plast Reconstr Surg 1999; 15(2):139–142.

260. Shields JA, Shields CL, Christian C, et al. Orbital nodular fasciitis simulating a dermoid cyst in an 8-month-old child. Case report and review of the literature. Ophthal Plast Reconstr Surg 2001; 17(2):144–148.

261. Thompson LD, Fanburg-Smith JC, Wenig BM. Nodular fasciitis of the external ear region: a clinicopathologic study of 50 cases. Ann Diagn Pathol 2001; 5(4):191–198.

262. Boddie DE, Distante S, Blaiklock CT. Cranial fasciitis of childhood: an incidental finding of a lytic skull lesion. Br J Neurosurg 1997; 11(5):445–447.

263. Gibson SE, Prayson RA. Primary skull lesions in the pediatric population: a 25-year experience. Arch Pathol Lab Med 2007; 131(5):761–766.

264. Hussein MR. Cranial fasciitis of childhood: a case report and review of literature. J Cutan Pathol 2008; 35(2):212–214.

265. Sarangarajan R, Dehner LP. Cranial and extracranial fasciitis of childhood: a clinicopathologic and immuno-histochemical study. Hum Pathol 1999; 30(1):87–92.

266. Sayama T, Morioka T, Baba T, et al. Cranial fasciitis with massive intracranial extension. Childs Nerv Syst 1995; 11 (4):242–245.

267. Takeda N, Fujita K, Katayama S, et al. Cranial fasciitis presenting with intracranial mass: a case report. Pediatr Neurosurg 2008; 44(2):148–152.

268. Ekinci S, Karnak I, Tanyel FC. Infantile fibromatosis of the sternocleidomastoid muscle mimicking muscular torticollis. J Pediatr Surg 2004; 39(9):1424–1425.

269. Kumar V, Prabhu BV, Chattopadhayay A, et al. Bilateral sternocleidomastoid tumor of infancy. Int J Pediatr Otorhinolaryngol 2003; 67(6):673–675.

270. Sharma S, Mishra K, Khanna G. Fibromatosis colli in infants. A cytologic study of eight cases. Acta Cytol 2003; 47(3):359–362.

271. Tyagi I, Syal R, Goyal A. Staging and surgical approaches in large juvenile angiofibroma—study of 95 cases. Int J Pediatr Otorhinolaryngol 2006; 70(9):1619–1627.

272. Marshall AH, Bradley PJ. Management dilemmas in the treatment and follow-up of advanced juvenile nasopharyngeal angiofibroma. ORL J Otorhinolaryngol Relat Spec 2006; 68(5):273–278.

273. Celik B, Erisen L, Saraydaroglu O, et al. Atypical angiofibromas: a report of four cases. Int J Pediatr Otorhinolaryngol 2005; 69(3):415–421.

274. Abraham SC, Montgomery EA, Giardiello FM et al. Frequent beta-catenin mutations in juvenile nasopharyngeal angiofibromas. Am J Pathol 2001; 158(3):1073–1078.

275. Carlson JW, Fletcher CD. Immunohistochemistry for beta-catenin in the differential diagnosis of spindle cell lesions: analysis of a series and review of the literature. Histopathology 2007; 51(4):509–514.

276. Ferouz AS, Mohr RM, Paul P. Juvenile nasopharyngeal angiofibroma and familial adenomatous polyposis: an

association? Otolaryngol Head Neck Surg 1995; 113 (4):435–439.

277. Guertl B, Beham A, Zechner R, et al. Nasopharyngeal angiofibroma: an APC-gene-associated tumor? Hum Pathol 2000; 31(11):1411–1413.

278. Valanzano R, Curia MC, Aceto G, et al. Genetic evidence that juvenile nasopharyngeal angiofibroma is an integral FAP tumour. Gut 2005; 54(7):1046–1047.

279. Hoos A, Lewis JJ, Urist MJ, et al. Desmoid tumors of the head and neck—a clinical study of a rare entity. Head Neck 2000; 22(8):814–821.

280. Wang CP, Chang YL, Ko JY, et al. Desmoid tumor of the head and neck. Head Neck 2006; 28(11):1008–1013.

281. Ferrari A, Gronchi A, Casanova M, et al. Synovial sarcoma: a retrospective analysis of 271 patients of all ages treated at a single institution. Cancer 2004; 101(3):627–634.

282. Harb WJ, Luna MA, Patel SR, et al. Survival in patients with synovial sarcoma of the head and neck: association with tumor location, size, and extension. Head Neck 2007; 29(8):731–740.

283. Okcu MF, Munsell M, Treuner J, et al. Synovial sarcoma of childhood and adolescence: a multicenter, multivariate analysis of outcome. J Clin Oncol 2003; 21(8):1602–1611.

284. Raney RB. Synovial sarcoma in young people: background, prognostic factors, and therapeutic questions. J Pediatr Hematol Oncol 2005; 27(4):207–211.

285. Abrosimov AY, LiVolsi VA. Spindle epithelial tumor with thymus-like differentiation (SETTLE) of the thyroid with neck lymph node metastasis: a case report. Endocr Pathol 2005; 16(2):139–143.

286. Carli M, Ferrari A, Mattke A, et al. Pediatric malignant peripheral nerve sheath tumor: the Italian and German soft tissue sarcoma cooperative group. J Clin Oncol 2005; 23(33):8422–8430.

287. Chan JK, Rosai J. Tumors of the neck showing thymic or related branchial pouch differentiation: a unifying concept. Hum Pathol 1991; 22(4):349–367.

288. de Saint Aubain Somerhausen N, Fletcher CD. Leiomyosarcoma of soft tissue in children: clinicopathologic analysis of 20 cases. Am J Surg Pathol 1999; 23(7):755–763.

289. Papi G, Corrado S, LiVolsi VA. Primary spindle cell lesions of the thyroid gland; an overview. Am J Clin Pathol 2006; 125(suppl):S95–S123.

290. Slater O, Shipley J. Clinical relevance of molecular genetics to paediatric sarcomas. J Clin Pathol 2007; 60(11):1187–1194.

291. Alaggio R, Ninfo V, Rosolen A, et al. Primitive myxoid mesenchymal tumor of infancy: a clinicopathologic report of 6 cases. Am J Surg Pathol 2006; 30(3):388–394.

292. Lyos AT, Goepfert H, Luna MA, et al. Soft tissue sarcoma of the head and neck in children and adolescents. Cancer 1996; 77(1):193–200.

293. Hawkins DS, Anderson JR, Paidas CN, et al. Improved outcome for patients with middle ear rhabdomyosarcoma: a children's oncology group study. J Clin Oncol 2001; 19(12):3073–3079.

294. Karcioglu ZA, Hadjistillianou D, Rozans M, et al. Orbital rhabdomyosarcoma. Cancer Control 2004; 11(5):328–333.

295. Raney RB, Meza J, Anderson JR, et al. Treatment of children and adolescents with localized parameningeal sarcoma: experience of the Intergroup Rhabdomyosarcoma Study Group protocols IRS-II through -IV, 1978–1997. Med Pediatr Oncol 2002; 38(1):22–32.

296. Simon JH, Paulino AC, Smith RB, et al. Prognostic factors in head and neck rhabdomyosarcoma. Head Neck 2002; 24(5):468–473.

297. Walterhouse DO, Pappo AS, Baker KS, et al. Rhabdomyosarcoma of the parotid region occurring in childhood and adolescence. A report from the Intergroup Rhabdomyosarcoma Study Group. Cancer 2001; 92(12):3135–3146.

298. Wurm J, Constantinidis J, Grabenbauer GG, et al. Rhabdomyosarcomas of the nose and paranasal sinuses: treatment results in 15 cases. Otolaryngol Head Neck Surg 2005; 133(1):42–50.

299. Kapadia SB, Meis JM, Frisman DM, et al. Fetal rhabdomyoma of the head and neck: a clinicopathologic and immunophenotypic study of 24 cases. Hum Pathol 1993; 24(7):754–765.

300. Rosenberg AS, Kirk J, Morgan MB. Rhabdomyomatous mesenchymal hamartoma: an unusual dermal entity with a report of two cases and a review of the literature. J Cutan Pathol 2002; 29(4):238–243.

301. Brehmer D, Overhoff HM, Marx A. Malignant ectomesenchymoma of the nose. Case report and review of the literature. ORL J Otorhinolaryngol Relat Spec 2003; 65 (1):52–56.

302. Ahmed S, Goel S, Khandwala M, et al. Neuroblastoma with orbital metastasis: ophthalmic presentation and role of ophthalmologists. Eye 2006; 20(4):466–470.

303. Lonergan GJ, Schwab CM, Suarez ES, et al. Neuroblastoma, ganglioneuroblastoma, and ganglioneuroma: radiologic-pathologic correlation. Radiographics 2002; 22(4):911–934.

304. Musarella MA, Chan HS, DeBoer G, et al. Ocular involvement in neuroblastoma: prognostic implications. Ophthalmology 1984; 91(8):936–940.

305. Schwab M, Westermann F, Hero B, et al. Neuroblastoma: biology and molecular and chromosomal pathology. Lancet Oncol 2003; 4(8):472–480.

306. Jethanamest D, Morris LG, Sikora AG, et al. Esthesioneuroblastoma: a population-based analysis of survival and prognostic factors. Arch Otolaryngol Head Neck Surg 2007; 133(3):276–280.

307. Kumar M, Fallon RJ, Hill JS, et al. Esthesioneuroblastoma in children. J Pediatr Hematol Oncol 2002; 24(6):482–487.

308. Agir H, Brasch HD, Tan ST. Extra-skeletal Ewing's sarcoma of the submandibular gland. J Plast Reconstr Aesthet Surg 2007; 60(12):1345–1348.

309. Lim TC, Tan WT, Lee YS. Congenital extraskeletal Ewing's sarcoma of the face: a case report. Head Neck 1994; 16(1):75–78.

310. Pfeiffer J, Boedeker CC, Ridder GJ. Primary Ewing sarcoma of the petrous temporal bone: an exceptional cause of facial palsy and deafness in a nursling. Head Neck 2006; 28(10):955–959.

311. Fanburg-Smith JC, Hengge M, Hengge UR, et al. Extrarenal rhabdoid tumors of soft tissue: a clinicopathologic and immunohistochemical study of 18 cases. Ann Diagn Pathol 1998; 2(6):351–362.

312. Madigan CE, Armenian SH, Malogolowkin MH, et al. Extracranial malignant rhabdoid tumors in childhood: the Childrens Hospital Los Angeles experience. Cancer 2007; 110(9):2061–2066.

313. White FV, Dehner LP, Belchis DA, et al. Congenital disseminated malignant rhabdoid tumor: a distinct clinicopathologic entity demonstrating abnormalities of chromosome 22q11. Am J Surg Pathol 1999; 23(3):249–256.

314. Bourdeaut F, Freneaux P, Thuille B, et al. hSNF5/INI1-deficient tumours and rhabdoid tumours are convergent but not fully overlapping entities. J Pathol 2007; 211 (3):323–330.

315. Oda Y, Tsuneyoshi M. Extrarenal rhabdoid tumors of soft tissue: clinicopathological and molecular genetic review and distinction from other soft-tissue sarcomas with rhabdoid features. Pathol Int 2006; 56(6):287–295.

316. Font RL, Jurco S III, Zimmerman LE. Alveolar soft-part sarcoma of the orbit: a clinicopathologic analysis of seventeen cases and a review of the literature. Hum Pathol 1982; 13(6):569–579.

317. Khan AO, Burke MJ. Alveolar soft-part sarcoma of the orbit. J Pediatr Ophthalmol Strabismus 2004; 41(4):245–246.

318. Simmons WB, Haggerty HS, Ngan B, et al. Alveolar soft part sarcoma of the head and neck. A disease of children and young adults. Int J Pediatr Otorhinolaryngol 1989; 17(2):139–153.

319. Needle MN, Cnaan A, Dattilo J, et al. Prognostic signs in the surgical management of plexiform neurofibroma: the Children's Hospital of Philadelphia experience, 1974–1994. J Pediatr 1997; 131(5):678–682.

320. Waggoner DJ, Towbin J, Gottesman G, et al. Clinic-based study of plexiform neurofibromas in neurofibromatosis 1. Am J Med Genet 2000; 92(2):132–135.

321. Wise JB, Cryer JE, Belasco JB, et al. Management of head and neck plexiform neurofibromas in pediatric patients with neurofibromatosis type 1. Arch Otolaryngol Head Neck Surg 2005; 131(8):712–718.

322. Knight DM, Birch R, Pringle J. Benign solitary schwannomas: a review of 234 cases. J Bone Joint Surg Br 2007; 89(3):382–387.

323. Baglaj M, Markowska-Woyciechowska A, Sawicz-Birkowska K, et al. Primary neurilemmoma of the thyroid gland in a 12-year-old girl. J Pediatr Surg 2004; 39(9):1418–1420.

324. Mazzoni A, Dubey SP, Poletti AM, et al. Sporadic acoustic neuroma in pediatric patients. Int J Pediatr Otorhinolaryngol 2007; 71(10):1569–1572.

325. Nakasato T, Kamada Y, Ehara S, et al. Multilobular neurilemmoma of the tongue in a child. AJNR Am J Neuroradiol 2005; 26(2):421–423.

326. Tang LF, Chen ZM, Zou CC. Primary intratracheal neurilemmoma in children: case report and literature review. Pediatr Pulmonol 2005; 40(6):550–553.

327. Nunes F, MacCollin M. Neurofibromatosis 2 in the pediatric population. J Child Neurol 2003; 18(10):718–724.

328. Ruggieri M, Iannetti P, Polizzi A, et al. Earliest clinical manifestations and natural history of neurofibromatosis type 2 (NF2) in childhood: a study of 24 patients. Neuropediatrics 2005; 36(1):21–34.

329. Collins MH, Chatten J. Lipoblastoma/lipoblastomatosis: a clinicopathologic study of 25 tumors. Am J Surg Pathol 1997; 21(10):1131–1137.

330. Sakaida M, Shimizu T, Kishioka C, et al. Lipoblastoma of the neck: a case report and literature review. Am J Otolaryngol 2004; 25(4):266–269.

331. Jung SM, Chang PY, Luo CC, et al. Lipoblastoma/lipoblastomatosis: a clinicopathologic study of 16 cases in Taiwan. Pediatr Surg Int 2005; 21(10):809–812.

332. Brandal P, Bjerkehagen B, Heim S. Rearrangement of chromosomal region 8q11-13 in lipomatous tumours: correlation with lipoblastoma morphology. J Pathol 2006; 208(3):388–394.

333. Lack EE. Extragonadal germ cell tumors of the head and neck region: review of 16 cases. Hum Pathol 1985; 16(1):56–64.

334. Martino F, Avila LF, Encinas JL, et al. Teratomas of the neck and mediastinum in children. Pediatr Surg Int 2006; 22(8):627–634.

335. Schneider DT, Calaminus G, Koch S, et al. Epidemiologic analysis of 1,442 children and adolescents registered in the German germ cell tumor protocols. Pediatr Blood Cancer 2004; 42(2):169–175.

336. Coppit GL III, Perkins JA, Manning SC. Nasopharyngeal teratomas and dermoids: a review of the literature and case series. Int J Pediatr Otorhinolaryngol 2000; 52(3):219–227.

337. De Backer A, Madern GC, van de Ven CP, et al. Strategy for management of newborns with cervical teratoma. J Perinat Med 2004; 32(6):500–508.

338. Jarrahy R, Cha ST, Mathiasen RA, et al. Congenital teratoma of the oropharyngeal cavity with intracranial extension: case report and literature review. J Craniofac Surg 2000; 11(2):106–112.

339. Kivela T, Tarkkanen A. Orbital germ cell tumors revisited: a clinicopathological approach to classification. Surv Ophthalmol 1994; 38(6):541–554.

340. Oka K, Okane M, Okuno S, et al. Congenital cervical immature teratoma arising in the left lobe of the thyroid gland. APMIS 2007; 115(1):75–79.

341. Shine NP, Sader C, Gollow I, et al. Congenital cervical teratomas: diagnostic, management and postoperative variability. Auris Nasus Larynx 2006; 33(1):107–111.

342. Thompson LD, Rosai J, Heffess CS. Primary thyroid teratomas: a clinicopathologic study of 30 cases. Cancer 2000; 88(5):1149–1158.

343. Yossuck P, Williams HJ, Polak MJ, et al. Oropharyngeal tumor in the newborn: a case report. Neonatology 2007; 91(1):69–72.

344. Dehner LP, Mills A, Talerman A, et al. Germ cell neoplasms of head and neck soft tissues: a pathologic spectrum of teratomatous and endodermal sinus tumors. Hum Pathol 1990; 21(3):309–318.

345. Kebudi R, Ayan I, Darendeliler E, et al. Non-midline endodermal sinus tumor in the head and neck region: a case report. Med Pediatr Oncol 1993; 21(9):685–689.

346. Kusumakumari P, Geetha N, Chellam VG, et al. Endodermal sinus tumors in the head and neck region. Med Pediatr Oncol 1997; 29(4):303–307.

347. Riedlinger WF, Lack EE, Robson CD, et al. Primary thyroid teratomas in children: a report of 11 cases with a proposal of criteria for their diagnosis. Am J Surg Pathol 2005; 29(5):700–706.

348. Carrizo F, Pineda-Daboin K, Neto AG, et al. Pharyngeal teratocarcinosarcoma: review of the literature and report of two cases. Ann Diagn Pathol 2006; 10(6):339–342.

349. Crazzolara R, Puelacher W, Ninkovic M, et al. Teratocarcinosarcoma of the oral cavity. Pediatr Blood Cancer 2004; 43(6):687–691.

350. Rotenberg B, El-Hakim H, Lodha A, et al. Nasopharyngeal teratocarcinosarcoma. Int J Pediatr Otorhinolaryngol 2002; 62(2):159–164.

351. Hostalet F, Hellin D, Ruiz JA. Tumefactive fibroinflammatory lesion of the head and neck treated with steroids: a case report. Eur Arch Otorhinolaryngol 2003; 260(4):229–231.

352. Olsen KD, DeSanto LW, Wold LE, et al. Tumefactive fibroinflammatory lesions of the head and neck. Laryngoscope 1986; 96(9 pt 1):940–944.

353. McDermott MB, Lind AC, Marley FF, et al. Deep granuloma annulare (pseudorheumatoid nodule) in children: clinicopathologic study of 35 cases. Pediatr Dev Pathol 1998; 1(4):300–308.

354. Grogg KL, Nascimento AG. Subcutaneous granuloma annulare in childhood: clinicopathologic features in 34 cases. Pediatrics 2001; 107(3):E42.

355. McNeal S, Daw JL Jr. Subcutaneous granuloma annulare: an unusual presentation in the eyelids and scalp. Ann Plast Surg 2005; 55(6):684–686.

356. Cancado CG, Vale FR, Bacchi CE. Subcutaneous (deep) granuloma annulare in children: a possible mimicker of epithelioid sarcoma. Fetal Pediatr Pathol 2007; 26(1):33–39.

357. Wick MR, Manivel JC. Epithelioid sarcoma and isolated necrobiotic granuloma: a comparative immunocytochemical study. J Cutan Pathol 1986; 13(4):253–260.

358. Blenc AM, Gomez JA, Lee MW, et al. Phakomatous choristoma: a case report and review of the literature. Am J Dermatopathol 2000; 22(1):55–59.

359. Ellis FJ, Eagle RC Jr., Shields JA, et al. Phakomatous choristoma (Zimmerman's tumor). Immunohistochemical

confirmation of lens-specific proteins. Ophthalmology 1993; 100(6):955–960.

360. Seregard S. Phakomatous choristoma may be located in the eyelid or orbit or both. Acta Ophthalmol Scand 1999; 77(3):343–346.

361. Thaung C, Bonshek RE, Leatherbarrow B. Phakomatous choristoma of the eyelid: a case with associated eye abnormalities. Br J Ophthalmol 2006; 90(2):245–246.

362. Daniel SJ, Al-Sebeih K, Al-Ghamdi SA, et al. Surgical management of nonmalignant parotid masses in the pediatric population: the Montreal Children's Hospital's experience. J Otolaryngol 2003; 32(1):51–54.

363. Guzzo M, Ferrari A, Marcon I, et al. Salivary gland neoplasms in children: the experience of the Istituto Nazionale Tumori of Milan. Pediatr Blood Cancer 2006; 47 (6):806–810.

364. Bentz BG, Hughes CA, Ludemann JP, et al. Masses of the salivary gland region in children. Arch Otolaryngol Head Neck Surg 2000; 126(12):1435–1439.

365. Childers EL, Furlong MA, Fanburg-Smith JC. Hemangioma of the salivary gland: a study of ten cases of a rarely biopsied/excised lesion. Ann Diagn Pathol 2002; 6(6): 339–344.

366. Weitzner S. Plexiform neurofibroma of major salivary glands in children. Oral Surg Oral Med Oral Pathol 1980; 50(1):53–57.

367. Hornigold R, Morgan PR, Pearce A, et al. Congenital sialolipoma of the parotid gland first reported case and review of the literature. Int J Pediatr Otorhinolaryngol 2005; 69(3):429–434.

368. Sinha DD, Joshi M, Sharma C, et al. Infantile congenital parotid lipomatosis: a rare case report. J Pediatr Surg 2005; 40(9):e15–e16.

369. Akata D, Akhan O, Akyuz C, et al. Involvement of the thyroid and the salivary glands in childhood non-Hodgkin's lymphomas at initial diagnosis. Eur J Radiol 2002; 44(3):228–231.

370. Bauer GP, Volk MS, Siddiqui SY, et al. Burkitt's lymphoma of the parapharyngeal space. Arch Otolaryngol Head Neck Surg 1993; 119(1):117–120.

371. Berrebi D, Lescoeur B, Faye A, et al. MALT lymphoma of labial minor salivary gland in an immunocompetent child with a gastric Helicobacter pylori infection. J Pediatr 1998; 133(2):290–292.

372. Ferry JA. Burkitt's lymphoma: clinicopathologic features and differential diagnosis. Oncologist 2006; 11(4):375–383.

373. Starek I, Mihal V, Novak Z, et al. Pediatric tumors of the parapharyngeal space. Three case reports and a literature review. Int J Pediatr Otorhinolaryngol 2004; 68 (5):601–606.

374. da Cruz Perez DE, Pires FR, Alves FA, et al. Salivary gland tumors in children and adolescents: a clinicopathologic and immunohistochemical study of fifty-three cases. Int J Pediatr Otorhinolaryngol 2004; 68(7):895–902.

375. Laikui L, Hongwei L, Hongbing J, et al. Epithelial salivary gland tumors of children and adolescents in west China population: a clinicopathologic study of 79 cases. J Oral Pathol Med 2008; 37(4):201–205.

376. Rutigliano DN, Meyers P, Ghossein RA, et al. Mucoepidermoid carcinoma as a secondary malignancy in pediatric sarcoma. J Pediatr Surg 2007; 42(7):E9–E13.

377. Vedrine PO, Coffinet L, Temam S, et al. Mucoepidermoid carcinoma of salivary glands in the pediatric age group: 18 clinical cases, including 11 second malignant neoplasms. Head Neck 2006; 28(9):827–833.

378. Brigger MT, Pearson SE. Management of parapharyngeal minor salivary neoplasms in children: a case report and review. Int J Pediatr Otorhinolaryngol 2006; 70(1): 143–146.

379. Ellies M, Schaffranietz F, Arglebe C, et al. Tumors of the salivary glands in childhood and adolescence. J Oral Maxillofac Surg 2006; 64(7):1049–1058.

380. Ogata H, Ebihara S, Mukai K. Salivary gland neoplasms in children. Jpn J Clin Oncol 1994; 24(2):88–93.

381. Sato T, Kamata SE, Kawabata K, et al. Acinic cell carcinoma of the parotid gland in a child. Pediatr Surg Int 2005; 21(5):377–380.

382. Tsang YW, Tung Y, Chan JK. Polymorphous low grade adenocarcinoma of the palate in a child. J Laryngol Otol 1991; 105(4):309–311.

383. Tatlidede S, Karsidag S, Ugurlu K, et al. Sialoblastoma: a congenital epithelial tumor of the salivary gland. J Pediatr Surg 2006; 41(7):1322–1325.

384. Brandwein M, Al-Naeif NS, Manwani D, et al. Sialoblastoma: clinicopathological/immunohistochemical study. Am J Surg Pathol 1999; 23(3):342–348.

385. Luna MA. Sialoblastoma and epithelial tumors in children: their morphologic spectrum and distribution by age. Adv Anat Pathol 1999; 6(5):287–292.

386. Williams SB, Ellis GL, Warnock GR. Sialoblastoma: a clinicopathologic and immunohistochemical study of 7 cases. Ann Diagn Pathol 2006; 10(6):320–326.

387. Ozdemir I, Simsek E, Silan F, et al. Congenital sialoblastoma (embryoma) associated with premature centromere division and high level of alpha-fetoprotein. Prenat Diagn 2005; 25(8):687–689.

388. Siddiqi SH, Solomon MP, Haller JO. Sialoblastoma and hepatoblastoma in a neonate. Pediatr Radiol 2000; 30 (5):349–351.

389. Brandwein-Gensler M. Sialoblastoma. In: Barnes L, Eveson JW, Reichart P, eds. Pathology and Genetics of Head and Neck Tumours. Lyon: IARC Press, 2005:253.

390. Scott JX, Krishnan S, Bourne AJ, et al. Treatment of metastatic sialoblastoma with chemotherapy and surgery. Pediatr Blood Cancer 2008; 50(1):134–137.

391. Shet T, Ramadwar M, Sharma S, et al. An eyelid sialoblastoma-like tumor with a sarcomatoid myoepithelial component. Pediatr Dev Pathol 2007; 10(4):309–314.

392. Millman B, Pellitteri PK. Nodular thyroid disease in children and adolescents. Otolaryngol Head Neck Surg 1997; 116(6 pt 1):604–609.

393. Niedziela M. Pathogenesis, diagnosis and management of thyroid nodules in children. Endocr Relat Cancer 2006; 13 (2):427–453.

394. Grigsby PW, Gal-or A, Michalski JM, et al. Childhood and adolescent thyroid carcinoma. Cancer 2002; 95(4):724–729.

395. Vasko V, Bauer AJ, Tuttle RM, et al. Papillary and follicular thyroid cancers in children. Endocr Dev 2007; 10:140–172.

396. Vassilopoulou-Sellin R, Goepfert H, Raney B, et al. Differentiated thyroid cancer in children and adolescents: clinical outcome and mortality after long-term follow-up. Head Neck 1998; 20(6):549–555.

397. Kouvaraki MA, Shapiro SE, Perrier ND, et al. RET protooncogene: a review and update of genotype-phenotype correlations in hereditary medullary thyroid cancer and associated endocrine tumors. Thyroid 2005; 15(6):531–544.

398. Nikiforov YE. RET/PTC rearrangement in thyroid tumors. Endocr Pathol 2002; 13(1):3–16.

399. Rabes HM, Klugbauer S. Molecular genetics of childhood papillary thyroid carcinomas after irradiation: high prevalence of RET rearrangement. Recent Results Cancer Res 1998; 154:248–264.

400. Zimmerman D. Thyroid neoplasia in children. Curr Opin Pediatr 1997; 9(4):413–408.

401. Alessandri AJ, Goddard KJ, Blair GK, et al. Age is the major determinant of recurrence in pediatric differentiated thyroid carcinoma. Med Pediatr Oncol 2000; 35(1):41–46.

402. Carney JA. Familial multiple endocrine neoplasia: the first 100 years. Am J Surg Pathol 2005; 29(2):254–274.

403. Lakhani VT, You YN, Wells SA. The multiple endocrine neoplasia syndromes. Annu Rev Med 2007; 58:253–265.

404. Szinnai G, Sarnacki S, Polak M. Hereditary medullary thyroid carcinoma: how molecular genetics made multiple endocrine neoplasia type 2 a paediatric disease. Endocr Dev 2007; 10:173–187.

405. Skinner MA, DeBenedetti MK, Moley JF, et al. Medullary thyroid carcinoma in children with multiple endocrine neoplasia types 2A and 2B. J Pediatr Surg 1996; 31(1):177–181; discussion 181–182.

406. Ashworth M. The pathology of preclinical medullary thyroid carcinoma. Endocr Pathol 2004; 15(3):227–231.

407. Yamashita S, Saenko V. Mechanisms of Disease: molecular genetics of childhood thyroid cancers. Nat Clin Pract Endocrinol Metab 2007; 3(5):422–429.

408. Buchmann L, Emami A, Wei JL. Primary head and neck Langerhans cell histiocytosis in children. Otolaryngol Head Neck Surg 2006; 135(2):312–317.

409. Dehner LP. Juvenile xanthogranulomas in the first two decades of life: a clinicopathologic study of 174 cases with cutaneous and extracutaneous manifestations. Am J Surg Pathol 2003; 27(5):579–593.

410. Janssen D, Harms D. Juvenile xanthogranuloma in childhood and adolescence: a clinicopathologic study of 129 patients from the Kiel pediatric tumor registry. Am J Surg Pathol 2005; 29(1):21–28.

411. Margulis A, Melin-Aldana H, Bauer BS. Juvenile xanthogranuloma invading the muscles in the head and neck: clinicopathological case report. Ann Plast Surg 2003; 50 (4):425–428.

412. Group FLCHS. A multicentre retrospective survey of Langerhans' cell histiocytosis: 348 cases observed between 1983 and 1993. Arch Dis Child 1996; 75(1):17–24.

413. al-Ammar AY, Tewfik TL, Bond M, et al. Langerhans' cell histiocytosis: paediatric head and neck study. J Otolaryngol 1999; 28(5):266–272.

414. Braier J, Chantada G, Rosso D, et al. Langerhans cell histiocytosis: retrospective evaluation of 123 patients at a single institution. Pediatr Hematol Oncol 1999; 16 (5):377–385.

415. Quraishi MS, Blayney AW, Walker D, et al. Langerhans' cell histiocytosis: head and neck manifestations in children. Head Neck 1995; 17(3):226–231.

416. Surico G, Muggeo P, Muggeo V, et al. Ear involvement in childhood Langerhans' cell histiocytosis. Head Neck 2000; 22(1):42–47.

417. Ahsan SF, Madgy DN, Poulik J. Otolaryngologic manifestations of Rosai-Dorfman Disease. Int J Pediatr Otorhinolaryngol 2001; 59(3):221–227.

418. Carbone A, Passannante A, Gloghini A, et al. Review of sinus histiocytosis with massive lymphadenopathy (Rosai-Dorfman disease) of head and neck. Ann Otol Rhinol Laryngol 1999; 108(11 pt 1):1095–1104.

419. Goodnight JW, Wang MB, Sercarz JA, et al. Extranodal Rosai-Dorfman disease of the head and neck. Laryngoscope 1996; 106(3 pt 1):253–256.

420. Guven G, Ilgan S, Altun C, et al. Rosai Dorfman disease of the parotid and submandibular glands: salivary gland scintigraphy and oral findings in two siblings. Dentomaxillofac Radiol 2007; 36(7):428–433.

421. Wenig BM, Abbondanzo SL, Childers EL, et al. Extranodal sinus histiocytosis with massive lymphadenopathy (Rosai-Dorfman disease) of the head and neck. Hum Pathol 1993; 24(5):483–492.

422. Gaitonde S. Multifocal, extranodal sinus histiocytosis with massive lymphadenopathy: an overview. Arch Pathol Lab Med 2007; 131(7):1117–1121.

21

Pathology of the Thyroid Gland

Lori A. Erickson and Ricardo V. Lloyd
Mayo Clinic College of Medicine, Rochester, Minnesota, U.S.A.

I. NORMAL THYROID GLAND

A. Embryology and Development

The thyroid anlage arises as a bilateral vesicular tissue in the foramen cecum of the tongue. It is visible by day 17 of fetal life as an endodermal structure in the pharynx in close association with the heart (1,2). The developing thyroid descends as part of the thyroglossal duct to the neck. After the thyroglossal duct atrophies, the thyroid anlage expands laterally. Between 9 and 12 weeks of development, follicle formation is ongoing, and colloid production can be detected starting around 12 weeks. Well-developed colloid follicles can be seen by 14 weeks of gestation (1,2).

The C cells migrate to the ultimobranchial bodies from the neural crest and are subsequently incorporated into the thyroid gland (3,4). The ultimobranchial bodies are derived from the branchial pouch complexes IV and V and develop during weeks 5 to 7 of fetal life. The ultimobranchial bodies are composed of a central and peripheral component with a stratified epithelial cyst and solid component of cells that transform into a cystic structure.

Anatomy

The adult thyroid consists of a bilobed organ in the midportion of the neck. It lies in front of the larynx and trachea, and the two lobes are joined by the isthmus in the middle. The lobes have a pointed superior pole and a more blunted inferior pole. The isthmus lies across the trachea anteriorly below the cricoid cartilage. The right lobe may be larger than the left lobe. About 40% of individuals have a pyramidal lobe, which is a vestige of the thyroglossal duct.

The adult thyroid weighs between 15 and 25 g. The weight varies with iodine intake, age, sex, size of the individual, and hormonal and functional status. It is generally larger and heavier in women and changes with the menstrual cycle and pregnancy (5–7). The left superior thyroid arteries, which are branches of the external carotid arteries, supply blood to the thyroid gland along with the right and left inferior thyroid arteries derived from the subclavian arteries. Venous outflow goes to the internal jugular, the brachycephalic, and sometimes the anterior jugular veins. The larger lymphatics exit the glands with the veins.

The nerve supply originates from the superior and middle cervical sympathetic ganglia. Adrenergic nerve fibers, which terminate in the vicinity of the thyroid follicle, may have an effect on thyroid secretion (8).

Histology

The thyroid gland is made up of lobules that are composed of 20 to 40 follicles. These are supplied by a branch of the thyroid artery. The follicles have an average size of 200 μm (range of 50–500 μm). Follicles have colloid in their lumens, which is made up mostly of thyroglobulin. Calcium oxalate crystals are present in normal colloid and allows distinction from colloid-like material in parathyroid gland tissue that is devoid of calcium oxalate (9). Normal thyroid may be present in soft tissues and skeletal muscle next to the thyroid as ectopic thyroid tissue (10).

Follicular cells. Follicular cells are the basic structural unit of the thyroid. They make up the acini with colloid in the central lumen, and the base of the follicle is associated with the basement membrane. Ultrastructural studies show microvilli at the apical portion of the cells with cilia projecting from the central portion of each cell (11). Follicular cells have well-developed desmosomes with terminal bars between cells, and the nuclei are round with diffuse chromatin.

Immunohistochemical studies show reactivity for thyroglobulin and low molecular weight keratin. The nuclei are positive for Thyroid transcription factor-I (TTF-1) (12,13). In situ hybridization studies show thyroglobulin mRNA in the follicular cells (14,15).

C cells. The calcitonin-producing C cells are usually difficult to identify on hematoxylin and eosin (H&E) sections. They are intrafollicular in location and have pale-to-clear cytoplasm and oval nuclei. C cells are most numerous in neonates and subsequently decrease in the adult thyroid gland. However, their numbers increase again in older adults as well (16).

Immunohistochemical stains are positive for calcitonin, chromogranin, synaptophysin, somatostatin, calcitonin-gene-related peptide, and bombesin in the C cells (16). Ultrastructural studies show secretory granules including type I (diameter of 280 nm) and type II (diameter of 130 nm) granules. Calcitonin is present in both types of granules. In situ hybridization studies have localized calcitonin mRNA in the C cells (17).

Solid cell nests. Solid cell nests can be seen in the thyroid gland. They probably represent ultimobranchial body rests (17,18). These small nests are usually less than 0.1 mm in diameter and consist of oval cells with fine granular chromatin. Nuclear grooves are sometimes prominent. They are found in about 3% of routinely examined thyroid glands (17). Immunohistochemical studies show staining for low molecular weight keratin and variable expression of calcitonin (19,20). Immunoreactivity for polyclonal carcinoembryonic antigen (CEA) is also present (16). Ultrastructural studies show prominent desmosomes, intermediate filaments, and intraluminal cytoplasmic projections.

B. Physiology

The hormones produced by thyroid follicular cells include thyroxine (T4) and triiodothyronine (T3) by the follicular cells and calcitonin by the C cells. One of the main functions of the thyroid is to produce thyroid hormones to meet the demands of peripheral tissues to help maintain homeostasis. Exogenous iodine is used for synthesis of T3 and T4. Once iodine is in the thyroid gland, it is oxidized to the organic form with catalysis by thyroid peroxidase. Thyroglobulin is synthesized and stored as colloid. Hydrolysis of thyroglobulin leads to release of T3 and T4. During thyroid hormone release, colloid from the follicular lumen is endocytosed. This process is regulated by thyroid-stimulating hormone (TSH). T4 is resorbed within the thyroid cells and then transferred to the plasma, which is also regulated by TSH (21). The breakdown of thyroglobulin and release of T3 and T4 are inhibited by various chemicals, including iodine, which inhibits the stimulation of thyroid adenylate cyclase by TSH. Calcitonin, which is produced by the C cells lowers serum calcium by acting on bone, kidney, and the gastrointestinal tract (22).

C. Effects of Various Drugs in the Thyroid

A variety of drugs can inhibit thyroid hormone synthesis. Antithyroid drugs can act by inhibiting thyroid iodine transport or organic binding and coupling reactions (16). (*i*) Chemicals in the first group include thiocyanate and perchlorate. (*ii*) The second group includes thioamides such as propylthiouracil, methimazole, and phenylbutazone. (*iii*) The third groups includes lithium, which inhibits organic-binding reactions and thyroid hormone release (23). Some natural foods such as members of the genus *Brassica*, which includes cabbage and turnips, have thiocyanates with antithyroid activity. The vegetable cassava has a cyanogenic glycoside linamarin, which can be metabolized to thiocyanate with antithyroid activity (16).

Amiodarone Toxicity

Amiodarone is used to treat patients with cardiac arrhythmias. It contains a large amount of iodine, so

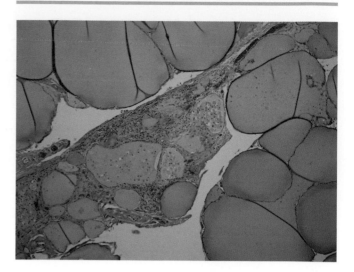

Figure 1 Amiodarone thyroid with follicular disruption, vacuolization of follicular epithelial cells, and degeneration of follicles with infiltration of macrophages and lymphocytes.

it can lead to hyperthyroidism (24–26). It also produces toxic effects in other organs such as the lungs and liver. Amiodarone probably interferes with thyroid hormone production and/or degradation, and effects can range from myxedema to hyperthyroidism. In patients with hyperthyroidism, the morphologic manifestations include follicular disruption, vacuolization of follicular epithelial cells, and degeneration of follicles with infiltration of macrophages and lymphocytes (Fig. 1). The release of colloid from the destroyed follicles probably leads to increased thyroid hormone levels and hyperthyroidism (16).

Diphenylhydantoin (Dilantin)

Diphenylhydantoin or Dilantin is an antiepileptic drug, which competes with thyroxin for thyroxinbinding globulin sites and decreases T4 production (27). Diphenylhydantoin can induce thyroiditis possibly by inducing an autoimmune reaction with the thyroid as the target organ (28).

D. Radiation Changes

The effects of radiation in the thyroid is dependent on the dosage and the radioactive isotope used (29–32). A dose of less than 15 grenz can lead to nodular hyperplasia of the gland. Such changes may be seen in the thyroid after radiation of the tonsils (Fig. 2). Acute changes after radiation include follicular disruption, hemorrhagic necrosis, and neutrophilic infiltration (31). Patients irradiated in the treatment of lymphomas show changes in the thyroid, including hypercellularity, cytologic atypia, increased nodular size, fibrosis, and chronic thyroiditis (29). It is well documented that external radiation can lead to an increased incidence of thyroid cancer (33,34). The

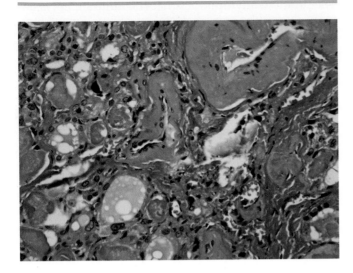

Figure 2 Radiation-induced changes characterized by nuclear pleomorphism and atypia. An associated vessel shows thickening of the wall.

latency period usually consists of several years. After the Chernobyl accident, there was a much shorter latency period for development of thyroid cancer, especially in younger children (35).

II. DEVELOPMENTAL AND HEREDITARY ABNORMALITIES

A. Aplasia and Hypoplasia

These conditions reflect a complete or partial absence of the thyroid gland and are the most common causes of congenital hypothyroidism (16). In North America, abnormalities leading to hypothyroidism occur in 1 in 3000 to 1 in 4000 live births (36). Patients with Di George's syndrome, which is associated with arrested development of the parathyroid and thymus glands associated with the third and fourth bronchial pouches, also have arrested C-cell development (37).

B. Ectopic Thyroid Tissue

Thyroid tissue may be located along the thyroglossal tract, in a lingual, sublingual region, or in the midline below the thyroid gland. Other abnormal locations such as the pericardium, heart, chest wall, vagina, inguinal region, and porta hepatis, have all been reported (38–43). The presence of normal-appearing thyroid tissue in lymph nodes most likely represent metastatic papillary thyroid carcinoma (PTC) to lymph nodes, especially if the lymph nodes are located lateral to the jugular vein (44–47).

C. Thyroglossal Duct Cyst

This is a persistent connection between the median anlage of the thyroid gland, the foramen cecum, and the descended thyroid gland. If the cyst becomes infected, a fistula may develop (48,49). Most thyroglossal duct cysts are between 1 and 4 cm in diameter. Fistulas may develop secondary to infection and may open into the pharynx or skin. The cysts are usually lined by ciliated respiratory epithelium and often undergo squamous metaplasia. Thyroid follicles may be present in the cyst wall. With chronic infection, the epithelial lining may be lost. Treatment is with surgical excision of the entire tract of the duct down to the foramen cecum to prevent recurrence (16). A significant complication in thyroglossal duct cysts is the development of carcinomas that are usually papillary carcinomas (45), although other types of carcinomas including anaplastic carcinomas have developed in these remnants (50).

D. Parasitic Nodule

A parasitic nodule is a thyroid nodule in the neck that is anatomically separate from the main thyroid gland. The thyroid gland is often a multinodular goiter (51,52). The parasitic nodule probably results from a colloid or hyperplastic nodule located outside of the thyroid gland, which becomes enlarged and migrates laterally in the neck. It may sometimes be connected to the thyroid gland by a thin strand of fibrovascular tissue, or it may be completely separate and obtain its blood supply from the surrounding tissues. The nodules may range from 1 to 4 cm in diameter (16). The histologic appearance is similar to normal thyroid tissue with hyperplastic or colloid-filled follicles. The presence of many lymphoid cells in a patient with Hashimoto's thyroiditis and a parasitic or sequestered nodule may lead to a mistaken diagnosis of metastatic carcinoma to a lymph node (53).

E. Hereditary Abnormalities

Transcription Factor Deficiency

Transcription factors are proteins produced by specific cell types, which regulate gene activity by interacting with nuclear DNA (16). They affect development and the regulation of specific genes in adults (54,55). Several transcription factors important for the development and regulation of thyroid follicular cells have been reported. These include TTF-1, TTF-2, and PAX8 (55,56). These genes are important for the regulation of thyroglobulin and thyroid peroxidase genes. They also influence the expression of TSH receptors (37,56–64). Deficiency of TTF-1 has been linked to congenital goiter (37).

Genetic Disorders of the Thyrotropin Receptor Gene

Genetic alterations of the thyrotropin receptor gene have been associated with nonautoimmune hyperthyroidism (61–63). Cases of congenital hyperthyroidism secondary to mutations of the thyrotropin receptor gene are very uncommon (61). This disorder has been reported in four family members with loss of function mutations of the *TSH receptor* gene (63).

III.   THYROID DISORDERS

A.   Autoimmune Thyroid Diseases

Hashimoto Disease

Hashimoto thyroiditis is an autoimmune disease characterized by a goiter and circulating antithyroglobulin and antithyroid peroxidase (antimicrosomal) antibodies. Hashimoto thyroiditis is more common in women and occurs in middle age. Patients are often hypothyroid and treated with thyroxine. Hashimoto thyroiditis is the most common thyroid disease in children and adolescents (65). Different human leukocyte antigen (HLA) haplotypes have been associated with Hashimoto disease (66). Hashimoto thyroiditis is associated with other autoimmune diseases (67). Individuals with Down syndrome have an increased susceptibility to autoimmune thyroid diseases, including Hashimoto thyroiditis (68).

Grossly, the thyroid is enlarged and firm with an irregular surface. Increasing fibrosis can be noted with increasing age. The cut surface of the gland may show areas of fibrosis and pale tan color because of the chronic inflammatory infiltrate, unlike the beefy red diffuse appearance of the thyroid in Graves disease, the parenchyma shows atrophic-appearing follicles intermixed with a marked lymphoid infiltrate with follicles and germinal center formation (Fig. 3). Cells are usually prominent, and foci of squamous metaplasia and fibrosis are usually present.

A number of variants of Hashimoto thyroiditis have been described, including: (*i*) a fibrous variant, (*ii*) a fibrous atrophy variant, (*iii*) a juvenile variant, and (*iv*) a cystic variant. The fibrous variant is particularly problematic as it can be confused with Riedel thyroiditis as well as carcinoma clinically and grossly because of its adherence to adjacent structures. Microscopically, the parenchyma retains its normal lobular architecture and lacks cytologic features of malignancy.

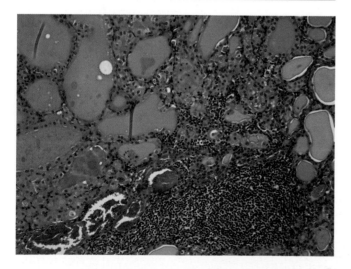

Figure 3   Hashimoto thyroiditis with a marked lymphocytic infiltrate with follicles and germinal centers and prominent Hurthle cells.

The prominent lymphoplasmacytic infiltrate in Hashimoto thyroiditis can be mistaken for malignant lymphoma. Because thyroid lymphomas usually arise in the setting of Hashimoto thyroiditis, a high index of suspicion is needed when examining thyroid tissues with atypical lymphocytes.

Graves Disease

Graves disease (diffuse hyperplasia) is the most common cause of hyperthyroidism. Graves disease is an autoimmune disease characterized by hyperthyroidism associated with circulating autoantibodies against the TSH receptor. Women are more commonly affected with a female to male ratio of 8:1. Patients usually present after age 20, but Graves disease may also occur in children. In the United States, Graves disease affects about one in every 2000 people. A study of Olmstead County, Minnesota, estimated the incidence to be 30 cases per 100,000 persons per year (69,70). Patients often have a family history of autoimmune diseases, particularly autoimmune thyroid diseases, and there is an association with HLA-B8 and DR3. Patients can present with signs and symptoms of hyperthyroidism including anxiety, insomnia, fatigue, tachycardia, diaphoresis, tremor, heat sensitivity, weight loss with normal eating, and goiter. Graves ophthalmopathy and dermopathy may develop in some patients with Graves disease. Graves disease is diagnosed clinically by physical examination and laboratory testing, including elevated serum thyroxine with low levels of thyroid-stimulating hormone and high radioactive iodine uptake. Untreated, Graves disease can cause severe thyrotoxicosis, thyroid storm, osteoporosis, catabolism of muscle and bone with myopathy, neonatal hyperthyroidism by transplacental transfer of thyroid-stimulating antibodies, among others complications. Graves disease is treated with β-blockers, which relieve signs and symptoms of hyperthyroidism such as tachycardia, agitation, and tremors, antithyroid medications (propylthiouracil and methimazole), radioactive iodine treatment, and surgery.

Grossly, thyroid glands are usually diffusely enlarged. Histologically, the follicular cells are columnar and hyperplastic, and colloid is decreased with scalloping of colloid seen around the apices of the epithelial cells within the follicle (Fig. 4). Papillae with fibrovascular cores can be seen and mistaken for PTC (Fig. 5). A lymphocytic infiltrate is commonly seen. Patients are often treated prior to surgery, which changes the histologic features. Patients treated with iodine before surgery show involution of the epithelium with cuboidal rather than columnar cells, increased colloid, and decreased vascularity. Antithyroid medications (propylthiouracil and methimazole) are associated with hyperplastic changes.

In most cases, the differential diagnosis between Graves disease and PTC is relatively easy, but on occasion Graves disease may simulate a PTC with papillary fronds and fibrovascular cores. The cytologic features of PTC with the cytoplasmic clearing, large nuclei with irregular nuclear membranes, nuclear clearing ("Orphan Annie" nuclei), nuclear grooves,

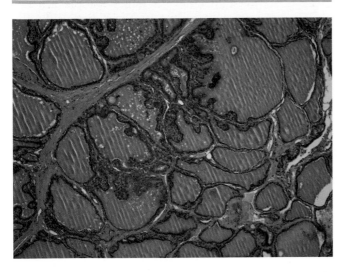

Figure 4 Graves disease characterized by columnar and hyperplastic follicular cells.

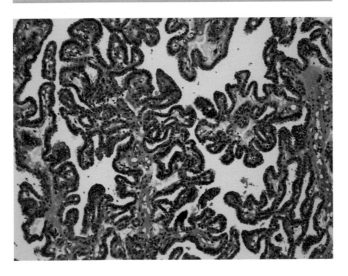

Figure 5 Graves disease with marked papillary formations that can be confused for papillary thyroid carcinoma.

and intranuclear holes are helpful in separating PTC from Graves. In difficult cases of Graves disease with papillary hyperplasia, p27 protein and HBME-1 may be used to separate these two lesions. p27 shows higher expression in Graves disease compared with PTC (71). Graves disease differs from toxic nodular goiters, which can also be associated with hyperthyroidism by the multinodular appearance of the gland in toxic multinodular goiters and the focal involvement histologically as opposed to the diffuse enlargement of the thyroid and diffuse involvement of the parenchyma in Graves disease. Hyperfunctioning follicular adenomas and carcinomas can also be associated with hyperthyroidism, but they are single nodules or tumors rather than diffuse involvement of the gland as in Graves disease.

Postpartum Thyroiditis

Postpartum thyroiditis is an autoimmune disorder, which occurs in approximately 7.5% of women (72), although incidences ranging from 1.9% to 16.7% have been reported (72,73). The thyroid dysfunction occurs in the first postpartum year, usually within the first six months, and is associated with microsomal antibodies in the serum (73). The early thyrotoxic phase may go unnoticed although laboratory testing shows low radioactive iodine or technetium in the thyroid as opposed to the high uptake seen in Graves disease (73). The hypothyroid phase lasts longer and is treated by short-term thyroxine replacement (73). Although thyroid dysfunction is usually transient, some patients may remain permanently hypothyroid, and there is a risk of recurrent disease with subsequent pregnancies (73). Histologically, postpartum thyroiditis is characterized by focal or diffuse chronic thyroiditis and resembles spontaneous silent thyroiditis (74). Follicular disruption and hyperplastic follicular change are seen in the hypothyroid phase and early recovery phase (74). In the late recovery phase, only focal lymphocytic infiltration is seen (74).

Focal Lymphocytic Thyroiditis

Focal lymphocytic thyroiditis (nonspecific thyroiditis, focal autoimmune thyroiditis) is characterized by dense lymphoid aggregates with or without germinal center formation in the fibrous tissue of the thyroid (75,76). Elderly patients are more commonly affected with autopsy studies showing approximately 20% of thyroids with focal lymphocytic thyroiditis (77). Women are affected more often then men (78). Focal lymphocytic thyroiditis is thought to be an incidental finding.

Riedel Thyroiditis

Riedel thyroiditis is a rare inflammatory condition in which the thyroid gland becomes densely fibrotic. The fibrosis replaces the normal thyroid parenchyma and can involve adjacent structures (79,80) and result in hypoparathyroidism (80,81), recurrent laryngeal involvement, esophageal compression (82), and airway obstruction (83,84). Most patients present with painless goiter. An autoimmune etiology has been suggested, and it can be a manifestation of multifocal fibrosclerosis (85–88), which can be associated with orbital involvement (86), idiopathic retroperitoneal fibrosis (87), sclerosing mediastenitis, sclerosing cholangitis (86), pituitary involvement (86), and testicular involvement (86). Riedel thyroiditis is more common in women and usually occurs in adults.

Grossly, the thyroid is enlarged, hard, and fibrotic. The fibrosis can extend beyond the thyroid into the soft tissues of the neck. This gross appearance correlates with the clinical differential diagnosis of Riedel thyroiditis versus high-grade fast growing malignancies such as anaplastic thyroid carcinoma and lymphoma. Histologically, the dense fibrous tissue diffusely effaces the normal thyroid parenchyma and a mixed inflammatory infiltrate is present (Fig. 6).

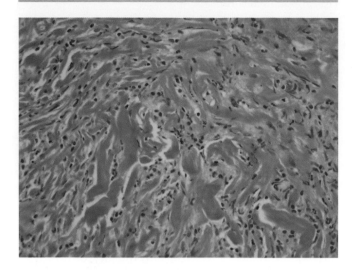

Figure 6 Reidel thyroiditis with dense fibrous tissue diffusely effacing the normal thyroid parenchyma.

The fibrosis can grossly or microscopically extend beyond the thyroid into adjacent soft tissue or anatomic structures. Occlusive phlebitis may also be seen (89). Giant cells are not prominent, which help in differentiating Riedel thyroiditis from granulomatous thyroiditis, although granulomatous thyroiditis lacks the extensive fibrosis seen in Riedel thyroiditis. The fibrous variant of Hashimoto thyroiditis may be confused with Riedel thyroiditis (90). Patients with the fibrous variant of Hashimoto thyroiditis are hypothyroid (although Riedel thyroiditis can also be associated with hypothyroidism), have high antibody titers, lack pressure symptoms, and often have diagnostic fine needle aspiration biopsies (90). Histologically, the fibrous variant of Hashimoto does not extend beyond the thyroid into the soft tissues as is seen in Riedel thyroiditis (90). Also, occlusive phlebitis and vasculitis may be seen in Riedel thyroiditis, but not in the fibrous variant of Hashimoto thyroiditis (90).

Riedel thyroiditis may be treated surgically if decompression is needed. Hypothyroidism, if present, is treated with levothyroxine therapy. Corticosteroids and tamoxifen are also used (91,92). Tamoxifen induces transforming growth factor-β, which inhibits fibroblast proliferation. Although the clinical and pathologic findings can be striking, Riedel thyroiditis is generally self-limiting and has a favorable prognosis.

B. Goiters

Simple and Multinodular Nontoxic Goiter

A goiter is an enlarged thyroid gland. There are many types of goiters, including simple nontoxic goiter, multinodular nontoxic goiter, dyshormonogenetic goiter, toxic multinodular goiter, and endemic goiter. Simple nontoxic goiters can be either sporadic or endemic. Endemic goiters occur in geographical

areas of iodine deficiency in which people are not able to get sufficient iodine in their diet. With the advent of iodized table salt, endemic goiters are very uncommon in most areas. Sporadic nontoxic goiter is the most common nontoxic goiter in the United States, affecting approximately 5% of the population. Sporadic goiters are more common in women and are very rare in children. Simple nontoxic goiters usually occur when the thyroid gland is unable to produce enough thyroid hormone, resulting in enlargement of the thyroid gland to overcome this deficiency. The cause of sporadic nonendemic goiters is unknown in most cases. Certain medications such as lithium and aminoglutethimide can be associated with nontoxic goiters. A hereditary component is also present in some patients (93).

Goiterous thyroids are usually slow-growing and painless. Pain may be associated with hemorrhage. A sudden increase in growth, or a new discrete nodule, is of concern as it may be the sign of a carcinoma developing in association with the goiter (94). A study from Italy identified carcinoma in 13.7% of patients operated for goiter and concluded that the risk of malignancy in multinodular goiter should not be underestimated and that a dominant nodule in this setting should be considered similar to a solitary nodule in an otherwise normal thyroid gland (95). Goiters may cause obstructive symptoms such as dyspnea and stridor with exertion due to tracheal compression. If the goiter extends posteriorly to compress the esophagus, then patients may experience dyspnea. Compression of the recurrent laryngeal nerve can cause change in voice, and compression of venous outflow through the thoracic inlet may result in dilated veins in the neck.

Grossly, the thyroid gland is enlarged in both simple and multinodular goiters. The normal thyroid gland weighs 15 to 20 g, while goiterous thyroid glands can weigh over a 100 g. Simple goiters are diffusely enlarged, while multinodular goiters show multiple nodules grossly (Fig. 7). Microscopically, simple and multinodular goiters are composed of a

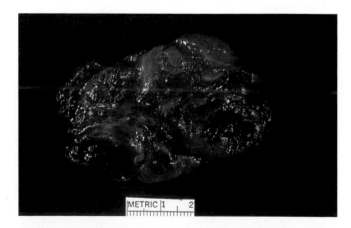

Figure 7 Multinodular goiter demonstrating enlargement of the thyroid by multiple nodules.

mixture of smaller follicles with cuboid lining cells and larger follicles with flattened lining cells. Cystic areas due to large distended follicles are also noted. In multinodular goiters, the parenchyma is organized into nodulesthat compress the adjacent thyroid parenchyma. In multinodular goiters, it can be difficult to distiniguish a follicular adenoma from a nodule, particularly a dominant nodule. Furthermore, clonality has been shown in adenomatous nodules also. Follicular carcinoma arising in the setting of a multinodular goiter must show a clearly invasive growth pattern.

Goiters are treated with thyroxine and radioactive iodine as well as surgery in symptomatic patients, although goiters can recur in a minority of patients.

Dyshormonogenetic Goiter

Dyshormonogenetic goiters are characterized by thyroid hyperplasias usually because of an autosomal recessive genetic defect in the pathways of thyroid hormone synthesis (96). Most dyshormonogenetic goiters develop in childhood, usually at birth or infancy with hypothyroidism or goiter. Patients may present with growth deficiencies. However, in a recent study of 56 patients with dyshormonogenetic goiters, the patients ranged in age newborn to 52 years, although the median age was 16 years, and 75% of the cases occurred before 24 years of age (96). Hypothyroidism is often present, although some patients may be euthyroid or have subclinical hypothyroidism.

Pendred's syndrome (PDS) is the association of congenital goiters with congenital sensorineural deafness and incidences as high as 7.5 to 20 in 100,000 individuals have been reported (97–99). This disorder is estimated to account for 10% of patients with hereditary deafness (97). The syndrome was first linked to chromosome 7q22–31.1, and the *PDS* gene has been cloned (97). The *PDS* gene encodes pendrin, an iodide/chloride transporter.

Histologically, dyshormonogenetic goiters are enlarged and multinodular and are markedly cellular (96,100). The nodules can show many patterns, but solid and microfollicular are common with minimal colloid (96,100). Marked nuclear atypia with nuclear enlargement, mitoses and fibrosis separating the nodules and resulting in an irregular growth pattern are features that can be confused with malignancy (96). In the study by Ghossein et al., 18% of cases showed such prominent hyperplasia and atypia that a mistaken diagnosis of follicular, papillary, medullary, or undifferentiated carcinoma was considered (96). Malignancies have been reported in dyshormonogenetic goiters (96,101–103). In Ghossein's series of 56 dyshormonogenetic thyroids, three showed a micropapillary carcinoma (96). Although papillary carcinomas have been reported by others as well (102), follicular carcinomas (103) are particularly noted, and metastases and anaplastic transformation have been documented (103).

Toxic Multinodular Goiter

Patients with multinodular thyroid glands can develop thyrotoxicosis, often insidiously and usually in goiters that have been present for many years. The symptoms of thyrotoxicosis are similar to that seen in Graves disease, but patients lack the ophthalmic changes seen in Graves disease. Plummer described thyrotoxicosis due to autonomous hyperfunction of a nodule within a multinodular thyroid gland. Multinodular goiters can also be associated with thyrotoxicosis. Grossly, toxic multinodular goiter is enlarged and composed of multiple nodules with fibrosis, appearing similar to that of nontoxic multinodular goiter. Histologically, the nodules in toxic multinodular goiter are composed of hypercellular nodules with tall columnar cells and may show papillary hyperplasia as well as nodules that appear more inactive with follicles lined by flattened epithelium. The pattern of hypercellularity of toxic multinodular goiter with areas or nodules of hypercellularity differ from that of dyshormonogenetic goiters, which show more diffuse hyperplasia throughout the gland. Patients with toxic multinodular goiters are usually treated with radioactive iodine and possibly surgery.

Endemic Goiter

Endemic goiters are most common in geographic areas of iodine deficiency. In these areas, people are not able to get sufficient iodine in their diet. With the advent of iodized table salt, endemic goiters are very uncommon in most areas, including the United States. Endemic goiters grossly and microscopically are similar to multinodular goiters.

Amyloid Goiter

Amyloid goiter can present as a diffuse enlargement of the thyroid gland or as a mass lesion. Patients may or may not be symptomatic. Symptomatic patients usually have a nontender, rapidly enlarging neck mass with compressive symptoms (104). Amyloid goiters are often associated with no clinical or laboratory thyroid dysfunction (104). It has been identified in patients with primary systemic amyloidosis (105,106) and secondary amyloidosis from a variety of conditions (107–109). Unlike the stromal amyloid seen in medullary thyroid carcinoma (MTC), the amyloid in these goiters is often in large masses or diffusely involving the gland. Amyloid often involves the thyroid in secondary amyloidosis, but amyloid goiters are not common (110). The masses of amyloid seen in amyloid goiters may be associated with a foreign body–type giant-cell response, and adipose tissue has also been described (104,111). The amyloid shows characteristic apple-green birefringence with Congo red stain. Thyroidectomy may be performed in symptomatic patients to alleviate compressive symptoms (104). There are a few case reports of thyroid carcinomas in association with amyloid goiters (112,113).

C. Infections and Granulomatous Diseases

Acute Thyroiditis

Acute thyroiditis is usually caused by bacteria, although fungi and viruses have also been implicated. In the majority of cases, the thyroid is secondarily involved by a systemic infection or local infection in the neck (114–117). Patients usually present with systemic symptoms of chills, fever, and malaise with an enlarged and painful thyroid. *Staphylococcus aureus, Streptococcus pyogenes, Streptococcus epidermidis,* and *Streptococcus pneumoniae* are gram-negative bacilli and *Peptostreptococcus* are common isolates (118). Trauma, ischemic necrosis, and thyroid tumoral embolism from visceral cancer, and aggressive malignant thyroid tumors can also present clinically as acute thyroiditis, although they would differ histologically (119–121). A study of 30 patients with similar clinical presentations of acute thyroiditis from Taiwan was reported (121). Most patients (i.e., 25) were subsequently diagnosed with acute thyroiditis and five with aggressive malignant thyroid tumor, and it was found that older age at diagnosis, dysphonia, large size of lesions, anemia, and sterile cultures from thyroid aspirates were significant features favoring malignancy over acute thyroiditis (121). Histologically, acute thyroiditis is characterized by acute inflammation of the thyroid gland with neutrophils and microabscess formation as well as foci of necrosis. Special stains for bacteria and fungal organisms can help identify the organism. Treatment with antimicrobials is usually effective with surgical drainage if abscesses are present.

Granulomatous Thyroiditis

Granulomatous inflammation occurs in the thyroid in a variety of conditions, including infection, sarcoidosis, foreign body reaction, reaction to hemorrhage, among others.

Granulomatous thyroiditis goes by a number of other names, including nonsuppurative thyroiditis, subacute thyroiditis (a clinical term), and De Quervain's thyroiditis. Granulomatous thyroiditis is usually associated with pain and systemic symptoms such as fever, malaise, and weakness. The clinical course of granulomatous thyroiditis has been divided into hyperthyroid phase, hypothyroid phase, and recovery phase. A study from the Mayo Clinic of Olmsted County, Minnesota showed an age- and sex-adjusted incidence of 4.9 cases per 100,000 per year with pain, which was the presenting symptom in 96% of patients, and recurrence in 4% (122). Granulomatous thyroiditis is more common in women. An Australian study found that subacute thyroiditis accounted for 9.9% of patients scanned for hyperthyroidism, with 84% of cases being painful (123). The etiology is unknown, but granulomatous thyroiditis is thought to be caused by a viral infection, either systemic or an infection of the thyroid itself. The majority of patients have recently had an upper respiratory infection (124). Epidemiologic studies have shown association of subacute thyroiditis with specific viruses such as mumps (125), Coxsackie (126), adenovirus (127), influenza (127), Epstein–Barr virus (EBV) (128), measles (129), mononucleosis (129), as well as in the setting of HIV infection (130) and hepatitis C infection (131). A case of subacute thyroiditis has recently been reported following influenza vaccine (132).

The term "subacute thyroiditis" has also been used to describe a painless form of thyroiditis referred to as subacute lymphocytic thyroiditis or painless subacute thyroiditis. These patients may present with a mass lesion and mimic a malignancy or mild thyromegaly (133). In these patients, thyroid glands usually show granulomatous thyroiditis. Histologically, granulomatous thyroiditis is characterized by patchy uneven involvement of the thyroid by neutrophils and microabscesses early on to noncaseating granulomas with colloid, lymphocytes, plasma cells, macrophages, and foreign body–type multinucleated giant cells and loss of follicular epithelium over time (134,135). Lymphoid follicles with and without germinal centers are also noted (135). Immunophenotypically, the giant cells are positive for CD68 and negative for thyroglobulin and keratin (135). The lymphocytes are positive for CD3 and CD8 (135). The overwhelming majority of patients recover in a few months. Mild cases are treated with aspirin, while prednisone is used in severe cases.

Palpation Thyroiditis

In 1975, Carney described palpation thyroiditis as multifocal granulomatous thyroiditis (136). Palpation thyroiditis was identified in greater than 80% of surgically resected thyroids (136). This histologic finding was associated with thyroids that were traumatized by palpation. The number of foci correlates with the vigor of the palpation (136). Single follicles or small groups of follicles are affected. The involved follicles show loss of epithelium and an inflammatory infiltrate with lymphocytes, plasma cells, and prominent histiocytes giving the foci a granulomatous quality.

Granulomatous Infections and Other Causes of Granulomatous Inflammation in the Thyroid

Tuberculosis usually manifests as necrotizing granulomas in the thyroid in patients with other sites of tuberculosis infection, particularly in disseminated tuberculosis and immunocompromised patients (137,138). Other granulomatous infections of the thyroid include fungal and syphilitic thyroiditis as well as disseminated aspergillosis and echinococcosis (137,138). Other noninfectious causes of granulomatous inflammation of the thyroid include sarcoidosis (139,140), Wegener's granulomatosis (141,142), and posttrauma such as surgery or fine needle aspiration.

D. Metabolic Diseases

Metabolic diseases can affect the thyroid gland, including glycogenosis, cystinosis, and lipidoses. Glycogenoses affecting the thyroid include Gierke disease (143) and Pompe disease (type II glycogenosis) (144). In addition to other endocrine organs, intralysosomal glycogen has been identified in the thyroid of patients with Pompe disease (144). Type II glycogenosis and thyroxine-binding globulin deficiency have also been reported in the same family, suggesting that thyroxine may play a role in the activation of acid maltase (145). Hypothyroidism is relatively common in patients with cystinosis (146,147), and abnormal pituitary resistance has been noted as feedback by thyroid hormone in patients with cystinosis (148). Cystine crystals have been associated with destruction and infiltration of epithelium in patients with nephropathic cystinosis (149). Thyroid involvement is reported in patients with the devastating Batten disease (juvenile amaurotic family idiocy) (150), with characteristic intracytoplasmic deposits classic of the disorder (151).

E. Pigment Deposition

Iron

Iron pigment can accumulate in the thyroid follicular cells from trauma with hemorrhage as well as in rare disorders of iron metabolism such as neonatal iron storage disease (152). Although iron pigment in the thyroid is usually not associated with function, patients can develop hypothyroidism.

Minocycline

The classic "black thyroid" seen in patients with chronic minocycline ingestion is another example of pigment accumulation in the thyroid. Grossly, the thyroid is dark brown to black and hence the name "black thyroid." Microscopically, the pigment in the thyroid in patients who take minocycline is dark brown to black and located at the apical portion of the follicular cells and in the colloid, unlike the golden hue of iron, which is usually in the stroma and macrophages. In patients with minocycline-associated black thyroids, ultrastructural studies have shown lysosomal accumulations of lipofuscin-like pigment and granular electron-dense material (153). Pigment accumulation is thought to occur by inhibition of thyroid peroxidase. Although the gross findings are remarkable, minocycline-associated changes are not associated with thyroid dysfunction or malignancy. In patients with black thyroids and malignancy, the tumor is usually not pigmented.

F. Crystals in the Thyroid

Crystals are identifiable in the majority of thyroids, normal or pathological (9,154). Calcium oxalate crystals generally appear during childhood and increase with age (9). Birefringent calcium oxalate crystals are even identifiable in the colloid in struma ovarii (155). Crystals have been recognized in the thyroid for more than 50 years (156). Historical reports exist of calcium oxalate crystals in the thyroid of leprosy patients (157) and in patients killed by hanging (158), among other unusual situations. Patients with chronic renal failure on long-term dialysis have been shown to have oxalate crystals deposition in the thyroid (159). Crystals are less common in Hashimoto's thyroiditis, and the granulomas seen in subacute thyroiditis are related more to colloid than to crystals (9). The presence of birefringent crystals in thyroid parenchyma has diagnostic utility in distinguishing thyroid from parathyroid gland (160).

G. Teflon

Teflon paste (polytef) has been injected for vocal cord paralysis. A pseudotumoral granulomatous foreign body reaction to Teflon can occur and simulate a thyroid tumor or nodule clinically (161–163). The lesion may present as a cold thyroid nodule or a clinical mass simulating carcinoma clinically (161,162). The lesion may present within months or years of the patients prior Teflon injection. Histologically, Teflon granulomas show a granulomatous reaction with refringent particles (162).

IV. THYROID TUMORS

A. Papillary Thyroid Carcinoma

Introduction

PTC is defined as a malignant epithelial tumor showing follicular differentiation and distinctive nuclear features (164). PTC is the most common endocrine malignancy, accounting for 80% of thyroid carcinomas (165).

Clinical Features

PTC is defined as a malignant epithelial tumor showing follicular differentiation and distinctive nuclear features (164). PTC is the most common endocrine malignancy, accounting for 80% of thyroid carcinomas (165). This tumor may occur at any age, with most tumors occurring from 20 to 50 years of age, and women are more commonly affected than men (164). PTC is the most common thyroid carcinoma in children (164). At least 90% of pediatric thyroid carcinomas are papillary carcinomas. Rare cases of congenital PTC have been reported. The overwhelming majority of cases occur sporadically, but familial cases have been identified. PTC has also been identified in association with ataxia telangiectasia (166–168), Gardner syndrome (169), and Cowden syndrome (169). PTC can arise in the thyroid gland as well as in ectopic thyroid tissue, such as struma ovarii. PTC has been identified with variety of thyroid disorders, including Graves disease, Hashimoto thyroiditis, hyperplastic nodules, and a history of radiation exposure.

A history of radiation exposure is frequently associated with PTC (170,171). The Chernobyl accident resulted in large amounts of radioactive iodine being released and was associated with an increase in the incidence of thyroid cancer in children in the Republic of Belarus (35,172–176). These post-Chernobyl pediatric PTCs were associated with a short latency, occurrence in young children, and an almost equal sex ratio (173). Additionally, these radiation-associated tumors were aggressive with intraglandular spread, capsular and soft tissue invasion, metastases, and a high frequency of solid growth pattern (35,172–176). Although radiation-induced tumors show a low prevalence of *BRAF* mutations, they frequently show *RET/PTC* rearrangements (177).

Imaging

PTCs are often identified by ultrasound as well as demarcated or irregular masses. PTC is typically a cold nodule on radioactive iodine scan.

Pathology

Gross features. PTCs are often ill-defined, infiltrative firm masses that are granular and whitish on cut section and may be associated with calcifications (Fig. 8) (165). These tumors can be extremely small and not discernable grossly, although the mean tumor size is about 2 to 3 cm. Papillary carcinomas can be single or multiple and bilateral.

Cytologic features. Fine needle aspiration biopsy shows a cellular aspirate in which follicular cells may be in papillary structures with a branching pattern or sheets. The cells are cuboidal or columnar and have cytologic features classic of PTC, including enlarged and irregular nuclei, nuclear grooves, and nuclear pseudoinclusions. Other features include ropy "bubble gum" colloid and psammoma bodies. Aspiration specimens are of limited utility in typing the variants of PCT because of overlapping features, but the columnar cell variant, tall cell and Hurthle cell variants can be differentiated to a degree, although there are overlapping features (178).

Microscopic features. PTCs are composed of fibrovascular papillae lined by follicular cells with characteristic cytologic features (Fig. 9). Cytologically, PTC shows enlarged, irregular nuclei, nuclear clearing ("Orphan Annie" nuclei), longitudinal nuclear grooves, and intranuclear holes (cytoplasmic invaginations into the nucleus). The colloid in PTC is often darker than that of the surrounding normal thyroid. Psammoma bodies, which are microcalcifications with concentric lamellations, are seen in approximately 50% of cases, most often in tumors with a prominent papillary growth pattern (165). The stroma is often abundant, fibrous, and sclerotic, and a lymphocytic infiltrate can be seen at the periphery of the tumor lobules. Cystic change is not uncommon. Classic cases usually show a predominance of papillary structures, although this feature can be extremely variable. Foci of more solid areas and squamous metaplasia can be seen. Mitotic figures are uncommon.

Numerous variants of PTC have been described (Fig. 10). The importance of these variants rests both in the recognition of the tumor as a PTC and the understanding that some of the variants, such as diffuse sclerosing variant, tall cell variant, columnar cell variant, and solid variant have more aggressive behavior than conventional PTC. Additionally, the cribriform morular variant can be associated with hereditary colonic polyposis and colon carcinoma.

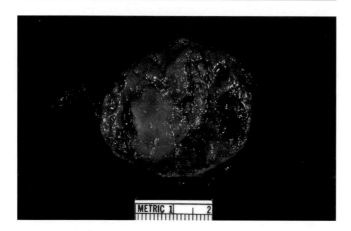

Figure 8 Papillary thyroid carcinoma showing a whitish, firm, infiltrative tumor.

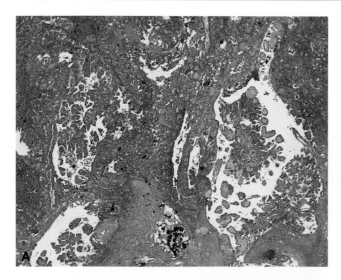
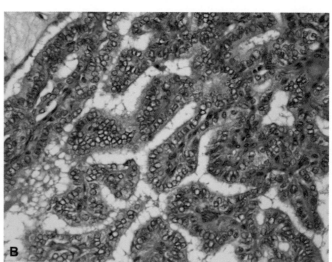

Figure 9 Papillary thyroid carcinoma. (**A**) Papillary thyroid carcinoma showing papillary architectural growth, focal cystic change, infiltrative growth, and calcifications. (**B**) A classic papillary thyroid carcinoma showing papillae with fibrovascular cores covered by epithelial cells with enlarged irregular nuclei with nuclear clearing, nuclear grooves, and intranuclear holes.

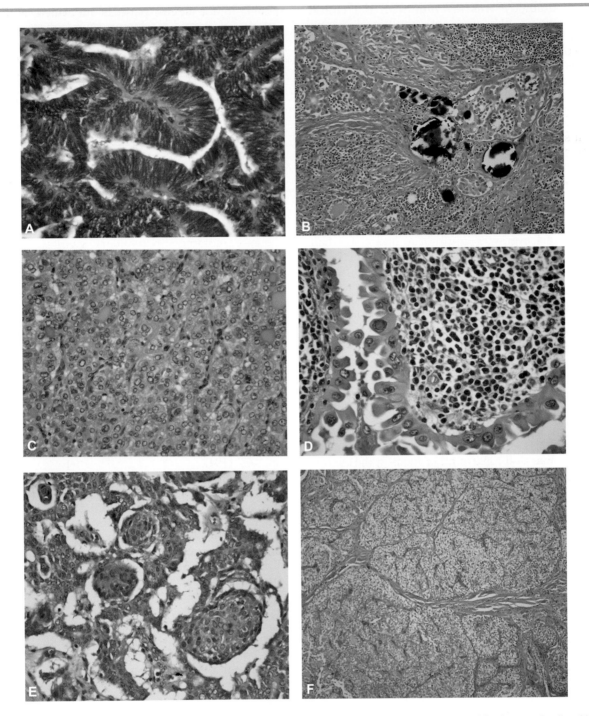

Figure 10 Variants of PTC. (**A**) Columnar variant of PTC—a prominent papillary architectural pattern with elongated cells with nuclear stratification. (**B**) Diffuse sclerosing variant of PTC. (**C**) Solid variant of PTC showing cytologic features of PTC but a solid architectural pattern. (**D**) Warthin-like variant of PTC with oxyphilic cells showing intranuclear holes and a prominent lymphocytic stroma. (**E**) Cribriform-morular variant of PTC with cribriform structures and areas of morular growth. (**F**) PTC with prominent clear cell change. *Abbreviation*: PTC, papillary thyroid carcinoma.

Variants of Papillary Thyroid Carcinoma

Papillary microcarcinoma. Papillary microcarcinoma is defined as a PTC measuring 1 cm or less. These tumors are usually indolent and often identified as an incidental finding in thyroids removed for benign clinical nodules or thyroiditis (179). The overwhelming majority are cured by lobectomy alone. In an autopsy study from Austria, 118 thyroid glands from adults ranging in age from 37 to 77 years were serially sectioned at 2- to 3-mm intervals and 10 (8.6%; 4 females and 6 males) were found to have PTCs (180).

The mean diameter was 4.9 mm with the largest tumor measuring 10.5 mm, with multifocal disease identified in three cases (30%) (180). Although goiters remain common in Austria, the incidence of these tumors is similar to that of nongoitrous regions, suggesting that the levels of iodine intake may only have a minor role in the early phase of the PTC carcinogenesis, but may be important in the progression of latent PTC to clinically evident PTC (180). A Brazilian study of 166 consecutive autopsies and 261 thyroids surgically resected for thyroid disease in general found papillary microcarcinomas in 7.8% of autopsies and 7.2% of surgical material (181). Another surgical series of 380 patients operated for presumably benign thyroid disease identified 27 (7.1%) incidentally discovered papillary microcarcinomas with a mean diameter of 4.4 mm, 40% multifocal, and about half were identified in both lobes (94). A study of 101 consecutive autopsies from Finland identified 52 foci of occult PTC from 36 thyroids (36 of 101, 35.6%) (182). Ten of the thyroids contained multiple (2 to 5) tumor foci (182). They suggested referring to tumors less than 0.5 cm as occult papillary tumors rather than carcinomas. Another author has recently proposed changing the name of papillary microcarcinomas ("the Porto proposal") (183).

The treatment for papillary microcarcinomas has been somewhat controversial. When papillary microcarcinomas present clinically as a lymph node metastasis or a neck mass, they are usually treated as a clinical cancer (179). Up to 15% to 20% of papillary microcarcinomas will have another focus in the contralateral lobe and that long-term recurrent disease may reach 20% or more in the absence of complete resection. Despite their small size, 5% or more of these tumors may be associated with invasion of the capsule or distant metastases (stage III or IV) (184). Papillary microcarcinomas can behave aggressively, with tumors presenting clinically as a solitary cutaneous metastasis (185) and skull metastasis with brain invasion (186). When papillary microcarcinomas present as an incidental finding or as clinically occult, their behavior appears to be different from those presenting clinically (187). In a series of 185 papillary microcarcinomas, most were clinically overt, while 75 were occult (187). Clinically overt tumors were larger and more often multifocal. Extrathyroidal extension, vascular invasion, nodal metastases, and postoperative recurrence occurred in overt papillary microcarcinomas only. The authors concluded that clinically overt PTC should be managed according to tumor risk profile and clinical presentation (187). Other reports have also concluded that clinically evident PTC may be distinctly different from solitary or multifocal papillary microcarcinomas in terms of etiology and behavior, supporting a conservative approach to management (188). However, the issue remains controversial.

Although papillary thyroid microcarcinomas are generally considered to have an excellent prognosis, in the setting of the familial papillary thyroid microcarcinomas, these tumors may behave aggressively (189). A study of 119 patients with papillary thyroid microcarcinoma found familial occurrence in 5.9% of cases (189). In the seven patients identified with family history of thyroid carcinoma, their tumors were multifocal in five cases, bilateral in three, and showed vascular invasion in three. One patient developed lung metastases and died in less than a year. This aggressive behavior in familial cases of papillary microcarcinoma led the authors to suggest more radical treatment and careful follow-up in this setting (189).

RET/PTC rearrangement is the most common genetic alteration in PTC. The prevalence of this rearrangement varies among geographical sites and tumor subtypes (190). *RET/PTC* is more common in PTC associated with radiation exposure. Although numerous *RET/PTC* rearrangments have been identified, *RET/PTC1* and *RET/PTC3* account for greater than 90% of the rearrangments. *RET/PTC1* tends to be more common in papillary microcarcinomas and tumors with typical papillary growth and a more benign clinical course, while *RET/PTC3* is more common in the solid variant of PTC and more aggressive tumor behavior (190).

Follicular variant of papillary thyroid carcinoma. Follicular variant of PTC is the most common variant of PTC and one of the most challenging to diagnose. Crile and Hazard (191) and Hazard et al. (192) are recognized for describing the features in 1953 and 1955, respectively, while the term "follicular variant" was used by Lindsay in 1960 (193). These tumors were originally classified as a type of follicular carcinoma. Chen and Rosai further described the histologic features of these "papillary carcinoma, follicular variant" in 1977 (194).

Numerous patterns have been identified in follicular variant of PTC, including a microfollicular pattern, a macrofollicular pattern, a diffuse pattern, as well as mixtures. Albores-Saavedra's group described 17 cases of the macrofollicular variant of PTC as a "distinctive variant of encapsulated papillary carcinoma that is likely to be confused with macrofollicular adenoma or goiter" (195). These tumors can be particularly difficult to diagnose on fine needle aspiration biopsy (196). Histologically, greater than 50% of the tumor shows a macrofollicular pattern, but foci of conventional follicular variant of PTC are also noted (195). All of the patients in the original description were women, ranging in age from 15 to 69 years. The tumors were relatively large in size with a mean diameter of 4.8 cm, but only two were associated with cervical lymph node metastases, both in tumors with aggressive histologic features including extrathyroidal extension and a widely invasive growth pattern, respectively (195). All patients with follow-up were alive and symptom free two months to six years following surgery (195). Encapsulated tumors can be particularly difficult to diagnose if a clearly identifiable infiltrative growth pattern is not identified or if the tumor shows only borderline features for PTC. The term "well-differentiated tumor of uncertain malignant potential" has been suggested for some of these difficult cases (197). The diffuse pattern of follicular variant of PTC targets younger patients, is often multicentric, shows extrathyroidal extension, nodal metastases, and vascular invasion (198,199).

Recognizing the follicular variant of PTC can be extremely difficult, particularly in differentiating the tumor from a follicular neoplasm as the tumors show architectural similarities. The cytologic features classic of PTC may only be focally noted in follicular variant of PTC, often near the capsule, making the diagnoses very problematic. Recent reports have suggested that this neoplasm may be frequently overdiagnosed by pathologists. A recent study of 87 FVPCA by 10 experienced thyroid pathologists noted that a concordant diagnosis of FVPCA was made by all 10 reviewers with a cumulative frequency of 39% (200). In the 21 cases (24%) with metastatic disease, a diagnosis of FVPCA was made by all 10 reviewers with a cumulative frequency of 66.7%, although seven of the reviewers made a diagnosis of FVPCA with a cumulative frequency of 100% (200). The most important criteria identified to diagnose FVPCA were nuclear pseudoinclusions (cytoplasmic invaginations into the nucleus), abundant nuclear grooves, and ground glass nuclei (200). Although diagnostic agreement among experienced pathologists varies, most diagnosed the tumor in cases that were associated with metastases (200). Follicular variant of PTC behaves similarly to conventional PTC.

Tall cell variant of papillary thyroid carcinoma. The tall cell variant of PTC was described by Hawk and Hazard in 1976 and comprised approximately 10% of the PTCs in their series (201). The tumor is more common in the elderly, and males are affected more commonly than in conventional PTC. The tumors are usually large at diagnosis (>6 cm). The tumors show prominent papillary structures lined by cells in which the height of a cell is at least twice the width. The nuclei are basally located, and the tumors have abundant eosinophilic, oxyphilic cytoplasm. Cytologic features are characteristic of PTC. A prominent lymphocytic infiltrate often accompanies the tumor. The tall cell variant of PTC is an aggressive tumor (202–204). This tumor is commonly associated with extrathyroidal disease, recurrent disease, vascular invasion, and metastases (202). These tumors are associated with shorter disease-free survival than conventional PTC (204), The lethality for these tumors has been reported to be between 20% and 25% (203). Because these tumors are so aggressive, it is important to recognize this variant so that the patients may receive more aggressive treatment and more extensive follow-up (204).

Columnar variant of papillary thyroid carcinoma. The columnar variant of PTC is an uncommon, aggressive variant of PTC that occurs over a wide age range (197,205–208). Histologically, the columnar variant of PTC is characterized by a prominent papillary architectural pattern with elongated cells with nuclear stratification. The nuclear stratification and scant cytoplasm are helpful in differentiating the columnar variant of PTC from the tall cell variant of PTC (203). However, PTCs with both tall cell and columnar features occur (209,210). The tumors show cytoplasmic clearing that has been noted to be similar to that seen in association with secretory-type endometrium (208). The tumors may also show areas of solid growth and organoid or glandular features (208). The tumors may also exhibit foci of solid spindle cells (205), microfollicular and follicular growth (211). The tumor may be encapsulated (212) or unencapsulated (205,206,211–213). Encapsulated columnar cell thyroid tumors are reported to have a more favorable prognosis than those that are unencapsulated and invasive into adjacent thyroid or extrathyroid tissue (211). There does not appear to be an increased incidence of DNA aneuploidy in columnar cell carcinomas to account for their more aggressive behavior (207); however, the proliferation index (MIB-1 index) has been noted to be extremely high in the columnar variant of PTC compared with that of ordinary papillary carcinoma (213). These tumors occur over a wide age range, can metastasize widely, and usually do not respond to radioactive iodine or chemotherapy (207).

Diffuse sclerosing variant of papillary thyroid carcinoma. The diffuse sclerosing variant of PTC was described by Vickery et al. in 1985 as a morphologic variant of PTC (214). This tumor is characterized by diffuse involvement of one or both lobes of the thyroid, extensive squamous metaplasia, numerous psammoma bodies, interstitial fibrosis, and a marked lymphocytic infiltrate (215,216). Diffuse sclerosing PTCs can show widespread intrathyroid lymphatic permeation (216). These tumors are more common in women and in younger individuals. When compared with conventional PTC, diffuse sclerosing PTC shows more aggressive features, including greater incidence of cervical lymph node involvement and lung metastases (216–218). However, the outcome for these patients has been controversial. Although some studies have shown a decreased probability of disease-free survival on follow-up (216) and a worse prognosis (197), others have found that in spite of aggressive histologic features, such as large tumor size and extensive lymph node metastases, overall survival is not significantly different from that of conventional PTC (217,219–221).

Solid variant of papillary thyroid carcinoma. The solid variant of PTC is uncommon, comprising only 2.6% (20 of 756) of PTCs at the Mayo Clinic between 1962 and 1989 (222). Although a variety of thyroid tumors may show focal solid areas of growth, the criteria for inclusion in this study were predominantly (>70%) solid growth pattern of primary tumor, retention of cytologic features typical of papillary carcinoma, and absence of tumor necrosis (222). The solid variant of papillary carcinoma was associated with a slightly higher frequency of distant metastases and less favorable prognosis than classical papillary carcinoma (222). This tumor needs to be distinguished from poorly differentiated thyroid carcinoma, which has a reported lower survival rate compared with the solid variant of papillary carcinoma (222). A study between variants of papillary carcinoma and AMES (age, metastasis, extent, and size) risk classification including 121 PTCs subclassified for cell type and risk groups according to AMES classification system, found that among variants of PTC, solid cell variant has the highest proportion of high-risk tumor classified by the AMES criteria (75%), followed by tall cell subtype with 33.3% of high-risk patients, while conventional PTC classifies only 8.3% as high-risk group (223).

Although the solid cell variant of PTC occurs more commonly in children, this variant was the most common subtype of *PTC* in the Belarussian children after the Chernobyl accident comprising 34% of the PTCs (173). These tumors were associated with lymph node metastases, extrathyroidal etension, and vascular invasion as well as a slightly higher incidence of distant metastases and less favorable prognosis than conventional PTC. Interestingly, two *RET* oncogene rearrangements resulting from inversion of part of chromosome 10 (*PTC1* and *PTC3*) accounted for the majority of RET rearrangements identified in the PTCs of the children post-Chernobyl, with *PTC1* being associated with papillary carcinomas of the classic and diffuse sclerosing variants and *PTC3* with the solid/follicular variant (224). A novel *BRAF* triplet deletion has recently been reported in a PTC displaying a predominantly solid growth pattern (225). The deletion leads to the replacement of a valine and a lysine by a glutamate in the *BRAF* activation segment [BRAF(VK600-1E)] (225).

Oxyphilic (oncocytic/Hurthle cell) variant of papillary thyroid carcinoma. The oxyphilic (oncocytic/Hurthle cell) variant of PTC is an uncommon variant in which the architectural pattern is papillary, the cytoplasm is oxyphilic, and nuclear features are characteristic of PTC. The papillae are lined by a single layer of oncocytic cells with nuclear features of PTC. While some have found that these tumors generally behave similarly to conventional PTC, others have suggested more aggressive behavior similar to that of Hurthle cell carcinomas for these tumors (226). Another study evaluated 1552 patients with thyroid carcinoma and found 42 cases of Hurthle cell variant of PTC (227). The 5-year and 10-year survivals were 94% and 87%, respectively; and the 5-year and 10-year disease-free intervals were 93% and 81%, respectively. Factors correlating with the survival in these tumors included age, extrathyroid extension, primary tumor stage, and regional and distant metastases. Although these tumors were frequently associated with extrathyroidal extension, the prognosis was generally favorable (227). Others have found that tumors with features of both oxyphilic (oncycytic/Hurthle cell) PTC and tall cell variant behave aggressively (228). Oxyphilic (oncocytic/Hurthle cell) PTC must be differentiated from Hurthle cell carcinomas showing papillary architectural features (papillary hyperplasia), but lacking the characteristic PTC nuclear features. This variant must also be distinguished from areas of papillary hyperplasia showing oxyphilic change as can be seen in Hashimoto thyroiditis and Graves disease.

Warthin-like variant of papillary thyroid carcinoma. In 1995, Apel et al. reported 13 cases of "a peculiar thyroid tumor of follicular epithelial differentiation with distinctly papillary architecture, oxyphilic cytology, and lymphocytic infiltrates in papillary stalks" (229). She described the tumor as papillary Hurthle cell carcinoma with lymphocytic stroma "Warthin-like tumor" of the thyroid. This variant of PTC resembles Warthin tumor (papillary cystadenoma lymphomatosum) of the salivary gland with its oxyphilic cells and lymphocytic stroma (229). Warthin-like tumors can be mistaken for benign lymphoepithelial lesions of the thyroid, Hurthle cell carcinoma, and tall cell variant of papillary carcinoma in both fine needle aspiration and histologic specimens (230). There is an association with chronic lymphocytic thyroiditis. Overall, these tumors behave similarly to conventional PTC. As has been documented with conventional PTC, a case of Warthin-like variant of PTC has been documented in association with an anaplastic thyroid carcinoma with an aggressive course as would be expected (231).

Cribriform-morular variant of papillary thyroid carcinoma. The cribriform-morular variant of PTC can occur as sporadic cases (232), but characteristically occurs in the setting of familial adenomatous polyposis (FAP) and germ-line mutations in the *APC* gene (232–236). Chan described a case of PTC with unusual cribriform structures, which was positive for thyroglobulin (233). The cribriform-morular variant of PTC may be solitary or multiple and occurs predominantly in women. Although the tumors are often well demarcated, because of the multicentricity total thyroidectomy has been advocated by some authors (234). The tumor cells have cytologic features of conventional PTC, but the architecture is characterized by cribriform, solid/trabecular, and morular growth. The cribriform areas show anastomosing bars and arches of cells in the absence of intervening fibrovascular stroma (235). Areas of follicular and papillary growth can also be seen. The morular areas are considered to be a helpful clue to the diagnosis and must be distinguished from squamous metaplasia (237). These tumors generally behave similarly to conventional PTC.

The association of the cribriform-morular variant of PTC with FAP is important to consider because patients with FAP may present with this variant of PTC before their colonic findings are known (234). Patients diagnosed with the cribriform-morular variant of PTC should be evaluated for the possibility of FAP. FAP is an autosomal dominantly inherited susceptibility to colonic adenomas and carcinomas as well as childhood medulloblastomas and the cribriform-morular variant of PTC. A recent pathologic and molecular genetic study of five young women with the cribriform-morular variant of PTC found two patients with attenuated FAP (236). Immunohistochemically, the tumor cells were positive for thyroglobulin, neuron-specific enolase, epithelial membrane antigen, high– and low–molecular weight cytokeratins, vimentin, Bcl-2, estrogen and progesterone receptors, and retinoblastoma protein. Germ-line *APC* mutation was identified in only one FAP patient. Somatic mutation analysis of exon 3 of the *β-catenin gene* (CTNNB1) revealed alterations in seven tumors from all five individuals, and two different tumors from two patients with the multicentric PTC had different somatic mutations of the *CTNNB1* gene, suggesting that accumulation of mutant β catenin contributes to the development of the cribriform-morular variant of PTC (236). A report of two FAP kindreds with thyroid cancer with two novel germ-line

APC mutations suggested that genetic alterations in FAP-associated thyroid cancer involve loss of function of APC along with the gain of function of *RET/PTC*, while alterations of *p53* were not common in early PTC (235).

Papillary thyroid carcinoma with nodular fasciitis-like stroma. PTC may rarely show a prominent nodular fasciitis-like stroma (238–240) that can be mistaken for a mesenchymal tumor, a carcinosarcoma, or an anaplastic thyroid carcinoma (238). The low-power appearance is often of a prominent spindle cell stromal component reminiscent of nodular fasciitis in which small tubules and nests of epithelioid cells are noted. The nuclear characteristics of the nested cells are characteristic of PTC. Foci of squamous differentiation and/or papillae may be present (238). When a fibroproliferative lesion is identified in the thyroid, a search should be made for islands of papillary carcinoma (238).

Papillary thyroid carcinoma with lipomatous stroma. PTC with lipomatous stroma (241–243) is an uncommon variant of PTC proposed by Vestfrid in 1986 (243). Mature adipose tissue was identified in numerous papillae in this case (243). Gnepp et al. evaluated 17 lipomatous thyroid lesions at the Armed Forces Institute of Pathology of which seven were PTC (242). The other lesions showing lipomatous change included four adenomatous nodules, one follicular adenoma, one minimally invasive follicular carcinoma, four amyloid goiters, two cases of lymphocytic thyroiditis, one dyshormonogenetic goiter, and one case of thyroid atrophy (242).

Clear cell variant of papillary thyroid carcinoma. The clear cell variant of PTC is uncommon, but appears to have similar behavior to conventional PTC (244–246). Of the 38 thyroid tumors with greater than 50% of the cells showing clear cell change evaluated by Carcangiu et al., seven were PTC (244). The others were follicular tumors (17 cases), Hurthle cell tumors (10 cases), and undifferentiated carcinomas (4 cases). The clear cell change was associated with formation of mitochondrial-derived vesicles, glycogen accumulation, and intracellular thyroglobulin. These tumors must be differentiated from other clear cell tumors, including renal cell metastases to the thyroid (244).

Immunohistochemistry

PTCs are positive for thyroglobulin, TTF-1, and cytokeratins. Immunohistochemical markers that have shown promise in helping to confirm a diagnosis of PTC include HMBE-1 (247, 248, 249–252), galectin-3 (247,248,251,253–255), cytokeratin 19 (247,248,251, 252,256), and CITED-1 (248,251,257), although these markers are not completely specific. PTCs are negative for chromogranin, synaptophysin, and calcitonin.

Electron Microscopy

PTCs show cytoplasmic invaginations in the nuclei (nuclear pseudoinclusions) as well as large nuclei with nuclear clearing. Ultrastructural studies have shown that the intraglandular dissemination typical of the diffuse sclerosing variant of PTC is due to massive lymphatic invasion (258). The cribriform-morular variant of PTC has numerous microfilaments approximately 100-nm long at the nuclear clearing area of the morular regions (259).

Molecular Genetics

RET/PTC rearrangement is a common genetic alteration in PTC. The prevalence of this rearrangement varies among geographical sites and tumor subtypes (190). Overall, approximately 20% to 30% of sporadic adult PTCs have *RET/PTC* rearrangement (164). Although numerous *RET/PTC* rearrangments have been identified, *RET/PTC1* and *RET/PTC3* account for greater than 90% of the rearrangments. *RET/PTC1* tends to be more common in papillary microcarcinomas and tumors with typical papillary growth and a more benign clinical course, while *RET/PTC3* is more common in the solid variant of PTC and more aggressive tumor behavior (190). *RET/PTC* is common in PTC associated with radiation exposure (260,261).

BRAF mutations and *RET/PTC* rearrangments are alternative events in the pathogenesis of PTC (262). *BRAF* mutations, specifically *BRAF(V600E)* is frequently detected in PTC (36–69%) (263). Some studies have found the frequencies of *BRAF* mutation to vary among different variants of PTC, with high frequency in PTC with a papillary or mixed papillary-follicular growth pattern, in Warthin-like PTCs, in micropapillary thyroid carcinomas, and in oncocytic/oxyphilic (Hurthle cell) variant of PTC (263,264). *BRAF* mutations are not common events in pediatric or radiation-associated PTCs (177,265,266). In addition to PTC, *BRAF* mutations are also present in poorly differentiated and anaplastic carcinomas arising from PTC (267).

Differential Diagnosis

PTC must be differentiated from Graves disease with papillary hyperplasia. In most cases, the differential diagnosis is relatively easy, but on occasion Graves disease may simulate a PTC with papillary fronds with fibrovascular cores. The cytologic features of PTC with the cytoplasmic clearing, large nuclei with irregular nuclear membranes, nuclear clearing ("Orphan Annie" nuclei), nuclear grooves, and intranuclear holes are helpful in separating PTC from Graves. In difficult cases of Graves disease with papillary hyperplasia, p27 protein expression has shown some promise in separating these entities, as it has shown significantly higher expression in papillary hyperplasia of Graves disease compared with PTC (71).

Separating the follicular variant of PTC from follicular thyroid neoplasms can be extremely difficult in some cases. Cytologic features classic of PTC may only be focally noted in follicular variant of PTC. One study found the most important criteria identified to diagnose follicular variant of PTC were nuclear pseudoinclusions (cytoplasmic invaginations into the nucleus), abundant nuclear grooves, and ground glass nuclei (200). Immunoperoxidase studies, as noted in the immunohistochemistry section above, including HBME-1, galectin-3, and cytokerain 19 can also be helpful in difficult cases.

The Warthin-like variant of PTC can be mistaken for benign lymphoepithelial lesions of the thyroid, Hurthle cell carcinoma, and tall cell variant of papillary carcinoma in both fine needle aspiration and histology specimens (230). Cytologic features, classic of PTC, are helpful in separating the Warthin-like variant of PTC from benign lymphoepithelial lesions of the thyroid. Cytologic features are also helpful in separating this tumor from Hurthle cell carcinoma. Additionally, the prominent lymphoplasmacytic infiltrate associated with the Warthin-like variant of PTC is a low-power clue to the diagnosis. Although the cells in the Warthin-like variant can be elongated, the height of the cells is not at least twice the width as is seen in the tall cell variant of PTC. The nuclear stratification and scant cytoplasm seen in the columnar variant of PTC are helpful in differentiating the columnar variant of PTC from the tall cell variant of PTC (203).

Treatment and Prognosis

PTCs are often treated by complete thyroidectomy and ipsilateral lymph node dissection. Radioactive iodine can also then be administered in an attempt to ablate any possible remaining tumor, including metastatic sites or suppression of TSH secretion without radioactive iodine. The overall prognosis for patients with PTC is excellent, with greater than 90% overall survival (164). PTCs can show multifocal involvement of the gland, extrathyroidal extension into soft tissues, and has a propensity to metastasize to cervical lymph nodes, particularly ipsilateral lymph nodes, and may spread to the lung (165). Unfavorable prognostic features include older age, male sex, large tumor size, multicentricity, blood vessel invasion, extrathyroidal extension, distant metastases, aneuploidy, high microscopic grade, progression to poorly differentiated carcinoma (165). Other poor prognostic features include tumor necrosis, vascular invasion, numerous mitoses, and marked nuclear atypia (268). Recognition of the variants of PTC is important as some of them, including the tall cell variant of PTC (202,204,243,269), the columnar variant of PTC (207), the solid variant of PTC, and Hurthle cell variant of PTC (227), may be more aggressive tumors. The tall cell variant of PTC is an aggressive tumor (202–204) commonly associated with extrathyroidal disease, recurrent disease, vascular invasion, and metastases (202). These tumors are associated with shorter disease-free survival than conventional PTC (204) and fatal in 20% to 25% (203). It is important to recognize this variant so the patients may receive more aggressive treatment and more extensive follow-up (204). The columnar variant is also aggressive, can metastasize widely, and may not respond to radioactive iodine or chemotherapy (207). A study between variants of papillary carcinoma and AMES risk classification included 121 PTCs subclassified for cell type and risk groups according to AMES classification system, found that among variants of PTC, solid cell variant has the highest proportion of high-risk tumor classified by the AMES criteria (75%), followed by tall cell subtype with 33.3% of high-risk patients, while conventional PTC classifies only 8.3% as high-risk group (223). The solid cell variant is common in children, particularly those who have been exposed to radiation, such as the Chernobyl accident (173). These tumors were associated with lymph node metastases, extrathyroidal extension, and vascular invasion as well as a slightly higher incidence of distant metastases and less favorable prognosis than conventional PTC. The oxyphilic (oncocytic/Hurthle cell) variant of PTC has also been found by some authors to behave more aggressively (228).

B. Hyalinizing Trabecular Tumor

Introduction and Clinical Features

In 1987, Carney et al. described "hyalinizing trabecular adenoma" as a unique thyroid tumor that can mimic medullary and papillary carcinoma microscopically (270). In their original series of 11 cases, all were from women of ages 27 to 72 (mean, 46 years). The tumors were originally diagnosed by other pathologists as carcinoma, adenoma, paraganglioma, and "indeterminate." None of the tumors recurred or metastasized with a mean follow-up of 10 years (270). Many additional case reports and small series followed (271–274). In 1994, Molberg and Albores-Saavedra described three cases of hyalinizing trabecular thyroid tumors with capsular invasion, two of which also showed vascular invasion and suggested that hyalinizing trabecular thyroid adenomas had a malignant counterpart (275). All three patients were free of disease at one to two years follow-up (275). A few additional cases showing capsular and vascular invasion have been reported (276). These lesions are now generally referred to as hyalinizing trabecular "tumors." Since most hyalinizing trabecular tumors in the literature are benign, they should probably only be considered malignant when there is obvious capsular or vascular invasion or metastasis (277).

Pathology

Gross features. Hyalinizing trabecular tumors are grossly yellow-tan, encapsulated, circumscribed nodules (270). The neoplasms measure from 0.3 to 4 cm in diameter (270).

Cytologic features. Aspirates of hyalinizing trabecular tumors have features overlapping with PTC, including cellularity, nuclear grooves, and intranuclear cytoplasmic inclusions (278). The Papanicolaou method highlights the intranuclear inclusions, nuclear grooves, and nuclear overlapping, while the Diff–Quik method highlights the hyaline material, perinucleolar clearing, and cytoplasmic bodies (278). Hyalinizing trabecular tumors generally lack papillary architecture and psammoma bodies (279). The presence of radially oriented cohesive cells, very frequent nuclear inclusions, frequent nuclear grooves, abundant cytoplasm, and hyalin in a bloody background

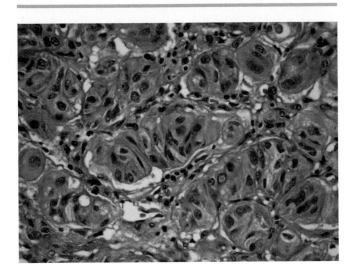

Figure 11 Hyalinizing trabecular tumor composed of sharply outlined polygonal and elongated cells arranged in trabeculae and clusters. The cells show frequent intranuclear cytoplasmic inclusions, a feature that causes confusion with PTC. *Abbreviation*: PTC, papillary thyroid carcinoma.

are features helpful in hyalinizing trabecular tumors in cytology specimens (278).

Microscopic features. Hyalinizing trabecular tumors are encapsulated or circumscribed and solid and composed of sharply outlined polygonal and elongated cells arranged in trabeculae and clusters (270). The cells have fine granular cytoplasm and oval nuclei with perinucleolar vacuoles, acidophilic nuclear inclusions, nuclear grooves, and infrequent mitotic figures (Fig. 11) (270). The tumors show frequent intranuclear cytoplasmic inclusions, a feature that causes diagnostic confusion with PTC (271). Extracellular eosinophilic hyaline fibrosis is noted particularly around vessels that can mimic amyloid, but is negative for Congo red (270). Cytoplasmic yellow bodies are frequently noted in hyalinizing trabecular tumors, but these may also be seen, although numerically infrequently, in papillary carcinoma and in follicular and Hurthle cell neoplasms (280). The diagnosis of hyalinizing trabecular tumor is based on a circumscribed neoplasm forming trabeculae or solid nests, markedly hyalinized stroma, elongated tumor cells with nuclear pseudoinclusions and prominent nuclear grooves, cytoplasmic and cell membrane staining for Ki67 with MIB-1 antibody, and cytoplasmic yellow bodies (277).

Immunohistochemistry

Immunophenotypically, hyalinizing trabecular tumors are positive for thyroglobulin and negative for calcitonin, chromogranin, and CEA, features helpful in differentiating this tumor from MTC (270,276). Hyalinizing trabecular tumors have been reported to be positive for simple epithelial-type keratins 4, 8, 18, and 19 and can show expression of stratified epithelial keratins 1, 5/6, and 13, while many other reports find a

heterogeneous keratin-staining pattern with little positivity for cytokeratin 19 (281–284). These tumors also show cytoplasmic and cell membrane staining for Ki67 with MIB-1 antibody, a feature not seen in PTC (285). Galectin-3 is a β-galactoside-binding lectin, which is overexpressed in many neoplasms and shows variable staining in hyalinizing trabecular tumors (253). A recent study showed variable expression of galectin-3 in hyalinizing trabecular tumors, intermediate between benign and malignant thyroid tumors (253). Hyalinizing trabecular tumors are generally negative for HBME1, a marker that is usually positive in papillary carcinomas, including follicular variant of papillary carcinoma with prominent hyalinization and trabeculation, a tumor that must be differentiated from hyalinizing trabecular adenoma (284).

Electron Microscopy

Ultrastructural studies show the frequent round, pale yellow, cytoplasmic inclusion bodies seen in histologic sections of hyalinizing trabecular tumors, which are consistent with giant lysosomes, with parallel whorled and arrayed membranes referred to as "fingerprint" bodies (286). Another interesting ultrastructural feature reported in hyalinizing trabecular tumors is accumulated basement membrane materials at the periphery of cell clusters (287). The basal aspect of the cells rest on this material, suggesting pseudointracytoplasmic deposits of basement membrane material from cytoplasmic infoldings (287). The material is described as having a mesh-like branching or frame-like appearance (287).

Molecular Genetics

The relationship between hyalinizing trabecular tumor to PTC has been controversial, including the molecular studies (277). *RET* proto-oncogene rearrangments are common in PTC, and reports of *RET* rearrangments detected by reverse transcription-polymerase chain reaction and immunohistochemistry have been published (288,289). However, these findings may not necessarily establish hyalinizing trabecular tumors as variants of PTCs, as *RET/PTC* rearrangements are not completely specific for PTC (277). *RET/PTC* rearrangements have been reported in Hashimoto thyroiditis (290,291), although others did not corroborate these findings (292). Additionally, the studies finding *RET* rearrangments in hyalinizing trabecular tumors included thyroids that also harbored PTCs (288,289), unlike the original study by Carney et al. in which hyalinizing trabecular tumors were not associated with PTCs (270,293). These studies suggest that the detection of *BRAF* mutations in a follicular thyroid tumor may be helpful in differentiating PTC from hyalinizing trabecular tumor (294).

Differential Diagnosis

In the original description of hyalinizing trabecular tumors, the authors noted that the tumor could mimic medullary and papillary carcinoma microscopically (270). A trabecular growth pattern can be seen in both MTC and hyalinizing trabecular tumor. Extracellular eosinophilic hyaline fibrosis in hyalinizing trabecular tumors can be confused with the amyloid of MTCs. Congo red is helpful in this differentiation. Cytologically, the nuclei in hyalinizing trabecular tumors are reminiscent of PTC, unlike the stippled neuroendocrine chromatin pattern seen in MTC. Hyalinizing trabecular tumors also show frequent intranuclear pseudoinclusions. MTC can show intranuclear pseudoinclusions, but they are sparse and uncommon. PTC, which characteristically shows nuclear pseudoinclusions, can be particularly difficult to differentiate from hyalinizing trabecular tumors. The nuclear pseudoinclusions in hyalinizing trabecular carcinoma are very prominent and numerous compared with those seen in most PTCs. The prominent trabecular growth pattern seen in hyalinizing trabecular tumors along with the extracellular eosinophilic hyaline fibrosis are helpful in distinguishing hyalinizing trabecular tumors from PTCs. The diagnosis of hyalinizing trabecular tumor is based on a circumscribed neoplasm forming trabeculae or solid nests, markedly hyalinized stroma, elongated tumor cells with nuclear pseudoinclusions and prominent nuclear grooves, cytoplasmic and cell membrane staining for Ki67 with MIB-1 antibody, and cytoplasmic yellow bodies (277).

Treatment and Prognosis

Although hyalinizing trabecular tumors have been controversial regarding their malignant potential, the overwhelming majority of these tumors behave in an indolent fashion. They should probably only be treated as a malignancy when there is obvious capsular or vascular invasion or metastasis.

C. Follicular Thyroid Tumors

Follicular Adenoma

Introduction. Follicular adenomas are benign, encapsulated thyroid tumors showing follicular differentiation (164).

Clinical features. Follicular adenomas are solitary thyroid nodules that generally present as a mass in the thyroid. These tumors are more common in females than in males, occur most commonly in adults, and are more common in iodine-deficient areas (164).

Imaging. Follicular adenomas are often identified by ultrasound as well as demarcated solitary nodules. Radioactive iodine scans usually show hypofunction (164).

Pathology.

Gross Features. Follicular adenomas are solitary, round to oval in shape, tan or brown in color, and usually measure 1 to 3 cm, although they can be larger (164). They are encapsulated, but the capsule is usually not as thick and irregular as follicular carcinomas.

Cytologic Features. Follicular adenoma aspirates are usually cellular specimens. The cells are usually arranged into microfollicles with little colloid. The follicular cells lack cytologic features diagnostic of PTC. Cytologic aspirates cannot be used to reliably separate follicular adenomas from follicular carcinomas. The

diagnosis of follicular adenoma is based on the lack of capsular and/or vascular invasion after thorough evaluation of histologic specimens.

Microscopic Features. By definition, capsular and vascular invasion are not identified. Follicular adenomas can show a variety of histologic patterns, including microfollicular, normofollicular, macrofollicular, and trabecular patterns. In addition to these patterns, variants of follicular adenoma can be seen. Follicular adenomas with bizarre nuclei, adenolipomas, adenochondromas, mucinous follicular adenomas, toxic adenomas, follicular adenomas with clear cell change, follicular adenoma with papillary hyperplasia, and signet ring cell adenomas are variants of follicular adenoma. Atypical adenomas are follicular neoplasms with high cellularity, nuclear atypia, or unusual histologic patterns, but without definitive vascular or capsular invasion (252). Atypical adenomas usually behave in an indolent fashion.

Immunohistochemistry. Follicular adenomas are positive for thyroglobulin, TTF-1, and low molecular weight cytokeratin (Cam5.2) (164).

Molecular genetics. Specific genetic markers diagnostic of follicular adenoma have not been identified. Follicular adenomas frequently show *RAS* mutations and a small percentage of tumor may show *PAX8* to *peroxisome proliferator-activated receptor gamma (PPARγ)* rearrangements (295,296).

Electron microscopy. Generally, ultrastructural features are not helpful in separating malignant follicular lesions from benign ones (297). Scanning electron microscopy has demonstrated that cilia are present in the center of the follicular surface of epithelial cells in the normal thyroid gland and in most goiters, but they are reduced in number in adenomas and differentiated carcinomas and usually absent in medullary carcinomas and anaplastic carcinomas (298).

Differential diagnosis. Follicular adenomas must be distinguished from follicular carcinomas by the lack of capsular and vascular invasion in the former. Follicular adenomas are differentiated from hyperplastic or adenomatous nodules by a well-defined capsule and a more frequent occurrence as a solitary nodule than the multiple nodules often seen in cases of hyperplastic or adenomatous nodules. One of the most difficult problems in thyroid pathology is differentiating follicular adenoma from follicular variant of PTC as the tumors show architectural similarities. In most cases, the cytologic features of PTC are classic in the follicular variant of PTC. But it is important to carefully evaluate the cytologic features in follicular lesions to rule out a follicular variant of PTC, as classic cytologic features of PTC may only be focally noted often near the capsule in follicular variant of PTC that makes the differential diagnosis difficult in some cases.

Treatment and prognosis. As follicular adenomas are benign, patients are treated with lobectomy and have an excellent prognosis.

Follicular Carcinoma

Introduction. Follicular carcinoma is defined as a malignant epithelial tumor showing follicular differentiation and lacking the diagnostic nuclear features of papillary carcinoma (164).

Clinical features. Follicular carcinomas account for approximately 10% to 15% of clinically evident thyroid carcinomas, is more common in women, most commonly occurs in the fifth decade (rare in children), and has a higher incidence in iodine-deficient regions (164). The tumors present as mass lesions and show infrequent (less than 5%) ipsilateral lymphadenopathy (164).

Imaging. Ultrasound is useful in determining the size and consistency of the tumor as well as guiding fine needle aspiration biopsies. The tumors are cold nodules on scintigraphic scans.

Pathology.

Gross Features. Follicular carcinomas form solid, encapsulated round to oval tumors, tan to brown in color. The capsule is often thicker and more irregular than in follicular adenoma. Minimally invasive follicular carcinomas can be difficult to distinguish from follicular adenomas grossly. Widely invasive tumors may show gross invasion of the capsule or visibly involved vascular structures.

Cytologic Features. Follicular carcinoma aspirates are cellular specimens with follicular cells usually showing a microfollicular pattern with little colloid. The follicular cells lack classic cytologic features of PTC. Aspiration cytology findings cannot reliably distinguish follicular carcinomas from follicular adenomas. Clinical findings associated with malignancy in thyroid aspirates reported as "suspicious for follicular neoplasm" include larger tumors, fixation of mass, and younger age of patient (299). Overall, the diagnosis of malignancy is based on finding capsular and/or vascular invasion in histologic specimens.

Microscopic Features. Follicular carcinomas are cellular tumors with a follicular or solid growth pattern. Rare cases may show clear or signet ring cell change (244). The follicular cells lack cytologic features of PTC. Invasion of the capsule and/or vessels is diagnostic of follicular carcinoma. Capsular invasion is defined as tumor penetrating through the capsule. Capsular invasion often shows a mushroom type of growth pattern through the capsule. Caution must be taken to avoid misdiagnosing fine needle aspiration sites from areas of capsular invasion. Vascular invasion must occur within or beyond the tumor capsule (Fig. 12). Tumors with capsular invasion only (no vascular invasion) tend to behave in a more indolent fashion than those that show vascular invasion (300). Follicular carcinomas have been divided into two major types on the basis of the invasiveness of the tumor, minimally invasive and widely invasive. Minimally invasive follicular carcinomas show focal capsular and/or vascular invasion. Histologic variants of follicular carcinoma include clear and signet ring cell change (244).

Immunohistochemistry. Follicular carcinomas are positive for thyroglobulin, TTF-1, and low molecular weight cytokeratin (Cam5.2) (164). These tumors are also positive for E-cadherin (301–303), with decreased expression a poor prognostic feature in some studies (302). HMBE-1 (304–306), galectin 3

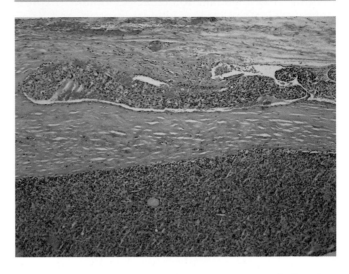

Figure 12 Follicular thyroid carcinoma showing vascular invasion.

(305), and focal cytokeratin 19 expression have been noted (307). PAX8 has also been studied in benign and malignant follicular thyroid neoplasms, and PAX8 is expressed mainly in benign rather than malignant thyroid lesions (308). Well-differentiated thyroid carcinomas express PAX8 more frequently than undifferentiated carcinomas (308).

Electron microscopy. Generally, ultrastructural features are not helpful in separating malignant follicular lesions from benign lesions (297). Scanning electron microscopy has demonstrated that cilia are present in the center of the follicular surface of epithelial cells in the normal thyroid gland and in most goiters, but they are reduced in number in adenomas and differentiated carcinomas and usually absent in medullary carcinomas and anaplastic carcinomas (298).

Molecular genetics. A chromosomal translocation t(2;3)(q13;p25), resulting in fusion of *PAX8* to *PPARγ* encoding a fusion oncoprotein, has been identified in a proportion of follicular thyroid carcinomas (309) and occasionally in follicular adenomas (295,296). *RAS* mutations are also seen in a proportion of follicular carcinomas and appear to be a different molecular pathway for follicular thyroid carcinogenesis from *PAX8–PPARγ* (296). A recent study has shown follicular carcinomas with *PAX8–PPARγ* tended to occur in younger patients with smaller, but overtly invasive, tumors that were usually positive for galectin-3 but not for HBME-1 (296). Follicular carcinomas with *RAS* mutations were often positive for HBME-1 and negative for galectin-3 and were either minimally or overtly invasive (296).

Differential diagnosis. Follicular carcinomas must be differentiated from follicular adenomas, follicular variant of PTC, and poorly differentiated carcinomas. Invasive growth separates follicular carcinoma from follicular adenoma. Follicular carcinomas show capsular and/or vascular invasion. Follicular carcinomas also tend to be larger and have a thicker, more irregular capsule than follicular adenomas. Expression of p27, a cell cycle inhibitory protein, and Ki-67 (MIB-1), a proliferation marker, showed follicular adenomas to have a higher p27-labeling index and a lower Ki67-labeling index than follicular carcinomas (310). Significantly higher expression of Ki67 is also seen in follicular carcinomas associated with metastases than those without metastases (310). Follicular variant of PTC shows cytologic features of PTC. Widely invasive follicular carcinomas need to be differentiated from poorly differentiated thyroid carcinomas. Poorly differentiated carcinomas often show a solid growth pattern with frequent mitoses and necrosis.

Treatment and prognosis. Follicular thyroid carcinomas are treated by total thyroidectomy. The prognosis is very good for minimally invasive tumors with a mortality as low as 3% to 5% in some studies (164). The prognosis is particularly good in those showing capsular invasion only (300). Widely invasive follicular carcinomas are aggressive tumors with a long-term mortality of 50% (164).

D. Hurthle Cell Tumors

Hurthle Cell Adenoma

Introduction. Hurthle cell adenomas are benign thyroid neoplasms composed exclusively or predominantly of Hurthle cells (oxyphil cells, oncocytes). The WHO considers Hurthle cell adenoma an oncocytic variant of follicular adenoma (164). Hurthle cell adenomas are more common than Hurthle cell carcinomas.

Clinical features. Hurthle cell adenoma usually presents as a mass lesion in the thyroid. Women are affected more often than men (311). Hurthle cell adenomas usually occur in adults with a mean age of 45 years, about 5 to 10 years younger than those with Hurthle cell carcinomas (311).

Imaging. Hurthle cell adenoma is often identified by ultrasound as well as demarcated solitary nodule. Ultrasound is useful in determining the size and consistency of the tumor as well as in guiding fine needle aspiration biopsies.

Pathology.

Gross Features. Hurthle cell adenomas are solitary, round to oval in shape, encapsulated, brown neoplasms (164). Infarction with fine needle aspiration biopsies is not uncommon.

Cytologic Features. Aspirates of Hurthle cell adenomas are cellular and usually show microfollicles of Hurthle cells with little colloid. The cells lack the cytologic features classic of PTC as would be seen in the oxyphilic/oncocytic (Hurthle cell) variant of PTC. Hurthle cell adenomas cannot be reliably distinguished from Hurthle cell carcinomas in cytologic specimens. The diagnosis of Hurthle cell adenoma is based on the lack of capsular and/or vascular invasion after thorough evaluation of histologic specimens.

Microscopic Features. Hurthle cell adenomas are encapsulated, but the capsule is usually not as thick and irregular as Hurthle cell carcinomas. By definition, capsular and vascular invasion are not identified. The tumors can show a variety of architectural patterns, including follicles, solid growth, trabecular growth, and areas of papillary growth. Hurthle cell adenomas are composed exclusively or predominantly with over 75% Hurthle cells (165). Hurthle cell adenomas have abundant granular eosinophilic cytoplasm and large nuclei with prominent nucleoli (164,165).

Immunohistochemistry. Hurthle cell adenomas are positive for thyroglobulin and TTF-1 and are negative for chromogranin, synaptophysin, and calcitonin.

Electron microscopy. Ultrastructurally, the abundant eosinophilic cytoplasm of the Hurthle cells is packed with mitochondria. By scanning electron microscopy Hurthle cells, both benign and neoplastic are distinct, smooth-surfaced cells are interspersed among cells rich in microvilli (298).

Differential diagnosis. Hurthle cell adenomas must be distinguished from Hurthle cell carcinomas by the lack of capsular and vascular invasion in the former. Hurthle cell adenomas are generally smaller than Hurthle cell carcinomas. The Ki67-labeling index in Hurthle cell adenomas is significantly lower than that in Hurthle cell carcinoma (312). Diffuse nuclear staining for cyclin D1 is much less common in Hurthle cell adenomas than in Hurthle cell carcinomas (312). Hurthle adenomas are differentiated from hyperplastic or adenomatous nodules often seen in Hashimoto thyroiditis by a well-defined capsule and a more frequent occurrence as a solitary nodule than the multiple nodules often seen in cases of Hashimoto thyroiditis. Hurthle cell adenomas showing papillary growth must be distinguished from the oncocytic/ oxyphilic (Hurthle cell) variant of PTC as the tumors show architectural similarities, although the oncocytic/oxyphilic (Hurthle cell) variant of PTC has cytologic features of PTC, which are not seen in Hurthle cell adenomas with papillary change.

Treatment and prognosis. As Hurthle cell adenomas are benign, patients are treated with lobectomy and have an excellent prognosis.

Hurthle Cell Carcinoma

Introduction. Hurthle cell carcinomas are malignant neoplasms are composed predominantly or exclusively of Hurthle (oncocytic/oxyphilic) cells. The WHO considers Hurthle cell carcinoma the oncocytic variant of follicular carcinoma (oncocytic follicular carcinoma) (164).

Clinical features. A study from Mayo Clinic found that between 1946 and 1971, Hurthle cell carcinoma accounted for 2% to 3% of thyroid carcinomas and approximately one-fifth of all follicular carcinomas (313). Women are more commonly affected than men, and the mean age at diagnosis is approximately 50 to 60 years.

Imaging. Hurthle cell carcinoma is often identified by ultrasound as well as demarcated solitary nodule. Ultrasound is useful in determining the size and consistency of the tumor as well as guiding fine needle aspiration biopsies.

Pathology.

Gross Features. Hurthle cell carcinomas form solid, encapsulated, round to oval tumors, brown in color. The capsule is often thicker and more irregular than in follicular adenoma. Hurthle cell carcinomas are generally larger than Hurthle cell adenomas (312). Minimally invasive Hurthle cell carcinomas can be difficult to distinguish from Hurthle cell adenomas grossly. Widely invasive tumors may show gross invasion of the capsule or visibly involved vascular structures.

Cytologic Features. Apirates of Hurthle cell carcinomas are cellular and usually show microfollicles of Hurthle cells with little colloid. The cells lack the cytologic features classic of PTC as would be seen in the oxyphilic/oncocytic (Hurthle cell) variant of PTC. Hurthle cell carcinomas cannot be reliably distinguished from Hurthle cell adenomas in cytologic specimens. The diagnosis of malignancy is based on finding capsular and/or vascular invasion in histologic specimens.

Microscopic Features. Hurthle cell carcinomas are cellular tumors with a follicular, solid, or trabecular growth pattern. Hurthle cell carcinomas are composed exclusively or predominantly of oncocytic cells in which ultrastructurally are packed with mitochondria. The Hurthle cells lack cytologic features of PTC. Invasion of the capsule and/or vessels is diagnostic of Hurthle cell carcinoma (Fig. 13). Capsular invasion is defined as tumor penetrating through the capsule. Capsular invasion often shows a mushroom type of growth pattern through the capsule. Caution must be taken to avoid misdiagnosing fine needle aspiration sites from areas of capsular invasion. Vascular invasion must occur within or beyond the tumor capsule. Tumors with capsular invasion only (no vascular invasion) tend to behave in a more indolent fashion than those that show vascular invasion (312).

Immunohistochemistry. Hurthle cell adenomas are positive for thyroglobulin and TTF-1 and are negative for chromogranin, synaptophysin, and calcitonin.

Electron microscopy. Ultrastructurally, the abundant eosinophilic cytoplasm of the Hurthle cells is packed with mitochondria. By scanning electron microscopy Hurthle cells, both benign and neoplastic are distinct, smooth-surfaced cells are interspersed among cells rich in microvilli (298).

Molecular genetics. Unlike follicular carcinomas, Hurthle cell tumors show a low prevalence of *PAX8–PPARγ* translocations (314). A recent study evaluating the molecular profile of Hurthle cell tumors and well-differentiated thyroid tumors, using DNA microarray and hierarchical cluster analysis showed the molecular profiles of Hurthle cell adenomas, and carcinomas are more similar to follicular carcinomas than benign lesions or PTC (315). Numeric chromosomal abnormalities, including changes in *p53* and *cyclin D1* have also been studied in Hurthle cell tumorigenesis. Interphase fluorescence in situ hybridization studies have shown chromosomal imbalances as gains are common in both benign and malignant Hurthle cell neoplasm, but Hurthle cell carcinomas tend to have more chromosome losses than adenomas (316). Among Hurthle cell carcinomas, chromosome losses are more frequent in patients who died of disease, particularly chromosome 22 (316). Hurthle cell tumors infrequently show *PAX8-PPARγ* rearrangement or *RAS* mutations (296). Recently, point mutation in *GRIM-19* was described in Hurthle cell neoplasms (317,318). The *GRIM-19* mutations are the first nuclear gene mutations specific to Hurthle cell tumors (318). *GRIM-19* mutations are proposed to be involved in the genesis of Hurthle cell tumors through both mitochondrial metabolism and cell death (318).

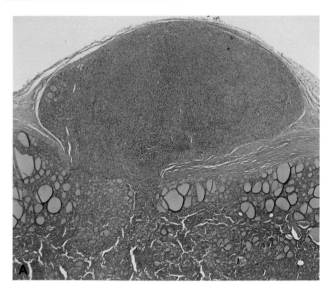 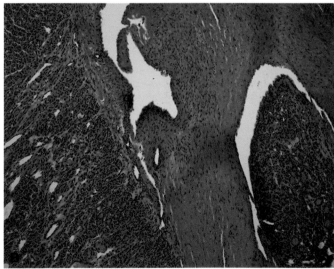

Figure 13 Hurthle cell carcinoma. **(A)** Hurthle cell carcinoma showing capsular invasion. **(B)** Vascular invasion in a Hurthle cell carcinoma.

Differential diagnosis. Hurthle cell carcinomas must be differentiated from Hurthle cell adenomas, the oncocytic/oxyphilic (Hurthle cell) variant of PTC, and the rare oncocytic/oxyphilic variant of MTC. Invasive growth, capsular or vascular, separates Hurthle cell carcinoma from adenoma. Hurthle cell carcinomas also tend to be larger and have a thicker and more irregular capsule than Hurthle cell adenomas. The Ki-67 labeling index in Hurthle cell carcinoma is significantly higher than that of Hurthle cell carcinoma (312). Diffuse nuclear staining for cyclin D1 is more often seen in Hurthle cell carcinoma than in Hurthle cell adenoma (312). Hurthle cell carcinomas are distinguished from the oncocytic/oxyphilic (Hurthle cell) variant of PTC by cytologic features classic of PTC in the latter. The oxyphilic variant of MTC has nuclear features characteristic of a neuroendocrine tumor. In difficult cases, immunoperoxidase studies can be helpful as Hurthle cell tumors are positive for thyroglobulin, while the oncocytic/oxyphilic variant of MTC is positive for chromogranin, synaptophysin, calcitonin, and CEA.

Treatment and prognosis. Hurthle cell carcinomas are slightly more aggressive than follicular carcinomas. The overall five-year survival for Hurthle cell carcinoma is 50% to 60% in many series (165). Hurthle cell carcinomas invade into adjacent soft tissues more frequently than follicular carcinomas (165,313). The most common sites of metastases are lung and bone, followed by regional lymph nodes, although lymph node involvement is more common in Hurthle cell carcinomas than in conventional follicular carcinomas (165). Among the Hurthle cell carcinomas, large tumor size and vascular invasion are associated with clinically aggressive tumors (312). Hurthle cell neoplasms with only equivocal capsular invasion and no vascular invasion usually behave in a less aggressive manner (312).

E. Poorly Differentiated Carcinoma

Introduction

Poorly differentiated carcinomas are follicular cell neoplasms that are in between well-differentiated follicular and papillary carcinomas and undifferentiated or anaplastic carcinomas. These tumors have been designated by various other names, including poorly differentiated follicular carcinomas, insular carcinomas, and poorly differentiated carcinomas with a primordial cell component (319–335).

The poorly differentiated thyroid carcinoma is diagnosed more often in some parts of the world such as Italy and Latin America (319), constituting 4% to 7% of thyroid carcinomas. It is diagnosed much less commonly in the United States. This subtype of thyroid carcinoma is more common in older patients beyond 50 years. It is also more common in women (319).

Clinical Features

Patients usually present with a solitary large thyroid mass. Radiologic studies usually show a cold nodule. Patients usually have a history of recent enlargement in the tumor, which may have been present for some years. They may sometimes present with a rapidly growing mass reminiscent of an anaplastic carcinoma or lymphoma (319). At the time of diagnosis, patients may have involvement of cervical lymph nodes, lung, and/or bone metastasis (319).

Imaging Studies

Only limited studies have been done on these tumors. MRI and fluorodeoxyglucose positron emission tomographic (FDG-PET) uptake have been used to localize poorly differentiated carcinoma (336).

Pathology

Gross features. Tumors are usually large and often measure over 3 cm in diameter. The cut surface is gray-white in areas. Necrosis is common. The tumors may have a pushing border with extrathyroidal extension and/or satellite nodules within the thyroid.

Cytologic features. Cytologic features include highly cellular neoplastic cells that are small to intermediate in size with microfollicles and scant amounts of colloid. The nuclei are bland with small nucleoli. However, necrosis and metastatic figures are frequently present (62,63,330,332,333).

Microscopic features. The histopathologic appearance of the tumors is variable. The most frequent patterns are insular, trabecular, and solid growth patterns (337). Necrosis and vascular invasion are frequently identified (Fig. 14). Oncocytic or clear-cell features may be present, and occasionally rhabdoid features can be seen (319). The insular pattern is most striking, and some authors refer to these tumors as insular carcinomas (Fig. 15) (320,321). It is characterized by nests of tumor cells surrounded by thin fibrovascular septa. The nests are made up of solid sheets of cells, but may sometimes contain small follicles. The tumor cells are small and uniform with vesicular or hyperchromatic nuclei containing small

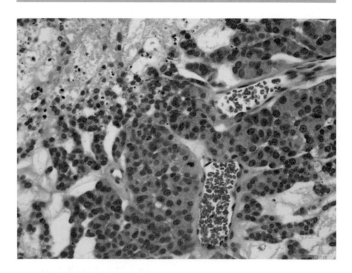

Figure 14 Poorly differentiated carcinoma with necrosis and prominent mitotic activity.

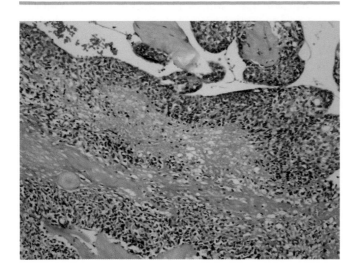

Figure 15 Insular thyroid carcinoma with an insular growth pattern, thin fibrovascular septae, and necrosis.

nucleoli. Mitotic figures are frequently present. A peritheliomatous growth pattern may be present admixed with fibrosis and/or necrosis (329). The trabecular pattern of growth is characterized by cells arranged in cords or ribbons. The solid pattern of growth consists of cells with sheets, which may have abortive follicles with colloid droplets. The tumors may contain areas resembling papillary or follicular carcinomas, and some of the nuclei may show cytologic features of PTC focally (319). Focal areas with marked nuclear pleomorphism reminiscent of anaplastic carcinoma may be present (319).

Immunohistochemistry

Poorly differentiated carcinomas show diffuse immunoreactivity for thyroglobulin and for TTF-1. The thyroglobulin immunostaining may be focal (334). TP53 nuclear staining, when present, may be focal (334). A high Ki-67 index is commonly present.

Electron Microscopy

Ultrastructural features include nests or trabeculae of tumor cells with well- to poorly developed junctions. The lumina are usually abortive and are lined by short microvilli. The nuclei have irregular contours and small nucleoli.

Molecular Genetics

Mutations of *TP53* are present in 20% to 30% of poorly differentiated carcinomas. Aberrant p53 overexpression is present in 40% to 50% of these tumors (328). Mutations of *H-, K-,* and *N-RAS* are present in around 50% of poorly differentiated carcinomas (325). Nuclear localization of β catenin is present in a small percentage of these tumors. Mutations of *BRAF* are also present in a small percentage of these tumors (328). Similarly, *RET/PTC* and *NTRK1* rearrangements may

be present in a small percentage of poorly differentiated carcinomas (328).

Differential Diagnosis

The differential diagnosis includes various lesions such as MTC, follicular carcinoma, solid variant of papillary carcinoma, and metastatic carcinoma to the thyroid. Immunohistochemical staining for thyroglobulin can help to separate poorly differentiated carcinomas from MTCs. TTF-1 can be used to separate poorly differentiated carcinomas from many metastatic tumors except for lung primaries. The solid variant of PTC usually has distinct and diffuse cytologic features that allow separation from poorly differentiated thyroid carcinomas.

Treatment and Prognosis

Treatment is usually by total thyroidectomy and resection of enlarged lymph nodes (329) followed by radioactive iodine therapy. The mean five-year survival is around 50% in most series (319). Most patients die in the first three years after diagnosis. Death is usually secondary to regional and distant metastases (319).

F. Anaplastic Carcinoma

Introduction

Anaplastic or undifferentiated thyroid carcinomas are highly malignant tumors that are composed in part or entirely of undifferentiated cells with immunohistochemical and ultrastructural features supporting epithelial differentiation (319). These tumors have also been referred to as sarcomatoid carcinomas, giant cell carcinomas, carcinosarcoma, metaplastic carcinoma, and dedifferentiated carcinomas.

These tumors usually occur mainly in older patients beyond 60 years. There is a female to male ratio of 1.5:1 (319). The mortality rate is over 90%. The mean survival is six months after the initial diagnosis (319,338–341).

Clinical Features

Patients usually present with a rapidly growing neck mass. They may have hoarseness (80%), dysphagia (60%), vocal cord paralysis (50%), or cervical pain (30%). The tumors are usually quite hard and may be composed of a single or multiple nodules (319). At the time of surgery, invasion of adjacent structures in the neck, including the neck muscles, trachea, esophagus, laryngeal nerve, and larynx are common. Almost half of all patients have distant metastases at diagnosis. The most common metastatic sites include the lungs, bones, and brain (319).

Imaging Studies

FDG-PET studies have been used to study primary anaplastic thyroid carcinomas as well as to localize metastatic lesions (342). In addition to ultrasound and CT studies, the use of Tc-99m sestamibi scans can help to outline the extent of tumor infiltration.

Pathology

Gross features. The tumors are white to tan and firm to hard (Fig. 16). Areas of hemorrhage and necrosis are commonly seen. Most tumors infiltrate the adjacent soft tissue and adjacent structures such as the esophagus and trachea.

Cytologic features. The aspirates are usually highly cellular but may be sparsely cellular depending on the subtype of anaplastic carcinoma. The highly fibrous paucicellular variant may yield a hypocellular aspirate. The cells are usually quite pleomorphic with a heterogeneous population of cells. Mitotic figures are usually abundant. Necrotic debris with neutrophilic cells may be present in the background.

Microscopic features. The tumors are usually composed of a mixture of various cell types, including spindle cells, pleomorphic multinucleated cells, and epithelial cells. Mitotic figures are readily seen, and necrosis may be abundant (Fig. 17). Angiolymphatic invasion is usually present. Some tumors may have predominantly giant cells, while others may be composed of mainly spindled cells. If the tumors are highly vascular, they may look like angiosarcomas or hemangiopericytomas.

Variants of anaplastic carcinoma include the osteoclastic variant with abundant multinucleated cells, the paucicellular variant, which is usually composed of hypocellular spindle cells and may suggest Riedel's thyroiditis. The lymphoepithelioma-like variant resembles the nasopharyngeal lymphoepithelioma, but these tumors are usually not EBV positive (319).

Immunohistochemistry

Immunohistochemical analysis is usually positive for keratins such as AE1/AE3. This is usually present in about 80% of cases. Most tumors are negative for thyroglobulin and TTF-1, but focal staining may be seen in the better-differentiated areas of dedifferentiated tumors. The tumors are usually positive for vimentin and for TP53 overexpression.

Electron Microscopy

Ultrastructural studies show epithelial differentiation with well-developed cell junctions and tonofilaments.

Molecular Genetics

Molecular alterations include overexpression of cyclin D1, decreased expression of p27, and inactivation of PTEN and p16 (343). Mutations of *TP53* and of

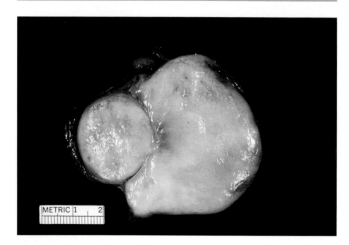

Figure 16 Anaplastic thyroid carcinoma involving the bulk of the thyroid.

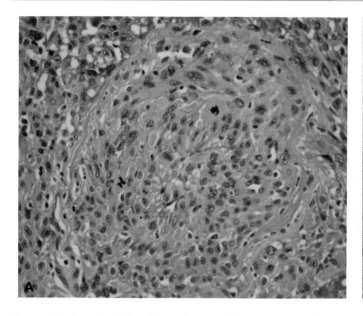
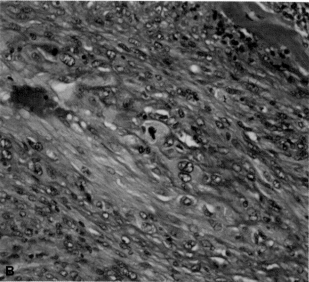

Figure 17 Anaplastic thyroid carcinoma with markedly atypical cells in a solid growth pattern and prominent mitotic activity.

the *β-catenin* gene (*CTNNB1*) have also been reported (344–346). Cytogenetic studies have shown complex chromosomal alterations with allelic losses of 1q, 1p, 5, 8, 9p, 11, 17p, 19p, 22q, 16p, and 18q (319).

Differential Diagnosis

The differential diagnosis includes Riedel's thyroiditis for the paucicellular variant of anaplastic carcinoma, especially in small biopsy specimens. The clinical differential diagnosis of a rapidly growing mass in the thyroid also includes a large B-cell lymphoma, which usually develops in a background of Hashimoto's thyroiditis. Histologically, distinction between a large B-cell lymphoma and an anaplastic carcinoma is readily made with adequate sections. The lymphoepithelioma-like variant may be confused with lymphoma in small biopsy specimens. Other lesions in the differential diagnosis would include metastatic poorly differentiated carcinomas to the thyroid since both of these tumors usually develop in older patients. Immunohistochemical staining for a series of markers should help to distinguish between some of these metastatic lesions.

Treatment and Prognosis

Patients are usually treated by biopsy followed by radiation and chemotherapy if the tumor is not amenable to surgical resection. The prognosis is related to the extent of disease at initial diagnosis. The overall five-year survival ranges from 0% to 14%, and the median survival is 2.5 to 6 months (319).

G. Tumors of C Cells

C-Cell Hyperplasia

Introduction. C-cell hyperplasia is defined by an increase in the total mass of C cells in the thyroid gland. The C cells are usually difficult to identify on H&E-stained sections, but are readily seen after immunostaining for calcitonin and chromogranin. The definition of increased numbers of C cells varies among investigators. One historical definition required 50 C cells per low-power field (10×) (347,348).

Clinical features. C-cell hyperplasia appears to be more common in men than in women (348). C-cell hyperplasia has been divided into physiologic and neoplastic types (347–349). Physiologic hyperplasia can be seen in neonates and elderly patients. It can be associated with other conditions such as follicular tumors, hyperparathyroidism, Hashimoto's thyroiditis, and hypergastrinemia (348,350–353). It has been suggested that physiologic C-cell hyperplasia may be associated with overstimulation by thyroid-stimulating hormone (350).

Neoplastic C-cell hyperplasia is associated with familial MTC [multiple endocrine neoplasia (MEN) type 2a and 2b]. Mutations of the RET proto-oncogene, which encodes a member of the tyrosine kinase family of transmembrane receptors is usually associated with germ-line mutations in familial MTC and in some sporadic tumors (354–357).

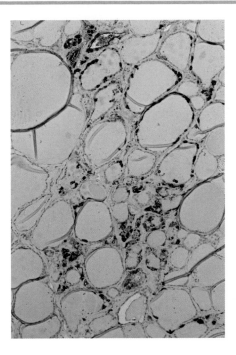

Figure 18 Calcitonin immunostain highlighting the increased numbers of C-cells (C-cell hyperplasia) in a patient with MEN2b.

Pathology.

Gross Features. The changes are usually very subtle and not generally appreciated on gross examination. Careful sectioning may show a few small 1- to 2-mm foci in the middle to upper portions of the thyroid lobes in familial disease.

Microscopic Features. There is an increase in C cells in the middle and upper lobes of the thyroid gland compared with age- and sex-matched controls. These should be at least 50 C cells per lower-power field (10×) (Fig. 18). The hyperplasia may be diffuse or nodular with the latter being more prominent in neoplastic C-cell hyperplasia (347–358).

Electron microscopy. The hyperplasic C cells contain dense core secretory granules similar to those seen in normal C cells and in MTC. There are two granule populations of 130 nm and 280 nm in these cells (359).

Immunohistochemistry. The hyperplasic C cells are positive for chromogranin A, synaptophysin, calcitonin, and calcitonin gene-related peptide (347).

Differential diagnosis. Distinguishing physiologic from neoplastic C-cell hyperplasia may be difficult. Family history should be helpful since in neoplastic C-cell hyperplasia, the nodular clusters are prominent. Nodular C-cell clusters should be distinguished from solid cell nests that represent remnants of the ultimobranchial bodies embedded in the thyroid (360). They usually stain for keratin and CEAs and may stain for calcitonin, which will make them more difficult to distinguish from C-cell hyperplasia. Ultrastructural studies show that they lack dense core secretory granules, which help in making the distinction.

Treatment and prognosis. Total thyroidectomy is usually the recommended treatment for C-cell hyperplasia, especially for neoplastic C-cell hyperplasia. Neoplastic C-cell hyperplasia will progress to invasive MTC if left untreated (361). Once a patient develops MTC, the five-year survival varies from 60% to 70%, and the 10-year survival rate ranges from 40% to 50%. Thus, early intervention with prophylactic surgery when the patient only has C-cell hyperplasia should markedly improve survival.

Medullary Thyroid Carcinoma

Introduction. MTC constitutes about 5% to 10% of thyroid malignancies. About 25% of MTCs are familial, while the other cases are sporadic (362). Familial tumors belong to the MEN2a and 2b and familial MTC (362–365). These conditions are inherited in an autosomal-dominant mode (348). Patients with sporadic tumors usually present with tumors around age 50 years, while patients with familial cancers develop tumors or C-cell hyperplasia during adolescence or young adulthood. Patients with familial MTC in which they do not have involvement with other endocrine tumors, such as pheochromocytomas, usually develop tumors around age 50 years. Patients with familial MTC usually have bilateral involvement of the thyroid, while those with sporadic disease have tumors involving only one lobe of the thyroid gland.

Clinical features. MTCs produce calcitonin, so patients usually have elevated serum levels of this hormone (366). Patients often present with a painless thyroid nodule. Some patients may have metastatic disease at the time of diagnosis (~50%), while a smaller percentage may present with metastatic disease (319). Some patients may present with diarrhea and flushing, especially if the tumor is large and produced cysts, abundant vasoactive amines, and peptides. Occasionally, patients may present with

Cushing's syndrome secondary to production of pro-opiomelanocortin proteolytic products such as adrenocorticotropic hormone (ACTH).

Medullary microcarcinomas are defined as tumors less than 1 cm in diameter. They may be associated with elevated serum calcitonin, but in many cases, they have been discovered as incidental findings during surgery for thyroid nodules (367).

Imaging studies. Tumors are usually biopsied under ultrasound guidance. Specialized studies such as meraiodobenzylguanidine (MIBG), scintigraphy with 111-In- or 99mTc-labeled somatostatin analogs, or FDG-PET have been used to image these tumors (368).

Pathology.

Gross Features. MTCs are usually gray-white tumors that are firm and gritty on cut section. They may be circumscribed or infiltrative. Sporadic tumors are usually unilateral, while familial tumors are often bilateral.

Cytologic Features. Aspirates are typically hypercellular, and the cells may be loosely cohesive. They may vary from spindle to epithelioid or plasmacytoid in shape. The nuclei are hyperchromatic with granular chromatin and moderate pleomorphism. Multinucleated tumor giant cells are frequently seen. Amyloid may be detected in up to 70% of the aspirate but may be very sparse.

Microscopic Features. MTCs are quite variable in their histologic features (369–371). The early tumors were recognized by their spindle and epithelioid shapes, and most tumors have amyloid (Fig. 19) (370). There are many histologic variants of MTCs (Fig. 20) (362,372–375). These include follicular tubular variant with solid growth and microcystic spaces, papillary variant that can simulate PTCs, small cell variant characterized by cells with hyperchromatic nuclei, and scanty amounts of cytoplasm. The giant cell variant is composed of tumors with clusters of multinucleated cells and may simulate an anaplastic

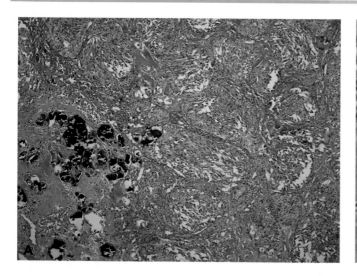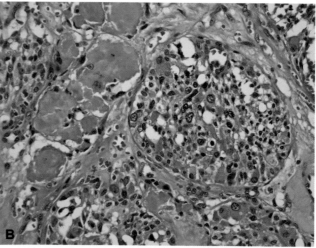

Figure 19 Medullary thyroid carcinoma. (**A**) Medullary thyroid carcinoma with spindled cells, amyloid, and calcifications. (**B**) Nested growth pattern in a medullary thyroid carcinoma with polygonal and spindled cells with stippled nuclear chromatin and amyloid.

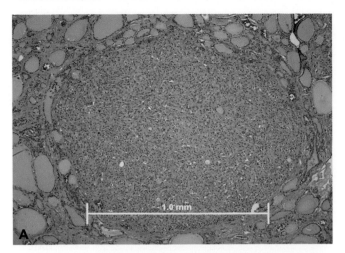

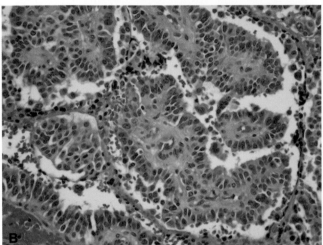

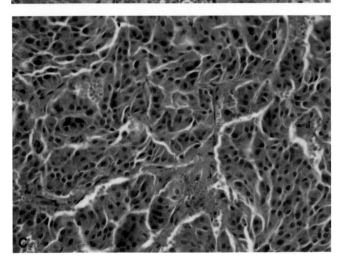

Figure 20 Variants of medullary thyroid carcinoma. (**A**) Micromedullary thyroid carcinoma. (**B**) Hurthle/oxyphilic variant of medullary thyroid carcinoma. (**C**) Papillary variant of medullary thyroid carcinoma.

carcinoma. Other variants include clear cell, melanotic or pigmented, oxyphilic, and squamous variants. Other tumors may produce abundant mucin (mucin-producing variant) or may look like paragangliomas

(paraganglioma-like variant). Almost all MTCs should be positive for calcitonin, chromogranin, and synaptophysin. Encapsulated MTCs are uncommon since most tumors are infiltrative. In contrast, MTCs with necrosis and squamous metaplasia and decreased immunoreactive calcitonin are associated with a worse prognosis (376).

Mixed Medullary-Follicular Carcinoma

These are rare tumors that may arise from the ultimobranchial bodies. They are composed of C cells and follicular cell-derived tumors and grow in a solid or follicular pattern. Amyloid is uncommon in this variant. They usually express both calcitonin and thyroglobulin on immunostaining. Ultrastructural studies show dual differentiation toward C cells and dense core granules as well as follicular cells (377,378)

Mixed Medullary-Papillary Carcinoma

These tumors are even less common than the mixed medullary-follicular carcinomas. Admixtures of papillary and medullary elements have been reported both in the primary and in the metastatic tumors (379).

Immunohistochemistry. The tumor cells are positive for calcitonin, chromogranin, synaptophysin, calcitonin gene-related peptides, keratin, as well as TTF-1. Other neuroendocrine peptides such as somatostatin, bombesin, and pro-opiomelanocortin may also be expressed.

Electron microscopy. The tumor cells usually have dense core secretory granules of two types. The type I granules are 280 nm, and type II granules are 130 nm in diameter. Other organelles such as prominent rough endoplasmic reticulin and Golgi are usually present.

Molecular genetics. Germline mutation of *RET* are seen in familial MTC (380,381). Some sporadic tumors show mutation within the tumor. Germline *RET* mutations in codon 768, 790, 791, and 804 have been associated with familial MTC and low penetrance (380–382).

Differential diagnosis. The differential diagnosis includes follicular carcinomas, hyalinizing trabecular tumors, paragangliomas, as well as parathyroid tumors and poorly differentiated thyroid carcinomas and metastatic neuroendocrine tumors to the thyroid. Immunohistochemical staining for calcitonin, keratin, TTF-1, thyroglobulin as well as broad-spectrum neuroendocrine markers usually help to sort out the lesions in the differential diagnosis.

Treatment and prognosis. Patients with MTC are treated with total thyroidectomy and central lymph node dissection to evaluate for metastatic disease (383). Micromedullary thyroid carcinomas are tumors less than 1 cm in diameter. The 10-year survival in these patients is much higher than with larger MTC, and lymph node metastasis is rarely present at the time of surgery (384). With the usual MTC, the 10-year survival is 73.7% (383). Reduced survival is noted in older patients, males, and patients with extensive metastatic disease (383). Widespread metastasis in

MTC is usually associated with systemic symptoms of diarrhea, bone pain, or flushing, and the five-year survival is relatively poor (<11%) (385). Patients with persistently elevated serum calcitonin without clinical or radiologic evidence of residual disease after curative surgery may have a good long-term survival in spite of the presence of occult MTC.

H. Uncommon Thyroid Tumors

Mucoepidermoid Carcinoma

Introduction. These are malignant epithelial tumors with epidermoid and mucinous components. The tumors comprise less than 1% of thyroid neoplasms. They are more frequent in women. Mucoepidermoid carcinomas have been associated with a history of childhood radiation exposure to the neck (386).

Clinical features. Patients usually present with a cold neck nodule that is painless (387). Extrathyroidal extension is present in about 20% of patients at diagnosis. These tumors can metastasize to lung and bone.

Pathology.

Gross Features. Tumors vary in size but may be very large, ranging up to 10 cm in diameter. Cut surface shows a rubbery, firm mass that may vary from tan brown to yellow. The tumors are usually well encapsulated. There may be involvement of neck lymph nodes at the time of surgery.

Cytologic Features. Fine needle aspiration shows epidermoid and mucus-secreting cells with vacuolated cytoplasm. Cells may have signet ring features.

Microscopic Features. The histologic appearance is distinct with anastomosing clusters of epidermal cells and mucus-producing cells in a fibrous stroma. There are variable amounts of extracellular mucin. Hyaline colloid-like PAS-positive hyaline bodies may be present. The tumor cells may have nuclear grooves and pseudoinclusions. Mitoses are uncommon (388).

Immunohistochemistry. The tumor cells are positive for polyclonal CEA and keratins. Positive staining for TTF-1 and thyroglobulin may be focal.

Differential diagnosis. The tumors may look like sclerosing mucoepidermoid carcinoma with eosinophilia, but the eosinophils are not as numerous as in this tumor.

Treatment and prognosis. These are low-grade tumors with an indolent biologic behavior. Reports of dedifferentiation to anaplastic carcinomas have been noted (387). Distant metastases are rare, but they may extend extrathyroidally or spread to regional lymph nodes.

Sclerosing Mucoepidermoid Carcinoma with Eosinophilia

Introduction. Sclerosing mucoepidermoid carcinoma with eosinophilia is a rare malignant tumor showing epidermal and glandular differentiation with prominent sclerosis, eosinophils, and lymphocytes. Patients are usually adults and are almost always women (387,389–391).

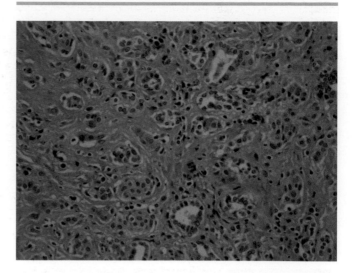

Figure 21 Sclerosing mucoepidermoid carcinoma with eosinophilia.

Clinical features. Most patients have a slowly growing thyroid mass, but they may sometimes develop rapidly. Imaging studies show cold or hypofunctioning nodules on radionuclide scans. About half of the cases may involve the parathyroidal soft tissues.

Pathology.

Gross Features. The tumors are usually well circumscribed with a firm, white-tan to yellow cut surface. Cystic changes may be seen occasionally.

Microscopic Features. The histologic appearance is distinct with a sclerotic stroma infiltrated by eosinophils, lymphocytes, and occasional plasma cells (Fig. 21). The tumor grows in nests and cords, and there is minimal nuclear pleomorphism. The tumors may assume a pseudoangiomatous appearance because of the loss of tumor cell cohesion. Perineural invasion is frequently noted. They may occasionally be associated with papillary thyroid carcinomas.

Immunohistochemistry. The tumor cells are positive for keratin and negative for calcitonin and thyroglobulin. About 50% of the cases are positive for TTF-1 (319).

Differential diagnosis. The tumors may look like benign squamous metaplasia. However, the presence of invasive growth in sclerosing mucoepidermoid carcinoma with eosinophilia helps to make this distinction. Squamous cell carcinoma and anaplastic carcinoma of the thyroid may look similar in small biopsies, but both of these lesions show more atypical cytologic features than the sclerosing mucoepidermoid carcinomas with eosinophilia.

Treatment and prognosis. Surgical excision is the usual treatment. About 50% of patients are disease free from three months to nine years after surgery, while the others show regional or distant metastasis (319).

Spindle Epithelial Tumor with Thymus-Like Differentiation

Introduction. Spindle cell tumor with thymus-like differentiation or spindle epithelial tumor with thymus-like differentiation (SETTLE) is an uncommon malignant thyroid tumor composed of spindle-shaped epithelial cells with a lobulated pattern admixed with glandular structures (392–396).

Clinical features. They are most commonly seen in children and young adults with a mean age of 19 years. There is also a slight male preponderance. Patients present with a thyroid mass. Occasionally, they may be rapidly enlarging with diffuse involvement of the entire thyroid gland. On imaging, they appear as cold nodules with heterogenous, solid, and cystic densities on CT scan. Patients are usually euthyroid.

Pathology.

Gross Features. The tumors can be circumscribed or infiltrative, usually between 1 and 3 cm in diameter. The cut surface is gray to white, and cystic spaces may be seen grossly.

Microscopic Features. The tumors have prominent fibrous septa and a cellular background. A biphasic pattern of spindle and glandular cells is common, but sheets of monophasic spindle cells may be the predominant pattern. Mitotic figures are uncommon, but focal necrosis and increased mitotic activity may be seen in some areas of the tumor. The glandular cells range from cuboidal to columnar, and the cells may be mucinous or ciliated. Squamous metaplasia may be present.

Immunohistochemistry. Cytokeratin is expressed in both the spindle cells and glandular elements. The tumor cells are negative for thyroglobulin, calcitonin, CEA, and S-100 protein (394,396).

Electron microscopy. Epithelial differentiation with tonofilaments, desmosomes, and basement membrane are usually present.

Molecular genetics. Very few studies have been done, but K-RAS mutation may be present. TP53 gene mutation has been reported to be absent (394).

Treatment and prognosis. Treatment is usually surgical. The tumors are slow growing, but the metastatic rate is over 60% after long-term follow-up (395).

Carcinoma Showing Thymus-Like Differentiation

Introduction. These tumors are also known as lymphoepithelioma-like carcinomas of the thyroid. They develop mainly in the lower poles of the gland but may also be present in the perithyroidal soft tissues. Carcinomas showing thymus-like differentiation (CASTLEs) develop mainly in middle-aged adults with a slight female preponderance (397–402).

Clinical features. Patients present with a painless thyroid mass and may have tracheal compression and hoarseness if the recurrent laryngeal nerve is involved. About a third of patients may have lymph node involvement at diagnosis (398).

Imaging. Imaging studies show a cold nodule on thyroid scan. The tumors appear hypoechoic and heterogenous on ultrasound. On CT scan, there is a soft tissue density with minimal contrast enhancement.

Pathology.

Gross Features. Cut sections show a gray-tan surface with a well-demarcated area between the normal thyroid and tumor.

Microscopic Features. Invasive growth into the adjacent thyroid is commonly present, and a prominent lobulated pattern reminiscent of thymoma or thymic carcinoma is seen. The tumor cells are squamoid or syncytial like with eosinophilic cytoplasm, and oval nuclei. Lymphocytes and plasma cells are occasionally present in the background.

Immunohistochemistry. The tumors were positive for keratin and CD5. EBV by in situ hybridization is absent in site of the lymphoepithelioma-like appearance (398,399).

Differential diagnosis. The differential diagnosis usually includes squamous cell carcinoma of the thyroid, anaplastic carcinoma, and metastatic carcinoma to the thyroid. Positive staining for CD5 is restricted to CASTLEs, which excludes the other lesions in this differential diagnosis. Follicular dendritic cell sarcoma may enter into the differential diagnosis, but it is usually keratin negative.

Treatment and prognosis. The tumors are treated surgically. They are usually slow growing, and recurrence may occur after a long period (402). Rare tumors may pursue a rapidly fatal course.

Squamous Cell Carcinoma

Introduction. Primary squamous cell carcinomas of the thyroid are uncommon malignant tumors.

Clinical features. These tumors occur in older patients with a female preponderance (403–408). These are rapidly growing tumors, and patients present with symptoms secondary to tracheal or esophageal compression. Some patients may have a history of goiter or Hashimoto's thyroiditis. Nodal metastasis may be present in up to 20% of patients (408).

Imaging. Imaging studies show a cold nodule, and such studies are important to exclude other possible primaries before performing surgery. X rays are used to exclude squamous cell carcinoma from the lung or other head and neck regions.

Pathology.

Gross Features. The tumors may involve one or both thyroid lobes, and satellite nodules are often present. Cut sections show a firm, gray-white tumor and areas of central necrosis may be prominent.

Cytologic Features. Fine needle aspiration biopsy is usually diagnostic with adequate specimens. Epithelial cells with keratinization, keratin pearls, and necrosis may be present.

Microscopic Features. Cells are composed of tumor cells with pure squamous cell differentiation (Fig. 22). Other types of thyroid tumors such as papillary and anaplastic carcinomas may show focal squamous cell differentiation, which helps to separate the tumor from pure squamous cell carcinoma of the thyroid. Infiltration of the perithyroidal soft tissue with vascular and perineurial invasion is often present.

Immunohistochemistry. The tumor cells are positive for various keratins, including CK19, CK18, and CK7. Stains for CK1, CK4, and CK20 are usually negative. Thyroglobulin is usually negative in the tumor.

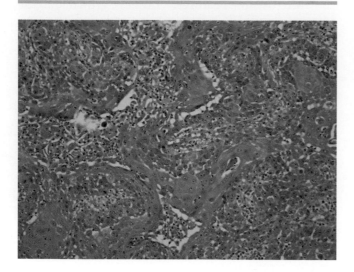

Figure 22 Squamous cell carcinoma of the thyroid. The tumor is composed of large epithelioid cells showing squamous differentiation and atypia with an infiltrative growth pattern.

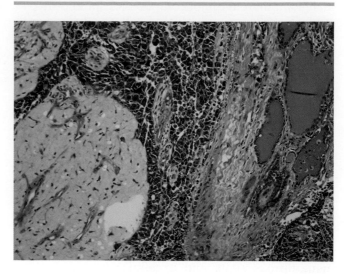

Figure 23 Immature teratoma of the thyroid.

Molecular studies. Overexpression of TP53 is seen in some cases. There is loss of expression of p21.

Treatment and prognosis. Treatment is usually surgical followed by radiation therapy. The prognosis is usually poor.

Teratoma

Introduction. These are tumors with mature and/or immature tissues from all three germ layers. Over 300 cases have been reported (409–413).

Clinical features. They can occur at any age but are most common in neonates. Most of the tumors in neonates are benign, while over 50% of the tumors in adults are malignant (156). Tumors may be in the thyroid or in direct continuity with the gland. Patients present with a neck mass. There may be dyspnea and/or stridor of variable duration at presentation.

Imaging. Imaging studies often show a multicystic mass in the thyroid, which may compress the airway.

Pathology.

Gross Features. The tumors usually average 6 cm in maximum diameter. They are cystic and multiloculated. Cut surface shows dark brown hemorrhagic fluid and necrosis. Brain tissue, bone, and cartilage may be seen grossly.

Cytologic Features. The cytologic findings can be quite variable. Neuroepithelial small round blue cells from the immature areas with neural elements may be present.

Microscopic Features. A wide spectrum of microscopic features may be seen. Neuroblastic elements arranged in sheets or rosette-like structures may be present (Fig. 23). Small cystic spaces with squamous, or columnar, or cuboidal cells, or transitional cells, or pseudostratified ciliated epithelium

may be present. The tumors are graded as completely mature (grade 0), predominantly mature (grades 1 and 2), and mostly immature (grades 3 or malignant). Areas with bone, cartilage, muscle, adipose tissue, and other mesenchymal elements admixed with neural and epithelial elements are often present (410–413).

Immunohistochemistry. A wide variety of antigens are expressed by teratomas, including S-100 protein and glial fibrillary acidic protein in a neural element.

Differential diagnosis. The differential diagnosis includes cystic lymphangiomas in neonates, thyroglossal duct cysts, and bronchial cleft cysts. Teratomas are usually located in the midline as are thyroglossal duct cysts. Other lesions in the differential diagnosis include Ewing's sarcoma, primitive neuroectodermal tumor (PNET), and other small round blue cell tumors, which may be mistaken for teratomas. Immunostaining and molecular studies are usually helpful in sorting out the differential diagnosis.

Treatment and prognosis. Surgical treatment followed by chemotherapy is usually done. Neonates usually have benign tumors, while adults have malignant tumors with recurrences in about 30% of cases. Although the tumors in neonates are usually benign, there is increased morbidity due to respiratory difficulties in these patients.

Primary Lymphomas and Plasmacytomas

Introduction. Thyroid lymphomas make up about 5% of thyroid tumors and 2.5% to 7% of all extranodal lymphomas. They are usually in older individuals with a female predominance (414–419). Most patients with thyroid lymphomas have a history of Hashimoto's thyroiditis. Most cases are B cell lymphomas associated with Hashimoto's thyroiditis. Non-Hodgkin's lymphomas are relatively uncommon.

The lymphomas develop in the setting of acquired mucosa-associated lymphoid tissue (MALT) as a result of an autoimmune or inflammatory process.

Clinical features. Patients present with a mass and variable symptoms that may include pain, dyspnea, hoarseness, coughing, and hemoptysis. Imaging studies show a cold area with ^{131}I scans (414).

Pathology.

Gross Features. The tumors are usually quite variable in size and may be very large, ranging up to 20 cm in maximum diameter. They may range from soft to firm on cut sections and are white-gray with "fish-flesh" appearance.

Cytologic Features. Aspirates are frequently hypercellular with noncohesive cells, which range from small to large. Crush artifacts may be present.

Microscopic Features. The microscopic features are quite variable, ranging from small cells with sparse cytoplasm of extranodal marginal zone B-cell lymphomas to much larger cells and diffuse large B-cell lymphomas. Follicular lymphomas of the thyroid are rare. Plasmacytomas or MALT lymphomas with prominent plasma cell differentiation may also be present. About half of the thyroid lymphomas have perithyroidal extension.

Immunohistochemistry. Immunostaining for CD45, CD20, CD79a, and CD3 are useful in the workup. Bcl-2 immunoreactivity in the neoplastic-colonizing B-cells may be present. CD43 may be coexpressed with CD20. Light chain restriction is often present in the B-cell lesions.

Molecular genetics. Clonal rearrangement of the heavy chain variable region and *Fas* gene mutations have been reported. Monoclonal rearrangements of the heavy chain genes may also be present.

Treatment and prognosis. Diagnosis is usually established by fine needle aspiration or biopsy. Treatment is by chemotherapy and radiation therapy (418,419). Localized tumors (stage IE) with low-grade histology usually have an excellent prognosis. Tumors with large B-cells have a worse prognosis. Perithyroidal extension, vascular invasion, and high mitotic activity are associated with a worse prognosis.

Sinus Histiocytosis with Massive Lymphadenopathy (Rosai–Dorfman Disease)

These are rare lesions of the thyroid seen mainly in adult women (420–422). The tumors are composed of histiocyte-like cells arranged in nodules showing emperipolesis. Lymphocytic thyroiditis is usually present in the background. The prognosis is usually very good.

Solitary Fibrous Tumor

These are rare tumors involved in the thyroid as a solitary circumscribed mass in middle-aged adults (423–426). The tumors are composed of spindle cells that may mimic other thyroid lesions. They may range from 2 to 8 cm in diameter. They are composed of cells with a wavy, storiform, or desmoids-like arrangement (Fig. 24). They usually arrange from hypocellular to hypercellular in other areas. Immunohistochemistry is

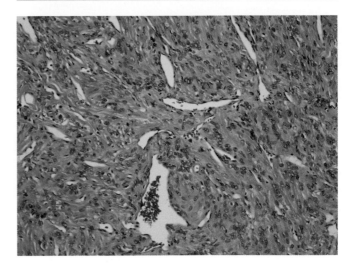

Figure 24 Solitary fibrous tumor of the thyroid.

usually positive for CD34, CD99, and Bcl-2. The thyroid lesions usually behave in a benign manner.

Langerhans Cell Histiocytosis

These tumors develop rarely in the thyroid and are characterized by proliferation of dendritic Langerhans cells with eosinophils in the background. Most patients are less than 20 years of age (427–432). Histologic examination shows diffuse or focal involvement. The characteristic Langerhans cells have eosinophilic cytoplasm and a vesicular nucleus with a lobulated folding groove and a vesicular appearance (Fig. 25). Eosinophils are abundant in the background, and there may be areas of necrosis. Ultrastructural features include the Birbeck or Langerhans granules with invagination of the plasma membrane arranged in a pentilaminar pattern. The cells are usually positive for S-100 protein and CD1a. Patients with localized thyroid disease do not usually develop subsequent systemic involvement.

Mesenchymal Tumors

Angiosarcoma. Although all cell types of mesenchymal tumors may occur in the thyroid, angiosarcomas are the most common (433–436). Angiosarcomas have been reported most commonly from the Alpine regions of central Europe. They develop most frequently in patients with long-standing nodular goiters. The tumors are usually cystic and variegated with intermixed solid areas. Hemorrhage and necrosis is often seen. The histologic appearances are similar to other angiosarcomas with solid areas showing extensive necrosis and anastomosing channels with papillary structures lined by endothelial cells (Fig. 26). Thyroid angiosarcomas are frequently epithelioid. Immunohistochemistry shows staining for CD31, CD34, and factor VIIIR-antigen (181). Ultrastructural studies show Weibel–Palade bodies with single

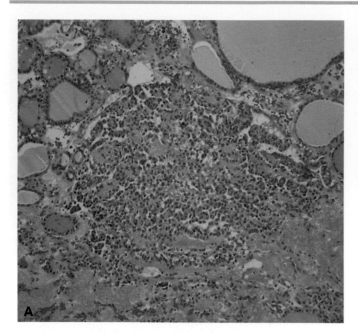
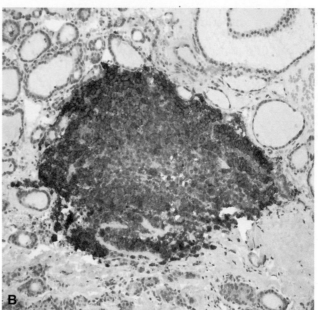

Figure 25 Langerhan cell histiocytosis involving the thyroid. (**A**) Tumifactive nodule of Langerhan cells on H&E. (**B**) CD1a immunostain highlighting the Langerhan cells.

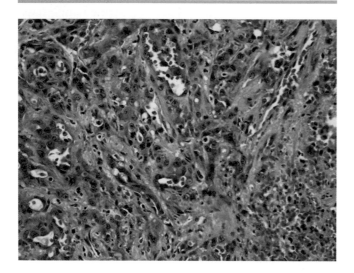

Figure 26 Angiosarcoma of the thyroid composed of cells with marked nuclear atypia forming vascular spaces.

membrane-bound rod-shaped structures in the cytoplasm of tumor cells. Most patients die from their tumors in less than six months after diagnosis, regardless of the treatment. A few patients have survived for five years.

Smooth muscle tumors. Leiomyomas occur in younger patients, while leiomyosarcomas occur in older patients in both sexes (437–442). The tumors vary from 1 cm up to very large tumors of 12 cm or larger. Histopathologic features show smooth muscle fibers arranged in bundles or fascicles. Cells are

spindled with blunt, cigar-shaped nuclei. Vascular invasion may be seen in the malignant tumors in the leiomyosarcomas. Immunohistochemical stains are positive for vimentin, smooth muscle actin, muscle-specific actin, and desmin. Stains for thyroglobulin are usually negative. These tumors are treated by surgical excision. Leiomyosarcomas usually have a poor clinical outcome.

Metastatic Tumors to the Thyroid

Introduction. Metastases to the thyroid are present in up to 25% of patients at autopsy who have disseminated disease.

Clinical. Patients present with a thyroid mass (443,444). They may have hoarseness, dysphagia, and/or neck pain. The most common metastatic sites include kidney (33%) (Fig. 27), lung (16%), and uterus (7%), followed by melanoma (5%) in one series. In an autopsy series, breast, lung, and melanomas were the most common sites of primary tumors involving the thyroid gland as secondary metastases.

Pathology.

Gross Features. Multifocal disease is common, and tumors vary in size.

Microscopic Features. Tumors involving the thyroid by direct extension include squamous cell carcinoma and malignant lymphomas. Metastatic tumors usually retain the histologic features of the primary tumors, so comparison with the primary tumor should be helpful.

Immunohistochemistry. Stains for TTF-1 are the most reliable way of distinguishing between a primary thyroid tumor and a breast tumor, with the exception of lung primaries.

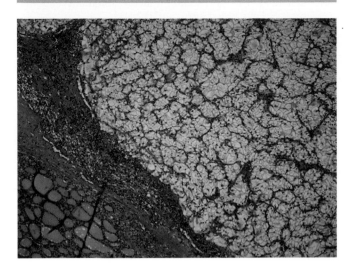

Figure 27 Metastatic renal cell carcinoma to the thyroid. The renal cell carcinoma is highly vascular and composed of clear cells.

Treatment and prognosis. Resection of solitary metastasis is usually recommended and may increase survival. The overall prognosis with metastasis to the thyroid is generally poor.

REFERENCES

1. Noris EH. The early morphogenesis of the human thyroid gland. Am J Anat 1918; 24:443–465.
2. Weller GL. Development of the thyroid, parathyroid, and thymus glands in man. Contrib Embryol Carnegie Institute 1933; 141:93–140.
3. Le Douarin N, Fontaine J, Le Lievre C. New studies on the neural crest origin of the avian ultimobranchial glandular cells—interspecific combinations and cytochemical characterization of C cells based on the uptake of biogenic amine precursors. Histochemistry 1974; 38(4):297–305.
4. Pearse AG, Polak JM. Cytochemical evidence for the neural crest origin of mammalian ultimobranchial C cells. Histochemie 1971; 27(2):96–102.
5. Eales JG. The influence of nutritional state on thyroid function in various vertebrates. Am Zool 1988; 20:351–362.
6. Hegedus L, Karstrup S, Rasmussen N. Evidence of cyclic alterations of thyroid size during the menstrual cycle in healthy women. Am J Obstet Gynecol 1986; 155 (1):142–145.
7. Hegedus L, Perrild H, Poulsen LR, et al. The determination of thyroid volume by ultrasound and its relationship to body weight, age, and sex in normal subjects. J Clin Endocrinol Metab 1983; 56(2):260–263.
8. Tice LW, Creveling CR. Electron microscopic identification of adrenergic nerve endings on thyroid epithelial cells. Endocrinology 1975; 97(5):1123–1129.
9. Reid JD, Choi CH, Oldroyd NO. Calcium oxalate crystals in the thyroid. Their identification, prevalence, origin, and possible significance. Am J Clin Pathol 1987; 87(4): 443–454.
10. Hanson GA, Komorowski RA, Cerletty JM, et al. Thyroid gland morphology in young adults: normal subjects versus those with prior low-dose neck irradiation in childhood. Surgery 1983; 94(6):984–988.
11. Gould VE, Johannesser JV, Sobrinho-Simoes M. The thyroid gland. In: Johannesser JV, ed. Electron Microscopy in Human Medicine. Vol. 10. New York: McGraw-Hill, 1981:29–107.
12. Dockhorn-Dworniczak B, Franke WW, Schroder S, et al. Patterns of expression of cytoskeletal proteins in human thyroid gland and thyroid carcinomas. Differentiation 1987; 35(1):53–71.
13. Kurata A, Ohta K, Mine M, et al. Monoclonal antihuman thyroglobulin antibodies. J Clin Endocrinol Metab 1984; 59(4):573–579.
14. Berge-Lefranc JL, Cartouzou G, De Micco C, et al. Quantification of thyroglobulin messenger RNA by in situ hybridization in differentiated thyroid cancers. Difference between well-differentiated and moderately differentiated histologic types. Cancer 1985; 56(2):345–350.
15. Papotti M, Negro F, Carney JA, et al. Mixed medullary-follicular carcinoma of the thyroid. A morphological, immunohistochemical and in situ hybridization analysis of 11 cases. Virchows Arch 1997; 430(5):397–405.
16. Lloyd RV, Douglas BR, Young WF. Parathyroid Gland—endocrine disease. Atlas of nontumor pathology (1st series, fascicle1). Washington DC: American Registry of Pathology and the Armed Forces Institute of Pathology in collaboration with Universities Associated for Research and Education in Pathology, 2002:91–169.
17. Harach HR. Solid cell nests of the thyroid. J Pathol 1988; 155(3):191–200.
18. Williams ED, Toyn CE, Harach HR. The ultimobranchial gland and congenital thyroid abnormalities in man. J Pathol 1989; 159(2):135–141.
19. Janzer RC, Weber E, Hedinger C. The relation between solid cell nests and C cells of the thyroid gland: an immunohistochemical and morphometric investigation. Cell Tissue Res 1979; 197(2):295–312.
20. Nadig J, Weber E, Hedinger C. C-cell in vestiges of the ultimobranchial body in human thyroid glands. Virchows Arch B Cell Pathol 1978; 27(2):189–191.
21. Ishii H, Inada M, Tanaka K, et al. Induction of outer and inner ring monodeiodinases in human thyroid gland by thyrotropin. J Clin Endocrinol Metab 1983; 57(3): 500–505.
22. Austin LA, Heath H, III. Calcitonin: physiology and pathophysiology. N Engl J Med 1981; 304(5):269–278.
23. Bocchetta A, Bernardi F, Pedditzi M, et al. Thyroid abnormalities during lithium treatment. Acta Psychiatr Scand 1991; 83(3):193–198.
24. Gammage MD, Franklyn JA. Amiodarone and the thyroid. Q J Med 1987; 62(238):83–86.
25. Hawthorne GC, Campbell NP, Geddes JS, et al. Amiodarone-induced hypothyroidism. A common complication of prolonged therapy: a report of eight cases. Arch Intern Med 1985; 145(6):1016–1019.
26. Smyrk TC, Goellner JR, Brennan MD, et al. Pathology of the thyroid in amiodarone-associated thyrotoxicosis. Am J Surg Pathol 1987; 11(3):197–204.
27. Oppenheimer JH, Tavernetti RR. Displacement of thyroxine from human thyroxine-binding globulin by analogues of hydantoin. Steric aspects of the thyroxinebinding site. J Clin Invest 1962; 41:2213–2220.
28. Kuiper JJ. Lymphocytic thyroiditis possibly induced by diphenylhydantoin. Jama 1969; 210(13):2370–2372.
29. Carr RF, LiVolsi VA. Morphologic changes in the thyroid after irradiation for Hodgkin's and non-Hodgkin's lymphoma. Cancer 1989; 64(4):825–829.
30. Favus MJ, Schneider AB, Stachura ME, et al. Thyroid cancer occurring as a late consequence of head-and-neck irradiation. Evaluation of 1056 patients. N Engl J Med 1976; 294(19):1019–1025.

31. Holten I. Acute response of the thyroid to external radiation. Acta Pathol Microbiol Immunol Scand Suppl 1983; 283:1–111.

32. Kennedy JS, Thomson JA. The changes in the thyroid gland after irradiation with 131I or partial thyroidectomy for thyrotoxicosis. J Pathol 1974; 112(2):65–81.

33. Fogelfeld L, Wiviott MB, Shore-Freedman E, et al. Recurrence of thyroid nodules after surgical removal in patients irradiated in childhood for benign conditions. N Engl J Med 1989; 320(13):835–840.

34. Schneider AB, Recant W, Pinsky SM, et al. Radiation-induced thyroid carcinoma. Clinical course and results of therapy in 296 patients. Ann Intern Med 1986; 105(3): 405–412.

35. Williams ED, Abrosimov A, Bogdanova T, et al. Thyroid carcinoma after Chernobyl latent period, morphology and aggressiveness. Br J Cancer 2004; 90(11):2219–2224.

36. Fisher DA, Klein AH. Thyroid development and disorders of thyroid function in the newborn. N Engl J Med 1981; 304(12):702–712.

37. Acebron A, Aza-Blanc P, Rossi DL, et al. Congenital human thyroglobulin defect due to low expression of the thyroid-specific transcription factor TTF-1. J Clin Invest 1995; 96(2):781–785.

38. Baughman RA. Lingual thyroid and lingual thyroglossal tract remnants. A clinical and histopathologic study with review of the literature. Oral Surg Oral Med Oral Pathol 1972; 34(5):781–799.

39. Block MA, Wylie JH, Patton RB, et al. Does benign thyroid tissue occur in the lateral part of the neck? Am J Surg 1966; 112(4):476–481.

40. deSouza FM, Smith PE. Retrosternal goiter. J Otolaryngol 1983; 12(6):393–396.

41. Neinas FW, Gorman CA, Devine KD, et al. Lingual thyroid. Clinical characteristics of 15 cases. Ann Intern Med 1973; 79(2):205–210.

42. Pollice L, Caruso G. Struma cordis. Ectopic thyroid goiter in the right ventricle. Arch Pathol Lab Med 1986; 110(5): 452–453.

43. Spinner RJ, Moore KL, Gottfried MR, et al. Thoracic intrathymic thyroid. Ann Surg 1994; 220(1):91–96.

44. LiVolsi V. Surgical pathology of the thyroid. Major problems in the pathology series. Philadelphia: WB Saunders Co., 1990:1–438.

45. LiVolsi VA, Perzin KH, Savetsky L. Carcinoma arising in median ectopic thyroid (including thyroglossal duct tissue). Cancer 1974; 34(4):1303–1315.

46. Meyer JS, Steinberg LS. Microscopically benign thyroid follicles in cervical lymph nodes. Serial section study of lymph node inclusions and entire thyroid gland in 5 cases. Cancer 1969; 24(2):302–311.

47. Moses DC, Thompson NW, Nishiyama RH, et al. Ectopic thyroid tissue in the neck. Benign or malignant? Cancer 1976; 38(1):361–365.

48. Jain SN. Lingual thyroid. Int Surg 1969; 52(4):320–325.

49. Jaques DA, Chambers RG, Oertel JE. Thyroglossal tract carcinoma. A review of the literature and addition of eighteen cases. Am J Surg 1970; 120(4):439–446.

50. Nussbaum M, Buchwald RP, Ribner A, et al. Anaplastic carcinoma arising from median ectopic thyroid (thyroglossal duct remnant). Cancer 1981; 48(12):2724–2728.

51. Hathong BM. Innocuous accessory thyroid nodules. Arch Surg 1965; 90:222–227.

52. Sisson JC, Schmidt RW, Beierwaltes WH. Sequestered Nodular Goiter. N Engl J Med 1964; 270:927–932.

53. Shimizu M, Hirokawa M, Manabe T. Parasitic nodule of the thyroid in a patient with Graves' disease. Virchows Arch 1999; 434(3):241–244.

54. Latchman DS. Transcription-factor mutations and disease. N Engl J Med 1996; 334(1):28–33.

55. Guazzi S, Price M, De Felice M, et al. Thyroid nuclear factor 1 (TTF-1) contains a homeodomain and displays a novel DNA binding specificity. Embo J 1990; 9(11):3631–3639.

56. Fabbro D, Di Loreto C, Beltrami CA, et al. Expression of thyroid-specific transcription factors TTF-1 and PAX-8 in human thyroid neoplasms. Cancer Res 1994; 54(17): 4744–4749.

57. Shimura H, Shimura Y, Ohmori M, et al. Single strand DNA-binding proteins and thyroid transcription factor-1 conjointly regulate thyrotropin receptor gene expression. Mol Endocrinol 1995; 9(5):527–539.

58. Sinclair AJ, Lonigro R, Civitareale D, et al. The tissue-specific expression of the thyroglobulin gene requires interaction between thyroid-specific and ubiquitous factors. Eur J Biochem 1990; 193(2):311–318.

59. Mitchell PJ, Tjian R. Transcriptional regulation in mammalian cells by sequence-specific DNA binding proteins. Science 1989; 245(4916):371–378.

60. Zannini M, Francis-Lang H, Plachov D, et al. Pax-8, a paired domain-containing protein, binds to a sequence overlapping the recognition site of a homeodomain and activates transcription from two thyroid-specific promoters. Mol Cell Biol 1992; 12(9):4230–4241.

61. Duprez L, Parma J, Van Sande J, et al. Germline mutations in the thyrotropin receptor gene cause non-autoimmune autosomal dominant hyperthyroidism. Nat Genet 1994; 7(3):396–401.

62. Fuhrer D, Holzapfel HP, Wonerow P, et al. Somatic mutations in the thyrotropin receptor gene and not in the Gs alpha protein gene in 31 toxic thyroid nodules. J Clin Endocrinol Metab 1997; 82(11):3885–3891.

63. Paschke R, Ludgate M. The thyrotropin receptor in thyroid diseases. N Engl J Med 1997; 337(23):1675–1681.

64. Rossi DL, Acebron A, Santisteban P. Function of the homeo and paired domain proteins TTF-1 and Pax-8 in thyroid cell proliferation. J Biol Chem 1995; 270(39):23139–23142.

65. Lorini R, Gastaldi R, Traggiai C, et al. Hashimoto's Thyroiditis. Pediatr Endocrinol Rev 2003; 1(suppl 2):205–211 (discussion 211).

66. Tandon N, Zhang L, Weetman AP. HLA associations with Hashimoto's thyroiditis. Clin Endocrinol (Oxf) 1991; 34(5):383–386.

67. Goudie RB, Anderson JR, Gray KG, et al. Autoimmune Associations of Hashimoto's Disease. Lancet 1965; 17: 322–323.

68. Nicholson LB, Wong FS, Ewins DL, et al. Susceptibility to autoimmune thyroiditis in Down's syndrome is associated with the major histocompatibility class II DQA 0301 allele. Clin Endocrinol (Oxf) 1994; 41(3):381–383.

69. Furszyfer J, Kurland LT, McConahey WM, et al. Graves' disease in Olmsted County, Minnesota, 1935 through 1967. Mayo Clin Proc 1970; 45(9):636–644.

70. Bartley GB, Fatourechi V, Kadrmas EF, et al. The incidence of Graves' ophthalmopathy in Olmsted County, Minnesota. Am J Ophthalmol 1995; 120(4):511–517.

71. Erickson LA, Yousef OM, Jin L, et al. p27kip1 expression distinguishes papillary hyperplasia in Graves' disease from papillary thyroid carcinoma. Mod Pathol 2000; 13 (9):1014–1019.

72. Stagnaro-Green A. Postpartum thyroiditis. Best Pract Res Clin Endocrinol Metab 2004; 18(2):303–316.

73. Terry AJ, Hague WM. Postpartum thyroiditis. Semin Perinatol 1998; 22(6):497–502.

74. Mizukami Y, Michigishi T, Nonomura A, et al. Postpartum thyroiditis. A clinical, histologic, and immunopathologic study of 15 cases. Am J Clin Pathol 1993; 100(3):200–205.

75. Weaver DR, Deodhar SD, Hazard JB. A characterization of focal lymphocytic thyroiditis. Cleve Clin Q 1966; 33(2): 59–72.

76. Harris M. The cellular infiltrate in Hashimoto's disease and focal lymphocytic thyroiditis. J Clin Pathol 1969; 22(3): 326–333.

77. Denham MJ, Wills EJ. A clinico-pathological survey of thyroid glands in old age. Gerontology 1980; 26(3):160–166.

78. Mitchell JD, Kirkham N, Machin D. Focal lymphocytic thyroiditis in Southampton. J Pathol 1984; 144(4):269–273.

79. Beahrs OH, McConahey WM, Woolner LB. Invasive fibrous thyroiditis (Riedel's struma). J Clin Endocrinol Metab 1957; 17(2):201–220.

80. Best TB, Munro RE, Burwell S, et al. Riedel's thyroiditis associated with Hashimoto's thyroiditis, hypoparathyroidism, and retroperitoneal fibrosis. J Endocrinol Invest 1991; 14(9):767–772.

81. Chopra D, Wool MS, Crosson A, et al. Riedel's struma associated with subacute thyroiditis, hypothyroidism, and hypoparathyroidism. J Clin Endocrinol Metab 1978; 46(6):869–871.

82. Malotte MJ, Chonkich GD, Zuppan CW. Riedel's thyroiditis. Arch Otolaryngol Head Neck Surg 1991; 117(2):214–217.

83. Yasmeen T, Khan S, Patel SG, et al. Clinical case seminar: Riedel's thyroiditis: report of a case complicated by spontaneous hypoparathyroidism, recurrent laryngeal nerve injury, and Horner's syndrome. J Clin Endocrinol Metab 2002; 87(8):3543–3547.

84. Sato K, Hanazawa H, Watanabe J, et al. Differential diagnosis and management of airway obstruction in Riedel's thyroiditis: a case report. Auris Nasus Larynx 2005; 32(4):439–443.

85. de Lange WE, Freling NJ, Molenaar WM, et al. Invasive fibrous thyroiditis (Riedel's struma): a manifestation of multifocal fibrosclerosis? A case report with review of the literature. Q J Med 1989; 72(268):709–717.

86. Brazier DJ, Sanders MD. Multifocal fibrosclerosis associated with suprasellar and macular lesions. Br J Ophthalmol 1983; 67(5):292–296.

87. Meijer S, Hoitsma HF, Scholtmeijer R. Idiopathic retroperitoneal fibrosis in multifocal fibrosclerosis. Eur Urol 1976; 2(5):258–260.

88. Comings DE, Skubi KB, Van Eyes J, et al. Familial multifocal fibrosclerosis. Findings suggesting that retroperitoneal fibrosis, mediastinal fibrosis, sclerosing cholangitis, Riedel's thyroiditis, and pseudotumor of the orbit may be different manifestations of a single disease. Ann Intern Med 1967; 66(5):884–892.

89. Meijer S, Hausman R. Occlusive phlebitis, a diagnostic feature in Riedel's thyroiditis. Virchows Arch A Pathol Anat Histol 1978; 377(4):339–349.

90. Papi G, Corrado S, Carapezzi C, et al. Riedel's thyroiditis and fibrous variant of Hashimoto's thyroiditis: a clinicopathological and immunohistochemical study. J Endocrinol Invest 2003; 26(5):444–449.

91. Pritchyk K, Newkirk K, Garlich P, et al. Tamoxifen therapy for Riedel's thyroiditis. Laryngoscope 2004; 114(10): 1758–1760.

92. Few J, Thompson NW, Angelos P, et al. Riedel's thyroiditis: treatment with tamoxifen. Surgery 1996; 120(6):993–998 (discussion 998–999).

93. Bignell GR, Canzian F, Shayeghi M, et al. Familial nontoxic multinodular thyroid goiter locus maps to chromosome 14q but does not account for familial nonmedullary thyroid cancer. Am J Hum Genet 1997; 61(5):1123–1130.

94. Sakorafas GH, Stafyla V, Kolettis T, et al. Microscopic papillary thyroid cancer as an incidental finding in patients treated surgically for presumably benign thyroid disease. J Postgrad Med 2007; 53(1):23–26.

95. Gandolfi PP, Frisina A, Raffa M, et al. The incidence of thyroid carcinoma in multinodular goiter: retrospective analysis. Acta Biomed 2004; 75(2):114–117.

96. Ghossein RA, Rosai J, Heffess C. Dyshormonogenetic goiter: a clinicopathologic study of 56 cases. Endocr Pathol 1997; 8(4):283–292.

97. Kopp P. Pendred's syndrome: identification of the genetic defect a century after its recognition. Thyroid 1999; 9(1): 65–69.

98. Kopp P. Pendred's syndrome and genetic defects in thyroid hormone synthesis. Rev Endocr Metab Disord 2000; 1(1–2):109–121.

99. Borck G, Roth C, Martine U, et al. Mutations in the PDS gene in German families with Pendred's syndrome: V138F is a founder mutation. J Clin Endocrinol Metab 2003; 88(6):2916–2921.

100. Kennedy JS. The pathology of dyshormonogenetic goitre. J Pathol 1969; 99(3):251–264.

101. Vickery AL Jr. The diagnosis of malignancy in dyshormonogenetic goitre. Clin Endocrinol Metab 1981; 10(2):317–335.

102. Yashiro T, Ito K, Akiba M, et al. Papillary carcinoma of the thyroid arising from dyshormonogenetic goiter. Endocrinol Jpn 1987; 34(6):955–964.

103. Medeiros-Neto G, Gil-Da-Costa MJ, Santos CL, et al. Metastatic thyroid carcinoma arising from congenital goiter due to mutation in the thyroperoxidase gene. J Clin Endocrinol Metab 1998; 83(11):4162–4166.

104. Hamed G, Heffess CS, Shmookler BM, et al. Amyloid goiter. A clinicopathologic study of 14 cases and review of the literature. Am J Clin Pathol 1995; 104(3):306–312.

105. Sinha RN, Plehn JF, Kinlaw WB. Amyloid goiter due to primary systemic amyloidosis: a diagnostic challenge. Thyroid 1998; 8(11):1051–1054.

106. Daoud F, Nieman RE, Vilter RW. Amyloid goiter in a case of generalized primary amyloidosis. Am J Med 1967; 43(4): 604–608.

107. Habu S, Watanobe H, Kimura K, et al. A case of amyloid goiter secondary to Crohn's disease. Endocr J 1999; 46(1): 179–182.

108. Duzgun N, Morris Y, Yildiz HI, et al. Amyloid goiter in juvenile onset rheumatoid arthritis. Scand J Rheumatol 2003; 32(4):253–254.

109. Cohan P, Hirschowitz S, Rao JY, et al. Amyloid goiter in a case of systemic amyloidosis secondary to ankylosing spondylitis. J Endocrinol Invest 2000; 23(11):762–764.

110. D'Antonio A, Franco R, Sparano L, et al. Amyloid goiter: the first evidence in secondary amyloidosis. Report of five cases and review of literature. Adv Clin Path 2000; 4(2): 99–106.

111. Goldsmith JD, Lai ML, Daniele GM, et al. Amyloid goiter: report of two cases and review of the literature. Endocr Pract 2000; 6(4):318–323.

112. Liftin AJ. Nonmedullary carcinoma of the thyroid gland in association with amyloid goiter: case report. Mt Sinai J Med 1985; 52(3):225–227.

113. Nessim S, Tamilia M. Papillary thyroid carcinoma associated with amyloid goiter. Thyroid 2005; 15(4):382–385.

114. Takai SI, Miyauchi A, Matsuzuka F, et al. Internal fistula as a route of infection in acute suppurative thyroiditis. Lancet 1979; 1(8119):751–752.

115. Miyauchi A, Matsuzuka F, Takai S, et al. Piriform sinus fistula. A route of infection in acute suppurative thyroiditis. Arch Surg 1981; 116(1):66–69.

116. Andres JC, Nagalla R. Acute bacterial thyroiditis secondary to urosepsis. J Am Board Fam Pract 1995; 8(2):128–129.

117. Yung BC, Loke TK, Fan WC, et al. Acute suppurative thyroiditis due to foreign body-induced retropharyngeal abscess presented as thyrotoxicosis. Clin Nucl Med 2000; 25(4):249–252.

118. Brook I. Microbiology and management of acute suppurative thyroiditis in children. Int J Pediatr Otorhinolaryngol 2003; 67(5):447–451.

119. Chen HW, Tseng FY, Su DH, et al. Secondary infection and ischemic necrosis after fine needle aspiration for a painful papillary thyroid carcinoma: a case report. Acta Cytol 2006; 50(2):217–220.

120. Jimenez-Heffernan JA, Perez F, Hornedo J, et al. Massive thyroid tumoral embolism from a breast carcinoma presenting as acute thyroiditis. Arch Pathol Lab Med 2004; 128(7):804–806.

121. Lin KD, Lin JD, Huang MJ, et al. Acute suppurative thyroiditis and aggressive malignant thyroid tumors: differences in clinical presentation. J Surg Oncol 1998; 67(1):28–32.

122. Fatourechi V, Aniszewski JP, Fatourechi GZ, et al. Clinical features and outcome of subacute thyroiditis in an incidence cohort: Olmsted County, Minnesota, study. J Clin Endocrinol Metab 2003; 88(5):2100–2105.

123. Kitchener MI, Chapman IM. Subacute thyroiditis: a review of 105 cases. Clin Nucl Med 1989; 14(6):439–442.

124. Stancek D, Stancekova-Gressnerova M, Janotka M, et al. Isolation and some serological and epidemiological data on the viruses recovered from patients with subacute thyroiditis de Quervain. Med Microbiol Immunol (Berl) 1975; 161(2):133–144.

125. Eylan E, Zmucky R, Sheba C. Mumps virus and subacute thyroiditis; evidence of a causal association. Lancet 1957; 272(6978):1062–1063.

126. Brouqui P, Raoult D, Conte-Devolx B. Coxsackie thyroiditis. Ann Intern Med 1991; 114(12):1063–1064.

127. Volpe R, Row VV, Ezrin C. Circulating viral and thyroid antibodies in subacute thyroiditis. J Clin Endocrinol Metab 1967; 27(9):1275–1284.

128. Volta C, Carano N, Street ME, et al. Atypical subacute thyroiditis caused by Epstein-Barr virus infection in a three-year-old girl. Thyroid 2005; 15(10):1189–1191.

129. Greene JN. Subacute thyroiditis. Am J Med 1971; 51(1):97–108.

130. Friedman ND, Spelman DW. Subacute thyroiditis presenting as pyrexia of unknown origin in a patient with human immunodeficiency virus infection. Clin Infect Dis 1999; 29(5):1352–1353.

131. Parana R, Cruz M, Lyra L, et al. Subacute thyroiditis during treatment with combination therapy (interferon plus ribavirin) for hepatitis C virus. J Viral Hepat 2000; 7(5):393–395.

132. Hsiao JY, Hsin SC, Hsieh MC, et al. Subacute thyroiditis following influenza vaccine (vaxigrip(r)) in a young female. Kaohsiung J Med Sci 2006; 22(6):297–300.

133. Rotenberg Z, Weinberger I, Fuchs J, et al. Euthyroid atypical subacute thyroiditis simulating systemic or malignant disease. Arch Intern Med 1986; 146(1):105–107.

134. Volpe R. The pathology of thyroiditis. Hum Pathol 1978; 9(4):429–438.

135. Kojima M, Nakamura S, Oyama T, et al. Cellular composition of subacute thyroiditis. an immunohistochemical study of six cases. Pathol Res Pract 2002; 198(12):833–837.

136. Carney JA, Moore SB, Northcutt RC, et al. Palpation thyroiditis (multifocal granulomatour folliculitis). Am J Clin Pathol 1975; 64(5):639–647.

137. Harach HR, Williams ED. The pathology of granulomatous diseases of the thyroid gland. Sarcoidosis 1990; 7(1):19–27.

138. Berger SA, Zonszein J, Villamena P, et al. Infectious diseases of the thyroid gland. Rev Infect Dis 1983; 5(1):108–122.

139. Cilley RE, Thompson NW, Lloyd RV, et al. Sarcoidosis of the thyroid presenting as a painful nodule. Thyroidology 1988; (1):61–62.

140. Gentilucci UV, Picardi A, Manfiini S, et al. Granulomatous thyroiditis: an unexpected finding leading to the diagnosis of sarcoidosis. Acta Biomed 2004; 75(1):69–73.

141. Ozdogu H, Boga C, Bolat F, et al. Wegener's granulomatosis with a possible thyroidal involvement. J Natl Med Assoc 2006; 98(6):956–958.

142. Schuerwegh AJ, Verhelst J, Slabbynck H, et al. Wegener's granulomatosis presenting as a thyroid mass. Clin Rheumatol 2007; 26(3):454–456.

143. Grassi A, Torcigliani A. [Galactose, glucagon, BZ 55 and thyroid in hepatic glycogenosis (Gierke's disease).]. Minerva Pediatr 1960; 12:907–911.

144. Hui KS, Williams JC, Borit A, et al. The endocrine glands in Pompe's disease. Report of two cases. Arch Pathol Lab Med 1985; 109(10):921–925.

145. Manta P, Kontoleon P, Panousopoulou A, et al. Type II glycogenosis and thyroxine binding globulin deficiency in the same family. Funct Neurol 1996; 11(2–3):105–110.

146. Chan AM, Lynch MJ, Bailey JD, et al. Hypothyroidism in cystinosis. A clinical, endocrinologic and histologic study involving sixteen patients with cystinosis. Am J Med 1970; 48(6):678–692.

147. Burke JR, El-Bishti MM, Maisey MN, et al. Hypothyroidism in children with cystinosis. Arch Dis Child 1978; 53(12):947–951.

148. Bercu BB, Orloff S, Schulman JD. Pituitary resistance to thyroid hormone in cystinosis. J Clin Endocrinol Metab 1980; 51(6):1262–1268.

149. Lucky AW, Howley PM, Megyesi K, et al. Endocrine studies in cystinosis: compensated primary hypothyroidism. J Pediatr 1977; 91(2):204–210.

150. Dayan AD, Trickey RJ. Thyroid involvement in juvenile amaurotic family idiocy (Batten's disease). Lancet 1970; 2(7667):296–297.

151. Armstrong D, VanWormer DE, Neville H, et al. Thyroid peroxidase deficiency in Batten-Spielmeyer-Vogt disease. Arch Pathol 1975; 99(8):430–435.

152. Goldfischer S, Grotsky HW, Chang CH, et al. Idiopathic neonatal iron storage involving the liver, pancreas, heart, and endocrine and exocrine glands. Hepatology 1981; 1(1):58–64.

153. Alexander CB, Herrera GA, Jaffe K, et al. Black thyroid: clinical manifestations, ultrastructural findings, and possible mechanisms. Hum Pathol 1985; 16(1):72–78.

154. Boniciolli B, Brollo A, Bianchi C. [Frequency and significance of intravesicular thyroid crystals]. Ann Anat Pathol (Paris) 1976; 21(3):339–346.

155. Robboy SJ, Scully RE. Strumal carcinoid of the ovary: an analysis of 50 cases of a distinctive tumor composed of thyroid tissue and carcinoid. Cancer 1980; 46(9):2019–2034.

156. Richter MN, Mc CK. Anisotropic crystals in the human thyroid gland. Am J Pathol 1954; 30(3):545–553.

157. Furuta M, Ozaki M. Calcium oxalate crystals in the kidney and thyroid of leprosy patients. Int J Lepr Other Mycobact Dis 1970; 38(3):286–293.

158. Nanetti L. [On the presence of intrafollicular crystals in the thyroid of persons killed by hanging]. Boll Soc Ital Biol Sper 1972; 48(3):50–52.

159. Fayemi AO, Ali M, Braun EV. Oxalosis in hemodialysis patients: a pathologic study of 80 cases. Arch Pathol Lab Med 1979; 103(2):58–62.

160. Isotalo PA, Lloyd RV. Presence of birefringent crystals is useful in distinguishing thyroid from parathyroid gland tissues. Am J Surg Pathol 2002; 26(6):813–814.

161. Walsh FM, Castelli JB. Polytef granuloma clinically simulating carcinoma of the thyroid. Arch Otolaryngol 1975; 101(4):262–263.

162. Wassef M, Achouche J, Guichard JP, et al. A delayed teflonoma of the neck simulating a thyroid neoplasm. ORL J Otorhinolaryngol Relat Spec 1994; 56(6):352–356.

163. Wilson RA, Gartner WS Jr. Teflon granuloma mimicking a thyroid tumor. Diagn Cytopathol 1987; 3(2):156–158.

164. DeLellis RA, Lloyd RV, Heitz PU, et al. Pathology and Genetics of Tumours of Endocrine Organs. Lyon, France: IARC Press, 2004:49–134.

165. Rosai J, Carcangiu ML, DeLellis RA. Tumors of the Thyroid Gland. Washington, DC: Armed Forces Institute of Pathology, 1992:1–182.

166. Narita T, Takagi K. Ataxia-telangiectasia with dysgerminoma of right ovary, papillary carcinoma of thyroid, and adenocarcinoma of pancreas. Cancer 1984; 54(6): 1113–1116.

167. Sandoval C, Schantz S, Posey D, et al. Parotid and thyroid gland cancers in patients with ataxia-telangiectasia. Pediatr Hematol Oncol 2001; 18(8):485–490.

168. Brasseur B, Beauloye V, Chantrain C, et al. Papillary thyroid carcinoma in a 9-year-old girl with ataxia-telangiectasia. Pediatr Blood Cancer 2006.

169. Alsanea O, Clark OH. Familial thyroid cancer. Curr Opin Oncol 2001; 13(1):44–51.

170. Albright EC, Allday RW. Thyroid carcinoma after radiation therapy for adolescent acne vulgaris. JAMA 1967; 199(4): 280–281.

171. Calandra DB, Shah KH, Lawrence AM, et al. Total thyroidectomy in irradiated patients. A twenty-year experience in 206 patients. Ann Surg 1985; 202(3):356–360.

172. Furmanchuk AW, Averkin JI, Egloff B, et al. Pathomorphological findings in thyroid cancers of children from the Republic of Belarus: a study of 86 cases occurring between 1986 ('post-Chernobyl') and 1991. Histopathology 1992; 21(5):401–408.

173. Nikiforov Y, Gnepp DR. Pediatric thyroid cancer after the Chernobyl disaster. Pathomorphologic study of 84 cases (1991–1992) from the Republic of Belarus. Cancer 1994; 74(2):748–766.

174. Unger K, Zurnadzhy L, Walch A, et al. RET rearrangements in post-Chernobyl papillary thyroid carcinomas with a short latency analysed by interphase FISH. Br J Cancer 2006; 94(10):1472–1477.

175. Nikiforov YE, Nikiforova MN, Gnepp DR, et al. Prevalence of mutations of ras and p53 in benign and malignant thyroid tumors from children exposed to radiation after the Chernobyl nuclear accident. Oncogene 1996; 13(4): 687–693.

176. Rabes HM. Gene rearrangements in radiation-induced thyroid carcinogenesis. Med Pediatr Oncol 2001; 36(5): 574–582.

177. Nikiforova MN, Ciampi R, Salvatore G, et al. Low prevalence of BRAF mutations in radiation-induced thyroid tumors in contrast to sporadic papillary carcinomas. Cancer Lett 2004; 209(1):1–6.

178. Gupta S, Sodhani P, Jain S, et al. Morphologic spectrum of papillary carcinoma of the thyroid: role of cytology in identifying the variants. Acta Cytol 2004; 48(6):795–800.

179. Baloch ZW, LiVolsi VA. Microcarcinoma of the thyroid. Adv Anat Pathol 2006; 13(2):69–75.

180. Neuhold N, Kaiser H, Kaserer K. Latent carcinoma of the thyroid in Austria: a systematic autopsy study. Endocr Pathol 2001; 12(1):23–31.

181. de Matos PS, Ferreira AP, Ward LS. Prevalence of papillary microcarcinoma of the thyroid in Brazilian autopsy and surgical series. Endocr Pathol 2006; 17(2):165–173.

182. Harach HR, Franssila KO, Wasenius VM. Occult papillary carcinoma of the thyroid. A "normal" finding in Finland. A systematic autopsy study. Cancer 1985; 56(3):531–538.

183. Rosai J, LiVolsi VA, Sobrinho-Simoes M, et al. Renaming papillary microcarcinoma of the thyroid gland: the Porto proposal. Int J Surg Pathol 2003; 11(4):249–251.

184. Haas SN. Management of papillary microcarcinoma of the thyroid. S D Med 2006; 59(10):425–427.

185. Lissak B, Vannetzel JM, Gallouedec N, et al. Solitary skin metastasis as the presenting feature of differentiated thyroid microcarcinoma: report of two cases. J Endocrinol Invest 1995; 18(10):813–816.

186. Lin KD, Lin JD, Huang HS, et al. Skull metastasis with brain invasion from thyroid papillary microcarcinoma. J Formos Med Assoc 1997; 96(4):280–282.

187. Lo CY, Chan WF, Lang BH, et al. Papillary microcarcinoma: is there any difference between clinically overt and occult tumors? World J Surg 2006; 30(5):759–766.

188. Piersanti M, Ezzat S, Asa SL. Controversies in papillary microcarcinoma of the thyroid. Endocr Pathol 2003; 14(3): 183–191.

189. Lupoli G, Vitale G, Caraglia M, et al. Familial papillary thyroid microcarcinoma: a new clinical entity. Lancet 1999; 353(9153):637–639.

190. Nikiforov YE. RET/PTC rearrangement in thyroid tumors. Endocr Pathol 2002; 13(1):3–16.

191. Crile G Jr., Hazard JB. Relationship of the age of the patient to the natural history and prognosis of carcinoma of the thyroid. Ann Surg 1953; 138(1):33–38.

192. Hazard JB, Crile G Jr., Dinsmore RS, et al. Neoplasms of the thyroid: classification, morphology, and treatment. AMA Arch Pathol 1955; 59(4):502–513.

193. Lindsay S. Natural history of thyroid carcinoma. Ariz Med 1960; 17:623–627.

194. Chen KT, Rosai J. Follicular variant of thyroid papillary carcinoma: a clinicopathologic study of six cases. Am J Surg Pathol 1977; 1(2):123–130.

195. Albores-Saavedra J, Gould E, Vardaman C, et al. The macrofollicular variant of papillary thyroid carcinoma: a study of 17 cases. Hum Pathol 1991; 22(12):1195–1205.

196. Fadda G, Fiorino MC, Mule A, et al. Macrofollicular encapsulated variant of papillary thyroid carcinoma as a potential pitfall in histologic and cytologic diagnosis. A report of three cases. Acta Cytol 2002; 46(3):555–559.

197. Muzaffar M, Nigar E, Mushtaq S, et al. The morphological variants of papillary carcinoma of the thyroid: a clinico-pathological study—AFIP experience. Armed Forces Institute of Pathology. J Pak Med Assoc 1998; 48(5):133–137.

198. Ivanova R, Soares P, Castro P, et al. Diffuse (or multinodular) follicular variant of papillary thyroid carcinoma: a clinicopathologic and immunohistochemical analysis of ten cases of an aggressive form of differentiated thyroid carcinoma. Virchows Arch 2002; 440(4):418–424.

199. Mizukami Y, Nonomura A, Michigishi T, et al. Diffuse follicular variant of papillary carcinoma of the thyroid. Histopathology 1995; 27(6):575–577.

200. Lloyd RV, Erickson LA, Casey MB, et al. Observer variation in the diagnosis of follicular variant of papillary thyroid carcinoma. Am J Surg Pathol 2004; 28(10):1336–1340.

201. Hawk WA, Hazard JB. The many appearances of papillary carcinoma of the thyroid. Cleve Clin Q 1976; 43(4): 207–215.

202. Johnson TL, Lloyd RV, Thompson NW, et al. Prognostic implications of the tall cell variant of papillary thyroid carcinoma. Am J Surg Pathol 1988; 12(1):22–27.

203. Hicks MJ, Batsakis JG. Tall cell carcinoma of the thyroid gland. Ann Otol Rhinol Laryngol 1993; 102(5):402–403.

204. Moreno Egea A, Rodriguez Gonzalez JM, Sola Perez J, et al. Prognostic value of the tall cell variety of papillary cancer of the thyroid. Eur J Surg Oncol 1993; 19(6): 517–521.

205. Evans HL. Columnar-cell carcinoma of the thyroid. A report of two cases of an aggressive variant of thyroid carcinoma. Am J Clin Pathol 1986; 85(1):77–80.

206. Sobrinho-Simoes M, Nesland JM, Johannessen JV. Columnar-cell carcinoma. Another variant of poorly differentiated carcinoma of the thyroid. Am J Clin Pathol 1988; 89(2):264–267.

207. Ferreiro JA, Hay ID, Lloyd RV. Columnar cell carcinoma of the thyroid: report of three additional cases. Hum Pathol 1996; 27(11):1156–1160.

208. Gaertner EM, Davidson M, Wenig BM. The columnar cell variant of thyroid papillary carcinoma. Case report and discussion of an unusually aggressive thyroid papillary carcinoma. Am J Surg Pathol 1995; 19(8):940–947.

209. Akslen LA, Varhaug JE. Thyroid carcinoma with mixed tall-cell and columnar-cell features. Am J Clin Pathol 1990; 94(4):442–445.

210. Putti TC, Bhuiya TA. Mixed columnar cell and tall cell variant of papillary carcinoma of thyroid: a case report and review of the literature. Pathology 2000; 32(4):286–289.

211. Evans HL. Encapsulated columnar-cell neoplasms of the thyroid. A report of four cases suggesting a favorable prognosis. Am J Surg Pathol 1996; 20(10):1205–1211.

212. Wenig BM, Thompson LD, Adair CF, et al. Thyroid papillary carcinoma of columnar cell type: a clinicopathologic study of 16 cases. Cancer 1998; 82(4):740–753.

213. Hirokawa M, Shimizu M, Fukuya T, et al. Columnar Cell Carcinoma of the Thyroid: MIB-1 Immunoreactivity as a Prognostic Factor. Endocr Pathol 1998; 9(1):31–34.

214. Vickery AL Jr., Carcangiu ML, Johannessen JV, et al. Papillary carcinoma. Semin Diagn Pathol 1985; 2(2): 90–100.

215. Chan JK, Tsui MS, Tse CH. Diffuse sclerosing variant of papillary carcinoma of the thyroid: a histological and immunohistochemical study of three cases. Histopathology 1987; 11(2):191–201.

216. Carcangiu ML, Bianchi S. Diffuse sclerosing variant of papillary thyroid carcinoma. Clinicopathologic study of 15 cases. Am J Surg Pathol 1989; 13(12):1041–1049.

217. Soares J, Limbert E, Sobrinho-Simoes M. Diffuse sclerosing variant of papillary thyroid carcinoma. A clinicopathologic study of 10 cases. Pathol Res Pract 1989; 185(2): 200–206.

218. Falvo L, Giacomelli L, D'Andrea V, et al. Prognostic importance of sclerosing variant in papillary thyroid carcinoma. Am Surg 2006; 72(5):438–444.

219. Fujimoto Y, Obara T, Ito Y, et al. Diffuse sclerosing variant of papillary carcinoma of the thyroid. Clinical importance, surgical treatment, and follow-up study. Cancer 1990; 66(11):2306–2312.

220. Schroder S, Bay V, Dumke K, et al. Diffuse sclerosing variant of papillary thyroid carcinoma. S-100 protein immunocytochemistry and prognosis. Virchows Arch A Pathol Anat Histopathol 1990; 416(4):367–371.

221. Thompson LD, Wieneke JA, Heffess CS. Diffuse sclerosing variant of papillary thyroid carcinoma: a clinicopathologic and immunophenotypic analysis of 22 cases. Endocr Pathol 2005; 16(4):331–348.

222. Nikiforov YE, Erickson LA, Nikiforova MN, et al. Solid variant of papillary thyroid carcinoma: incidence, clinical-pathologic characteristics, molecular analysis, and biologic behavior. Am J Surg Pathol 2001; 25(12):1478–1484.

223. Keelawat S, Poumsuk U. Association between different variants of papillary thyroid carcinoma and risk-group according to AMES (age, metastasis, extent and size) classification system. J Med Assoc Thai 2006; 89(4):484–489.

224. Santoro M, Thomas GA, Vecchio G, et al. Gene rearrangement and Chernobyl related thyroid cancers. Br J Cancer 2000; 82(2):315–322.

225. Trovisco V, Soares P, Soares R, et al. A new BRAF gene mutation detected in a case of a solid variant of papillary thyroid carcinoma. Hum Pathol 2005; 36(6):694–697.

226. Herrera MF, Hay ID, Wu PS, et al. Hurthle cell (oxyphilic) papillary thyroid carcinoma: a variant with more aggressive biologic behavior. World J Surg 1992; 16(4):669–674 (discussion 774–665).

227. Besic N, Hocevar M, Zgajnar J, et al. Aggressiveness of therapy and prognosis of patients with Hurthle cell papillary thyroid carcinoma. Thyroid 2006; 16(1):67–72.

228. Mai KT, Thomas J, Yazdi HM, et al. Pathologic study and clinical significance of Hurthle cell papillary thyroid carcinoma. Appl Immunohistochem Mol Morphol 2004; 12(4):329–337.

229. Apel RL, Asa SL, LiVolsi VA. Papillary Hurthle cell carcinoma with lymphocytic stroma. "Warthin-like tumor" of the thyroid. Am J Surg Pathol 1995; 19(7):810–814.

230. Baloch ZW, LiVolsi VA. Warthin-like papillary carcinoma of the thyroid. Arch Pathol Lab Med 2000; 124(8):1192–1195.

231. Lam KY, Lo CY, Wei WI. Warthin tumor-like variant of papillary thyroid carcinoma: a case with dedifferentiation (anaplastic changes) and aggressive biological behavior. Endocr Pathol 2005; 16(1):83–89.

232. Cameselle-Teijeiro J, Chan JK. Cribriform-morular variant of papillary carcinoma: a distinctive variant representing the sporadic counterpart of familial adenomatous polyposis-associated thyroid carcinoma? Mod Pathol 1999; 12(4):400–411.

233. Chan JK, Loo KT. Cribriform variant of papillary thyroid carcinoma. Arch Pathol Lab Med 1990; 114(6):622–624.

234. Harach HR, Williams GT, Williams ED. Familial adenomatous polyposis associated thyroid carcinoma: a distinct type of follicular cell neoplasm. Histopathology 1994; 25(6): 549–561.

235. Soravia C, Sugg SL, Berk T, et al. Familial adenomatous polyposis-associated thyroid cancer: a clinical, pathological, and molecular genetics study. Am J Pathol 1999; 154(1): 127–135.

236. Xu B, Yoshimoto K, Miyauchi A, et al. Cribriform-morular variant of papillary thyroid carcinoma: a pathological and molecular genetic study with evidence of frequent somatic mutations in exon 3 of the beta-catenin gene. J Pathol 2003; 199(1):58–67.

237. Hirokawa M, Kuma S, Miyauchi A, et al. Morules in cribriform-morular variant of papillary thyroid carcinoma: immunohistochemical characteristics and distinction from squamous metaplasia. Apmis 2004; 112(4–5):275–282.

238. Chan JK, Carcangiu ML, Rosai J. Papillary carcinoma of thyroid with exuberant nodular fasciitis-like stroma. Report of three cases. Am J Clin Pathol 1991; 95(3):309–314.

239. Michal M, Chlumska A, Fakan F. Papillary carcinoma of thyroid with exuberant nodular fasciitis-like stroma. Histopathology 1992; 21(6):577–579.

240. Basu S, Nair N, Shet T, et al. Papillary thyroid carcinoma with exuberant nodular fasciitis-like stroma: treatment outcome and prognosis. J Laryngol Otol 2006; 120(4): 338–342.

241. Akslen LA, Maehle BO. Papillary thyroid carcinoma with lipomatous stroma. Am J Surg Pathol 1997; 21(10): 1256–1257.

242. Gnepp DR, Ogorzalek JM, Heffess CS. Fat-containing lesions of the thyroid gland. Am J Surg Pathol 1989; 13(7):605–612.

243. Vestfrid MA. Papillary carcinoma of the thyroid gland with lipomatous stroma: report of a peculiar histological type of thyroid tumour. Histopathology 1986; 10(1):97–100.

244. Carcangiu ML, Sibley RK, Rosai J. Clear cell change in primary thyroid tumors. A study of 38 cases. Am J Surg Pathol 1985; 9(10):705–722.

245. Variakojis D, Getz ML, Paloyan E, et al. Papillary clear cell carcinoma of the thyroid gland. Hum Pathol 1975; 6(3): 384–390.

246. Dickersin GR, Vickery AL Jr., Smith SB. Papillary carcinoma of the thyroid, oxyphil cell type, "clear cell" variant: a light- and electron-microscopic study. Am J Surg Pathol 1980; 4(5):501–509.

247. Casey MB, Lohse CM, Lloyd RV. Distinction between papillary thyroid hyperplasia and papillary thyroid carcinoma by immunohistochemical staining for cytokeratin 19, galectin-3, and HBME-1. Endocr Pathol 2003; 14(1): 55–60.

248. Prasad ML, Pellegata NS, Huang Y, et al. Galectin-3, fibronectin-1, CITED-1, HBME1 and cytokeratin-19 immunohistochemistry is useful for the differential diagnosis of thyroid tumors. Mod Pathol 2005; 18(1):48–57.

249. van Hoeven KH, Kovatich AJ, Miettinen M. Immunocytochemical evaluation of HBME-1, CA 19-9, and CD-15 (Leu-M1) in fine-needle aspirates of thyroid nodules. Diagn Cytopathol 1998; 18(2):93–97.

250. Mai KT, Ford JC, Yazdi HM, et al. Immunohistochemical study of papillary thyroid carcinoma and possible papillary thyroid carcinoma-related benign thyroid nodules. Pathol Res Pract 2000; 196(8):533–540.

251. Scognamiglio T, Hyjek E, Kao J, et al. Diagnostic usefulness of HBME1, galectin-3, CK19, and CITED1 and evaluation of their expression in encapsulated lesions with questionable features of papillary thyroid carcinoma. Am J Clin Pathol 2006; 126(5):700–708.

252. Cheung CC, Ezzat S, Freeman JL, et al. Immunohistochemical diagnosis of papillary thyroid carcinoma. Mod Pathol 2001; 14(4):338–342.

253. Gaffney RL, Carney JA, Sebo TJ, et al. Galectin-3 expression in hyalinizing trabecular tumors of the thyroid gland. Am J Surg Pathol 2003; 27(4):494–498.

254. Cvejic D, Savin S, Petrovic I, et al. Galectin-3 expression in papillary microcarcinoma of the thyroid. Histopathology 2005; 47(2):209–214.

255. Herrmann ME, LiVolsi VA, Pasha TL, et al. Immunohistochemical expression of galectin-3 in benign and malignant thyroid lesions. Arch Pathol Lab Med 2002; 126 (6):710–713.

256. Nasr MR, Mukhopadhyay S, Zhang S, et al. Immunohistochemical markers in diagnosis of papillary thyroid carcinoma: utility of HBME1 combined with CK19 immunostaining. Mod Pathol 2006; 19(12):1631–1637.

257. Prasad ML, Pellegata NS, Kloos RT, et al. CITED1 protein expression suggests Papillary Thyroid Carcinoma in high throughput tissue microarray-based study. Thyroid 2004; 14(3):169–175.

258. Gomez-Morales M, Alvaro T, Munoz M, et al. Diffuse sclerosing papillary carcinoma of the thyroid gland: immunohistochemical analysis of the local host immune response. Histopathology 1991; 18(5):427–433.

259. Kameyama K, Mukai M, Takami H, et al. Cribriform-morular variant of papillary thyroid carcinoma: ultrastructural study and somatic/germline mutation analysis of the APC gene. Ultrastruct Pathol 2004; 28(2):97–102.

260. Bounacer A, Wicker R, Caillou B, et al. High prevalence of activating ret proto-oncogene rearrangements, in thyroid tumors from patients who had received external radiation. Oncogene 1997; 15(11):1263–1273.

261. Nikiforov YE, Rowland JM, Bove KE, et al. Distinct pattern of ret oncogene rearrangements in morphological variants of radiation-induced and sporadic thyroid papillary carcinomas in children. Cancer Res 1997; 57(9): 1690–1694.

262. Soares P, Trovisco V, Rocha AS, et al. BRAF mutations and RET/PTC rearrangements are alternative events in the etiopathogenesis of PTC. Oncogene 2003; 22(29): 4578–4580.

263. Trovisco V, Vieira de Castro I, Soares P, et al. BRAF mutations are associated with some histological types of papillary thyroid carcinoma. J Pathol 2004; 202(2):247–251.

264. Trovisco V, Soares P, Preto A, et al. Type and prevalence of BRAF mutations are closely associated with papillary thyroid carcinoma histotype and patients' age but not with tumour aggressiveness. Virchows Arch 2005; 446(6): 589–595.

265. Lima J, Trovisco V, Soares P, et al. BRAF mutations are not a major event in post-Chernobyl childhood thyroid carcinomas. J Clin Endocrinol Metab 2004; 89(9): 4267–4271.

266. Kumagai A, Namba H, Saenko VA, et al. Low frequency of BRAFT1796A mutations in childhood thyroid carcinomas. J Clin Endocrinol Metab 2004; 89(9):4280–4284.

267. Nikiforova MN, Kimura ET, Gandhi M, et al. BRAF mutations in thyroid tumors are restricted to papillary carcinomas and anaplastic or poorly differentiated carcinomas arising from papillary carcinomas. J Clin Endocrinol Metab 2003; 88(11):5399–5404.

268. Akslen LA, LiVolsi VA. Prognostic significance of histologic grading compared with subclassification of papillary thyroid carcinoma. Cancer 2000; 88(8):1902–1908.

269. Michels JJ, Jacques M, Henry-Amar M, et al. Prevalence and prognostic significance of tall cell variant of papillary thyroid carcinoma. Hum Pathol 2007; 38(2):212–219.

270. Carney JA, Ryan J, Goellner JR. Hyalinizing trabecular adenoma of the thyroid gland. Am J Surg Pathol 1987; 11(8):583–591.

271. Katoh R, Jasani B, Williams ED. Hyalinizing trabecular adenoma of the thyroid. A report of three cases with immunohistochemical and ultrastructural studies. Histopathology 1989; 15(3):211–224.

272. Chan JK, Tse CC, Chiu HS. Hyalinizing trabecular adenoma-like lesion in multinodular goitre. Histopathology 1990; 16(6):611–614.

273. Cerasoli S, Tabarri B, Farabegoli P, et al. Hyalinizing trabecular adenoma of the thyroid. Report of two cases, with cytologic, immunohistochemical and ultrastructural studies. Tumori 1992; 78(4):274–279.

274. Chetty R, Beydoun R, LiVolsi VA. Paraganglioma-like (hyalinizing trabecular) adenoma of the thyroid revisited. Pathology 1994; 26(4):429–431.

275. Molberg K, Albores-Saavedra J. Hyalinizing trabecular carcinoma of the thyroid gland. Hum Pathol 1994; 25 (2):192–197.

276. McCluggage WG, Sloan JM. Hyalinizing trabecular carcinoma of thyroid gland. Histopathology 1996; 28(4): 357–362.

277. Lloyd RV. Hyalinizing trabecular tumors of the thyroid: a variant of papillary carcinoma? Adv Anat Pathol 2002; 9(1):7–11.

278. Casey MB, Sebo TJ, Carney JA. Hyalinizing trabecular adenoma of the thyroid gland: cytologic features in 29 cases. Am J Surg Pathol 2004; 28(7):859–867.

279. Kaleem Z, Davila RM. Hyalinizing trabecular adenoma of the thyroid. A report of two cases with cytologic, histologic and immunohistochemical findings. Acta Cytol 1997; 41(3):883–888.

280. Rothenberg HJ, Goellner JR, Carney JA. Prevalence and incidence of cytoplasmic yellow bodies in thyroid neoplasms. Arch Pathol Lab Med 2003; 127(6):715–717.

281. Fonseca E, Nesland JM, Sobrinho-Simoes M. Expression of stratified epithelial-type cytokeratins in hyalinizing trabecular adenomas supports their relationship with papillary carcinomas of the thyroid. Histopathology 1997; 31(4):330–335.

282. Hirokawa M, Carney JA, Ohtsuki Y. Hyalinizing trabecular adenoma and papillary carcinoma of the thyroid gland express different cytokeratin patterns. Am J Surg Pathol 2000; 24(6):877–881.

283. Papotti M, Riella P, Montemurro F, et al. Immunophenotypic heterogeneity of hyalinizing trabecular tumours of the thyroid. Histopathology 1997; 31(6):525–533.

284. Galgano MT, Mills SE, Stelow EB. Hyalinizing trabecular adenoma of the thyroid revisited: a histologic and immunohistochemical study of thyroid lesions with prominent trabecular architecture and sclerosis. Am J Surg Pathol 2006; 30(10):1269–1273.

285. Hirokawa M, Carney JA. Cell membrane and cytoplasmic staining for MIB-1 in hyalinizing trabecular adenoma of the thyroid gland. Am J Surg Pathol 2000; 24(4):575–578.

286. Rothenberg HJ, Goellner JR, Carney JA. Hyalinizing trabecular adenoma of the thyroid gland: recognition and characterization of its cytoplasmic yellow body. Am J Surg Pathol 1999; 23(1):118–125.

287. Katoh R, Kakudo K, Kawaoi A. Accumulated basement membrane material in hyalinizing trabecular tumors of the thyroid. Mod Pathol 1999; 12(11):1057–1061.

288. Papotti M, Volante M, Giuliano A, et al. RET/PTC activation in hyalinizing trabecular tumors of the thyroid. Am J Surg Pathol 2000; 24(12):1615–1621.

289. Cheung CC, Boerner SL, MacMillan CM, et al. Hyalinizing trabecular tumor of the thyroid: a variant of papillary carcinoma proved by molecular genetics. Am J Surg Pathol 2000; 24(12):1622–1626.

290. Sheils O, Smyth P, Finn S, et al. RET/PTC rearrangements in Hashimoto's thyroiditis. Int J Surg Pathol 2002; 10(2):167–168. (author reply 168–169).

291. Wirtschafter A, Schmidt R, Rosen D, et al. Expression of the RET/PTC fusion gene as a marker for papillary carcinoma in Hashimoto's thyroiditis. Laryngoscope 1997; 107(1):95–100.

292. Nikiforova MN, Caudill CM, Biddinger P, et al. Prevalence of RET/PTC rearrangements in Hashimoto's thyroiditis and papillary thyroid carcinomas. Int J Surg Pathol 2002; 10(1):15–22.

293. Nakamura N, Carney JA, Jin L, et al. RASSF1A and NORE1A methylation and BRAFV600E mutations in thyroid tumors. Lab Invest 2005; 85(9):1065–1075.

294. Salvatore G, Chiappetta G, Nikiforov YE, et al. Molecular profile of hyalinizing trabecular tumours of the thyroid: high prevalence of RET/PTC rearrangements and absence of B-raf and N-ras point mutations. Eur J Cancer 2005; 41(5):816–821.

295. Marques AR, Espadinha C, Catarino AL, et al. Expression of PAX8-PPAR gamma 1 rearrangements in both follicular thyroid carcinomas and adenomas. J Clin Endocrinol Metab 2002; 87(8):3947–3952.

296. Nikiforova MN, Lynch RA, Biddinger PW, et al. RAS point mutations and PAX8-PPAR gamma rearrangement in thyroid tumors: evidence for distinct molecular pathways in thyroid follicular carcinoma. J Clin Endocrinol Metab 2003; 88(5):2318–2326.

297. Johannessen JV, Sobrinho-Simoes M. The fine structure of follicular thyroid adenomas. Am J Clin Pathol 1982; 78(3):299–310.

298. Nesland JM, Sobrinho-Simoes M, Johannessen JV. Scanning electron microscopy of the human thyroid gland and its disorders. Scanning Microsc 1987; 1(4):1797–1810.

299. Schlinkert RT, van Heerden JA, Goellner JR, et al. Factors that predict malignant thyroid lesions when fine-needle aspiration is "suspicious for follicular neoplasm". Mayo Clin Proc 1997; 72(10):913–916.

300. van Heerden JA, Hay ID, Goellner JR, et al. Follicular thyroid carcinoma with capsular invasion alone: a non-threatening malignancy. Surgery 1992; 112(6):1130–1136 (discussion 1136–1138).

301. Scheumman GF, Hoang-Vu C, Cetin Y, et al. Clinical significance of E-cadherin as a prognostic marker in thyroid carcinomas. J Clin Endocrinol Metab 1995; 80(7):2168–2172.

302. Brecelj E, Frkovic Grazio S, Auersperg M, et al. Prognostic value of E-cadherin expression in thyroid follicular carcinoma. Eur J Surg Oncol 2005; 31(5):544–548.

303. Motti ML, Califano D, Baldassarre G, et al. Reduced E-cadherin expression contributes to the loss of p27kip1-mediated mechanism of contact inhibition in thyroid anaplastic carcinomas. Carcinogenesis 2005; 26(6):1021–1034.

304. Ito Y, Yoshida H, Tomoda C, et al. HBME-1 expression in follicular tumor of the thyroid: an investigation of whether it can be used as a marker to diagnose follicular carcinoma. Anticancer Res 2005; 25(1A):179–182.

305. Papotti M, Rodriguez J, De Pompa R, et al. Galectin-3 and HBME-1 expression in well-differentiated thyroid tumors with follicular architecture of uncertain malignant potential. Mod Pathol 2005; 18(4):541–546.

306. Miettinen M, Karkkainen P. Differential reactivity of HBME-1 and CD15 antibodies in benign and malignant thyroid tumours. Preferential reactivity with malignant tumours. Virchows Arch 1996; 429(4–5):213–219.

307. Schelfhout LJ, Van Muijen GN, Fleuren GJ. Expression of keratin 19 distinguishes papillary thyroid carcinoma from follicular carcinomas and follicular thyroid adenoma. Am J Clin Pathol 1989; 92(5):654–658.

308. Puglisi F, Cesselli D, Damante G, et al. Expression of Pax-8, p53 and bcl-2 in human benign and malignant thyroid diseases. Anticancer Res 2000; 20(1A):311–316.

309. Kroll TG, Sarraf P, Pecciarini L, et al. PAX8-PPARgamma1 fusion oncogene in human thyroid carcinoma [corrected]. Science 2000; 289(5483):1357–1360.

310. Erickson LA, Jin L, Wollan PC, et al. Expression of p27kip1 and Ki-67 in benign and malignant thyroid tumors. Mod Pathol 1998; 11(2):169–174.

311. Chen HY, Benjamin LB, Chen MF. Hurthle cell tumor. Int Surg 1996; 81(2):168–170.

312. Erickson LA, Jin L, Goellner JR, et al. Pathologic features, proliferative activity, and cyclin D1 expression in Hurthle cell neoplasms of the thyroid. Mod Pathol 2000; 13(2):186–192.

313. Watson RG, Brennan MD, Goellner JR, et al. Invasive Hurthle cell carcinoma of the thyroid: natural history and management. Mayo Clin Proc 1984; 59(12):851–855.

314. Volante M, Bozzalla-Cassione F, DePompa R, et al. Galectin-3 and HBME-1 expression in oncocytic cell tumors of the thyroid. Virchows Arch 2004; 445(2):183–188.

315. Finley DJ, Zhu B, Fahey TJ 3rd, . Molecular analysis of Hurthle cell neoplasms by gene profiling. Surgery 2004; 136(6):1160–1168.

316. Erickson LA, Jalal SM, Goellner JR, et al. Analysis of Hurthle cell neoplasms of the thyroid by interphase fluorescence in situ hybridization. Am J Surg Pathol 2001; 25(7):911–917.

317. Fusco A, Viglietto G, Santoro M. Point mutation in GRIM-19: a new genetic lesion in Hurthle cell thyroid carcinomas. Br J Cancer 2005; 92(10):1817–1818.

318. Maximo V, Botelho T, Capela J, et al. Somatic and germline mutation in GRIM-19, a dual function gene involved in mitochondrial metabolism and cell death, is linked to mitochondrion-rich (Hurthle cell) tumours of the thyroid. Br J Cancer 2005; 92(10):1892–1898.

319. DeLellis RA, Lloyd RV, Heitz PU, eds. WHO Classification of Tumours—Pathology and Genetics. Lyon, France: IARC Press, 2004.

320. Carcangiu ML, Zampi G, Rosai J. Poorly differentiated ("insular") thyroid carcinoma. A reinterpretation of Langhans' "wuchernde Struma". Am J Surg Pathol 1984; 8(9): 655–668.

321. Rosai J. Poorly differentiated thyroid carcinoma: introduction to the issue, its landmarks, and clinical impact. Endocr Pathol 2004; 15(4):293–296.

322. Sakamoto A, Kasai N, Sugano H. Poorly differentiated carcinoma of the thyroid. A clinicopathologic entity for a high-risk group of papillary and follicular carcinomas. Cancer 1983; 52(10):1849–1855.

323. Sakamoto A. Definition of poorly differentiated carcinoma of the thyroid: the Japanese experience. Endocr Pathol 2004; 15(4):307–311.

324. Akslen LA, LiVolsi VA. Poorly differentiated thyroid carcinoma—it is important. Am J Surg Pathol 2000; 24(2): 310–313.

325. Albores-Saavedra J, Carrick K. Where to set the threshold between well differentiated and poorly differentiated follicular carcinomas of the thyroid. Endocr Pathol 2004; 15(4):297–305.

326. Ashfaq R, Vuitch F, Delgado R, et al. Papillary and follicular thyroid carcinomas with an insular component. Cancer 1994; 73(2):416–423.

327. Hiltzik D, Carlson DL, Tuttle RM, et al. Poorly differentiated thyroid carcinomas defined on the basis of mitosis and necrosis: a clinicopathologic study of 58 patients. Cancer 2006; 106(6):1286–1295.

328. Nikiforov YE. Genetic alterations involved in the transition from well-differentiated to poorly differentiated and anaplastic thyroid carcinomas. Endocr Pathol 2004; 15(4): 319–327.

329. Papotti M, Botto Micca F, Favero A, et al. Poorly differentiated thyroid carcinomas with primordial cell component. A group of aggressive lesions sharing insular, trabecular, and solid patterns. Am J Surg Pathol 1993; 17(3):291–301.

330. Papotti M, Torchio B, Grassi L, et al. Poorly differentiated oxyphilic (Hurthle cell) carcinomas of the thyroid. Am J Surg Pathol 1996; 20(6):686–694.

331. Pilotti S, Collini P, Mariani L, et al. Insular carcinoma: a distinct de novo entity among follicular carcinomas of the thyroid gland. Am J Surg Pathol 1997; 21(12):1466–1473.

332. Pilotti S, Collini P, Manzari A, et al. Poorly differentiated forms of papillary thyroid carcinoma: distinctive entities or morphological patterns? Semin Diagn Pathol 1995; 12(3):249–255.

333. Sobrinho-Simoes M, Sambade C, Fonseca E, et al. Poorly differentiated carcinomas of the thyroid gland: a review of the clinicopathologic features of a series of 28 cases of a heterogeneous, clinically aggressive group of thyroid tumors. Int J Surg Pathol 2002; 10(2):123–131.

334. Volante M, Landolfi S, Chiusa L, et al. Poorly differentiated carcinomas of the thyroid with trabecular, insular, and solid patterns: a clinicopathologic study of 183 patients. Cancer 2004; 100(5):950–957.

335. Volante M, Cavallo GP, Papotti M. Prognostic factors of clinical interest in poorly differentiated carcinomas of the thyroid. Endocr Pathol 2004; 15(4):313–317.

336. Diehl M, Graichen S, Menzel C, et al. F-18 FDG PET in insular thyroid cancer. Clin Nucl Med 2003; 28(9): 728–731.

337. Volante M, Collini P, Nikiforov YE, et al. Poorly differentiated thyroid carcinoma. The Turin proposal for the use of uniform diagnostic criteria and an algorithmic diagnostic approach. Am J Surg Pathol 2007; 31(8):1256–1264.

338. Giuffrida D, Gharib H. Anaplastic thyroid carcinoma: current diagnosis and treatment. Ann Oncol 2000; 11(9): 1083–1089.

339. Karavitaki N, Vlassopoulou V, Tzanela M, et al. Recurrent and/or metastatic thyroid cancer: therapeutic options. Expert Opin Pharmacother 2002; 3(7):939–947.

340. Ordonez NG, El-Naggar AK, Hickey RC, et al. Anaplastic thyroid carcinoma. Immunocytochemical study of 32 cases. Am J Clin Pathol 1991; 96(1):15–24.

341. Venkatesh YS, Ordonez NG, Schultz PN, et al. Anaplastic carcinoma of the thyroid. A clinicopathologic study of 121 cases. Cancer 1990; 66(2):321–330.

342. Khan N, Oriuchi N, Higuchi T, et al. Review of fluorine-18-2-fluoro-2-deoxy-D-glucose positron emission tomography (FDG-PET) in the follow-up of medullary and anaplastic thyroid carcinomas. Cancer Control 2005; 12(4):254–260.

343. Gimm O, Perren A, Weng LP, et al. Differential nuclear and cytoplasmic expression of PTEN in normal thyroid tissue, and benign and malignant epithelial thyroid tumors. Am J Pathol 2000; 156(5):1693–1700.

344. Fagin JA, Matsuo K, Karmakar A, et al. High prevalence of mutations of the p53 gene in poorly differentiated human thyroid carcinomas. J Clin Invest 1993; 91(1):179–184.

345. Farid NR. P53 mutations in thyroid carcinoma: tidings from an old foe. J Endocrinol Invest 2001; 24(7):536–545.

346. Garcia-Rostan G, Tallini G, Herrero A, et al. Frequent mutation and nuclear localization of beta-catenin in anaplastic thyroid carcinoma. Cancer Res 1999; 59(8): 1811–1815.

347. de Lellis RA, Wolfe HJ. The pathobiology of the human calcitonin (C)-cell: a review. Pathol Annu 1981; 16(pt 2): 25–52.

348. Rosai J, Carcangiu ML, de Lellis RA. Tumors of the Thryoid Gland. Washington, DC: Armed Forces Institute of Pathology 1992:207–258.

349. Perry A, Molberg K, Albores-Saavedra J. Physiologic versus neoplastic C-cell hyperplasia of the thyroid: separation of distinct histologic and biologic entities. Cancer 1996; 77(4):750–756.

350. Albores-Saavedra J, Monforte H, Nadji M, et al. C-cell hyperplasia in thyroid tissue adjacent to follicular cell tumors. Hum Pathol 1988; 19(7):795–799.

351. Libbey NP, Nowakowski KJ, Tucci JR. C-cell hyperplasia of the thyroid in a patient with goitrous hypothyroidism and Hashimoto's thyroiditis. Am J Surg Pathol 1989; 13(1):71–77.

352. Lips CJ, Leo JR, Berends MJ, et al. Thyroid C-cell hyperplasia and micronodules in close relatives of MEN-2A patients: pitfalls in early diagnosis and reevaluation of criteria for surgery. Henry Ford Hosp Med J 1987; 35 (2–3):133–138.

353. LiVolsi VA, Feind CR, LoGerfo P, et al. Demonstration by immunoperoxidase staining of hyperplasia of parafollicular cells in the thyroid gland in hyperparathyroidism. J Clin Endocrinol Metab 1973; 37(4):550–559.

354. Eng C. Seminars in medicine of the Beth Israel Hospital, Boston. The RET proto-oncogene in multiple endocrine neoplasia type 2 and Hirschsprung's disease. N Engl J Med 1996; 335(13):943–951.

355. Eng C, Thomas GA, Neuberg DS, et al. Mutation of the RET proto-oncogene is correlated with RET immunostaining in subpopulations of cells in sporadic medullary thyroid carcinoma. J Clin Endocrinol Metab 1998; 83(12): 4310–4313.

356. Lloyd RV. RET proto-oncogene mutations and rearrangements in endocrine diseases. Am J Pathol 1995; 147(6): 1539–1544.

357. Komminoth P, Kunz EK, Matias-Guiu X, et al. Analysis of RET protooncogene point mutations distinguishes heritable from nonheritable medullary thyroid carcinomas. Cancer 1995; 76(3):479–489.

358. Wolfe HJ, Melvin KE, Cervi-Skinner SJ, et al. C-cell hyperplasia preceding medullary thyroid carcinoma. N Engl J Med 1973; 289(9):437–441.

359. DeLellis RA, Nunnemacher G, Wolfe HJ. C-cell hyperplasia. An ultrastructural analysis. Lab Invest 1977; 36 (3):237–248.

360. Yamaoka Y. Solid cell nest (SCN) of the human thyroid gland. Acta Pathol Jpn 1973; 23(3):493–506.

361. Lallier M, St-Vil D, Giroux M, et al. Prophylactic thyroidectomy for medullary thyroid carcinoma in gene carriers of MEN2 syndrome. J Pediatr Surg 1998; 33(6):846–848.

362. Albores-Saavedra J, LiVolsi VA, Williams ED. Medullary carcinoma. Semin Diagn Pathol 1985; 2(2):137–146.

363. Carney JA, Sizemore GW, Tyce GM. Bilateral adrenal medullary hyperplasia in multiple endocrine neoplasia, type 2: the precursor of bilateral pheochromocytoma. Mayo Clin Proc 1975; 50(1):3–10.

364. DeLellis RA, Rule AH, Spiler I, et al. Calcitonin and carcinoembryonic antigen as tumor markers in medullary thyroid carcinoma. Am J Clin Pathol 1978; 70(4):587–594.

365. Mendelsohn G, Eggleston JC, Weisburger WR, et al. Calcitonin and histaminase in C-cell hyperplasia and medullary thyroid carcinoma. A light microscopic and immunohistochemical study. Am J Pathol 1978; 92(1): 35–43.

366. Gagel RF, Tashjian AH Jr., Cummings T, et al. The clinical outcome of prospective screening for multiple endocrine neoplasia type 2a. An 18-year experience. N Engl J Med 1988; 318(8):478–484.

367. Pacini F, Fontanelli M, Fugazzola L, et al. Routine measurement of serum calcitonin in nodular thyroid diseases allows the preoperative diagnosis of unsuspected sporadic medullary thyroid carcinoma. J Clin Endocrinol Metab 1994; 78(4):826–829.

368. Iagaru A, Masamed R, Singer PA, et al. Detection of occult medullary thyroid cancer recurrence with 2-deoxy-2-[F-18]fluoro-D-glucose-PET and PET/CT. Mol Imaging Biol 2007; 9(2):72–77.

369. Hazard JB, Hawk WA, Crile G Jr. Medullary (solid) carcinoma of the thyroid; a clinicopathologic entity. J Clin Endocrinol Metab 1959; 19(1):152–161.

370. Papotti M, Sambataro D, Pecchioni C, et al. The pathology of medullary carcinoma of the thyroid: review of the literature and personal experience on 62 cases. Endocr Pathol 1996; 7(1):1–20.

371. Uribe M, Fenoglio-Preiser CM, Grimes M, et al. Medullary carcinoma of the thyroid gland. Clinical, pathological, and immunohistochemical features with review of the literature. Am J Surg Pathol 1985; 9(8):577–594.

372. Beerman H, Rigaud C, Bogomoletz WV, et al. Melanin production in black medullary thyroid carcinoma (MTC). Histopathology 1990; 16(3):227–233.

373. Beskid M, Lorenc R, Rosciszewska A. C-cell thyroid adenoma in man. J Pathol 1971; 103(1):1–4.

374. Mendelsohn G, Baylin SB, Bigner SH, et al. Anaplastic variants of medullary thyroid carcinoma: a light-microscopic and immunohistochemical study. Am J Surg Pathol 1980; 4(4):333–341.

375. Harach HR, Bergholm U. Medullary (C cell) carcinoma of the thyroid with features of follicular oxyphilic cell tumours. Histopathology 1988; 13(6):645–656.

376. Franc B, Rosenberg-Bourgin M, Caillou B, et al. Medullary thyroid carcinoma: search for histological predictors of survival (109 proband cases analysis). Hum Pathol 1998; 29(10):1078–1084.

377. Hales M, Rosenau W, Okerlund MD, et al. Carcinoma of the thyroid with a mixed medullary and follicular pattern: morphologic, immunohistochemical, and clinical laboratory studies. Cancer 1982; 50(7):1352–1359.

378. Ljungberg O, Bondeson L, Bondeson AG. Differentiated thyroid carcinoma, intermediate type: a new tumor entity with features of follicular and parafollicular cell carcinoma. Hum Pathol 1984; 15(3):218–228.

379. Albores-Saavedra J, Gorraez de la Mora T, de la Torre-Rendon F, et al. Mixed medullary-papillary carcinoma of the thyroid: a previously unrecognized variant of thyroid carcinoma. Hum Pathol 1990; 21(11):1151–1155.

380. Gimm O, Marsh DJ, Andrew SD, et al. Germline dinucleotide mutation in codon 883 of the RET proto-oncogene in multiple endocrine neoplasia type 2B without codon 918 mutation. J Clin Endocrinol Metab 1997; 82(11):3902–3904.

381. Gimm O, Niederle BE, Weber T, et al. RET proto-oncogene mutations affecting codon 790/791: a mild form of multiple endocrine neoplasia type 2A syndrome? Surgery 2002; 132(6):952–959 (discussion 959).

382. Eng C, Clayton D, Schuffenecker I, et al. The relationship between specific RET proto-oncogene mutations and disease phenotype in multiple endocrine neoplasia type 2. International RET mutation consortium analysis. JAMA 1996; 276(19):1575–1579.

383. Bhattacharyya N. A population-based analysis of survival factors in differentiated and medullary thyroid carcinoma. Otolaryngol Head Neck Surg 2003; 128(1):115–123.

384. Beressi N, Campos JM, Beressi JP, et al. Sporadic medullary microcarcinoma of the thyroid: a retrospective analysis of eighty cases. Thyroid 1998; 8(11):1039–1044.

385. Kebebew E, Ituarte PH, Siperstein AE, et al. Medullary thyroid carcinoma: clinical characteristics, treatment, prognostic factors, and a comparison of staging systems. Cancer 2000; 88(5):1139–1148.

386. Bondeson L, Bondeson AG, Thompson NW. Papillary carcinoma of the thyroid with mucoepidermoid features. Am J Clin Pathol 1991; 95(2):175–179.

387. Baloch ZW, Solomon AC, LiVolsi VA. Primary mucoepidermoid carcinoma and sclerosing mucoepidermoid carcinoma with eosinophilia of the thyroid gland: a report of nine cases. Mod Pathol 2000; 13(7):802–807.

388. Tanda F, Massarelli G, Bosincu L. Primary mucoepidermoid carcinoma of the thyroid gland. Surg Pathol 1990; 3: 317–324.

389. Cavazza A, Toschi E, Valcavi R, et al. [Sclerosing mucoepidermoid carcinoma with eosinophilia of the thyroid: description of a case]. Pathologica 1999; 91(1):31–35.

390. Chan JK, Albores-Saavedra J, Battifora H, et al. Sclerosing mucoepidermoid thyroid carcinoma with eosinophilia. A distinctive low-grade malignancy arising from the metaplastic follicles of Hashimoto's thyroiditis. Am J Surg Pathol 1991; 15(5):438–448.

391. Chung J, Lee SK, Gong G, et al. Sclerosing mucoepidermoid carcinoma with eosinophilia of the thyroid glands: a case report with clinical manifestation of recurrent neck mass. J Korean Med Sci 1999; 14(3):338–341.

392. Chetty R, Goetsch S, Nayler S, et al. Spindle epithelial tumour with thymus-like element (SETTLE): the predominantly monophasic variant. Histopathology 1998; 33(1): 71–74.

393. Kloboves-Prevodnik V, Jazbec J, Us-Krasovec M, et al. Thyroid spindle epithelial tumor with thymus-like differentiation (SETTLE): is cytopathological diagnosis possible? Diagn Cytopathol 2002; 26(5):314–319.

394. Xu B, Hirokawa M, Yoshimoto K, et al. Spindle epithelial tumor with thymus-like differentiation of the thyroid: a case report with pathological and molecular genetics study. Hum Pathol 2003; 34(2):190–193.

395. Cheuk W, Jacobson AA, Chan JK. Spindle epithelial tumor with thymus-like differentiation (SETTLE): a distinctive malignant thyroid neoplasm with significant metastatic potential. Mod Pathol 2000; 13(10):1150–1155.

396. Su L, Beals T, Bernacki EG, et al. Spindle epithelial tumor with thymus-like differentiation: a case report with cytologic, histologic, immunohistologic, and ultrastructural findings. Mod Pathol 1997; 10(5):510–514.

397. Berezowski K, Grimes MM, Gal A, et al. CD5 immunoreactivity of epithelial cells in thymic carcinoma and CASTLE using paraffin-embedded tissue. Am J Clin Pathol 1996; 106(4):483–486.

398. Chan JK, Rosai J. Tumors of the neck showing thymic or related branchial pouch differentiation: a unifying concept. Hum Pathol 1991; 22(4):349–367.

399. Dorfman DM, Shahsafaei A, Miyauchi A. Immunohistochemical staining for bcl-2 and mcl-1 in intrathyroidal epithelial thymoma (ITET)/carcinoma showing thymus-like differentiation (CASTLE) and cervical thymic carcinoma. Mod Pathol 1998; 11(10):989–994.

400. Dorfman DM, Shahsafaei A, Miyauchi A. Intrathyroidal epithelial thymoma (ITET)/carcinoma showing thymus-like differentiation (CASTLE) exhibits CD5 immunoreactivity: new evidence for thymic differentiation. Histopathology 1998; 32(2):104–109.

401. Namba H, Gutman RA, Matsuo K, et al. H-ras protooncogene mutations in human thyroid neoplasms. J Clin Endocrinol Metab 1990; 71(1):223–229.

402. Mizukami Y, Kurumaya H, Yamada T, et al. Thymic carcinoma involving the thyroid gland: report of two cases. Hum Pathol 1995; 26(5):576–579.

403. Lam KY, Lo CY, Liu MC. Primary squamous cell carcinoma of the thyroid gland: an entity with aggressive clinical behaviour and distinctive cytokeratin expression profiles. Histopathology 2001; 39(3):279–286.

404. Chaudhary RK, Barnes EL, Myers EN. Squamous cell carcinoma arising in Hashimoto's thyroiditis. Head Neck 1994; 16(6):582–585.

405. Cook AM, Vini L, Harmer C. Squamous cell carcinoma of the thyroid: outcome of treatment in 16 patients. Eur J Surg Oncol 1999; 25(6):606–609.

406. Lam KY, Lui MC, Lo CY. Cytokeratin expression profiles in thyroid carcinomas. Eur J Surg Oncol 2001; 27(7):631–635.

407. Lam KY, Lo CY, Chan KW, et al. Insular and anaplastic carcinoma of the thyroid: a 45-year comparative study at a single institution and a review of the significance of p53 and p21. Ann Surg 2000; 231(3):329–338.

408. Booya F, Sebo TJ, Kasperbauer JL, et al. Primary squamous cell carcinoma of the thyroid: report of ten cases. Thyroid 2006; 16(1):89–93.

409. Jordan RB, Gauderer MW. Cervical teratomas: an analysis. Literature review and proposed classification. J Pediatr Surg 1988; 23(6):583–591.

410. Buckley NJ, Burch WM, Leight GS. Malignant teratoma in the thyroid gland of an adult: a case report and a review of the literature. Surgery 1986; 100(5):932–937.

411. Tapper D, Lack EE. Teratomas in infancy and childhood. A 54-year experience at the Children's Hospital Medical Center. Ann Surg 1983; 198(3):398–410.

412. Thompson LD, Rosai J, Heffess CS. Primary thyroid teratomas: a clinicopathologic study of 30 cases. Cancer 2000; 88(5):1149–1158.

413. Ueno NT, Amato RJ, Ro JJ, et al. Primary malignant teratoma of the thyroid gland: report and discussion of two cases. Head Neck 1998; 20(7):649–653.

414. Aozasa K, Tsujimoto M, Sakurai M, et al. Non-Hodgkin's lymphomas in Osaka, Japan. Eur J Cancer Clin Oncol 1985; 21(4):487–492.

415. Freeman C, Berg JW, Cutler SJ. Occurrence and prognosis of extranodal lymphomas. Cancer 1972; 29(1):252–260.

416. Derringer GA, Thompson LD, Frommelt RA, et al. Malignant lymphoma of the thyroid gland: a clinicopathologic study of 108 cases. Am J Surg Pathol 2000; 24(5):623–639.

417. Ghazanfar S, Quraishy MS, Essa K, et al. Mucosa associated lymphoid tissue lymphoma (Maltoma) in patients with cold nodule thyroid. J Pak Med Assoc 2002; 52(3):131–133.

418. Pedersen RK, Pedersen NT. Primary non-Hodgkin's lymphoma of the thyroid gland: a population based study. Histopathology 1996; 28(1):25–32.

419. Pledge S, Bessell EM, Leach IH, et al. Non-Hodgkin's lymphoma of the thyroid: a retrospective review of all patients diagnosed in Nottinghamshire from 1973 to 1992. Clin Oncol (R Coll Radiol) 1996; 8(6):371–375.

420. Cocker RS, Kang J, Kahn LB. Rosai-Dorfman disease. Report of a case presenting as a midline thyroid mass. Arch Pathol Lab Med 2003; 127(4):e197–e200.

421. Larkin DF, Dervan PA, Munnelly J, et al. Sinus histiocytosis with massive lymphadenopathy simulating subacute thyroiditis. Hum Pathol 1986; 17(3):321–324.

422. Tamouridis N, Deladetsima JK, Kastanias I, et al. Cold thyroid nodule as the sole manifestation of Rosai-Dorfman disease with mild lymphadenopathy, coexisting with chronic autoimmune thyroiditis. J Endocrinol Invest 1999; 22(11):866–870.

423. Brunnemann RB, Ro JY, Ordonez NG, et al. Extrapleural solitary fibrous tumor: a clinicopathologic study of 24 cases. Mod Pathol 1999; 12(11):1034–1042.

424. Cameselle-Teijeiro J, Lopes JM, Villanueva JP, et al. Lipomatous hemangiopericytoma of the thyroid. Pathologica 2002; 94:74.

425. Cameselle-Teijeiro J, Varela-Duran J, Fonseca E, et al. Solitary fibrous tumor of the thyroid. Am J Clin Pathol 1994; 101(4):535–538.

426. Deshmukh NS, Mangham DC, Warfield AT, et al. Solitary fibrous tumour of the thyroid gland. J Laryngol Otol 2001; 115(11):940–942.

427. Behrens RJ, Levi AW, Westra WH, et al. Langerhans cell histiocytosis of the thyroid: a report of two cases and review of the literature. Thyroid 2001; 11(7):697–705.

428. Dey P, Luthra UK, Sheikh ZA. Fine needle aspiration cytology of Langerhans cell histiocytosis of the thyroid. A case report. Acta Cytol 1999; 43(3):429–431.

429. el-Halabi DA, el-Sayed M, Eskaf W, et al. Langerhans cell histiocytosis of the thyroid gland. A case report. Acta Cytol 2000; 44(5):805–808.

430. Kitahama S, Iitaka M, Shimizu T, et al. Thyroid involvement by malignant histiocytosis of Langerhans' cell type. Clin Endocrinol (Oxf) 1996; 45(3):357–363.

431. Wang WS, Liu JH, Chiou TJ, et al. Langerhans' cell histiocytosis with thyroid involvement masquerading as thyroid carcinoma. Jpn J Clin Oncol 1997; 27(3):180–184.

432. Ornvold K, Ralfkiaer E, Carstensen H. Immunohistochemical study of the abnormal cells in Langerhans cell histiocytosis (histiocytosis x). Virchows Arch A Pathol Anat Histopathol 1990; 416(5):403–410.

433. Chan YF, Ma L, Boey JH, et al. Angiosarcoma of the thyroid. An immunohistochemical and ultrastructural study of a case in a Chinese patient. Cancer 1986; 57(12):2381–2388.

434. Hedinger C. Geographic pathology of thyroid diseases. Pathol Res Pract 1981; 171(3–4):285–292.

435. Eusebi V, Carcangiu ML, Dina R, et al. Keratin-positive epithelioid angiosarcoma of thyroid. A report of four cases. Am J Surg Pathol 1990; 14(8):737–747.

436. Beer TW. Malignant thyroid haemangioendothelioma in a non-endemic goitrous region, with immunohistochemical evidence of a vascular origin. Histopathology 1992; 20(6):539–541.

437. Ladurner D, Totsch M, Luze T, et al. [Malignant hemangioendothelioma of the thyroid gland. Pathology, clinical aspects and prognosis]. Wien Klin Wochenschr 1990; 102(9):256–259.

438. Biankin SA, Cachia AR. Leiomyoma of the thyroid gland. Pathology 1999; 31(1):64–66.

439. Andrion A, Bellis D, Delsedime L, et al. Leiomyoma and neurilemoma: report of two unusual non-epithelial tumours of the thyroid gland. Virchows Arch A Pathol Anat Histopathol 1988; 413(4):367–372.

440. Chetty R, Clark SP, Dowling JP. Leiomyosarcoma of the thyroid: immunohistochemical and ultrastructural study. Pathology 1993; 25(2):203–205.

441. Takayama F, Takashima S, Matsuba H, et al. MR imaging of primary leiomyosarcoma of the thyroid gland. Eur J Radiol 2001; 37(1):36–41.

442. Thompson LD, Wenig BM, Adair CF, et al. Primary smooth muscle tumors of the thyroid gland. Cancer 1997; 79(3):579–587.

443. Nakhjavani MK, Gharib H, Goellner JR, et al. Metastasis to the thyroid gland. A report of 43 cases. Cancer 1997; 79(3):574–578.

444. Heffess CS, Wenig BM, Thompson LD. Metastatic renal cell carcinoma to the thyroid gland: a clinicopathologic study of 36 cases. Cancer 2002; 95(9):1869–1878.

22

Pathology of the Parathyroid Glands

Raja R. Seethala, Mohamed A. Virji, and Jennifer B. Ogilvie

University of Pittsburgh Medical Center, Pittsburgh, Pennsylvania, U.S.A.

I. INTRODUCTION

While the parathyroid glands were likely recognized as early as 1850 by English anatomist Sir Richard Owen in an Indian rhinoceros (1), the first detailed description of these glands is generally attributed to Ivar Sandström in 1880 (2). He dubbed these structures *glandulae parathyreoideae*, though their function was unknown until Gley demonstrated that removal of these glands with experimental thyroidectomy in dogs resulted in tetany, while preservation did not (3,4). The subsequent discovery in the 1900s that parathyroid extract was able to reverse postthyroidectomy tetany ultimately led to the characterization of parathyroid hormone (PTH) (5). Ever since the first parathyroidectomy for tumor was performed by Mandl in 1924 (4), management of parathyroid disease has required close communication between the pathologist and surgeon. Over the next several decades, the introduction of advances such as rapid intraoperative PTH measurement and Sestamibi nuclear scanning have only served to reinforce the multimodal approach to management of parathyroid disease (5). Today, the pathologist needs to be aware of the uses and limitations of clinical, laboratory, and imaging parameters to correlate the histologic findings and arrive at an appropriate *clinicopathologic* diagnosis.

II. NORMAL PARATHYROID GLAND

A. Embryology

The paired superior parathyroid glands originate from the fourth pharyngeal (branchial) pouch along with the parafollicular C cells and the lateral lobes of the thyroid gland, after the fourth week of gestation. In the adult, the superior parathyroids glands usually occupy a posterior position adjacent to the posterior superior aspect of the thyroid gland, most commonly within 1 cm of the intersection of the inferior thyroid artery and recurrent laryngeal nerve. The paired inferior parathyroid glands arise from the more cephalad third pharyngeal pouch with the thymus gland. They migrate through fetal development into a more anterior and usually more caudal position in the neck.

Because of their shared embryologic origin with the thymus gland, the inferior parathyroids also may be found in the thyrothymic ligament or deeper within the thymus in the anterior superior mediastinum.

Norris described five distinct stages of parathyroid embryogenesis on the basis of evaluation of 137 human embryos and fetuses (6). The preprimordial stage (embryo length 4–8 mm) is characterized by dorsal third and fourth pharyngeal pouches. The third tube-like pouch contacts the pharyngeal cleft ectoderm and migrates in a ventral direction. The early primordial stage (9 mm) is characterized by proliferation of large, clear polygonal parathyroid precursor cells in the third and fourth pharyngeal pouches. The branchial complex stage (18–20 mm) is defined by separation of the pouches from the embryologic pharynx into the third and fourth branchial complexes. The third branchial complex migrates caudally and ventrally into the lower neck and anterior superior mediastinum, where it forms the thymus and inferior parathyroid glands. The fourth branchial complex is composed of the lateral lobes of the thyroid and the superior parathyroid glands. The isolation stage (20 mm) is when each branchial complex separates into distinct glands, with the thymus overlying the pericardium and the lateral lobes of the thyroid fused with the median thyroid, which has descended from the foramen cecum at the base of the tongue. The superior and inferior parathyroids are at this stage located in their final positions. The definitive form stage is characterized by the parathyroid glands assuming their ultimate shape, which is determined by their position relative to adjacent cervical structures.

B. Gross Anatomy

The majority of normal individuals have four parathyroid glands. Two paired superior and inferior glands. Autopsy studies have demonstrated supernumerary parathyroid glands in 2% to 13% of normal individuals, most commonly a fifth gland located in the cervical thymus (7,8). Approximately, 1% to 3% have only three identifiable parathyroid glands, and 0.6% have six glands. The final location of the inferior parathyroids is more variable than the superior parathyroid glands, possibly due to their longer path of embryologic descent. Inferior glands are most commonly located on the lower pole of the thyroid gland or in the thyrothymic ligament. Less commonly, inferior parathyroid glands are found lateral to the lower pole of the thyroid gland, in the anterior mediastinum, or in a high, undescended position, usually associated with a small ectopic thymic remnant.

The distribution of parathyroid glands is depicted in Figure 1. Superior parathyroid glands are most commonly located near the cricothyroid junction, posterior to the mid-superior pole of the thyroid at the level of the ligament of Berry, or posterior to the superior pole. Rarely, superior parathyroid glands may be found in the posterior mediastinal, retropharyngeal, or retroesophageal positions. Both superior and inferior parathyroid glands can also be located inside the capsule of the thyroid gland. True intrathyroidal parathyroid glands are found in 3% of individuals with primary hyperparathyroidism, all in the lower third of the thyroid gland, consistent with inferior embryologic origin (6). Supernumerary parathyroid glands have been identified in up to 13% of normal individuals on autopsy studies (6,8,9).

Normal parathyroid glands are often associated with or surrounded by a small amount of normal fat. They have a distinct, delicate connective tissue capsule and a fine network of vessels on the surface. The average weight of a normal parathyroid gland is generally accepted as 30 to 40 mg. However, the upper limit of normal in some series is as high as 103 mg (10). The distribution of normal parathyroid gland weights is actually skewed toward the upper weight ranges (11). Thus, the traditional assumption that any parathyroid gland over 40 mg is abnormal is likely not accurate (12). Parathyroid glands in the 40–80-mg range should be correlated with histologic, clinical, and laboratory findings. Gross appearance ranges from ovoid to flattened, to bean shaped, with an average long axis diameter of less than 0.6 mm, although apparently, normal glands measuring up to 1.2 cm in length have been reported in autopsy series. Normal parathyroid tissue is soft, with a fine granular texture and golden tan color.

The vascular supply to the parathyroid glands is derived from both the superior and inferior thyroid arteries. An arterial injection study in cadavers demonstrated that at least one-third of parathyroid glands were supplied by two or more distinct arteries, and in close to one half, the parathyroid artery arose from an anastomotic branch between the superior and inferior thyroid arteries. Injection of the superior parathyroid artery identified 98% of superior and 50% of inferior parathyroid glands (13). Occlusion of either the superior or inferior thyroid artery produced a 30% reduction in blood flow to the parathyroids, demonstrated by laser Doppler flowmetry (14). Venous drainage of the parathyroids follows the thyroid veins, with contralateral cross flow through the thyroid plexus, vertebral venous plexus, and anterior jugular veins, as documented by venous sampling (15).

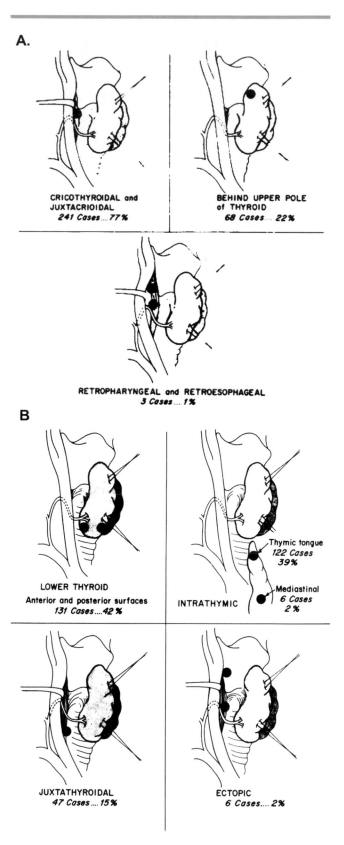

Figure 1 (**A**) Anatomic distribution of superior and (**B**) inferior parathyroid glands *Source*: Adapted from Figs.1 and 2 and Ref. 8.

C. Microscopic Anatomy

The parathyroid glands are thinly encapsulated by delicate layers of fibrous connective tissue. Strands from this capsule penetrate into the glands and carry a rich vascular supply (Fig. 2). These fibrous septations impart a vaguely lobulated appearance at low magnification (10,12). Unencapsulated parathyroid cell nests are occasionally noted outside the parathyroid gland proper in the surrounding soft tissue and even within the thyroid gland or thymus (16). Occasionally, cystic structures are seen adjacent to or within the parathyroid gland (Fig. 3). These structures are lined by flattened cuboidal parenchymal cells and may represent remnants of Kursteiner's canals (17,18). Some authors postulate that these structures give rise to parathyroid cysts (17).

The stroma of the parathyroid gland consists of adipocytes, vessels, and fibroconnective tissue. These elements, particularly the adipose component, generally increase with age. In adults, the proportion of stromal fat is an important histologic parameter used to correlate with functional status, with hyperfunctional states having less stromal fat secondary to increased parenchymal cell mass (10,12,19). This parameter when used alone, however, has little

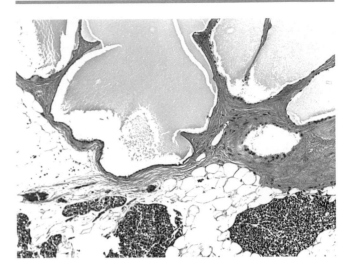

Figure 3 Presumed remnants of Kursteiner's canals with adjacent parathyroid nests below (H&E, 100×). *Abbreviation*: H&E, hematoxylin and eosin.

A

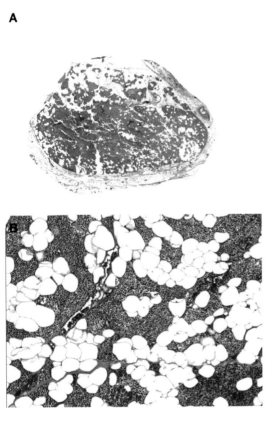

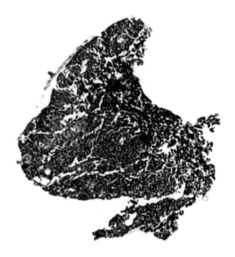

Figure 4 A 17-mg parathyroid gland with no fatty stroma in an elderly patient (H&E, whole slide scan). This was unintentionally removed during a thyroid lobectomy from a euparathryoid patient with thyroid nodules. *Abbreviation*: H&E, hematoxylin and eosin.

Figure 2 (**A**) Normal parathyroid gland comprising small nests of parenchymal cells interspersed in a fatty stroma (H&E, whole slide scan). (**B**) The nests and cords of chief cells are separated by delicate fibrovascular septae (H&E, 100×). *Abbreviation*: H&E, hematoxylin and eosin.

practical utility, especially when assessing shave biopsies or partial gland excisions. This can be attributed to two major considerations:

First, the prevailing dogma is that normal adult parathyroid glands consist of 50% stromal fat (16,19). However, more rigorous morphometric approaches have suggested a lower percentage (16,20,21). Additional confounding variables include advanced age, nutritional status, and underlying chronic disease states, all of which result in connective tissue atrophy and a subsequently lower stromal fat percentage (Fig. 4). On the basis of autopsy studies, the mean stromal fat percentage in normal glands is less than 20% (20–22)!

However, patients undergoing autopsy may have an underlying disease state that implicates stromal atrophy as a confounding variable. More recent studies on fairly healthy euparathyroid patients with parathyroid glands removed during thyroidectomy for thyroid lesions suggest a fat percentage of 35% to 38%, though still, a significant proportion of these were even less than 15% (23,24).

Second, the distribution of stromal fat even within an individual parathyroid gland is not uniform or predictable. The polar regions of the gland tend to have more adipose tissue than the center; however, Grimelius et al. (22) suggested that roughly 10 serial sections or levels are required to arrive at a reliable stromal fat proportion for a given gland. This degree of effort is both time consuming and costly, and most authorities would argue against assessment of cellularity on small parathyroid biopsies (22,25).

The three cell types that comprise the parathyroid parenchyma are chief cells, oxyphil cells, and clear cells, although the latter two "types" are basically modified chief cells (10,19). Chief cells, which comprise the majority of most normal parathyroid glands, are small polygonal cells measuring roughly 8 μm with pale amphophilic vacuolated cytoplasm (26) (Fig. 5). The nuclei are round and centrally located with coarse chromatin and indistinct nucleoli. Chief cells are arranged in thin nests and small cords with interspersed stromal adipose tissue. In the normal gland, the parathyroid parenchyma has a "compressed" appearance with each nest tapering as if crushed by the surrounding fibrous septae or stromal fat. In addition to the nests and cords, chief cells may form acini or even follicles with dense periodic acid–Schiff (PAS) positive secretions that resemble colloid seen in thyroid follicles. This material may represent an intrafollicular localized amyloid containing PTH, and a small percentage of hyperplasias have this as a prominent feature (12,27,28). Clear cells are

essentially chief cells with abundant glycogen (Fig. 6). During embryologic development, this is the most common cell type. However, the percentage of these cells declines after birth and is only a minor constituent in adults (26). The clear cells are not equivalent to the "water-clear (wasserhelle) cells" seen in clear cell hyperplasia, since the latter have a clear appearance as a result of abundant cytoplasmic vacuoles rather than glycogen and have not been described in normal glands (29). Oxyphil cells are slightly larger and less isomorphic ranging from 12 to 20 μm (12) (Fig. 7).

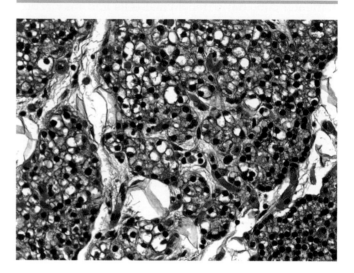

Figure 6 Glycogenated chief cells (clear cells) (H&E, 400×). Cells are slightly larger with clear cytoplasm transitioning from typical chief cells (*bottom right*). Nuclear characteristics are identical to chief cells. *Abbreviation*: H&E, hematoxylin and eosin.

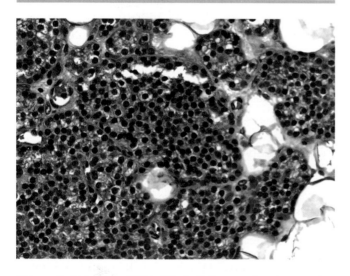

Figure 5 Chief cells (H&E, 400×). Cells contain pale vacuolated amphophilic cytoplasm with small dark round nuclei with indistinct nucleoli. *Abbreviation*: H&E, hematoxylin and eosin.

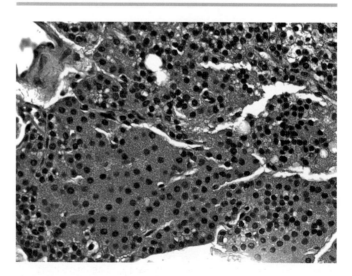

Figure 7 Oxyphil cells (H&E, 400×). These cells have abundant granular eosinophilic cytoplasm. Transitional cells with a resemblance to chief cells, but with slightly more granular eosinophilic cytoplasm are present on top. *Abbreviation*: H&E, hematoxylin and eosin.

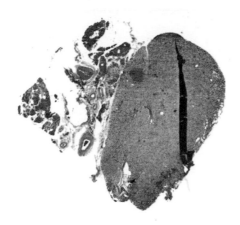

Figure 8 A nodule in a 42-mg parathyroid gland found on a thyroidectomy specimen in a euparathyroid patient (H&E, whole slide scan). *Abbreviation*: H&E, hematoxylin and eosin.

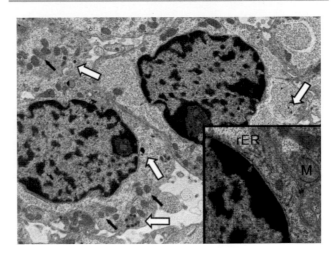

Figure 9 Electron micrograph of parathyroid tissue (5330×). Note the moderate number of mitochondria (*small black arrows*) dense core secretory granules (*white arrows*). The granules are sparse, and the lipid vacuoles are not seen, suggesting an active secretory state. (*Inset*, 17700×) Additional organellar structures. *Abbreviations*: rER, perinuclear rough endoplasmic reticulum stacks; M, mitochondria from neighboring cell.

These cells are oncocytes akin to those seen at other sites such as the thyroid, adrenal, and salivary glands and as such are characterized by abundant granular eosinophilic cytoplasm. Additionally, the nuclei are slightly enlarged with more size variation with respect to chief cells. A transitional cell type with less pronounced oxyphilic change can be seen in association with or separate from mature oxyphils (12). This cell constituent is generally thought to increase with age, forming clusters or nodules (Fig. 8) (26). However, as with most histologic variation in parathyroid glands, this association is not strong or reproducible (16).

D. Ultrastructural Anatomy

Cords and nests of parathyroid parenchymal cells are separated from the interstitium by a well-developed basal lamina. The surrounding capillaries are similar to those of other endocrine organs in that they comprise fenestrated endothelial cells (10,12,29–31). Chief cells contain moderate numbers of mitochondria, perinuclear endoplasmic reticulum, and electron-dense secretory granules measuring up to 0.3 μm in diameter (Fig. 9). Prosecretory granules can also be seen forming near the Golgi apparatus and are only moderately electron dense as compared with mature secretory granules.

Only about 20% of chief cells are actively producing PTH (i.e., in secretory phase) at a given time (10). As such many ultrastructural characteristics are determined by functional state; active cells have more tortuous, convoluted membranes and well-developed Golgi with numerous vesicles and prosecretory granules than inactive cells. Similarly, the amount of glycogen and lipid is inversely proportional to the secretory activity of a chief cell.

As mentioned previously, the clear cell type often seen in fetal development contains abundant glycogen stores. In contrast, the water-clear cell is not a normal parathyroid cell constituent, and in contrast to the aforementioned glycogenated clear cells, the ultrastructural correlate to the clear light microscopic appearance is the presence of multiple large electron-lucent vacuoles derived from the Golgi apparatus (32). Oxyphils are characteristically filled almost entirely with mitochondria. Additionally, these mitochondria are increased in size, often with morphologic abnormalities. Oxyphils also have fewer secretory granules and lipid vacuoles (12,31).

E. Histochemistry/Immunohistochemistry

Normal parathyroid chief cells contain glycogen and neutral lipid stores. As noted above, these stores are inversely proportional to a given cell's secretory activity (12). Hence, the heavy glycogenation seen in clear cells of fetal parathyroid glands reflects their inactivity. This concept also forms the basis for the use of histochemical stains to assess functional status of parathyroids since hyperfunctioning glands will have a higher proportion of actively secreting cells. The routine histochemical stain PAS will highlight glycogen stores in these cells, while intracytoplasmic lipid will be highlighted by stains such as oil red O or Sudan IV (Fig. 10). It is important to note that oxyphil cells normally have less glycogen and lipid than chief cells (12). Reflective of their abundant often-abnormal mitochondria, oxyphil cells are rich in oxidative enzymes (33). The mitochondria can be highlighted by histochemical techniques such as phosphotungstic acid–hematoxylin (PTAH) (34) or immunocytochemical techniques directed against generic mitochondrial epitopes. Some studies have identified cytochrome *c* oxidase defects in oxyphil cells of both normal and hyperfunctioning glands, particularly nodular hyperplasia, suggesting that this

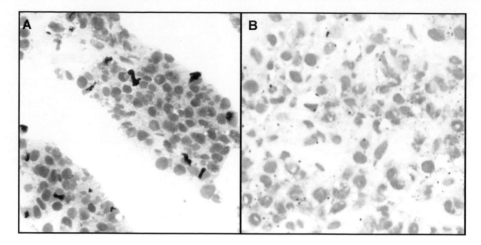

Figure 10 (**A**) Normal intracytoplasmic lipid seen as coarse thick orange globules in a normal parathyroid gland (oil red O, 400×). (**B**) Absent intracytoplasmic lipid in a hyperfunctioning gland (oil red O, 400×).

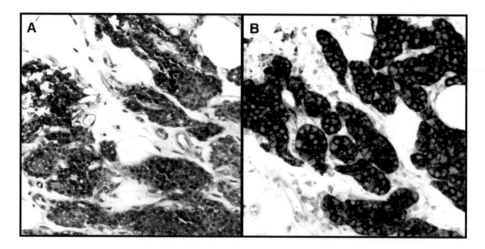

Figure 11 (**A**) Immunohistochemical staining for chromogranin (200×). (**B**) Immunohistochemical staining for PTH (200×). *Abbreviation*: PTH, parathyroid hormone.

change may be an age-related mitochondrial cytopathy (35,36).

The immunophenotype of normal parathyroid cells is mainly of descriptive interest with only a few practical applications. Miettinen et al. (37) described the intermediate filament staining characteristics of parathyroid cells and found that they are positive for low–molecular weight keratins such as cytokeratin 8, 18, and 19, but negative for glial fibrillary acidic protein, vimentin, and neurofilaments.

Perhaps the most useful application of immunohistochemistry on parathyroid glands, both normal and abnormal, is for conformation of its identity as parathyroid tissue, particularly when the follicular pattern predominates or if it is in an abnormal location. To this end, antibodies to both PTH and chromogranin A have been used (Fig. 11). Chromogranin A is a constituent of neurosecretory granules in many neuroendocrine organs throughout the body (38) and colocalizes with PTH (39,40). The limiting aspect of chromogranin A is the lack of specificity in the situation where the differential diagnosis includes a metastatic neuroendocrine neoplasm from another site. Initially, anti-PTH immunohistochemistry had been hampered both technically and by the low concentration within chief cells (41). However, improved antigen retrieval methods for paraffin tissue have made anti-PTH immunostaining routine in most laboratories, superseding chromogranin immunohistochemistry for identification of parathyroid tissue in most cases. The intensity of staining for both chromogranin A and PTH in normal glands is typically higher than that of hyperfunctioning glands, and typically higher in chief cells than in oxyphil cells (42).

The parathyroid gland expresses several receptors. Among the more relevant receptors are the calcium-sensing receptor (CaSR) and vitamin D receptor (VDR). CaSR is a G-protein-coupled receptor (120 kD) that modulates PTH secretion in response to fluctuations in extracellular Ca^{2+} concentrations (43). VDR is an intracellular receptor (48.3 kD) that is structurally related to thyroid hormone receptor and binds the active form of vitamin D (1,25-dihydroxy-vitamin D3) and controls PTH secretion via transcriptional regulation (44). CaSR is a cell surface receptor and accordingly shows immunoreactivity on the surface, while VDR is expressed in nucleus. The intensity of staining for both these receptors is generally higher in normal parathyroid glands than in hyperfunctioning glands (45–48).

Interestingly, parathyroid chief cells show immunoreactivity to certain clones of anti-CD3 and anti-CD4, which are directed toward T-cell antigens. These CD3 and CD4-like moieties expressed in parathyroid glands may play a role in PTH release (49–51). From a practical standpoint, awareness of this phenomenon will prevent misinterpretation of this reactivity as indicative of a lymphoid process.

F. Molecular Biology

The human *PTH* gene maps chromosome 11p15.3–15.1 and consists of three exons. Exon 1 is untranslated, while exons 2 and 3 encode the precursor molecule, pre-pro-PTH (52,53). Repressor DNA response elements are in close proximity to promoter elements of the human *PTH* gene (54). VDR is a major repressor of *PTH* transcription (55). An increased extracellular Ca^{2+} negatively regulates PTH by increasing ref-1, a repressor of PTH expression (56), as well as modulation via CaSR-dependent mechanisms (57). In humans, CaSR has more rapid kinetics and broader effects and is thus dominant over VDR in its modulation of PTH (57). Enhanced expression of PTH, on the other hand, may be mediated by an SP1 family DNA element in the promoter region of PTH, suggesting that SP1 and SP3 promote PTH transcription (58). Nuclear factor Y is also thought to promote PTH transcription and may act synergistically with SP1 (59). The promoter region of PTH also has a cAMP response element (60). Since CaSR is a G-protein-coupled receptor, which affects cAMP concentrations; this element may indirectly mediate the CaSR's effect on PTH secretion (57,61). Of recent interest is the characterization of the Glial Cells Missing gene (*GCMB*) on chromosome 6p23–24. *GCMB* is a transcription factor that appears to be a master regulator of parathyroid development. While the effect of GCMB on PTH is not entirely clear, GCMB has been noted to be upregulated in hyperfunctioning parathyroid tissue as compared with normal and mutated in rare cases of familial hypoparathyroidism (62–65).

PTH messenger RNA (mRNA) in situ hybridization can be performed on paraffin-embedded tissue sections. Normal parathyroid gland shows mRNA expression in a limited set of chief cells, while hyperfunctioning parathyroid glands express PTH mRNA more diffusely. Oxyphils, on the other hand, have a low level of expression (66–68). In contrast, CaSR and VDR mRNA are decreased in hyperfunctioning parathyroid glands (69).

G. PHYSIOLOGY AND BIOCHEMISTRY

PTH is synthesized by the parathyroid glands as an inactive precursor protein pre-pro-PTH, comprising 115 amino acids. This precursor undergoes postsynthesis modification, first with removal of the pre- or the lead sequence of 25 amino acids, as the nascent peptide is transferred from the ribosome to the endoplasmic reticulum and then through removal of six pro-peptide amine terminal sequences as the protein transits through the Golgi, resulting in the formation of biologically active 84 amino acid protein that is stored in secretory granules in the chief cells of the parathyroid gland (Fig. 12). The secretory granules also contain proteases that cleave the PTH molecule to generate fragments that are biologically inactive. The active hormone secreted from the parathyroid glands is a single chain molecule comprising 84 amino acids.

The secretion of the hormone is regulated by ionized calcium concentration in blood through a calcium sensor in the parathyroid cell membrane. There is an inverse relationship between the ionized calcium concentration and the secretion of PTH, and

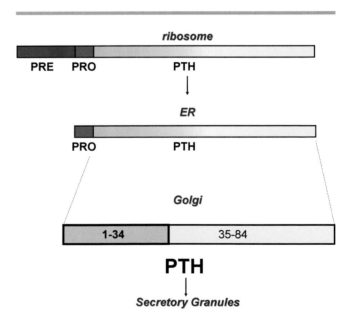

Figure 12 Transition from pre-pro-PTH to pro-PTH and finally PTH. The N-terminal region (*orange*, comprising amino acids 1–34) constitutes the bioactive portion of the hormone. Immunoassays used to measure serum PTH concentration need to recognize this portion, particularly beginning amino acids, to accurately measure the "intact PTH." *Abbreviation*: PTH, parathyroid hormone.

the threshold calcium concentrations for release or for suppression of PTH is within the range defined by the lower and the upper physiological reference limits for blood-ionized calcium. The ionized calcium concentration regulation of PTH secretion impacts the hormone action on bone mineral metabolism, modulating bone formation or resorption, renal tubular calcium resorption, and through regulation of vitamin D synthesis, absorption of dietary calcium from intestines. The net effect is maintenance of blood calcium concentration within a defined narrow concentration range. The PTH synthesis and secretion is especially sensitive to low ionized calcium concentrations as the set point for parathyroid stimulation favors rapid response to lowering of calcium. Other regulators of PTH secretion with lesser impact than calcium include vitamin D and phosphate. Mutations in the calcium sensor alter the parathyroid gland response to calcium concentrations and may present as syndromes of parathyroid dysfunction. Inactivating mutations of the sensor are associated with familial hypocalciuric hypercalcemia (FHH) (see sect. "FHH").

The biologically active hormone binds to specific receptors located primarily in osteoblasts, renal tubular cells, and the endothelial cells lining the small intestine. The binding is dependent on the amino acids 1–14 at the aminoterminal of the hormone, and the peptide consisting of the amino acid sequence 1–34 has hormone potency equivalent to the full length 1–84 protein. This bioactive portion of the hormone comprising amino acid sequence 1–14 is critical for all tissue actions of PTH, and therefore it is important that the assays measuring blood concentration of the hormone detect the entire intact PTH molecule, including the bioactive portion. Most of the immunoassays available currently recognize the entire PTH molecule by the use of two antibody sandwich techniques, but differ from one another in the use of PTH preparation to calibrate the assay and the specificity of the antibodies in recognition of epitopes in the amino and the carboxy portion of the PTH molecule. The carboxyterminal portion of the hormone has a role in the avidity of hormone binding, but does not activate the receptor to generate the intracellular signal cascade. PTH has a direct effect on osteoblasts, one of the target cells, and an effect on the osteoclasts through its action on the osteoblasts. The hormone action through specific receptors on osteoblasts results in synthesis of proteins that localize to the osteoblast surface and interact with osteoclasts via receptors affecting the maturation and activity of osteoclasts (10,12).

The action of PTH on renal tubular cells is primarily in regulation of calcium reabsorption from the distal nephron. Though this comprises only 10% of the total renal calcium reabsorption, PTH modulation has an impact on the dynamic calcium concentration in blood. PTH also inhibits phosphate reabsorption through effects on the proximal and the distal portions of the renal tubules. The impact on vitamin D synthesis is primarily at the proximal tubule by upregulation of the enzyme for converting 25-hydroxy-vitamin D to 1, 25-dihydroxy-vitamin D and downregulation of the enzymes that form inactive metabolites of the vitamin D.

PTH is cleared rapidly from blood after secretion from the parathyroid glands. Binding to target tissues in bone and kidney account for only a very small portion of the hormone, and the hormone is mainly degraded in the liver by the action of cathepsins. The half-life of the intact hormone in circulation is approximately two minutes. The fragments generated include aminoterminal, midmolecule, and carboxyterminal segments, which have a variable half-life. Glomerular filtration also accounts for a proportion of PTH elimination. PTH is metabolized in the renal tubules, and the fragments generated are eliminated in the urine. Carboxyterminal fragments have a prolonged half-life in circulation, and concentrations of the fragments may exceed intact PTH concentrations by several folds. The concentration of these fragments is markedly elevated in renal failure and indicates decreased elimination. Though the fragments do not have biological activity of PTH and do not bind to the cell receptors for the hormone, carboxyterminal fragments have as yet incompletely characterized actions that have been speculated to be opposite of the intact hormone (10,12).

PTH Assay

Ideally, the analytic methods for PTH should recognize and measure the entire intact molecule, including the aminoterminal sequence that contains the receptor-binding portion of PTH. There are several fragments of PTH that are produced through metabolism in the liver and kidney. The major fragments represent the amine, the midmolecule, and the carboxyterminal sequences of PTH. The various molecular fragments may be detected by immunoassays that are not designed specifically for recognition of the intact, bioactive hormone. Though there is as yet no standardization of the immunoassays for PTH, increasingly with the recognition of the importance to measure specifically the biologically active hormone, most manufacturers are designing the assays to be specific for the intact 1–84 amino acid–containing PTH molecule. There are, however, differences in the assays from different manufacturers especially in the recognition of the aminoterminal end of the molecule, leading to terms that designate the assays variously as being specific for "intact" or "bioactive" molecule (70,71).

The assays currently in use are mostly enzyme-linked immunosorbent assays (ELISA) that are based on binding of the intact PTH by a capture antibody linked to a solid substrate like polystyrene beads. The PTH-antibody then forms a complex upon exposure to a second antibody directed preferably to a recognition site at the other end of the molecule. The second antibody is conjugated to a signal that enzymatically activates color generation, fluorescence or chemiluminescence, which is proportional to the concentration of the hormone and can be adapted for automated immunoassay analyzers. This has resulted in wide availability of the assays for PTH and also modifications for use of the analysis for guiding completion of parathyroidectomies.

The serum concentrations obtained with these assays for intact PTH are comparable, providing a normal reference range of 10 to 65 pg/mL (70,71).

III. PRIMARY HYPERPARATHYROIDISM

A. Definition

Primary hyperparathyroidism is defined as an excessive production of PTH from one of several distinct pathologic entities: adenoma, hyperplasia, and carcinoma. At least 85% of patients with primary hyperparathyroidism have a single parathyroid adenoma, approximately 10% have parathyroid hyperplasia, 5% have double adenoma, and less than 1% have parathyroid carcinoma.

B. Epidemiology

The age and sex-adjusted incidence of primary hyperparathyroidism is approximately 20 to 30 per 100,000 person-years in North America (72,73). The disease is 2 to 3 times higher in women, and the incidence increases to close to 100 per 100,000 person-years after age 65. A population-based screening in Sweden found a 2.1% prevalence of primary hyperparathyroidism in women aged 55 to 75 years (74). In the majority of cases of primary hyperparathyroidism, no etiologic cause can be identified. A small number of cases are associated with a history of prior head and neck irradiation, genetic mutations, or familial endocrinopathies. Significantly, less than 1% of patients with primary hyperparathyroidism have parathyroid carcinoma, which accounts for 0.005% of all cancers in the United States (75). A recent population-based study demonstrated a 60% increase in the incidence of parathyroid carcinoma in the United States from 1988–2003.

External ionizing radiation exposure to the head and neck was first associated with the subsequent development of hyperparathyroidism in the mid 1970s (76). Radiation treatment for benign head and neck conditions, including hirsutism, acne, hemangioma, cervical lymphadenopathy, and thymus or tonsillar enlargement was common in the middle third of the 20th century, until it was noted that radiation exposure was associated with a higher risk of benign and malignant tumors of the thyroid, salivary, and parathyroid glands. Multiple retrospective reports confirmed this association (77–82), and almost fourfold increased rates of parathyroid tumors have also been described among atomic bomb survivors in Hiroshima (83,84). Long-term follow-up of 2795 patients treated with radiation for benign head and neck conditions found an overall rate of hyperparathyroidism in 2.5%, most cases occurring after 30 to 40 years of follow-up (approaching 5% after 50 years of follow-up), for a 2.9-fold overall increased risk relative to the general population (85–87). Therapeutic radioactive iodine treatment has neither been associated with an increased rate of hyperparathyroidism (88) nor has environmental exposure to iodine-131 from the Hanford Nuclear Reservation (89).

Genetic mutations have been described in sporadic parathyroid tumors as well as parathyroid tumors associated with familial endocrinopathies, including multiple endocrine neoplasia type I (MEN I) and multiple endocrine neoplasia type IIA (MEN IIA), hyperparathyroidism-jaw tumor (HPT-JT) syndrome, and familial isolated hyperparathyroidism (FIHP). The salient features of each are summarized in Table 1.

In MEN I, patients typically present in the third to fifth decade. Hyperparathyroidism is almost invariably present (90%) and is usually the first presenting

Table 1 Common Familial Hyperparathyroidism Syndromes

Syndrome	Pattern of inheritance	Gene	Locus	Clinical features
MEN1	AD	MEN1	11q13	Multigland parathyroid disease (>90%) Gastrointestinal and pancreatic endocrine tumors Pituitary adenomas Facial angiofibromas Collagenomas
MEN2A	AD	RET	10q21	Single or multigland disease (20–30%) C-cell tumors of thyroid Pheochromocytomas
HPT-JT	AD	HRPT2	1q21–32	Cystic parathyroid adenomas Parathyroid carcinoma (10–15%) Fibro-osseous lesions of jaws Kidney—renal cysts Wilm's tumor mixed epithelial-stromal tumor Uterine—leiomyoma Atypical polypoid adenomyoma Adenosarcoma
FIHP	AD	MEN1 CaSR	11q13 19p13.3	Benign multiglandular parathyroid disease Carcinomas of breast, colon, endometrium, and other

Abbreviations: AD, autosomal dominant; HPT-JT, hyperparathyroidism-jaw tumor syndrome; FIHP, familial isolated hyperparathyroidism.
Source: From Refs. 91–103.

endocrinopathy (90). As a rule, hyperparathyroidism in MEN I is a multigland disease. Even supranumery glands (prominent in up to 20% of MEN I patients) (91) and normal-appearing glands may be hyperfunctioning and a potential cause of recurrent hypercalcemia. However, unlike most sporadic multigland disease, MEN-1-associated hyperparathyroidism is oligoclonal and has a gene expression profile more similar to adenomas (92,93). The mutated gene *MEN1* is a tumor-suppressor gene on chromosome 11q13, which encodes menin. Menin is a nuclear protein that interacts with SMAD3 to suppress transforming growth factor beta (94).

Hyperparathyroidism is less common in MEN IIA, present in only 20% to 30% of cases. The age distribution is similar to MEN I, and the typical presentation is milder and may be single- or multigland disease (95). The mutated gene *RET*, on chromosome 10q11, encodes proto-oncogene tyrosine kinase. To some degree, mutation type reflects disease manifestation. Mutations at codon 634 may correlate with a hyperparathyroidism phenotype (93), though there is conflicting data regarding this (96). Similar to MEN I disease, MEN IIA parathyroid glands tend to be mono- or oligoclonal.

In HPT-JT, the parathyroid tumors are typically adenomas and are notoriously cystic (97). However, parathyroid carcinomas are seen in as many as 15% of HPT-JT patients (as compared with <1% in patients with hyperparathyroidism in general) (98,99). The development of this syndrome is rooted in the gene *HRPT2*, which was mapped to the chromosomal region 1q21–32 (100,101). The gene was subsequently found to encode parafibromin, a protein involved in RNA polymerase II/Paf-1 complex–presumed histone deacetylation role (101,102).

FIHP may very well be a heterogenous group of disorders from a clinical and genetic standpoint. Distinguished from other syndromes by the absence of extraparathyroidal manifestations, mutations in *MEN1*, *HRPT2*, and *CaSR* have all been described in kindreds of FIHP. In many instances, the mutated gene is not identified (103).

C. Clinical Presentation

Primary hyperparathyroidism is characterized by hypercalcemia in the setting of an inappropriately elevated PTH level. Since serum calcium is commonly ordered as part of a metabolic panel, for most patients today, the initial presentation is a chemical rather than a clinical finding. However, after a careful clinical history is taken, patients with apparently asymptomatic primary hyperparathyroidism often complain of nonspecific symptoms of fatigue, weakness, musculoskeletal or abdominal aches and pains, anorexia, constipation, polydipsia, polyuria, nocturia, cognitive dysfunction, and depression (104). Other manifestations of primary hyperparathyroidism include loss of bone mineral density, osteitis fibrosa cystica, pathologic fractures, nephrolithiasis, nephrocalcinosis, renal insufficiency, peptic ulcer disease, hypertension, gout, and pancreatitis. Physical examination is often noncontributory, as enlarged parathyroids are most commonly located posterior to the thyroid gland and are not palpable. Occasionally, examination of the eyes reveals band keratopathy, deposition of calcium phosphate in the limbus of the cornea. Rarely, patients present with acute hypercalcemic crisis, associated with mental status changes, abdominal pain, nausea, vomiting, peptic ulcer, or pancreatitis.

Laboratory studies reveal hypercalcemia, hyperparathormonemia, hypophosphatemia, normal or increased calcitriol with low or low-normal calcidiol, and hypercalciuria (105). PTH assay has gained acceptance as a part of the evaluation for parathyroid dysfunction specifically for glandular hyperfunction due to adenoma or hyperplasia. The interpretation of serum concentration takes into account either the total serum calcium or ionized blood calcium. The relationship between the PTH and calcium concentrations provides guidance in differentiating various causes for increased serum PTH concentrations. In parathyroid hyperfunction due to adenoma or hyperplasia, serum calcium and intact PTH are both elevated, and there is increase in urinary excretion of calcium. In renal failure and renal osteodystrophy, there is increase in serum PTH, but the calcium concentration is usually within the reference range. In hypercalcemia of malignancy, serum PTH concentration is not increased, but the calcium concentration may be markedly elevated. In renal failure and also in malignancy-related hypercalcemia, the urinary loss of calcium is increased. FHH is accompanied by elevation of serum calcium without an increase in the PTH concentration. Therefore, serum PTH concentration should at the minimum be interpreted together with serum calcium concentration. Evaluation of parathyroid hyperfunction due to hyperplasia or adenoma may require determination of 24-hour urinary calcium excretion (calcium unrestricted diet, <300 mg/day, and restricted diet, <200 mg/day).

Primary hyperparathyroidism caused by parathyroid carcinoma is characterized by marked elevation of PTH, 3 to 10 times the upper limit of normal, with severe associated hypercalcemia, typically over 14 mg/dL (106). Patients with parathyroid carcinoma present with a higher rate of nephrolithiasis, renal insufficiency, and osteoporosis (107). They may also present with vocal cord paralysis or a palpable neck mass, which are rare in adenomas. Lymph node metastases may be present in up to 6%.

The clinical differential diagnosis of primary hyperparathyroidism includes other causes of hypercalcemia (see sect. "Miscellaneous Conditions"), such as cancer, benign FHH, milk alkali syndrome, and sarcoidosis. Thiazide diuretics and lithium decrease urine calcium excretion and can also be associated with hypercalcemia or may unmask mild cases of primary hyperparathyroidism. The majority of nonparathyroid carcinomas causing hypercalcemia produce excess PTH-related protein (PTHrP), others are associated with calcitriol production or widespread lytic bony metastases (108,109). The milk alkali syndrome is caused by excess exogenous calcium supplementation and is associated with an appropriately

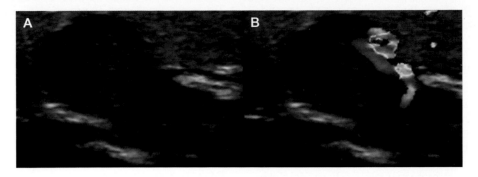

Figure 13 (**A**) Ultrasonogram of an abnormal parathyroid present as a hypoechoic mass. (**B**) Doppler flow demonstrates prominent vascularity and a hilar vessel.

suppressed PTH level. FHH is an autosomal dominant condition characterized by a normal or slightly elevated PTH level, is asymptomatic, and is not associated with the skeletal or renal complications of hyperparathyroidism (110). This will be discussed in more detail in the section "Parathyroid Cysts."

D. Preoperative Localization

Imaging

With the development of minimally invasive surgical approaches to parathyroid surgery, the use of accurate, noninvasive preoperative parathyroid imaging is vital to ensure effective surgical treatment of primary hyperparathyroidism. Parathyroid imaging is also critical to localize ectopic parathyroid glands or the remaining abnormal parathyroid glands after failed parathyroid exploration. The two most widely used imaging modalities for preoperative parathyroid localization are ultrasound and Technetium 99m-sestamibi scintigraphy with single-photon emission computed tomography (Tc99m sestamibi SPECT). Localization accuracy is improved when both modalities are used, especially if there is concordant demonstration of a single abnormal gland in the same location (111,112). Cross-sectional imaging with computed tomography (CT) and magnetic resonance imaging (MRI) can also be helpful for parathyroid localization but are more often used to localize ectopic glands after failed parathyroid exploration. Four-dimensional CT, a new technique, which uses contrast perfusion characteristics to distinguish abnormal parathyroid glands from surrounding structures, has been shown to have improved sensitivity over sestamibi and ultrasound, but is not yet widely available (113). Fusion SPECT/CT allows precise anatomic localization of abnormal parathyroid glands that localize with Tc99m sestamibi SPECT, especially in the presence of concomitant multinodular goiter or with ectopic parathyroid glands (114).

Parathyroid ultrasound is typically performed with a high-frequency linear transducer (10–15 MHz), using gray-scale imaging as well as power and color Doppler imaging. Abnormal parathyroid glands are typically hypoechoic with a characteristic hilar vessel and peripheral vascularity (Fig. 13) (115). Advantages of ultrasound include the ability to accurately locate the abnormal parathyroid gland relative to cervical surface anatomy to plan the most effective operative approach. Ultrasound also facilitates an examination of the thyroid gland and can be combined with ultrasound-guided fine-needle aspiration (FNA) of concomitant thyroid nodules as indicated. Disadvantages of ultrasound are that it is operator dependent and is not effective for imaging ectopic parathyroid glands in the mediastinum. The overall accuracy of ultrasound for preoperative parathyroid localization is 72% to 79% and is most accurate for single parathyroid adenomas (116–118).

Tc99m sestamibi scintigraphy SPECT is the most well-documented and commonly used imaging modality for preoperative parathyroid localization (Fig. 14). Increased radiotracer uptake on early and delayed images can be reconstructed with three-dimensional SPECT imaging to increase depth visualization and contrast. Like ultrasound, Tc99m Sestamibi SPECT is most accurate for single large parathyroid adenomas (88–95%), but much less accurate for double adenomas or hyperplasia (30–73%)

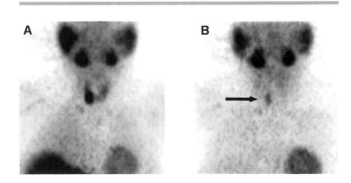

Figure 14 Tc99m sestamibi SPECT of a right inferior parathyroid adenoma. (**A**) Initial scan showing uptake in the thyroid region. (**B**) Delayed imaging showing a focus of persistent uptake compatible with abnormal thyroid tissue.

(119). Tc99m sestamibi SPECT combined with ultrasound has been shown to be complementary, providing increased accuracy of parathyroid localization (120).

Selective Venous Sampling

Selective venous sampling (SVS) for PTH levels is an invasive, technically challenging modality that is reserved for difficult cases of persistent or recurrent hyperparathyroidism, when all noninvasive imaging is negative. It has been shown to have higher sensitivity than sestamibi or ultrasound in patients with recurrent or persistent hyperparathyroidism after previous parathyroid exploration (121). SVS was found to be false positive or indeterminate in 17% of patients with recurrent or persistent hyperparathyroidism (122). The utility of SVS is also limited in that it does not directly image the abnormal gland. Instead, SVS provides functional data that approximates the location of PTH hypersecretion.

FNA: PTH Level Vs. Cytology

Ultrasound-guided FNA for parathyroid disease assessment was initially described in 1981 in which a single enlarged gland was successfully localized and cytologically confirmed (123). Soon after, the use of PTH measurements on aspirates for the successful localization was described (124). The combination of preoperative imaging modalities yields an accuracy of detection of single-gland disease that is as high as 95% (112,125). However, the assessment of parathyroid disease after prior surgery and enlarged glands in ectopic locations is still problematic. Hence, these are the cases in which FNA may be of benefit. Assessment of aspirate PTH levels has been shown to be a highly specific and sensitive test in such cases with three studies showing a specificity of 100% and a sensitivity ranging from 70% to 94%. There is not yet a standardized PTH level to be considered diagnostic of parathyroid tissue, but most negative aspirates are less that 20 pg/mL, while most parathyroids are in the hundreds or thousands (126–128). An additional application of aspirate PTH measurements is in the evaluation of possible parathyroid cysts. Parathyroid cyst aspirates are characterstically clear, watery, and nearly acellular, and it is critical to send this fluid for PTH evaluation to confirm the diagnosis (129,130).

However, the role of preoperative evaluation of parathyroid disease by FNA cytology is still unclear. In fact, much of the literature regarding parathyroid cytology consists of case reports of incidental parathyroid lesions masquerading as thyroid lesions or other neck masses (131–134). Several authors suggest that cytologic evaluation may be useful in confirmation of parathyroid tissue (135–139). The major difficulty in the cytologic interpretation of parathyroid aspirates is the discrimination from thyroid follicular cells, and occasionally, medullary thyroid carcinoma. Parathyroid tissue may be misinterpreted as thyroid in 8% to almost 92%, especially if no history of hypercalcemia or hyperparathyroidism is noted (140–142).

Table 2 A Comparison of Key Cytologic Features of Thyroid Tissue and Parathyroid Tissue on FNA

Parameter	Thyroid	Parathyroid
Architectural		
3-D fibrovascular fragments with attached epithelial cells	+	+++
Papillae	+++	++
Follicles	+++	++
Stripped nuclei/lymphoid pattern	+	+++
Cytologic		
Nuclear molding	+	+++
Coarse (salt and pepper) chromatin	+	+++
Paravacuolar granulation	++[a]	++[a]
Background		
Colloid/colloid-like material	+++	+
Macrophages	+++	+
Mast cells	+/−	+

[a]Paravacuolar granules in thyroid are typically brown on H&E stain and blue on Diff-Quik, whereas the granules in parathyroid are typically clear lipid vacuoles. *Abbreviation*: FNA, fine-needle aspiration.
Source: From Refs. 135,136,140,141,143,146.

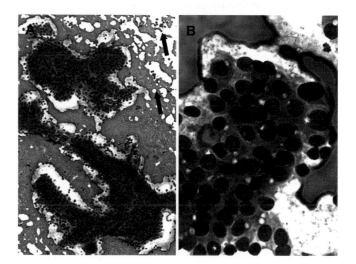

Figure 15 (**A**) Characteristic architectural pattern of a parathyroid aspirate showing a three-dimensional fragment with underlying vasculature and scattered naked nuclei (*arrows*) (Diff-Quik 100×). (**B**) On high magnification, the parathyroid chief cells show scant granular cytoplasm, round dark nuclei with indistinct nucleoli, and characteristic paranuclear lipid vacuoles throughout (Diff-Quik 600×).

A comparison of key cytoarchitectural parameters found in thyroid and parathyroid aspirates is summarized in Table 2. No single morphologic parameter alone can separate parathyroid tissue from thyroid, though a constellation of findings may support a parathyroid origin. A useful architectural finding to suggest parathyroid is the presence of three-dimensional fibrovascular fragments lined by epithelial cells in cords (Fig. 15); thyroid nodules tend to form two-dimensional honeycomb sheets. However, a recent review by Dimashkieh and Krishnamurthy (135) noted that while this architectural feature is useful, most parathyroid aspirates actually show two-dimensional aggregates. Cytologically, parathyroid chief cells are smaller and typically have more pronounced stippled "salt and pepper chromatin" than thyroid follicular cells, though these findings may be rather subtle. Rarely, parathyroid cells will have nucleoli, particularly if they are oxyphilic (140,143) and may be mistaken for Hurthle cell lesions of the thyroid (131). The cytoplasm is more likely to be stripped from the nuclei in parathyroid cells than in thyroid follicular epithelial cells, though even thyroid tissue may have "naked nuclei" as well. In parathyroid glands, the nuclei are more likely to show molding (140). Typically, in intact chief cells, the cytoplasm is amphophilic to pink, vacuolated to granular. On Romanowsky or Diff-Quik stains, fat vacuoles that may indent the nucleus may be seen as well (Fig. 15), more commonly in normal parathyroid than in hyperfunctioning parathyroid cells (135,141,143). One interesting finding by Bondeson et al. (143) in their review of 120 parathyroid aspirates is the frequent presence of mast cells in 22% of parathyroid aspirates versus only 1 of 50 follicular thyroid lesions. This finding was substantiated by Absher et al. in 2002 (140), and mast cells have been documented in the histologic sections of parathyroid glands of chronic renal failure patients (144).

Features that have been historically deemed useful in separating these two tissue types cannot be applied with absolute certainty. For instance, the presence of follicular or even papillary patterned areas can be seen in both tissue types. Furthermore, parathyroid aspirates may also contain colloid-like material in up to 15% of cases making the distinction even more difficult (141,143). While the presence of macrophages suggests thyroid tissue, parathyroid tissue may also contain significant numbers in up to 18% of cases (135) (Fig. 16). Similarly, coarse paravacuolar

granulation, a finding thought to be specific for thyroid tissue (139), may be seen in up to 13% of parathyroid aspirates (143).

Medullary thyroid carcinoma may also enter into the differential diagnosis for parathyroid cells. On aspirate, both have overlap in chromatin characteristics and architecture. However, medullary thyroid carcinoma does not typically have stripped nuclei. Additionally, medullary thyroid carcinoma will tend to have eccentrically located nuclei (a plasmacytoid appearance) and a mixture of spindled and ovoid cells (135,139).

It is ultimately prudent to confirm the morphologic impression of parathyroid tissue with immunohistochemical staining, whenever possible. Reports of sensitivity using anti-PTH immunohistochemistry range from 60% to 100% (135,138,145). Rare cases of misleading immunostains may be due to the use of air-dried smear preparations (133). Hence, ethanol fixed smears or paraffin sections of the cell block are recommended for immunohistochemical staining.

Thus, the main utility of cytologic evaluation is that, in the recognition of key morphologic parameters on FNA, the possibility that a given thyroid nodule or neck mass may actually be a parathyroid lesion may be raised. But when used as a tool to localize parathyroid tissue in the select cases of hyperparathyroidism mentioned above, it is not clear whether cytomorphology has added benefit beyond that of an aspirate PTH level. For instance, in the study by Stephen et al. (128), the cytology was less sensitive than PTH aspirate levels, and there was no case in which the cytology was read as positive for parathyroid tissue, and the aspirate PTH levels were negative. Furthermore, in the evaluation of parathyroid cysts, the cytologic smears may show only rare epithelial cells or none at all, and the definitive diagnosis rests on the fluid PTH levels (130).

Regarding the ability of FNA to distinguish between various parathyroid disease states, some authors state that nuclear pleomorphism in an aspirate distinguishes adenoma from hyperplasia (137,141). However, others claim that this is not a robust discriminatory feature showing no significant differences in morphologic parameters (135,146). We heavily favor this latter opinion since the aforementioned differences between adenoma and hyperplasia were noted only retrospectively (137,141) and are of dubious validity prospectively, considering the histologic spectrum of hyperplasia (see section "Pathology of Specific Disease Entities"). Similarly, the distinction between parathyroid carcinoma, which is typically defined by architectural rather than cytologic features, and other benign parathyroid lesions is nearly impossible on FNA. Only two of the eight cases reported that describe the cytologic features in detail demonstrated marked pleomorphism (147–153).

Complications of parathyroid FNA are rare and typically consist of a local infection (128). While there is a theoretical concern of parathyromatosis secondary to FNA, this has yet to be documented in the literature in benign disease (154). However, there have been two

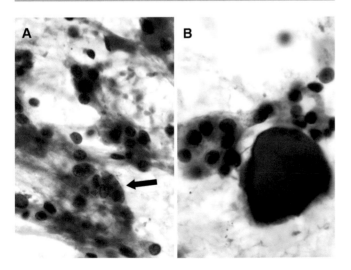

Figure 16 Features that may rarely be seen in parathyroid aspirates that mimic a thyroid aspirate. (**A**) Hemosiderin is seen among these chief cells (*arrow*) (Papanicolou, 400×). (**B**) Rare parathyroid aspirates also show colloid-like material (Papanicolou, 600×).

Table 3 Characteristics of FNA in Parathyroid Disease Pre-operative Evaluation

-FNA in preoperative localization of parathyroid glands is mainly reserved for cases in which there was prior surgery in the neck region, or if imaging studies suggest an unusual or ectopic location. In these cases, FNA aspirate analysis for PTH levels appears superior to cytolomorphogic evaluation.

-During FNA evaluation of a neck or thyroid mass, it is important to recognize cytologic parameters that may raise the possibility of a parathyroid tissue, though it may be impossible to definitively distinguish parathyroid from thyroid tissue without immunohistochemical stains. These should always be performed on a cell block or ethanol-fixed smears, if available.

-Cytologic evaluation cannot reliably distinguish between normal, hyperplasia, adenoma, and carcinoma, despite some literature to the contrary.

-The complication rate of FNA is low, and mainly that of infection, though rare cases of seeding of needle tract by parathyroid carcinoma have been reported.

Abbreviation: FNA, fine-needle aspiration.
Source: From Refs. 126–127,128,135,136,140,141,143,146.

case reports of seeding of a parathyroid carcinoma along a fine-needle tract (152,155).

Table 3 summarizes the characteristics of FNA in preoperative parathyroid evaluation.

IV. SECONDARY AND TERTIARY HYPERPARATHYROIDISM

A. Definition

Secondary hyperparathyroidism is defined by compensatory PTH hypersecretion in response to low serum calcium. Causes of secondary hyperparathyroidism are most commonly due to low vitamin D levels, either from malabsorption, nutritional deficiency, or lack of 1α-hydroxylase in chronic renal failure, resulting in low calcitriol levels. Chronic renal failure also leads to increased serum phosphorus levels, which act as a direct stimulus to PTH synthesis and secretion. Chronic parathyroid stimulation eventually results in multiple gland parathyroid hyperplasia. Elevated PTH levels lead to increased calcium and phosphorus release from bone, which worsens hyperphosphatemia and leads to renal osteodystrophy. Over time, hyperplastic parathyroid glands become resistant to regulation by calcium and calcitriol (156). Less common causes of secondary hyperparathyroidism include hypomagnesemia and pseudohyperparathyroidism.

Tertiary hyperparathyroidism is defined as the autonomous function of parathyroid glands in the setting of chronically overstimulated parathyroid glands in secondary hyperparathyroidism. The end result is hypercalcemia even after the stimulus for parathyroid hypersecretion is removed. Hypercalcemia can be observed in patients after successful renal transplantation, but is also seen in patients still on hemodialysis. A rare cause of tertiary hyperparathyroidism is X-linked hypophosphatemic rickets (157).

B. Epidemiology

Over 336,000 patients were treated with dialysis for end-stage renal disease in the United Stated in 2006 (158). All patients with end-stage renal disease have abnormal calcium, vitamin D, and phosphorus metabolism. The majority of patients on dialysis for end-stage renal disease will have some degree of compensatory secondary hyperparathyroidism (159).

C. Clinical Presentation

Patients with secondary and tertiary hyperparathyroidism are usually identified by biochemical testing during dialysis. Symptoms of secondary hyperparathyroidism include fatigue, bone pain, muscle weakness, skeletal deformity, cardiovascular disease, pathologic fractures, and pruritus.

Skeletal abnormalities are a common finding in secondary and tertiary hyperparathyroidism. Patients with PTH levels more than 800 pg/mL or less than 195 pg/mL have significantly increased risk of pathologic fractures (160,161). High PTH levels in secondary hyperparathyroidism lead to high turnover bone disease, including osteitis fibrosa cystica and mixed uremic osteodystrophy. Renal osteodystrophy occurs in 75% to 100% of patients with a glomerular filtration rate (GFR) less than 60 mL/min/1.73 m^2 and is associated with poorly mineralized and structurally inferior bone (162).

Cardiovascular complications are fairly common in secondary and tertiary hyperparathyroidism as well. Hemodialysis patients with elevated PTH levels more than 495 pg/mL have a higher rate of sudden cardiac death compared with patients with PTH levels between 91 and 197 pg/mL (163). Elevated PTH levels are also associated with a significantly higher risk of thrombosis of vascular access grafts (164). An increased calcium-phosphorus product has been associated with higher rates of cardiovascular calcification (165). An increased calcium-phosphorus product of more than 72 mg^2/dL^2 imparts a 34% increased relative risk of mortality compared with a calcium-phosphorus product of less than 52 mg^2/dL^2 (166). Increased PTH levels also activate cardiomyocyte–protein kinase C, leading to left ventricular hypertrophy (167,168).

A rare but also often fatal complication of secondary hyperparathyroidism in patients with a high calcium-phosphorus product is calciphylaxis, characterized by painful purpuric skin lesions and extensive vascular and soft tissue calcification.

D. Preoperative Localization

Imaging

Preoperative parathyroid imaging has not traditionally been widely used for secondary or tertiary hyperparathyroidism, as most patients have multiple gland involvement requiring traditional bilateral parathyroid exploration. However, parathyroid localization studies including Tc99m sestamibi SPECT and ultrasound can be very helpful to identify supernumerary or ectopic parathyroid glands. Supernumerary parathyroid glands have been identified in up to 16% of patients with secondary hyperparathyroidism and cause postoperative recurrent or persistent hyperparathyroidism in 2% (169). Neck ultrasound can also be used to diagnose concomitant thyroid pathology, cervical lymphadenopathy, or intrathyroidal parathyroid glands.

Selective Venous Sampling

SVS for PTH can be used to localize enlarged parathyroid glands before reoperative parathyroid exploration for recurrent or persistent secondary/tertiary hyperparathyroidism, with 90% sensitivity (170). Because it is an invasive and technically challenging technique, it is typically used only in cases where noninvasive localizing studies are negative or equivocal.

V. INTRAOPERATIVE EVALUATION

A. PTH Assay

PTH determination during parathyroid surgery to guide complete removal of hyperfunctioning glands came into use in the early 1990s with the introduction of assays that provided blood concentrations of the hormone through modification of an assay available at the time for routine analysis. These more rapid assays, with performance times between 5 and 20 minutes, are available from some manufacturers and are in use for guidance during surgery for completion of removal of hyperfunctioning parathyroid glands.

The impact of this development has been on the reoperation rate for parathyroid adenoma and hyperplasia, which decreased from 4% to less than 0.5% at institutions where experienced surgeons perform the procedure. The availability of rapid PTH assay during surgery has also resulted in limited exploration of the neck with the procedure now being performed as a same-day surgery. In combination with sestamibi scan performed preoperatively in nuclear medicine to locate hyperfunctioning parathyroid tissue, in most patients the surgery is limited to the side of the neck where the scan has identified the adenoma. In cases where there is no significant decline in the blood concentration of PTH following removal of one gland identified by scan, the indication is that of remaining hyperfunctional tissue, either in the usual anatomic location of the parathyroid glands, or location at an aberrant site, or the presence of supernumery glands.

There is an established protocol that is in use currently with minor variations that are based on the experience and preferences at a particular institution. The blood samples are drawn in the following order: (*i*) after neck incision and exposure of the gland to serve as the baseline, (*ii*) 10 minutes after excision of the gland identified visually as that located previously on sestamibi scan. The blood samples are obtained either from the jugular vein or from the peripheral vein. A decline of more than 50% from the elevated baseline value indicates complete removal of the hyperfunctioning tissue. If this concentration of PTH is not within the reference range or if the PTH did not drop sufficiently, a third sample may be obtained to ensure that there is a further decline in the PTH concentration. The experience of the surgeon guides the decision for the third sample.

B. Pathologic Assessment

Advances in preoperative localization and the advent of the rapid intraoperative PTH level assessment have greatly diminished the role of intraoperative pathologic examination in hyperparathyroidism. In the minds of some, intraoperative (and even final) pathologic assessment of parathyroid glands yields little other than confirmation of parathyroid tissue (171). However, pathologic assessement remains a critical component of parathyroid disease management in the setting of equivocal imaging studies, prior surgery, ectopic or intrathyroidal locations, and concomitant thyroid nodules. There is a surprisingly wide arsenal of techniques available for pathologic assessment of parathyroid glands, ranging from simple gross assessment to fat stains on frozen sections. Regardless of methodology, the primary objective at the time of frozen section is the confirmation of tissue identity. A secondary objective is the determination of whether the parathyroid tissue removed is normal or abnormal.

Gross Assessment

Gross abnormalities are an outward manifestation of hyperfunctional status, but enlargement by size or weight does not always equate with functional abnormality (172). Hence, some consider the drop in intraoperative PTH values, which is a functional assessment, to take precedence over gross abnormalities (171). Nonetheless, as the difficulty in preoperative localization and the surgery itself increases, each available parameter becomes more and more critical, and for this reason, grossing standards should not become lax or viewed as a simple academic exercise.

All parathyroid specimens should be measured in three dimensions (i.e., *x by y by z cm*). Though abnormal parathyroid glands are typically larger than normal glands, ranging from 0.5 to 8.0 cm in greatest dimension, the lower limit overlaps with normal parathyroid tissue (which may be up to 0.9 cm along its long axis) (10). However, abnormal parathyroid glands are often more rounded than the bean-shaped normal parathyroid glands and will be relatively larger along the second and third axes than a normal parathyroid gland. Hence, the three-dimensional measurement conveys valuable information to the pathologist, especially if they did not grossly examine the specimen themselves as is often the case at busy centers.

All parathyroid glands should be weighed. Gland weight is a simple, yet high yield parameter that may be more discriminatory than size, and possibly even cellularity in the distinction between normal and abnormal parathyroid glands. However, overlap between normal and abnormal parathyroid tissue may still exist. Normal parathyroid glands typically weigh 30 to 40 mg, and almost all parathyroid glands over 80 mg are abnormal. But while glands larger than 40 mg are often considered abnormal, practically speaking, glands between 40 and 80 mg should be interpreted in the context of clinical, laboratory, and histologic findings since normal glands are often seen within this weight range as well (10–12,16,25). Parathyroid glands are often excised with surrounding adipose tissue. This adipose tissue should be trimmed prior to weighing the gland (173). Ideally, the trimmed fat should also be weighed in the event that it also contains parathyroid tissue on permanent section evaluation.

An even more accurate assessment of parathyroid cell mass that was performed in the past involved the use of density-gradient techniques, using a solution such as Percoll or mannitol solution (174–179). Parenchyma and fat are of different densities, the density of a parathyroid gland is linearly related to parenchymal cell content. If total weight is known, parenchymal cell mass can also be calculated. An adaptation of this technique has been applied intraoperatively in which the qualitative difference in gland densities is reflected by how deep a gland sinks in the solution (175,180). For instance, if one gland sinks and one gland floats, the suggestion is that the sunken gland is an adenoma. The utility of the density testing is ultimately unclear since studies did not have long-term follow-up (181). Additionally, the result of the density testing may depend on heterogeneity within the gland leading to inaccuracies, especially if only a sliver of gland is assessed in this manner (182). Finally, density-gradient measurement for parathyroid tissue assessment is cumbersome, requires additional technical expertise, and presumably, additional quality control requirements. Hence, without substantial proven benefit, this test has become largely one of historical significance only.

The qualitative gross assessment is important in the confirmation of parathyroid tissue.

Tissue fragments that are less than 0.5 cm in thickness can be grossly examined as is, while those that are larger should be sliced serially as thinly as possible (usually at 0.2–0.3-cm intervals) along the longest axis. This allows visualization of the greatest cross-sectional area and thus control for glandular heterogeneity. Parathyroid parenchyma is a characteristic red-brown. Normal parathyroid tissue is typically paler or more yellow than abnormal parathyroid tissue reflecting the higher amount of stromal fat. Oxyphil-rich parathyroid tissue may display a dark mahogany brown appearance typical to mitochondria rich or "oncocytic" lesions at other sites, including thyroid, salivary gland, and kidney (10,12). The cut surfaces are homogenous and slightly glistening as a result of a thin, clear, watery surface exudate. Abnormal gland cut surfaces will tend to "bulge" to varying degrees.

The gross differential diagnosis of parathyroid tissue can be challenging especially on smaller fragments and includes thymus, lymph node, and thyroid tissue. The distinction between these tissue types is often subtle but can be made with reasonable accuracy by surgeons and pathologist alike (183). In fact, the "clinical intraoperative impression" that is so highly touted (171) is comprised in part by gross pathologic evaluation, except that it is performed by a surgeon. In a review of 50 cases, gross assessment was reported to be 91.4% accurate in identifying parathyroid tissue (184). However, in this study, all specimens assessed were greater than 100 mg and all were abnormal, hence this accuracy may not apply to more difficult, yet common situations, such as smaller specimens in the setting of prior surgery. Nonetheless, the surgeon may not necessarily request a frozen section on a specimen with a classic gross appearance of parathyroid tissue, especially if preoperative imaging is concordant with the gross impression.

Abnormal parathyroid tissue is typically firmer than normal parathyroid tissue, but softer and more friable than lymph node tissue. This subtle difference in consistency is best appreciated in the tactile sensation from slicing the specimen, since parathyroid tissue cuts with less resistance than a lymph node. Additionally, as compared with a lymph node, and most thyroid nodules, a parathyroid gland cut surface has more of a brown hue. Anthracosis may be helpful, if present, since it is indicative of lymph node tissue and effectively excludes parathyroid tissue. Another subtle finding to distinguish between thyroid and parathyroid tissue grossly is the presence of a slightly stickier, more heavily glistening surface, which is more typical of thyroid tissue. The gross distinction between thymic tissue and parathyroid tissue is, in our experience, extremely difficult and unreliable. In fact, both tissue types may actually be intermingled. Thymic tissue in adults is more fatty, hence more yellow than parathyroid, particularly abnormal parathyroid tissue (185), but in younger patients, this may not be as useful a distinguishing criterion. Cases of parathyromatosis have been noted in grossly normal-appearing thymic tissue (12). Another unreliable gross distinction is between brown fat and a normal parathyroid tissue—both can be of the same size and may have the same tan-yellow appearance. Interestingly, brown fat deposits may have uptake on radionuclide studies, hence preoperatively mimicking parathyroid tissue as well (186).

Frozen Section and Intraoperative Imprint Cytology

Despite the rise in popularity of intraoperative parathyroid aspirates for PTH level, frozen section still remains an important tool in the intraoperative confirmation of parathyroid tissue. In most cases, the frozen section discriminates between normal and abnormal parathyroid tissue, though this portion of the assessment has in large part been superseded by assessment of intraoperative PTH levels. Accuracy rates for frozen section are as high as 99.4% in the identification of parathyroid tissue (187). This near perfect accuracy is vital to minimizing postoperative failures (183). However, errors in frozen section interpretation have been historically cited among the most common reasons of parathyroid surgery failure (188,189). Hence, it is important to be aware of the pitfalls of frozen section interpretation to minimize error and know when to defer to permanent histologic and possibly immunophenotypic evaluation.

The use of intraoperative cytologic smear preparations made from the main specimens stained either by Diff-Quik or hematoxylin and eosin stains is controversial. Intraoperative cytologic evaluations are cheaper and quicker, typically completed in two to seven minutes (190–192). Additionally, a touch imprint of a small fatty biopsy may yield diagnostic material, whereas a frozen section of the same specimen may be limited by various frozen section artifacts. However, accuracy ranges from less than 70% to almost 100%, suggesting wide variation based on technique and pathologist's experience among other variables (190–194). The lower end of this range of accuracy is clearly not acceptable (183). Intraoperative cytologic preparations are subject to the same pitfalls as preoperative parathyroid cytology. Namely, parathyroid tissue can be readily confused with thyroid tissue. Hence, cytology as a stand-alone intraoperative assessment may thus only be appropriate if a pathology practice can demonstrate accuracy comparable to that of frozen section, otherwise the speed and cost effectiveness is diminished by the results of the increased rate of misdiagnosis. Perhaps the approach by Shidham et al. (192) is the most logical, using cytology to complement frozen section for an improved accuracy over either technique alone, particularly with regard to small fatty specimens.

Frozen section interpretation of parathyroid is typically straightforward. The sample procedural approach to parathyroid frozen section is summarized in Table 4.

A key grossing technique that should be implemented is the trimming of surrounding fat prior to sectioning. Trimming the excess fat not only provides a more accurate weight but also minimizes technical difficulty in generating frozen sections. In a review of 1579 frozen sections by Westra et al. (187), sampling error and frozen artifact/technical difficulty were both common reasons for frozen section misinterpretation. Hence, frozen section from a technical standpoint should be optimized to reduce this component of error. Additionally, a touch imprint of fatty or small specimens as recommended above may help since significant tissue dropout on frozen section may be anticipated. As on permanent sections, parathyroid tissue is often arranged in a nested or corded pattern with delicate fibrovascular septation. Abnormal glands may be composed of solid or nodular growth patterns and thicker cords/trabeculae as well. Hence, correct identification of parathyroid tissue is typically not challenging. The problem arises when the follicular pattern of growth predominates, mimicking a thyroid follicular lesion, or in oxyphil-predominant areas, mimicking a thyroid oncocytic (Hurthle) lesion. In the review by Westra et al. (187), these pitfalls were the most common source of misdiagnosis and deferral. The follicles in parathyroid with this growth pattern often contain colloid-like material adding further to the difficulty (Fig. 17). Conversely, thyroid tissue with stromal edema may mimic permeation

Table 4 Sample Approach to Intraoperative Frozen Section/Cytologic Assessment of Parathyroid Glands

-After gross examination, the specimen can be entirely frozen if less than 0.5 cm in greatest dimension, or representatively frozen if larger.
-For predominantly fatty yellow specimens or small specimens less than 0.2 cm in greatest dimension, a scrape or touch imprint can be performed depending on the pathologist's proficiency in cytologic evaluation.
-For larger specimens, the largest slice when serially sectioned along the long axis as recommended above should be the section that is frozen for histologic evaluation.
-Prior to embedding in OCT media, excess fluid should be removed from the specimen to be frozen by (very) gentle blotting to minimize ice crystal formation.
-Another important component to minimizing crystal formation is rapid even freezing to the optimal cutting temperature. Using a wider cooling surface area and precooled "chucks" achieves this objective more readily.
-The appropriate cutting temperature may vary from cryostat to cryostat, but relative to other head and neck specimens (margins, upper aerodigestive tract lesions), "soft" parenchymal types such as parathyroid glands and lymph nodes cut more evenly at temperatures that are ~3°C–5°C warmer (typically –19°C–22°C as compared to –25°C–28°C), though for fatty specimen types, cooler temperatures are optimal. Colder temperatures seem to induce "chatter artifact." If feasible, one cryostat should be kept at this slightly warmer temperature, but otherwise, simply pressing the cutting surface of the frozen OCT block with a thumb for 1–2 sec will achieve similar warmth.
-Sections should be cut at 5–7 μm in thickness for histologic evaluation. Thinner sections give a reliable two-dimensional plane of view with minimal cell overlap and often superior cytologic quality. However, thicker sections may be required in fatty specimens to minimize tissue dropout. Hence, section thickness should be modulated according to need.

Source: From Ref. 412.

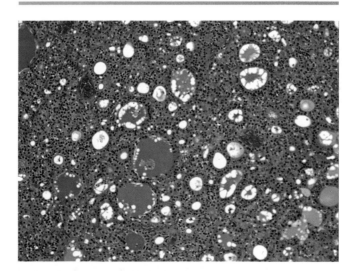

Figure 17 Follicular pattern and pseudocolloid in parathyroid tissue may mimic thyroid on frozen section (H&E, 100×). *Abbreviation*: H&E, hematoxylin and eosin.

by fatty stroma on frozen section and falsely imply parathyroid tissue. If other areas that are classic for parathyroid tissue are not observed in an oxyphilic- or follicular-patterned nodule, it is best to defer and convey the uncertainty to the surgeon. Such cases may need immunohistochemistry on the formalin-fixed material for definitive confirmation of parathyroid tissue (187).

The assessment of abnormal parathyroid versus normal parathyroid tissue can often be performed by integration with clinical and gross findings, including specimen weight, but is generally not a required component of a frozen section diagnosis. And in fact, some have argued against the utility of frozen section in distinguishing normal from abnormal para-thyroid tissue with error rates in either direction of up to almost 30% (195). As mentioned in the section "Normal Parathyroid Gland," normal parathyroid glands can have a range of cellularity that overlaps with abnormal glands (20,21,24). In addition to bio-logic variation, on frozen section, because of fat drop-out, the remaining parathyroid nests may become compressed together and appear artifactually hyper-cellular. Acknowledging the fact that the surgeon may care only that parathyroid tissue is present, we report hypercellularity on frozen section when there is an enlarged gland by size and weight and the cellularity is unequivocally high with less than 10% stromal fat, that is, in situations where there is a low risk of being incorrect. Along similar lines, we conversely report normocellularity in the context of a normal gland by size and weight with the frozen section showing roughly 30% to 50% stromal fat. Outside of these categories, we simply confirm the presence of para-thyroid tissue.

Fat Stains

Assessment of intracytoplasmic neutral lipids in para-rthyroid parenchyma, using a fat stain such as oil red O or Sudan IV, is in principle a closer reflection of functional status than size and cellularity. Normal or suppressed parathyroid tissue will have numerous fine and coarse lipid vacuoles. Hyperfunctioning glands will have far less intracytoplasmic lipid vacuoles, usually of the finer type, if present. The accuracy of fat stains in predicting functional status is typically over 80% (20,196–198). Generally, fat stains should not be used for distinction between adenoma and hyperplasia on the basis of the findings in one gland alone. Distribution of intracytoplasmic lipid within a gland may be heterogeneous. An adenoma may have a normal rim of parathyroid tissue, which has greater amounts of intracytoplasmic lipid, but similarly, an enlarged gland from nodular hyperplasia may mimic this pattern in that the nodules tend to have less intracytoplasmic lipid than the surrounding nonnodular parenchyma (196,198).

Results may vary based on the fat stain used, though a large-scale methodical comparison of vari-ous fat stains has never been performed. The original Sudan IV mixture used by Roth and Gallagher (199) was thought to be less discriminatory because of poor staining contrast between normal and abnormal as compared with oil red O (200). Monchik et al. (201) claim that both oil red O and Sudan IV have organic solvent components that may leach lipid and thus favor aqueous osmium carmine as the lipid stain of choice.

Fat stains can be performed in the intraoperative setting and have historically been used for this pur-pose (199,201,202). Intraoperative PTH levels have superseded the intraoperative impact of fat stains, but these stains may yield valuable information when considered in the final interpretation of find-ings. Some degree of inaccuracy is noted with fat stains, and like any other parameter in parathyroid disease, these should be interpreted within the context of all other findings (20,196–198). Additionally, even when correct, it is debatable whether fat stains add useful information (197). However, fat stains may still have utility in the assessment of clinically and histo-logic borderline cases, in which every available parameter may help in patient management (10). In our practice, fat stains have the highest impact in the interpretation of small or shave biopsies of parathy-roid glands. These are often performed on normal glands for confirmation of parathyroid tissue. As a result of heterogeneity, these biopsies may appear to be hypercellular, though clinically noted to be taken from a normal-sized gland. In these situations, the presence of abundant intracytoplasmic lipid within the hypercellular-appearing biopsy is reassuring of the fact that the hypercellularity is a result of hetero-geneity within normal gland and/or compression artifact rather than a functional disturbance.

VI. PATHOLOGY OF SPECIFIC DISEASE ENTITIES

A. General

The pathologic hallmarks of hyperfunctioning parathy-roid glands are enlargement and hypercellularity. As mentioned in the section "Intraoperative Evaluation," in addition to being enlarged (typically ≥100 mg) hyperfunctioning parathyroid glands are more roun-ded and homogeneous red tan than normal glands. They are softer than lymph nodes and less gelatinous than thyroid tissue. Histologically, hyperfunction para-thyroid glands have an increased parathyroid paren-chymal mass typically accompanied by a decrease in stromal fat. However, the distinction between various disease states of hyperparathyroidism is more difficult and typically impossible when relying on histology alone. In other words, *there are no reliable histologic criteria to separate adenoma from hyperplasia*, especially when examining only one gland.

B. Single-Gland Disease

Adenoma

Adenomas range from less than 100 mg to several grams, and range from 6 mm to several centimeters. The average weight is about 500 mg. Small adenomas (microadenomas) may constitute up to 3% of adenomas (203,204). We delineate microadenomas as adenomas that are less than 200 mg. Grossly, the classic parathyroid adenoma is a rounded nodule of red tan tissue with a tail of paler tan tissue, often at one pole (Fig. 18). However, the demonstration of a rim of normal is only possible in 50% to 60% of cases. Cystic change may be present to varying degrees and is estimated to be present in about 10% of adenomas (Fig. 19) (205,206). Conversely, parathyroid cysts are functional (thus best regarded as cystic adenomas) in 10% to 15% of cases as well. Cystic change in adenomas is more frequent in patients with familial HPT-JT syndrome (98). Larger lesions may demonstrate degenerative changes, including fibrosis, hemorrhage, and calcification.

The histologic correlate to the classic finding of a red-brown nodule with a rim of tan tissue is the presence of well-demarcated or even encapsulated hypercellular parathyroid tissue with a compressed rim of normal parathyroid (Fig. 20). The chief cells of the adenoma are typically larger and more anisomorphic than those of the normal rim, though the chromatin characteristics are typically maintained. The cells can be arranged in a variety of architectural patterns: purely solid, confluent nests and cords, follicular/glandular, or a mixture of these three (Fig. 21). The stroma is highly vascular, comprising a delicate arborizing capillary network. Some adenomas may have perivascular hyalinization and even localized amyloid deposition (10,12). True papillae formation is rare (207). Occasionally, marked degenerative nuclear atypia with large hyperchromatic cells with "smudgy" chromatin can be seen but should not be confused for malignancy (208). Mitotic activity is

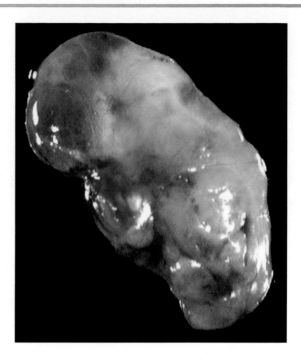

Figure 19 Cystic change in an adenoma. Note the translucent appearance.

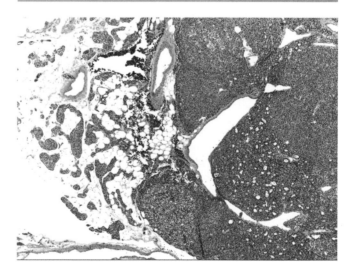

Figure 20 Parathyroid adenoma and adjacent rim of normal parathyroid tissue (H&E, 40×). There is a rounded well-demarcated solid proliferation of chief cells devoid of adipocytes with an adjacent rim of normal parathyroid tissue (*left*). *Abbreviation*: H&E, hematoxylin and eosin.

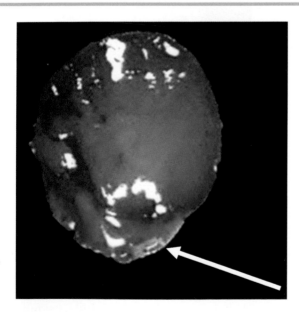

Figure 18 Typical gross appearance of an adenoma. A rounded tan nodule with a paler rim of normal parathyroid and fat at one pole (*arrow*).

generally minimal to absent, but may occasionally be as high as 4 per 10 high-power fields (209–211). Some of these more proliferative cases may be more accurately categorized as "atypical adenomas" (see below). Historically, Ghandur-Mnaymneh and Kimura (212) required the following histologic criteria to be fulfilled for the diagnosis of adenoma: (*i*) pushing border with

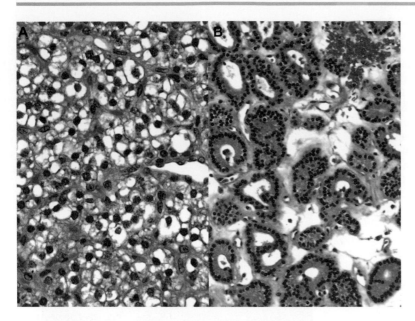

Figure 21 (**A**) Solid pattern in an adenoma consisting of a proliferation of variably glycogenated chief cells (H&E, 200×). (**B**) Follicular pattern in an adenoma (H&E, 100×). *Abbreviation*: H&E, hematoxylin and eosin.

no intralesional stromal fat, (*ii*) complete demarcation, and (*iii*) absence of lobularity. These represent the most stringent criteria for adenoma, and actually, most single-gland disease would fail these criteria. The current proposed criterion standard for the diagnosis of adenoma is *not solely histologic*. Instead, it is outcome based, namely, the removal of a single enlarged gland with long-term cure (171). Hence, cases, which do not fulfill the classic criteria, are still accepted by Ghandur-Mnaymneh and Kimura as adenomas, using clinical and laboratory criteria, if only a single gland is enlarged and the intraoperative PTH levels drop appropriately.

While the majority of adenomas comprise chief cells, about 3% to 8% may be oxyphilic (34,213,214). Oxyphilic adenomas classically present in the sixth or seventh decade (213) and are noted to be more readily detected on sestamibi scan as compared with chief cell predominant adenomas (215,216). Grossly, these may assume a mahogany brown appearance (Fig. 22). Despite the indication of a senescent cell type in normal parathyroid gland, the majority of oxyphil-rich adenomas are hyperfunctioning, and there is no significant difference between oxyphil adenomas and chief cell adenomas with regard to size or serum calcium levels (215). Ordonez et al. (217) demonstrated immunohistochemically and ultrastructurally that oxyphils are indeed functional. Criteria recommended by Wolpert et al. (213) to define oxyphil adenoma are as follows: (*i*) greater than 90% oxyphils, (*ii*) the confirmation that the other glands are normal, and (*iii*) resolution of hypercalcemia postoperatively (Fig. 23).

Clear cell change in chief cell adenomas as a result of glycogenation is relatively common and underreported. However, "water-clear" adenomas are extremely rare with only six cases mentioned in the literature (218–223). Of these, one case was that of double adenomas. Each "adenoma" was shown to be

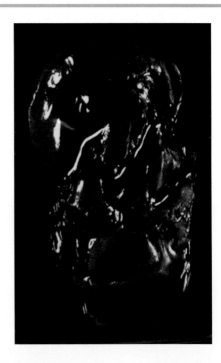

Figure 22 Gross appearance of an oxyphilic adenoma. Similar to other oncocytic lesions of other sites, the classic appearance is a mahogany brown.

monoclonal using inactivation pattern of the human androgen receptor gene, though even the authors caution that they were unable to exclude asymmetric hyperplasia (223). Water-clear cell adenomas consist of cells that are larger and more polygonal than glycogenated chief cells and often show some microvacuolization. Ultrastructurally, numerous electron-lucent

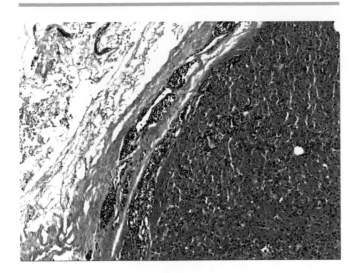

Figure 23 An oxyphilic adenoma that is thinly encapsulated with a compressed rim of paler and smaller chief cells (H&E, 100×). *Abbreviation*: H&E, hematoxylin and eosin.

vacuoles are noted. Microscopic details of water-clear cells will be further delineated below (section "Single-Gland Disease").

Lipoadenomas are also rare variants with fewer than 50 cases reported (73,224–251). Initially, this entity was thought to be a hamartomatous process since the original report was that of a nonfunctioning process, but the majority are indeed hyperfunctioning (242). The size of lipoadenomas varies greatly, ranging from 500 to 480,000 mg (245). The gross appearance may vary as well, ranging from that of a conventional parathyroid adenoma to a lobulated yellow mass resembling a lipoma. The characteristic histologic findings are an increase in stromal and glandular elements (Fig. 24). The stroma may be lipomatous or

myxoid and ranges from constituting 30% to 90% of the cross-sectional area of an adenoma (241). One recent series defines the minimal stromal fat percentage as 50% (229). The parathyroid parenchymal constituents are usually chief cells arranged in a corded-to-nodular pattern. These cords are often compressed, resembling the pattern in normal parathyroid. However, there is greater variation in cord/trabecular width in lipoadenomas, and there is a tendency for these cords to coalesce into nodular aggregates. One case of an oxyphilic lipoadenoma has been reported (229), and one case with thymic tissue, a "lipothymoadenoma," has been described (249).

Atypical Adenoma

The term "atypical adenoma" is used to describe parathyroid adenomas with features that are worrisome, but not diagnostic of malignancy. It is neither a universally accepted term nor are there unanimously agreed upon criteria (12,252–254). Atypical parathyroid adenomas tend to be grossly larger than typical adenomas and are more similar in size to carcinomas (255). Fibrosis and cystic change may be noted as well, and intraoperatively, they may exhibit some degree of firmness and/or tissue adherence (255,256). Histologically, criteria for inclusion in the category of atypical adenoma are shown in Table 5 (12,252–256). Other than the absence of the bottom criteria (which would indicate malignancy), there is no specific requirement for number of positive criteria to designate a tumor as an atypical adenoma. Equivocal/incomplete capsular invasion, fibrous bands, mitosis, nonsecondary necrosis, and trabecular growth pattern (not to be confused with short thin cords/trabeculae in normal parathyroid gland) are the most common reasons for designation as atypical adenoma (252,255–257). Usually, atypical adenomas contain at least two of these criteria.

There are some criteria that are controversial in terms of their importance. Among these is the presence of abnormal mitoses. Most would consider a single abnormal mitotic form diagnostic of malignancy (12,252). At the very least, this should be considered sufficient for the diagnosis of atypical adenoma. We have also encountered a few cases with unusual

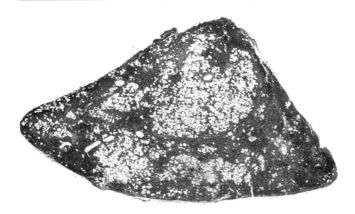

Figure 24 A lipoadenoma appears superficially to resemble a normal parathyroid gland. However, this particular gland weighed 3800 mg (H&E, whole slide scan). *Abbreviation*: H&E, hematoxylin and eosin.

Table 5 Histologic Criteria for Designation of Atypical Adenoma

Presence (2 or more of the following)
  Clinically adherent without soft tissue invasion
  Incomplete or equivocal capsular invasion
  Fibrous bands
  Pronounced back-to-back trabecular growth pattern
  Mitotic activity >1 per 10 HPF
  Tumor necrosis without secondary explanation

Absence
  Metastasis
  Angiolymphatic invasion
  Perineural invasion
  Unequivocal invasion

Source: From Refs. 12,252–256.

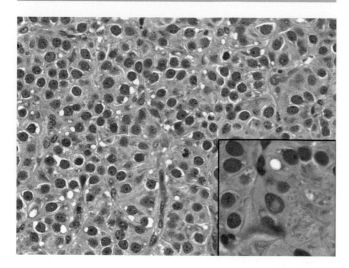

Figure 25 Atypical parathyroid adenoma (H&E, 400×). This adenoma has increased mitoses, open vesicular chromatin with prominent nucleoli, but no vascular, perineural, or capsular invasion. Occasional intranuclear inclusions were noted (*inset*, H&E, 600×). This adenoma had a fractional allelic loss of 50%, but no evidence of recurrence or metastasis. *Abbreviation*: H&E, hematoxylin and eosin.

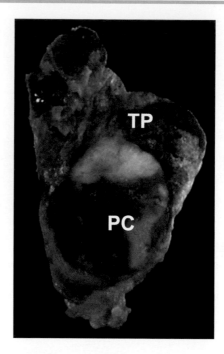

Figure 26 The gross appearance of a PC pushing into the adjacent red-brown TP. The tumor is white tan with central hemorrhage. *Abbreviations*: PC, parathyroid carcinoma; TP, thyroid parenchyma.

nuclear features (Fig. 25): (*i*) clearing, elongation, and grooves mimicking papillary thyroid carcinoma nuclei and (*ii*) diffuse large cell change with prominent nucleoli and high nuclear-to-cytoplasmic ratios rather than the random degenerative nuclear atypia that is acceptable in conventional adenomas. The significance of these unusual nuclear features is unclear, but a designation as atypical adenoma is supported by the molecular profile in at least a few cases (see below).

Carcinoma

Parathyroid carcinomas are usually larger than adenomas and range in weight from 2 to 10 g and measure on average 3 cm (75,258). Parathyroid carcinomas are typically firmer and more grayish white (Fig. 26) (259,260), though many can have a gross appearance that is very similar to adenoma (261). Occasionally an en bloc excision of a parathyroid gland may include a cuff of surrounding soft tissue or thyroid lobe if the clinical suspicion is high. In such instances, the gross impression of tissue infiltration is critical to document, as this may not be maintained after gross and histologic processing. In any en bloc excision or suspected carcinoma, margins should be inked prior to sectioning. Prior surgery, however, will mitigate the reliability of fibrosis and adherence to surrounding structures as a criterion for malignancy.

Histologically, parathyroid carcinomas range from well differentiated or adenoma -like to frankly anaplastic tumors. Most will share several features of atypical adenomas, namely, fibrous bands (in up to 90%), trabecular growth, mitotic activity (Fig. 27) and,

in addition, will have one or more definitive features of malignancy, namely, soft tissue/skeletal muscle, thyroid gland or large vessel infiltration, angiolymphatic invasion, perineural invasion, and/or metastases. Oxyphil-rich carcinomas, tumors with greater than 80% oxyphils, are rare (262). The original criteria noted by Schantz and Castleman (260) listed capsular invasion as diagnostic of malignancy. However, we consider small foci of incomplete capsular invasion without soft tissue invasion sufficient only for the diagnosis of atypical adenoma. In unencapsulated lesions, a slightly irregular border with minimal protrusion does not constitute tissue invasion. The problem of subjectivity is apparent with this criterion since a minimal extension beyond the contour of the gland has not been established for diagnosis of carcinoma. Nonetheless, tissue infiltration is among the most common diagnostic features present in at least 60% to 70% of cases (Fig. 28) (107,252,255). Vascular invasion is noted commonly to varying degrees ranging from 15% to over 80% (Fig. 29) (107,252,255,256). Perineural invasion, on the other hand, is uncommon, present in 0% to 19% of cases (Fig. 30) (252).

Differential Diagnosis and Molecular Pathology

Within the context of single-gland disease, the differential diagnosis is generally between the three classes: adenoma, atypical adenoma, and carcinoma. Occasionally, entities outside this spectrum are considered. Follicular-patterned parathyroid adenomas may resemble thyroid lesions, particularly in the intrathyroidal

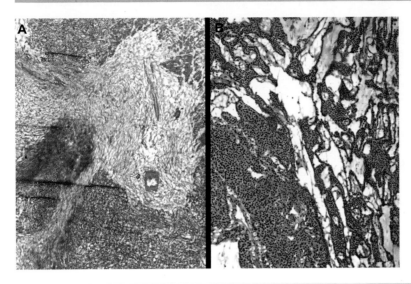

Figure 27 Common histologic features of parathyroid carcinomas. (**A**) Broad-based fibrosis (H&E frozen section, 100×). (**B**) long trabeculae (H&E frozen section, 100×). *Abbreviation*: H&E, hematoxylin and eosin.

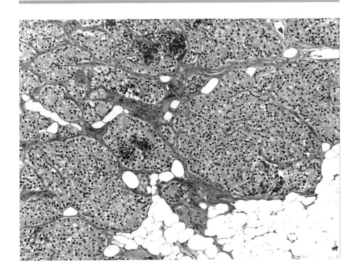

Figure 28 Extension of a parathyroid carcinoma into fat (H&E, 200×). *Abbreviation*: H&E, hematoxylin and eosin.

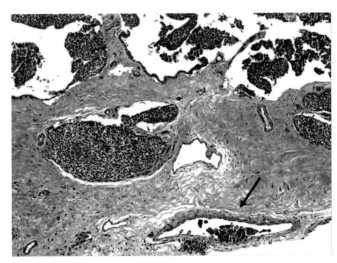

Figure 29 This parathyroid carcinoma with broad bands of fibrosis also shows angiolymphatic invasion (H&E, 100×). *Abbreviation*: H&E, hematoxylin and eosin.

region. Morphologically, parathyroid adenomas, even follicular patterned ones will tend to have a more delicate vasculature, nested growth, and smaller darker nuclei (263). When colloid-like material is present in parathyroid follicles, scalloping is usually not present. Another useful feature is the presence of oxalate crystals in follicles, which is indicative of thyroid tissue. Similarly, oxyphilic parathyroid adenomas may resemble oncocytic thyroid nodules and in rare instances also raise the possibility of medullary thyroid carcinoma as well. Here, the majority of an oxyphilic adenoma may show a solid growth pattern, but there will be scattered areas of transitional cell types that show more of a nested pattern, typical of parathyroid tissue. Medullary thyroid carcinoma, while sharing some cytologic similarities, will often show an infiltrative growth

with sclerosis and amyloid deposition more prominent than that seen in intrathyroidal parathyroids. Some micromedullary thyroid carcinomas have areas of C-cell hyperplasia that maintain the parafollicular growth pattern, which should not be seen in parathyroid adenomas, which are well delineated from surrounding thyroid tissue (264,265). Ultimately, immunohistochemical stains may be necessary in difficult cases. Table 6 summarizes the immunophenotypic characteristics using a simple panel of markers: PTH, TTF-1, thyroglobulin, calcitonin, and chromogranin. Generally, the bare minimum requirements to distinguish parathyroid from thyroid are anti-PTH and anti-TTF-1 immunohistochemistry, though the panel should be modified depending on in-house staining performance characteristics and on a case-by-case basis.

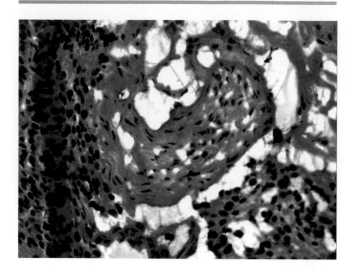

Figure 30 Perineural invasion in parathyroid carcinoma is quite rare (H&E frozen section, 400×). *Abbreviation*: H&E, hematoxylin and eosin.

Table 6 Immunophenotypic distinction between Parathyroid Tissue, Thyroid Nodules, and Medullary Carcinoma

Antigen	Parathyroid tissue	Thryoid nodule	Medullary carcinoma
PTH	+	−	−
TTF-1	−	+	+/−
Thyroglobulin	−	+	−
Calcitonin	−	−	+
Chromogranin	+	−	+

Abbreviations: PTH, parathyroid hormone; TTF-1, thyroid transcription factor 1.
Source: From Ref. 257.

Chromogranin is a useful surrogate when PTH is negative, which is a rare situation with improvement in antigen retrieval methods.

In addition to the histologic criteria noted above, several immunohistochemical biomarkers have been employed for the delineation of adenoma from carcinoma. However, generally there is some degree of overlap in immunophenotype between adenoma and carcinoma limiting the utility of immunohistochemistry. Table 7 lists biomarkers commonly employed for the distinction between adenoma and carcinoma. Ki-67 labeling indices may have some utility (Fig. 31). A proliferation index of greater than 6% generally correlates with a more aggressive behavior. However, a low Ki-67 index does not exclude parathyroid carcinoma as a diagnosis. Interestingly atypical adenomas tend to cluster with conventional adenomas with regard to Ki 67. The cyclin-dependent kinase inhibitor p27 and the retinoblastoma (Rb) protein are more often decreased in carcinomas than in adenomas. The marker CaSR is reported to be further decreased in carcinomas than adenomas, but considerable overlap exists. We have found that CaSR immunoexpression in atypical adenomas clusters with carcinomas

Table 7 Immunophenotypic Distinction Between Adenoma and Carcinoma

Antigen	Parathyroid adenoma	Parathyroid carcinoma
Potential utility		
Ki-67	+/− as a rule <6%	++ usually >8%
p27	+++	+
Rb	+++	+
CaSR	++/+ (can be negative)	+/−
Parafibromin	+ in nucleus[a]	− in nucleus
No utility		
Cyclin D1		
Bcl-2		
p53		

[a]Hyperparathyroidism-jaw tumor syndrome adenomas are negative as well.
Abbreviations: Rb, retinoblastoma protein; CaSR, calcium-sensing receptor.
Source: From Refs. 102,252,266–270,271.

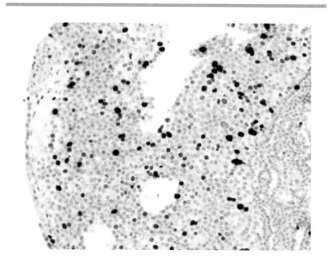

Figure 31 Ki-67 is elevated in this parathyroid carcinoma (200×).

instead of conventional adenomas. Parafibromin, a protein that has a presumed histone deacetylase role, is lost from the nuclei of parathyroid carcinomas. This marker is promising, showing a high degree of sensitivity and specificity, with one caveat: since this is the product of the *HRPT-2* gene, which is mutated in familial HPT-JT, parafibromin will be lost in adenomas found in HPT-JT kindreds (see below for further discussion). Markers generally not deemed useful in the differential diagnosis between parathyroid adenoma and carcinoma are p53 (rarely mutated in parathyroid disease), Bcl-2, and cyclin D1 (expressed in both adenomas and carcinomas) (102,252,266–271).

Understanding of the molecular pathogenesis of single-gland disease is evolving and reveals both similarities and differences between multigland diseases. As noted above, single-gland disease by convention is considered adenoma (or carcinoma if malignancy criteria are met), while multigland disease is generally considered hyperplasia. These clinicopathologic determinants imply that single-gland disease is mono-clonal, thus neoplastic, while multigland disease is polyclonal, thus reactive. However, molecular studies have shown conflicting data with regard to these assumptions, particularly in the case of multigland disease. Studies using various X-linked inactivation-based methodologies have demonstrated that at least 75% of adenomas had a monoclonal pattern of hybrid-ization. However, clonal patterns may be demonstrated in hyperplasias as well, particularly in the nodular form (272–275).

Among the first gene abnormalities detected in adenomas were pericentromeric rearrangements in the *PTH* gene, which placed its regulatory sequences near *CCND1/PRAD1* (chromosome 11q13), which encodes cyclin D1. This and other mechanisms result in cyclin D1 overexpression in 20–40% of adenomas (272,276,277). Another major gene involved in para-thyroid tumorigenesis is the tumor-suppressor gene *MEN1*, also on chromosome 11q13, which encodes menin. In addition to its role in familial hyperpara-thyroidism, loss of heterozygosity at chromosome 11q13 in this region can be seen in 15% to 30% of sporadic adenomas (278–280). Hemmer and col-leagues also noted a loss of 11q23 as a common event in parathyroid adenoma by comparative geno-mic hybridization (CGH) (281). In addition to the losses mentioned above, losses on chromosomes 1, 6q, 13q, and 15q are recurrent in the CGH literature (282,283).

There is emerging gene array data on the com-parative expression profiles of adenoma, hyperplasia, and normal. Haven et al. (92) demonstrated three clusters of parathyroid disease: hyperplasia, sporadic adenomas /MEN1 and MEN2A tumors/tertiary hyperplasia, and parathyroid carcinomas/ adenomas in the setting of HRPT2 mutations. Schachter and colleagues (284) demonstrated differential kinase expression profiles between adenomas and hyperpla-sias using a custom-built complementary DNA (cDNA) array consisting of 359 kinases.

Microsatellite instability is not thought to play a role in parathyroid disease (285). While abnormally expressed, several candidate genes: *CaSR*, *VDR*, *SMAD3* (a candidate tumor-suppressor gene related to the menin pathway), and *RET* are not mutated in sporadic parathyroid adenomas (286–289).

Parathyroid carcinomas appear to have a molec-ular pathogenesis that is distinct from adenoma. Loss of 11q13, which is fairly common in adenomas, is essentially absent in carcinomas (290). Furthermore, recent gene array data based on the pattern of cluster-ing suggest that carcinomas do not arise from adeno-mas, with the exception of adenomas in HP-JTS and rare cystic sporadic adenomas (92,97). Among the most significant advances in the understanding of parathyroid carcinoma is the characterization of *HRPT2* mutations in carcinomas. *HRPT2* is mapped to chromosome 1q21–23 (100,101). It encodes parafi-bromin, which is involved in the RNA polymerase/ Paf-1 complex and thus has a presumed histone deacetylation role. In addition to its role in HP-JTS, *HRPT2* is inactivated in most sporadic carcinomas

(291,292). Parathyroid carcinomas often have abnor-malities of chromosome 13q and loss of heterozygosi-ty at the Rb locus (293). However, roughly 30% of adenomas will show similar losses (281). As noted above, parafibromin and phospho-retinoblastoma protein (pRb) immunohistochemistry can thus be applied in the differential diagnosis between adenoma and carcinoma. On the basis of this available molecular data, an assay based on loss of heterozygosity, which can be readily performed on paraffin-embedded tissue, has been successfully applied to a very small set of tumors to effectively discriminate carcinoma from ade-noma and hyperplasia. An additional useful discrimi-nating variable derived from this study was the fractional allelic loss which was on average 63% in carcinomas, but only 11% in adenomas and 15% in hyperplasias (294). Atypical adenomas, however, do show significant overlap between both conventional adenoma and carcinoma in terms of fractional allelic loss (unpublished results, institutional experience). Hence this loss of heterozygosity panel should be used only as an ancillary rather than a defining test.

C. Multigland and Multifocal Disease

This category consists of hyperplasia: primary (chief cell, water clear, and lipohyperplasia), secondary and tertiary; the controversial "double adenomas"; and parathyromatosis, which is technically multifocal rather than multigland. The gross appearance of glands in hyperplasia cannot be reliably distinguished from adenoma except for the fact that multiple glands are involved. Enlargement may be diffuse with some maintenance of the "bean shape" of a normal para-thyroid gland or nodular, with an appearance similar to an adenoma. Not all glands are affected symmetri-cally or even synchronously. Black and Haff (295) recognized three major patterns of gross disease—classic in which all glands are symmetrically involved, pseudoadenomatous in which there is marked varia-tion in size with minimal enlargement of some glands, and "occult" in which there was only minimal enlargement of glands. Actually, Akerstrom et al. found symmetric four-gland enlargement in only 15% of parathyroid hyperplasia patients, usually in MEN syndromes or water-clear cell hyperplasia (7). In secondary and tertiary hyperplasia, parathyroid glands tend to be symmetrically enlarged initially (12,296) but more varied in size in advanced-stage disease (297). Gland size correlates with duration of renal disease, but not with chemical markers such as serum calcium, phosphate or alkaline phosphatase (296). Debruyne et al. (298) report about a 4:1 ratio between the largest and smallest gland weights in hyperparathyroidism as well as a predilection of size enlargement toward the superior glands. Of note, water-clear hyperplasia often results in massive glands with total gland weights ranging from 10 to 60 g! Cut surfaces of hyperplastic glands are similar to adenomas; however, secondary and tertiary hyper-parathyroidism-associated glands tend to have more fibrosis and degenerative changes (299). Calcification

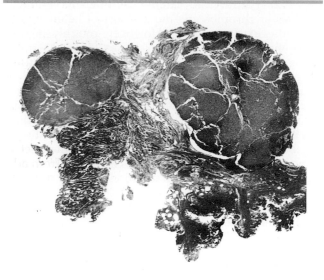

Figure 32 Parathyromatosis in an autograft extending along skeletal muscle of the forearm manifesting as multiple nodules (H&E, whole slide scan). *Abbreviation*: H&E, hematoxylin and eosin.

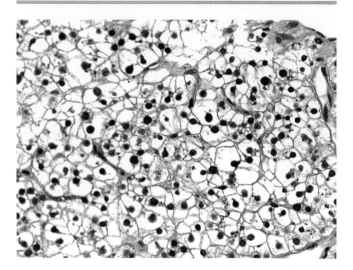

Figure 33 Water-clear hyperplasia (400×). Cells are large with thick cytoplasmic membranes and a microvacuolar appearance.

of the glands is more common in secondary/tertiary disease. Parathyromatosis manifests as numerous nodules of parathyroid tissue throughout the neck or mediastinum. Rarely parathyromatosis manifest in forearm autografts (Fig. 32). When parathyromatosis results from iatrogenic causes, it may have significant fibrosis from previous surgery, making management of disease especially difficult (255). The parathyroid tissue has a gross appearance that is similar to hyperplastic glands, but there may be considerable variation in size. Occasionally, fibrosis or intrathymic location may mask the appearance of smaller parathyroid nests (12). Double adenomas by definition grossly manifest as two enlarged parathyroids, though pathologically it is essentially impossible to distinguish between double adenomas and asymmetric or metachronous hyperplasia in which two glands are involved, which would be ultimately defined by long-term cure after removal of enlarged glands only (300). Double adenomas appear to have a predilection for affecting both superior glands, leading some to suggest that it is a fourth brancial cleft type "field effect" or "parathyroid IV distribution (301)."

Histologically, parathyroids in hyperplasia show hypercellularity. The pattern may be diffuse or nodular. Nodular hyperplasia is more common in advanced secondary or tertiary hyperparathyroidism and correlates clinically with more severe hyperparathyroidism and decreased vitamin D levels (275). Lipohyperplasia is a rare disease in which there are multiple glands that show increased parenchyma and stromal fat with only six reported cases (227,302). A similar histologic appearance is noted in some cases of FHH (see below) (303). The vast majority of hyperplasias are of the chief cell type. Occasionally, particularly in secondary and tertiary hyperparathyroidism,

oxyphil areas may predominate (10). Wasserhelle or water-clear cell hyperplasia (Fig. 33) is a vanishingly rare disease that appears to be decreasing in incidence without any clear explanation. On light microscopy, water-clear cells are distinguished from glycogenated clear cells by several characteristics: (*i*) water-clear cells are larger with thick cell membranes (reminiscent to one of the authors of "chromophobe renal cell carcinoma"), (*ii*) the cytoplasm on higher magnification has a "bubbly" or microvacuolar appearance, and (*iii*) within a nest of cells, nuclei are hyperchromatic and polarized toward the supporting blood vessel, leading to a "bunches of berries" appearance. Ultrastructurally, water-clear cells are defined by their multiple small vacuoles rather than abundant glycogen deposits.

Differential Diagnosis and Molecular Pathology

The differential diagnosis between multigland and single-gland disease rests on the clinical, intraoperative, and/or pathologic findings in all glands. It is important again to reiterate that, *for a given gland, there are no criteria that distinguish between hyperplasia and adenoma.* While hyperplasia tends to be more diffuse with preservation of lobular architecture, single-gland enlargement with a similar configuration occurs. Conversely, nodular hyperplasia may mimic adenoma with some nodules even containing a capsule (Fig. 34). The differential diagnosis between parathyromatosis, secondary/tertiary hyperplasia, and parathyroid carcinoma may often be challenging. In these instances, fibrosis and mitotic activity may be common in secondary/tertiary hyperplasia. The multifocality of parathyromatosis may mimic tissue invasion. Clinical features such as markedly elevated calcium and palpable neck mass are, however, uncommon in hyperplasias and parathyromatosis (255). Very rarely, a true carcinoma may arise in the setting of multigland

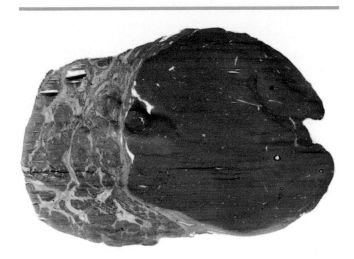

Figure 34 Nodular hyperplasia with an encapsulated nodule mimicking adenoma (H&E frozen section, whole slide scan). This patient had renal failure and multigland disease. The non-nodular tissue is still diffusely hyperplastic without much stromal fat. *Abbreviation*: H&E, hematoxylin and eosin.

disease. While some of these reported cases may simply represent exuberant tertiary hyperparathyroidism, others in which there is vascular, perineural invasion, or nodal metastasis may be *bona fide* examples. Immunohistochemical studies have little value in the distinction between single-gland and multigland disease. Decreases in CaSR, VDR, p21, and p27 are noted, however, to correlate with nodular progression in secondary hyperparathyroidism.

VII. TREATMENT AND PROGNOSIS

A. Primary Hyperparathyroidism

Surgery is the only effective treatment for primary hyperparathyroidism. Successful parathyroid surgery is associated with excellent long-term clinical outcomes, and long-term normocalcemia in 98% to 100%. The nonspecific symptoms of fatigue, weakness, musculoskeletal or abdominal aches and pains, anorexia, constipation, polydipsia, polyuria, nocturia, cognitive dysfunction, and depression associated with primary hyperparathyroidism have been shown to significantly improve in most patients following successful parathyroid surgery (304–306). Nephrolithiasis is significantly decreased after parathyroidectomy (307). Successful parathyroid surgery leads to increased bone mineral density (308) and decreased fracture risk (309). Retrospective studies of patients with untreated mild hyperparathyroidism have documented an increased risk of premature death from cardiovascular causes or cancer (310–312), although a smaller study found an increased mortality risk only in patients with severe hypercalcemia (72).

Since 1925, bilateral parathyroid exploration has been considered the gold standard for treatment of primary hyperparathyroidism, with long-term

postoperative cure rates of at least 95% (313–316). Minimally invasive parathyroid surgery has developed over the past decade to replace bilateral four-gland parathyroid exploration in select patients with a single parathyroid gland detected on preoperative localization studies. Minimally invasive techniques include focused parathyroid exploration, video-assisted parathyroidectomy, and videoscopic parathyroidectomy. All minimally invasive techniques involve removing the abnormal gland(s) identified on preoperative localization studies, using small incision(s). Most minimally invasive techniques employ intraoperative parathyroid hormone testing (IOPTH) to determine the extent of resection and predict ultimate surgical success. An alternative technique uses a Tc99m sestamibi radioguided gamma probe to facilitate identification of abnormal parathyroid glands (317), although many have found that the radioguided probe does not improve outcomes over preoperative Tc99m sestamibi scintigraphy (120,318). Minimally invasive parathyroid exploration in patients with adequate preoperative localization studies and IOPTH monitoring has been shown to have outcomes equal to conventional bilateral exploration (319–324).

Conventional bilateral four-gland exploration is nonetheless an acceptable alternative to minimally invasive exploration and is a requisite for multigland disease. The hyperparathyroidism associated with MEN-1 syndrome is particularly aggressive. Recurrence on long-term follow-up is as high as 61% (91) and is deemed inevitable if follow-up is extended indefinitely. While direct comparision via randomized prospective study has not been made, it appears that the extent of parathyroid exploration correlates with a lower rate of recurrence. Thus, many advocate an aggressive approach, including exploration of common sites of ectopic parathyroid tissue (i.e., paraesophageal, mediastinal, carotid sheath), in MEN-1 patients, although the extent of surgery also imparts an increased risk of hypocalcemia (93). Current recommendations in MEN-1 are a subtotal parathyroidectomy leaving a 20- to –30-mg remnant of the most normal-appearing parathyroid, though total parathyroidectomy with heterotopic autotransplantation of 15 to 20 mg of parathyroid tissue is an alternative treatment (93).

Ectopic parathyroid glands are most commonly accessible through standard cervical incision. Approximately, 2% of ectopic parathyroid glands are found in the deep mediastinum and can be effectively and safely resected with video-assisted thoracoscopic mediastinal parathyroid exploration, guided by IOPTH to assess the completeness of resection, and avoiding the morbidity of median sternotomy (325).

Parathyroid carcinoma has a 10-year cancer-related mortality of 12.4%. The majority of patients (78.6%) are treated with parathyroidectomy alone, and more extensive en bloc resection is not associated with increased survival. Factors associated with improved survival include absence of distant metastases, young age, and female gender (326). Early surgical resection is the only available curative treatment for parathyroid carcinoma. Histologic and cytometric parameters have been assessed for prognosis as well. While aneuploidy, mitoses, atypia, and necrosis were important prognosticators in one series of 95 cases, by multivariate analysis, only mitotic count was statistically significant. However, clinical variables were not evaluated (209). Additionally, several ''equivocal cases'' were included, which obscures the significance of this finding.

B. Secondary And Tertiary Hyperparathyroidism

Medical Management

Standard medical treatment of secondary hyperparathyroidism includes vitamin D analogues, calcium supplements, and phosphate-binding agents. In 2003, the National Kidney Foundation published guidelines with revised targets for calcium, phosphorus, Ca $\times$ P (calcium-phosphorus product), and PTH levels in patients with end-stage renal disease on hemodialysis (327). However, standard medical therapy has been inadequate in conforming to these guideline recommendations. Recent studies found that only 8% to 11% of patients on hemodialysis in the United States had laboratory values within the aforementioned guideline ranges (328,329). A relatively new class of pharmaceutical agents, the calcimimetics, increases parathyroid gland calcium receptor sensitivity and reduces PTH, calcium, and phosphorus levels in patients with secondary hyperparathyroidism (330). However, to date, there have been no long-term studies demonstrating reduced rates of cardiovascular mortality, renal osteodystrophy, or pathologic fracture with calcimimetic treatment (331).

Surgical Management

Indications for surgical management of secondary hyperparathyroidism are somewhat controversial, but most agree that parathyroid exploration is indicated for symptomatic disease refractory to medical treatment, high turnover renal osteodystrophy, or osteitis fibrosa cystica. Analysis of over 4500 adult patients undergoing parathyroidectomy for secondary hyperparathyroidism, matched to similar controls treated with medical management, demonstrated a 13% decreased long-term mortality in patients treated surgically. This study also observed a 3.1% 30-day postoperative mortality rate, similar to published perioperative surgical mortality rates among dialysis patients. Mortality was highest in patients with diabetes, patients on hemodialysis for less than one year, and African-American patients (332). Both subtotal parathyroidectomy with cryopreservation and total parathyroidectomy with autotransplantation are accepted surgical treatments for secondary hyperparathyroidism, with similar rates of recurrent hyperparathyroidism, usually less than 10% (333,334).

Indications for surgery in tertiary hyperparathyroidism are the same as those in primary and secondary hyperparathyroidism. The standard operative approach to tertiary hyperparathyroidism is bilateral parathyroid exploration and subtotal parathyroidectomy versus total parathyroidectomy with autotransplantation. Less than subtotal parathyroidectomy has been described as successful in a limited group of patients, (335,336) but was associated with a fivefold increased risk of recurrent or persistent hyperparathyroidism over long-term follow-up in another large retrospective study (337).

VIII.   MISCELLANEOUS CONDITIONS

A. Parathyroid Cysts

Clinical Features

Parathyroid cysts are uncommon lesions that may be present in the neck or mediastinum. They generally stratify into two groups: nonfunctioning and functioning, both of which are most common in the fourth and fifth decades. The functional cysts comprise 15% to 57% of all parathyroid cysts, and some may in fact be adenomas with extensive cystic change (205,338,339). In a relatively large series of 14 cases, functioning parathyroid cysts were more common in males and older patients (340); however, other series show no such differences (336). The clinical presentation is that neck mass is often mistaken for a thyroid nodule (205,338).

Pathologic Features

Cysts on average measure 4 cm, but may be as large as 10 cm. Grossly, cyst walls are thin, typically a pale tan white and semitranslucent (Fig. 35) (12,338). There are generally no nodularities or excrescences, though the associated parathyroid gland may be occasionally embedded or attached to the cyst wall. Parathyroid

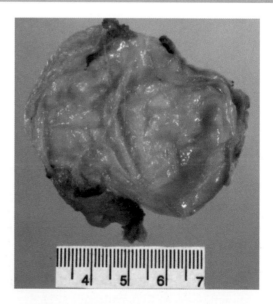

Figure 35 Gross appearance of an opened parathyroid cyst with a thin smooth tan wall.

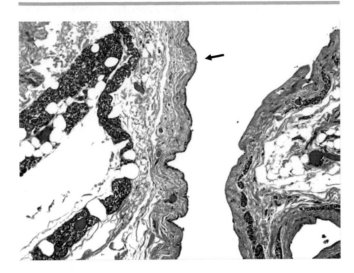

Figure 36 Parathyroid cyst walls (H&E, 100×) comprising an attenuated single layer of cuboidal cells (*arrow*). The walls may often contain normal parathyroid tissue. *Abbreviation*: H&E, hematoxylin and eosin.

cyst aspirates are characterstically clear, watery, and nearly acellular (12). Occasionally, when a prior aspiration was performed, the cyst fluid would be bloody. Opaque or purulent fluid is exceptionally rare. It is critical to send this fluid for PTH evaluation to confirm the diagnosis since the lining of cyst walls may be completely denuded (129,130). Histologically, the cyst wall is composed mainly of paucicellular fibroconnective tissue. Parathyroid nests may be present within the cyst wall. The lining when intact is typically a single layer of flattened cuboidal epithelium with vacuolated clear cells (Fig. 36).

Differential Diagnosis

The most common differential diagnostic consideration is a colloid cyst of the thyroid glands. Colloid may be translucent, but it is typically stickier than parathyroid cyst fluid. Histologically, instead of parathyroid tissue in the cyst wall, there is thyroid tissue. Other diagnostic considerations grossly include cervical thymic cysts and branchial cleft cysts. However, both of these cysts tend to occur in children and young adults. Histologically, thymic cysts may have parathyroid tissue in their cyst wall, but they will also have thymic tissue with Hassal's corpuscles, and the lining will be squamous (341). Similarly, branchial cleft cysts are lined by squamous epithelium. Second pouch–derived cysts are associated with lymphoid tissue, and third and fourth pouch derivatives are more commonly sinuses rather than cysts and are typically complicated by suppurative inflammation (342). These are detailed further in chapter 18. Recently, Carney has described a set "salivary heterotopia-cyst complexes" with cyst walls lined by cuboidal lining very similar to that of a parathyroid cyst. However, these are surrounded by

salivary tissue, and by immunohistochemistry, the cyst wall linings are negative for PTH (18).

Molecular Biology

The pathogenesis is not well understood. Possible explanations include a branchial cleft anomaly or dilation of persistent Kursteiner canals (12). Other explanations include cystic change in an adenoma. Patients with HP-JTS and rare cystic sporadic adenomas show evidence of *HRPT2* mutations (92,97). It must be noted, that most tumors designated as "cystic adenomas" have cysts that are usually smaller (<1.0 cm) (97) than those designated as "parathyroid cysts," hence contributory role of these mutations in the latter category is unclear.

Treatment and Prognosis

Treatment options range from therapeutic fluid aspiration to injection with sclerosing agents to surgical excision. Functional cysts should be treated surgically, similar to adenomas. Fluid aspiration may not be curative, as even nonfunctioning cysts may recur. Injection with sclerosing agents may induce fibrosis and impinge on the recurrent laryngeal nerve (343).

B. FHH

Clinical Features

FHH is an autosomal dominant disorder that mimics primary hyperparathyroidism (344–346). About one-third of patients with this disorder are asymptomatic, while the remainder may have vague mild symptoms such as arthralgias, headaches, polyuria, and polydypsia (344). Only rare cases of chondrocalcinosis, cholelithiasis, and pancreatitis have been reported, and the association with the latter is debatable (347,348). Affected patients have a mild hypercalcemia, hypermagnesemia, and hypophosphatemia. PTH levels are normal- to mildly elevated (349). The classic laboratory finding is that of hypocalciuria, with low 24-hour urine calcium excretion. The calcium-creatinine clearance (Ca/Cr) ratio is low as well.

Pathologic Features

Parathyroid glands in FHH are slightly enlarged or within the upper limits of normal weight. Law et al. (350) reported a mean weight of 60 mg for each gland. Regarding parenchymal area/hypercellularity, early literature shows conflicting results. While Law et al. (350) reported normocellularity and a normal-to-decreased parenchymal area as compared with matched controls, Thorgeirsson et al. (351) reported an increase in parenchymal area. Other investigators have reported chief cell hyperplasia as well (352). More recently, a subset of FHH patients were described as having histologic features identical to parathyroid lipohyperplasia in which both parenchyma and fatty stroma are increased (303,353).

Differential Diagnosis

The main clinical differential diagnostic consideration is primary hyperparathyroidism with multigland disease or hyperplasia. Urine calcium levels are of critical importance in making this distinction. The Ca/Cr ratio of less than 0.01 is 80% sensitive and 88% specific for FHH, while a value of more than 0.02 essentially excludes the possibility of FHH (354). Lithium-associated hyperparathyroidism may rarely present in a similar fashion with hypocalciuria as well. A history of chronic lithium is a distinguishing feature. As noted above, the histologic spectrum ranges from normal to hyperplasia to lipohyperplasia; the underlying etiology, if not primary, must be separated on the basis of clinical and laboratory findings. For instance, primary hyperplasia/lipohyperplasia will have elevated urinary calcium and an increased Ca/Cr ratio.

Molecular Biology

Pollak et al. (355) first demonstrated the presence of inactivating mutations in the *CaSR* gene in FHH. As of 2004, 64 different inactivating mutations had been described, 17 of which are recurring in the literature (356). Mutations are typically missense mutations and cluster at exons 3, 4, and 7. Structurally, these mutations tend to affect the extracellular and transmembrane domains (356).

Treatment and Prognosis

Patients with FHH do not require parathyroid surgery, and since symptoms are absent to mild, only surveillance is necessary (354). In fact, patients who have undergone surgery will still have persistently elevated calcium. Historically, misdiagnosed FHH has represented up to 9% of "failed" parathyroid surgeries (345), though this number is lower in a more recent review (357), presumably because of the more routine inclusion of urine calcium levels in the work-up of hypercalcemia.

C. Neonatal Hyperparathyroidism

Clinical Features

Neonatal hyperparathyroidism is a severe disease described prior to FHH (358). It has also been noted to be related to FHH (359). More recently, it has been shown that both copies of the *CaSR* gene show mutations in neonatal hyperparathyroidism (360). Neonatal hyperparathyroidism typically presents during the first weeks of life with hypotonia, failure to thrive, skeletal defects, including pathologic fractures (361). Hypercalcemia is typically severe as is the elevation in PTH levels (354,360,362). Milder forms have been described (361).

Pathologic Features

The histologic features are essentially identical to diffuse chief cell hyperplasia (12,361).

Differential Diagnosis

The differential diagnosis is limited. Occasionally, a "secondary" neonatal hyperparathyroidism may arise when a mother with hypoparathyroidism or pseudohypoparathyroidism is inadequately treated (361). Hence, serum and urine metabolite levels should be measured in the mother as well. An additional radiologic diagnostic consideration is Murk Jansen's chondrodysplasia, which is an autosomal dominant short-limbed dwarfism caused by alterations in the *PTH/PTHrP* receptor gene (361,363). The classic laboratory findings here are elevated PTH and decreased 1-25 dihydroxy-vitamin D3. Pathologic features of the parathyroid glands in these patients have not been described.

Molecular Biology

The molecular biology of neonatal hyperparathyroidism is similar to FHH in that the key alterations are in *CaSR*. Classic neonatal hyperparathyroidism is seen in FHH kindreds where the affected infant inherits mutations from both parents. The child may be truly homozygous for a mutation or doubly heterozygous for two different mutations (364,365). Rare cases of singly heterozygous mutations have been described in neonatal hyperparathyroidism. These are more often sporadic and often have a milder phenotype. The postulated mechanism in these mutations is a dominant negative one—the altered receptor heterodimerizes with the normal receptor impairing its function (361,365).

Treatment and Prognosis

Left untreated, this is a rapidly fatal disease, hence early recognition and aggressive management is important (354,360,362). Early management is also critical to prevent irreversible growth and mental retardation (366). While some milder cases may be treated supportively with fluid and electrolyte management, subtotal parathyroidectomy may be necessary (354). Surgical treatment has a positive impact on remineralization and healing of bone lesions (361).

D. Lithium-Associated Hypercalcemia/ Hyperparathyroidism

Clinical Features

Chronic lithium therapy for bipolar disorder has been linked to hyperparathyroidism. Estimates of the prevalence of hyperparathyroidism in patients on chronic lithium therapy range from less than 3% to 35% (367–369). The incidence of hypercalcemia with lithium therapy increases if treatment has been for more than 15 years (370). The majority of patients with lithium-associated hyperparathyroidism reported that they have presented with signs and symptoms of hypercalcemia (367,371).

Pathologic Features

Counterintuitively, a large proportion of lithium-associated hyperparathyroidism cases have been reported to be adenomas, which comprised the majority of cases in one series (367). However, follow-up was not presented in this series, and their criteria for adenoma versus hyperplasia were purely histologic, which is inappropriate. Nonetheless, even using intraoperative PTH criteria to determine completeness of excision, a more recent study demonstrated single-gland enlargement in 50% (6/12) cases, though on follow-up, only two of these cases showed unequivocal cure (371). Hence, with adequate follow-up, the incidence of hyperplasia in lithium-induced hyperparathyroidism may be much higher with "adenomas" representing metachronously evolving hyperplasia.

Differential diagnosis

The differential diagnosis is mainly clinical and includes primary hyperparathyroidism without lithium exposure and FHH. The distinction between lithium-associated hyperparathyroidism and sporadic primary hyperparathyroidism is primarily based on the history of long-term lithium exposure. Additionally, lithium-induced hyperparathyroidism may present with hypocalciuria in contrast to sporadic primary hyperparathyroidism. As mentioned previously, FHH is distinguished by the absence of lithium treatment and a known family history. There are no distinctive histologic features for lithium-associated hyperparathyroidism.

Molecular Biology

The pathogenesis in lithium-induced hyperparathyroidism is largely speculative. In vitro, lithium has been shown to induce PTH secretion short term (372). However, the incidence of parathyroid disease clinically correlates with long-term exposure. Additionally, most cases of lithium-induced hyperparathyroidism do not resolve after cessation of lithium treatment, suggesting additional mechanisms to perpetuate parathyroid disease. One theory is that lithium serves as a mitogen for adenoma formation (367). However, as mentioned above, it is not entirely clear using modern clinicopathologic criteria as to what percentage of cases actually represent adenomas. There is indirect evidence that lithium may competitively bind to CaSR. Clinically, the presentation is often similar to FHH, particularly with regard to hypocalciuria. Additionally, there have been a few reported cases in which Cinalcet, an allosteric activator of CaSR successfully treated lithium-associated hyperparathyroidism (370,373).

Treatment and Prognosis

As noted above, cessation of lithium therapy does not often cause resolution of hyperparathyroidism, and thus, parathyroidectomy is often necessary (370,373). Hundley et al. (371) note limitations in intraoperative PTH in predicting surgical success and recommend a bilateral neck exploration in the setting of lithium-associated hyperparathyroidism.

Table 8 Non-PTH Causes of Hypercalcemia

Malignancy associated
Lytic bony metastases
HHM
Vitamin D mediated
Vitamin D intoxication
Increased 1,25-dihydroxy-vitamin D3 synthesis
Vitamin A intoxication
Other endocrinopathies
Hyperthyroidism
Hypoadrenalism
Milk-alkali syndrome
Immobilization with bone turnover
Sarcoidosis
Multiple myeloma

Abbreviations: PTH, parathyroid hormone; HHM, humoral hypercalcemia of malignancy.
Source: From Ref. 372.

E. Parathyroid Glands in Non-PTH-Related Hypercalcemia.

Clinical Features

Non-PTH-related hypercalcemia is far less common, and of these, the most common cause is nonparathyroid malignancy. Discussion of each specific etiology associated with non-PTH hypercalcemia is beyond the scope of this chapter. A summary of relatively common non-PTH causes of hypercalcemia is presented in Table 8. Malignancy-associated hypercalcemia may be a result of lytic metastases that induce increased bone turnover, notably in hematopoietic malignancies or breast carcinoma (12), or as a result of secretion of PTHrP, so-called humoral hypercalcemia of malignancy (HHM) (374). Squamous cell carcinomas of the upper aerodigestive tract and renal cell carcinomas are the most common tumors to be associated with HHM, though a variety of other tumor types have been described as well (12). The combination of increased urinary cyclic AMP and normal-to-low PTH in the setting of malignancy and hypercalcemia suggest HHM (12,374).

Pathologic Features

The parathyroid glands in non-PTH hypercalcemia are histologically normal with intracytoplasmic lipid demonstrable by fat stains, suggesting normal function as well. Occasional vacuolar change with displaced nuclei has been noted, but this can be seen in other disease states as well (375).

Differential Diagnosis

The differential diagnosis of hypercalcemia can be found in several texts and reviews and will not be discussed in detail here. Classically, non-PTH-related causes of hypercalcemia are defined by their normal or low PTH levels. Immunochemical assays for PTHrP are available as well (374).

Treatment and Prognosis

For the majority of the non-PTH-related hypercalcemia etiologies, treatment of the underlying disease is the only definitive treatment. Medical management of fluids and electrolytes can serve as a short-term solution (374).

Molecular Biology

Each etiologic factor for non-PTH-related hypercalcemia will not be discussed here. The following is a brief mention of the characteristics of PTHrP, the hormone involved in HHM. The *PTHrP* gene is located on chromosome 12 and encodes a 144–amino acid protein that shares significant homology with PTH in the first 13 amino acids. PTHrP also binds to the PTH receptor (also known as the PTH/PTHrP receptor) and has effects that are identical to PTH. Physiologically, it may be involved in chondrogenesis and enchondral ossification (374).

F. Noniatrogenic Hypoparathyroidism and Pseudohypoparathyroidism

Clinical Features

Generically, hypoparathyroidism is characterized by hypocalcemia, hyperphosphatemia, and a decreased PTH. Clinical features range from subtle to overt. In subclinical disease, Chvostek's sign, facial muscle contractions, may be elicited by tapping the facial nerve, and Trousseau's sign, carpal flexure contractions, may be induced by a blood pressure cuff. In overt disease, paresthesias, tetany, central nervous system defects, and cardiac arrythmias (prolonged QT interval and T-wave changes) may ensue. The most common cause of hypoparathyroidism, both transient and long term, is surgical exploration of the neck. The following discussion will focus on noniatrogenic causes of hyperparathyroidism. These can be divided into developmental, autoimmune, PTH molecule defects, and PTH secretion defects. Also included with these entities are the syndromes of PTH resistance or pseudohyperparathyroidism. In these, PTH may actually be elevated, but the patients will be hypocalcemic (376).

The main developmental abnormality associated with hypoparathyroidism is DiGeorge syndrome, which is classified along with velocardiofacial syndrome and conotruncal anomaly syndrome as a chromosome 22q11 microdeletion syndrome, and results in agenesis or dysgenesis of some or all of the components of the third and fourth branchial pouches (376). Clinically, infants may present with severe hypoparathyroidism as well as cell-mediated immune defects and cardiac and craniofacial defects (377). Another more rare genetic developmental abnormality is X-linked idiopathic hypoparathyroidism, which is characterized by an isolated PTH deficiency, which presents before six months of age as severe hypocalcemia (378). An autosomal recessive form of idiopathic hypoparathyroidism has been described in which glial cells missing-B *(GCMB)*, a regulator of parathyroid development, is altered (62,379). Two syndromes exist in which the mechanisms for hypoparathyroidism are unclear, though the genes are known: (*i*) the autosomal dominant syndrome, hypoparathyroidism-deafness-renal dysplasia syndrome (380) and (*ii*) the autosomal recessive syndrome in the Middle Eastern population, Kenny–Caffey syndrome characterized by hypoparathyroidism, growth failure, osteosclerosis, and facial dysmorphism (381).

Autoimmune hypoparathyroidism typically affects children and young adults and is typically seen as a part of the autoimmune polyendocrinopathy-candidiasis-ectodermal dystrophy (APECED) syndrome (also known as autoimmune polyglandular syndrome-1). The classic clinical presentation begins typically with mucocutaneous candidiases, usually by age 5 years followed by hypoparathyroidism, prior to age 10 years, and Addison's disease by age 15 years (382). This disease is often accompanied by other autoimmune endocrinopathies as well. Antibodies to CaSR have been noted in some patients with APECED as well as some patients with isolated hypoparathyroidism (383,384).

Nonimmune, nonagenic causes of hypoparathyroidism include both PTH gene and PTH secretion defects (as a result of CaSR) and have a heterogeneous clinical presentation, and depending on mutation type may present with autosomal dominant or autosomal recessive pattern (356,385).

The main pseudohypoparathyroidism syndromes are characterized by defects in the G protein, which lead to a blunted response or resistance of tissues to PTH. Pseudohypoparathyroidism type 1a is characterized by the syndrome Albright's hereditary osteodystrophy. These patients are short, stocky with round facies, mental retardation, cataracts, and soft tissue calcinosis. These patients are often resistant to thyroid stimulating hormone (TSH) and gonadotropins as well. In pseudohypoparathyroidism type 1b, patients have PTH resistance but not hereditary osteodystrophy (386).

Pathologic Features

DiGeorge syndrome, X-linked idiopathic hypoparathyroidism, and Kenny–Caffey syndrome are characterized by the partial or complete absence of parathyroid tissue (10,378,381). In autoimmune hypoparathyroidism, parathyroids may not be identifiable on postmortem examination or may have total fatty replacement (387). Other cases show chronic parathyroiditis with fibrosis, gland atrophy, and a lymphoplasmacytic infiltrate (10). *It must be noted that histologic evidence of parathyroiditis or lymphoid infiltrates in parathyroid parenchyma does not equate with hypoparathyroidism.* Parathyroids in pseudohypoparathyroidism range from normal to hyperplastic (10,388).

Differential Diagnosis

The differential diagnosis between the various causes of hypoparathyroidism requires an accurate characterization of family history/inheritance pattern, clinical findings, particularly the presence of extraparathyroid manifestations, and ultimately the molecular characterization. Histologic examination does not have a role in discrimination between these causes.

Table 9 Gene Alterations in Hypoparathyroidism and Pseudohypoparathyroidism Syndromes

Syndrome	Inheritance	Chromosome	Gene(s)
Presumed developmental			
DiGeorge		22q11.2	?*TBX1, CRKL1*
Idiopathic hypoparathyroidism	X-linked	Xq26–27	?*SOX3*
Familial isolated hypoparathyroidism	Autosomal recessive	6p23–24	*GCMB*
Hypoparathyroidism-deafness-renal dysplasia	Autosomal dominant	10p15	*GATA3*
Kenny–Caffey	Autosomal recessive	1q42.3	*TBCE*
Autoimmune			
Autoimmune polyendocrinopathy-candidiasis-ectodermal dystrophy	Autosomal recessive	21q22.3	*AIRE*
PTH function/secretion			
Familial isolated hypoparathyroidism	Autosomal recessive	11p15.3–15.1	(pre-pro)-*PTH*
Familial isolated hypoparathyroidism	Autosomal dominant	3q13.3–21	*CaSR*
Pseudohypoparathyroidism			
Type 1A	Autosomal dominant (maternal allele)	20q13.2	*GNAS*
Pseudo-pseudo hypoparathyroidism	Autosomal dominant (paternal allele)	20q13.2	*GNAS*
Type 1B	Imprinting pattern (maternally inherited)	20q13.2	*GNAS*

Source: From Refs. 354,375,376,379,380,383,387,388.

Molecular Biology

Gene alterations and syndromic associations are summarized in Table 9. The 22q11 deletion is the most common microdeletion syndrome in humans. The most common form (90%) is a 3-Mb deletion of chromosome 22q11.2 spanning over 30 genes. Genes such as *TBX-1* and *CRKL-1* are thought to be key factors involved in the pathogenesis of Digeorge syndrome (377). In X-linked idiopathic hypoparathyroidism, Thakker et al. (378,389) mapped the responsible gene to Xq26–27 using linkage analysis. More recently, the same group implicated *SOX-3* as the developmental modulator that is perturbed in this syndrome. The *GCMB* mutations in some autosomal recessive isolated hypoparathyroidism cases reflect an alteration of DNA binding (379). The autosomal dominant hypoparathyroidism-deafness-renal dysplasia syndrome is found in the setting of *GATA3* (encoding a double-zinc finger transcription factor) mutations (381). No cases of isolated hypoparathyroidism have been reported with this mutation, suggesting that the effect of *GATA3* is more global and not parathyroid specific (390). The *TCBE* mutations in Kenny–Chaffey syndrome affect tubulin assembly, but the mechanism for its effect in parathyroid is unclear (381).

The autoimmune regulator (*AIRE*) gene in the autoimmune polyendocrinopathy, APECED is normally expressed in the hematolymphoid/reticuloendothelial system and presumed to be associated with immune tolerance based on distribution and structure (382). Alterations in the *PTH* gene are typically autosomal recessive (384), while *CaSR* mutations are autosomal dominant. The localization of *CaSR* mutations in hypoparathyroidism is similar to FHH, namely, exons 3, 4, and 7 but are instead activating rather than inactivating mutations (356).

The molecular biology of pseudohypoparathyroidism is complex and in part explained by genomic imprinting. Inactivating mutations of the G-protein alpha subunit (*GNAS*) gene lead to Albright's hereditary osteodystrophy, pseudohypoparathyroidism type 1A, and multihormone resistance if the maternal allele is the one that carries the mutation. If the paternal allele carries the mutation, only the hereditary osteodystrophy component is evident (in so-called pseudohypoparathyroidism). In some paternally inherited cases, progressive osseous heteroplasia defined by ectopic ossification will be evident. This is explained by the fact that the GNAS is primarily expressed from the maternal allele in endocrine target tissues (renal proximal tubules, thyroid glands, and ovaries), while other tissues have an equal contribution of both alleles (386). The skeletal abnormalities may be linked to misexpression of osteoblast-specific transcription factor *Cbfa1/RUNX2* (391). In pseudohypoparathyroidism type 1B, as a result of a methylation defect (exon 1A DMR), the maternal imprinting pattern is lost, hence only the paternal pattern is present in both alleles. This results in a phenotype of endocrine resistance only since paternal pattern is actually normal in other tissues (386).

Treatment and Prognosis

Treatment and prognosis involve supplementation with calcium, vitamin D, and thiazide diuretics. All cases of decreased or absent PTH will have decreased 1,25 dihydroxy vitamin D and decreased hypocalciuric response, which is the rationale for the later two therapeutic agents. In theory, parathyroid transplant is appealing, but the immunosuppression required for an allograft (autografts are essentially impossible in this set of hypoparathyroid patients) is currently prohibitive. However, allotransplantation of cultured nonimmunogenic parathyroid cells has been performed successfully and holds promise (392). The use of recombinant PTH (1-34) or teriparatide also shows promise as an alternative to calcium/vitamin D/thiazide supplementation (393).

G. Secondary Tumor Involvement of Parathyroid Glands

Clinical Features

Parathyroid glands may be involved secondarily by tumors via local extension or by distant metastasis (394). These patients occasionally present with

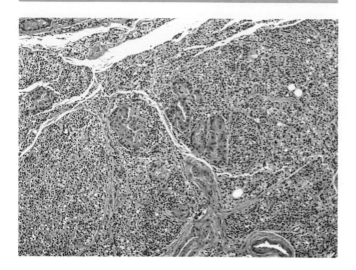

Figure 37 Metastatic papillary thyroid carcinoma to a parathyroid gland (H&E, 200×). Note the abrupt transition in morphology from the bland parathyroid chief cells to the atypical nests of metastatic carcinoma in the center. *Abbreviation*: H&E, hematoxylin and eosin.

hypoparathyroidism (395), though this requires a loss of greater than 70% of total parathyroid parenchyma (394).

Pathologic Features

Papillary thyroid carcinoma is one of the most frequent cancers to involve the parathyroid glands (Fig. 37). Parathyroid involvement may be present as a result of direct extension or angiolymphatic spread in as many as 7.9% of cases in which the parathyroid glands are histologically examined (396,397). In one complete autopsy series of 187 cases, widely disseminated breast carcinoma involved the parathyroid glands in 6% of cases (398). Similarly, the same study noted parathyroid gland involvement by disseminated melanoma in 8.9% of cases. In one historical series of 160 patients dying of metastatic disease, 11.9% had parathyroid gland involvement, with breast being the most common site. Leukemia, melanoma, lung, and soft tissue were the other primary sites (394).

Differential Diagnosis

A metastasis may, in theory, invoke parathyroid carcinoma as a diagnostic consideration. However, metastatic tumors are usually pleomorphic with high cytologic grade and will have a "lymphangitic" pattern with haphazard nests of tumor scattered throughout bland parathyroid parenchyma showing an abrupt transition in morphology (394). Parathyroid carcinomas usually have low-grade nuclear features, and the morphologic transition between more bland appearing areas is more gradual. Immunohistochemical stains for PTH in conjunction with markers frequently found in the metastasis (i.e., thyroglobulin, TTF-1 in papillary thyroid carcinoma, S-100, HMB-45 in melanoma) in question may be helpful, though there is little experience noted in the literature.

Treatment and Prognosis

Secondary involvement of parathyroid glands by carcinoma is typically indicative of advanced disease, although in the case of papillary thyroid carcinoma, small primaries have been described with parathyroid gland involvement (397). Parathyroid gland involvement by papillary thyroid carcinoma has been correlated with distant metastases and shorter disease-free survival (396), at least by univariate analysis.

H. Secondary Systemic Disease Involvement of Parathyroid Glands

Clinical Features

Parathyroid glands may be secondarily involved by storage diseases, though patients only rarely have parathyroid-related clinical findings such as hypoparathyroidism (10,399).

Pathologic Features

Cases of Pompe's disease involving endocrine organs, including the parathyroid glands, have been described (400). Rare cases of hemochromatosis or secondary iron storage disease have been reported to involve parathyroid glands, with stainable iron present in the parenchyma (399,401).

IX. PARATHYROID CRYOPRESERVATION AND AUTOTRANSPLANTATION

Autotransplantation of parathyroid glands was first performed in humans in 1926 by Lahey (402), and cryopreservation of parathyroid tissue for subsequent implantation was described as early as 1974 by Wells and colleagues (403,404). Both immediate heterotopic autotransplantation of parathyroid tissue into the forearm and delayed autotransplantation are considered viable options for prevention/treatment of hypoparathyroidism. Generically, crypopreservation of parathyroid tissue for autotransplantation is advocated for patients undergoing near total parathyroidectomy for multigland disease and for patients undergoing surgery for recurrent hyperparathyroidism, where the risk of hypoparathyroidism may be as high as 30% (405–407).

The success of reimplanted parathyroid tissue in full restoration of parathyroid function is 37%, and for full or partial restoration, 53%. In 5%, there will be hyperfunction (405–409). In contrast, the success of immediate heterotopic implantation of parathyroid tissue is 80% to 95%. The reasons for this disparity are not entirely clear. Wagner et al. (410) suggested that the main determinant was the degree of necrosis in the reimplanted tissue rather than the functionality of the viable cells. Cohen et al. (407) indicate in their series that the average cryopreservation time for functional autografts is significantly less than nonfunctional autografts, suggesting decreased functionality over time even in cryopreserved tissue. However, Ulrich et al. (411), using an elegant in vitro cell culture–testing model, found that viability did not decrease as the duration of cryopreservation increased. Hence, other mechanisms may be involved in this observed time dependency.

The pathologist's role in the process of cryopreservation varies greatly depending on institution. If the pathology department participates in the collection, transport, and processing of the specimen, it is critical for the surgical team to clearly designate when a specimen is to be sent for cryopreservation both verbally and on the requisition form. Additionally, it is important for the pathologist responsible for the case to be familiar with their institutional policies for cryopreservation to help prevent any procedural breakdowns that may result in parathyroid designated for cryopreservation being mistakenly processed for routine pathologic examination.

While there are minor variations, the general procedure for cryopreservation of parathyroid tissue is as follows (406,407):

1. The parathyroid tissue will be morcellated into fragments 1 to 3 mm in greatest dimension and placed into a sterile saline container and immediately placed on ice. At the same time, a clot tube for preparation of autologous serum is also placed on ice. At this point, if the surgical pathology laboratory mistakenly receives this specimen on ice, the specimen container should not be opened. Transport to the appropriate laboratory (typically a tissue typing/immunology laboratory) should be arranged as soon as possible.

2. On transport to the laboratory responsible for processing and storing, the parathyroid slices will be placed into vials containing freezing solution, typically a mixure of chilled 10% dimethyl sulfoxide (DMSO), 10% to 30% chilled autologous serum (made from the collected clot tube), and 60% to 80% tissue culture media RPMI-1640 that is filtered through a 0.2-μm syringe filter. Prior to freezing, many laboratories use the prepared freezing solution as a "wash"—the tissue and mixture are agitated for 10 minutes, and the freezing solution is replaced by a portion of the unused solution. This process may be repeated two to three times before the specimen is finally frozen in the freezing solution from the last "wash" cycle.

3. The tissue is finally frozen at –70°C to –80°C overnight and subsequently stored long term in liquid nitrogen at –170°C to –200°C.

4. For reimplantation, the parathyroid tissue is rapidly thawed in a 37°C water bath and rinsed with a solution of 70% to 90% RPMI-1640 and 10% to 30% autologous or pooled human sera.

REFERENCES

1. Owen R. On the anatomy of the Indian rhinoceros (Rh unicornis, L.). Trans Zool Soc Lond 1862; 4:31–38.
2. Sandström I. Om en ny körtel hos menniskan och àtskilliga däggdjur. Ups Läk Forh 1880; 15:441–471.
3. Albright F. A page out of the history of hyperparathyroidism. J Clin Endocrinol 1948; 8:649–658.
4. Carney JA. The glandulae parathyroideae of Ivar Sandstrom. Contributions from two continents. Am J Surg Pathol 1996; 20(9):1123–1144.
5. Irvin GL, 3rd. The William H. Harrige memorial lecture. Parathormone and the disease. Am J Surg 2007; 193(3): 301–304.
6. Norris EH. The parathyroid glands and the lateral thyroid in man: their morphogenesis, histogenesis, topographic anatomy and prenatal growth. Contrib Embryol 1937; 159:249.
7. Akerstrom G, Bergstrom R, Grimelius L, et al. Relation between changes in clinical and histopathological features of primary hyperparathyroidism. World J Surg 1986; 10(4): 696–702.
8. Wang C. The anatomic basis of parathyroid surgery. Ann Surg 1976; 183(3):271–275.
9. Akerstrom G, Malmaeus J, Bergstrom R. Surgical anatomy of human parathyroid glands. Surgery 1984; 95(1):14–21.
10. Apel RL, Asa SL. The parathyroid glands. In: Barnes EL, ed. Surgical Pathology of the Head and Neck. 2nd ed. New York, NY: Marcel Dekker Inc; 2001:1719–1792.
11. Dufour DR, Wilkerson SY. Factors related to parathyroid weight in normal persons. Arch Pathol Lab Med 1983; 107 (4):167–172.
12. DeLellis RA. Tumors of the Parathyroid Glands. 3rd ed. Bethesda: Armed Forces Institute of Pathology, 1993.
13. Nobori M, Saiki S, Tanaka N, et al. Blood supply of the parathyroid gland from the superior thyroid artery. Surgery 1994; 115(4):417–423.
14. Johansson K, Ander S, Lennquist S, et al. Human parathyroid blood supply determined by laser-Doppler flowmetry. World J Surg 1994; 18(3):417–420 (discussion 420–411).
15. Dunlop DA, Papapoulos SE, Lodge RW, et al. Parathyroid venous sampling: anatomic considerations and results in 95 patients with primary hyperparathyroidism. Br J Radiol 1980; 53(627):183–191.
16. Saffos RO, Rhatigan RM, Urgulu S. The normal parathyroid and the borderline with early hyperplasia: a light microscopic study. Histopathology 1984; 8(3):407–422.
17. Gilmour JR. The embryology of the parathyroid glands, the thymus and certain associated rudiments. J Pathol Bacteriol 1937; 45:507–522.
18. Carney JA. Salivary heterotopia, cysts, and the parathyroid gland: branchial pouch derivatives and remnants. Am J Surg Pathol 2000; 24(6):837–845.
19. Nelson SD. Pathology of the Parathyroid Gland. In: Fu YS, Wenig BM, Abemayor E, et al. eds. Head and Neck Pathology with Clinical Correlation. New York: Churchill-Livingstone; 2001. p. 646–667.
20. Dekker A, Dunsford HA, Geyer SJ. The normal parathyroid gland at autopsy: the significance of stromal fat in adult patients. J Pathol 1979; 128(3):127–132.
21. Dufour DR, Wilkerson SY. The normal parathyroid revisited: percentage of stromal fat. Hum Pathol 1982; 13(8): 717–721.
22. Grimelius L, Akerstrom G, Johansson H, et al. Estimation of parenchymal cell content of human parathyroid glands using the image analyzing computer technique. Am J Pathol 1978; 93(3):793–800.

23. Iwasaki A, Shan L, Kawano I, et al. Quantitative analysis of stromal fat content of human parathyroid glands associated with thyroid diseases using computer image analysis. Pathol Int 1995; 45(7):483–486.
24. Obara T, Fujimoto Y, Aiba M. Stromal fat content of the parathyroid gland. Endocrinol Jpn 1990; 37(6):901–905.
25. Grimelius L, Akerstrom G, Bondeson L, et al. The role of the pathologist in diagnosis and surgical decision making in hyperparathyroidism. World J Surg 1991; 15(6):698–705.
26. Gilmour JR. The normal histology of the parathyroid glands. J Pathol Bacteriol 1939; 48:187–222.
27. Leedham PW, Pollock DJ. Intrafollicular amyloid in primary hyperparathyroidism. J Clin Pathol 1970; 23(9):811–817.
28. Pollock DJ, Leedham PW. Hyperparathyroidism with local amyloid deposition. J Pathol 1970; 100(2):vi.
29. Altenahr E. Ultrastructural pathology of parathyroid glands. Curr Top Pathol 1972; 56:2–54.
30. Nilsson O. Studies on the ultrastructure of the human parathyroid glands in various pathological conditions. Acta Pathol Microbiol Scand Suppl 1977; (263):1–88.
31. Roth SI, Capen CC. Ultrastructure and functional correlations of the parathyroid gland. Int Rev Exp Pathol 1974; 13:161–221.
32. Roth SI. The ultrastructure of primary water-clear cell hyperplasia of the parathyroid glands. Am J Pathol 1970; 61(2):233–248.
33. Bedetti CD. Immunocytochemical demonstration of cytochrome c oxidase with an immunoperoxidase method: a specific stain for mitochondria in formalin-fixed and paraffin-embedded human tissues. J Histochem Cytochem 1985; 33(5):446–452.
34. Bedetti CD, Dekker A, Watson CG. Functioning oxyphil cell adenoma of the parathyroid gland: a clinicopathologic study of ten patients with hyperparathyroidism. Hum Pathol 1984; 15(12):1121–1126.
35. Muller-Hocker J. Random cytochrome-C-oxidase deficiency of oxyphil cell nodules in the parathyroid gland. A mitochondrial cytopathy related to cell ageing? Pathol Res Pract 1992; 188(6):701–706.
36. Muller-Hocker J, Aust D, Napiwotzky J, et al. Defects of the respiratory chain in oxyphil and chief cells of the normal parathyroid and in hyperfunction. Hum Pathol 1996; 27(6):532–541.
37. Miettinen M, Clark R, Lehto VP, et al. Intermediate-filament proteins in parathyroid glands and parathyroid adenomas. Arch Pathol Lab Med 1985; 109(11):986–989.
38. O'Connor DT, Burton D, Deftos LJ. Chromogranin A: immunohistology reveals its universal occurrence in normal polypeptide hormone producing endocrine glands. Life Sci 1983; 33(17):1657–1663.
39. Cohn DV, Morrissey JJ, Shofstall RE, et al. Cosecretion of secretory protein-I and parathormone by dispersed bovine parathyroid cells. Endocrinology 1982; 110(2):625–630.
40. Arps H, Dietel M, Lauritzen B, et al. Co-localization of parathyroid hormone and secretory protein-I in bovine parathyroid glands: a double immunocytochemical study at the electron microscopical level. Bone Miner 1987; 2(3):175–183.
41. Futrell JM, Roth SI, Su SP, et al. Immunocytochemical localization of parathyroid hormone in bovine parathyroid glands and human parathyroid adenomas. Am J Pathol 1979; 94(3):615–622.
42. Tomita T. Immunocytochemical staining patterns for parathyroid hormone and chromogranin in parathyroid hyperplasia, adenoma and carcinoma. Endocr Pathol 1999; 10:145–156.
43. Brown EM, Gamba G, Riccardi D, et al. Cloning and characterization of an extracellular Ca(2+)-sensing receptor from bovine parathyroid. Nature 1993; 366(6455):575–580.
44. Baker AR, McDonnell DP, Hughes M, et al. Cloning and expression of full-length cDNA encoding human vitamin D receptor. Proc Natl Acad Sci U S A 1988; 85(10):3294–3298.
45. Grzela T, Chudzinski W, Lasiecka Z, et al. The calcium-sensing receptor and vitamin D receptor expression in tertiary hyperparathyroidism. Int J Mol Med 2006; 17(5):779–783.
46. Sudhaker Rao D, Han ZH, Phillips ER, et al. Reduced vitamin D receptor expression in parathyroid adenomas: implications for pathogenesis. Clin Endocrinol (Oxf) 2000; 53(3):373–381.
47. Yano S, Sugimoto T, Tsukamoto T, et al. Association of decreased calcium-sensing receptor expression with proliferation of parathyroid cells in secondary hyperparathyroidism. Kidney Int 2000; 58(5):1980–1986.
48. Yano S, Sugimoto T, Tsukamoto T, et al. Decrease in vitamin D receptor and calcium-sensing receptor in highly proliferative parathyroid adenomas. Eur J Endocrinol 2003; 148(4):403–411.
49. Faure GC, Tang JQ, Mathieu P, et al. A CD4-like molecule can be expressed in vivo in human parathyroid. J Clin Endocrinol Metab 1990; 71(3):656–660.
50. Hellman P, Juhlin C, Karlsson-Parra A, et al. Expression and function of a CD3-like molecule on normal and abnormal human parathyroid cells. Surgery 1995; 118(6):1055–1061; (discussion 1062).
51. Hellman P, Karlsson-Parra A, Klareskog L, et al. Expression and function of a CD4-like molecule in parathyroid tissue. Surgery 1996; 120(6):985–992.
52. Goswami R, Mohapatra T, Gupta N, et al. Parathyroid hormone gene polymorphism and sporadic idiopathic hypoparathyroidism. J Clin Endocrinol Metab 2004; 89(10):4840–4845.
53. Tonoki H, Narahara K, Matsumoto T, et al. Regional mapping of the parathyroid hormone gene (PTH) by cytogenetic and molecular studies. Cytogenet Cell Genet 1991; 56(2):103–104.
54. Demay MB, Kiernan MS, DeLuca HF, et al. Sequences in the human parathyroid hormone gene that bind the 1,25-dihydroxyvitamin D3 receptor and mediate transcriptional repression in response to 1,25-dihydroxyvitamin D3. Proc Natl Acad Sci U S A 1992; 89(17):8097–8101.
55. Buchwald PC, Westin G, Akerstrom G. Vitamin D in normal and pathological parathyroid glands: new prospects for treating hyperparathyroidism (review). Int J Mol Med 2005; 15(4):701–706.
56. Okazaki T, Chung U, Nishishita T, et al. A redox factor protein, ref1, is involved in negative gene regulation by extracellular calcium. J Biol Chem 1994; 269(45):27855–27862.
57. Quarles LD. Extracellular calcium-sensing receptors in the parathyroid gland, kidney, and other tissues. Curr Opin Nephrol Hypertens 2003; 12(4):349–355.
58. Alimov AP, Langub MC, Malluche HH, et al. Sp3/Sp1 in the parathyroid gland: identification of an Sp1 deoxyribonucleic acid element in the parathyroid hormone promoter. Endocrinology 2003; 144(7):3138–3147.
59. Alimov AP, Park-Sarge OK, Sarge KD, et al. Transactivation of the parathyroid hormone promoter by specificity proteins and the nuclear factor Y complex. Endocrinology 2005; 146(8):3409–3416.
60. Rupp E, Mayer H, Wingender E. The promoter of the human parathyroid hormone gene contains a functional cyclic AMP-response element. Nucleic Acids Res 1990; 18(19):5677–5683.

61. Brown EM, Pollak M, Seidman CE, et al. Calcium-ion-sensing cell-surface receptors. N Engl J Med 1995; 333(4): 234–240.

62. Ding C, Buckingham B, Levine MA. Familial isolated hypoparathyroidism caused by a mutation in the gene for the transcription factor GCMB. J Clin Invest 2001; 108 (8):1215–1220.

63. Kebebew E, Peng M, Wong MG, et al. GCMB gene, a master regulator of parathyroid gland development, expression, and regulation in hyperparathyroidism. Surgery 2004; 136(6):1261–1266.

64. Kronenberg HM. GCMB–another serendipitous gift from evolution to clinical investigators. J Clin Endocrinol Metab 2004; 89(1):6–7.

65. Maret A, Bourdeau I, Ding C, et al. Expression of GCMB by intrathymic parathyroid hormone-secreting adenomas indicates their parathyroid cell origin. J Clin Endocrinol Metab 2004; 89(1):8–12.

66. Baba H, Kishihara M, Tohmon M, et al. Identification of parathyroid hormone messenger ribonucleic acid in an apparently nonfunctioning parathyroid carcinoma transformed from a parathyroid carcinoma with hyperparathyroidism. J Clin Endocrinol Metab 1986; 62(2):247–252.

67. Kendall CH, Potter L, Brown R, et al. In situ correlation of synthesis and storage of parathormone in parathyroid gland disease. J Pathol 1993; 169(1):61–66.

68. Kendall CH, Roberts PA, Pringle JH, et al. The expression of parathyroid hormone messenger RNA in normal and abnormal parathyroid tissue. J Pathol 1991; 165(2):111–118.

69. Bas S, Aguilera-Tejero E, Bas A, et al. The influence of the progression of secondary hyperparathyroidism on the set point of the parathyroid hormone-calcium curve. J Endocrinol 2005; 184(1):241–247.

70. Gao P, D'Amour P. Evolution of the parathyroid hormone (PTH) assay—importance of circulating PTH immunoheterogeneity and of its regulation. Clin Lab 2005; 51(1–2): 21–29.

71. Potts JT, Gardella TJ. Progress, paradox, and potential: parathyroid hormone research over five decades. Ann N Y Acad Sci 2007; 1117:196–208.

72. Wermers RA, Khosla S, Atkinson EJ, et al. Incidence of primary hyperparathyroidism in Rochester, Minnesota, 1993–2001: an update on the changing epidemiology of the disease. J Bone Miner Res 2006; 21(1):171–177.

73. Heath H, 3rd, Hodgson SF, Kennedy MA. Primary hyperparathyroidism. Incidence, morbidity, and potential economic impact in a community. N Engl J Med 1980; 302 (4):189–193.

74. Lundgren E, Rastad J, Thrufjell E, et al. Population-based screening for primary hyperparathyroidism with serum calcium and parathyroid hormone values in menopausal women. Surgery 1997; 121(3):287–294.

75. Hundahl SA, Fleming ID, Fremgen AM, et al. Two hundred eighty-six cases of parathyroid carcinoma treated in the U.S. between 1985–1995: a National Cancer Data Base Report. The American College of Surgeons Commission on Cancer and the American Cancer Society. Cancer 1999; 86(3):538–544.

76. Rosen IB, Strawbridge HG, Bain J. A case of hyperparathyroidism associated with radiation to the head and neck area. Cancer 1975; 36(3):1111–1114.

77. Tisell LE, Carlsson S, Lindberg S, et al. Autonomous hyperparathyroidism: a possible late complication of neck radiotherapy. Acta Chir Scand 1976; 142(5):367–373.

78. Tisell LE, Carlsson S, Fjalling M, et al. Hyperparathyroidism subsequent to neck irradiation. Risk factors. Cancer 1985; 56(7):1529–1533.

79. Prinz RA, Paloyan E, Lawrence AM, et al. Radiation-associated hyperparathyroidism: a new syndrome? Surgery 1977; 82(3):296–302.

80. Beard CM, Heath H, 3rd, O'Fallon WM, et al. Therapeutic radiation and hyperparathyroidism. A case-control study in Rochester, Minn. Arch Intern Med 1989; 149(8):1887–1890.

81. Russ JE, Scanlon EF, Sener SF. Parathyroid adenomas following irradiation. Cancer 1979; 43(3):1078–1083.

82. Rao SD, Frame B, Miller MJ, et al. Hyperparathyroidism following head and neck irradiation. Arch Intern Med 1980; 140(2):205–207.

83. Takeichi N, Dohi K, Yamamoto H, et al. Parathyroid tumors in atomic bomb survivors in Hiroshima: epidemiological study from registered cases at Hiroshima Prefecture Tumor Tissue Registry, 1974–1987. Jpn J Cancer Res 1991; 82(8):875–878.

84. Fujiwara S, Sposto R, Ezaki H, et al. Hyperparathyroidism among atomic bomb survivors in Hiroshima. Radiat Res 1992; 130(3):372–378.

85. Mihailescu D, Shore-Freedman E, Mukani S, et al. Multiple neoplasms in an irradiated cohort: pattern of occurrence and relationship to thyroid cancer outcome. J Clin Endocrinol Metab 2002; 87(7):3236–3241.

86. Schneider AB, Gierlowski TC, Shore-Freedman E, et al. Dose-response relationships for radiation-induced hyperparathyroidism. J Clin Endocrinol Metab 1995; 80(1): 254–257.

87. Cohen J, Gierlowski TC, Schneider AB. A prospective study of hyperparathyroidism in individuals exposed to radiation in childhood. JAMA 1990; 264(5):581–584.

88. Rasmuson T, Tavelin B. Risk of parathyroid adenomas in patients with thyrotoxicosis exposed to radioactive iodine. Acta Oncol 2006; 45(8):1059–1061.

89. Hamilton TE, Davis S, Onstad L, et al. Hyperparathyroidism in persons exposed to iodine-131 from the Hanford Nuclear Site. J Clin Endocrinol Metab 2005; 90(12):6545–6548.

90. Skogseid B, Rastad J, Oberg K. Multiple endocrine neoplasia type 1. Clinical features and screening. Endocrinol Metab Clin North Am 1994; 23(1):1–18.

91. Hellman P, Skogseid B, Oberg K, et al. Primary and reoperative parathyroid operations in hyperparathyroidism of multiple endocrine neoplasia type 1. Surgery 1998; 124(6):993–999.

92. Haven CJ, Howell VM, Eilers PH, et al. Gene expression of parathyroid tumors: molecular subclassification and identification of the potential malignant phenotype. Cancer Res 2004; 64(20):7405–7411.

93. Carling T, Udelsman R. Parathyroid surgery in familial hyperparathyroid disorders. J Intern Med 2005; 257(1): 27–37.

94. Kaji H, Canaff L, Lebrun JJ, et al. Inactivation of menin, a Smad3-interacting protein, blocks transforming growth factor type beta signaling. Proc Natl Acad Sci U S A 2001; 98(7):3837–3842.

95. Raue F, Kraimps JL, Dralle H, et al. Primary hyperparathyroidism in multiple endocrine neoplasia type 2A. J Intern Med 1995; 238(4):369–373.

96. Schuffenecker I, Virally-Monod M, Brohet R, et al. Risk and penetrance of primary hyperparathyroidism in multiple endocrine neoplasia type 2A families with mutations at codon 634 of the RET proto-oncogene. Groupe D'etude des Tumeurs a Calcitonine. J Clin Endocrinol Metab 1998; 83(2):487–491.

97. Villablanca A, Farnebo F, Teh BT, et al. Genetic and clinical characterization of sporadic cystic parathyroid tumours. Clin Endocrinol (Oxf) 2002; 56(2):261–269.

98. Haven CJ, Wong FK, van Dam EW, et al. A genotypic and histopathological study of a large Dutch kindred with hyperparathyroidism-jaw tumor syndrome. J Clin Endocrinol Metab 2000; 85(4):1449–1454.

99. Teh BT, Farnebo F, Kristoffersson U, et al. Autosomal dominant primary hyperparathyroidism and jaw tumor syndrome associated with renal hamartomas and cystic kidney disease: linkage to 1q21-q32 and loss of the wild type allele in renal hamartomas. J Clin Endocrinol Metab 1996; 81:4204–4211.

100. Szabo J, Heath B, Hill VM, et al. Hereditary hyperparathyroidism-jaw tumor syndrome: the endocrine tumor gene HRPT2 maps to chromosome 1q21-q31. Am J Hum Genet 1995; 56(4):944–950.

101. Carpten JD, Robbins CM, Villablanca A, et al. HRPT2, encoding parafibromin, is mutated in hyperparathyroidism-jaw tumor syndrome. Nat Genet 2002; 32(4):676–680.

102. Gill AJ, Clarkson A, Gimm O, et al. Loss of nuclear expression of parafibromin distinguishes parathyroid carcinomas and hyperparathyroidism-jaw tumor (HPT-JT) syndrome-related adenomas from sporadic parathyroid adenomas and hyperplasias. Am J Surg Pathol 2006; 30(9): 1140–1149.

103. Carling T. Molecular pathology of parathyroid tumors. Trends Endocrinol Metab 2001; 12(2):53–58.

104. Lundgren E, Ljunghall S, Akerstrom G, et al. Case-control study on symptoms and signs of "asymptomatic" primary hyperparathyroidism. Surgery 1998; 124(6):980–985 (discussion 985–986).

105. Bondeson AG, Bondeson L, Thompson NW. Clinicopathological peculiarities in parathyroid disease with hypercalcaemic crisis. Eur J Surg 1993; 159(11–12):613–617.

106. Shane E. Clinical review 122: Parathyroid carcinoma. J Clin Endocrinol Metab 2001; 86(2):485–493.

107. Wynne AG, van Heerden J, Carney JA, et al. Parathyroid carcinoma: clinical and pathologic features in 43 patients. Medicine (Baltimore) 1992; 71(4):197–205.

108. Ikeda K, Mangin M, Dreyer BE, et al. Identification of transcripts encoding a parathyroid hormone-like peptide in messenger RNAs from a variety of human and animal tumors associated with humoral hypercalcemia of malignancy. J Clin Invest 1988; 81(6):2010–2014.

109. Ratcliffe WA, Hutchesson AC, Bundred NJ, et al. Role of assays for parathyroid-hormone-related protein in investigation of hypercalcaemia. Lancet 1992; 339(8786):164–167.

110. Fuleihan Gel H. Familial benign hypocalciuric hypercalcemia. J Bone Miner Res 2002; 17(Suppl 2):N51–N56.

111. Purcell GP, Dirbas FM, Jeffrey RB, et al. Parathyroid localization with high-resolution ultrasound and technetium Tc 99m sestamibi. Arch Surg 1999; 134(8):824–828 (discussion 828–830).

112. Lumachi F, Zucchetta P, Marzola MC, et al. Advantages of combined technetium-99m-sestamibi scintigraphy and high-resolution ultrasonography in parathyroid localization: comparative study in 91 patients with primary hyperparathyroidism. Eur J Endocrinol 2000; 143(6):755–760.

113. Rodgers SE, Hunter GJ, Hamberg LM, et al. Improved preoperative planning for directed parathyroidectomy with 4-dimensional computed tomography. Surgery 2006; 140(6):932–940 (discussion 940–931).

114. Serra A, Bolasco P, Satta L, et al. Role of SPECT/CT in the preoperative assessment of hyperparathyroid patients. Radiol Med (Torino) 2006; 111(7):999–1008.

115. Reeder SB, Desser TS, Weigel RJ, et al. Sonography in primary hyperparathyroidism: review with emphasis on scanning technique. J Ultrasound Med 2002; 21(5):539–552; quiz 553–534.

116. Haber RS, Kim CK, Inabnet WB. Ultrasonography for preoperative localization of enlarged parathyroid glands in primary hyperparathyroidism: comparison with (99m) technetium sestamibi scintigraphy. Clin Endocrinol (Oxf) 2002; 57(2):241–249.

117. Siperstein A, Berber E, Mackey R, et al. Prospective evaluation of sestamibi scan, ultrasonography, and rapid PTH to predict the success of limited exploration for sporadic primary hyperparathyroidism. Surgery 2004; 136(4):872–880.

118. Solorzano CC, Carneiro-Pla DM, Irvin GL, 3rd. Surgeon-performed ultrasonography as the initial and only localizing study in sporadic primary hyperparathyroidism. J Am Coll Surg 2006; 202(1):18–24.

119. Moka D, Voth E, Dietlein M, et al. Technetium 99m-MIBI-SPECT: A highly sensitive diagnostic tool for localization of parathyroid adenomas. Surgery 2000; 128(1):29–35.

120. Perrier ND, Ituarte PH, Morita E, et al. Parathyroid surgery: separating promise from reality. J Clin Endocrinol Metab 2002; 87(3):1024–1029.

121. Reidel MA, Schilling T, Graf S, et al. Localization of hyperfunctioning parathyroid glands by selective venous sampling in reoperation for primary or secondary hyperparathyroidism. Surgery 2006; 140(6):907–913 (discussion 913).

122. Jones JJ, Brunaud L, Dowd CF, et al. Accuracy of selective venous sampling for intact parathyroid hormone in difficult patients with recurrent or persistent hyperparathyroidism. Surgery 2002; 132(6):944–950 (discussion 950–941).

123. Clark OH, Gooding GA, Ljung BM. Locating a parathyroid adenoma by ultrasonography and aspiration biopsy cytology. West J Med 1981; 135(2):154–158.

124. Doppman JL, Krudy AG, Marx SJ, et al. Aspiration of enlarged parathyroid glands for parathyroid hormone assay. Radiology 1983; 148(1):31–35.

125. Johnson NA, Tublin ME, Ogilvie JB. Parathyroid imaging: technique and role in the preoperative evaluation of primary hyperparathyroidism. AJR Am J Roentgenol 2007; 188(6):1706–1715.

126. MacFarlane MP, Fraker DL, Shawker TH, et al. Use of preoperative fine-needle aspiration in patients undergoing reoperation for primary hyperparathyroidism. Surgery 1994; 116(6):959–964 (discussion 964–955).

127. Sacks BA, Pallotta JA, Cole A, et al. Diagnosis of parathyroid adenomas: efficacy of measuring parathormone levels in needle aspirates of cervical masses. AJR Am J Roentgenol 1994; 163(5):1223–1226.

128. Stephen AE, Milas M, Garner CN, et al. Use of surgeon-performed office ultrasound and parathyroid fine needle aspiration for complex parathyroid localization. Surgery 2005; 138(6):1143–1150 (discussion 1150–1141).

129. Lerud KS, Tabbara SO, DelVecchio DM, et al. Cytomorphology of cystic parathyroid lesions: report of four cases evaluated preoperatively by fine-needle aspiration. Diagn Cytopathol 1996; 15(4):306–311.

130. Silverman JF, Khazanie PG, Norris HT, et al. Parathyroid hormone (PTH) assay of parathyroid cysts examined by fine-needle aspiration biopsy. Am J Clin Pathol 1986; 86 (6):776–780.

131. Giorgadze T, Stratton B, Baloch ZW, et al. Oncocytic parathyroid adenoma: problem in cytological diagnosis. Diagn Cytopathol 2004; 31(4):276–280.

132. Ruf J, Seehofer D, Nadjari B, et al. Incidental parathyroid adenoma mimicking tumor recurrence in a patient with follicular thyroid carcinoma. Clin Nucl Med 2006; 31(2): 74–76.

133. Odashiro AN, Nguyen GK. Fine-needle aspiration cytology of an intrathyroid parathyroid adenoma. Diagn Cytopathol 2006; 34(11):790–792.

134. Ren R, Gong Y. Fine-needle aspiration of a parathyroid hyperplasia with unusual clinical and cytologic presentation. Diagn Cytopathol 2007; 35(4):250–251.

135. Dimashkieh H, Krishnamurthy S. Ultrasound guided fine needle aspiration biopsy of parathyroid gland and lesions. Cytojournal 2006; 3:6.

136. Mincione GP, Borrelli D, Cicchi P, et al. Fine needle aspiration cytology of parathyroid adenoma. A review of seven cases. Acta Cytol 1986; 30(1):65–69.

137. Liu F, Gnepp DR, Pisharodi LR. Fine needle aspiration of parathyroid lesions. Acta Cytol 2004; 48(2):133–136.

138. Winkler B, Gooding GA, Montgomery CK, et al. Immunoperoxidase confirmation of parathyroid origin of ultrasound-guided fine needle aspirates of the parathyroid glands. Acta Cytol 1987; 31(1):40–44.

139. Abati A, Skarulis MC, Shawker T, et al. Ultrasound-guided fine-needle aspiration of parathyroid lesions: a morphological and immunocytochemical approach. Hum Pathol 1995; 26(3):338–343.

140. Absher KJ, Truong LD, Khurana KK, et al. Parathyroid cytology: avoiding diagnostic pitfalls. Head Neck 2002; 24 (2):157–164.

141. Tseng FY, Hsiao YL, Chang TC. Ultrasound-guided fine needle aspiration cytology of parathyroid lesions. A review of 72 cases. Acta Cytol 2002; 46(6):1029–1036.

142. Tseleni-Balafouta S, Gakiopoulou H, Kavantzas N, et al. Parathyroid proliferations: a source of diagnostic pitfalls in FNA of thyroid. Cancer 2007; 111(2):130–136.

143. Bondeson L, Bondeson AG, Nissborg A, et al. Cytopathological variables in parathyroid lesions: a study based on 1,600 cases of hyperparathyroidism. Diagn Cytopathol 1997; 16(6):476–482.

144. Yong JL, Vrga L, Warren BA. A study of parathyroid hyperplasia in chronic renal failure. Pathology 1994; 26(2): 99–109.

145. Chang TC, Tung CC, Hsiao YL, et al. Immunoperoxidase staining in the differential diagnosis of parathyroid from thyroid origin in fine needle aspirates of suspected parathyroid lesions. Acta Cytol 1998; 42(3):619–624.

146. Davey DD, Glant MD, Berger EK. Parathyroid cytopathology. Diagn Cytopathol 1986; 2(1):76–80.

147. Guazzi A, Gabrielli M, Guadagni G. Cytologic features of a functioning parathyroid carcinoma: a case report. Acta Cytol 1982; 26(5):709–713.

148. Hara H, Oyama T, Kimura M, et al. Cytologic characteristics of parathyroid carcinoma: a case report. Diagn Cytopathol 1998; 18(3):192–198.

149. Ikeda K, Tate G, Suzuki T, et al. Cytologic comparison of a primary parathyroid cancer and its metastatic lesions: a case report. Diagn Cytopathol 2006; 34(1):50–55.

150. de la Garza S, Flores de la Garza E, Hernandez Batres F. Functional parathyroid carcinoma. Cytology, histology, and ultrastructure of a case. Diagn Cytopathol 1985; 1(3):232–235.

151. Du SD, Chang TC, Chen YL, et al. Ultrasonography and needle aspiration cytology in the diagnosis and management of parathyroid lesions. J Formos Med Assoc 1994; 93 (2):153–159.

152. Agarwal G, Dhingra S, Mishra SK, et al. Implantation of parathyroid carcinoma along fine needle aspiration track. Langenbecks Arch Surg 2006; 391(6):623–626.

153. Sulak LE, Brown RW, Butler DB. Parathyroid carcinoma with occult bone metastases diagnosed by fine needle aspiration cytology. Acta Cytol 1989; 33(5):645–648.

154. Kendrick ML, Charboneau JW, Curlee KJ, et al. Risk of parathyromatosis after fine-needle aspiration. Am Surg 2001; 67(3):290–293 (discussion 293–294).

155. Spinelli C, Bonadio AG, Berti P, et al. Cutaneous spreading of parathyroid carcinoma after fine needle aspiration cytology. J Endocrinol Invest 2000; 23(4):255–257.

156. Rodriguez M, Canalejo A, Garfia B, et al. Pathogenesis of refractory secondary hyperparathyroidism. Kidney Int Suppl 2002; (80):155–160.

157. Savio RM, Gosnell JE, Posen S, et al. Parathyroidectomy for tertiary hyperparathyroidism associated with X-linked dominant hypophosphatemic rickets. Arch Surg 2004; 139 (2):218–222.

158. (USRDS) UDS. USRDS 2006 Annual Data Report Reference Tables. Bethesda, MD: National Institute of Health, National Institute of Diabetes Digestive and Kidney Diseases; 2006.

159. Salem MM. Hyperparathyroidism in the hemodialysis population: a survey of 612 patients. Am J Kidney Dis 1997; 29(6):862–865.

160. Kim HC, Cheigh JS, David DS, et al. Long term results of subtotal parathyroidectomy in patients with end-stage renal disease. Am Surg 1994; 60(9):641–649.

161. Coco M, Rush H. Increased incidence of hip fractures in dialysis patients with low serum parathyroid hormone. Am J Kidney Dis 2000; 36(6):1115–1121.

162. Elder G. Pathophysiology and recent advances in the management of renal osteodystrophy. J Bone Miner Res 2002; 17(12):2094–2105.

163. Ganesh SK, Stack AG, Levin NW, et al. Association of elevated serum PO(4), Ca × PO(4) product, and parathyroid hormone with cardiac mortality risk in chronic hemodialysis patients. J Am Soc Nephrol 2001; 12 (10):2131–2138.

164. Grandaliano G, Teutonico A, Allegretti A, et al. The role of hyperparathyroidism, erythropoietin therapy, and CMV infection in the failure of arteriovenous fistula in hemodialysis. Kidney Int 2003; 64(2):715–719.

165. Goodman WG, Goldin J, Kuizon BD, et al. Coronary-artery calcification in young adults with end-stage renal disease who are undergoing dialysis. N Engl J Med 2000; 342(20):1478–1483.

166. Block GA, Hulbert-Shearon TE, Levin NW, et al. Association of serum phosphorus and calcium × phosphate product with mortality risk in chronic hemodialysis patients: a national study. Am J Kidney Dis 1998; 31 (4):607–617.

167. Schluter KD, Piper HM. Cardiovascular actions of parathyroid hormone and parathyroid hormone-related peptide. Cardiovasc Res 1998; 37(1):34–41.

168. Ha SK, Park HS, Kim SJ, et al. Prevalence and patterns of left ventricular hypertrophy in patients with predialysis chronic renal failure. J Korean Med Sci 1998; 13(5):488–494.

169. Numano M, Tominaga Y, Uchida K, et al. Surgical significance of supernumerary parathyroid glands in renal hyperparathyroidism. World J Surg 1998; 22(10):1098–1102 (discussion 1103).

170. Seehofer D, Steinmuller T, Rayes N, et al. Parathyroid hormone venous sampling before reoperative surgery in renal hyperparathyroidism: comparison with noninvasive localization procedures and review of the literature. Arch Surg 2004; 139(12):1331–1338.

171. Elliott DD, Monroe DP, Perrier ND. Parathyroid histopathology: is it of any value today? J Am Coll Surg 2006; 203 (5):758–765.

172. Mun HC, Conigrave A, Wilkinson M, et al. Surgery for hyperparathyroidism: does morphology or function matter most? Surgery 2005; 138(6):1111–1120 (discussion 1120).

173. Johnson SJ, Sheffield EA, McNicol AM. Best practice no 183. Examination of parathyroid gland specimens. J Clin Pathol 2005; 58(4):338–342.

174. Akerstrom G, Grimelius L, Fridh C, et al. Estimation of parenchymal cell mass of parathyroid glands using a volumeter technique. Ups J Med Sci 1979; 84(3):255–258.

175. Wang CA, Rieder SV. A density test for the intraoperative differentiation of parathyroid hyperplasia from neoplasia. Ann Surg 1978; 187(1):63–67.

176. Akerstrom G, Grimelius L, Johansson H. A density test for the intraoperative differentiation of parathyroid hyperplasia from neoplasia. Ann Surg 1980; 191(3):387–388.

177. Akerstrom G, Grimelius L, Johansson H, et al. Estimation of the parenchymal-cell content of the parathyroid gland, using density-gradient columns. Preliminary report. Acta Pathol Microbiol Scand [A] 1977; 85(4):555–557.

178. Akerstrom G, Grimelius L, Johansson H, et al. Estimation of the parathyroid parenchymal cell mass by density gradients. Am J Pathol 1980; 99(3):685–694.

179. Akerstrom G, Pertoft H, Grimelius L, et al. Density determinations of human parathyroid glands by density gradients. Acta Pathol Microbiol Scand [A] 1979; 87A(2):91–96.

180. Welsh CL, Taylor GW. The density test for the intraoperative differentiation of single or multigland parathyroid disease. World J Surg 1984; 8(4):522–526.

181. Rothmund M. The density test for the intraoperative differentiation of single or multiglandular parathyroid disease. World J Surg 1984; 8:525–526.

182. Lockett LJ. A source of false results in the intraoperative parathyroid density test. Am J Clin Pathol 1982; 78(5):781–783.

183. Roth SI, Faquin WC. The pathologist's intraoperative role during parathyroid surgery. Arch Pathol Lab Med 2003; 127(1):15.

184. Dewan AK, Kapadia SB, Hollenbeak CS, et al. Is routine frozen section necessary for parathyroid surgery? Otolaryngol Head Neck Surg 2005; 133(6):857–862.

185. Anton RC, Wheeler TM. Frozen section of thyroid and parathyroid specimens. Arch Pathol Lab Med 2005; 129(12):1575–1584.

186. Higuchi T, Kinuya S, Taki J, et al. Brown adipose tissue: evaluation with 201Tl and 99mTc-sestamibi dual-tracer SPECT. Ann Nucl Med 2004; 18(6):547–549.

187. Westra WH, Pritchett DD, Udelsman R. Intraoperative confirmation of parathyroid tissue during parathyroid exploration: a retrospective evaluation of the frozen section. Am J Surg Pathol 1998; 22(5):538–544.

188. Levin KE, Clark OH. The reasons for failure in parathyroid operations. Arch Surg 1989; 124(8):911–914 (discussion 914–915).

189. Roslyn JJ, Mulder DG, Gordon HE. Persistent and recurrent hyperparathyroidism. Am J Surg 1981; 142(1):21–25.

190. Geelhoed GW, Silverberg SG. Intraoperative imprints for the identification of parathyroid tissue. Surgery 1984; 96(6):1124–1131.

191. Silverberg SG. Imprints in the intraoperative evaluation of parathyroid disease. Arch Pathol 1975; 99(7):375–378.

192. Shidham VB, Asma Z, Rao RN, et al. Intraoperative cytology increases the diagnostic accuracy of frozen sections for the confirmation of various tissues in the parathyroid region. Am J Clin Pathol 2002; 118(6):895–902.

193. Rohaizak M, Munchar MJ, Meah FA, et al. Prospective study comparing scrape cytology with frozen section in the intraoperative identification of parathyroid tissue. Asian J Surg 2005; 28(2):82–85.

194. Yao DX, Hoda SA, Yin DY, et al. Interpretative problems and preparative technique influence reliability of intraoperative parathyroid touch imprints. Arch Pathol Lab Med 2003; 127(1):64–67.

195. Saxe AW, Baier R, Tesluk H, et al. The role of the pathologist in the surgical treatment of hyperparathyroidism. Surg Gynecol Obstet 1985; 161(2):101–105.

196. Dufour DR, Durkowski C. Sudan IV stain. Its limitations in evaluating parathyroid functional status. Arch Pathol Lab Med 1982; 106(5):224–227.

197. Kasdon EJ, Rosen S, Cohen RB, et al. Surgical pathology of hyperparathyroidism. Usefulness of fat stain and problems in interpretation. Am J Surg Pathol 1981; 5(4):381–384.

198. Bondeson AG, Bondeson L, Ljungberg O, et al. Fat staining in parathyroid disease—diagnostic value and impact on surgical strategy: clinicopathologic analysis of 191 cases. Hum Pathol 1985; 16(12):1255–1263.

199. Roth SI, Gallagher MJ. The rapid identification of "normal" parathyroid glands by the presence of intracellular fat. Am J Pathol 1976; 84(3):521–528.

200. Ljungberg O, Tibblin S. Peroperative fat staining of frozen sections in primary hyperparathyroidism. Am J Pathol 1979; 95(3):633–641.

201. Monchik JM, Farrugia R, Teplitz C, et al. Parathyroid surgery: the role of chief cell intracellular fat staining with osmium carmine in the intraoperative management of patients with primary hyperparathyroidism. Surgery 1983; 94(6):877–886.

202. Farnebo LO, von Unge H. Peroperative evaluation of parathyroid glands using fat stain on frozen sections. Advantages and limitations. Acta Chir Scand Suppl 1984; 520:17–24.

203. Sarfati E, Lavergne A, Le Charpentier Y, et al. Parathyroid microadenomas. Ann Med Interne (Paris) 1987; 138(8):604–606.

204. Rasbach DA, Monchik JM, Geelhoed GW, et al. Solitary parathyroid microadenoma. Surgery 1984; 96(6):1092–1098.

205. Gough IR. Parathyroid cysts. Aust N Z J Surg 1999; 69(5):404–406.

206. Villablanca A, Farnebo F, Teh BT, et al. Genetic and clinical characterization of sporadic cystic parathyroid tumours. Clin Endocrinol (Oxf) 2002; 56(2):261–269.

207. Sahin A, Robinson RA. Papillae formation in parathyroid adenoma. A source of possible diagnostic error. Arch Pathol Lab Med 1988; 112(1):99–100.

208. Lawrence DA. A histological comparison of adenomatous and hyperplastic parathyroid glands. J Clin Pathol 1978; 31(7):626–632.

209. Bondeson L, Sandelin K, Grimelius L. Histopathological variables and DNA cytometry in parathyroid carcinoma. Am J Surg Pathol 1993; 17(8):820–829.

210. Grimelius L, Johansson H. Pathology of parathyroid tumors. Semin Surg Oncol 1997; 13(2):142–154.

211. Snover DC, Foucar K. Mitotic activity in benign parathyroid disease. Am J Clin Pathol 1981; 75(3):345–347.

212. Ghandur-Mnaymneh L, Kimura N. The parathyroid adenoma. A histopathologic definition with a study of 172 cases of primary hyperparathyroidism. Am J Pathol 1984; 115(1):70–83.

213. Wolpert HR, Vickery AL, Jr., Wang CA. Functioning oxyphil cell adenomas of the parathyroid gland. A study of 15 cases. Am J Surg Pathol 1989; 13(6):500–504.

214. Poole GV, Jr., Albertson DA, Marshall RB, et al. Oxyphil cell adenoma and hyperparathyroidism. Surgery 1982; 92(5):799–805.

215. Bleier BS, LiVolsi VA, Chalian AA, et al. Technetium Tc 99m sestamibi sensitivity in oxyphil cell-dominant parathyroid adenomas. Arch Otolaryngol Head Neck Surg 2006; 132(7):779–782.

216. Mehta NY, Ruda JM, Kapadia S, et al. Relationship of technetium Tc 99m sestamibi scans to histopathological features of hyperfunctioning parathyroid tissue. Arch Otolaryngol Head Neck Surg 2005; 131(6):493–498.

217. Ordonez NG, Ibanez ML, Mackay B, et al. Functioning oxyphil cell adenomas of parathyroid gland: immunoperoxidase evidence of hormonal activity in oxyphil cells. Am J Clin Pathol 1982; 78(5):681–689.

218. Kovacs K, Horvath E, Ozawa Y, et al. Large clear cell adenoma of the parathyroid in a patient with MEN-1

syndrome. Ultrastructural study of the tumour exhibiting unusual RER formations. Acta Biol Hung 1994; 45(2–4): 275–284.

219. Dundar E, Grenko RT, Akalin A, et al. Intrathyroidal water-clear cell parathyroid adenoma: a case report. Hum Pathol 2001; 32(8):889–892.

220. Grenko RT, Anderson KM, Kauffman G, et al. Water-clear cell adenoma of the parathyroid. A case report with immunohistochemistry and electron microscopy. Arch Pathol Lab Med 1995; 119(11):1072–1074.

221. Roth SI. Water-clear cell 'adenoma'. A new entity in the pathology of primary hyperparathyroidism. Arch Pathol Lab Med 1995; 119(11):996–997.

222. Prasad KK, Agarwal G, Krishnani N. Water-clear cell adenoma of the parathyroid gland: a rare entity. Indian J Pathol Microbiol 2004; 47(1):39–40.

223. Kuhel WI, Gonzales D, Hoda SA, et al. Synchronous water-clear cell double parathyroid adenomas a hitherto uncharacterized entity? Arch Pathol Lab Med 2001; 125(2):256–259.

224. Abul-Haj SK, Conklin H, Hewitt WC. Functioning lipoadenoma of the parathyroid gland. Report of a unique case. Nord Hyg Tidskr 1962; 26:121–123.

225. Attie JN, Wise L, Mir R, et al. The rationale against routine subtotal parathyroidectomy for primary hyperparathyroidism. Am J Surg 1978; 136(4):437–444.

226. Aukee S, Meurman LO. Hormonal inactivity in a case of parathyroid tumour. Acta Chir Scand 1971; 137(5):478–482.

227. Auriol M, Malki B, Koulibaly M, et al. Parathyroid lipoadenoma and lipomatous hyperplasia. 3 cases. Arch Anat Cytol Pathol 1985; 33(4):205–208.

228. Bleiweiss IJ, Harpaz N, Strauchen JA, et al. Functioning lipoadenoma of the parathyroid: case report and literature review. Mt Sinai J Med 1989; 56(2):114–117.

229. Chow LS, Erickson LA, Abu-Lebdeh HS, et al. Parathyroid lipoadenomas: a rare cause of primary hyperparathyroidism. Endocr Pract 2006; 12(2):131–136.

230. Coen G, Bondatti F, de Matteis A, et al. Severe vitamin D deficiency in a case of primary hyperparathyroidism caused by parathyroid lipoadenoma, effect of 25OHD3 treatment. Miner Electrolyte Metab 1989; 15(6):332–337.

231. Daboin KP, Ochoa-Perez V, Luna MA. Adenolipomas of the head and neck: analysis of 6 cases. Ann Diagn Pathol 2006; 10(2):72–76.

232. Daroca PJ, Jr., Landau RL, Reed RJ, et al. Functioning lipoadenoma of the parathyroid gland. Arch Pathol Lab Med 1977; 101(1):28–29.

233. de Leacy EA, Axelsen RA, Kleinman DS, et al. Functioning lipoadenoma of the parathyroid gland. Pathology 1988; 20(4):377–380.

234. Ducatman BS, Wilkerson SY, Brown JA. Functioning parathyroid lipoadenoma. Report of a case diagnosed by intraoperative touch preparations. Arch Pathol Lab Med 1986; 110(7):645–647.

235. Fischer I, Wieczorek R, Sidhu GS, et al. Myxoid lipoadenoma of parathyroid gland: a case report and literature review. Ann Diagn Pathol 2006; 10(5):294–296.

236. Frennby B, Nyman U, Aspelin P, et al. CT of a parathyroid lipoadenoma. Case report. Acta Radiol 1993; 34(4): 369–371.

237. Gabbert H, Rothmund M, Hohn P. Myxoid lipoadenoma of the parathyroid gland. Pathol Res Pract 1980; 170(4): 420–425.

238. Grimelius L, Johansson H, Lindquist B. A case of unusual stromal development in a parathyroid adenoma. Acta Chir Scand 1972; 138(6):628–629.

239. Hargreaves HK, Wright TC Jr. A large functioning parathyroid lipoadenoma found in the posterior mediastinum. Am J Clin Pathol 1981; 76(1):89–93.

240. Legolvan DP, Moore BP, Nishiyama RH. Parathyroid hamartoma: report of two cases and review of the literature. Am J Clin Pathol 1977; 67(1):31–35.

241. Obara T, Fujimoto Y, Ito Y, et al. Functioning parathyroid lipoadenoma–report of four cases: clinicopathological and ultrasonographic features. Endocrinol Jpn 1989; 36(1): 135–145.

242. Ober WB, Kaiser GA. Hamartoma of the parathyroid. Cancer 1958; 11(3):601–606.

243. Rastogi A, Jain M, Agarawal T, et al. Parathyroid lipoadenoma: case report and review of the literature. Indian J Pathol Microbiol 2006; 49(3):404–406.

244. Saik RP, Gmelich JT. Hyperparathyroidism from a hamartoma. Am Surg 1979; 45(8):542–543.

245. Seethala RR, Yim JH, Hunt JL. Pathology quiz case 2. Parathyroid lipoadenoma. Arch Otolaryngol Head Neck Surg 2006; 132(12):1391–1393.

246. Sheikh SS, Massloom HS. Lipoadenoma: is it arising from thyroid or parathyroid? A diagnostic dilemma. ORL J Otorhinolaryngol Relat Spec 2002; 64(6):448–450.

247. Turner WJ, Baergen RN, Pellitteri PK, et al. Parathyroid lipoadenoma: case report and review of the literature. Otolaryngol Head Neck Surg 1996; 114(2):313–316.

248. Uden P, Berglund J, Zederfeldt B, et al. Parathyroid lipoadenoma: a rare cause of primary hyperparathyroidism. Case report. Acta Chir Scand 1987; 153(10):635–639.

249. van Hoeven KH, Brennan MF. Lipothymoadenoma of the parathyroid. Arch Pathol Lab Med 1993; 117(3):312–314.

250. Weiland LH, Garrison RC, ReMine WH, et al. Lipoadenoma of the parathyroid gland. Am J Surg Pathol 1978; 2(1):3–7.

251. Wolff M, Goodman EN. Functioning lipoadenoma of a supernumerary parathyroid gland in the mediastinum. Head Neck Surg 1980; 2(4):302–307.

252. Stojadinovic A, Hoos A, Nissan A, et al. Parathyroid neoplasms: clinical, histopathological, and tissue microarray-based molecular analysis. Hum Pathol 2003; 34(1):54–64.

253. Levin KE, Galante M, Clark OH. Parathyroid carcinoma versus parathyroid adenoma in patients with profound hypercalcemia. Surgery 1987; 101(6):649–660.

254. Levin KE, Chew KL, Ljung BM, et al. Deoxyribonucleic acid cytometry helps identify parathyroid carcinomas. J Clin Endocrinol Metab 1988; 67(4):779–784.

255. Fernandez-Ranvier GG, Khanafshar E, Jensen K, et al. Parathyroid carcinoma, atypical parathyroid adenoma, or parathyromatosis? Cancer 2007; 110(2):255–264.

256. Ippolito G, Palazzo FF, Sebag F, et al. Intraoperative diagnosis and treatment of parathyroid cancer and atypical parathyroid adenoma. Br J Surg 2007; 94(5): 566–570.

257. DeLellis RA. Parathyroid carcinoma: an overview. Adv Anat Pathol 2005; 12(2):53–61.

258. Rodgers SE, Perrier ND. Parathyroid carcinoma. Curr Opin Oncol 2006; 18(1):16–22.

259. Wang CA, Gaz RD. Natural history of parathyroid carcinoma. Diagnosis, treatment, and results. Am J Surg 1985; 149(4):522–527.

260. Schantz A, Castleman B. Parathyroid carcinoma. A study of 70 cases. Cancer 1973; 31(3):600–605.

261. Hakaim AG, Esselstyn CB, Jr. Parathyroid carcinoma: 50-year experience at The Cleveland Clinic Foundation. Cleve Clin J Med 1993; 60(4):331–335.

262. Erickson LA, Jin L, Papotti M, et al. Oxyphil parathyroid carcinomas: a clinicopathologic and immunohistochemical study of 10 cases. Am J Surg Pathol 2002; 26(3):344–349.

263. Livolsi VA. Unusual tumors and tumorlike conditions of the thyroid. In: Livolsi VA, ed. Surgical Pathology of the Thyroid. Philadelphia: W.B. Saunders Company, 1990: 323–350.

264. Guyetant S, Dupre F, Bigorgne JC, et al. Medullary thyroid microcarcinoma: a clinicopathologic retrospective study of 38 patients with no prior familial disease. Hum Pathol 1999; 30(8):957–963.

265. Beressi N, Campos JM, Beressi JP, et al. Sporadic medullary microcarcinoma of the thyroid: a retrospective analysis of eighty cases. Thyroid 1998; 8(11):1039–1044.

266. Lloyd RV, Carney JA, Ferreiro JA, et al. Immunohistochemical Analysis of the Cell Cycle-Associated Antigens Ki-67 and Retinoblastoma Protein in Parathyroid Carcinomas and Adenomas. Endocr Pathol 1995; 6(4):279–287.

267. Abbona GC, Papotti M, Gasparri G, et al. Proliferative activity in parathyroid tumors as detected by Ki-67 immunostaining. Hum Pathol 1995; 26(2):135–138.

268. Vargas MP, Vargas HI, Kleiner DE, et al. The role of prognostic markers (MiB-1, RB, and bcl-2) in the diagnosis of parathyroid tumors. Mod Pathol 1997; 10(1):12–17.

269. Erickson LA, Jin L, Wollan P, et al. Parathyroid hyperplasia, adenomas, and carcinomas: differential expression of p27Kip1 protein. Am J Surg Pathol 1999; 23(3):288–295.

270. Tan MH, Morrison C, Wang P, et al. Loss of parafibromin immunoreactivity is a distinguishing feature of parathyroid carcinoma. Clin Cancer Res 2004; 10(19):6629–6637.

271. Cetani F, Ambrogini E, Viacava P, et al. Should parafibromin staining replace HRTP2 gene analysis as an additional tool for histologic diagnosis of parathyroid carcinoma? Eur J Endocrinol 2007; 156(5):547–554.

272. Arnold A, Staunton CE, Kim HG, et al. Monoclonality and abnormal parathyroid hormone genes in parathyroid adenomas. N Engl J Med 1988; 318(11):658–662.

273. Miedlich S, Krohn K, Lamesch P, et al. Frequency of somatic MEN1 gene mutations in monoclonal parathyroid tumours of patients with primary hyperparathyroidism. Eur J Endocrinol 2000; 143(1):47–54.

274. Imanishi Y, Tahara H, Palanisamy N, et al. Clonal chromosomal defects in the molecular pathogenesis of refractory hyperparathyroidism of uremia. J Am Soc Nephrol 2002; 13(6):1490–1498.

275. Tominaga Y, Kohara S, Namii Y, et al. Clonal analysis of nodular parathyroid hyperplasia in renal hyperparathyroidism. World J Surg 1996; 20(7):744–750 (discussion 750–742).

276. Arnold A, Shattuck TM, Mallya SM, et al. Molecular pathogenesis of primary hyperparathyroidism. J Bone Miner Res 2002; 17(suppl 2):N30–N36.

277. Mallya SM, Arnold A. Cyclin D1 in parathyroid disease. Front Biosci 2000; 5:D367–D371.

278. Heppner C, Kester MB, Agarwal SK, et al. Somatic mutation of the MEN1 gene in parathyroid tumours. Nat Genet 1997; 16(4):375–378.

279. Farnebo F, Teh BT, Kytola S, et al. Alterations of the MEN1 gene in sporadic parathyroid tumors. J Clin Endocrinol Metab 1998; 83(8):2627–2630.

280. Carling T, Correa P, Hessman O, et al. Parathyroid MEN1 gene mutations in relation to clinical characteristics of nonfamilial primary hyperparathyroidism. J Clin Endocrinol Metab 1998; 83(8):2960–2963.

281. Hemmer S, Wasenius VM, Haglund C, et al. Deletion of 11q23 and cyclin D1 overexpression are frequent aberrations in parathyroid adenomas. Am J Pathol 2001; 158(4):1355–1362.

282. Agarwal SK, Schrock E, Kester MB, et al. Comparative genomic hybridization analysis of human parathyroid tumors. Cancer Genet Cytogenet 1998; 106(1):30–36.

283. Palanisamy N, Imanishi Y, Rao PH, et al. Novel chromosomal abnormalities identified by comparative genomic hybridization in parathyroid adenomas. J Clin Endocrinol Metab 1998; 83(5):1766–1770.

284. Schachter PP, Ayesh S, Matouk I, et al. Differential expression of kinase genes in primary hyperparathyroidism: adenoma versus normal and hyperplastic parathyroid tissue. Arch Pathol Lab Med 2007; 131(1):126–130.

285. Mallya SM, Gallagher JJ, Arnold A. Analysis of microsatellite instability in sporadic parathyroid adenomas. J Clin Endocrinol Metab 2003; 88(3):1248–1251.

286. Cetani F, Pinchera A, Pardi E, et al. No evidence for mutations in the calcium-sensing receptor gene in sporadic parathyroid adenomas. J Bone Miner Res 1999; 14(6):878–882.

287. Samander EH, Arnold A. Mutational analysis of the vitamin D receptor does not support its candidacy as a tumor suppressor gene in parathyroid adenomas. J Clin Endocrinol Metab 2006; 91(12):5019–5021.

288. Shattuck TM, Costa J, Bernstein M, et al. Mutational analysis of Smad3, a candidate tumor suppressor implicated in TGF-beta and menin pathways, in parathyroid adenomas and enteropancreatic endocrine tumors. J Clin Endocrinol Metab 2002; 87(8):3911–3914.

289. Uchino S, Noguchi S, Nagatomo M, et al. Absence of somatic RET gene mutation in sporadic parathyroid tumors and hyperplasia secondary to uremia, and absence of somatic Men1 gene mutation in MEN2A-associated hyperplasia. Biomed Pharmacother 2000; 54(suppl 1):100s–103s.

290. Kytola S, Farnebo F, Obara T, et al. Patterns of chromosomal imbalances in parathyroid carcinomas. Am J Pathol 2000; 157(2):579–586.

291. Shattuck TM, Valimaki S, Obara T, et al. Somatic and germ-line mutations of the HRPT2 gene in sporadic parathyroid carcinoma. N Engl J Med 2003; 349(18):1722–1729.

292. Howell VM, Haven CJ, Kahnoski K, et al. HRPT2 mutations are associated with malignancy in sporadic parathyroid tumours. J Med Genet 2003; 40(9):657–663.

293. Cetani F, Pardi E, Viacava P, et al. A reappraisal of the Rb1 gene abnormalities in the diagnosis of parathyroid cancer. Clin Endocrinol (Oxf) 2004; 60(1):99–106.

294. Hunt JL, Carty SE, Yim JH, et al. Allelic loss in parathyroid neoplasia can help characterize malignancy. Am J Surg Pathol 2005; 29(8):1049–1055.

295. Black WC, Haff RC. The surgical pathology of parathyroid chief cell hyperplasia. Am J Clin Pathol 1970; 53(5):565–579.

296. Malmaeus J, Grimelius L, Johansson H, et al. Parathyroid pathology in hyperparathyroidism secondary to chronic renal failure. Scand J Urol Nephrol 1984; 18(2):157–166.

297. Takagi H, Tominaga Y, Uchida K, et al. Polymorphism of parathyroid glands in patients with chronic renal failure and secondary hyperparathyroidism. Endocrinol Jpn 1983; 30(4):463–468.

298. Debruyne F, Ostyn F, Delaere P. Weight characteristics of the parathyroid glands in renal hyperparathyroidism. Head Neck 2000; 22(5):509–512.

299. Roth SI, Marshall RB. Pathology and ultrastructure of the human parathyroid glands in chronic renal failure. Arch Intern Med 1969; 124(4):397–407.

300. Tezelman S, Shen W, Shaver JK, et al. Double parathyroid adenomas. Clinical and biochemical characteristics before and after parathyroidectomy. Ann Surg 1993; 218(3):300–307 (discussion 307–309).

301. Milas M, Wagner K, Easley KA, et al. Double adenomas revisited: nonuniform distribution favors enlarged superior parathyroids (fourth pouch disease). Surgery 2003; 134(6):995–1003 (discussion 1003–1004).

302. Straus FH, 2nd, Kaplan EL, Nishiyama RH, et al. Five cases of parathyroid lipohyperplasia. Surgery 1983; 94(6):901–905.

303. Yamauchi M, Sugimoto T, Yamaguchi T, et al. Familial hypocalciuric hypercalcemia caused by an R648stop mutation in the calcium-sensing receptor gene. J Bone Miner Res 2002; 17(12):2174–2182.

304. Ambrogini E, Cetani F, Cianferotti L, et al. Surgery or surveillance for mild asymptomatic primary hyperparathyroidism: a prospective, randomized clinical trial. J Clin Endocrinol Metab 2007; 92(8):3114–3121.

305. Pasieka JL, Parsons LL, Demeure MJ, et al. Patient-based surgical outcome tool demonstrating alleviation of symptoms following parathyroidectomy in patients with primary hyperparathyroidism. World J Surg 2002; 26(8):942–949.

306. Talpos GB, Bone HG, 3rd, Kleerekoper M, et al. Randomized trial of parathyroidectomy in mild asymptomatic primary hyperparathyroidism: patient description and effects on the SF-36 health survey. Surgery 2000; 128(6):1013–1020 (discussion 1020–1011).

307. Mollerup CL, Vestergaard P, Frokjaer VG, et al. Risk of renal stone events in primary hyperparathyroidism before and after parathyroid surgery: controlled retrospective follow up study. BMJ 2002; 325(7368):807.

308. Silverberg SJ, Shane E, Jacobs TP, et al. A 10-year prospective study of primary hyperparathyroidism with or without parathyroid surgery. N Engl J Med 1999; 341(17):1249–1255.

309. Vestergaard P, Mosekilde L. Fractures in patients with primary hyperparathyroidism: nationwide follow-up study of 1201 patients. World J Surg 2003; 27(3):343–349.

310. Hedback G, Oden A, Tisell LE. The influence of surgery on the risk of death in patients with primary hyperparathyroidism. World J Surg 1991; 15(3):399–405 (discussion 406–397).

311. Hedback G, Tisell LE, Bengtsson BA, et al. Premature death in patients operated on for primary hyperparathyroidism. World J Surg 1990; 14(6):829–835 (discussion 836).

312. Palmer M, Adami HO, Bergstrom R, et al. Survival and renal function in untreated hypercalcaemia. Population-based cohort study with 14 years of follow-up. Lancet 1987; 1(8524):59–62.

313. van Heerden JA, Grant CS. Surgical treatment of primary hyperparathyroidism: an institutional perspective. World J Surg 1991; 15(6):688–692.

314. Low RA, Katz AD. Parathyroidectomy via bilateral cervical exploration: a retrospective review of 866 cases. Head Neck 1998; 20(7):583–587.

315. Kaplan EL, Yashiro T, Salti G. Primary hyperparathyroidism in the 1990s. Choice of surgical procedures for this disease. Ann Surg 1992; 215(4):300–317.

316. Schell SR, Dudley NE. Clinical outcomes and fiscal consequences of bilateral neck exploration for primary idiopathic hyperparathyroidism without preoperative radionuclide imaging or minimally invasive techniques. Surgery 2003; 133(1):32–39.

317. Norman J, Chheda H, Farrell C. Minimally invasive parathyroidectomy for primary hyperparathyroidism: decreasing operative time and potential complications while improving cosmetic results. Am Surg 1998; 64(5):391–395 (discussion 395–396).

318. Inabnet WB, 3rd, Kim CK, Haber RS, et al. Radioguidance is not necessary during parathyroidectomy. Arch Surg 2002; 137(8):967–970.

319. Grant CS, Thompson G, Farley D, et al. Primary hyperparathyroidism surgical management since the introduction of minimally invasive parathyroidectomy: Mayo Clinic experience. Arch Surg 2005; 140(5):472–478 (discussion 478–479).

320. Bergenfelz A, Lindblom P, Tibblin S, et al. Unilateral versus bilateral neck exploration for primary hyperparathyroidism: a prospective randomized controlled trial. Ann Surg 2002; 236(5):543–551.

321. Aarum S, Nordenstrom J, Reihner E, et al. Operation for primary hyperparathyroidism: the new versus the old order. A randomised controlled trial of preoperative localisation. Scand J Surg 2007; 96(1):26–30.

322. Russell CF, Dolan SJ, Laird JD. Randomized clinical trial comparing scan-directed unilateral versus bilateral cervical exploration for primary hyperparathyroidism due to solitary adenoma. Br J Surg 2006; 93(4):418–421.

323. Miccoli P, Berti P, Materazzi G, et al. Endoscopic bilateral neck exploration versus quick intraoperative parathormone assay (qPTHa) during endoscopic parathyroidectomy: A prospective randomized trial. Surg Endosc 2008; 22(2):398–400.

324. Beyer TD, Solorzano CC, Starr F, et al. Parathyroidectomy outcomes according to operative approach. Am J Surg 2007; 193(3):368–372 (discussion 372–363).

325. Weigel TL, Murphy J, Kabbani L, et al. Radioguided thoracoscopic mediastinal parathyroidectomy with intraoperative parathyroid hormone testing. Ann Thorac Surg 2005; 80(4):1262–1265.

326. Lee PK, Jarosek SL, Virnig BA, et al. Trends in the incidence and treatment of parathyroid cancer in the United States. Cancer 2007; 109(9):1736–1741.

327. Eknoyan G, Levin A, Levin NW. National Kidney Foundation: Bone metabolism and disease in chronic kidney disease. Am J Kidney Dis 2004; 42(S3):S1–S202.

328. Kim J, Pisoni RL, Danese MD. Achievement of proposed NKF-K/DOQI bone metabolism and disease guidelines: results from the Dialysis Outcomes and Practice Patterns Study (DOPPS). J Am Soc Nephrol 2003; 14(14):269A–270A.

329. Walters BAJ, Danese MD, Kim JJ, et al. Patient prevalence within proposed NKF-K/DOQI guidelines for bone metabolism and disease. J Am Soc Nephrol 2003; 14:473A–474A.

330. Block GA, Martin KJ, de Francisco AL, et al. Cinacalcet for secondary hyperparathyroidism in patients receiving hemodialysis. N Engl J Med 2004; 350(15):1516–1525.

331. Strippoli GFM, Tong A, Palmer SC, et al. Calcimimetics for secondary hyperparathyroidism in chronic kidney disease patients. Cochrane Database Syst Rev 2006; 4:CD006254.

332. Kestenbaum B, Andress DL, Schwartz SM, et al. Survival following parathyroidectomy among United States dialysis patients. Kidney Int 2004; 66(5):2010–2016.

333. Gasparri G, Camandona M, Abbona GC, et al. Secondary and tertiary hyperparathyroidism: causes of recurrent disease after 446 parathyroidectomies. Ann Surg 2001; 233(1):65–69.

334. Dotzenrath C, Cupisti K, Goretzki E, et al. Operative treatment of renal autonomous hyperparathyroidism: cause of persistent or recurrent disease in 304 patients. Langenbecks Arch Surg 2003; 387(9–10):348–354.

335. Nichol PF, Starling JR, Mack E, et al. Long-term follow-up of patients with tertiary hyperparathyroidism treated by resection of a single or double adenoma. Ann Surg 2002; 235(5):673–678 (discussion 678–680).

336. Nichol PF, Mack E, Bianco J, et al. Radioguided parathyroidectomy in patients with secondary and tertiary hyperparathyroidism. Surgery 2003; 134(4):713–717 (discussion 717–719).

337. Triponez F, Kebebew E, Dosseh D, et al. Less-than-subtotal parathyroidectomy increases the risk of persistent/recurrent hyperparathyroidism after parathyroidectomy in tertiary hyperparathyroidism after renal transplantation. Surgery 2006; 140(6):990–997 (discussion 997–999).

338. Ujiki MB, Nayar R, Sturgeon C, et al. Parathyroid cyst: often mistaken for a thyroid cyst. World J Surg 2007; 31(1):60–64.

339. Clark OH. Parathyroid cysts. Am J Surg 1978; 135(3): 395–402.

340. Rosenberg J, Orlando R, 3rd, Ludwig M, et al. Parathyroid cysts. Am J Surg 1982; 143(4):473–480.

341. Nguyen Q, deTar M, Wells W, et al. Cervical thymic cyst: case reports and review of the literature. Laryngoscope 1996; 106(3 Pt 1):247–252.

342. Rea PA, Hartley BE, Bailey CM. Third and fourth branchial pouch anomalies. J Laryngol Otol 2004; 118(1):19–24.

343. Fortson JK, Patel VG, Henderson VJ. Parathyroid cysts: a case report and review of the literature. Laryngoscope 2001; 111(10):1726–1728.

344. Marx SJ, Attie MF, Levine MA, et al. The hypocalciuric or benign variant of familial hypercalcemia: clinical and biochemical features in fifteen kindreds. Medicine (Baltimore) 1981; 60(6):397–412.

345. Marx SJ, Spiegel AM, Brown EM, et al. Divalent cation metabolism. Familial hypocalciuric hypercalcemia versus typical primary hyperparathyroidism. Am J Med 1978; 65 (2):235–242.

346. Marx SJ, Stock JL, Attie MF, et al. Familial hypocalciuric hypercalcemia: recognition among patients referred after unsuccessful parathyroid exploration. Ann Intern Med 1980; 92(3):351–356.

347. Stuckey BG, Gutteridge DH, Kent GN, et al. Familial hypocalciuric hypercalcaemia and pancreatitis: no causal link proven. Aust N Z J Med 1990; 20(5):718–719, 725.

348. Heath H, 3rd. Familial benign (hypocalciuric) hypercalcemia. A troublesome mimic of mild primary hyperparathyroidism. Endocrinol Metab Clin North Am 1989; 18 (3):723–740.

349. Herfarth KK, Wells SA, Jr. Parathyroid glands and the multiple endocrine neoplasia syndromes and familial hypocalciuric hypercalcemia. Semin Surg Oncol 1997; 13 (2):114–124.

350. Law WM, Jr., Carney JA, Heath H, 3rd. Parathyroid glands in familial benign hypercalcemia (familial hypocalciuric hypercalcemia). Am J Med 1984; 76(6):1021–1026.

351. Thorgeirsson U, Costa J, Marx SJ. The parathyroid glands in familial hypocalciuric hypercalcemia. Hum Pathol 1981; 12(3):229–237.

352. Lyons TJ, Crookes PF, Postlethwaite W, et al. Familial hypocalciuric hypercalcaemia as a differential diagnosis of hyperparathyroidism: studies in a large kindred and a review of surgical experience in the condition. Br J Surg 1986; 73(3):188–192.

353. Fukumoto S, Chikatsu N, Okazaki R, et al. Inactivating mutations of calcium-sensing receptor results in parathyroid lipohyperplasia. Diagn Mol Pathol 2001; 10(4):242–247.

354. Schwartz SR, Futran ND. Hypercalcemic hypocalciuria: a critical differential diagnosis for hyperparathyroidism. Otolaryngol Clin North Am 2004; 37(4):887–896, xi.

355. Pollak MR, Brown EM, Chou YH, et al. Mutations in the human Ca(2+)-sensing receptor gene cause familial hypocalciuric hypercalcemia and neonatal severe hyperparathyroidism. Cell 1993; 75(7):1297–1303.

356. Pidasheva S, D'Souza-Li L, Canaff L, et al. CASRdb: calcium-sensing receptor locus-specific database for mutations causing familial (benign) hypocalciuric hypercalcemia, neonatal severe hyperparathyroidism, and autosomal dominant hypocalcemia. Hum Mutat 2004; 24(2): 107–111.

357. Arnalsteen L, Quievreux JL, Huglo D, et al. Reoperation for persistent or recurrent primary hyperparathyroidism. Seventy-seven cases among 1888 operated patients. Ann Chir 2004; 129(4):224–231.

358. Hillman DA, Scriver CR, Pedvis S, et al. Neonatal Familial Primary Hyperparathyroidism. N Engl J Med 1964; 270:483–490.

359. Marx SJ, Fraser D, Rapoport A. Familial hypocalciuric hypercalcemia. Mild expression of the gene in heterozygotes and severe expression in homozygotes. Am J Med 1985; 78(1):15–22.

360. Chattopadhyay N, Brown EM. Role of calcium-sensing receptor in mineral ion metabolism and inherited disorders of calcium-sensing. Mol Genet Metab 2006; 89(3): 189–202.

361. Doria AS, Huang C, Makitie O, et al. Neonatal, severe primary hyperparathyroidism: a 7-year clinical and radiological follow-up of one patient. Pediatr Radiol 2002; 32 (9):684–689.

362. D'Souza-Li L. The calcium-sensing receptor and related diseases. Arq Bras Endocrinol Metabol 2006; 50(4): 628–639.

363. Silverthorn KG, Houston CS, Duncan BP. Murk Jansen's metaphyseal chondrodysplasia with long-term followup. Pediatr Radiol 1987; 17(2):119–123.

364. Pearce SH, Trump D, Wooding C, et al. Calcium-sensing receptor mutations in familial benign hypercalcemia and neonatal hyperparathyroidism. J Clin Invest 1995; 96 (6):2683–2692.

365. Hendy GN, D'Souza-Li L, Yang B, et al. Mutations of the calcium-sensing receptor (CASR) in familial hypocalciuric hypercalcemia, neonatal severe hyperparathyroidism, and autosomal dominant hypocalcemia. Hum Mutat 2000; 16(4):281–296.

366. Chikatsu N, Fukumoto S, Suzawa M, et al. An adult patient with severe hypercalcaemia and hypocalciuria due to a novel homozygous inactivating mutation of calcium-sensing receptor. Clin Endocrinol (Oxf) 1999; 50 (4):537–543.

367. Awad SS, Miskulin J, Thompson N. Parathyroid adenomas versus four-gland hyperplasia as the cause of primary hyperparathyroidism in patients with prolonged lithium therapy. World J Surg 2003; 27(4):486–488.

368. Bendz H, Sjodin I, Toss G, et al. Hyperparathyroidism and long-term lithium therapy–a cross-sectional study and the effect of lithium withdrawal. J Intern Med 1996; 240(6):357–365.

369. Presne C, Fakhouri F, Noel LH, et al. Lithium-induced nephropathy: Rate of progression and prognostic factors. Kidney Int 2003; 64(2):585–592.

370. Sloand JA, Shelly MA. Normalization of lithium-induced hypercalcemia and hyperparathyroidism with cinacalcet hydrochloride. Am J Kidney Dis 2006; 48(5):832–837.

371. Hundley JC, Woodrum DT, Saunders BD, et al. Revisiting lithium-associated hyperparathyroidism in the era of intraoperative parathyroid hormone monitoring. Surgery 2005; 138(6):1027–1031 (discussion 1031–1022).

372. Birnbaum J, Klandorf H, Giuliano A, et al. Lithium stimulates the release of human parathyroid hormone in vitro. J Clin Endocrinol Metab 1988; 66(6):1187–1191.

373. Lions C, Precloux P, Burckard E, et al. Important hypercalcaemia due to hyperparathyroidism induced by lithium. Ann Fr Anesth Reanim 2005; 24(3):270–273.

374. Hristkova EN, Henry JB. Metabolic intermediates, inorganic ions and biochemical markers of bone metabolism. In: Henry JB, ed. Clinical diagnosis and management by laboratory methods. 20th ed ed. Philadelphia: W.B. Saunders, 2001:180–210.

375. Dufour DR, Marx SJ, Spiegel AM. Parathyroid gland morphology in nonparathyroid hormone-mediated hypercalcemia. Am J Surg Pathol 1985; 9(1):43–51.

376. Marx SJ. Hyperparathyroid and hypoparathyroid disorders. N Engl J Med 2000; 343(25):1863–1875.

377. Wurdak H, Ittner LM, Sommer L. DiGeorge syndrome and pharyngeal apparatus development. Bioessays 2006; 28(11):1078–1086.

378. Thakker RV, Davies KE, Whyte MP, et al. Mapping the gene causing X-linked recessive idiopathic hypoparathyroidism to Xq26-Xq27 by linkage studies. J Clin Invest 1990; 86(1):40–45.

379. Sticht H, Hashemolhosseini S. A common structural mechanism underlying GCMB mutations that cause hypoparathyroidism. Med Hypotheses 2006; 67(3): 482–487.

380. Nesbit MA, Bowl MR, Harding B, et al. Characterization of GATA3 mutations in the hypoparathyroidism, deafness, and renal dysplasia (HDR) syndrome. J Biol Chem 2004; 279(21):22624–22634.

381. Parvari R, Hershkovitz E, Grossman N, et al. Mutation of TBCE causes hypoparathyroidism-retardation-dysmorphism and autosomal recessive Kenny-Caffey syndrome. Nat Genet 2002; 32(3):448–452.

382. Vogel A, Strassburg CP, Obermayer-Straub P, et al. The genetic background of autoimmune polyendocrinopathy-candidiasis-ectodermal dystrophy and its autoimmune disease components. J Mol Med 2002; 80(4):201–211.

383. Goswami R, Brown EM, Kochupillai N, et al. Prevalence of calcium sensing receptor autoantibodies in patients with sporadic idiopathic hypoparathyroidism. Eur J Endocrinol 2004; 150(1):9–18.

384. Gavalas NG, Kemp EH, Krohn KJ, et al. The calcium-sensing receptor is a target of autoantibodies in patients with autoimmune polyendocrine syndrome type 1. J Clin Endocrinol Metab 2007; 92(6):2107–2114.

385. Sunthornthepvarakul T, Churesigaew S, Ngowngarmratana S. A novel mutation of the signal peptide of the preproparathyroid hormone gene associated with autosomal recessive familial isolated hypoparathyroidism. J Clin Endocrinol Metab 1999; 84(10):3792–3796.

386. Weinstein LS, Liu J, Sakamoto A, et al. Minireview: GNAS: normal and abnormal functions. Endocrinology 2004; 145(12):5459–5464.

387. Steinberg H, Waldron BR. Idiopathic hypoparathyroidism; an analysis of fifty-two cases, including the report of a new case. Medicine (Baltimore) 1952; 31(2):133–154.

388. Chen EM, Mishkin FS. Parathyroid hyperplasia may be missed by double-phase Tc-99m sestamibi scintigraphy alone. Clin Nucl Med 1997; 22(4):222–226.

389. Trump D, Dixon PH, Mumm S, et al. Localisation of X linked recessive idiopathic hypoparathyroidism to a 1.5 Mb region on Xq26-q27. J Med Genet 1998; 35(11):905–909.

390. Ali A, Christie PT, Grigorieva IV, et al. Functional characterization of GATA3 mutations causing the hypoparathyroidism-deafness-renal (HDR) dysplasia syndrome: insight into mechanisms of DNA binding by the GATA3 transcription factor. Hum Mol Genet 2007; 16(3):265–275.

391. Yeh GL, Mathur S, Wivel A, et al. GNAS1 mutation and Cbfa1 misexpression in a child with severe congenital platelike osteoma cutis. J Bone Miner Res 2000; 15 (11):2063–2073.

392. Nawrot I, Wozniewicz B, Tolloczko T, et al. Allotransplantation of cultured parathyroid progenitor cells without immunosuppression: clinical results. Transplantation 2007; 83(6):734–740.

393. Winer KK, Ko CW, Reynolds JC, et al. Long-term treatment of hypoparathyroidism: a randomized controlled study comparing parathyroid hormone-(1–34) versus calcitriol and calcium. J Clin Endocrinol Metab 2003; 88 (9):4214–4220.

394. Horwitz CA, Myers WP, Foote FW Jr. Secondary malignant tumors of the parathyroid glands. Report of two cases with associated hypoparathyroidism. Am J Med 1972; 52(6):797–808.

395. Mariette X, Khalifa P, Boissonnas A, et al. Hypocalcaemia due to parathyroid metastases. Eur J Med 1993; 2(4):242–244.

396. Kakudo K, Tang W, Ito Y, et al. Parathyroid invasion, nodal recurrence, and lung metastasis by papillary carcinoma of the thyroid. J Clin Pathol 2004; 57(3):245–249.

397. Tang W, Kakudo K, Nakamura MY, et al. Parathyroid gland involvement by papillary carcinoma of the thyroid gland. Arch Pathol Lab Med 2002; 126(12):1511–1514.

398. de la Monte SM, Hutchins GM, Moore GW. Endocrine organ metastases from breast carcinoma. Am J Pathol 1984; 114(1):131–136.

399. Mautalen CA, Kvicala R, Perriard D, et al. Case report: hypoparathyroidism and iron storage disease. Treatment with 25-hydroxy-vitamin D3. Am J Med Sci 1978; 276(3): 363–368.

400. Hui KS, Williams JC, Borit A, et al. The endocrine glands in Pompe's disease. Report of two cases. Arch Pathol Lab Med 1985; 109(10):921–925.

401. Macdonald RA, Mallory GK. Hemochromatosis and hemosiderosis. Study of 211 autopsied cases. Arch Intern Med 1960; 105:686–700.

402. Lahey FH. The transplantation of parathyroids in partial thyroidectomy. Surg Gynecol Obstet 1926; 62:508–509.

403. Wells SA, Jr., Burdick JF, Hattler BG, et al. The allografted parathyroid gland: evaluation of function in the immunosuppressed host. Ann Surg 1974; 180(6):805–813.

404. Wells SA, Jr., Christiansen C. The transplanted parathyroid gland: evaluation of cryopreservation and other environmental factors which affect its function. Surgery 1974; 75(1):49–55.

405. Herrera M, Grant C, van Heerden JA, et al. Parathyroid autotransplantation. Arch Surg 1992; 127(7):825–829 (discussion 829–830).

406. Feldman AL, Sharaf RN, Skarulis MC, et al. Results of heterotopic parathyroid autotransplantation: a 13-year experience. Surgery 1999; 126(6):1042–1048.

407. Cohen MS, Dilley WG, Wells SA Jr., et al. Long-term functionality of cryopreserved parathyroid autografts: a 13-year prospective analysis. Surgery 2005; 138(6):1033–1040 (discussion 1040–1031).

408. Saxe A. Parathyroid transplantation: a review. Surgery 1984; 95(5):507–526.

409. Wells SA, Jr., Farndon JR, Dale JK, et al. Long-term evaluation of patients with primary parathyroid hyperplasia managed by total parathyroidectomy and heterotopic autotransplantation. Ann Surg 1980; 192(4):451–458.

410. Wagner PK, Rumpelt HJ, Krause U, et al. The effect of cryopreservation on hormone secretion in vitro and morphology of human parathyroid tissue. Surgery 1986; 99 (3):257–264.

411. Ulrich F, Steinmuller T, Rayes N, et al. Cryopreserved human parathyroid tissue: cell cultures for in vitro testing of function. Transplant Proc 2001; 33(1–2):666–667.

412. Peters S. http://www.pathologyinnovations.com/frozen_section_technique.htm. (accessed 2007).

23

Pathology of Selected Skin Lesions of the Head and Neck

Kim M. Hiatt, Shayesteh Pashaei, and Bruce R. Smoller
*Department of Pathology, University of Arkansas for Medical Sciences,
Little Rock, Arkansas, U.S.A.*

I. BENIGN EPITHELIAL NEOPLASMS

A. Seborrheic Keratosis

Synonym: stucco keratosis.

Clinical Features

Seborrheic keratoses (SKs) are common benign cutaneous neoplasms seen most frequently in adults and the elderly without a gender predilection. With the exception of palms, soles, and mucosal surfaces, SKs may be seen on any site. They present as scaly, greasy, raised growths that range from several millimeters to a centimeter in diameter and are described as having a "stuck-on" appearance, suggesting that they could be simply lifted from the surrounding skin. Many SKs are hyperpigmented, occasionally causing some difficulty in distinction from primary cutaneous melanoma. The variant known as stucco keratosis tends to occur more commonly as verrucous plaques on the extremities. Multiple small SKs may be seen on the face, in particular, the cheeks of dark-skinned patients. This condition, referred to as dermatosis papulosis nigra, is seen twice as frequently in women than in men. Inverted follicular keratosis has been considered a variant of an irritated SK. Recent research shows distinct antigenic expression, which may ultimate in classifying these lesions as distinct entities (1,2).

Imaging

As SKs are benign and not believed to undergo malignant transformation, imaging studies are not required in the diagnosis and treatment of this neoplasm. The surface features of SKs gives them a unique pattern, referred to as "fat fingers" on dermoscopy, and has been helpful clinically in distinguishing pigmented SKs from melanoma (3).

Histologic Features

While there are many histologic variants of SK, each of these shares certain basic histologic characteristics. Each variant demonstrates acanthosis with an expansion of the basaloid keratinocytes, overlying hyperkeratosis without parakeratosis, an abrupt transition from normal adjacent epidermis and a flat horizontal base to the lesion (Fig. 1). The basaloid keratinocytes are uniform in size and appearance and have bland cytologic features. Other variants demonstrate a reticulated growth pattern (Fig. 2) showing numerous interlacing strands of basaloid cells extending from the overlying epidermis, or small intraepidermal basaloid "clones" (Fig. 3), but no atypical keratinocytes. In the so-called clonal variant of SK, foci of parakeratosis may be present overlying the clones of basaloid keratinocytes. Cytologic atypia is present only in very irritated SKs. Except when irritated or markedly inflamed, mitoses are scant. Atypical mitoses are not seen. In most types of SKs, there is a very flat base to the lesion with underlying papillary dermal fibrosis. Some SKs have a papillomatous growth pattern, the stucco keratoses (Fig. 4), while in others the surface is relatively smooth. Hyperpigmentation of basal keratinocytes is variably present. The SKs with concomitant banal-appearing melanocytic proliferations are sometimes designated as melanoacanthomas. A histologic variant with basilar clear cells, mimicking melanoma, has also been described (4). The keratinocytes in SKs may take on spindle-shaped morphology. This is most common when there is marked inflammation and irritation. Focal parakeratosis and spongiosis may also be present in this situation. These commonly described histologic patterns, namely, acanthotic, reticulated, clonal, papillomatous, irritated, and melanoacanthoma, are of interest only in so much as one is able to recognize the pattern to make the diagnosis. The histologic features of dermatosis papulosis nigra cannot be distinguished from other SKs. Clinical implications are not imparted in diagnosing any of the variants.

Immunohistochemistry

Immunohistochemical studies are not required to make a diagnosis of SK. Research has demonstrated that the neoplastic cells express keratins 5 and 14, similar to the normal keratin expression of basal keratinocytes.

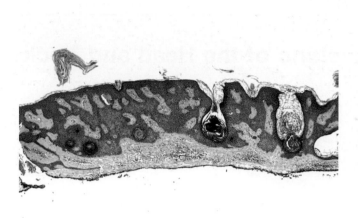

Figure 1 Seborrheic keratosis. There is expansion of basaloid keratinocytes that are uniform in size and have bland cytologic features. The epidermis is acanthotic with overlying hyperkeratosis, no parakeratosis, and a flat horizontal base to the lesion.

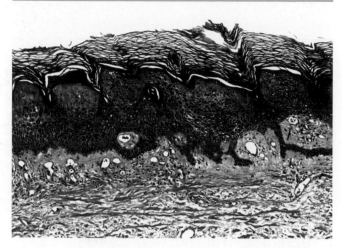

Figure 3 Seborrheic keratosis, clonal. The epidermis has small intraepidermal basaloid "clones." Foci of parakeratosis may be present overlying these clones. Horn cysts are also present.

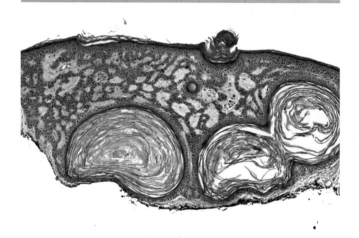

Figure 2 Seborrheic keratosis, reticulated. The epidermis has numerous interlacing strands of basaloid cells extending from the overlying epidermis and enveloping several horn cysts.

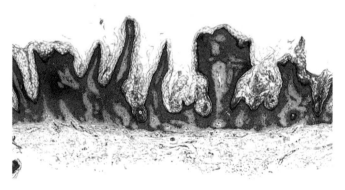

Figure 4 Seborrheic keratosis, stucco keratosis. The epidermis is mildly acanthotic with a papillomatous growth pattern.

Differential Diagnosis

The histologic differential diagnosis includes epidermal nevus, verruca vulgaris, and less commonly, eccrine poroma and squamous cell carcinoma in situ (SCCIS). Epidermal nevi are histologically identical to SKs and can only be distinguished on the basis of a clinical history of appearance during early childhood (as opposed to SKs that are growths associated with middle to later life). Verruca vulgaris can sometimes be distinguished on the basis of the presence of overlying columns of parakeratosis, clumping of keratohyaline granules, and dilated vessels within the papillary dermal tips. Papillary dermal fibrosis and horn cysts are not usually seen in verruca vulgaris. In other cases, such a distinction may be virtually impossible. Eccrine poromas demonstrate a similar growth pattern but are characterized by the presence of small intraepithelial ducts and by the absence of horn cysts. Further, vascular ectasia within the dermis and reduplicated basement membrane, resulting in foci of eosinophilic "hyaline," are seen in poromas, but not in SKs. Cytologic atypia that characterizes SCCIS is only present in markedly inflamed and irritated SKs, in which case, differentiation can be quite difficult. Care should be taken not to overcall carcinoma in cases with brisk, destructive inflammatory infiltrates. This is especially difficult when there is a spindle cell configuration to the neoplastic keratinocytes in the setting of mitotic activity and marked inflammation. However, true cytologic atypia and pleomorphism are not present in SKs, in contrast to squamous cell carcinomas (SCCs).

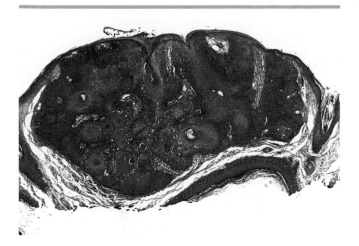

Figure 5 Inverted follicular keratosis. There is an endophytic growth pattern with a central, keratin-filled dell and abundant squamous eddies toward the periphery of the dermal nodule.

Inverted follicular keratosis may also show a marked similarity to SK. Some investigators believe these lesions to be variants of SK; the distinction is not a clinically important one. Inverted follicular keratoses are characterized by an invaginated growth pattern with a central, keratin-filled dell and abundant squamous eddies (Fig. 5). While squamous eddies may be seen in very inflamed and irritated SKs, they do not demonstrate the same architectural features as are seen in inverted follicular keratoses.

Associated Syndromes

The rapid eruption of numerous SKs has been associated with internal malignancies in a syndrome known as Leser-Trelat. This is a very controversial syndrome. Those who believe it exists suggest that the SKs represent a paraneoplastic process, perhaps induced by epidermal growth factor (or other growth factors) in a manner analogous to the onset of acanthosis nigricans in patients with certain carcinomas.

Treatment and Prognosis

SKs do not require any medical treatment. In some cases, they are removed with simple shave excisional biopsies for cosmetic reasons. In other situations, the clinical resemblance to malignant melanoma results in a surgical excision to exclude the latter condition. These are benign tumors, with no tendency for infiltrative growth or metastasis and only a slight chance for local recurrence if not fully excised.

B. Pilar Cyst

Synonyms: trichilemmal cyst and isthmus-catagen cyst.

Introduction

Ninety percent of pilar cysts (PCs) occur on the scalp, often as multiple lesions, with a small percentage also developing on the face, trunk, or extremities. There is a strong female predominance with an autosomal dominant inheritance pattern (2). PCs are solitary in only 30% of cases, with 10% having more than 10 cysts (3).

PC walls recapitulate outer root sheath epithelium at the level of the isthmus.

Clinical Features

PCs are solitary or multiple intradermal or subcutaneous lesions with firm and smooth cyst walls containing semisolid, cheesy, and keratin material. Clinically, PCs can be misdiagnosed as epidermal/infundibular cysts. However, they differ from the latter not only by the fact that they are easily excised and lack a punctum but also by their distribution. PCs are almost exclusively on the scalp, whereas epidermal inclusion cysts are more commonly on the face and trunk. The sharp circumscription enables easy, complete excision.

Imaging

As benign and almost exclusively dermal proliferations, imaging studies are rarely necessary.

Pathology

PCs arise from the isthmus of anagen hairs, an area where the inner root sheath is absent. They are lined by stratified squamous epithelium showing trichilemmal keratinization in which the individual cells increase in size toward the lumen, at which point there is an abrupt transition to homogeneous, compact, eosinophilic keratotic material (Fig. 6). This transition from keratinocyte to keratin, without granular cell formation, is trichilemmal keratinization, and characterizes follicular isthmus-type keratinization. Calcification and cholesterol clefts may also be seen within the luminal

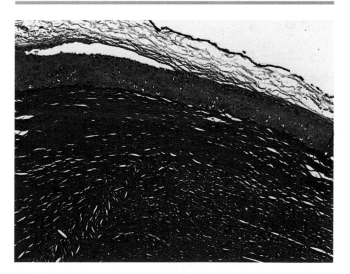

Figure 6 Pilar cyst. The cyst is lined by stratified squamous epithelium in which the individual cells increase in size toward the lumen, at which point there is an abrupt transition, without a granular cell layer, to homogeneous, compact, eosinophilic keratotic material.

keratin. Cysts showing combined isthmus and infundibular keratinization patterns are called hybrid cysts, as originally described. However, the use of this term has evolved to encompass cysts with any combination of histologic patterns to additionally include pilomatrical, vellus hair cyst, and steatocystoma (5).

Immunohistochemistry

Although not necessary for diagnostic purposes, immunohistochemical studies demonstrate expression of both cytokeratins (CKs) 5 and 6 in 97% of neoplasms of cutaneous adnexae (6). Expression of CK 10 and 17, similar to steatocystoma, has also been reported (7).

Electron Microscopy

Ultrastructural examination of the epithelial lining of PC shows that the epithelial cells have an increasing number of cytoplasmic filaments from periphery to the luminal aspect of cysts. Despite the absence of a granular cell layer, a few small keratohyaline granules are seen in addition to spherical particles with lipid droplets and desmosomal structures (8). There is loss of all cytoplasmic organelles in the anucleate lining cells.

Molecular-Genetic Data

An autosomal dominant inheritance pattern has been suggested (9), and more recently, the gene locus for these hereditary PCs has been localized to a chromosome 3p10 gene, termed "TRICY1" (10).

Differential Diagnosis

None of the other cystic structures that may enter into the histologic differential diagnosis show the abrupt keratinization of a PC. Accordingly, the diagnosis is typically without dilemma. A proliferating PC shows significantly more acanthotic epithelial lining with keratinocyte atypia, as described below.

Treatment and Prognosis

Excision is the treatment of choice for PCs. They typically "deliver" themselves through an incision without rupture more easily than do epidermal cysts. PCs are associated with minimal morbidity and no mortality.

C. Proliferating Pilar Cyst

Synonyms: proliferating tricholemmal cyst, proliferating tricholemmal tumor, and proliferating follicular-cystic neoplasm.

Introduction

Proliferating pilar cyst (PPC) is a lesion showing features similar to PC, along with a proliferative epithelium with variable cytologic atypia and mitoses that can be so extreme as to resemble SCC. The malignant potential of PPC is controversial because of the lack of a significant number of case reports of

lesions with clinically malignant behavior. However, it is generally agreed that the classic PPC, which is a well-circumscribed dermal nodule on the scalp and lacking prominent cytologic atypia, is a benign lesion. While cytologic atypia alone does not confer malignant behavior (11), it has been suggested that those lesions that are greater than 5 cm, in an atypical location, with recent rapid growth, and histologically have an infiltrative pattern with numerous mitoses in addition to significant cytologic atypia, be classified as malignant (12).

Clinical Features

PPCs are slow-growing lobulated dermal tumors that present in adults, have a female predominance, and are typically located on the scalp. The mean size at presentation is 3.5 cm, but can be as large as 16 cm (12). Ulceration, in particular with a report of recent growth, is also seen. Recurrence after incomplete excision is not uncommon.

Imaging

Imaging studies are generally not necessary. However, should imaging be performed for other reasons, as is more often the case, computer tomography (CT) scans will reveal rim-enhancing soft tissue masses, with or without cyst formation. When cystic, it tends to be a complex cyst. Intralesional mineralization can be detected by this procedure (13).

Pathology

PPCs are circumscribed lobular dermal tumors that may show extension into the subcutaneous tissue. They are composed of intermediate-sized keratinocytes that show the same outer root sheath differentiation with central tricholemmal keratinization as is seen in PC (Fig. 7). PPC additionally shows a

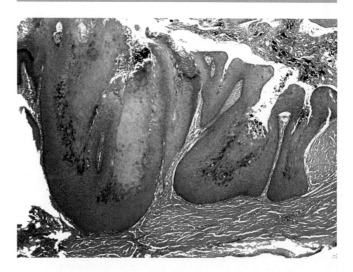

Figure 7 Proliferating pilar cyst. This is a well-circumscribed, lobular, dermal-based lesion showing abrupt keratinization on the luminal suface and a proliferative, but not infiltrating, epithelium.

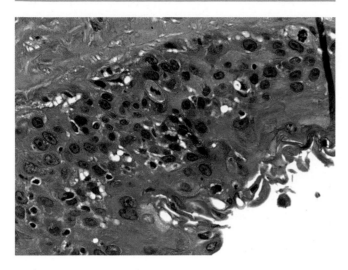

Figure 8 Proliferating pilar cyst. The proliferative epithelial component in this specimen shows focal cytologic atypia and mitoses, resembling squamous cell carcinoma.

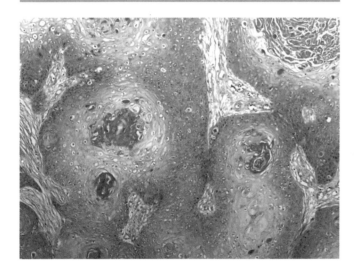

Figure 9 Proliferating pilar cyst. The cyst lining shows proliferative epithelium with squamous eddies and apoptotic cells.

proliferative epithelial component with variable cytologic atypia and mitoses, generally less than 2 in 10 high-power fields (HPFs), which can be striking in some foci, resembling SCC (Fig. 8) (12). Squamous eddies and apoptotic cells may be present as well (Fig. 9).

Stratification of histologic features to determine lesions with benign behavior and locally aggressive and metastatic potential has been proposed (14). On the basis of this proposal, metastatic potential is determined by the presence of an invasive growth pattern, marked nuclear atypia, atypical mitotic forms, and geographic necrosis. An additional report of five cases includes large size (>5 cm), atypical location,

and history of recent growth as clinical features of malignancy (12). Consistent among these reports of metastasizing PPCs are lesions with an infiltrative growth pattern and striking cytologic atypia and mitoses; those without an infiltrative growth pattern but in which foci of striking cytologic atypia and mitoses should be regarded with caution and considered as having malignant potential, and all others, i.e., those lacking invasion, cytologic atypia, and numerous mitoses, are best classified as benign.

Immunohistochemistry

Evaluation of antigen expression is not typically employed for these lesions and is not helpful in differentiating this from its histologic simulatant. However, as in most neoplasms of cutaneous adnexae, there is expression of CK 5/6.

Electron Microscopy

Electron microscopy is not diagnostically useful.

Molecular-Genetic Data

There have been no reports of a genetic association. One study evaluating argyrophilic nucleolar organizer regions (AgNORs) showed a progressive increase in AgNORs from one per nucleus in PCs to 1.5 to 2 in benign pilar tumors, 2.8 in atypical pilar tumors, and 3.5 in malignant pilar tumors, suggesting, as is indicated in the variable histologic expression, that there is a continuum between benign PCs and pilar tumors with metastatic potential (15).

Differential Diagnosis

The differential diagnosis includes SCC for which PPC may show similar cytologic atypia and mitoses. SCC is not well circumscribed and does not show tricholemmal keratinization as is seen in PPC. Trichilemmal carcinoma (TLC) is an additional consideration as it may be solid or cystic, show outer root sheath differentiation, and show nuclear atypia. TLC is a folliculocentric lesion that will show continuity to the attached epidermis, features not seen in PPC. As there are no reports of metastasizing TLC, the distinction is important.

Treatment and Prognosis

For conventional PPC, complete excision is curative. Recurrences are reported in transected lesions. Close clinical follow-up for lesions with any atypical features is clearly warranted.

D. Pilomatricoma

Synonyms: calcifying epithelioma of Malherbe and pilomatrixoma.

Introduction

Pilomatricoma is a benign neoplasm with differentiation toward the hair follicle matrix. They typically present as a solitary lesion on the head, neck, or upper extremities of patients. There is an equal gender predilection (16). Although they can occur at any age, the majority are diagnosed in the first two decades of life (16,17). Pilomatricomas are usually solitary, but multiple tumors have been described as part of an autosomal dominant disorder and in patients with Turner's syndrome, trisomy 9, and spina bifida (18–21). Pilomatricomas have been reported as a cutaneous presentation of systemic diseases, such as myotonic dystrophy and Gardner's syndrome (22–24), and internal malignancy, in particular colon cancer (25). Familial inheritance of multiple pilomatricomas, in otherwise healthy patients, has also been reported (26,27).

Clinical Features

Pilomatricoma is an asymptomatic, slow-growing, firm nodule measuring between 0.5 and 7.0 cm in diameter, or larger. The skin overlying the lesion can be clinically unremarkable or erythematous and, on stretching, may show the "tent sign," with multiple facets and angles. Occasionally, pilomatricomas may have a bluish surface.

Imaging

As benign and almost exclusively dermal proliferations, imaging studies are rarely necessary.

Pathology

Pilomatricoma is a sharply demarcated, multilobulated dermal mass with a surrounding rim of compressed dermal connective tissue (Fig 10). The lobules consist of variably sized nests of peripherally located basaloid epithelial cells and centrally placed

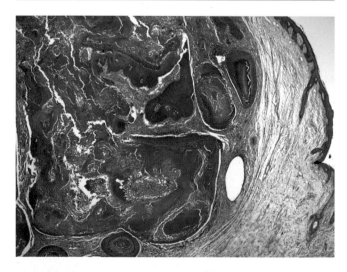

Figure 10 Pilomatricoma. This is a sharply demarcated, multilobulated dermal mass with a surrounding rim of compressed dermal connective tissue. The lobules consist of peripherally located basaloid epithelial cells and centrally placed eosinophilic cellular remnants, referred to as "ghost cells" or "shadow cells."

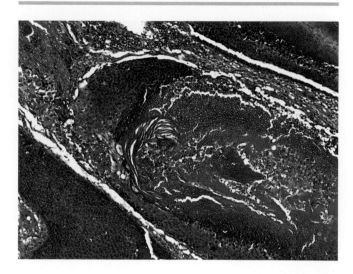

Figure 11 Pilomatricoma. When present, the basophilic cells are usually present at the periphery of nests and have little cytoplasm and hyperchomatic nuclei.

eosinophilic cellular remnants, referred to as "ghost cells" or "shadow cells" (Fig. 11). The eosinophilic cell remnants have abundant cytoplasm and distinct cell borders and have lost their nuclear material. The basophilic cells, which may be absent in 20% of cases and are the predominant cell types in early lesions, are usually present at the periphery of nests and have little cytoplasm and hyperchomatic nuclei (17,28). Mitoses, especially in the early lesions, may be seen. However, atypical mitoses are not characteristic. Between the lobules is fibrous connective tissue intermixed with chronic inflammatory cells (including foreign body giant cells), bone, and, rarely, amyloid (29). Tumors with a predominance of basophilic cells, resembling basal cell carcinoma (BCC), are referred to as proliferating pilomatricomas, a variant necessary to acknowledge because of its higher rate of recurrence (12). Proliferating pilar tumors usually arise in elderly patients (12). Pilomatricomas may arise from an epidermal cyst or a hair follicle. Pilomatricoma-like changes may be seen in the epidermal cysts in Gardner's syndrome (24).

Immunohistochemistry

Immunohistochemistry is usually not used for diagnostic purposes, as the diagnosis is usually made by routine histologic examination. Keratin 15 expression in BCC may be useful in differentiating them from proliferating pilomatricoma, which does not expresss keratin 15 (30).

Electron Microscopy

In pilomatricomas, the cells differentiate and keratinize similar to the cells that form the cortex of the hair. The eosinophilic shadow cells contain cytoplasmic sworls of keratin that surround the nuclear remnants (31).

Molecular-Genetic Data

β-Catenin, an intracellular protein that provides a link between adherens junctions and the actin cytoskeleton and mediates transcriptional activation of target genes such as c-myc and cyclin D1 as part of Wnt/wingless signal transduction pathway (28,32), has been implicated as a key molecule in the molecular pathogenesis of pilomatricoma. Wnt signaling prevents phosphorylation of β-catenin, leading to its cytosolic accumulation. β-Catenin stabilization, caused by truncating mutations in its N-terminus (which prevents phosphorylation), has been shown to result in the formation of pilomatricoma in a mouse model (33). Numerous studies on keratin and gene expression demonstrate that differentiation of pilomatricoma toward the hair matrix involves β-catenin and apoptosis pathways, leading to the formation of shadow cells (34,35).

Differential Diagnosis

Histologically, pilomatricoma should be distinguished from BCC with extensive follicular differentiation. In the former, there is presence of ghost cells and follicular matrical differentiation. BCCs typically show peripherhal palisading of cells and retraction artifact in addition to mucin production. Although ghost cells are characteristic of pilomatricoma, they can also be seen in other follicular neoplasms, including infundibular cysts and trichoepitheliomas (36). Pilomatricoma can show a locally aggressive pattern of growth (20). The most commonly used criteria to distinguish pilomatricoma from pilomatrical carcinoma are infiltrative borders of the tumor, the degree of cytological atypia, and the high mitotic activity in the carcinoma (37). Zonal necrosis may also be more common in the malignant tumors with pilomatrical differentiation.

Treatment and Prognosis

As a benign neoplasm, pilomatricoma is usually treated by simple enucleation (16). With the exception of some proliferating pilomatricomas, most tumors will not recur. However, local recurrence and aggressive forms have been documented (17,38). Wide local excision is the treatment of choice for these cases.

E. Trichilemmoma

Introduction

Trichilemmomas (TLs) are benign neoplasms originating from the outer root sheath of the hair follicle. Earlier reports of an association of these lesions with human papilloma virus have not yet been substantiated (39,40). TLs may develop within nevus sebaceus, and multiple TLs develop in the setting of Cowden disease, a syndrome that is associated with adenocarcinomas, most commonly of the breast, thyroid, and gastrointestinal tract.

Clinical Features

TLs may present anywhere, except on palms and soles, but in particular on the central face, and, most commonly, in adults. The lesions are small, solitary or multiple, skin-colored papules with a smooth or warty surface. In the setting of Cowden disease, there may also be involvement of the oral mucosa, including the lips, palate, tongue, and buccal mucosa.

Imaging

Imaging studies are needed only to further evaluate the patient for complications of Cowden disease.

Pathology

Histologically, TL is a well-circumscribed endophytic lobular proliferation extending from follicular epithelium or the overlying epidermis (Fig. 12). The lobules are composed of cells with abundant glycogenated cytoplasm with small monomorphic nuclei (Fig. 13). Nuclear atypia, mitoses, and apoptosis are not seen. There is peripheral palisading and often a prominent PAS-D positive thickened basement membrane. Desmoplastic TL shows similar cytology; however, there are angulated nests resesmbling infiltrative carcinoma, set in a fibrotic stroma (41). The epithelial nests may show central desmoplasia, potentially as a result of tenascin secretion by the neoplastic cells (Fig. 14) (42). Often in this setting, there are areas of conventional TL.

Immunohistochemistry

Involucrin expression is seen in TL, as it is in other tumors of the hair follicle (43).

Expression of CK 1, 10, 14, 15, 16, and 17 suggests that TLs are of follicular infundibulum origin (44). CK 5/6 expression is noted in most (97%) benign and malignant neoplasms of cutaneous adnexal origin, which includes TL; strong diffuse CK 5/6 expression is seen in 13% of metastatic carcincomas. This is helpful to the extent that it is useful as part of a

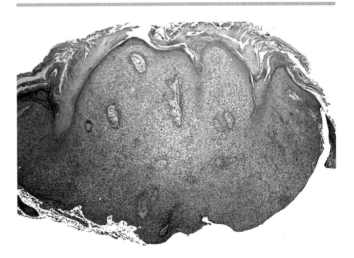

Figure 12 Trichilemmoma. This is a well-circumscribed, endophytic, and lobular proliferation extending from the follicular epithelium or the overlying epidermis.

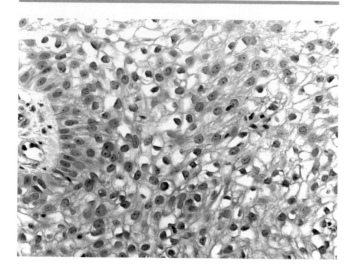

Figure 13 Trichilemmoma The lobules are composed of cells with abundant glycogenated cytoplasm and small monomorphic nuclei.

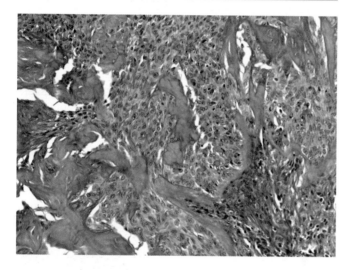

Figure 14 Desmoplastic trichilemmoma. The epithelial nests may show central desmoplasia.

panel of markers used to assist in differentiating primary cutaneous lesions from metastatic histologic mimics (6).

Electron Microscopy

Electron Microscopy sections have been studied, and they have failed to reveal viral particles (40).

Molecular-Genetic Data

Germ line mutations in chromosome 10q22-23, the locus for the tumor suppressor gene PTEN, are seen in those cases associated with Cowden disease.

Differential Diagnosis

Lack of eccrine differentiation and the presence of peripheral palisading of nuclei are useful features in differentiating TL from eccrine poroma, which also extends from the overlying epidermis and is composed of banal cells lacking nuclear pleomorphism and mitoses. Irritated SK enters the histologic differential diagnosis because of its endophytic growth pattern and presence of squamatization, which may on occasion be seen in the superficial portion of TL. Irritated SK, however, lacks glycogenation, peripheral palisading, and prominent basement membrane that characterize TL.

Treatment and Prognosis

Simple excision is curative of this benign adnexal neoplasm.

F. Cutaneous Lymphadenoma

Synonyms: lymphoepithelial tumor and benign lymphoepithelial tumor of the skin.

Introduction

Cutaneous lymphadenoma (CL) is a rare basaloid tumor, which was first recognized as a lymphoepithelial tumor in 1987 and later named "cutaneous lymphadenoma" in 1991 (45,46). The etiology is uncertain and, over time, has been presented as a variant of trichoblastoma, a neoplasm of eccrine or pilosebaceous origin, or a BCC with adnexal differentiation (47–50).

Clinical Features

CL presents on the face, with rare exceptions reported on the legs (46). Patients are typically adults, 20 to 50 years old, with an equal gender distribution. The lesions are asymptomatic, slow growing, erythematous to skin-colored papules or nodules, and less than 1 cm in diameter, which have been present for months to years. Clinically, CLs are most often mistaken for dermatofibroma (DF), sebaceous hyperplasia (SH), or BCC.

Imaging

Imaging studies are not necessary.

Pathology

CLs are well-defined unencapsulated dermal nodules, classically composed of three histologic elements: dermal nests, a fibrotic stroma, and an inflammatory infiltrate (Fig. 15). The dermal nests are irregularly shaped lobules of epithelial cells composed of large glycogenated cells with peripheral palisading. The cells have large vesicular nuclei with prominent nucleoli and rare mitoses (Fig. 16). The larger cells may demonstrate squamatization, sebaceous differentiation, or follicular differentiation (46,47). The inflammatory infiltrate consists of a mixed population of small, mature T and B lymphocytes with scattered

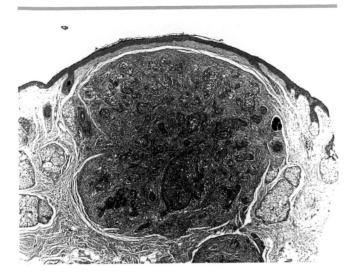

Figure 15 Lymphadenoma. The tumor is composed of well-defined, unencapsulated dermal nodules, classically consisting of three histologic elements: epithelial nests, a fibrotic stroma, and an inflammatory infiltrate.

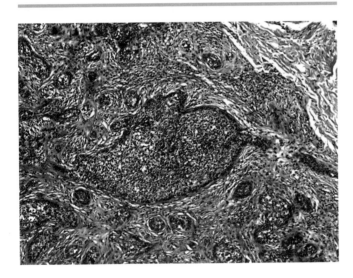

Figure 16 Lymphadenoma. The nests of epithelial cells are irregularly shaped and have peripheral palisading. The cells have large vesicular nuclei with prominent nucleoli and an infiltrate of small, mature T and B lymphocytes.

CD30 expression in large activated cells with abundant cytoplasm, vesicular nuclei, and prominent nucleoli (51). Germinal center formation may be seen adjacent to the nodules.

Immunohistochemistry

The glycogenated cells making up the epithelial islands express CKs (AE1-3) (48). CLs demonstrate CK 20-positive Merkel cells (49), and immunohistochemical staining for S-100 protein reveals a dendritic

cell infiltrate (52). Some lesions also show CD1a expression, supporting the hypothesis of a Langerhans cell infiltrate (49). Additionally, bcl-2 expression is seen in the peripheral epithelial layer. Epithelial membrane antigen (EMA) may be expressed, and carcinoembryonic antigen (CEA) is negative. The stroma may show CD34 expression (49).

Electron Microscopy

CL has not been studied ultrastructurally.

Molecular-Genetic Data

A chromosomal aberration has not been identified, and CLs are not associated with syndromes or other genetic anomalies.

Differential Diagnosis

The main consideration in the histologic diferential diagnosis is a lymphoepithelioma-like carcinoma (LE-LC), which is hypothesized to originate from adnexal structures; the World Health Organization classification includes this as an SCC. LE-LC arises most commonly in the nasopharynx. However, lesions in the skin, salivary glands, stomach, lung, and thymus have also been reported (53). In the skin, it presents as a nodule almost exclusively on the head and neck of elderly adults and has an equal gender distribution, and unlike those in the nasopharynx, an association with Epstein-Barr virus (EBV) has not been established (53). Histologically, LE-LC is a dermal or subcutaneous nodule composed of infiltrating lobules and cords of eosinophilic epithelioid cells with a surrounding dense lymphoplasmacytic infiltrate. The lobules of LE-LC do not have peripheral palisading (Fig. 17). Like CL, the cells comprising these lobules

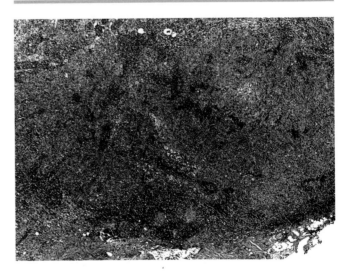

Figure 17 Lymphoepithelioma-like carcinoma (LE-LC). This dermal nodule is composed of infiltrating lobules and cords of epithelioid cells with a surrounding dense lymphoplasmacytic infiltrate. The lobules of LE-LC do not have peripheral palisading.

express CK and EMA and have vesicular nuclei with prominent nucleoli. Unlike CL, they demonstrate numerous mitoses and do not show squamatization.

Treatment and Prognosis

Simple excision is curative of the benign CL. Recurrence and metastasis have not been reported.

G.   Hidrocystoma

Synonyms: cystadenoma and Moll's gland cyst.

Introduction

Traditionally, hidrocystomas have been classified as apocrine or eccrine on the basis of their histologic features. Eccrine hidrocystomas are believed to represent obstructed and subsequently dilated eccrine sweat ducts, whereas apocrine hidrocystomas are believed to represent a benign neoplasm of the apocrine sweat gland. Though the presence of solitary eccrine hidrocystomas has been questioned, one study using an antigen specific for the secretory portion of the eccrine gland showed expression in all eccrine neoplasms studied, including eccrine hidrocystomas; lack of expression in all apocrine lesions studied, however, did not include apocrine hidrocystoma (54,55). Those with a purported eccrine pathogenesis may increase in size during exposure to heat such as during the summer months, after exercise, or a hot bath. Multiple eccrine hidrocystomas with seasonal size variations are a distinct type, referred to as Robinson type; solitary lesions have been referred to as Smith type. The conventional classification based solely on histologic features is not without debate, as there are reports of histologically eccrine lesions that express apocrine antigens and lesions that have combined apocrine and eccrine morphology. Multiple eccrine hidrocystomas have also been seen as the presenting sign in a patient with Grave's disease who additionally complained of hyperhidrosis. The cutaneous lesions resolved with successful treatment of the thyroid disease and implicated the thyroid as one possible mechanism in multiple eccrine hidrocystomas (56). Multiple apocrine hidrocystomas may be seen in Schopf-Schulz-Passarge syndrome, a variant of ectodermal dysplasia that also presents with palmoplantar keratoderma, hypodontia, and abnormalities of other ectodermally derived structures (57). Multiple epidermally derived neoplasms have also been reported in patients with this genodermatosis. However, a stastically significant correlation has not yet been established (58).

Clinical Features

Hidrocystomas may be solitary or multiple and are most commonly located on the face, with a predilection for the periocular areas, although many sites have been reported, including the scalp, penis, and finger (59–61). Only 9% of apocrine hidrocystomas occur in sites with apocrine glands, i.e., the axilla and groin (62). Both apocrine and eccrine hidrocystomas present as a translucent dome-shaped papule, which may be skin colored or have a blue hue. They often are 1 to 3 mm in diameter; those measuring greater than 2 cm are referred to as giant hidrocystomas and often result in mechanical obstruction of neighboring structures (63,64). These lesions are more common in adults, but cases in patients younger than 20 years are reported (62). There is no gender predilection, with the exception of a female prevalence in Robinson-type multiple eccrine hidrocystomas. Clinically, because of the discoloration imparted by the cyst, these lesions may be mistaken for a pigmented lesion, in particular a blue nevus, which imparts a similar color, or other melanocytic neoplasm (65). Because of its smooth dome shape, clinical confusion with a BCC is also common.

Imaging

While typically not necessary, should imaging studies be performed because of uncertainity of the nature of the lesion, a hidrocystoma will show a circumscribed echolucent mass by ultrasound (65). For deeper masses, magnetic resonance imaging (MRI) may be employed and will reveal a cystic lesion (64).

Pathology

Histology shows a cystically dilated structure in the superficial to mid dermis. The eccrine lesions are typically unilocular with two layers of cuboidal cells (Fig. 18), characteristic of eccrine duct morphology. Apocrine hidrocystomas show a cystically dilated space, often multilocular, lined by columnar cells with apical decapitation (Fig. 19). Flattened cuboidal cells, presumably as a result of intraluminal mechanical compression, may also be seen. Lesions that are inadequately sampled may show exclusively this flattened epithelilum, leading to a misdiagnosis of eccrine hidrocystoma rather than the correct apocrine type.

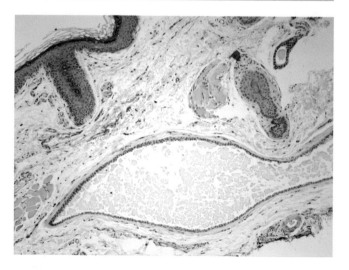

Figure 18   Eccrine hidrocystoma. A unilocular cyst showing two layers of cuboidal cells, characteristic of eccrine ducts, is present in the superficial dermis.

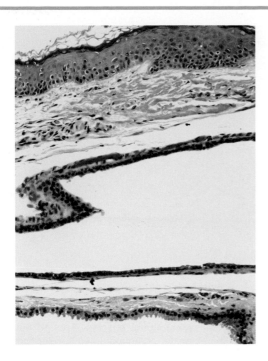

Figure 19 Apocrine hidrocystoma. A cystically dilated space lined by cells with apical decapitation, characteristic of apocrine cells, is present in the lower portion of the image. Note also the presence of a flattened cuboidal epithelium lining in the upper portion.

Papillary projections into the cystic spaces are also commonly seen in the apocrine lesions. PAS-positive diastase-resistant cytoplasmic granules are found in the luminal cells.

Immunohistochemistry

CK expression in apocrine hidrocystoma correlates with the expression in the normal apocrine and eccrine glands. That is to say, there is expression of AE1/AE3 (CK 1–8, 10, 14–16, and 19) in all portions (flattened and secretory) of apocrine and eccrine types (66,67). Additionally, in the apocrine hidrocystoma, involucrin is not expressed, smooth muscle actin is seen focally in the basal cells of the flattened epithelium and in the outermost cell of the secretory portion, and human milk fat globulin-1 (HMFG1) is seen in the luminal cells, most pronounced in the areas with decapitation secretion (66). The secretory cells and myoepithelial cells express S-100 protein, and the epithelial cells of the cyst wall show CEA expression (56). Antigen expression analysis on a vulvar pigmented eccrine hidrocystoma showed CA19-9 and CK 7, 8, and 19 expression with no reactivity for HMFG1 (68). In one study differentiating primary cutaneous adnexal neoplasms from metastatic breast carcinoma, 1 of 17 hidrocystomas showed membraneous Her-2 expression (69).

Electron Microscopy

Pigmented hidrocystomas ultrastructurally show melanosomes in various stages (68). Electron microscopy is otherwise not used in the diagnostic evaluation of these lesions.

Molecular-Genetic Data

DNA aneuploidy has not been detected in these lesions (70), and an inheritance pattern has not been established.

Differential Diagnosis

As BCC may show differentiation toward adnexal structures, cystic BCC enters high on the histologic differential diagnosis, especially, if the specimen represents a superficial biopsy of the lesion. Cytologic atypia, not typically seen in hidrocystoma, may be the only clue to suggest a BCC and recommend complete excision (71).

Superficially biopsied apocrine hidrocystomas may show only flattened cuboidal epithelium, and, as suggested above, may be histologically misdiagnosed as an eccrine hidrocystoma.

Treatment and Prognosis

Simple excision is adequate for solitary lesions of both eccrine and apocrine etiology. However, this is not a practical approach for those rare patients with multiple lesions. Multiple lesions have been successfully treated with a 595-nm pulsed dye laser after a topical application of 1% atropine sulfate was unsuccessful because of poor patient compliance due to intolerable side effects (72). Botulinum toxin interferes with cholinergic ends of the parasympathetic system and, accordingly, sweat gland secretion. It has been used effectively to treat multiple eccrine hidrocystomas (73). In a similar fashion, 1% topical atropine, an anticholinergic, has been shown to be effective, safe, and well tolerated in treating the eruption of multiple eccrine hidrocystomas during warm weather (74). For multiple apocrine hidrocystomas, a single session of carbon dioxide laser vaporization using a continuous, defocused mode at 5 J/cm² has been effective (75).

H. Syringoma

Introduction

Syringoma is a benign eccrine neoplasm most commonly presenting in adolescents and young adult women (76). Eruptive syringomas have been proposed to be a reactive proliferative response to inflammation, rather than a neoplasm (77). Multiple syringomas have been reported in Costello syndrome (78). Familial cases have been reported, and there is an increased incidence in patients with Down syndrome, although a specific genetic alteration has not been found in syringoma (79).

Clinical Features

Syringomas are 1 to 3 mm, skin-colored or slightly yellow, closely set, soft papules. While many sites have been reported, there is a strong predilection for cheeks

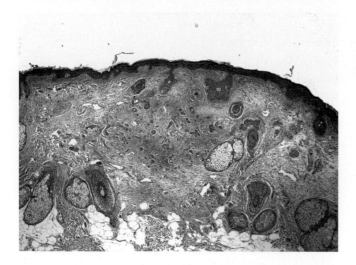

Figure 20 Syringoma. On low power, syringoma is unencapsulated. In an adequate biopsy, the lesion is well demarcated.

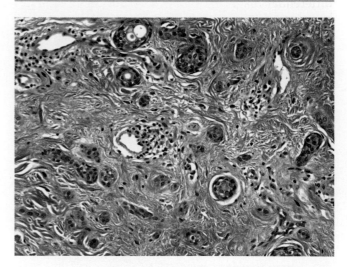

Figure 21 Syringoma. Higher-power evaluation of syringoma shows aggregates of monomorphous small cells set in a densely fibrous stroma. These cells are in tubular formation, often showing central lumina and luminal cuticles. Though not always present, the characteristic comma-shaped tubular structure is seen here.

and periocular distribution. The lesions may be multiple or solitary. A clear cell variant is seen in association with diabetes mellitus (80). In some instances, they may be found in unilateral or linear groupings. Generalized eruptive variant of syringomas have been reported in Down syndrome as a familial trait (81).

Imaging

As benign and almost exclusively dermal proliferations, imaging studies are rarely necessary.

Pathology

On scanning magnification, syringoma has a well-demarcated contour and usually assumes a platelike configuration in the dermis (Fig. 20). Small comma-shaped tubular aggregates, many of which have central lumens and luminal cuticles, are distributed in a densely fibrous stroma (Fig. 21). The small ducts are composed of one or two cuboidal cell layers. Small nests and strands of cells having a basaloid appearance may be present. In the clear cell variant, the clear cells contain abundant glycogen (Fig. 22).

Immunohistochemistry

Syringomas have been shown to express EKH-6, a marker of eccrine secretory elements (82), as well as CK 1, 5, 10, 11, 14, and 19 (66). Immunoreactivity for CEA and progesterone receptors supports the view that they are under hormonal control (83,84).

Electron Microscopy

There are numerous microvilli on the cells bordering the lumina and a band of periluminal tonofilaments. Intracytoplasmic lumen formation and keratohyaline granules in the luminal cells have also been reported (85).

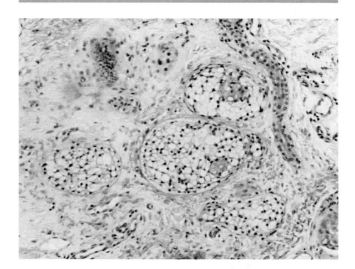

Figure 22 Syringoma. In this clear cell type, the cytoplasm is expanded with glycogen. The nuclei are small and hyperchromatic, the same as in a conventional syringoma.

Molecular-Genetic Data

Despite familial reports and associations with syndromes such as Down and Costello, a specific genetic aberration has not yet been found.

Differential Diagnosis

Microcystic adnexal carcinoma (MAC), a locally aggressive neoplasm with eccrine and follicular features, is the most significant lesion in the histologic differential diagnosis. MAC may appear deceptively bland, histologically, with keratinizing cysts lined by squamoid cells in the superficial portion of the neoplasm with subjacent strands and nests of epithelial cells with ductal differentiation. As in syringoma, these ducts may contain amorphous eosinophilic material. MAC is ill defined and may extend into the deep dermis, resulting in difficulty making the diagnosis with a superficial biopsy in which the specimen transects the deep aspect of the lesion. In such instances, the histology of MAC and syringoma can be identical, and a definitive diagnosis should be reserved for a complete excision for evaluation of the base (86). Syringomas differ from MAC by their lack of deep extension and of perineural infiltration (87). The dense fibrous stroma present in syringomas may also help to make this differentiation.

Treatment and Prognosis

Syringomas are benign and have negligible proliferative capacity. Accordingly, no further surgical intervention is indicated. The best available therapeutic approach to eruptive syringomas is laser ablation. Lesional pretreatment with trichloracetic acid may be helpful in limiting scarring (76).

I. Sebaceous Hyperplasia

Introduction

SH is a common benign lesion, which develops as a consequence of sun exposure, aging, and immunosuppression. Although sebaceous development is directly affected by androgens, this mode of action in SH has not yet been determined. Rare variants include SH overlying DF, isolated otophyma, presentation as an intraoral polyp, and a diffuse form (88–90). Increased prevalence has been observed in renal transplant patients (91). Recent studies investigating telomerase activity of sebaceous neoplasms showed consistent strong expression in the nucleoli of the germinative cells in all sebaceous lesions and negative expression in mature sebocytes by immunohistochemical staining for human telomerase reverse transcriptase, indicating that telomerase expression does not differentiate hyperplastic from neoplastic sebaceous lesions (92).

Clinical Features

SH presents most commonly on the faces of adult men as an asymptomatic solitary or multiple yellow-hued papules. The follicular ostia may be seen as a central depression. While ectopic intraoral sebaceous glands are common, intraoral SH is rarely reported (90).

Imaging

There is no need for imaging studies, as this lesion represents a benign dermal proliferation.

Pathology

Histologic sections show large, mature sebaceous lobules opening into a central duct, which is

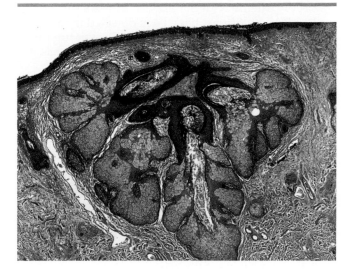

Figure 23 Sebaceous hyperplasia. This dermal tumor has mature sebaceous lobules opening into a central duct, which is commonly dilated. The lobules have a single peripheral layer of basaloid, geminative cells. The remainder of the lobule has fully mature sebocytes with hyperchromatic, indented nuclei and multivacuolated cytoplasm.

commonly dilated and often filled with debris. The sebaceous lobules have a single layer of basaloid, geminative cells with fully mature sebocytes, demonstrating hyperchromatic, indented nuclei and multivacuolated cytoplasm, composing the remainder of the lobule (Fig. 23). Fibrous septa are present, but may not demonstrate the invaginations seen in nonhyperplastic sebaceous glands. The overlying epidermis is usually unremarkable.

Immunohistochemistry

Immunohistochemistry is not necessary to make the diagnosis of SH and will not help in the differential diagnosis of SH and other sebaceous neoplasms.

Electron Microscopy

Ultrastructural evaluation is not needed for diagnostic purposes.

Molecular-Genetic Data

Premature SH in five generations has been reported, suggesting an autosomal dominant inheritance (93). A genetic locus has not been identified. Unlike sebaceous neoplasms, SH is not associated with Muir-Torre syndrome.

Myosin heavy chain genes, MYH, clustered on chromosome 17p, are responsible for encoding the multiple isoforms of myosin (94). Inherited defects in missense mutation variants (Tyr165Cys and GLY382Asp) of MYH, in areas known to function in mismatch repair, have been associated with familial adenocarcinoma of the colon (95). MYH-associated polyposis, an autosomal recessive disease, presents with multiple colonic adenomas and cancer. In a cohort of patients with SH and MYH-associated polyposis, BRAF mutations have been detected in their SH. BRAF mutations found in melanocytic skin tumors is linked to early tumorigenesis; a similar study has not yet been done for BRAF mutations in SH (96).

Differential Diagnosis

SH is frequently clinically misdiagnosed as BCC. Histologically, this entity should be distinguished from sebaceous adenoma (SA), as the latter could be associated with the Muir-Torre syndrome. SA is distinguished from SH by showing a larger basaloid germinative component (up to half of the sebaceous lobules) than is observed in SH. Other considerations include sebaceous trichofolliculoma and folliculosebaceous cystic hamartoma, both of which feature the presence of more complex pilar epithelial proliferation than that associated with SH.

Treatment and Prognosis

Treatment is unnecessary for these lesions. Unfavorable cosmetic appearance generally leads patients to desire treatment. There is evidence that treatment with 5-aminolevulinic acid and photodynamic therapy is safe and effective without rapid recurrence of lesions (97,98).

J. Sebaceous Adenoma

Introduction

SA is a benign tumor occurring predominantly on the head and neck of older individuals (99). Occasionally, lesions have been described on the trunk and leg (99). Rarely, SA may develop intraorally, in association with Fordyce papules (100,101). In keeping with the increased neoplasms seen in immunosuppressed patients, a solitary, large SA has been reported in association with AIDS (102). SA is a characteristic lesion seen in Muir-Torre syndrome, an autosomal dominant condition characterized by the presence of cutaneous sebaceous neoplasms in association with visceral malignancies, particularly of the colon, endometrium, urogenitalia, and upper gastrointestinal tract (103).

Clinical Features

SA presents as a slowly enlarging, yellowish nodule that usually measures up to several centimeters in diameter. The face and scalp of elderly people are the most common presentation. Occasionally, they ulcerate and bleed or become tender. Clinically, these lesions are often mistaken for BCC.

Imaging

There is no need for imaging studies, as this lesion represents a benign dermal proliferation.

Pathology

SA is a multilobulated and circumscribed dermal neoplasm that often attenuates the overlying epidermis

(Fig. 24). The individual lobules have a peripheral rim of basaloid cells, which may be a simple layer at the outermost portion of the lobule or several layers thick. The remainder of the lobule is composed of mature sebaceous cells. Compression of the surrounding stroma by the enlarging sebaceous neoplasm gives the appearance of a collagenous capsule, which in fact is just a pseudocapsule. The sebaceous lobules in SA open directly to the epidermis or to the follicular epithelium (Fig. 25).

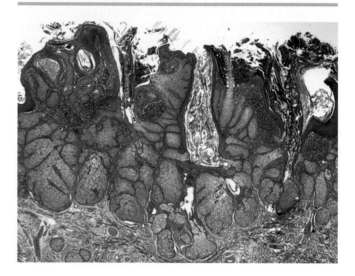

Figure 24 Sebaceous adenoma. This sebaceous tumor is composed of a well-circumscribed, multilobulated dermal neoplasm. The sebaceous lobules open directly to the epidermis or follicular epithelium.

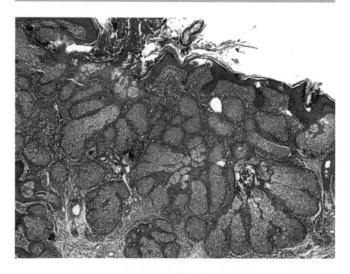

Figure 25 Sebaceous adenoma. The individual lobules have a peripheral rim of basaloid cells. The remainder of the lobule is composed of mature sebaceous cells. A pseudocapsule resulting from compression of the surrounding stoma by the enlarging sebaceous neoplasm is often noticed. The sebaceous lobules in SA open directly to the epidermis or to the follicular epithelium.

Immunohistochemistry

Immunohistochemistry is not necessary to make the diagnosis of SA or aid in the histologic differential diagnosis.

Electron Microscopy

There are no published studies regarding the ultrastructural characteristics of this entity.

Molecular-Genetic Data

SAs that are seen in the setting of Muir-Torre syndrome demonstrate microsatellite instability, which is characteristic of the syndrome. These lesions will have defects in DNA mismatch repair genes, most commonly hMLH-1 and hMSH-2 (Fig. 26) (104).

Differential Diagnosis

SH is differentiated from SA by its lack of the proliferative basaloid layer that is seen in SA. Additionally, SH recapitulates the normal sebaceous lobule by opening into ducts that empty into the follicular lumen. Sebaceous carcinoma (SC), when infiltrative, is not difficult to differentiate. However, if the specimen is fragmented or the lesion is only partially sampled, the distinction is more challenging. SC demonstrates atypia in the basaloid layer, which occupies significantly more of the lobule than is typically seen in SA. Additionally, the ordered maturation of basaloid to sebocyte that is seen in SA is lacking in SC.

Treatment and Prognosis

If completely excised, no further treatment is necessary. However, if the lesion is only partially sampled, circumscription and cytologic features cannot be adequately assessed. Accordingly, conservative reexcision to ensure comprehensive histologic evaluation is recommended.

K. Actinic Keratosis

Synonyms: solar keratosis, senile keratosis, precancerous keratosis, and keratinocytic intraepithelial neoplasia (KIN).

Introduction

Actinic keratoses (AKs) have a direct relationship to cumulative long-term sun exposure. They tend to be most prevalent in sun-exposed areas of patients with types I and II skin tones (fair-skinned complexions). For this reason, AKs are uncommon in younger patients or in those with darker skin tones. The frequency with which AKs progress to invasive SCC is currently a topic under intense investigation (105,106). For many years, it was generally accepted that approximately 1% of AKs progressed to in situ carcinomas, and perhaps another 1% of these actually ultimately invaded the basement membrane. However, recent data have suggested higher frequencies

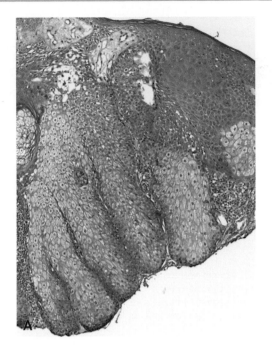

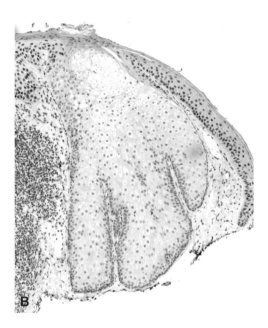

Figure 26 Sebaceous adenoma. (**A**) Showing normal maturation of sebocytes in a lobule (H&E) and (**B**) loss of expression of MLH-1 compared with normal expression in the basilar epithelial cells.

of progression, with some studies citing almost an incidence of progression approaching 20%.

Clinical Features

AKs present as flat or exophytic papules or macules on sun-exposed body sites. They are usually covered by a hyperkeratotic scale and are erythematous. They always occur in the setting of sun-damaged skin that

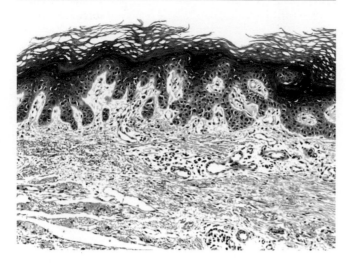

Figure 27 Actinic keratosis. Increased nuclear and cytoplasmic size, noted first in the basilar keratinocytes, results in the infolding and an apparent increase in rete ridge-like downward projections. This is often detected at low power.

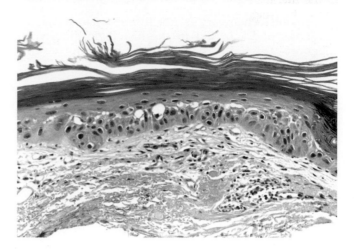

Figure 28 Actinic keratosis, acantholytic. In some cases, the dysmaturation results in extensive acantholysis, resulting in separation of the basilar from the suprabasilar keratinocytes.

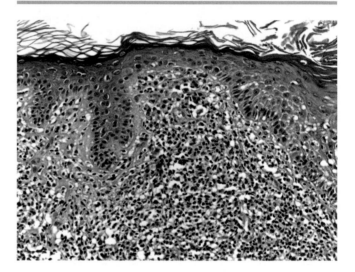

Figure 29 Actinic keratosis, lichenoid. A marked inflammatory response may be present along the basilar epithelium. Distinction from reactive atypia may be difficult unless evaluation of the lateral, uninflammed portion is interpreted.

is often atrophic, with telangiectasias and increased wrinkling. There is frequently a "cutaneous horn." The clinical differential diagnosis often includes verruca vulgaris, SK, BCC, and SCC.

Histologic Features

Cytologically, atypical keratinocytes are the primary histologic feature of an AK. The atypia is usually first detected in basal layer keratinocytes, which display increased and disordered nuclei and cellular enlargement. This is often detected at low power. As the proliferation of atypical cells continues, there is an increased amount of infolding, resulting in an apparent increase in rete ridge-like downward projections (Fig. 27). With progression, the cytologic atypia extends to cells above the basal layer to involve much of the epidermis. The cutaneous appendages are often spared until the latest stages of the process. This is easily reflected in the presence of parakeratosis, which is seen overlying the areas with disordered maturation, but is absent in areas overlying cutaneous appendages. Solar elastosis is a required histologic feature of AK, and the diagnosis cannot be made in the absence of significant sun damage. AKs may be hyperplastic, with elongation of rete ridges and extension deep into the papillary dermis, or atrophic, with pronounced thinning of the epidermis. In some cases, the dysmaturation results in extensive acantholysis (Fig. 28). In many cases, a marked inflammatory response may be present (Fig. 29), and this has been associated with increased p53 and bcl-2 expression, suggesting a higher malignant potential (107).

Imaging

AKs are intraepidermal growths that are, by definition, confined by a basement membrane. Thus, there is no ability for invasive growth or metastatic potential, and imaging studies are not required to make the diagnosis or for assessing treatment options.

Immunohistochemistry

Immunohistochemical studies have demonstrated aberrant CKexpression patterns, similar to those seen in cutaneous SCCs; however, these studies are not useful or necessary for diagnostic purposes.

Differential Diagnosis

The major differential diagnosis of AK is SCC, either invasive or in situ. There is currently much controversy in the literature as to whether these represent a spectrum of a single entity or are discrete entities. While there is not yet a consensus, many diagnosticians believe that "full-thickness" atypia is required to support a diagnosis of SCCIS and that atypia that does not reach fully to the granular layer keratinocytes is best regarded as an AK. (This is somewhat analogous to the grading scale used in cervical intraepithelial neoplasia that requires full thickness atypia to make a diagnosis of SCCIS.) It should be noted, however, that some cutaneous SCCs become invasive without demonstrating full-thickness atypia or an in situ component. In these cases, it is often quite difficult to distinguish an early invasive SCC from a hyperplastic AK.

In cases with a brisk inflammatory response, especially those with a lichenoid pattern, it can be difficult, if not impossible, to distinguish a lichenoid keratosis from an AK. Reactive atypia secondary to marked inflammation can often be impossible to separate from the primary keratinocyte atypia required for the diagnosis of AK. However, in most cases, there are no differences in treatment, and the distinction is purely academic. Arsenical keratoses can also be difficult to distinguish from AK. However, the location and lack of solar elastosis help in this differential diagnosis.

Chemotherapy-induced atypia is often more pronounced than that seen in AK. Further, clinical history usually serves to separate these entities, as would the lack of solar elastosis in many cases of chemotherapy-induced atypia.

Discoid lupus erythematosus, especially when occurring on sun-exposed body sites, can be difficult to distinguish from AK. Clinical history is often invaluable in this situation. The presence of mucin and follicular plugging, along with an inflammatory infiltrate surrounding deeper cutaneous appendageal structures, would favor a diagnosis of lupus erythematosus.

In acantholytic AKs, the acantholysis can be so extensive as to make distinction from pemphigus vulgaris or warty dyskeratoma difficult. Neither of these two entities demonstrates true keratinocyte atypia, thus enabling accurate distinction in most cases.

Treatment and Prognosis

AKs are often removed with cryosurgery. Other techniques include shave excisions and electrodessication and curretage. In most cases, simple locally destructive therapy is sufficient. By definition, these growths are confined to the epidermis and, since they are above the basement membrane, usually do not possess the ability for invasive growth or metastatic potential. Topical application of antineoplastic agents, in particular 5-fluorouracil, has been effective in treating patients with numerous or confluent AKs that would not be amenable to surgical removal (108,109).

The incidence of malignant transformation to invasive SCC is unknown, but is generally believed to be from 1% to 7% in large series (110). It is very difficult to assess the exact incidence of AKs and probability of evolving into SCC, as most of these lesions do not come to medical attention. Further, even with those that do, there remains some inconsistency with regard to diagnostic criteria and the distinction from SCC.

II. MALIGNANT EPITHELIAL NEOPLASMS

A. Squamous Cell Carcinoma

Synonyms: Bowen's disease.

Introduction

SCC is the second most common cancer among whites and constitutes approximately 20% of all nonmelanoma skin cancers (111). As incidence and mortality data of SCC are not collected by the National Cancer Institute, epidemiologic data cannot be determined accurately. SCC is associated with long-standing sun exposure in the vast majority of cases, with ultraviolet (UV) B radiation being the principal factor and UV A adding to the risk (112). The tumors arise on sun-exposed sites in patients with fair complexions and an extensive cumulative lifetime sun exposure. In a study out of Nigeria, it was shown that SCC is the most common nonmelanocytic skin cancer in blacks, in contrast to BCC, which is the most common skin cancer in Caucasians. In that population, most SCC was due to poorly treated chronic wounds and chronic burn scars (113). Immunosuppressed patients form another group of individuals with a markedly increased risk for developing cutaneous SCC. The incidence of SCC in this population is increased upto 250-fold over a control population (114,115). Additionally, the SCCs that develop in this setting tend to be more aggressive. Increased cutaneous SCCs are also seen in patients with DNA-repair anomalies, such as those with xeroderma pigmentosum (116). Chronic nonhealing wounds have long been purported to give rise to increased numbers of cutaneous SCC, with a more aggressive clinical course and a higher rate of metastasis (117,118). However, a recent large study of 16,903 Danish patients with up to 25 years of follow-up showed no increase in cutaneous SCC inthose with the most severe burns or in the longest follow-up periods (119). Patients with SCC of the head and neck with a primary lesion measuring greater than 4 mm in thickness and in proximity to the parotid gland are at high risk for metastatic disease (120).

Clinical Features

Cutaneous SCC presents as an exophytic growth with overlying hyperkeratosis. There is frequently associated ulceration. The most common presentation is of such a growth occurring on a background of extensively sun-damaged atrophic skin in typically affected body sites. Less common presentations include ulcerations at sites of long-standing nonhealing wounds.

Imaging

Imaging studies are not generally employed in establishing the diagnosis of cutaneous SCC.

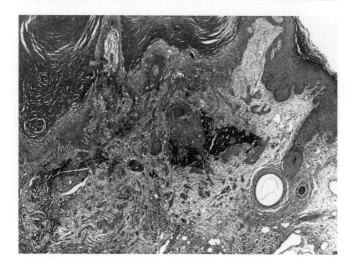

Figure 30 Squamous cell carcinoma, invasive. There are angulated nests of keratinocytes infiltrating the dermis. These nests show enlarged nuclei, nuclear pleomorphism, and varying degrees of differentiation, seen as eosinophilic cytoplasm and keratin pearls.

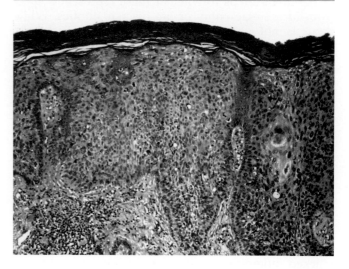

Figure 31 Squamous cell carcinoma, in situ. Full-thickness keratinocyte atypia often with overlying confluent parakeratosis.

Pathology

Cutaneous SCCs are histologically identical to SCC occurring at other body sites. Primary lesions grow down from the overlying epidermis, and in most cases, foci of keratinocyte atypia (AK) can be identified in areas adjacent to the fully transformed tumor. In SCCs that arise on sun-damaged skin, degenerative solar elastosis is present throughout the superficial dermis. Atypical keratinocytes proliferate downward, extending into the dermis as small nests and even single cells (Fig. 30). The tumor cells demonstrate abundant eosinophilic cytoplasm in most cases. Foci of acantholysis are common. As is the case with SCC arising in other organ systems, the malignant cells demonstrate variable degrees of differentiation. Well-differentiated SCC may largely recapitulate the cytologic features of the surrounding epidermis, with abundant keratinization. With lesser degrees of differentiation, keratinization becomes less pronounced, intercellular bridges may be progressively more difficult to identify, and nuclear anaplasia is more apparent. (There is no convincing evidence that degree of differentiation serves as an effective prognostic indicator for SCC developing within the skin.) A variable host immune response is present. Depth of invasion as a prognostic indicator remains controversial. The presence of neural and vascular invasion may be associated with higher rates of local recurrence and metastasis and should be commented on in the pathology report.

Variants of cutaneous SCC.

SCC In Situ. SCCIS (Bowen's disease) arises as a slow-growing, flat, scaly patch, most commonly on sun-exposed body sites. It may clinically resemble superficial BCC, psoriasis, or nummular eczema. SCCIS demonstrates full-thickness keratinocyte atypia with overlying confluent parakeratosis. The histologic changes are analogous to carcinoma in situ at other body sites such as the cervix. In most cases, the rete ridges do not become elongated, and the lesion retains its relatively flat architecture (Fig. 31). The relationship between in situ SCCs and invasive tumors is not fully established. Frequently, partial thickness cytologic atypia (AK) is present lateral to the most floridly atypical sections of the tumor. The vast majority of in situ lesions do not appear to invariably progress to invasive processes.

Verrucous Carcinoma. Verrucous carcinomas represent an exophytic, indolent variant of SCC. These neoplasms represent a specific type of cutaneous SCC, characterized by lack of significant cytologic atypia and a protruding, rather than invasive, growth pattern. Elongated rete ridges with blunt borders extend deeply into the reticular dermis without ever becoming overtly invasive (Fig. 32). If cytologic atypia is present, these proliferations are best regarded as SCC and not specifically as verrucous carcinomas.

Spindle Cell Carcinoma (Sarcomatoid SCC). Rarely, SCCs display a purely spindle-celled morphology. These tumors extend down from the overlying epidermis, though the connection may not be readily apparent on routine histologic sections. The spindled cells course through the dermis in fascicles and may produce very little keratin. There is a variable degree of cytologic atypia, and mitotic activity is relatively brisk in most cases (Fig. 33). Perineural invasion may be present. In these cases, it is difficult, if not impossible, to distinguish SCC from other neoplastic processes on routine sections, and keratin expression in these lesions may not be consistently strong. Increasing evidence points to the spindled cell component representing dedifferentiations along mesenchymal lines, with mesenchymal morphology and antigen expression characteristic of mesenchyme and epithelium (121–123).

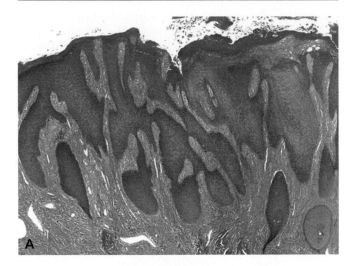

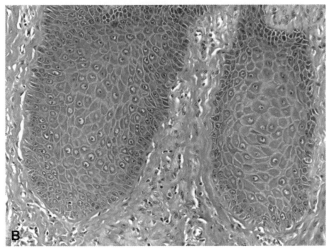

Figure 32 Verrucous carcinoma. (**A**) This is characterized by protruding, not infiltrating, down growths that lack significant cytologic atypia. (**B**) Additionally, the elongated rete ridges have blunt borders that extend deeply into the reticular dermis without ever becoming overtly invasive.

Keratoacanthoma. Keratoacanthoma is a controversial entity. Some authors regard this neoplasm as a "benign" tumor, with a rapid period of growth followed by spontaneous involution. Another, currently more popular, view is that this tumor represents a variant of SCC. The clinical appearance is that of a symmetrical, cup-shaped growth that appears almost always on sun-exposed skin. There is also a high incidence of keratoacanthomas in immunosuppressed patients, and these tumors have been associated with the Muir-Torre syndrome (in conjunction with sebaceous neoplasms and internal malignancies).

The histologic appearance is that of a well-differentiated SCC. Large keratinocytes with abundant pale-staining eosinophilic cytoplasm form a cuplike invagination with a central keratin-filled center. The nests of keratinocytes extend downward into the dermis and may separate from the epidermis, giving

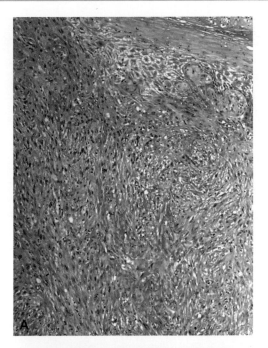

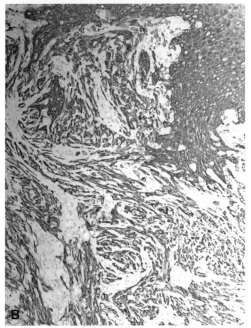

Figure 33 Sarcomatoid carcinoma. (**A**) Because of their spindled nature, the connection to the overlying epidermis may not be readily apparent on routine histologic sections. The cells course through the dermis in fascicles and often produce very little keratin to indicate their etiology. There is a variable degree of cytologic atypia, and mitotic activity is relatively brisk in most cases (H&E). (**B**) A panel of cytokeratins may be necessary to identify any expression, and some may be only focal (cytokeratin 5/6).

rise to the appearance of an invasive growth pattern. Perineural invasion has been described. Mitotic activity is usually brisk, and atypical forms may be observed (Fig. 34). Neutrophilic abscesses are present

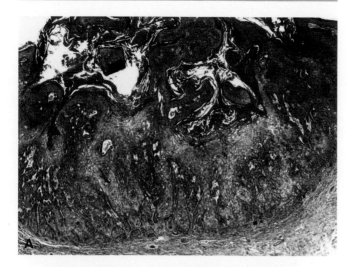

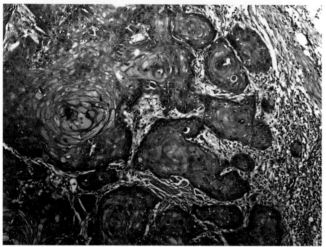

Figure 34 Keratoacanthoma. (**A**) These lesions resemble a well-differentiated squamous cell carcinoma that forms a cuplike invagination with a central keratin-filled center. They characteristically have large keratinocytes with abundant pale-staining eosinophilic cytoplasm. (**B**) The nests of keratinocytes extend downward into the dermis and may separate from the epidermis, giving rise to the appearance of an invasive growth pattern. Often a dense lymphocytic infiltrate is also present.

within the islands of proliferating keratinocytes in many cases. There is usually a brisk underlying inflammatory response, and, in later cases, underlying fibrosis and regressive changes are present.

Immunohistochemistry

Immunostains are very helpful in resolving the differential diagnosis of SCC in cases that are not straightforward. CK 5/6 are expressed by the vast majority of spindle cell SCC (124). Careful inspection of spindled SCCs is prudent as they often will show only focal CK expression, and several CK markers, including CK 5/6, AE1/3, and K903, should be included in the initial immunohistochemical panel to ensure detection of epithelial differentiation (124). All SCC variants are

negative for S-100 protein (124). Other tumors in the differential diagnosis include atypical fibroxanthoma (AFX), spindle cell or desmoplastic melanoma, angiosarcoma, and leiomyosarcoma. Each of these tumors fails to express CK 5/6, but is characteristically marked by other immunostains including CD68, S100 protein, CD34, and smooth muscle actin. Vimentin is not usually helpful, in that it is expressed by all of the tumors in this differential diagnosis, including a significant percentage of spindle cell SCC. For better-differentiated SCC, pan-CK cocktails will be positive in virtually all cases and will not be observed in most of the other tumors in the differential diagnosis.

Electron Microscopy

Electron microscopy is rarely required for establishing a diagnosis of cutaneous SCC. It is possible to detect intercellular bridges, desmosomes, and keratin tonofilaments with electron microscopy in the rare cases when the diagnosis cannot be established with routine histologic sections and immunostains (125). Additionally, poorly differentiated SCCs have accumulations of less-dense cytoplasmic intermediate filaments (126).

Molecular-Genetic Data

There is abundant literature regarding the genetic mutations that result in UV light–induced SCCs (127). Specifically, failure to repair thymidine dimers in the p53-tumor suppressor gene that are caused by UV radiation exposure is known to lead to tumor formation (128). Overexpression of p53 is seen in 40% of primary SCCs and 60% of their lymph node metastasis (126). However, while this information is vital to understanding the pathogenesis of this very common tumor, it is not useful in diagnostic pathology.

Differential Diagnosis

The major differential diagnosis of well-differentiated SCC is pseudoepitheliomatous or pseudocarcinomatous-reactive epidermal hyperplasia (PEH) (129). In some cases, this distinction is of vital importance, and extreme care should be taken to prevent overdiagnosis of cutaneous SCC. Reactive atypia can be seen in cases of florid epidermal hyperplasia, especially in situations with an extensive underlying inflammatory reaction. This situation can be seen in deep fungal infections such as blastomycosis, chromomycosis, and sporotrichosis, in infections by other fungi such as aspergillus and alternaria, and in bacterial infections (130–132). PEH is also seen in halogenodermas and overlying some dermal neoplasms such as granular cell tumors and DF, overlying lymphomatoid papulosis type A and cutaneous lymphoma (133–135), and rarely overlying cutaneous and oral mucosal melanoma (136–138) and oral Spitz nevi (SNs) (139). Similar epidermal hyperplasia, often with striking cytologic atypia, can be found at the edges of long-standing chronic ulcers and in cutaneous sinuses and fistulas (140). In these settings, distinction of SCC can be very difficult or even impossible. Squamous eddies and kekratin pearls may be seen in both. Mitoses may be seen in both; however, atypical forms are not seen in reactive hyperplasia. Apoptosis and dyskeratosis are uncommon in reactive proliferations (129). Complete excision to rule out one of these underlying processes may be indicated.

Poorly differentiated SCC presents a wider differential diagnosis. Marked nuclear anaplasia and lack of obvious keratinization are features shared with AFX, another neoplasm that occurs primarily on sun-damaged skin in elderly patients. Careful attention to the relationship between the epidermis and the neoplasm may help differentiate these entities in many cases; AFXs arise from within the dermis, but may push up against the epidermis. Multinucleated giant cells, xanthomatous cytoplasm, and an admixed inflammatory infiltrate may be more prominent in AFXs than in SCC, but these are not absolute criteria for distinction.

Angiosarcomas, leiomyosarcomas, and malignant melanomas may also present difficulties in making the distinction from poorly differentiated SCC. In these cases, attention to vascular spaces, fascicular growth pattern, or nesting (with or without melanin pigment) may be helpful in excluding these histologic mimics. However, in many cases, immunostains are the most effective way to arrive at a definitive diagnosis.

It may be difficult to definitively distinguish an SCC from a BCC with squamous differentiation. This distinction is of little clinical significance, as both tumors are treated with complete excision. BCCs demonstrate squamous differentiation following trauma or ulceration or in situations with marked inflammation. Thus, it is important to examine the deepest sections of the tumor most closely, looking for the characteristic findings of BCC described below. Peripheral palisading, cleft formation between the epithelial islands and myxoid, cellular tumor stroma are found in most BCCs, but are not features of SCC. Similarly, small, angulated nests of cells interspersed between collagen bundles are found more commonly in infiltrative or sclerosing type, also referred to as morpheic, morpheaform, and desmoplastic, BCCs than in SCC.

Treatment and Prognosis

The overall incidence of metastasis from cutaneous SCC that is related to sun exposure is on the order of 1% to 3%, though it is difficult to get an accurate estimate of this rate (141). The rate is higher for SCCs that develop in patients with tumors greater than 2 cm, invasion greater than 4 to 5 mm, incomplete excision, recurrent lesions, poorly differentiated tumors, perineural invasion, and lesions on or around the ears or lips, on mucous membranes, or with immunosuppression, and approaches 40% in tumors arising within long-standing ulcers (120). The current tumor-node-metastasis (TNM) staging only assigns size as a prognostic factor for patients without muscle or cartilage involvement and does not specifically address cutaneous SCC of the head and neck. Accordingly, this system

is inadequate for SCC of the head and neck and for use in patients in the high-risk groups listed above (142). Mohs surgery continues to provide the highest cure rate (143). However, this is often reserved for those with a high risk of tumors or with the highest risk of disfigurement. For others with a low risk of tumors, local excision with a 4-mm margin is the treatment of choice to achieve a 95% chance of clearance (111). A 6-mm margin is recommended for tumors greater than 2 cm or occurring on high-risk anatomical sites (111). For nonsurgical candidates with superficial tumors, topical chemotherapeutics, retinoids, and biologic–immune response modifiers provide an alternative to radiation therapy and its associated side effects (143). Radiation and/or lymph node dissection is used for treatment of nodal disease and regional disease with a five-year cure rate approaching 40%.

B. Basal Cell Carcinoma

Introduction

BCC is the most common cutaneous malignancy, especially among fair-skinned people (phototype I and II), and the incidence continues to increase (144,145). Women younger than 40 years have a greater increase in BCC than do men of the same age group (146). The lesions are slow growing and locally invasive with rare cases progressing to metastatic disease (147). Its association with UV light, both from environmental exposure as well as from tanning bed use, is clearly established, with intermittent and cumulative exposure showing an important causal relationship (148–150). Immunosuppressed organ transplant recipients are 65 to 250 times more likely to develop epithelial carcinomas, of which BCC is the most common (151). As in immunosuppressed organ transplant recipients, patients infected with HIV show increased rates of BCC. However, unlike SCC, the biologic behavior of the BCC does not show a more aggressive course (152). BCC that develops at the site of local irradiation has a more aggressive behavior and requires more aggressive surgical resection (153). Variations in biologic behavior have been associated with various subtypes of BCC. Accordingly, it is appropriate to classify BCC into five subtypes: nodular, infiltrative, sclerosing (morpheic, morpheaform, desmoplastic), superficial, and micronodular. Superficial BCC presents in a slightly younger age group than the other subtypes. The relative incidence of these subtypes varies with the amount of sun exposure (154). In a population with high sun exposure, in Queensland, Australia, the nodular subtype is the most common (48%), followed by superficial (26%), infiltrative (14%), and micronodular (8%) (154). The sclerosing type represents 6% in one report confined to BCC on the eyelid (155). While the absolute numbers change, the ranking remains the same in a similar study out of France (156). Nodular, infiltrative, and micronodular BCC predominate on the head and neck, while superficial BCC tends to present on the back in men and on the upper extremities in women (154).

Clinical Features

The classic presentation of BCC is on sun-exposed skin of elderly adults with a male predominance. However, that classic presentation is rapidly evolving to include younger patients and disproportionately more women (146). BCC presents as a pearly papule with overlying telangectasia. While typically asymptomatic, a history of bleeding is not uncommon (157), especially in the nodular subtype. In contrast, superficial BCC more often presents as an erythematous plaque or patch (158).

Imaging

Because of their locally aggressive nature, some patients with BCC present for surgical excision with a lesion much further advanced than was initially appreciated (159). Recent studies indicate that high-resolution MRI using a microscopy surface coil is an effective technique to stage BCC of the face for bone involvement (160).

Pathology

Predominant histologic features have been recognized and acknowledged in BCC because of the varying biologic behavior. *Nodular* BCC is by far the most common subtype, showing one or multiple nodules of basaloid cells in the dermis. The nodules are relatively well circumscribed and composed of cells having vesicular nuclei, large nuclei with less abundant cytoplasm, nuclear pleomorphism, and mitoses. The outermost layer of cells in each lobule is composed of cells with nuclei lining up perpendicular to the lobular border, a feature referred to as palisading (Fig. 35).

Because of histologic processing retraction artifact, clefting between the neoplastic lobules and the surrounding stroma is characteristic. Mucin deposition is also common in and around the lobules of BCC and helpful in differentiating this lesion from other basaloid proliferations in which mucin deposition would be uncommon. By nature of the germinative properties of the basilar keratinocytes, differentiation toward adnexal structures or keratinizing cells is commonly encountered in BCC. The surrounding stroma varies from loose to compact, and the overlying epidermis may be attenuated or ulcerated by the enlarging dermal mass. Multiple sections may need to be evaluated to find an epidermal connection.

The second most common type is *superficial*, or *multifocal*, BCC composed of multiple nodules of basaloid cells projecting from the epidermis into the subjacent dermis. Varying extents of uninvolved epidermis may separate these nodules (Fig. 36).

Infiltrative BCC, in contrast to the rounded lobules of the more common nodular and superficial BCC, is characterized by angulated basaloid nests with harsh contours extending into the dermis (Fig. 37). *Sclerosing type* BCC has a collagenous stroma with small islands and elongated strands of basaloid cells percolating between collagen bundles. In some cases, the elongated strands are only one cell layer thick. Palisading of peripheral nuclei and clefting between basaloid cells and the surrounding stroma will be seen focally in this variant, but typically not in the majority of the lesion; careful inspection is required (Fig. 38).

Micronodular BCC is characterized by multiple small dermal nests of basaloid cells. The nests may be so small as to be composed of only a peripheral rim of cells, without any cells in the center of the nodule. Peripheral palisading is less prominent in this variant (Fig. 39).

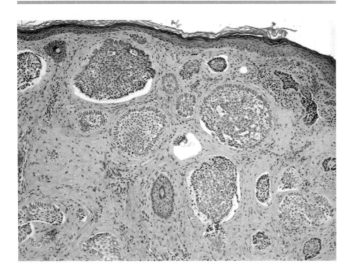

Figure 35 Basal cell carcinoma, nodular type. This is the most common variant and shows a relatively well-circumscribed nodule extending into the dermis from the overlying epidermis. It is composed of cells with large, vesicular nuclei with nuclear pleomorphism and mitoses. The nuclei of the cells in the outermost layer of each lobule align perpendicular to the lobular border, a feature referred to as palisading.

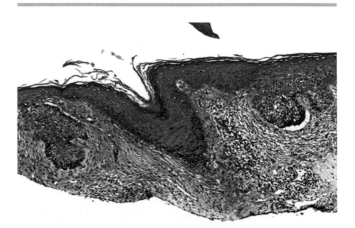

Figure 36 Basal cell carcinoma, superficial type. This type shows multiple nodules of basaloid cells projecting from the epidermis into the subjacent dermis. The amount of uninvolved epidermis separating these nodules varies considerably.

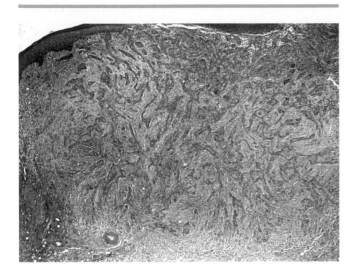

Figure 37 Basal cell carcinoma, infiltrative type. Angulated basaloid nests with sharp contours extending into the dermis characterize this variant.

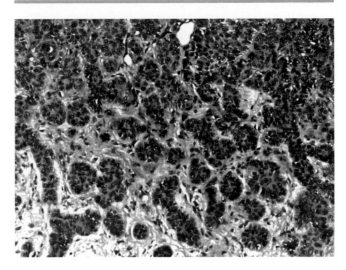

Figure 39 Basal cell carcinoma, micronodular type. Multiple small nests of basaloid cells are seen in the dermis. Often these nests are so small as to not have a center.

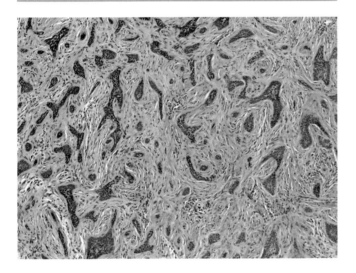

Figure 38 Basal cell carcinoma, sclerosing type. A collagenous stroma with small islands and elongated strands of basaloid cells are present intercalating between collagen bundles.

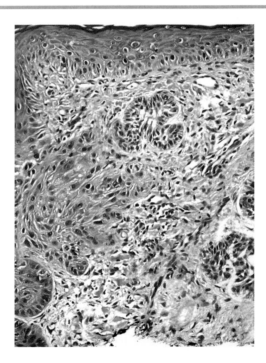

Figure 40 Basal cell carcinoma, metaypical type. This variant shows nests that lack peripheral palisading and have cells with more abundant cytoplasm and enlarged nuclei (*arrows*), along with more conventional basaloid nests with peripheral palisading (*arrowhead*).

And finally, *metatypical* BCC is composed of basaloid nests that lack peripheral palisading and have foci of enlarged cells with more abundant cytoplasm and enlarged nuclei (Fig. 40). This entity is often confused with basosquamous cell carcinoma (BSCC), and, in some reports, used interchangeably (161,162). However, if the terminology is used in the purest form, metatypical variant of BCC is reserved for those features mentioned above, while BSCC is used for lesions with basaloid, squamous, and intermediate cells types as described below. Both entities have an aggressive behavior and metastatic potential (163).

Immunohistochemistry

As the tumor is composed of epithelial keratinocytes, strong expression for CK 5/6 is present. Immunohistochemical staining with Ki-67, p53, and bcl-2 did not differentiate between conventional nonaggressive

BCCs and those more aggressive BCCs with metastatic potential (147). Additionally, BCCs, but not SCCs, stain with antibodies to BerEP4, and, with the exception of some aggressive variants, BCCs also express bcl-2 (164–166).

Electron Microscopy

Electron microscopy does not play a role in the diagnosis or differential diagnosis of BCC.

Molecular-Genetic Data

Development of BCC is closely linked to mutations in PTCH1 gene on chromosome 9q22.3. These mutations in both sporadic and familial cases are most commonly due to loss of heterozygosity at this locus. The aberrations are all inactivating mutations, lending support to the theory that PTCH1 is a tumor suppressor gene. PTCH1 codes for a protein that binds to the protein product of the smoothened (SMO) gene to form a receptor complex for the sonic hedgehog protein (167). Mutational inactivation of PTCH1 interferes with the inhibition of SMO signaling. Congential aberrations in this pathway are the basis of nevoid basal cell carcinoma syndrome (NBCCS), or Gorlin-Goltz syndrome, which is an uncommon, autosomal dominant disorder characterized by multiple BCC, especially at an early age. Additional features of NBCCS are palmar/plantar pits, bifid rib and other rib and spine abnormalities, odontogenic cysts, and calcification of the falx cerebri (168,169).

Differential Diagnosis

Other basaloid tumors form the differential diagnosis for BCC. These include predominantly tumors of follicular origin. Differentiating follicular neoplasms from BCC with follicular differentiation can be impossible at times. However, association with overlying epidermis, tumor-stromal clefting, and mucin deposition would favor a diagnosis of BCC. Whereas association with the follicular unit, lack of clefting, and lack of mucin favor an adnexal neoplasm, which is then further classified on the basis of the noeoplasm's efforts at recapitulating adnexal structures.

Basaloid hyperplasia, such as is seen secondary to DFs, presumably as an effect of syndecan-1 and/or other secreted cytokines I, is distinguished by its lack of cytoplasmic enlargement or nuclear atypia (170).

Sclerosing type BCC needs to be differentiated from desmoplastic trichoepithelioma by histologic features alone, as no antigen expression profile has proven unique to one lesion (171). Desmoplastic trichoepithelioma shows strands of basaloid cells with horn cysts in a sclerotic stroma. The horn cysts are unique to trichoepithelioma and help in the differential diagnosis. Mitoses, single-cell aptosis, mucinous stroma, and stromal clefting would also not be seen in desmoplastic trichoepithelioma. Sclerosing BCC must also be differentiated from infiltrating carcinomas of other etiologies, in particular breast carcinoma.

Careful searching will often result in more typical nodules of basaloid cells to support a diagnosis of BCC. Immunohistochemical staining patterns may also be helpful. With the exception of breast carcinoma with basaloid differentiation, CK 5/6 expression is unique to BCC (172,173).

Treatment and Prognosis

Complete excision is effective in eradicating most BCCs with less than 2% recurrence at five years (151). Thity-eight percent recurrence is reported with BCC involvement of the surgical margins (151). When treating the more aggressive subtypes, micronodular, infiltrative, and sclerosing, special attention is warranted to ensure complete removal and to avoid subsequent recurrences and metastasis (174). For nonsurgical candidates with low-risk variants, topical 5% imiquimod, an immune response modifier that targets toll-like receptroe 7 and 8, has shown good results, in particular when used as adjunctive therapy to curettage (175). For patients with xeroderma pigmentosum, NBCC syndrome, and solid organ or bone marrow transplants, systemic retinoids show promise as effective chemotherapeutic agents (176).

C. Basosquamous Cell Carcinoma

Introduction

While considered intermittently as a variant of BCC, BSCC is now recognized as a unique entity (177). Unequivocal evidence does not yet exist to confirm whether BSCC arises de novo or evolves from a preexisting lesion. Regardless, categorization into its own entity is supported by the significantly increased aggressive behavior over conventional BCC and SCC (178,179). In this same fashion, BSCCs require significantly more stages during Mohs micrographic surgery to establish clear margins and are more likely to present with pulmonary metastasis than either BCC or SCC (179). Interestingly, in patients with metastasis, both basaloid and squamous elements were present (177,179).

The rarity of this lesion makes epidemiologic data scarce, while discrepancy exists regarding which histologic features constitute BSCC. If BSCC is used for those lesions that contain discrete, admixed components of BCC and SCC, then this lesion represents 0.5% to 2.7% of all BCCs. BSCC is used synonymously with metatypical BCC in some reports (179,180), whereas others identify the two lesions separately. We prefer the latter nomenclature, reserving BSCC for those lesions showing mixed BCC and SCC elements.

Clinical Features

Virtually all BSCCs in one study of 27 lesions occurred on the face or ears with rare occurrences on the scalp and axilla (179). As this report analyzes patients presenting for Mohs repair, it is likely biased to those sites most treated by this technique: the head and neck. There are reports of other sites such as dorsum of the foot (177). There is a 2:1 male predominance, with an age at presentation ranging in the sixth to ninth decade. The lesions are typically flat to slightly raised with indistinct borders and rusty pigmentation, differentiating them clinically from the raised lesions with elevated borders and pearly appearance of the nodular BCC.

Imaging

Imaging studies are only needed for evaluating for distant metastasis in the staging workup of these patients. Diagnostic imaging studies are not useful.

Pathology

BSCCs have an infiltrative neoplasm consisting of basaloid cells extending from the overlying epidermis into the dermis and composed of cells with nuclei larger than conventional BCC nuclei. Within the clusters of these basaloid cells, there are aggregates of cells showing variable features of squamatization. In addition to the BCC and SCC comparable foci, BSCC has cells representing a transition between the basaloid and squamous elements; these cells are referred to as intermediate cells or transition cells.

Immunohistochemistry

BSCC has an antigenic profile similar to both BCC and SCC. The expression of Ber-EP4 in the basaloid cells, but not in the intermediate or squamous cells, supports the theory of tumor differentiation rather than of a collision of the two epithelial types (180). AE1/AE3, bcl-2, transforming growth factor (TGF)-α, and p53 are not helpful in differentiating this entity from SCC and BCC (180).

Electron Microscopy

Ultrastructural studies have not been used for this neoplasm.

Molecular-Genetic Data

A genetic association has not been established for this lesion.

Differential Diagnosis

Collision tumors, consisting of a focus of SCC abutting against a focus of BCC, are a major consideration in the histologic differential diagnosis and are distinctly different from the admixed nature of BSCC. The distinction is important because of the potentially aggressive behavior of BSCC over the others.

Keratinizing BCCs show a pattern of conventional, typically nodular BCC with keratin pearls. These foci of keratinization lack nuclear and cytologic atypia that characterizes BSCC.

Treatment and Prognosis

Positive surgical margins, lymphatic invasion, perineural invasion, and male gender are the most significant prognosticators. The most appropriate treatment is wide local excision with evaluation of the nodal basins and distant sites for metastasis. 5-fluorourocil adjuvant chemotherapy and radiation have been successfully used.

D. Microcystic Adnexal Carcinoma

Synonyms: sclerosing sweat duct carcinoma, ductal eccrine carcinoma, and malignant syringoma.

Introduction

MAC was first reported in 1982 by Goldstein and colleagues (181). It is an indolent, yet locally aggressive, malignant adnexal tumor with a high rate of recurrence and occasional distant metastasis (181–184). There are reports of these lesions being present for years prior to diagnosis (185). Biopsies, which are typically a small punch or superficial shave because of the location of the lesions on the face, lead to diagnostic difficulties as differentiating MAC from other benign entities, in particular syringoma, is impossible, or at best challenging in these inadequate specimens (186). MACs have been associated with previous radiation therapy for adolescent acne or cancers as well as primary immunodeficiency syndrome (187–190). In the United States, their predilection for the left side of the face, the side that gets most exposure to UV rays during driving, adds further support to radiation exposure as an etiologic factor (191). Similar studies have not been done in countries where driving and UV exposure occur on the right to confirm these data.

Clinical Features

The lesions present in young to middle-aged adults, often reported with a female predominance, though some studies show no gender predilection (192). The mean age at presentation is 61, with a range of 19 to 90 years (191). They begin as a slowly expanding papule. At presentation, MAC is typically a 0.5- to 2.0-cm, firm, pale yellow or erythematous plaque with indistinct orders. Periocular and perioral are common sites, but MAC may also involve the scalp, breast, auditory canal, genitalia, axilla, and extremities (191,193–195). Although lesions are often asymptomatic, they may become tender when perineural invasion is present.

Imaging

Imaging studies are unnecessary for the diagnosis or differential diagnosis of MAC.

Pathology

Histologically, MAC is a poorly circumscribed dermal tumor that may extend into the subcutis and skeletal muscle. It is composed of deceptively bland epithelial components demonstrating both follicular and sweat duct differentiations with a desmoplastic stroma (Fig. 41). The glandular structures are lined by two layers of cuboidal cells and may have amorphous, eosinophilic, PAS-positive material within the

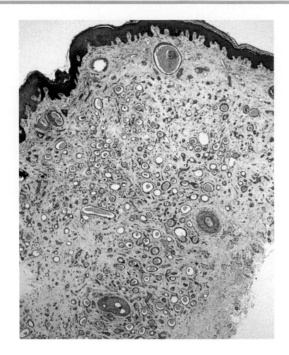

Figure 41 Microcystic adnexal carcinoma. MAC is characterized by a poorly circumscribed and deeply infiltrative dermal tumor composed of deceptively bland epithelial components and a desmoplastic stroma.

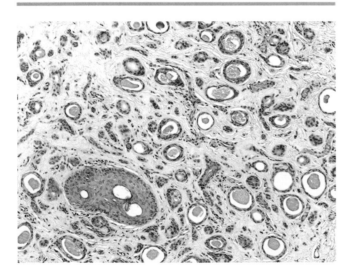

Figure 42 Microcystic adnexal carcinoma. The glandular structures are lined by two layers of cuboidal cells and may have amorphous, eosinophilic, PAS-positive material within the lumen.

lumen (Fig. 42). The superficial portion is often composed of keratinizing cysts lined by squamoid cells. Abortive adnexal structures make up the deeper portion of this infiltrate, with the deepest portion consisting of small islands and strands of epithelial cells. Cells with clear, glycogen-rich

cytoplasm may be present, with occasional sebaceous differentiation (196). Mitoses are usually rare or absent. Perineural invasion is frequently seen.

Immunohistochemistry

Antigen expression can be a helpful means of differentiating MAC from histologically similar entities. EMA, CEA, CK 7, and S-100 protein expression can be detected in the epithelial component (197–199). This can be useful in delineating the extent of tumor involvement, particularly in the deep aspect of the infiltrate where epithelial elements can be difficult to identify and in highlighting the presence of perineural involvement. As in other cutaneous adnexal neoplasms, CK 5/6 expression is seen in MAC (6).

Electron Microscopy

Ultrastructural studies confirm the presence of ductal differentiation (200).

Molecular-Genetic Data

Although there is one report documenting familial incidence in two sisters, MACs do not carry any specific genetic aberration (185).

Differential Diagnosis

Syringoma is the major entity in the differential diagnosis, and superficial biopsies may preclude the ability to give a definitive diagnosis. Syringoma has a similar clinical presentation and, histologically, is composed of bland-appearing ducts and keratinous cysts set in a desmoplastic stroma. The distinction is made on obtaining an adequately deep biopsy that allows for evaluation of a shallow specimen without an infiltrative base; deep extension and perineural invasion are not features of syringoma. Desmoplastic trichoepithelioma is a benign adnexal neoplasm with a superficial dermal growth pattern. It too is composed of thin strands of bland epithelial cells and a desmoplastic stroma (Fig. 43). Desmoplastic trichoepithelioma will not show expression of CEA, CK 7, EMA, or S-100, as would be seen in MAC. Additionally, infiltrative growth pattern and perineural invasion are not characteristic of desmoplastic trichoepithelioma.

The sclerosing variant of BCC will demonstrate nests extending from the overlying epidermis, a feature not seen in MAC. And, while ductal differentiation may be seen in BCC, it is not to the extent seen in MAC. Additionally, the epithelial elements in BCC display larger nuclei, mitoses, and cytologic atypia, none of which characterize MAC.

Treatment and Prognosis

MAC is a locally aggressive adnexal carcinoma with significant deep tissue infiltration, which at times is not amenable to surgical excision (201). Misdiagnosis

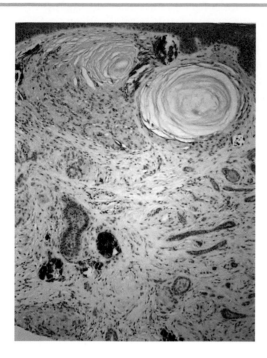

Figure 43 Desmoplastic trichoepithelioma. This lesion, which enters the differential diagnosis of MAC, shows narrow strands of tumor cells and keratocysts, some with calcification, in a sclerotic stroma.

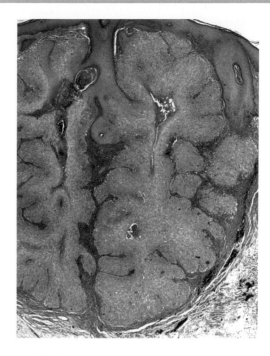

Figure 44 Tricholemmal carcinoma. This lesion is characterized by a multilobulated dermal growth pattern with infiltrative extensions. There is connection to the epidermis or pilosebaceous structures.

is reported in 30% of cases, leading to delay in proper management (191). Local recurrence occurs in nearly 50% of cases without adequate excision margins. More recent series have described high cure rates with maximum tissue sparing, using Mohs micrographic surgery (191,202). Radiation therapy has been contemplated for cases not deemed a surgical candidate because of poor patient health or tumor extent. This has resulted in initial clearing of the tumor, which subsequently recurred more extensively and, histologically, more aggressively (203). In a study of 48 patients with MAC, the 10-year local recurrence rate is 18%, and metastases were not seen (191). However, rare cases with metastasis in the scalp, lymph node, lung, liver, and bone were reported (182–184,190). Because of the rarity of the neoplasm and, even more rare, the metastasis, statistical data regarding metastatic rate are not available.

E. Trichilemmal Carcinoma

Introduction

Trichilemmal carcinoma (TLC) is the malignant counterpart of trichilemmoma, the benign counterpart of this outer root sheath neoplasm. The neoplasm has an indolent clinical course with no reports of recurrence (204). There have been rare reports of metastasis, and only three cases have been reported with lymph node metastasis, and all the three have been from primary lesions on the thigh (204–207).

Clinical Features

TLC presents on sun-exposed surfaces, most commonly the head and neck and dorsum of the hands, although the trunk and extremities have been described (208). The classic age distribution is in patients aged 60 to 80 years. A nine-year-old with xeroderma pigmentosum has been reported with TLC, as has a renal transplant patient, highlighting the role of cancer immune surveillance and DNA repair in this malignancy, as in other malignancies (209). Other rare reports include TLC in a burn scar (210,211). The lesions present as erythematous nodules, less than 2 cm, and often have become ulcerated. Most commonly, they are diagnosed clinically as a BCC (212).

Imaging

Imaging studies are not necessary for diagnosis.

Pathology

TLC has a dermal growth pattern with connection to the epidermis or pilosebaceous structures. The dermal tumor is multilobulated with infiltrative extensions (Fig. 44). The lobules show peripheral palisading and are composed of cells with large glycogenated cytoplasm showing differentiation toward the outer root sheath. Large cells with varying degrees of cytologic atypia, large pleomorphic nuclei, prominent nucleoli, and variable numbers of mitoses can be identified (Fig. 45). The pale or clear cytoplasm is PAS-positive and diastase sensitive. Keratinization, when present,

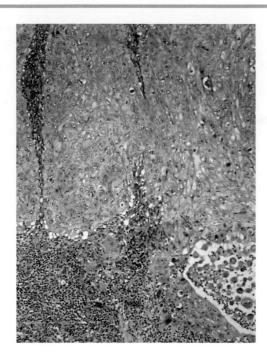

Figure 45 Tricholemmal carcinoma. The lobules lack peripheral palisading and are composed of cells with large glycogenated cytoplasm with differentiation toward the outer root sheath. The nuclei are large and pleomorphic with variable numbers of mitoses. A plasma cell-rich infiltrate is present at the periphery of the lobules.

is tricholemmal, and a hyaline basement memebrane can be identified around the tumor lobules. A plasma cell-rich lymphocytic infiltrate is often present at the periphery of the lobules.

Immunohistochemistry

TLC shows expression of CK 1,10,14, and 17, similar to TL. TLs additionally demonstrate expression of CK 15 and 16, the loss of which in TLC may be related to their malignant transformation (213).

Electron Microscopy

Ultrastructural studies have not been reported.

Molecular-Genetic Data

No genetic, syndromic, or familial associations have been made.

Differential Diagnosis

Clear cell SCC demonstrates an infiltrate border, rather than the pushing border of TLC, and does not have peripheral palisading or cytoplasmic glycogen. Keratinization, when present, is infundibular. A keratoacanthoma has very similar low-power architecture, but does not arise from the follicular epithelium, and most commonly has a central keratin-filled cavity. The basal layer of a keratoacanthoma maintains the

cuboidal morphology of basilar epithelium and does not demonstrate peripheral palisading. A SC also has an endophytic growth pattern, is composed of cells with clear cytoplasm, and may be seen associated with the follicular unit. However, the basaloid cells that comprise the periphery of the lobule are distinctly different from the palisaded periphery of TLC. Additionally, the cleared cytoplasm of SC is due to a finely vesicular cytoplasm, rather than glycogen, and sebaceous differentiation has not been described in TLC.

Treatment and Prognosis

Wide excision and Mohs micrographic surgery are the recommended treatment options because of the locally aggressive behavior of these lesions (209). Topical 5% imiquimod cream has also been used successfully to treat TLC (214).

F.   Merkel Cell Carcinoma

Synonyms: neuroendocrine carcinoma, and trabecular carcioma.

Introduction

Merkel cell carcinoma (MCC) was first reported in 1972 by Toker as trabecular carcinoma (215). Later, based on the ultrastructural findings of neurosecretory granules, the designation "primary (small cell) neuroendocrine carcinoma of the skin" became commonplace. MCC is an aggressive tumor with 30% mortality and whose incidence has increased dramatically over the past decades (216). Interestingly, in the setting of solid organ transplant, there is an increase in incidence of many malignancies, presumably due to immunosuppression and loss of surveillance abilities. However, organ transplant recipients have a lower rate of MCC, although those that do appear have unusual histologic features (217).

Clinical Features

MCC usually arises on sun-exposed skin of elderly patients and has a male predilection. These tumors present most commonly on the head and neck (37%), followed by the extremities (32%) (218). Only rare cases occur on sun-protected sites, such as the oral and nasal mucosa (219). MCCs have rarely been associated with chronic lymphocytic leukemia (220), sarcoidosis (221), autoimmuno hepatitis (222), treatment with anti-CD20 monoclonal antibody (223), and AFX (224). Clinically, the tumors are indistinguishable from other malignant cutaneous neoplasms. They present as a firm, raised painless nodule, often with an erythematous or violaceous overlying surface. They usually measure 2 cm or less.

Imaging

As they are dermal-based neoplasms, there is no need for complementary imaging to diagnose MCCs.

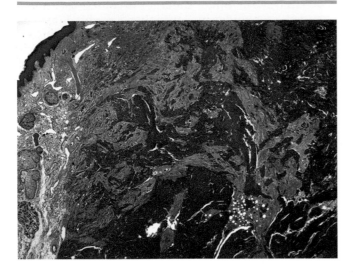

Figure 46 Merkel cell carcinoma. The lesion presents as a poorly defined dermal mass composed of small cells with minimal cytoplasm.

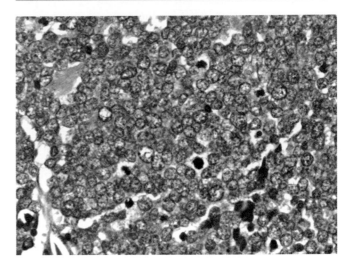

Figure 47 Merkel cell carcinoma. The tumor cells are uniformly round with vague cell borders, a small amount of amphophilic cytoplasm, and a speckled nuclear chromatin pattern. Nucleoli are not prominent. Mitosis and apoptotic bodies are easily identified.

Pathology

MCC appears as a poorly defined dermal mass, frequently infiltrating the subcutaneous fat (Fig. 46). Three histologic subtypes have been described. The trabecular variant is the least common and consists of ribbons of monotonous cells. The intermediate variant, which is the most common, has a nodular growth pattern. And, the small cell type resembles oat cell carcinoma of the lung (225). Cytologically, the tumor cells are round to oval and of uniform size with a so-called salt and pepper nuclear chromatin and multiple small and inconspicuous nucleoli. There are numerous mitoses and apoptotic bodies with small amount of amphophilic cytoplasm (Fig. 47). The cell borders are vaguely defined, and marked crush artifact may be present. In up to 10% of cases, there is intraepidermal spread, including Pautrier-like microabscess formation, and, therefore, cutaneous T-cell lymphoma and superficial spreading melanoma enter the differential diagnosis. MCC with associated SCC correlates with an increased risk of recurrence, although metastatic rates and overall survival figures are not affected (226,227).

Immunohistochemistry

The immunophenotypic characteristics of MCC resemble those of neuroendocrine carcinoma in other tissue sites. Keratin is uniformly expressed; neuroendocrine carcinomas demonstrate a perinuclear dotlike staining pattern of reactivity (228,229). CK 20 is expressed in approximately 85% of MCC (230). Nearly all MCCs express neuron-specific enolase. These tumors are also immunoreactive for neurofilament protein, EMA, and CD56 (231). Other neuroendocrine markers such as chromogranin and synaptophysin are detectable with variable frequency (232). Immunostaining for CK 20, especially when combined with thyroid transcription factor (TTF)-1, can be used to

distinguish between MCC and small cell carcinoma (both pulmonary and extrapulmonary). A recent study evaluated the immunophenotypic characteristics of 21 MCCs and 33 small cell carcinomas of lung using TTF-1 and CK 20. TTF-1 was 100% specific for the diagnosis of small cell carcinoma of lung associated with a diagnostic sensitivity of 85%. CK 20 was present in 95% of MCCs; however, 33% of small cell carcinoma of lung were also positive (229,233).

Electron Microscopy

Ultrastructurally, the tumor cells contain membrane-bound neurosecretory granules in their cytoplasm, which are located peripherally along the basement membrane and dendritic processes (234). Complex intercellular junctions and cytoplasmic spinous processes can also be seen (235).

Molecular-Genetic Data

Cytogenetic studies may also be useful. Primitive neuroectodermal tumors demonstrate t(11;22) chromosomal translocation, whereas in MCCS, the most common chromosomal abnormality is located on chromosome 1 (236). Trisomy 6 is seen in nearly 50% of MCCs (237).

Differential Diagnosis

Because of the histologically undifferentiated small blue cell appearance of MCCs, considerations must be given to other so-called small blue cell tumors such as lymphomas, neuroendocrine carcinomas metastatic to the skin, small cell malignant melanoma, and primitive neuroectodermal tumors (PNETs or Ewing sarcoma). Lymphomas fail to show the cellular patterning seen within MCCs. Melanomas most commonly demonstrate intraepidermal proliferations, though, as noted above, this finding is also rarely present in MCCs. The nesting pattern and pigment deposition may be helpful features in arriving at a diagnosis of melanoma. Rosette formation, characteristic of PNETs, is not seen in MCC. Immunohistologic analysis is the most informative method for separating these entities (see "Immunohistochemistry" section). Malignant melanomas and lymphomas express S-100 and CD45 (LCA: leukocyte common antigen), respectively. CD99 expression is common in PNET, but not seen in MCC.

Treatment and Prognosis

MCC has an aggressive clinical course with frequent locoregional recurrence and distant metastasis. Margin negative excision, whether by wide local excision or Mohs surgery, is the recommended treatment. Lymph node status is useful in identifying patients who may develop recurrence; however, lymph node dissection itself does not offer a survival advantage (238). A recent study identifying 251 patients, who had been treated between 1970 and 2002, reported a five-year disease-specific survival rate of 64%. Disease stage was the only independent predictor of survival (stage I, 81%; stage II, 67%; stage III, 52%; stage IV, 11%; $p = 0.001$). Pathologic nodal staging was associated with improved stage-specific survival probabilities (239). Recent studies show that patients treated with surgery plus adjuvant locoregional radiotherapy experience a better disease-free survival than those undergoing surgery alone (216,240). Adjuvant chemotherapy has not found a role treatment of MCC. Mucosal MCC is aggressive, and there is a high risk for local recurrence and regional and distant metastasis (241). Visceral involvement (the lungs, bone, brain, liver, and deep lymph nodes) has been observed in approximately 35% to 40% of patients, almost all of whom die within an average of six months.

III. MELANOCYTIC NEOPLASMS

A. Spitz Nevus

Synonyms: spindle and epithelioid cell nevus and benign juvenile melanoma.

Introduction

Conventional benign nevomelanocytic nevi of the head and neck are no different than those on other body sites. The same is true for the SN. However, as SN is commonly located on the head and neck, special attention will be given to it here. SN was originally named benign juvenile melanoma by Sophie Spitz in recognition of this cutaneous lesion composed of distinct pleomorphic cells, pagetoid spread, and dermal mitoses that histologically resembles malignant melanoma (242). It was recognized early that, despite its nomenclature, SN had an excellent prognosis

compared with other melanomas, and the name changed to avoid the confusion provided by the term "melanoma" (243). SN evolves, just as conventional nevi do, with junctional, compound, and intradermal phases (244). With the publication of cases of SN with pagetoid spread, and cases with metastasis and lymphatic invasion, it has become apparent that the entity we label SN not only has a wide range of histologic parameter but also has a wide range of clinical behaviors (245–247). Lymphatic invasion has been reported in 14% of cases in one study (247). In that report, all patients were doing well for years after excision. In addition to the diverse biologic behavior displayed by these lesions, there is a lack of objective criteria leading to diagnostic difficulties, even among experts (248).

Clinical Features

Both classic and atypical SN typically present in children and adolescents, rarely presenting in those older than 30 years (249). SN is a red-to-brown, dome-shaped nodule, which is often clinically mistaken for a hemangioma. The surface can range from smooth to verrucoid and may be slowly or rapidly growing. They present predominantly in Caucasians and have a slight female predominanc (249). These asymptomatic lesions are commonly located on the trunk, head, and neck, lower extremity, and upper extremity in decreasing order (249).

Imaging

Imaging studies are not necessary for the diagnosis and have not been reported.

Pathology

Conventional SN are symmetrical melanocytic proliferations composed of varying proportions of epithelioid cells and spindled cells. An evolution from junctional to compound to intradermal melanocytic proliferations occurs as in conventional nevi (244). An acanthotic or attenuated epidermis with spongiosis, hyperkeratosis, and occasional parakeratosis may overly the lesion (Fig. 48). The junctional component is composed of nests of melanocytes along the basilar layer. The melanocytes are large and pigmented with vesicular and typically large nuclei. Loss of cohesion from the surrounding epidermis is characteristically seen in these junctional nests (Fig. 49). This results in clefting, separating the nest from the overlying keratinocytes in contradistinction from conventional melanocytic nevi and melanoma, in which this cleft does not typically exist. The mechanism of the clefting has not been elucidated. Upwarding migrating single and clustered melanocytes may be seen in SN, with clusters or small groups predominating over single melanocytes (Fig. 50). Despite rare reports, fully evolved pagetoid proliferation is not characteristic (242) These junctional melanocytes have abundant cytoplasm and take on epithelioid or spindled morphology. The nuclei are slightly larger than those of typical melanocytes, but do not demonstrate pleomorphism.

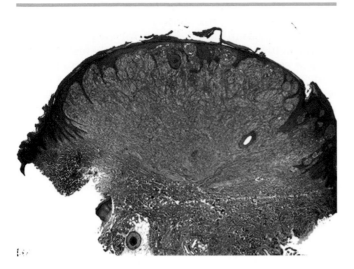

Figure 48 Spitz nevus. This melanocytic neoplasm is characterized by a symmetrical proliferation of melanocytes that have both spindled and/or epithelioid morphology. The clinical lesion is often dome-shaped, as seen in this image.

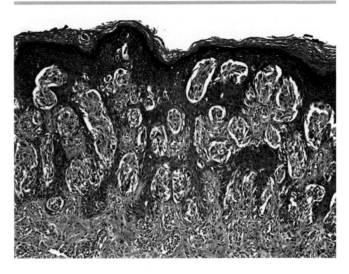

Figure 50 Spitz nevus. Upwarding migrating single and clustered melanocytes may be seen; however, clusters or small groups predominate over single melanocytes.

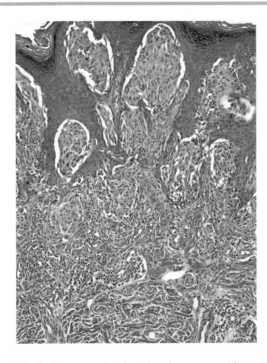

Figure 49 Spitz nevus. The junctional component is composed of nests of melanocytes that primarily maintain their orientation along the basilar layer. The melanocytes are large and pigmented with vesicular and typically large nuclei. Loss of cohesion from the surrounding epidermis, causing a cleft between the melanocytic nest and the overlying epidermis, is characteristically seen in these junctional nests.

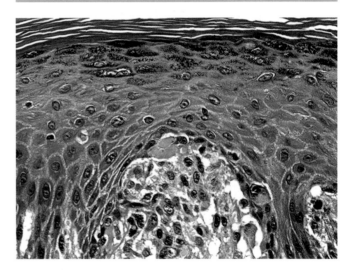

Figure 51 Spitz nevus. Eosinophilic globules of basement membrane material are present along the junction and, while not specific, are characteristic of SN.

Classically, amorphous, PAS-positive, diastase-resistant eosinophilic deposits, or Kamino bodies have been described along the junctional layer of SN (Fig. 51) (250). These eosinophilc globules, while rare,

may also be seen in melanoma and benign conventional nevi (250). However, the globules found in other nevi and melanoma are negative for PAS and trichrome stains (250). These globules represent basement membrane accumulations of collagen type IV and laminin, and not apoptotic material (251,252). In SN with a dermal component, as in conventional melanocytic nevi, the melanocytes demonstrate maturation with progression into the subjacent dermis. This maturation, comparable to conventional nevi, is recognized by decreases in nest size, nuclear size, cytoplasm, and pigmentation. The dermal component is composed of a varying mixture of large polygonal cells and spindle cells with large vesicular nuclei and prominent acidophilic nucleoli. Dermal mitoses may be present in SN; however, these are most commonly in the superficial and mid portion of the infiltrate and are not numerous. Mitoses in the deep portion of the dermal infiltrate and atypical forms should raise concern for a more worrisome lesion. There is significant overlap in the histologic features of SN and malignant melanoma, and, as in the rest of pathology, relying on any single feature to make this diagnosis can result in over- or underdiagnosis of SN. Variations from these diagnostic guidelines lead to a diagnosis of atypical SN. There is a histologic spectrum comprising SN at one end, atypical SN in the middle, and melanoma at the other extreme. A lack of objective histologic features that neatly distinguish SN from melanoma exists, even among experts (248). A suggestion has been proposed that stratification of SN into low-, intermediate-, and high-risk categories, based on a combination of clinical and histologic features, resolves the difficulties in attempting to issue one diagnosis for an entity that appears to comprise a spectrum of histologic findings and clinical behaviors (253).

Adult SN tend to be intradermal and have more dermal fibroplasia than the SN obtained from children (254).

Immunohistochemistry

The expression of numerous immunohistochemical markers, including S100A6, Mart-1, Melan A, CD99, CD117, e-cadherin, matrix metalloprotein 2 and 9, and vascular endothelial growth factor have been evaluated to help assist in differentiating SN, atypical SN, and melanoma (255–261). None have yet proven to be a useful independent marker, but suggest more promise when used as a panel examining antigenic expression.

Evaluation of cell cycle regulation shows that SN highly express p-27, p-16, and bcl-2, have limited expression of Ki-67, Rb, p-53, cyclin A, and bax, and moderate expression of cyclin D1 and p-21, a pattern of expression that parallels that of conventional nevi and is notably different from the cell cycle regulators expressed in melanoma (262). Another study showed that cytoplasmic expression of fatty acid synthase progressively increased from SN to atypical SN to melanoma, supporting the theory that these lesions are all part of a spectrum (254). Currently, there is no unique marker to identify SN from other melanocytic neoplasms or to differentiate unequivocally a benign from malignant SN.

Electron Microscopy

Electron microscopy may be useful only to the extent of identifying melanosomes in a lesion that is difficult to characterize. There is no role for electron microscopy in helping with the most troublesome diagnostic dilemma of SN versus melanoma.

Molecular-Genetic Data

Both acquired nevi and small congenital nevi have been shown to have BRAF mutations, a mutation that has not been found in large congenital nevi or SN (263). SN, do however show HRAS mutations, most commonly manifestated as an increase in 11p263. Microsatellite instability and loss of heterozygosity studies show similarities between SN and melanoma and, though not helpful in differentiating these lesions, may suggest biologic similarities that redirect us to the original term coined by Sophie Spitz: "melanoma of childhood" (242,264).

Differential Diagnosis

The most challenging differential diagnosis is with malignant melanoma. If all the features of SN are present, then the diagnosis can be made confidently. However, lack of symmetry, single upwardly migrating melanocytes outnumbering clusters, lack of maturation, and atypical or deep dermal mitoses are all features that would warrant consideration of melanoma. From the discussion above, it is clear that the diagnosis of SN or melanoma is made after considering the entire constellation of histologic findings.

Epithelioid histiocytoma enters the differential diagnosis. Clinically, it is characterized as a solitary nodule, often mistaken to be a vascular lesion, which most commonly presents on the lower extremities. The patients are older, ranging from 23 to 63 years, with a mean age of 42 years. Histologically, the lesion is composed of a dermal proliferation of cells with abundant eosinophilic cytoplasm. An epidermal collarette may be present. Nuclear atypia, hyperchromatism, and mitoses are not seen in epithelioid histiocytoma. An antigen expression profile that resembles histiocytoma with weak expression of factor XIIIa and negativity for S-100 protein and HMB-45 is helpful in distinguishing these large epithelioid cells from the epithelioid melanocytes of SN (265).

Treatment and Prognosis

Because of the uncertainty in clinical behavior, in particular for those lesions with atypical histologic features, and compounded by the challenge of interpreting the biopsy of a recurrent SN, reexcision with negative margins is the current recommendation at the time of initial diagnosis (266–268). There is lack of uniformity to the extent of margins necessary; however, conservative, narrow margins (2 mm) are commonly employed (267). In one study, patients aged 7 to 46 years with atypical SN underwent sentinel node biopsy. Five of the ten patients had positive sentinel nodes. At follow-up intervals of 1 to 54 months, all patients were free of disease (269). While, arguably, nodal involvement is indicative of a malignant neoplasm, in this instance, nodal nests of benign nevus cells have been documented in 3% to 22% of lymph nodes removed for melanoma staging (270). Their presence is associated with congenital cutaneous nevi in some cases (271). The extensive disease-free period in the cohort of patients with SN lymph node involvement suggests that this nodal involvement may be a feature of the congenital onset of the lesions, rather than an indication of the biologic behavior of the primary lesion. Regardless, nodal involvement adds further uncertainty to the understanding of biologic behavior in this lesion that has conventionally been considered benign despite its histologically malignant feature.

B. Melanoma

Introduction

The head and neck have been reported to have a higher density of melanomas than other body sites (272). Because of increased exposure to UV radiation on the head and neck, it has been proposed that melanomas of this area are notably different than those on body sites with less UV exposure. In particular, melanomas of the head and neck are associated with chronic sun exposure compared with the intermittent sun exposure classically associated with melanomas of the trunk (273). When compared with other body sites, head and neck melanomas are more common, occur more frequently in men, and present in an older patient. Melanomas on the scalp tend to be thicker and are more often ulcerated than melanomas at other body sites. Additionally, lentigo maligna melanomas are more common on the head and neck than other sites, and, of head and neck melanomas, nodular melanomas are more common on the scalp and neck. Outcome data for primary cutaneous melanomas of the head and neck are controversial; studies range from indicating an overall poorer prognosis to no variance in prognosis as compared with that of melanomas of comparable stage at other sites (274,275).

Of the head and neck melanomas, tumors of the scalp had the highest rate of recurrence and were associated with greater mortality than those on the face (276).

A recent population-based study on Caucasians living in Hawaii confirmed the conventional theories of melanoma risk being positively associated with Celtic and English ancestry, fair complexion, inability to tan, family history of skin cancer, duration of summer sun exposure, blistering sunburns before adulthood, and nevi (277).

Evidence continues to build, showing divergent pathways for the development of melanoma. The majority of these data are based on genetic alterations that are appearing to characterize not only types of melanoma but also the extent of sun exposure associated with melanoma (272), showing BRAF or N-RAS mutations on most non-UV-related melanomas, but not in acral or mucosal melanomas or in melanomas on sun-exposed sites. The BRAF/N-RAS-negative melanomas most commonly have increased copies of RAS-BRAF downstream components: cyclin-dependent kinase 4 and cyclin D1. Despite these differences, the 10-year survival rates for head and neck melanomas do not differ significantly from melanomas of other sites (272).

Clinical Features

Melanomas of the head and neck, like those on other sites, present as irregularly pigmented and irregularly shaped lesions, often with a history of growth or change in color. In addition, lesions greater than 6 mm and those that are irritated or bleeding are concerning features. Melanoma in situ is typically a flat lesion, whereas nodularity is an indication of invasion. Lentigo maligna and lentigo maligna melanoma present as an expanding patch of variably pigmented skin, most commonly on the temple, forehead, nose, and malar area. Superficial spreading melanoma is most common on the legs and back, but can occur on the head. Like lentigo maligna, it presents as an expanding plaque. Pigmentation is more variable, presenting with shades of black or blue, in addition to brown, and epidermal changes such as scaling may also be noted. Nodular melanoma lacks a radial growth phase and accordingly is nodular or polypoid at presentation. Ulceration, a recently added prognostic factor, is more common in nodular melanomas. Desmoplastic melanoma presents as an indurated lesion, with or without pigmentation, on sun-damaged skin, and is often clinically not thought to be melanoma.

With the support of a prospective database of 17,600 melanoma patients, American Joint Committee on Cancer (AJCC) issued an update on the staging guidelines for melanoma in 2002 (278). Melanoma staging uses both clinical as well as pathologic staging guidelines, a separation that is based on regional lymph nodes assessment being staged by radiologic/clinical criteria or by pathologic examination. One of the major changes in the updated guidelines with respect to pathologic features includes loss of the use of level of invasion (Clark level) for all except melanomas less than 1 mm in depth. For these melanomas, Clark level of invasion is determined by the *anatomic* level of extension of the deepest component of the invasive front. Clark levels are as follows:

1. Malignant melanocytes are confined to the epidermis, i.e., in situ melanoma.
2. Malignant melanocytes are in the papillary dermis.
3. Malignant melanocytes fill and expand the papillary dermis.
4. Malignant melanocytes extend beyond the superficial vascular plexus, i.e., into the reticular dermis.
5. Malignant melanocytes extend into the subcutaneous tissue.

For melanoma greater than 1 mm in depth, the tumor thickness (Breslow depth), defined as the depth of the invasion measured from the top of the granular cell layer to the deepest invasive component, is used to the exclusion of the Clark level. Tumor thickness determines T classification in the TNM classification scheme as follows:

- Tx—the primary melanoma cannot be assessed (regressed lesions and lesions extending to the base of a shallow biopsy)
- T0—a primary tumor is not identified
- Tis—melanoma in situ
- T1—less than or equal to 1-mm tumor depth
- T2—1.01- to 2-mm tumor depth

- T3—2.01- to 4-mm tumor depth
- T4—greater than 4-mm tumor depth

Ulceration, a relatively recent addition to the list of prognostic histologic features, upstages patients with stages I, II, and III disease from "A" to "B" subgroup. Additionally, satellite metastasis around the primary lesion and in-transit metastasis are included in the same prognostic category and grouped into stage III disease, regardless of the depth of the primary lesion. Additional major changes in the AJCC 2002 melanoma staging are the inclusion of the number of involved lymph nodes, rather than the dimensions, and an indication of clinically apparent (macroscopic) versus clinically occult (microscopic) lymph node involvement. Patients with no evidence of regional or distant metastases are grouped in pathologic stages I and II, whereas stage III patients have pathologic evidence of regional nodal or intralymphatic involvement, and stage IV patients have pathologic evidence of distant metastases. Advances in sentinel node evaluation are affecting previously understaged patients, offering an explanation for the extreme clinical variation in the previously classified stage II patients.

Imaging

Imaging studies are typically not necessary in the diagnosis of melanoma. Dermoscopy, a process of evaluating skin in vivo with a magnifying lens and a fluid substance to decrease refractiveness of the overlying stratum corneum, has shown some benefit in determining the overall architecture of melanocytic lesions (279–281). This technique has provided assistance in increasing or decreasing the level of concern in determining the appropriateness of removing any given lesion for histologic evaluation.

Pathology

Head and neck melanomas are characterized using the same subtypes of melanomas as on other body sites: lentigo maligna, superficial spreading, nodular, and desmoplastic/spindle cell. Normal skin has a regular distribution of melanocytes along the basilar layer. Extreme aberrations from this normal pattern characterize melanoma. Radial growth phase, in which the malignant (aberrant) population of melanocytes is wholly or predominanty confined to the epidermis, has significantly less metastatic potential compared with vertical growth phase melanoma. Vertical growth phase is characterized by expansion of the malignant melanocytes into the dermis. This phase of growth confers metastatic potential to the lesion.

For all variants of melanoma, a constellation of histologic features is necessary to render the correct diagnosis. Of these features, the concept of melanocytic maturation is the overriding theme. As melanocytes drop into the dermis from their position along the basilar layer of the epidermis, the melanocytes of benign nevi mature. This maturation is expressed as a gradual transition from larger cells with larger nuclei clustered in larger nests in the papillary dermis to

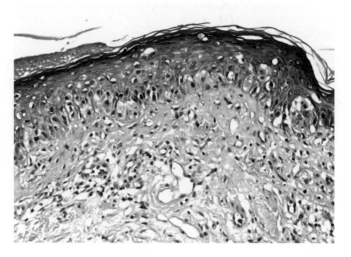

Figure 52   Melanoma in situ. A lentiginous proliferation of back-to-back melanocytes along the basilar layer without extension into the subjacent dermis.

smaller cells, with smaller nuclei and single dispersion in the deeper dermis. Additionally, a gradual loss of pigmentation is typically noted. Loss of this normal dermal maturation characterizes invasive melanoma. In addition, dermal mitoses are an ominous, however not diagnostic, feature.

Melanoma in situ/lentigo maligna.   Melanoma in situ shows a disorderly proliferation of melanocytes, both singly and in nests, within the epidermis. This disorderly proliferation may present as a back-to-back proliferation along the basilar layer, a pattern refered to as lentiginous proliferation (Fig. 52). Because of lack of desmosomes in melanocytes, this lentiginous proliferation, not uncommonly, causes clefting of the skin at the dermal-epidermal junction. As the melanocytes lose their normal function, the malignant melanocytes can lose their orientation along the basilar layer and migrate to higher levels of the epidermis, along with the maturing keratinocytes. This upward migration of melanocytes describes the pattern of pagetoid proliferation (Fig. 53). Lentigo maligna (Hutchinson's melanotic freckle), the most common subtype in this anatomic region (272), is defined by a lentiginous proliferation of melanocytes on atrophic sun-damaged skin (Fig. 54).

Lentigo Maligna Melanoma.   This subtype represents lentigo maligna, which has progressed from a nearly entirely intraepidermal lesion to one in which nests of similarly atypical melanocytes are seen within the dermis. As in nodular melanoma (see below), this dermal component lacks maturation.

Superficial spreading melanoma.   Superficial spreading melanoma, like lentigo maligna, is characterized by a disorderly proliferation of intraepidermal melanocytes with pagetoid and/or lentiginous proliferation patterns. These melanocytes show prominent cytologic atypia and do not demonstrate maturation with progression into the subjacent dermis. In this

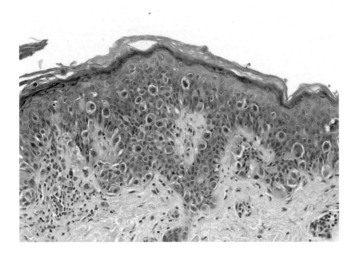

Figure 53 Melanoma in situ, pagetoid proliferation. Upward migration of melanocytes describes the pattern of pagetoid proliferation.

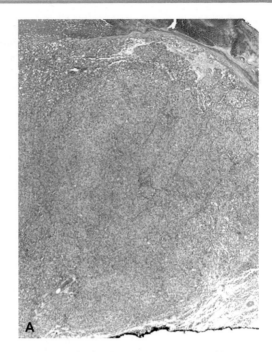

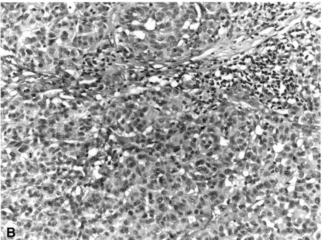

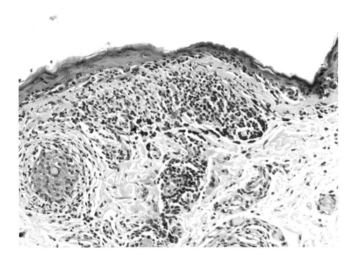

Figure 54 Melanoma in situ, lentigo maligna type. Lentiginous proliferation of melanocytes on atrophic, sun-damaged skin.

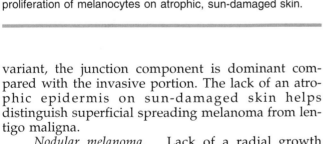

Figure 55 Melanoma, nodular type. This pattern is dominated by (**A**) a dermal proliferation of melanocytes that lack features of maturation; (**B**) the dermal infiltrate is associated with a variable host lymphocytic infiltrate.

variant, the junction component is dominant compared with the invasive portion. The lack of an atrophic epidermis on sun-damaged skin helps distinguish superficial spreading melanoma from lentigo maligna.

Nodular melanoma. Lack of a radial growth phase, by definition, characterizes nodular melanoma. The histology of this type of melanoma is dominated by a dermal proliferation of melanocytes that lack features of maturation. Dermal nests of melanocytes with variable cytologic and nuclear atypia, including prominent nucleoli and rare to numerous mitoses, are noted throughout the depth of the lesion (Fig. 55).

Spindle cell/desmoplastic melanoma. There is considerable histologic variability in the spectrum of lesions referred to as spindle cell or desmoplastic melanoma, a variability that is a reflection of the extent of stromal reaction as well as on the extent of the spindled nature of the infiltrate. Cells ranging from plump to fine, nearly dendritic, and spindled make up the extremes of this lesion (Fig. 56). These lesions are characteristically neurotropic and merit close inspection for neural involvement. Spindled melanomas are poorly circumscribed, making the involvement of margins difficult to assess. Accordingly, this variant has a high rate of local recurrence.

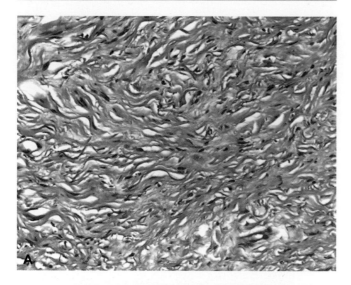

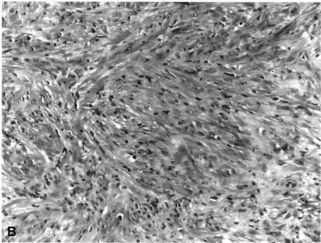

Figure 56 Melanoma, spindle cell type. Spindled melanomas are poorly circumscribed with variable amounts of stroma, as seen (**A**) in this lesion with a thick collagenous stroma (**B**) to lesions with more cellularity and less collagenous stroma.

Despite their locally aggressive nature, patients with desmoplastic melanomas have survival rates similar to patients with other melanomas of comparable thickness (282).

The spindled nature of this lesion makes it prone to misdiagnosis if not viewed with the benefit of antigen expression profiling using immunohistochemical markers.

Immunohistochemistry

Though rare exceptions exist, melanomas express S-100 protein. Spindled melanomas are notoriously negative for the more specific markers of melanocytic differentiation (MHB-45, melan A, Mart-1) that are classically positive in all other types of melanoma. A word of caution is warranted in using the cytoplasmic melanocytic markers for intrepidemral melanocytic

proliferations. As the melanocytic dendritic processes can be rather elaborate and extensive, these cytoplasmic markers, which also highlight these dendritic processes, may give the appearance of a fully evolved lentiginous melanocytic proliferation when one does not truly exist. In this regard, microphthalmia-associated transcription factor (Mitf) is a nuclear marker that is simpler to interpret than the conventional markers of melanocytic differentiation, as it provides crisp nuclear staining that highlights the melanocytic proliferation in a way that is not confounded by the extensive dendritic processes. Mitf also marks osteoclasts and mast cells, entities that are not typically confused histologically for melanocytes.

Electron Microscopy

While not a routine aspect of melanoma diagnoses, in rare circumstances, electron microscopy may be the tool needed to definitely diagnose the cell of orgin. In melanomas that are amelanotic, poorly differentiated, or lacking expression of antigens detected by traditional immunohistochemical markers, the electron microscope can help identify melanosomes.

Molecular-Genetic Data

Mutations in cyclin-dependent kinase inhibitor 2A (CDKN2A), a gene on chromosome 9p that encodes tumor suppressor proteins p16 and p14, are seen in 25% to 40% of familial cases of melanoma (283,284). A small number of familial cases are also known to have mutations in cyclin-dependent kinase 4, also a tumor suppressor gene (285). Nonfamilial melanomas show a high rate, 25% to 50%, of inactivating mutations in phosphatase and tensin homologue (PTEN), another tumor suprossor gene (286). In animal models, mutations in either of the genes is not sufficient to lead to progression to melanoma (287). Accordingly, these mutations represent only one step, in a presumed multistep tumorigenesis process ultimating in melanoma.

In support of the theories of divergent etiologies for melanomas on sun-exposed sites compared with those on sun-protected sites, it has been shown that activating mutations of BRAF and N-RAS, components of the mitogen-activated protein (MAP) kinase pathway, are more commonly seen in melanomas arising on sites without signs of chronic sun damage when compared with melanoms arising on mucosa, acral sites, or sites with evidence of chronic UV exposure (288,289). These later three sites have also been shown to have an increased frequency (28–39%) of KIT mutations compared with no KIT mutations in melanomas arising on skin without evidence of sun damage (290). BRAF mutations are seen in benign acquired nevi as well as in nevi continguous with melanoma (263,288), suggesting that this mutation is part of the common pathway of melanocytic neoplasia, benign and malignant, for which an additional step, most probably an inhibitory alteration, is required for further progression to malignancy.

Differential Diagnosis

Histologically, the spindle cell proliferation of desmoplastic/spindle cell melanoma needs to be differentiated from sarcomatoid (spindle cell) SCC, spindled BCC, leiomyosarcoma, and fibromatosis. The differential diagnosis for nodular melanoma adds AFX to the list. Immunohistochemical profiling is critical in making an accurate diagnosis (291). Sarcomatoid SCC may have only focal CK expression and a CK immunohistochemical panel, as mentioned above, is the most effective technique for detecting this expression. Spindled BCC will often have focal areas with classic basal cell histology showing a nodular growth pattern with peripheral palisading of nuclei, clefting between tumor and stroma and myxoid stroma. Like SCC, it will express CK, a feature not seen in melanomas. The fasicular pattern of leiomyosarcoma may be mistaken for the nodular pattern of melanocytic neoplasms. The nuclei of leiomyosarcoma typically have an open chromatin pattern, but lacks the prominent nucleoli seen in melanoma. Additionally, desmin expression will be seen in leiomyosarcoma, but not in melanoma. The elongated spindle cells in melanoma may mimic fibromatosis. However, fibromatosis is negative for melanocytic markers.

Treatment and Prognosis

Because of the typical lack of excess cutaneous tissue on the head and neck, melanomas of this region are often treated with Mohs micrographic surgery (120).

Although lentigo maligna is a type of melanoma in situ, standard excision with 0.5-cm margins appears to be inadequate, resulting in 8% to 20% recurrence rates (292). This high recurrence rate is attributed to the difficulty in assessing margins clinically as well as to the difficulty in evaluating histologic sections that commonly have numerous background atypical melanocytes as the skin's response to UV radiation exposure. Mohs micrographic surgery offers a lower recurrence rate of 4% to 5% (292).

Primary melanomas are excised with 1 to 2 cm margins (293). For patients with desmoplastic melanoma, wide local excision is reported to have a favorable outcome (294). Sentinel lymph node biopsy is the standard of care for melanomas greater than 1 mm thick. The unpredictable lymphatic drainage of this area poses problems in giving accurate clinical data. However, sensitive studies, with a low number of false negatives can be achieved with a combination of preoperative lymphoscintigrams, intraoperative blue dye injection, and hand-held gamma probes (295).

For those melanomas with KIT mutations, 69% are in domains presumed to result in activating mutations; the same mutations are found in gastrointestinal stromal tumors that are highly sensitive to imatinib therapy. Initial studies showing poor response to imatinib are difficult to interpret as they did not specifically include patients with the highly imatinib-sensitive KIT aberrations (296–298). While in vitro drug testing of stabilized cell lines with KIT mutation have shown specific drug sensitivities, other studies have shown that despite the presence of intense c-kit (CD117) immunoreactivity in some melanomas, they are not responsive to targeted c-kit receptor therapy (299,300). Imatinib therapy in c-kit-expressing melanomas shows promise as a therapeutic target. However, further work in this area is clearly indicated. Additional targeted therapy has focused on antiangiogenesis, immunomodulatory drugs, and bcl-2 antisense therapy, with further options on the horizon.

Prognosis, as with other malignancies, is closely tied to tumor stage at the time of diagnosis. The latest staging criteria, outlined by the AJCC Melanoma Staging Committee in 2002, indicate a 100% 10-year survival for melanoma in situ, or stage 0. Stage 1A and 1B have a 10-year survival of 88% and 79%, respectively (301). The 10-year survival declines through the stages with metastasis to the skin/subcutaneous, lung, and viscera, reporting only 16%, 3%, and 6%, respectively. Many studies suggesting prognostic significance of various markers and evaluation of antigenic expression to target therapies have been performed. Most recently, in a small study on metastatic melanoma, the presence of Fas ligand (CD95L) in primary melanoma was associated with significantly prolonged overall survival compared with Fas ligand-negative melanomas (302).

IV. MESENCHYMAL TUMORS

A. Keloid

Introduction

Keloids are benign overgrowths of thickened collagen bundles, usually occurring after trauma from inflammation such as in follculitis, acne, or herpes zonster, or at the site of cutaneous injury from procedures such as surgeries, body piercing, and vaccinations (303,304). Spontaneous occurances have also been reported in the setting of Ehlers-Danlos syndrome type IV, Rubenstein-Taybi and Goeminne syndromes, and scleroderma (305–308). Keloids are characterized by extending beyond the boundaries of the original wound and are the result of excess deposition of types I and III collagen (309,310). In keloids, 95% of the total collagen is due to type I collagen, compared with 75% type I collagenin normal skin (309). Increased factor XIIIa dermal dendritic cells are seen in the overlying dermal area of keloids when compared with the overlying dermal area of hypertrophic and mature scars (311). And immunoelectromicroscopic interpretation shows factor XIIIa immunoreactivity at the cytoplasm periphery, suggesting that factor XIIIa has an active role in keloid formation (311). In addition, there is increased histamine and proline-4-hydroxylase compared with hypertrophic scars or normal skin (312,313). One immunohistochemical study demonstrated that β-catenin protein levels are elevated in hypertrophic scar and keloids (314). As TGF-β induces activation of β-catenin-mediated transcription in human dermal fibroblasts, this finding may be relevant to the pathogenesis of hypertrophic scars and keloids. Recent years have seen an increased understanding in the molecular and biologic mechanisms of keloidal scar formation. IL-6, a proinflammatory cytokine, has been shown to have a primary role in keloid formation (315,316). Additionally, the role of epithelial-mesenchymal interactions as the primary process is gaining more support in the pathogenesis of keloids (317). In these models, the secretory function of keratinocytes is integrated in a system whereby normal dermal fibroblasts are responding to abnormal extracellular signals. The gli-1 oncogene, secreted by keratinocytes, has been proposed to be integral in this pathway (318,319). Advances such as these are allowing for the development of more specific therapeutic options for these lesions. Despite these developments, keloids are poorly understood and remain difficult to manage.

Clinical Features

Keloids are firm, variably pruritic or painful, smooth nodules that may be skin colored in their early stage and pale appearing later in their development. They typically develop during the late teens and early adult life and occur more frequently in black individuals than whites (320). By definition, they extend beyond the confines of the original wound, a feature that usually permits distinction from hypertrophic scars. They may develop as early as one to three months or, unlike hypertrophic scars, as late as one year following injury (321). Also, in contrast to hypertrophic scars, they do not undergo spontaneous regression and may continue to grow. Sites of predilection include the ear lobes, the upper part of back, and the presternal areas. Rarely, there is involvement of the genitalia, eyelids, palms, and soles.

Imaging

As benign and almost exclusively dermal proliferations, imaging studies are rarely necessary.

Pathology

Keloids are composed of broad, homogeneous, brightly eosinophilic collagen fibers arranged in haphazard array (Fig. 57). Fibroblasts are increased in number and are also arranged haphazardly (322). Formation of keloidal collagen typically occurs centrally in the fibroblastic proliferation. Depending on the age of the lesion, these unique collagen fibers may only be seen focally. Abundant mucopolysaccharides are also seen between collagenous bundles. Keloids have reduced vascularity when compared with hypertrophic scars and normal-healing wounds (323). The overlying epidermis may be normal or atrophic. Keloidal collagen is polarizable.

Immunohistochemistry

Keloids are sufficiently distinctive; thus, the routine light microscopy diagnosis is straightforward. Therefore, immunohistochemistry is rarely used as a diagnostic tool.

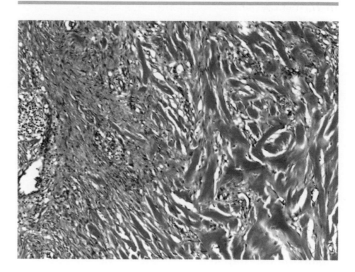

Figure 57   Keloid. This image demonstrates the broad, homogeneous, brightly eosinophilic collagen fibers haphazardly arranged, adjacent to a fibroblastic proliferation.

Electron Microscopy

Keloids exhibit numerous fibroblasts with abundant Golgi complexes and prominent rough endoplasmic reticulum (324). Although myofibroblasts have been suggested to be present in early lesions (325), they are usually not been demonstrated by electron microscopy (324).

Molecular-Genetic Data

Familial clustering suggests a genetic predisposition (326). In a study of 14 pedigrees, including 341 family members of which 96 had keloids, the pattern of expression shows autosomal dominance with incomplete penetrance and variable expression (327). Differential expression of one isoform of p63, a transcription factor that appears to be predominantly expressed in epidermis, is overexpressed in fibroblasts of keloids and hypertrophic scars, in comparison with normal skin fibroblasts, and there is increasing support for the role of TGF-β family members in the pathogenesis of keloids (328,329). There is a lower rate of apoptosis and p53 mutations in keloidal fibroblasts than in hypertrophic scars (330,331).

Differential Diagnosis

Hypertrophic scars can be differentiated from keloids clinically in that they are confined to the original wound boundaries, and they frequently regress over time. Microscopically, hypertrophic scars lack the thick, densely packed, and hyalinized collagen bundles of keloids. Instead, they are more likely to have a pattern of growth composed of vessels that are arranged perpendicular to the surface epidermis, horizontally arrayed fibroblasts, and fine collagen.

Collagenoma, a connective tissue nevus with an autosomal dominant inheritance pattern, is an intradermal fibrous nodule that microscopically resembles a hypertrophic scar or keloid, but has no antecedent history of trauma or skin wounding.

Sclerotic fibromas, fibrous papule of the face, and keloidal DFs are among entities that can be clinically confused with keloids. However, they can be differentiated from keloids by specific microscopic features. Fibrous papules demonstrate concentric dermal perivascular and perifollicular fibrosis, vascular ectasia, and stellate fibroblasts. Overlying epidermal hyperplasia and marked cellularity are usually present in DFs. Additionally, the spindled cells in DF are factor XIIIa positive. The nodular configuration and the "wood grain" pattern of a paucicellular collagen proliferation is characteristic of a sclerotic fibroma.

Treatment and Prognosis

Treatment of keloids is often ineffective, with 50% recurrence of excised lesions (332). A meta-analysis of 70 treatments showed a 70% chance of improvement (333). Topical application of 5% imiquimod cream reduces recurrences after surgery, and intralesional injection of triamcinolone suspension has also been reported as effective (332,334). Immediate postexcision intralesional injection of triamcinolone acetonide shows dermal suppression of type I collagen gene expression (335). Radiation, used alone or in combination with surgery, has also been used to prevent recurrence of keloids following excision (336). In a retrospective study reviewing the outcome of 126 keloids in 83 patients receiving postoperative radiation, Klumpar et al. reported an overall improvement rate of 83% (337). Other treatments such as topical tacrolimus and application of silicone gel sheeting have been proposed, but the beneficial effect remains unproven (338,339). Despite the variety of treatment options available and the progresses made in understanding the cytokines involved in wound healing, the amount of improvement one may expect for any give treatment plan is 60% (333).

B. Fibrous Papule

Synonyms: cutaneous angiofibroma, periungual fibroma, and pearly penile papule.

Introduction

Fibrous papules (FPs) are benign nodules presumed to be of dermal dendrocytic origin. Dermal dendrocytes are antigen-presenting dermal cells, are phenotypically distinct from dermal macrophages, and have both CD34- and factor XIIIa-expressing populations. These cells have stabilizing plaques that fix their location within the dermis and, at least with regard to the superficial dermal population, have an association with mast cells (340). The exact histogenesis of FPs is uncertain, however, a proliferative reactive process and involuted melanocytic nevi have been proposed (341,342). In addition to the isolated lesions presenting on the mid-face of adults, the most common setting, multiple FPs around the nose, cheek, and chin are seen in 75% of patients with tuberous sclerosis. In this

setting, these lesions are referred to as angiofibromas. Multiple FPs may also be seen closely aggregated around the corona of the glans penis. In this latter setting, they are referred to as pearly penile papules. The histology of the lesions, despite their various anatomical locations, is identical. FPs are often biopsied because of their clinical confusion for more worrisome entities such as BCC.

Clinical Features

FPs are 2- to 5-mm smooth dome-shaped nodules, most commonly presenting on the mid-face of adults. They are asymptomatic and may be skin colored or slightly erythematous. Clinically, they are often mistaken for intradermal nevi, neurofibromas, or BCCs. Isolated lesions are most common, however, multiple lesions are seen in the setting of tuberous sclerosis and multiple endocrine neoplasia.

Imaging

Imaging studies are not necessary for the diagnosis or follow-up care.

Pathology

FPs have a normal to mildly atrophic epidermis. Within the dermis, there are increased thin-walled ectatic vessels with an increase in fibroblasts, demonstrating plump, stellate, or multinucleate morphology. Collagen bundles forming concentric layers around follicular units and the small ectatic vessels are also characteristic (Fig. 58). Several histologic variations of FP have been recognized: hypercellular, clear cell, pigmented, pleomorphic, inflammatory, and granular cell (343–345).

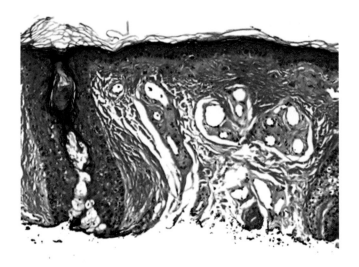

Figure 58 Fibrous papule. Skin with an atrophic epidermis, increased stellate fibroblasts in the papillary dermis, collagen deposition forming concentric layers around follicular units and small ectatic vessels characterize fibrous papules.

Immunohistochemistry

Consistent with a dermal dendrocytic etiology, the stromal cells express factor XIIIa and are negative for Mart-1, CKs, epithelial membrane antigen, and CEA (345). Reports on S-100 expression in FP have been conflicting. S-100 expression has been reported in the superficial dermis of some cases, while other reports failed to reveal S-100 expression (346,347). There is no increased expression in the vascular marker UEA-1 or in the macrophage marker MAC 387347. The clear cell variant is strongly and diffusely positive for NK1/C3. A case of CD34-positive FP has been reported (347).

Electron Microscopy

The fibroblastic nature of FP has been confirmed by several ultrastructural analyses. These evaluations have not been able to support a neural or melanocytic origin to FP (348–350).

Molecular-Genetic Data

A genetic association has not been established, and molecular studies of FP have not been performed.

Differential Diagnosis

Multinucleate cell angiohistiocytoma (MCHA) presents as papules or nodules, most commonly on the arms. Histologically, it too has stellate or multi-nucleate fibroblasts and small ectatic vessels. However, the characteristic perivascular and periadnexal collagen deposition seen in FP are not present in MCHA. Additionally, MCHA tends to have a more diffuse histologic pattern and not the nodular pattern seen in FP.

A scar shows a collagenous stroma, but not in a perivascular and periadnexal pattern of FP. Additionally, a scar does not express factor XIIIa (351).

While not typically in the histologic differential diagnosis, the case report of a CD34-expressing FP brings dermatofibrosarcoma protuberans (DFSP) into consideration. DFSP is typically located on the trunk and proximal extremities of young adults (347). It is a CD34-expressing spindle cell tumor (see below) with an aggressive behavior, and, if sampled only superficially, may be impossible to distinguish from a CD34-expressing FP.

Treatment and Prognosis

Shave excision is adequate for removal, and recurrences have not been described.

C. Nuchal-Type Fibroma

Synonym: collagenosis nuchae.

Introduction

Nuchal-type fibroma is an uncommon benign fibro-collagenous proliferation that typically arises in the nape of the neck. Other locations such as the extremities, buttock, and lumbosacral areas have also been

reported (352). Because these extranuchal lesions are histologically indistinguishable from the nuchal examples, the designation nuchal-type fibroma was proposed (353). In one series, 44% of patients with nuchal fibroma had diabetes mellitus (353). Identical lesions, when multiple and arising in children, are seen in the setting of Gardner syndrome and termed "Gardner fibroma" (354,355). Recent studies reported an association of this entity with scleroderma (356) and DFSP (357).

Clinical Features

Nuchal fibromas have a predilection for the nuchal and interscapular regions; the face and shoulder, forearm, anterior neck, knee, and trunk are other reported sites (353,358). Nuchal fibroma is more common in men than women (4:1). There is a broad age distribution, 3 to 74 years (mean, 40 years), with a peak incidence during the third through fifth decades (353,358). Clinically, it consists of an asymptomatic 2.5 to 8.0 cm firm nodule with associated erythema often thought to be subcutaneous clinically (358,359). Involvement of deep soft tissue and periosteum have been reported (353). Rarely, they can infiltrate the superficial skeletal muscle (359). Although benign, there is a potential for recurrence; 20% of patients in one study had one to three recurrences (353).

Imaging

As benign dermal and, rarely, subcutaneous proliferations, imaging studies are rarely required. In case of involvement of deeper soft tissue elements, complementary imaging studies such as CT could be helpful to better delineate the lesion (360).

Pathology

Nuchal fibroma is an unencapsulated, densely collagenized, hypocellular, subcutaneous mass with extension into the dermis and occasionally into subjacent skeletal muscle. The collagenous bundles are haphazardly arranged with a vague lobular architecture. The lobules have scattered mature fibroblasts between collagen bundles. Centrally, in the lobules, vague intersecting bundles may be seen (353). Focal entrapped mature adipose tissue, small thin-walled vessels, and traumatic neuroma-like small nerves are frequently seen. Additionally, some cases show large peripheral nerves with perineural fibrosis. The extra-nuchal lesions have identical histologic features (353).

Immunohistochemistry

The spindled cells of nuchal fibromas express CD34 and CD99. They are negative for desmin and actin (361). These findings are not specific and are rarely required for diagnosis.

Electron Microscopy

There are no published studies regarding the ultrastructural characteristics of this entity. Electron microscopy is not required for diagnosis.

Molecular-Genetic Data

No characteristic molecular or genetic data are available to this date.

Differential Diagnosis

Clinically, lipoma represents the most common differential diagnosis with nuchal fibroma. Histologically, the most difficult distinction is from fibrolipoma. Unlike nuchal fibroma, fibrolipomas are encapsulated, have a greater proportion of mature adipose tissue, and lack entrapped nerves. The nuchal fibrocartilagenous pseudotumor arises in the posterior aspect of the base of the neck with attachment to the nuchal ligament. Nuchal fibromas, however, are more superficial and lack association with ligaments (362). This distinction is best established at the time of surgery. Nuchal fibromas can be distinguished from extra-abdominal fibromatosis by their subcutaneous location and their hypocellular/acellular nature. Elastofibroma also enters the differential diagnososis. It has a similar clinical presentation, and, histologically, is also composed of an unencapsulated proliferation of collagen bundles with entrapped mature fat. The distinction is made by recognizing the presence of elastic fibers, which will stain with Verhoff elastic stain.

Treatment and Prognosis

Local recurrences do occur, but are nondestrucive and controlled with complete reexcision. Metastases have not been reported.

D. Dermatofibroma

Synonyms: fibrous histiocytoma and sclerosing hemangioma.

Introduction

DFs are benign proliferations of dermal dendrocytes with both fibroblastic and histiocytic differentiation. Whether DF is a reactive process or a neoplastic growth has not yet been definitively settled. Some authorities have suggested that DF is a fibrosing inflammatory process. Recent studies suggest that IL-1 may be involved in the fibrotic process in DF at the transcriptional level and may play a role as an autocrine factor in the fibroblast proliferation (363). This theory is further supported by the fact that multiple DFs occasionally develop in patients with immune disorders or under immunosuppressive therapy (i.e., HIV positivity and patients with systemic lupus erythematosus) (364). Others believe in the neoplastic nature of these lesions, citing monoclonality in histiocytoid or mixed-type DFs as evidence (365). Fibrous histiocytoma of the face is a DF variant that, in addition to having a different histologic pattern, has a more locally aggressive clinical behavior (366). Such lesions, with a clinical behavior, histologic pattern, and antigenic expression that vary from the classic DF, have been proposed to represent a group of indeterminant lesions that provide evidence for DF

and DFSP, being lesions at opposite ends of a spectrum; DF of the face is intermediate to these (367).

Clinical Features

DFs are common and account for almost 3% of specimens received in one dermatopathology laboratory (368). They are slow-growing, firm dermal nodules, usually less than 1 cm in diameter. There is a predilection for the lower extremities of young adult females. They impart a red or red-brown color to the overlying skin, but occasionally appear blue or black as a result of excessive deposits of hemosiderin. Such lesions may be confused clinically with malignant melanoma. The presence of a central dimple on lateral compression ("Fitzpatrick" sign) is a helpful clinical finding in distinguishing between the two entities. Deeply situated lesions are less common. Other clinical variants include the aneurysmal type and the rare annular hemosiderotic histiocytoma in which multiple brown papules in annular configurations are present on the buttocks. DF of the face is also more common in women, presents as a firm ill-defined nodule 0.3 to 1.9 cm, and is rarely thought to be a DF, clinically (366).

Imaging

As benign and almost exclusively dermal proliferations, imaging studies are rarely necessary.

Pathology

DFs are well-demarcated, unencapsulated dermal proliferations of spindle cells composed of a variable admixture of fibroblast-like cells and histiocytes. Most DFs consist of short, interlacing fascicles of fibroblast-like cells that usually form a loose crisscross pattern or a vague storiform pattern. The overlying epidermis frequently shows psoriasiform acanthosis and hyperpigmentation of basal keratinocytes. The stroma consists of a dense collagen network surrounding individual cells. The collagen bundles are more prominent at the periphery of the lesion (Fig. 59). Rare cases exhibit striking vascular proliferation and hemorrhage. These lesions were found to be reminiscent of a burned-out vascular lesion referred to as "sclerosing hemangioma" (369). Occasional rounded "histiocytic" cells accompany the spindle cells. When the former cell type predominates, the lesion is referred to as "histiocytoma" or "fibrous histiocytoma." Lymphocytes and xanthoma cells can also be present throughout the lesion. When cystic areas of hemorrhage are prominent with accumulation of hemosiderin, the lesions have been referred to as "aneurysmal" DFs (Fig. 60). Other histologic variants are lipidized, myxoid, keloidal, and atrophic DFs, as well as DFs with monster cells (Fig. 60). Each of these variants, however, has in common a dermally located proliferation of fibroblasts and histiocytes. DF of the face shows less circumscription, has a diffuse growth pattern, and often extends into the subcutaneous fat (Fig. 61) and occasionally into muscle (366). The dermal cells are predominantly spindled and may show a growth pattern reminiscent of typical DF, a storiform pattern

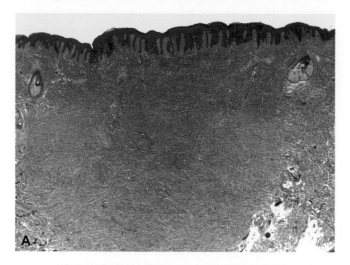

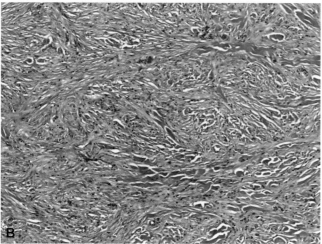

Figure 59 Dermatofibroma. (**A**) The low power image shows a well-demarcated, unencapsulated dermal proliferation of spindle cells in the dermis. The overlying epidermis shows psoriasiform hyperplasia and hyperpigmentation of basal keratinocytes. (**B**) The dermal infiltrate has short, interlacing fascicles composed of a variable admixture of fibroblast-like cells and histiocytes intercalating dense collagenous bundles at the periphery of the lesion.

is nearly always seen at least focally. As in classic DF, hyalinized collagen surrounded by tumor cells is a common feature in these lesions, and most lesions expresss factor XIIIa and are negative for CD34, S-100 protein, CK, and desmin (366).

Immunohistochemistry

Characteristically, DFs immunoreact with factor XIIIa but fail to express CD34. This finding is useful in differentiating between deep, cellular DFs and DFSP in histologically challenging cases. Unfortunately, some overlap occurs. In a study of the immunohistochemical properties of DF and DFSP, CD34 was strongly expressed in 25% of DFs and 80% of DFSPs, whereas factor XIIIa was strongly expressed in 95% of

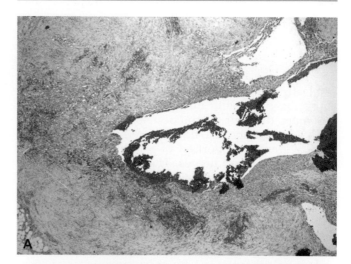

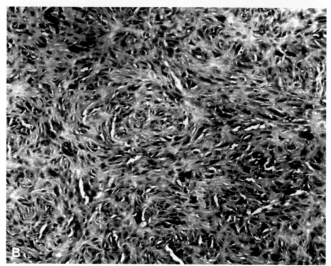

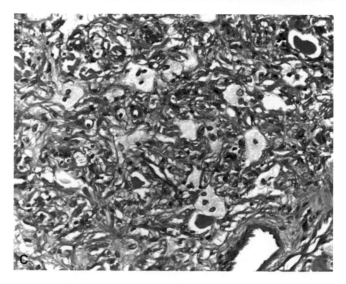

Figure 60 Dermatofibroma variants. (**A**) Aneurysmal DF has cystic areas of hemorrhage and prominent accumulations of hemosiderin. (**B**) DF with giant (monster) cells shows scattered large multinucleate cells in the background of conventional histologic features of DF. (**C**) This lipidized variant has scattered large polygonal cells with a small nucleus and a large vacuolated cytoplasm.

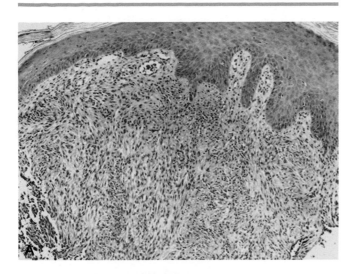

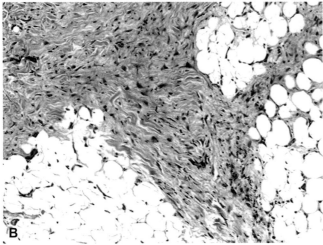

Figure 61 Dermatofibroma of the face. **(A)** This variant shows a diffuse growth pattern with less circumscription, **(B)** and often extends into the subcutaneous fat as is seen in this image.

DFs and 15% of DFSPs (370). CD44, the cell surface receptor for hyaluronate, has shown promise as a differentiating marker, as all classic DFs in one study showed strong CD44 reactivity, and was significantly reduced or absent in DFSP (371). Caution in interpreting the staining pattern is crucial as this study evaluated classic DFs; the authors subsequently showed that myxoid DF does not show strong CD44 expression (372).

Electron Microscopy

Ultrastructural studies have given conflicting results, with the cells variously reported as resembling fibroblasts, histiocytes, endothelial cells, and even myofibroblasts (373). These discrepancies no doubt reflect sampling differences. More recent ultrastructural evaluation revealed that DFs are composed of spindle cells, which lack cellular processes, and are in close approximation to capillary vessels with prominent endothelium. They have abundant cytoplasm and intracytoplasmic lipid droplets and lipolysosomes. These ultracturctural findings show DFs to have phagocytic and fibroblastic elements supporting the hypothesis of a perivascular dermal dendritic cell origin for this lesion (374).

Molecular-Genetic Data

There is no known specific genetic aberration seen in DFs. Genetics may help to differentiate DFs from DFSP in challenging cases. The overrepresentation of 17q22-qter and 22q13 is seen in DFSP but not in DDF (375). In a recent cytogenetic and fluorescent in situ hybridization (FISH) study on a single case of DF with clear cell change, deletion of p12 was shown (376).

Differential Diagnosis

Clinically, hyperpigmented DF can resemble a melanocytic proliferation (see clinical features). Otherwise, DFs are most frequently confused with other benign lesions, including neurofibroma, dermatomyofibroma, hypertrophic scar, and leiomyoma. The use of immunoperoxidase stains helps to differentiate between these entities. Neurofibroma, a Schwann cell proliferation, expresses S-100 protein. Smooth muscle actin can be used to highlight the myogenic differentiation seen in leiomyoma and dermatomyofibroma. The distinction between DF and DFSP is discussed above (see section "Immunohistochemistry").

Treatment and Prognosis

DFs usually persist, but, with time, may undergo partial regression, especially centrally. DFs may be biopsied or excised to exclude a melanocytic proliferation or other mesenchymal neoplasms. Excision for cosmetic purposes is of questionable value, as the resultant scar is often quite evident (363). DFs of the face, on the other hand, need to be excised with wider margins because of their high rate of recurrence, infiltrative pattern, and involvement of deeper structures (366). All local recurrences, on one study, involved those lesions that were only marginally excised (366).

E. Dermatofibrosarcoma Protuberans

Introduction

DFSP is a relatively uncommon tumor with borderline malignancy arising on the trunk and proximal extremities of young adults. It is a dermal-based, slow-growing, and locally aggressive sarcoma that often recurs but infrequently metastasizes. Ring chromosomes and reciprocal translocations involving chromosomes 17 and 22, leading to the fusion of collagen-1α1 (COL1A1) gene to platelet-derived growth factorβ (PDGFB) chain has been identified as the main genetic abnormality in DFSP (375,377). The same chromosomal abnormality t(17;22) has been described in giant cell fibroblastoma (GCF), a lesion arising on the back or thigh of children younger than 10 years (378). Both GCF and DFSP have a male predominance. GCF has been shown to recur with combined GCF and DFSP patterns, and fibrosarcomatous transformation, similar to that described in DFSP, has been described in GCF. On the basis of these parallels in the clinical behavior, histologic pattern, immunohistochemical reactions, and cytogenetics, it has been proposed that GCF and DFSP represent variation of the same entity (378,379). Overlapping histologic and immunohistologic features of DF and DFSP have led some to propose that these two lesions reside on a spectrum as well (367).

Clinical Features

DFSPs are tumors that have a predilection for the trunk and proximal extremities; however, up to 15% of cases occur in the head and neck, representing 1% of head and neck soft tissue sarcomas (380). There is a wide age distribution with a peak in young and middle-aged men. Fully developed lesions are solitary or multiple polypoid nodules. At initial presention, they appear as an asymptomatic, skin-colored, indurated plaque. Ultimately, they become slightly erythematous to violaceous, measuring from one to several centimeters in diameter (380,381). The lesions are slow growing and often ignored by the patient. On palpation, it is firm and attached to the subcutaneous tissue. There are case reportes of accelerated growth during pregnancy. This finding is supported by the fact that DFSPs appear to express low levels of hormone receptors (382).

Imaging

While not necessary for diagnosis, imaging studies for treatment planning are helpful. The extent of tumor involvement can be determined by CT imaging and further enhanced with MRI. T1- and T2-weighted MRIs offer the advantage of localizing atypical tumors prior to surgery. On T1-weighted MRI, DFSP is a well-defined lesion with a low signal, and on T2-weighted images, it has a signal higher than fat (383). For lesions with signal intensity similar to subcutaneous tissue, short tau inversion recovery (STIR) sequences, with an inversion time of 150 msec, provides clearer tumor definition (384). Although unnecessary, in patients who receive gadolinium, the lesions are enhanced. These imaging studies do not detect either the infiltrative strands of tumor extending in horizontal fashion through the dermis or the extension of fine fascicles into the subcutaneous tissue. Complete histologic evaluation of all surgical margins is necessary to detect these extensions.

Pathology

Macroscopically, the cut surface of the tumor appears firm and gray-white. Histologically, DFSP is a dermal-based spindle cell tumor that invariably extends to the subcutis. The tumor is composed of interlacing bundles of rather bland and uniform-appearing, small spindle cells with plump nuclei forming a storiform or cartwheel pattern (Fig. 62). No significant nuclear pleomorphism is noted, and mitoses are extremely

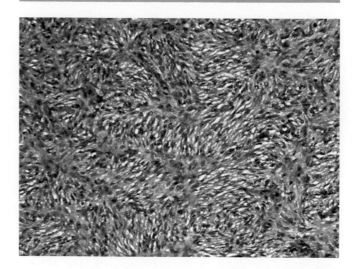

Figure 62 Dermatofibrosarcoma protuberans. The tumor is composed of interlacing bundles of rather bland, uniform-appearing, small spindle cells with plump nuclei forming a storiform or cartwheel pattern.

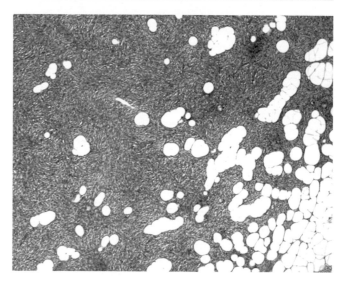

Figure 63 Dermatofibrosarcoma protuberans. The deep aspect of the tumor infiltrates the subcutaneous tissue, intercalating around adipocytes.

rare. Entrapment, but not invasion, of adnexal structures is seen. The deep aspect of the tumor infiltrates the subcutaneous tissue, intercalating around adipocytes (Fig. 63). The pigmented counterpart of DFSP is referred to as ''Bednar'' tumor. These tumors are rare and thought to represent the colonization of the tumor by melanocytes. In this subtype, scattered pigmented melanocytes are admixed with spindled tumor cells throughout the dermis. A myxoid DFSP has been described with greater than 50% myxoid stroma. These lesions have a similar site distribution:

most common on the extremities (40%), followed by the head and neck (30%) and trunk (17%). The cellular component has morphologic and immunohistochemical features similar to the conventional DFSP (385).

Giant cells, similar to those in GCF, can be identified in a small percentage of otherwise typical dermatofibrosarcomas. As both entities possess a similar cytogenetic abnormality (see section "Molecular-Genetic Data"), it is believed that GCF is a juvenile variant of DFSP (377). In 10% to 15% of cases, DFSP contains areas of sarcomatous change resembling conventional fibrosarcoma, malignant fibrous histiocytoma, or myxofibrosarcoma (386,387). Fibrosarcomatous change arises de novo, most commonly; however, it may arise in a recurrence (388). These areas have nuclear atypia and a higher mitotic rate. These fibrosarcomatous areas were originally believed to be more common in recurrent lesions, but recent studies have shown that a sarcomatous component occurred de novo in 15 of 18 cases and in a recurrence in three of those 18 cases (389). Other studies have shown similar data confirming a higher rate of fibrosarcomatous change de novo than in recurrent lesions (388,389).

Immunohistochemistry

The conventional immunuhistochemical marker used for diagnosing DFSP is CD34, a human progenitor cell antigen, which stains over 90% of these tumors and is helpful in differentiating DFSP from DF, which is characteristically negative for CD34 (370). Factor XIIIa, which stains most DFs, is only focally positive in a small number of DFSPs. However, as there is considerable overlap in the immunhistochemical staining patterns, these two markers have fallen out of favor with some laboratories. One study shows CD34 immunoreactivity in 92% of DFSPs and 40% of DFs and factor XIIIa immunoreactivity in 97% of DFs and 75% of DFSPs. The extent of staining in the lesions is significant such that the DFSPs tend to be diffusely positive for CD34, while CD34 in DF is weak and patchy. Accordingly, if one can accept some CD34-positive cells in DF and some factor XIIIa-positive cells in DFSP, these antibodies can be very helpful (370). CD44, a cell surface rceptor for extracellular matrix hyaluronic acid, has shown strong expression in DF and negative expression in DFSP, while hyaluronic acid was weak in the stroma of DF and strong in the stroma of DFSP (371). Focal loss of CD34 expression may be seen in transformed (fibrosarcomatous) DFSP.

Electron Microscopy

Although histology and immunohistochemistry are successful in identifying most cases of DFSP, those cases that pose a challenge may benefit from ultrastructural evaluation. DFSPs frequently have subplasmalemmal densities in their cellular processes and multivesicular buds containing microvesicles abutting from the cell membrane (390). DF, on the other hand, has a vascular proliferation with prominent endothelium and perivascular spindle cells that lack cell processes; multivesicular buds are absent, and subplasmalemmal densities are only rarely present (390).

Molecular-Genetic Data

Cytogenetic analysis may help to differentiate DFSPs from other dermal spindle cell neoplasms in challenging cases. DFSP and its juvenile variant (GCF) are characterized by reciprocal translocation t(17;22)(q22; q13) and a supernumerary ring chromosome derived from the translocation r(17;22), which results in fusion between the PDGFB (PDGFB-chain locus) gene and the COL1A1 (type 1 collagen) (391). These recent findings have given rise to new therapeutic options in locally recurrent and metastatic DFSPs (392). Overexpression of p53 has been found in the fibrosarcomatous foci of DFSP, associated with higher proliferative activity and aneuploidy (393).

Differential Diagnosis

The clinical differential diagnosis includes keloid, large and deep (cellular) DF, dermatomyofibroma, and morphea. Histologically, however, deep DF is the main concern and may be extremely difficult to differentiate from DFSP, in particular for small or superficial biopsies. The absence of overlying epidermal acanthosis and subcutaneous lymphoid nodules as well as the presence of nonpolarizable collagen is helpful in distinguishing DFSP. Additionally, DFSPs tend to lack the heterogenous cell population consisting of lymphocytes, foamy macrophages, and siderophages that are often seen in DF.

Treatment and Prognosis

Complete surgical excision, including Mohs micrographic surgery, remains the treatment of choice for DFSP (381). Resection with wide margins results in local control in greater than 90% of patients (386). Tumors excised with negative margins, on the basis of complete histologic evaluation, benefit from a 97% cure rate (394). Incompletely excised or narrowly excised tumors have an increased risk of local recurrence. However, these patients benefit from a greater than 85% control when postoperative radiotherapy is added to the treatment regimen (386). Unresectable gross disease also benefits from radiotherapy intervention. With the identification of chromosomal fusion leading to deregulated expression of PDGFB, the doors were opened for targeted therapy. As the tumor results from a genetic translocation that causes overactivation of a protein kinase, imatinib, a potent inhibitor of protein kinases, has been used in clinical trial with some efficacy, despite immunohistochemical negativity for CD117 or KIT receptor, a protein kinase homologue (395,396). Imatinib has also been used with dramatic results in patients with metastatic DFSP (392). Sarcomas arising in DFSP have conventionally been regarded as having a higher risk of metastasis. This convention was refuted in one study of 18 cases of sarcoma arising in DFSP. The sarcomatous portion represented 20% to 80% of the tumor mass. All patients were treated with wide local excision with negative margins with or without additional radiation (389). In a follow-up period of up to 17 years, there were no metastatic events; 22% of patients developed recurrences. A similar study of 41 patients with 5% to 95% of the DFSP demonstrating fibrosarcomatous change showed 20%, with recurrence 6 to 72 months after diagnosis and 10% (4/41) with metastatic disease to the bones and lungs at an interval of 36 to 72 months after diagnosis. Two of those patients died of their disease. Fibrosarcomatous change is a form of tumor progression that increases the risk of metastasis over DFSP. Neither the extent of fibrosarcomatous change nor the number of mitoses and the status of the surgical margins played prognostic significance (388).

F. Atypical Fibroxantoma

Synonyms: pseudosarcomatous DF and paradoxical fibrosarcoma of the skin.

Introduction

AFX, first described by Helwig in 1963, refers to a group of usually indolent cutaneous tumors on sun-exposed skin of the elderly. There is a predilection for Caucasian men (397). Although considered by most to have low malignant potential, cases with metastasis have been reported (398–400). Clinically, AFX may be confused with BCC or SCC. The lesion consists of an unencapsulated proliferation of pleomorphic cells with disputed histiogenesis. Recently, suggestions that AFX represents a variant of SCC have been presented in the literature, although immunohistochemical staining has not supported this proposal (401).

Clinical Features

AFX presents as a solitary, rapidly enlarging, exophytic polyp on sun-damaged skin of the elderly, most commonly on the head or neck, but many other sites have been reported (402). Most lesions are 1 to 2 cm, but can be as much as 8 cm, in diameter and attenuate the overlying epidermis, occasionally resulting in ulceration (402). An association with previous trauma or irradiation has been reported. Another clinical variant occurs in younger patients whose lesions are located typically on non-sun-exposed areas (403). As in other cutaneous malignancies, increased numbers have been reported in transplant recipients, presumably as an effect of immunosuppression (404,405). AFX has also been reported in children with xeroderma pigmentosum (406,407).

Imaging

As these are benign and almost exclusively dermal proliferations, imaging studies are rarely necessary.

Pathology

AFXs are usually well-circumscribed, nonencapsulated, highly cellular dermal-based tumors, which

may extend into the subcutis. Although neoplastic cells may appear to stream into the dermis from the basal layer, most lesions are separated from the overlying epidermis by a thin zone of collagen or Grenz zone (Fig. 64). AFX may have haphazard, storiform, or fascicular patterns composed of polygonal and spindled cells with striking cytologic atypia admixed with various numbers of giant cells. The cytoplasm, which is usually abundant and eosinophilic to amphophilic, may be filled with microvesicular lipid (Fig. 65). True

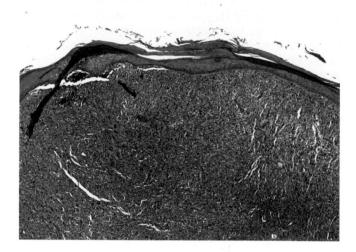

Figure 64 Aytpical fibroxanthoma. Pleomorphic neoplastic cells efface the epidermis and are separated from it by a thin zone of collagen.

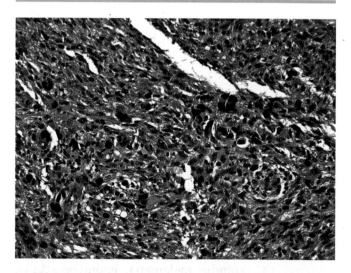

Figure 65 Atypical fibroxanthoma. This image shows the characteristic infiltrate of polygonal and spindled cells with striking cytologic atypia admixed with giant cells. Numerous mitoses, including atypical forms, may also be present. The cytoplasm, which is usually abundant and eosinophilic to amphophilic, may be filled with microvesicular lipid.

xanthoma cells are uncommon. The nuclei are hyperchromatic and pleomorphic with many atypical mitotic figures. Clear cell, pigmented, and granular variants have been described (408–410).

Immunohistochemistry

AFXs can be confused not only clinically but also histologically, with a variety of malignant dermal-based spindle cell neoplasms. Immunohistochemistry is mandatory to differentiate between the clinically indolent AFX and much more aggressive and potentially fatal tumors such as melanoma. AFXs are immunorective for vimentin, α-1 antitrypsin, and α-1 antichymotrypsin in almost all cases. In one study, 41% of cases stained for muscle-specific actin or smooth muscle actin, 57% expressed CD68, but no cases expressed CD34 (411). CD99 expression has been reported in two-thirds of cases (412). Procollagen-1 has been promoted as a sensitive marker for AFX, but a significant number of desmoplastic melanomas and desmoplastic SCCs also express this marker (413). Adding to the confusion are reports of aberrant CK expression in AFX, which not only confounds the attempt at arriving at a definitive diagnosis but also adds credence to the theories of AFX representing a dedifferentiated SCC (401,414). A specific marker for AFX remains elusive; however, the use of additional immunohistochemical stains such as CK 5/6, S-100, smooth muscle actin, and CD31 is essential for an accurate final histologic diagnosis (415). These markers should be used routinely to rule out spindle SCC, melanoma, leiomyosarcoma, and angiosarcoma respectively.

Electron Microscopy

Ultrastructurally, the cells have abundant cytoplasm with filopodia, numerous lysosomes, abundant rough endoplasmic reticulum, and variable amount of intracytoplasmic filaments (416,417). These findings suggest a fibrohistiocytic or myofibroblastic origin. There is no basal lamina, nor are there pinocytotic vesicles or inclusion bodies.

Molecular-Genetic Data

Although no specific genetic aberration characterizes AFXs, the DNA analysis by flow cytometry has shown mostly diploid DNA in AFXs, in contract with malignant fibrous histiocytomas, which are usually aneuploid (418).

Differential Diagnosis

The histologic differential diagnosis of AFXs includes other spindle cell neoplasms: sarcomatoid SCC, sarcomatoid BCC, spindle melanoma, leiomyosarcoma, malignant peripheral nerve sheath tumor, and poorly differentiated angiosarcoma. Spindled melanomas may not have an overlying in situ component and may not stain with specific melanocytic markers. S-100 is the most useful stain in this regard. AFX has been reported to express S-100 protein, however, not in the diffuse strong pattern typically seen in melanoma

(419). Sarcomatoid SCC usually demonstrates keratinocyte atypia in the overlying epidermis. It may not show diffuse strong CK expression, however, focal staining is typically noted, whereas AFX would be negative except for rare cases that show weak aberrant expression (420). Accurate diagnosis requires the use of multiple immunohistochemical stains in conjunction with routine histologic evaluation.

Treatment and Prognosis

Even though AFXs are considered indolent tumors, recurrences develop in approximately 5% of cases and metastases in even fewer. The superficial cases rarely recur. Spontaneous regression of incompletely removed tumor has been reported. To conserve tissue and improve the likelihood of cure, Mohs micrographic surgery has been used for treatment of AFX without superior cure rates (397).

V. VASCULAR PROLIFERATIONS

A. Vascular Tumors and Malformations

Introduction

Significant progress in understanding the biologic behavior of vascular lesions led to the currently accepted 1996 International Society for the Study of Vascular Anomalies (ISSVA), updated classification of vascular anomalies. This system broadly classifies vascular lesions as malformations, either simple (capillary, lymphatic, venous, and arterial) or combined, and tumors. The essence of the separation is based on the recognition that vascular tumors, which include hemangioma of infancy (HOI), tufted angioma, kaposiform hemangioendothelioma (KHE), hemangiopericytoma, pyogenic granuloma, spindle cell hemangioendothelioma, angiosarcoma, kaposi sarcoma (KS), and other rare tumors, demonstrate proliferative activity on the basis of 3H-thymidine uptake of endothelium and expression of proliferative markers such as proliferating cell nuclear antigen, type IV collagenase, vascular endothelial growth factor, and basic fibroblastic growth factor (421). On the other hand, vascular malformations lack 3H-thymidine uptake and markers of endothelial proliferation. Distinguishing vascular malformation from vascular tumors is crucial for the purposes of determining clinical course and treatment options.

Vascular Malformations

Synonyms: capillary malformation (CM)—telangectasia, port-wine stain, salmon patch, angel kiss, stork bite, cherry angioma, and capillary angioma; venous malformation (VM)—venous angioma, cavernous hemangioma, and cavernous angioma; lymphatic malformation (LM)—lymphangioma and cystic hygroma.

The ISSVA classification has clarified the lesions included in this category, yet confusion and misuse of nomenclature are rampant in the literature. On the basis of this classification scheme, capillary hemangioma is an inappropriate term and should be referred to as capillary malformation, and the same holds true for cavernous hemangioma, which should be referred to as a venous malformation. Vascular malformations are the result of a fault in embryonic or fetal development of hematologic or lymphatic vascular channels. Those malformations with an arterial component are "fast-flow" lesions, while all others are "slow-flow," a designation that may relate to the lesions' response rate to particular therapeutic options (422).

Vascular malformations may be seen associated with numerous syndromes, the more common of which are outlined in Table 1. Thorough review of all, common and uncommon, sydromes are covered elsewhere (423).

Clinical. Malformations have no gender predilection. They are often noted at birth and grow proportionately with the growth of the child. Malformations may be of any size and range, from small focal lesions to extensive lesions, involving an entire organ or body site.

Capillary Malformations. These are the most common of the malformations. Mild cutaneous erythema or red-brown discoloration, which may be seen at birth, darkens and develops texture with age. These lesions are commonly located on the face where they may be centrally located (glabella, nose, upper lip, and eyelid) or have a dermatomal distribution. Involvement of the oral mucosa, gingival, and lips may also be noted. Those that are centrally located have a tendency to fade over time.

Venous Malformations. These are relatively rare. They are common on the head and neck but may be located on any site with focal or extensive involvement, including extension into the subcutaneous tissue and underlying muscle. These lesions enlarge as the patient ages, with the most rapid period of growth ending with the onset of puberty (424). The ectatic venous spaces correlate to a clinically blue lesion. Ulceration, bleeding, and thrombosis are not uncommon.

Lymphatic Malformations (LMs). These may be primary or secondary, with secondary lymphedema being most commonly a result of traumatic or infectious disruption of the normal lymphatic system. Primary LMs are very rare and usually noted at birth. Large lesions may be detected with routine prenatal ultrasound. LMs are typically spongy, have a blue hue, and have no involvement of the overlying epidermis. Whether primary or secondary, the lesions range from a focal spongy mass to involvement of an entire organ or body site. Facial LMs, as with involvement of other body sites, can cause significant dysmorphism. Proptosis, ptosis, and interference with range of motion are all reported with high frequency in LMs of the orbit (422).

Imaging. Imaging studies including MRI, CT, arteriography, positron emission tomography, and single photon emission CT all have a role in delineating the extent of involvement of the underlying soft tissue, visceral organs, and central nervous system (424). In hereditary hemorrhagic telangiectasia or Rendu-Osler-Weber syndromes, the liver, lung, and brain are the most common extracutaneous sites of involvement of capillary and arteriovenous malformations. Ultrasonography provides a useful screening tool, but multidetector row helical CT and MRI provide rapid, thorough, and high-qulity images for comprehensive assessment of extent of involvement (425).

Pathology. CMs have increased ectatic vascular spaces in the papillary and reticular dermis. The endothelium has small nuclei with compressed cytoplasm, as is seen in normal capillaries (Fig. 66). While antigenic expression, as determined by immunohistochemical stains, shows a normal profile, additional studies reveal a decrease in the density of cutaneous nerves (426). Whether this represents a primary process or is secondary to decreased vascularity of the tissue is not clear.

VMs reveal a poorly circumscribed nodule composed of ectatic, interconnecting spaces with irregular luminal outlines. The endothelium is unremarkable, and the vascular walls are thin without a smooth muscle layer (Fig. 67). Thrombi and phleboliths are commonly noted.

LMs show multiple ectatic spaces with thin endothelium and varying amounts of smooth muscle in the wall. The vascular spaces vary from small to cisternal and are filled with paucicellular to acellular eosinophilic fluid (Fig. 68).

Immunohistochemistry. Factor VIII, ICAM-1, and ELAM-1 expression in CM is identical to normal capillaries. The most significant antigenic marker is GLUT-1, which is not expressed in malformations, reliably distinguishing all vascular malformations from vascular tumors (427,428).

Electron microscopy. VMs have been shown by electron microscopic evaluation to lack basement membrane. Pericytes are rarely seen (429). Electron microscopy also shows the presence of thin abluminal endothelial cell processes anastomosing to form electron-lucent blebs (430).

Genetics. CMs are typically sporadic, although familial cases with an autosomal dominant inheritance pattern have been recognized. In those cases, genetic susceptibility is conferred by a gene RASA1 on chromosome 5q, which encodes a p120-rasGTPase-activating protein (431,432). A subset of families with this mutation additionally have arteriovenous malformations, afteriovenous fistulas, or Parkes-Wever syndrome. The defect in hereditary benign telangectasia has been mapped to the same locus (433). Familial cases of VMs have revealed a defect in the endothelial cell receptor Tie2 on chromonsome 9p21, also noted in cerebral arteriovenous malformations (434,435).

Differential diagnosis. The histologic differential diagnosis is primarily differentiating a vascular malformation from a vascular tumor. The histologic features are typically straightforward. However, in difficult cases, GLUT-1 expression has been reliable (436,427). Acroangiodermatitis (AAD) could potentially cause some challenge; however, AAD has a proliferation of small vessels in the papillary dermis that are lined by plump endothelium, not the small endothelium of vascular malformations. Additionally,

Table 1 Syndromes Associated with Vascular Proliferations

Malformation/tumor	Syndrome	Select other associations
Capillary malformation	Sturge-Weber	• leptomeningeal anomalies • facial hypertrophy • glaucoma • epilepsy
	Klippel-Trenaunay	• hypertrophy of bone and soft tissue
	Osler-Rendu-Weber	• visceral and mucocutaneous telangectasias
	Ataxia-telangiectasia	• cerebellar degeneration • immunodeficiency • malignancies • growth retardation
	Beckwith-Wiedemann	• gigantism • omphalocele • macroglossia
	Proteus	
Venous malformation	Blue rubber bleb	• visceral VMs • anemia • coagulopathy
	Maffucci	• oral and/or intra-abdominal VMs • enchondromas, with risk of malignant transformation • short stature • bone irregularities
Arterial malformation	Parkes-Weber	• multiple arteriovenous fistulas • tissue hypertrophy
Lymphatic malformation	Congenital hereditary lymphedema	• infections • hydroceles • atrial septal defect
	Meige disease	• extradural cysts • vertebral anomalies • cerebrovascular malformations • sensorineural hearing loss
	Turner syndrome	• short stature • webbed neck • pectus excavatum • no ovarian development • heart defects • kidney abnormalities • diabetes
	Noonan syndrome	• short stature • webbed neck • pectus excavatum • delayed puberty • ptosis • hypertelorism
Kaposiform hemangioendothelioma Tufted angioma	Kassabach-Merrit	• thrombocytopenia • coagulopathy
hemangiomas	PHACE	• posterior fossa malformation • arterial anomalies • coarctaion of the aorta • eye abnormalities
Spindle cell hemangioma	Maffucci	• as above
Glomeruloid hemangioma	POEMS	• polyneuropathy • organomegaly • endocrinopathy • monoclonal gammopathy • skin changes
Angiokeratoma	Fabry's syndrome	• corneal opacity • neuropathic pain • sensorineural deafness • renal failure

Abbreviations: VMs, venous malformations; POEMS, polyneuropathy, organomegaly, endocrinopathy, monoclonal gammopathy, and skin changes.

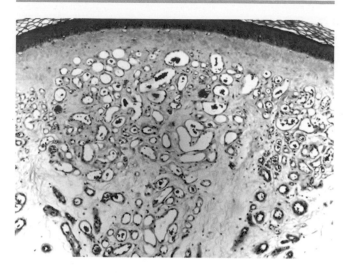

Figure 66 Capillary malformation. Numerous ectatic thin-walled vascular spaces fill the papillary and reticular dermis. The endothelium has small nuclei with compressed cytoplasm, as is seen in normal capillaries.

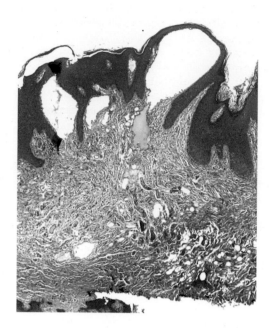

Figure 68 Lymphatic malformation. Multiple ectatic spaces with thin endothelium and varying amounts of smooth muscle in the wall. The vascular spaces, varying from small to cisternal, are filled with paucicellular to acellular eosinophilic fluid.

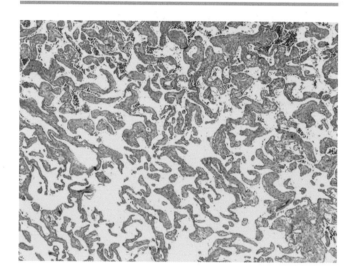

Figure 67 Venous malformation. A poorly circumscribed nodule composed of ectatic, interconnecting spaces with irregular luminal outlines. The endothelium is unremarkable, and the vascular walls are thin, without a smooth muscle layer.

AAD has an edematous stroma, which would be unusual in vascular malformations.

    Treatment and prognosis. Nonintervention is the primary mode of management for capillary lesions. Pulse dye lasers of wavelengths that target oxyhemoglobin (577, 585, and 595 nm) are effective in decreasing the vascular lesions with intraluminal erythrocytes such as CMs. It has been noted that CMs on the limb do not respond as well to this modality as do those on the head and neck. This poor response has been attributed to the lower blood flow in these lesions of the leg as well as to the lower blood flow at all tested ambient temperatures, which effectively provides less hemoglobin (the target chromophobe) for laser destruction (437). VMs, on the other hand, benefit from surgical intervention and/or sclerotherapy, with the goal of preserving function and limiting destruction of underlying structures (424).

Vascular Tumors

Vascular tumors represent the other large division of vascular proliferations, as outlined by the classification of ISSVA. The more common hemangiomas will be covered here. As addressed above, excluded from these hemangiomas are the capillary and cavernous hemangiomas, which currently are considered to be malformations and discussed in that section. Common syndromes associated with vascular tumors are listed in Table 1 (438,439).

B. Infantile Hemangioma

Synonyms: hemangioma of infancy, juvenile hemangioma, and cellular hemangioma of infancy.

Introduction

Infantile hemangioma (IH) does not appear to have a predominant genetic influence on the basis of a large study of twins with IH. This study showed no statistically significant difference in the prevalence of IH between monozygotic and dizygotic twins, suggesting hereditary factors are not the dominant factor in development of IH (440). Mapping of 177 focal IH of the head and neck showed a pattern of presentation at lines of mesenchymal-ectodermal embryonic fusion (441). Supporting the vascular tumor classification of hemangiomas of infancy is the demonstration of clonal expression in the endothelial cells of the proliferative phase (442). DNA microarray analysis of IH in distinct phases of evolution has identified insulin-like growth factor 2 (IGF-2) as a prominent regulator of the proliferative phase (443). Quantitative reverse transcription polymerase chain reaction (PCR) and immunohistochemical staining confirmed high expression of IGF-2 in the proliferative phase of IH and significant decreased expression in the involutional phase. This, along with the already established upregulation of expression of basic fibroblast growth factor and vascular endothelial growth factor in proliferative IH, opens the door for exploring new treatment options through modulation of these angiogenic cytokines during proliferation of the lesion, thus promoting cessation of proliferation and encouraging an earlier onset of the involutional stage (421).

Clinical Features

IH presents at birth, or within the ensuing weeks, as mild cutaneous dyspigmentation that becomes increasingly prominent over the next year and then undergoes a period of spontaneous involution that can last up to 10 years or more. During this maturation, the cutaneous surface evolves from flat to verrucoid to nodular. The final involuted lesion has a fibrofatty infiltrate that typically does not require intervention. Approximately 4% to 12% of children have IH, and 60% of them present on the head and neck (436,444,445). They are typically solitary and are more comomon in infants who are female, Caucasian, premature, the product of a multiple gestation, and in association with preeclampsia and placenta previa (446). As in the malformations, these lesions vary considerably in size. A small number of children develop complications because of their size and/or site. Ulceration, bleeding, infection, and involvement of adjacent structures are the most common direct complications. Disturbance of visual fields from periorbital lesions can cause astigmatism, strabismus, and amblyopia (447,448). Depending on the extent of the underlying vascular proliferation and interference with other associated structures, treatment of the lesions prior to their natural period of involution may be necessary.

Imaging

While not necessary for diagnosis, imaging studies are invaluable in determining the full extent of any vascular proliferation. This information is crucial to determining the appropriate treatment plan, if necessary. Doppler ultrasound is noninvasive and cost-effective in the initial evaluation and can be helpful in differentiating vascular malformations from vascular tumors on the basis of the vessel density and systolic Doppler shift (449). CT scan or MRI is the best tool for determining the extent of the vascular infiltrate (449). MRI, with or without MR angiography, allows characterization of hemangiomas with typical features (450).

Pathology

Early in their course, these lesions are composed of a sheetlike or lobular dermal proliferation of plump endothelial cells. The lumens are small and may not be apparent; the vascular etiology can be difficult to determine in the early proliferative phase. Eythrocytes may be the only clue (Fig. 69). Mitoses may be numerous; abnormal mitoses should raise concern for an alternative diagnosis. The vascular formation becomes more apparent in the later proliferative phase (Fig. 70). These vessels are small with plump endothelial lining. With evolution, the lumen becomes more obvious, and the endothelial lining becomes flatter (Fig. 71). As would be expected, during the involuting phase, apoptotic bodies are seen in increasing numbers. Additionally, increased mast cells are noted in the involuting stage, lower in the involuted lesion, and lowest in the proliferative phase (451). Mast cells elaborate mediators of angiogenesis as well as antiangiogenesis. It is proposed that both functions of mast cells are elaborated on in differing stages of evolution of IH; the mechanism by which one role or the other is functional has not been elucidated. The differing roles of the mast cell throughout the evolution of the lesions are highlighted by the observation that throughout the evolution, virtually all mast cells express biogenic amines, whereas the the proportion of chymase-postive mast cells decreases

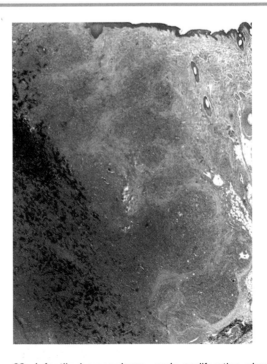

Figure 69 Infantile hemangioma, early proliferative phase. A sheetlike dermal proliferation of plump endothelial cells with small, nearly imperceptible lumina.

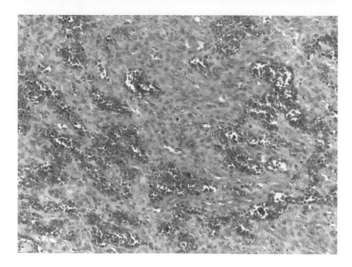

Figure 70 Infantile hemangioma, mid proliferative phase. Sheets of plump endothelial cells with apparent vascular formation.

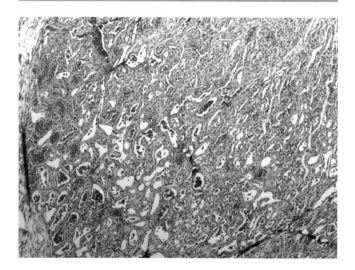

Figure 71 Infantile hemangioma, late proliferative phase. These vessels are small with flattened endothelial lining. Vascular lumens are patent.

with lesional evolution (452). Unless ulcerated, an inflammatory infiltrate in not characteristic. An entirely involuted IH has only a fatty infiltrate with scattered capillaries of normal capillary morphology.

Immunohistochemistry

The classic vascular antigens such as CD31, CD34, and factor VIII are expressed in IH. GLUT-1 is the most helpful marker in identifying IH, as its expression is seen at all stages of evolution and not seen in vascular malformations or other benign vascular tumors.

Electron Microscopy

Ultrastructurally, there are plump endothelial cells and a multilaminated basement membrane enveloping plump pericytes. There is abundant rough endoplasmic reticulum (436).

Molecular-Genetic Data

Allelic loss of 13q14 and 17p13 are seen in 60% of hemangiomas and of 11p13 in 20%, the same alleleic losses that are seen in angiosarcoma. No allelic loss is seen in granulation tissue (453).

Differential Diagnosis

For therapeutic options, vascular malformations present an important differential diagnosis, and without the assistance of GLUT-1, a marker for IH, the distinction cannot always be made on histologic features alone (454).

The lobular growth pattern of pyogenic granuloma can make distinction from an established IH difficult. The epithelial collarette at the margins of the lobular infiltrate differentiates it from IH, which lacks the collarette. Additionally, mast cells are not seen in pyogenic granuloma.

KHE is an aggressive vascular proliferation in children. Because of the rarity of the lesion, it is often mistaken clinically for IH (455). However, it typically presents later in life than IH, has a progressive clinical behavior, without involution, and a densely cellular spindle cell proliferation, more closely mimicking KS than the proliferative phase of IH.

Treatment and Prognosis

For the 20% of IHs that require treatment because of interference with other structures or because of significant social implications, steroids, topically, intralesionally, or systemically, are the first option in most instances (456,457). Intralesional triaminolone increases the mast cell infiltrate and decreases the expression of PDGF A and B, IL-6, and TGF-β-1 and β-3, while the expression of basic fibroblastic growth factor and vascular endothelial cell growth factor remain unaffected (456). For nonresponsive lesions, interferon-α, cyclophosphamide, and vincristine provide alternatives (458). Vincristine is effective in clinical trials for treating complicated lesions. Interferon is a negative regulator of angiogenesis and is effective in induction of the involutional phase. However, because of complications due to neurotoxicity, interferon is used as a last resort, especially in children younger than 1 year (459).

C. Kaposiform Hemangioendothelioma

Synonyms: congenital hemangioendothelioma and kaposi-like infantile hemangioendothelioma.

Introduction

KHE is a rare vascular tumor of childhood associated with Kasabach-Merritt phenomenon (KMP) and lymphangiomatosis (460,461). Along with tufted angioma, KHE is the only other lesion associated with KMP, which is a life-threatening consumptive coagulopathy characterized by profound thrombocytopenia, presumably due to architectural features that favor turbulent blood flow and platelet destruction (462,463). Despite the similar histologic features and clinical presentation, KMP is not seen in association with IH (464). KHE does not express GLUT-1 or LeY, reinforcing the endothelial differences, morphologic and functional, between the KHE and IH (465). KHE is locally aggressive, with two reports of local nodal involvement, but no distant metastasis. Unlike IH, KHE does not regress. Mortality is due to KMP and not metastatic disease, which appears limited to regional perinodal soft tissue. Given this behavior, its continued classification as a vascular tumor of intermediate malignancy is warranted (463). Both vascular and lymphatic components make up KHE.

Clinical Features

KHE is a solitary tumor that develops primarily in children. Historically, an equal gender predilection has been reported, distinguishing these lesions from IH. However, in the largest study to date, there is a 2:1 male predominance (463). The mean age of presention is 48 months, older than the presention of IH (463), although adult cases have been reported (461). KHE presents as a rapidly growing, tender plaque, papule, nodule, or telangectatic area, but most commonly as a blue-red soft tissue mass (463,466). Tumors are most common on the extremities, followed by the head and neck and then rare presentations at other sites. Rare patients developed regional perinodal soft tissue involvement, none developed distant metastases, and 40% of the patients developed KMP (460,463).

Imaging

Doppler ultrasound is useful in differentiating hemangioendotheliomas from other soft tissue tumors of infancy on the basis of the presence of an ill-defined focus with a moderate vessel density and a Doppler shift exceeding 2 kHz (467). In contrast to IH, MRI shows diffuse enhancement with ill-defined margins, cutaneous thickening, stranding of subcutaneous fat resembling LM or edema secondary to lymphatic obstruction, hemosiderin deposits, and dilated superficial feeding and draining vessels, indicative of fast flow (468).

Pathology

KHE lesions are composed of a lobular dermal infiltrate of irregular, infiltrating nodules of spindled endothelial cells intimately associated with small slit-like vessels. A hyalinized stroma with hemosiderin deposits surrounds the nodules. At the center of the nodule, the vessels are compressed resembling KS, whereas at the periphery, the vessels are open and more closely resemble those vessels in a CM. Epithelioid cells with finely granular hemosiderin, hyaline droplets, and cytoplasmic vacuoles can be identified

in some KHE. Small vascular spaces may have microthrombi. Nuclear atypia is not prominent, and mitoses are sparse, averaging 2 to 3 out of 10 HPF, but ranging from 0 to 7 out of 10 HPF (460,461). Small and large lymphatic channels may be seen peripheral or deep to the main tumor mass.

Immunohistochemistry

Well-formed capillaries in KHE express CD31, CD34, and FLI1; however, there is lack of expression of von Willebrand factor in the areas of spindled cells with slitlike vascular spaces (461,463). Additionally, the endothelial cells do not express GLUT1 or LeY, markers that characterize IH (463). Clusters of plump pericytes, which are seen surrounding the vessels, stain with smooth muscle actin. Human herpesvirus (HHV)-8 has not been identified in any lesions of KHE (463,469).

Electron Microscopy

Electron microscopy of KHE reveals wide endothelial intercellular gaps and incomplete basement membranes (468).

Molecular-Genetic Data

A genetic association has not been determined for these lesions.

Differential Diagnosis

On the basis of clinical and histologic features, distinguishing KHE from IH is the most problematic as well as the most significant, as KHE has a relatively high mortalitity (20–30%) (422). IH has a similar clinical presentation, though KHE most often presents in a slightly older age. The multinodular growth pattern can help in differentiating KHE from the proliferative phase of IH. The GLUT-1 and LeY antigen expression in IH is not found in KHE (463). HHV-8, once again, is very helpful, as this virus has only been determined in lesions of KS.

Treatment and Prognosis

In a review of 21 patients with a mean follow-up of two years (range 8 months–15 years), 10 were alive without residual disease, 8 were alive with disease, and 3 died of their disease. With the exception of one patient who refused treatment, those that were alive without residual disease had undergone complete excision, sometimes multiple and extensive, including one patient who required amputation. In this group, only two of the patients presented with KMP and five had received treatment with steroids, interferon, and/or chemotherapy. Of three patients that died of disease, all three presented with KMP and were all younger than six months at presentation: one patient succumbed to respiratory compromise secondary to lymphangiomatosis, one from sepsis and respiratory distress syndrome, and the third from severe coagulopathy and anemia. The fourth patient died of unrelated causes (463). In another report on 14 infants with

KHE who were treated with interferon-α2a, six had accelerated regression, two were stabilized, and six had no response. With this treatment, the mortality rate was 24% (5 of 21) (468). One child with an inoperable lesion causing significant morbidity was successfully treated with a chemotherapy regimen of vicristine, cyclophosphamide, and actinomycin D (470). Variable response to current pharmacologic therapy underscores our inadequate knowledge of the pathogenesis of thrombocytopenia in KHE (468).

D. Angiolymphoid Hyperplasia with Eosinophilia

Synonyms: epithelioid hemangioma, histiocytoid hemangioma, and atypical pyogenic granuloma.

Introduction

Angiolymphoid hyperplasia with eosinophilia (ALHE) is an uncommon vascular lesion originally proposed to represent a variant, or final stage, of Kimura's disease; these two diseases are now recognized to be separate entities. Wells and Whimster, in 1969, first reported ALHE under the name "subcutaneous angiolymphoid hyperplasia with eosinophilia" (471). There has been considerable controversy as to whether ALHE is a reactive process or a true neoplasm. Currently, in view of its local recurrence rate, ALHE is believed to be a benign vascular tumor. The alternative view that this is a reactive process is supported by a predilection for superficial soft tissue sites overlying bones coupled with a history of trauma and a pronounced inflammatory reaction accompanying the lesion.

Clinical Features

ALHE occurs during early to mid adult life (age 20–40 years). The subcutaneous lesions, as originally presented, have a male predominance; however, the purely cutaneous lesions have a female predominance. The majority of patients present with a mass of a year or less in duration. Typically, these masses are located in the head and neck, especially the forehead, preauricular area, scalp (often in the distribution of the superficial temporal artery), and distal extremities, especially the digits. They are small, red, pruritic plaques, papules, or nodules. About half of the patients have multiple lesions in the same area (472). Microscopic metastases to a regional lymph node has been reported but, after five years of follow-up, had no adverse effect on patient outcome (473). Other than this report of local nodal spread, there have been no reports of metastasis.

Imaging

Because of its superficial location, imaging is rarely necessary. Only sporadic cases have been reported in the radiologic literature related to their atypical, noncutaneous locations: striated muscles, bones, colon, blood vessels, and deep soft tissue of the head, neck, and extremities (474). In these cases, angiography and CT demonstrate a well-circumscribed hypervascular mass suspicious for a highly aggressive neoplasm. Positron emission tomography shows moderate to high metabolism by ALHE, presumably related to high vascularity of this lesion. The vascularity is confirmed by contrast enhancement on MR examination (474).

Pathology

ALHE nodules are typically 0.5 to 2.0 cm in diameter, with rare giant lesions exceeding 5 cm (472). The nodules are well-circumscribed dermal or subcutaneous lesions, occasionally involving or arising from a vessel (475). This histology shows a lobular proliferation of variable-sized capillaries, venules, and arterioles lined by plump, epithelioid, and vacuolated endothelial cells. The plump endothelium may be difficult to detect on low power, as they may be so epithelioid in nature as to obscure the lumen. In other cases, the endothelial cells may protrude into the lumen (tombstones) (Fig. 72). In some lesions, the vascular etiology is challenging to ascertain, and only with immunohistochemical staining can the vessels be identified. An inflammatory infiltrate is invariably present. However, despite the lesion's name, the proportion of eosinophils varies widely from infiltrates almost exclusively composed of eosinophils to those infiltrates in which the stereotypic cells are sparse and difficult to locate. Occasionally, lymphoid follicle formation is present. Mast cells and plasma cells may also be seen in the vicinity of the vessels (Fig. 73). An intravascular form of this tumor is reported by Rosai and Ackerman who described such lesions as "intravenous atypical vascular proliferation" (472).

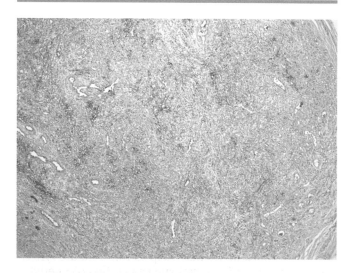

Figure 72 Angiolymphoid hyperplasia with eosinophilia. A lobular proliferation of variably sized capillaries, venules, and arterioles are lined by plump, epithelioid, and vacuolated endothelial cells that may tombstone into the vascular lumen.

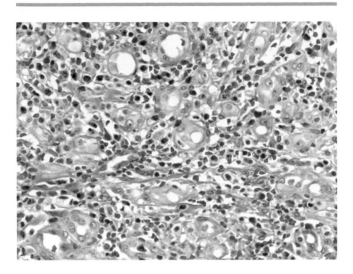

Figure 73 Angiolymphoid hyperplasia with eosinophilia. The epithelioid endothelial cells with narrow lumens are noted in these images. This case shows an inflammatory infiltrate composed of numerous eosinophils; other cases have sparse eosinophilia with a dominant lymphocyte population.

Immunohistochemistry

The epithelioid endothelial cells, characteristic of ALHE, are immunoreactive for CD31 and factor VIII. Immunoreactivity for CD34 is also present, though often to a lesser extent. Sometimes, a limited pankeratin expression is detected. Smooth muscle actin is helpful in demonstrating an intact myopericytic layer around the immature vessels. Actin-positive myopericytes are present to a much lesser extent in malignant vascular tumors such as epithelioid hemangioendothelioma and epithelioid angiosarcoma (476).

Electron Microscopy

The neoplastic cells of ALHE have many of the ultrastructural features of endothelium such as antiluminal basal lamina and Weibel-Palade bodies, in addition to large gaps between adjacent endothelial cells. Electron microscopy, in some cases, shows clusters of endothelial cells forming immature vascular lumens with numerous microvilli (477). Organelles such as mitochondria, smooth and rough endoplasmic reticulum, free ribosomes, and thin cytofilaments are more abundant in these cells.

Molecular-Genetic Data

There is no known specific genetic aberration seen in these lesions. Genetics may help to differentiate ALHE from vascular malignancies such as epithelioid hemangioendothelioma. The latter is a rare vascular tumor arising in either superficial or deep soft tissue of the extremities with a characteristic translocation involving chromosomes 1 and 3: t(1,3)(p36.3;q2). This finding has been reported in two of three cytogenetically analyzed

soft tissue epithelioid hemangioendotheliomas (478). No consistent, recurring chromosomal abnormality has yet been identified in epithelioid angiosarcoma. In one study, five of seven ALHE patients displayed a clonal T-cell population and proliferative T-cell activity in lesional tissue. Most of these cases followed a protracted and therapy-resistant course with recurrences, suggesting that ALHE or at least a subset of ALHE harboring a clonal T-cell population may represent a T-cell lymphoproliferative disorder of a benign or low-grade malignant nature (479).

Differential Diagnosis

ALHE is most likely to be confused with other benign and low-grade vascular proliferations such as epithelioid hemangioendothelioma. The latter is an angiocentric vascular tumor with metastatic potential, composed also of epithelioid endothelial cells, but with distinctive myxohyaline stroma. As discussed above, genetic studies might be helpful when morphologic distinction between ALHE and this entity is challenging.

Epithelioid angiosarcomas occur as cutaneous tumors, most likely in deep soft tissue. Even though no consistent, recurring chromosomal abnormality has yet been identified in this subtype of angiosarcomas, many of these lesions display characteristic histologic and immunohistochemical features such as their pancytokeratin expression, which, in difficult cases, might be helpful in further classifying the nature of the lesion.

Other differential diagnoses include a florid arthropod bite reaction, cutanous lymphoid hyperplasias, and lymphomas. Histologically, arthropod bites display more florid-mixed inflammatory infiltrate of lymphocytes and eosinophils with occasional lymphoid follicule and germinal center formation. While the endothelium may be reactive and plump, a vascular proliferation is not present, and the overall morphology of the arthropod bite reaction is wedge shaped, with the base of the wedge parallel to the epidermis.

Cutaneous lymphoid hyperplasia and cutaneous lymphomas should also be considered and appropriate immunohistochemical/molecular and cytogenetic studies should be performed if clinically indicated.

Treatment and Prognosis

Despite the recurrence of up to one-third of cases, surgical excision, including Mohs micrographic surgery when indicated, is the primary treatment option (480). For recalcitrant cases, numerous therapeutic approaches have been tried, including electrodesiccation, cryotherapy, surgery, radiotherapy, glucocorticoids (topical or intralesional), retinoids, sclerosing injections, pentoxifylline, pulse dye laser, argon laser, interferon-α2a and cytotoxic agents. Refractory ALHE has been reported to respond to topical application of imiquimod cream (481–483). There is a rare report of complete spontaneous regression of ALHE after just 10 weeks (484).

E. Kaposi Sarcoma

Introduction

KS is a neoplasm composed of endothelial-like spin-dled cells of disputed etiology and has traditionally been divided into four separate categories on the basis of the clinical presentation: endemic or African, classic or Mediterranean, iatrogenic or posttransplant, and epidemic or HIV associated. Although the patho-genesis and histology are identical to all variants, this division is not just for academic purposes, as the clinical course differs among the subtypes, tradition-ally being indolent in classic KS and more aggressive in the epidemic and iatrogenic variants. Classic KS develops primarily on the lower extremities of elderly men of Mediterranean and eastern European descent and runs an indolent course. Mean survival for classic KS is 10 to 15 years, with patients often dying of unrelated causes. Endemic KS is seen in young men and children in Africa. Immunosuppression, especial-ly in transplant patients, is responsible for iatrogenic KS, and immunosuppression along with coinfective properties of HIV is responsible for epidemic KS. The risk for acquiring KS in the HIV-positive population varies among the risk groups, with homosexual men at the highest risk and hemophilic patients in the lowest-risk group (485). Visceral involvement is higher in both immunosuppressed groups than it is in the immunocompetent groups.

HHV-8, a gamma herpes virus with 40% homol-ogy to EBV, has been detected in all forms of KS, as well as B-cell body cavity-based lymphoma, multi-centric Castleman's disease, non-Hodgkins lympho-ma, and sensory ganglia of HIV-positive patients with KS. In fact, the worldwide distribution of HHV-8 infection parallels the worldwide distribution of KS486. HHV-8 can be isolated from saliva and blood. Routes of HHV-8 transmission are similar to other herpes viruses such as cytomegalovirus and EBV. In endemic and high-risk groups, the most common route for horizontal HHV-8 transmission appears to be through saliva (486). In homosexual individuals, HHV-8 appears to be sexually transmit-ted (487). Transmission via blood, injection drugs, transfusion with nonleukocyte-reduced blood, and infected transplant organs has been documented (488,489). HHV-8 infection with seroconversion and subsequent immunosuppression, either through transplant treatment protocols or HIV infectivity, are the necessary steps prior to eruption of KS. Mild immunosuppression associated with aging and with particular HLA loci, physiologic stress, and malnutri-tion are proposed factors that lead to a level of immunosuppression in other populations that allows for the emergence of KS (490). Recently, aqueous natural products from KS endemic regions have been shown to cause HHV-8 reactivation. Particular plant extracts from Africa, where there is high preva-lence of HHV-8, caused the greatest level of reactiva-tion (491).

In the past, there were conflicting reports relat-ing an increased rate of second malignancies, mostly solid tumors and in particular lymphoma, as either the presenting tumor or subsequent to the presenta-tion KS (492–496). The most recent investigations in this regard include two large studies, representing 204 and 741 patients, respectively, with classic KS. Both these studies demonstrated that these patients are not at increased risk of cancer in general. The larger of the two studies uncovered some malignancies that arose at a higher than anticipated rate. In particular, cancer of the buccal cavity, pharynx, and colon occurred in excess among women, but not men. And, an increased incidence of lymphomas occurred in the first year of follow-up, but no new lymphomas in the subsequent years (495,496). Interpretation of these data without an adequate follow-up, or as isolated cases, may be the source of the conflicting reports, and, in the past decade, a link between increased malignancies and KS has not been reported.

The spindled cells of KS express endothelial antigens. However, their expression of antigens com-mon to smooth muscle, macrophages, and dendritic cells support a pluripotent precursor cell as the cell or origin. While the reactive versus neoplastic nature of KS has long been debated, telomerase activity in KS parallels that in other cutaneous neoplasms and sup-ports a neoplastic origin to KS (497). The overriding hypothesis is that an initially polyclonal, reactive proliferation is followed by an acquired clonal change because of chromosomal instability, which offers an acceptable explanation for the conflicting reports of polyclonality, oligoclonalilty, and monoclonality detected in these lesions. Clonal abnormalities have been detected in KS-derived cell lines (498–500).

Clinical Features

KS is a solitary or multifocal vascular tumor arising more commonly in men. Though it may arise in nearly any organ, skin is the most common site, with involve-ment being limited to dermis and subcutaneous tis-sue. Visceral involvement is more commonly seen in HIV-associated KS. With the exception of secondary ulceration, the epidermis is not involved. KS lesions evolve from a macular-papular lesion to a plaque and ultimately a tumor nodule and vary considerably in size. They present clinically as a violaceous to brown lesion, reflecting their vascularity and presence of hemosiderin, with typically a smooth or shiny surface. Lymphangioma-like or bullous KS is a rare variant that presents as multiple spongy, compressible, smooth nodules (501).

A large study on KS in women showed this cohort to be predominantly older than 60 years, with only clinically evident cutaneous lesions that were predominantly acral; visceral involvement was rare (502). Although limited, the clinical follow-up, along with this presentation, indicate a benign course, signi-fying that the majority of women who develop KS fit the epidemiologic classification of classic KS.

Imaging

Imaging studies may be required for staging, in par-ticular for iatrogenic KS and AIDS-related KS, which are frequently disseminated. Radiographic studies have been helpful in detecting visceral lesions, which are seen as nodular-filling defects (503). In the evaluation of patients with HIV infection, abdominal CT detected abnormalities in 95% of the patients, including visceral KS, further supporting a role for imaging studies as part of the workup (504).

Pathology

KS is composed of spindled cells forming slit-like vascular spaces with extravasated erythrocytes. In early patch-stage lesions (Fig. 74), an inflammatory infiltrate and the host vasculature predominate over the neoplastic infiltrate and can be challenging to distinguish these neoplastic spindles cells from normal dermal stroma. The tumor cells proliferate around

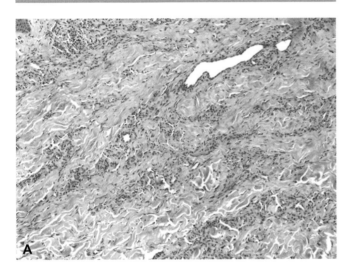

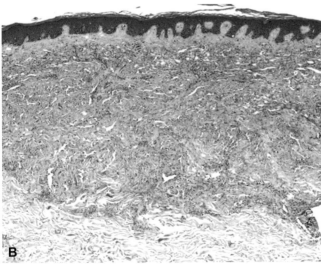

Figure 74 Kaposi sarcoma. (**A**) Early patch and (**B**) plaque lesions, which can be impossible to differentiate on histologic features alone, show a mild lymphoplasmacytic inflammatory infiltrate. The host vasculature predominates over the neoplastic infiltrate and can be challenging to distinguish. The tumor cells proliferate around preexisting vessels, leading to the classic "promontory sign."

preexisting vessels, leading to the classic "promontory sign," and form pseudovascular spaces with extravasated erythrocytes. As the neoplasm progresses, these spindled cells form a sheet and ultimately a nodule that may ulcerate. Prominent nuclear pleomorphism is typically lacking, however, mitoses may be seen. Keloidal-type collagen is also noted, most often in the earlier stages, interspersed amid the spindle cells. A mild to moderate inflammatory infiltrate may be seen coursing through the tumor. The inflammatory cells are lymphocytic with a very characteristic plasma cell component. Cytoplasmic and extracellular PAS-positive diastase-resistant eosinophilic globules are seen in the, plaque- and tumor-stage lesions, rarely in the patch stage, and are thought to represent erythrocyte breakdown products (Fig. 75) (505). These globules are also highlighted with phosphotungstic acid hematoxylin (506). Hemosiderin-laden macrophages may be seen in the tumor. The lymphangioma-like variant shows anastomosing dilated vascular spaces free of erythrocytes. These spaces are lined by bland endothelium. Papillary projections may be seen extending into the vascular lumen.

Immunohistochemistry

The spindled cells can be detected with the progenitor cell marker CD34, but are typically negative for factor VIII. Many other markers such as CD31, E-cadherin, CD68, and PAM-1 have been evaluated and have shown inconsistent expression patterns. Antibodies against HHV-8 antigens have provided for immuno-histochemical evaluation for HHV-8, a less sensitive but much more rapid detection method than the routinely used PCR analysis. Identification of HHV-8 confirms the diagnosis of KS in spindled vascular

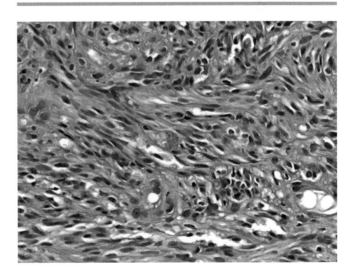

Figure 75 Kaposi sarcoma. Cytoplasmic and extracellular PAS-positive, diastase-resistant, eosinophilic globules are seen most often in plaque and tumor stage lesions, rarely in patch stage, and are thought to represent erythrocyte breakdown products.

lesions, as the virus has not been identified in any other histologic mimics (469).

Electron Microscopy

Ultrastructurally, the spindled cells of KS have many features in common with endothelium. Additionally, KS lesions show intracytoplasmic lumen formation and membrane-bound lysosomes with phagocytized erythrocytes, pinocytic vesicles, and rough endoplasmic reticulum (505). These electron microscopy findings, in conjunction with the histologic features, support the eosinophilic globules seen on routine sections of plaque, and nodular-stage KS represent erythrocyte breakdown products.

Molecular-Genetic Data

Although established KS cell lines have shown various complex chromosomal aberrations, the primary spindle cells are diploid, have a low mitotic rate, and have not been found to have a characteristic abnormalitiy.

Differential Diagnosis

The histology of the patch-stage lesion needs to be distinguished from AAD, stasis dermatitis, and pigmented purpuric dermatitis, all of which involve the vessels of the papillary dermis. Stasis dermatitis is seen on the lower legs of adults. Histology reveals a proliferation of thin-walled vessels in the papillary dermis, a mild lymphocytic infiltrate, and hemosiderin deposition throughout the dermis. The overlying epidermis is spongiotic. Pigmented purpuric dermatosis also presents most commonly on the lower extremities of adults and shows a superficial perivascular lymphocytic infiltrate around slightly ecstatic vessels. Plasma cells are not commonly seen. Erythrocyte extravasation and siderophages are present. These changes are limited to the papillary dermis. The overlying epidermis may be spongiotic.

AAD also arises on the legs of adults. Histology reveals a lobular proliferation of dilated thin-walled vessels in an edematous stroma. These vessels lack the irregular outlines that characterize KS and do no have endothelial atypia. Erythrocyte extravasation and hemosiderin depositions are often seen, but a plasma cell infiltrate would be uncharacteristic of AAD.

Additionally included in the histologic differential diagnosis are other vascular neoplasms, in particular angiosarcoma and KHE. The clinical presentation of KHE differs significantly in that it is an aggressive lesion that occurs almost exclusively in children and adolescents on the extremities (507). The histology is elaborated above. Angiosarcoma most often present on the head and neck of adults; however, many other sites, often with an accompanying history of remote radiation therapy or as a complication of lymphedema, have been described (508–511). Histology, regardless of the etiology, reveals an ill-defined dermal infiltrate of irregular vascular channels with striking endothelial atypia. Similar to KS, angiosarcoma may be multifocal and may infiltrate the subcutaneous

tissue. A lymphocytic infiltrate may be seen, but plasma cells would not be typical of angiosarcoma. Some lesions may not be distinguishable on histology alone. HHV-8 has been very helpful in these circumstances, as HHV-8 has been shown to be found only in KS but not in angiosarcoma or KHE (512). The same holds true for all vascular lesions in the differential diagnosis; HHV-8 is the most helpful marker in distinguishing KS from any of the histologic mimics (469).

Treatment and Prognosis

For patients with classic KS, the prognosis is good. One large study showed that for patients with localized disease, death was attributed to other causes, including associated malignancies (513). For patients with disseminated disease, systemic chemotherapy with vinblastine is very effective (514). With the introduction of highly active antiretroviral therapy (HAART) for AIDS patients, a significant clinical response was noted in KS patients, making HAART treatment a standard approach for HIV-related KS patients (515). While current treatment option for HHV-8-associated diseases remains ineffective, there are accumulating data regarding applications of antiviral treatments. HAART alone or in combination with systemic and local therapy remains an option for AIDS-KS (516). Current management for local disease includes radiotherapy, intralesional chemotherapy, and cryotherapy. Angiogenesis inhibitors are on the horizon as a treatment option (516).

VI. INFLAMMATORY LESIONS

A. Rosacea/Rhinophyma

Introduction

A brief discussion on rosacea must preceed a discussion on rhinophyma. Rosacea is a common disorder affecting approximately 13 million adults in the United States (517). The pathogenesis is not well understood; however, vascular hyperreactivity with exacerbations from factors such as heat, alcohol, stress, vitamin deficiencies, androgenic hormones, and perhaps even the demodex mite have all been associated with rosacea. Rhinophyma, a benign exuberant hypertrophy of the sebaceous glands and connective tissue, is a subtype of rosacea. Although rhinophyma may extend onto the cheeks and chin, it classically involves the distal nose. Increasingly, studies suggest that fibrosis plays a central role in the pathogenesis of these lesions (518,519). When compared with normal nasal tissue, the fibrogenic cytokines TGF-β-1 and β-2 showed significantly more expression in rhinophyma (518,519). Additionally, mRNA expression of TGF β-1 is fivefold higher in rhinophyma than in normal controls (519).

Clinical Features

The clinical presentation varies on the basis of the subtype, from simple rosy cheeks in vascular rosacea to a pustular eruption on the central face in the inflammatory variant and thickening of the skin on the nose and cheeks in rhinophyma, the SH variant. In vascular rosacea, the patient reports a long history of easy and recurrent blushing. Telangectasias become clinically apparent first on the nasal ala, then on the distal nose. The inflammatory variant of rosacea has facial lesions ranging from small papules and pustules to deep nodules. These lesions are erythematous and not necessarily centered around an inflamed follicle. The rosacea variant that involves SH is the variant that results in rhinophyma. It most commonly affects men in their fourth through seventh decade. The nose is most commonly involved; however, the cheeks, chin, forehead, and ears may also be affected. Initially, the skin becomes smooth and slightly indurated. As this process evolves, the pores become more pronounced, and the nose develops a bumpy surface, ultimately resulting in overgrowth and dimorphism of the nose.

Imaging

Imaging studies are unnecessary.

Pathology

In vascular rosacea, there are ectatic vessels in the superficial and mid-dermis and a perifollicular and perivascular lymphohistiocytic infiltrate. Exocytosis and spongiosis of the follicular epithelium may also be present (Fig. 76). Inflammatory rosacea shows more pronounced ectasia and a more exuberant perifolliculitis and perivasculitis with accumulation of a neutrophilc infiltrate, occasionally forming pustules.

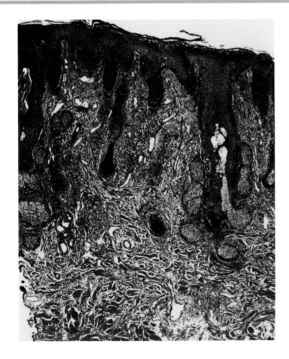

Figure 76 Rosacea, vascular variant. This image shows mild epithelial acanthosis with telangectatic vessels in the superficial dermis.

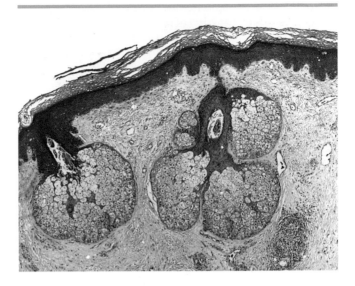

Figure 77 Rocasea, sebaceous hyperplasia. This image shows acanthosis, hyperkeratosis, sebaceous hyperplasia, a mild perivascular lymphohistiocytic infiltrate, and dermal fibrosis.

The SH variant, which leads to rhinophyma, shows enlarged sebaceous glands with patent infundibula, telangectasia, and dermal cysts (Fig. 77). Plasma cells may be seen in the perifollicular infiltrate admixed. The end stage is marked by dermal fibrosis and reduced sebaceaous units.

Immunohistochemistry

There is no role for immunohistochemistry in the evaluation or treatment planning of rosacea and its variants.

Electron Microscopy

A role for electron microscopy has not yet been found in the study of rosacea.

Molecular-Genetic Data

With the exception of a recent report of rosacea in monozygotic twins, reports of a genetic susceptibility are sparse (520). Other evidence for genetic susceptibility lies in the association between glutathione S-transferase isoforms, GSTT1, and GSTM1, and rosacea (521).

Differential Diagnosis

Clinically, rhinophyma may be mistaken for SH or BCC. The histology can easily make the distinction between these entities.

Treatment and Prognosis

Treatment is sought primarily for cosmetic reasons. Rosacea has been treated with topical and oral antibiotics; however, treatment regimens for combating an acute flare or for long-term maintenance lead to antibiotic-resistant organisms. Tetracycline in "anti-inflammatory" doses, rather than antibiotic doses, is also highly effective (522). The anti-inflammatory properties of tetracycline include suppression of neutrophils migration and inhibition of lymphocyte proliferation. Doxycycline, a tetracycline derivative, has similar anti-inflammatory properties and additionally inhibits phospholipase A2 and nitric oxide synthetase expression. A combination of immediate and delayed release deoxycycline in anti-inflammatory doses does not lead to drug resistance and has shown success in clinical trials (517). An evaluation of the efficacy of 29 treatment regimens revealed inadequate study designs with some evidence that topic metronidazole and azelaid acid are effective as are oral mtronidazole and tetracycline (523).

Rhinophyma is often treated for esthetic purposes as well. However, occasionally, functional problems such as nasal obstruction are the reason the patient seeks medical intervention. Isotretinoin is used with some success in decreasing the volume of the sebaceous glands, but as a treatment for the end-stage fibrotic condition, it is ineffective. For this later condition, there are multiple surgical options, including dermabrasion, cryosurgery, electrocautery, CO_2 laser, argon laser, and erbium laser. For mild to moderate rhinophyma, four treatments at four-week intervals, with a 1450-nm diode laser, have most recently shown good results with no complications. Radiotherapy, 40 Gy in 20 treatments over 32 days, resulted in a smooth nose with decreased pitting and pustules for 18 months of follow-up (524).

The detection of elevated levels of TGF-β-1 in rhinophyma provides an opportunity to treat medically if intervention can be started before the fibrosis has been established. Tamoxifen, a nonsteroidal antiestrogen, downregulates TGF-β. In vitro tamoxifen application to cultured rhinophyma fibroblasts decreased the production of TGF-β and the fibroblast function (525).

B. Chondrodermatitis Nodularis Helicis

Synonyms: chondrodermatitis nodularis chronica helicis, Winkler's disease, and ear corn.

Introduction

Chondrodermatitis nodularis helicis (CNH) is a degenerative process whose etiology is uncertain, but is likely due to local tissue ischemia secondary to poor structural support of the stroma, trauma, or pressure. The classic older patient reports sleeping on the same side in which the lesion develops.

Clinical Features

CNH is a painful papule, nodule, or ulcer on the helix or antihelix of the ear, typically occurring in patients older than 50 years with a male: female ratio of 10:1 (526). The pain is often disproportionate to the extent of the clinical lesion. Rare cases in the pediatric population have been reported (527,528). Up to 10% of patients have bilateral lesions. Risk factors include

actinic damage, cold exposure, and local trauma. CNH has been suggested to be an indication of underlying systemic diseases that are primarily associated with vascular injury, including immune-mediated disease and granuloma annular-associated conditions. Those patients with underlying disease tend to be younger than the average CNH patient (529–531).

Imaging

Imaging studies are not necessary in CNH.

Histologic Features

CNH has an acanthotic epidermis that is very often centrally ulcerated. Spongiosis may also be present (Fig. 78). In the dermis, there is a mild proliferation of superficial vessels. These vessels are ectatic and have a perivascular lymphocytic infiltrate. Mild fibrosis is also characteristic (Fig. 79). Inflammation and fibrinoid deposition may extend to the cartilage; however, biopsies are typically too shallow to evaluate for this effect. When present in the specimen, cartilage degeneration may be seen in the form of basophilia (532). In support of the disproportionate pain, a recent study revealed large nerves near the cartilage or ulcer bed in 22% of the cases and increased small neurites in 95% of the cases (533).

Immunohistochemistry

Immunohistochemical studies are not required to make a diagnosis of CNH.

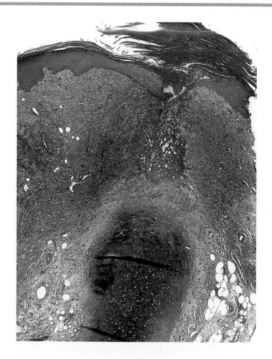

Figure 78 Chondrodermatitis nodularis helicis. This unusually deep specimen shows the characteristic acanthotic, ulcerated epidermis with extension of fibrinoid deposit and inflammation to the subjacent cartilage.

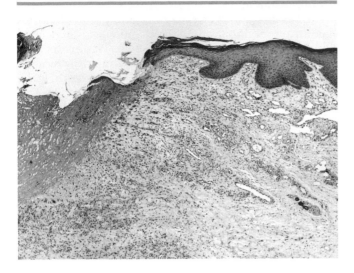

Figure 79 Chondrodermatitis nodularis helicis. Away from the ulceration, there is mild fibrosis of the superficial dermis and a proliferation of small, ectatic vessels with a lymphocytic perivascular infiltrate.

Differential Diagnosis

The clinical differential diagnosis includes weathering nodule of the ear (WNE), which is a painless hyperkeratotic nodule or cluster of nodules on the helical rim and consists of a fibrous nodule with chondroid metaplasia. Elastotic nodules of the ear also occur in the background of actinic damage and may be located on the helix or antihelix (534).

The histologic differential diagnosis includes AK and ulcerated epithelial neoplasms, specifically SCC and BCC. In such cases, close histologic inspection of the intact epidermis adjacent to the ulcer can give clues to the underlying process.

Treatment and Prognosis

Surgical wedge excision is the traditional treatment modality (535). Removal of cartilage only has also been promoted recently to be effective and spares the patient the large defect that may result after wedge resection (536,537). However, CNH is prone to recurrence. Some authors have suggested that a nonsurgical approach that relieves pressure on the affected ear is curative in most cases, and a surgical approach should not be the first line of care (538). A conservative approach, using a doughnut pillow has been successful, or even more successful, as measured by pain relief, in a population of patients with CNH (538,539).

C. Weathering Nodule of the Ear

Introduction

WNE is a newly recognized entity based on a report of 25 cases of these unique ear nodules (540). The etiology of WNE has not yet been elucidated, but does appear to have an association with chronic UV exposure.

Clinical Features

Invariably, WNE presents on the helical rim with a striking male predominance, presumably because women tend to wear their hair longer, thus protecting them from UV insult (541). The lesions are asymptomatic in contrast to the exquisitely tender helical lesions of CNH and are often multiple and bilateral, presenting as smooth, white- or skin-colored, 1- to 3-mm nodules. Elastotic nodules of the ear are also bilateral with a male predominance and a response to UV radiation damage. However, they tend to be painful and present with a different histologic pattern (534).

Imaging

Imaging has not proven to be necessary for diagnosis or further workup of these lesions.

Pathology

WNE is composed of a paucicellular nodule of fibrous tissue with cartilaginous metaplasia in the superficial dermis (Fig. 80). There may be focal cartilaginous metaplasia with focal connection to the underlying cartilage. An inflammatory infiltrate is not present (540). The epidermis is normal to atrophic and not ulcerated. Actinic change in the epidermis may be noted, but is not necessary for the diagnosis.

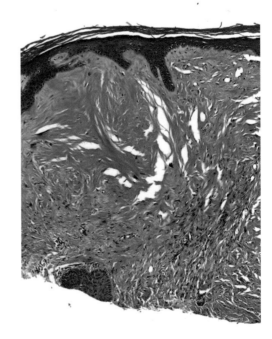

Figure 80 Weathering nodule of the ear. The lesion consists of a paucicellular, noninflammatory nodule of fibrous tissue in the superficial dermis. The epidermis is intact and atrophic.

Immunohistochemistry

While not needed for the diagnosis or differential diagnosis, the dermal nodule may have sparse spindled cells that are negative for factor XIIIa and S-100 protein (540).

Electron Microscopy

Ultrastructural studies have not been performed on WNE.

Molecular-Genetic Data

A genetic association has not been established, and molecular studies have not been performed on WNE.

Differential Diagnosis

The clinical differential diagnosis includes elastotic nodule of the ear, which has a similar clinical presentation; however, it may be painful, a feature not associated with WNE. Histologically, elastotic nodules show clumped, degenerated elastic fibers. Chondrodermatitis is also an ear nodule; however, the painful presentation is uncharacteristic of WNE. Histologically, epidermal acanthosis, spongiosis, ectatic vessels, and cartilage degeneration are unique to CNH. Stromal nodular fibrosis is typically not seen in CNH.

Treatment and Prognosis

Malignant potential has not been established, and the lesions are thought to be reactive in nature. Accordingly, simple excision is curative.

VII. HAMARTOMAS

A. Nevus Sebaceus of Jadassohn

Synonyms: organoid nevus.

Introduction

Nevus sebaceous of Jadassohn (NSJ) is a hamartomatous lesion of epithelial and nonepithelial elements. They have a well-documented morphogenesis from infancy to young adulthood, attributed to the influence of pubertal hormones, in particular androgens. Androgen receptors are known to be present in lesional prepubertal sebaceous glands as well as in the eccrine glands and some keratinocytes (542). Equally well recognized is the potential for neoplasms, both benign and malignant, to develop within 10% to 20% of NSJ (543). Benign tumors are far more common than malignant tumors in most studies (544). In one of the largest series, syringocystadenoma papilliferum (*n* = 30) and trichoblastoma (*n* = 28) were the most common neoplasms arising in the cohort of 596 cases (544). BCC, the most common malignant neoplasm, occurs in less than 1% of all lesions. Mucoepidermoid carcinoma and apocrine carcinoma are other malignant neoplasms that have been reported to arise in NSJ, futher supporting prophylactic excision of NSJ (545,546). Most cases of NSJ with associated neoplasms arise on the scalp. Additional tumors arising in NSJ include SC, syringoma, and trichoadenoma. Not uncommonly, more than one neoplasm may arise within the same NSJ lesion (547,548). With respect to SC arising in NSJ, they tend to arise in adult women with a mean age of 62 years (549). Although DNA mismatch repair defects were not assessed in this cohort, with the exception of one patient with a history of invasive ductal carcinoma of the breast, none of the patients had an underlying carcinoma of gastrointestinal or visceral organs (547,549). This is in contrast to patients with SCs in the setting of Muir-Torre syndrome (549). Extensive parasaggital lesions should raise concern for linear nevus sebaceous syndrome, also called organoid nevus syndrome or Schimmelpenning-Feuerstein syndrome, and is characterized by NSJ lesions, seizures, mental retardation, and ocular abnormalities among many other clinical manifestations (550).

Clinical Features

NSJ is a relatively common congenital lesion, most commonly presenting as a flat, round, well-circumscribed lesion. Ninety-three percent of NSJs arise on the scalp, most commonly in the parietal area (551). The earliest lesions may be difficult to recognize, clinically, except on hair-bearing sites, where they are noted by the lack of terminal hair growth. At this stage, they are often clinically mistaken for cutis aplasia. As the patient matures, the lesion develops texture, changing from flat to smooth and bumpy, with the most significant changes occurring during adolescence when pubertal hormones trigger marked growth of the lesion, which develops a waxy surface. In support of the hypothesis that hormones derive the morphologic changes during adolescence, androgen receptor expression was found in sebaceous glands, eccrine glands, and rarely in keratinocytes of NSJ without significant alteration in the distribution of these receptors between genders or across the age distribution (542). Any change in the lesion during adulthood is generally attributed to development of a neoplasm with the NSJ lesion. NSJ is usually brought to medical attention because of the associated alopecia.

Imaging

CT and ultrasound evaluation is helpful to rule out the presence of posterior osseous and/or cartilatinous ocular choristomas in linear NSJ syndrome (552).

Pathology

The histologic features of NSJ evolve with maturation of the lesion, likely as an effect of hormonal influence. The earliest lesions have a relatively normal epidermis. In the dermis, there is a focal striking absence of fully developed follicular units. This is typically juxtaposed to normal follicular units of normal hair-bearing skin. In the areas devoid of fully formed hair follicles, there may be abortive follicular structures ranging from none to numerous. These structures

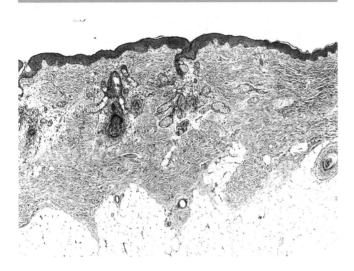

Figure 81 Nevus sebaceus of Jadassohn. Lesions in young patients show a relatively normal epidermis. In the dermis, there is an absence of fully developed follicular units. Instead, there are variable numbers of abortive follicular structures with an infundibulum and primitive sebaceous lobules.

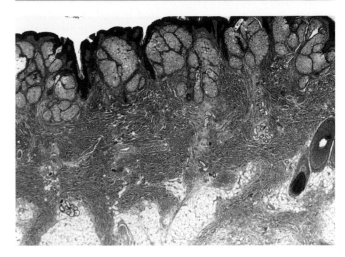

Figure 83 Nevus sebaceus of Jadassohn. At adolescence, the sebaceous glands of the abortive follicles become more pronounced with hypertrophy and hyperplasia of the lobules. Ectopic eccrine structures are noted, as in the earlier stages.

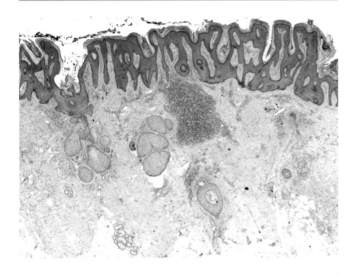

Figure 82 Nevus sebaceus of Jadassohn. As the patient, and hence the lesion, mature, the epidermis becomes acanthotic and papillomatous. The abortive follicular structures have more pronounced sebaceous lobules. Ectopic eccrine structures may be noted in the deeper portion of the specimen.

have an infundibulum with primitive sebaceous lobules (Fig. 81). Additionally, ectopic eccrine structures may be noted, more commonly in the deeper portion of the specimen. With age, the epidermis becomes acanthotic and papillomatous (Fig. 82). The sebaceous glands become more pronounced with hypertrophy and hyperplasia of the lobules (Fig. 83). The malignant neoplasms arising at the site of NSJ have recently come into question. Historically, BCC

has been the most common malignant neoplasm, though arising only in less than 1% of all NSJ. However, with refinement of diagnostic features for basaloid neoplasms, including trichoepithelioma and trichoblastoma, a review of previously diagnosed BCCs in NSJ was completed. NSJs seen over 19 years in one practice were reevaluated. As a result, many of the previously diagnosed BCCs were reclassified to trichoblastoma, a lesion with many similar histologic features but etiologically more consistent with the hamartomatous nature of NSJ (553). As a result, benign lesions arising in NSJ still far outweigh malignant lesions, and BCC, now much less common than previously documented, is still the most common malignant neoplasm arising in NSJ.

Molecular-Genetic Data

Although sporadic occurrence of NSJ is the most common presentation, several reports of familial presentations have suggested various inheritance patterns including dominant and paradominant (554–557).

Differential Diagnosis

Aplasia cutis congenital (ACC) has a similar clinical presentation in infants; however, with maturation, ACC does not evolve in the way NSJ does. Additionally, histologically, ACC shows a very thin epidermis, occasionally only two to three layers thick. The dermis may be fibrotic but will not show the primitive follicular units seen in NSJ.

Treatment and Prognosis

Prophylactic surgical excision during childhood is generally practiced because of the malignant transformations that may arise within the lesions (543). The recent study reclassifying many NSJ-associated BCCs as trichoblastomas has supported the practice of close clinical observation rather than surgical intervention (553). This is complemented by another large series of NSJ, confirming that the overall rate of neoplastic development is very low and most of those tumors are benign and occur in adults older than 40 years, also supporting the practice of clinical follow-up, rather than prophylactic pediatric surgery (544).

REFERENCES

1. Ko CJ, Kim J, Phan J, et al. Bcl-2-positive epidermal dendritic cells in inverted follicular keratoses but not squamous cell carcinomas or seborrheic keratoses. J Cutan Pathol 2006; 33:498.
2. Ko CJ, Shintaku P, Binder SW. Comparison of benign keratoses using p53, bcl-1, and bcl-2. J Cutan Pathol 2005; 32:356.
3. Kopf AW, Rabinovitz H, Marghoob A, et al. "Fat fingers": a clue in the dermoscopic diagnosis of seborrheic keratoses. J Am Acad Dermatol 2006; 55:1089.
4. Neuhaus IM, LeBoit PE, McCalmont TM. Seborrheic keratosis with basal clear cells: a distinctive microscopic mimic of melanoma in situ. J Am Acad Dermatol 2006; 54:132.
5. May SA, Quirey R, Cockerell CJ. Follicular hybrid cysts with infundibular, isthmic-catagen, and pilomatrical differentiation: a report of 2 patients. Ann Diagn Pathol 2006; 10:110.
6. Plumb SJ, Argenyi ZB, Stone MS, et al. Cytokeratin 5/6 immunostaining in cutaneous adnexal neoplasms and metastatic adenocarcinoma. Am J Dermatopathol 2004; 26: 447.
7. Tomkova H, Fujimoto W, Arata J. Expression of keratins (K10 and K17) in steatocystoma multiplex, eruptive vellus hair cysts, and epidermoid and trichilemmal cysts. Am J Dermatopathol 1997; 19:250.
8. Nakamura M, Toyoda M, Kagoura M, et al. Ultrastructural characteristics of trichilemmal cysts: report of two cases. Med Electron Microsc 2001; 34:134.
9. Leppard BJ, Sanderson KV, Wells RS. Hereditary trichilemmal cysts. Hereditary pilar cysts. Clin Exp Dermatol 1977; 2:23.
10. Eiberg H, Hansen L, Hansen C, et al. Mapping of hereditary trichilemmal cyst (TRICY1) to chromosome 3p24-p21.2 and exclusion of beta-CATENIN and MLH1. Am J Med Genet A 2005; 133:44.
11. Brownstein MH, Arluk DJ. Proliferating trichilemmal cyst: a simulant of squamous cell carcinoma. Cancer 1981; 48:1207.
12. Folpe AL, Reisenauer AK, Mentzel T, et al. Proliferating trichilemmal tumors: clinicopathologic evaluation is a guide to biologic behavior. J Cutan Pathol 2003; 30:492.
13. Chang SJ, Sims J, Murtagh FR, et al. Proliferating trichilemmal cysts of the scalp on CT. AJNR Am J Neuroradiol 2006; 27:712.
14. Ye J, Nappi O, Swanson PE, et al. Proliferating pilar tumors: a clinicopathologic study of 76 cases with a proposal for definition of benign and malignant variants. Am J Clin Pathol 2004; 122:566.
15. Shet T, Modi C. Nucleolar organizer regions (NORs) in simple and proliferating trichilemmal cysts (pilar cysts and pilar tumors). Indian J Pathol Microbiol 2004; 47:469.
16. Lan MY, Lan MC, Ho CY, et al. Pilomatricoma of the head and neck: a retrospective review of 179 cases. Arch Otolaryngol Head Neck Surg 2003; 129:1327.
17. Kaddu S, Soyer HP, Cerroni L, et al. Clinical and histopathologic spectrum of pilomatricomas in adults. Int J Dermatol 1994; 33:705.
18. Matsuura H, Hatamochi A, Nakamura Y, et al. Multiple pilomatricoma in trisomy 9. Dermatology 2002; 204:82.
19. Noguchi H, Kayashima K, Nishiyama S, et al. Two cases of pilomatrixoma in Turner's syndrome. Dermatology 1999; 199:338.
20. Marrogi AJ, Wick MR, Dehner LP. Pilomatrical neoplasms in children and young adults. Am J Dermatopathol 1992; 14:87.
21. Pielop JA, Metry D. Multiple pilomatricomas in association with spina bifida. Pediatr Dermatol 2005; 22:178.
22. Geh JL, Moss AL. Multiple pilomatrixomata and myotonic dystrophy: a familial association. Br J Plast Surg 1999; 52:143.
23. Graells J, Servitje O, Badell A, et al. Multiple familial pilomatricomas associated with myotonic dystrophy. Int J Dermatol 1996; 35:732.
24. Pujol RM, Casanova JM, Egido R, et al. Multiple familial pilomatricomas: a cutaneous marker for Gardner syndrome? Pediatr Dermatol 1995; 12:331.
25. Baglioni S, Melean G, Gensini F, et al. A kindred with MYH-associated polyposis and pilomatricomas. Am J Med Genet A 2005; 134:212.
26. Hubbard VG, Whittaker SJ. Multiple familial pilomatricomas: an unusual case. J Cutan Pathol 2004; 31:281.
27. Karpuzoglu T, Elpek GO, Alpsoy E, et al. Multiple familial pilomatrixomas. J Eur Acad Dermatol Venereol 2003; 17:358.
28. Kaddu S, Soyer HP, Hodl S, et al. Morphological stages of pilomatricoma. Am J Dermatopathol 1996; 18:333.
29. Sano Y, Mihara M, Miyamoto T, et al. Simultaneous occurrence of calcification and amyloid deposit in pilomatricoma. Acta Derm Venereol 1990; 70:256.
30. Jih DM, Lyle S, Elenitsas R, et al. Cytokeratin 15 expression in trichoepitheliomas and a subset of basal cell carcinomas suggests they originate from hair follicle stem cells. J Cutan Pathol 1999; 26:113.
31. McGavran M. Ultrastructure of pilomatrixoma (calcifying epithelioma). Cancer 1965; 18:1445.
32. Kurokawa I, Kusumoto K, Bessho K, et al. Immunohistochemical expression of bone morphogenetic protein-2 in pilomatricoma. Br J Dermatol 2000; 143:754.
33. He TC, Sparks AB, Rago C, et al. Identification of c-MYC as a target of the APC pathway. Science 1998; 281:1509.
34. Moreno-Bueno G, Gamallo C, Perez-Gallego L, et al. beta-catenin expression in pilomatrixomas. Relationship with beta-catenin gene mutations and comparison with beta-catenin expression in normal hair follicles. Br J Dermatol 2001; 145:576.
35. Gat U, DasGupta R, Degenstein L, et al. De Novo hair follicle morphogenesis and hair tumors in mice expressing a truncated beta-catenin in skin. Cell 1998; 95:605.
36. Kishimoto S, Nagata M, Takenaka H, et al. Detection of apoptosis by in situ labeling in pilomatricoma. Am J Dermatopathol 1996; 18:339.
37. Panico L, Manivel JC, Pettinato G, et al. Pilomatrix carcinoma. A case report with immunohistochemical findings, flow cytometric comparison with benign pilomatrixoma and review of the literature. Tumori 1994; 80:309.
38. Saussez S, Mahillon V, Blaivie C, et al. Aggressive pilomatrixoma of the infra-auricular area: a case report. Auris Nasus Larynx 2005; 32:407.
39. Leonardi CL, Zhu WY, Kinsey WH, et al. Trichilemmomas are not associated with human papillomavirus DNA. J Cutan Pathol 1991; 18:193.

40. Halevy S, Sandbank M, Pick AI, et al. Cowden's disease in three siblings: electron-microscope and immunological studies. Acta Derm Venereol 1985; 65:126.

41. Hunt SJ, Kilzer B, Santa Cruz DJ. Desmoplastic trichilemmoma: histologic variant resembling invasive carcinoma. J Cutan Pathol 1990; 17:45.

42. Massi D, Franchi A. Desmoplastic trichilemmoma: a case report with immunohistochemical characterization of the extracellular matrix components. Acta Derm Venereol 1997; 77:347.

43. Hashimoto T, Inamoto N, Nakamura K, et al. Involucrin expression in skin appendage tumours. Br J Dermatol 1987; 117:325.

44. Kurokawa I, Nishijima S, Kusumoto K, et al. Trichilemmoma: an immunohistochemical study of cytokeratins. Br J Dermatol 2003; 149:99.

45. Santa Cruz D, Barr R. Lymphoepithelial tumour of the skin. J Cutan Pathol 1987; 14:369.

46. Santa Cruz DJ, Barr RJ, Headington JT. Cutaneous lymphadenoma. Am J Surg Pathol 1991; 15:101.

47. Pujol RM, Matias-Guiu X, Taberner R, et al. Benign lymphoepithelial tumor of the skin ("cutaneous lymphadenoma"). Dermatol Online J 1999; 5:5.

48. Diaz-Cascajo C, Borghi S, Rey-Lopez A, Carretero-Hernandez G. Cutaneous lymphadenoma. A peculiar variant of nodular trichoblastoma. Am J Dermatopathol 1996; 18:186.

49. McNiff JM, Eisen RN, Glusac EJ. Immunohistochemical comparison of cutaneous lymphadenoma, trichoblastoma, and basal cell carcinoma: support for classification of lymphadenoma as a variant of trichoblastoma. J Cutan Pathol 1999; 26:119.

50. Aloi F, Tomasini C, Pippione M. Cutaneous lymphadenoma. A basal cell carcinoma with unusual inflammatory reaction pattern? Am J Dermatopathol 1993; 15:353.

51. Rodriguez-Diaz E, Roman C, Yuste M, et al. Cutaneous lymphadenoma: an adnexal neoplasm with intralobular activated lymphoid cells. Am J Dermatopathol 1998; 20:74.

52. Inaloz HS, Chowdhury MM, Knight AG. Cutaneous lymphadenoma. J Eur Acad Dermatol Venereol 2001; 15:481.

53. Ferlicot S, Plantier F, Rethers L, et al. Lymphoepithelioma-like carcinoma of the skin: a report of 3 Epstein-Barr virus (EBV)-negative additional cases. Immunohistochemical study of the stroma reaction. J Cutan Pathol 2000; 27:306.

54. Simon RS, Sanches Yus E. Does eccrine hidrocystoma exist? J Cutan Pathol 1998; 25:182.

55. Ishihara M, Mehregan DR, Hashimoto K, et al. Staining of eccrine and apocrine neoplasms and metastatic adenocarcinoma with IKH-4, a monoclonal antibody specific for the eccrine gland. J Cutan Pathol 1998; 25:100.

56. Kim YD, Lee EJ, Song MH, et al. Multiple eccrine hidrocystomas associated with Graves' disease. Int J Dermatol 2002; 41:295.

57. Mallaiah U, Dickinson J. Photo essay: bilateral multiple eyelid apocrine hidrocystomas and ectodermal dysplasia. Arch Ophthalmol 2001; 119:1866.

58. Gira AK, Robertson D, Swerlick RA. Multiple eyelid cysts with palmoplantar hyperkeratosis—quiz case. Arch Dermatol 2004; 140:231.

59. Matsushita S, Higashi Y, Uchimiya H, et al. Case of giant eccrine hidrocystoma of the scalp. J Dermatol 2007; 34:586.

60. Mataix J, Banuls J, Blanes M, et al. Translucent nodular lesion of the penis. Apocrine hidrocystoma of the penis. Arch Dermatol 2006; 142:1221.

61. Numata Y, Okuyama R, Sasai S, et al. Apocrine hidrocystoma on the finger. Acta Derm Venereol 2006; 86:188.

62. Anzai S, Goto M, Fujiwara S, et al. Apocrine hidrocystoma: a case report and analysis of 167 Japanese cases. Int J Dermatol 2005; 44:702.

63. Sheth HG, Raina J. Giant eccrine hidrocystoma presenting with unilateral ptosis and epiphora. Int Ophthalmol 2007 Oct 6; (Epub ahead of print).

64. Vignes JR, Franco-Vidal V, Eimer S, et al. Intraorbital apocrine hidrocystoma. Clin Neurol Neurosurg 2007; 109:631.

65. Furuta M, Shields CL, Danzig CJ, et al. Ultrasound biomicroscopy of eyelid eccrine hidrocystoma. Can J Ophthalmol 2007; 42:750.

66. Ohnishi T, Watanabe S. Immunohistochemical analysis of keratin expression in clear cell syringoma. A comparative study with conventional syringoma. J Cutan Pathol 1997; 24:370.

67. Ohnishi T, Watanabe S. Immunohistochemical analysis of cytokeratin expression in multiple eccrine hidrocystoma. J Cutan Pathol 1999; 26:91.

68. Kamishima T, Igarashi S, Takeuchi Y, et al. Pigmented hidrocystoma of the eccrine secretory coil in the vulva: clinicopathologic, immunohistochemical and ultrastructural studies. J Cutan Pathol 1999; 26:145.

69. Hiatt KM, Pillow JL, Smoller BR. Her-2 expression in cutaneous eccrine and apocrine neoplasms. Mod Pathol 2004; 17:28.

70. Vogelbruch M, Bocking A, Rutten A, et al. DNA image cytometry in malignant and benign sweat gland tumours. Br J Dermatol 2000; 142:688.

71. Buckel TB, Helm KF, Ioffreda MD. Cystic basal cell carcinoma or hidrocytoma? The use of an excisional biopsy in a histopathologically challenging case. Am J Dermatopathol 2004; 26:67.

72. Lee HW, Lee DK, Lee HJ, et al. Multiple eccrine hidrocystomas: successful treatment with the 595 nm long-pulsed dye laser. Dermatol Surg 2006; 32:296.

73. Blugerman G, Schavelzon D, D'Angelo S. Multiple eccrine hidrocystomas: a new therapeutic option with botulinum toxin. Dermatol Surg 2003; 29:557.

74. Sanz-Sanchez T, Dauden E, Perez-Casas A, et al. Efficacy and safety of topical atropine in treatment of multiple eccrine hidrocystomas. Arch Dermatol 2001; 137:670.

75. del Pozo J, Garcia-Silva J, Pena-Penabad C, et al. Multiple apocrine hidrocystomas: treatment with carbon dioxide laser vaporization. J Dermatolog Treat 2001; 12:97.

76. Lee JH, Chang JY, Lee KH. Syringoma: a clinicopathologic and immunohistologic study and results of treatment. Yonsei Med J 2007; 48:35.

77. Guitart J, Rosenbaum MM, Requena L. 'Eruptive syringoma': a misnomer for a reactive eccrine gland ductal proliferation? J Cutan Pathol 2003; 30:202.

78. Nguyen V, Buka RL, Roberts BJ, et al. Cutaneous manifestations of Costello syndrome. Int J Dermatol 2007; 46:72.

79. Draznin M. Hereditary syringomas: a case report. Dermatol Online J 2004; 10:19.

80. Singh A, Mishra S. Clear cell syringoma—association with diabetes mellitus. Indian J Pathol Microbiol 2005; 48:356.

81. Schepis C, Siragusa M, Palazzo R, et al. Palpebral syringomas and Down's syndrome. Dermatology 1994; 189:248.

82. Suzuki Y, Hashimoto K, Kato I, et al. A monoclonal antibody, SKH1, reacts with 40 Kd sweat gland-associated antigen. J Cutan Pathol 1989; 16:66.

83. Wallace ML, Smoller BR. Progesterone receptor positivity supports hormonal control of syringomas. J Cutan Pathol 1995; 22:442.

84. Landau-Price D, Barnhill RL, Kowalcyzk AP, et al. The value of carcinoembryonic antigen in differentiating

sclerosing epithelial hamartoma from syringoma. J Cutan Pathol 1985; 12:8.

85. Hashimoto K, Gross BG, Lever WF. Syringoma. Histochemical and electron microscopic studies. J Invest Dermatol 1966; 46:150.

86. Beyer G, Hiatt K. Microcystic Adnexal Carcinoma: a case report and discussion of the histologic differential diagnosis. Pathol Case Rev 2007; 12:70.

87. Henner MS, Shapiro PE, Ritter JH, et al. Solitary syringoma. Report of five cases and clinicopathologic comparison with microcystic adnexal carcinoma of the skin. Am J Dermatopathol 1995; 17:465.

88. Schirren CG, Jansen T, Lindner A, et al. Diffuse sebaceous gland hyperplasia. A case report and an immunohistochemical study with cytokeratins. Am J Dermatopathol 1996; 18:296.

89. Davis TT, Calilao G, Fretzin D. Sebaceous hyperplasia overlying a dermatofibroma. Am J Dermatopathol 2006; 28:155.

90. Ekmekci TR, Koslu A, Sakiz D. A case of otophyma. Clin Exp Dermatol 2005; 30:441.

91. Salim A, Reece SM, Smith AG, et al. Sebaceous hyperplasia and skin cancer in patients undergoing renal transplant. J Am Acad Dermatol 2006; 55:878.

92. Olsen SH, Su LD, Thomas D, et al. Telomerase expression in sebaceous lesions of the skin. J Cutan Pathol 2007; 34:386.

93. Boonchai W, Leenutaphong V. Familial presenile sebaceous gland hyperplasia. J Am Acad Dermatol 1997; 36:120.

94. Yoon SJ, Seiler SH, Kucherlapati R, et al. Organization of the human skeletal myosin heavy chain gene cluster. Proc Natl Acad Sci U S A 1992; 89:12078.

95. Al-Tassan N, Chmiel NH, Maynard J, et al. Inherited variants of MYH associated with somatic G:C–>T:A mutations in colorectal tumors. Nat Genet 2002; 30:227.

96. Ponti G, Venesio T, Losi L, et al. BRAF mutations in multiple sebaceous hyperplasias of patients belonging to MYH-associated polyposis pedigrees. J Invest Dermatol 2007; 127:1387.

97. Perrett CM, McGregor J, Barlow RJ, et al. Topical photodynamic therapy with methyl aminolevulinate to treat sebaceous hyperplasia in an organ transplant recipient. Arch Dermatol 2006; 142:781.

98. Richey DF. Aminolevulinic acid photodynamic therapy for sebaceous gland hyperplasia. Dermatol Clin 2007; 25:59.

99. Massa MC, Medenica M. Cutaneous adnexal tumors and cysts: a review. Part I. Tumors with hair follicular and sebaceous glandular differentiation and cysts related to different parts of the hair follicle. Pathol Annu 1985; 20(pt 2): 189.

100. Kaminagakura E, Andrade CR, Rangel AL, et al. Sebaceous adenoma of oral cavity: report of case and comparative proliferation study with sebaceous gland hyperplasia and Fordyce's granules. Oral Dis 2003; 9:323.

101. Izutsu T, Kumamoto H, Kimizuka S, et al. Sebaceous adenoma in the retromolar region: report of a case with a review of the English literature. Int J Oral Maxillofac Surg 2003; 32:423.

102. Frantz S, Greiner A, Schoen C, et al. A sebaceous tumor in a patient with acquired immunodeficiency syndrome. Eur J Med Res 2002; 7:135.

103. Ponti G, Ponz de Leon M. Muir-Torre syndrome. Lancet Oncol 2005; 6:980.

104. Machin P, Catasus L, Pons C, et al. Microsatellite instability and immunostaining for MSH-2 and MLH-1 in cutaneous and internal tumors from patients with the Muir-Torre syndrome. J Cutan Pathol 2002; 29:415.

105. Anwar J, Wrone DA, Kimyai-Asadi A, et al. The development of actinic keratosis into invasive squamous cell carcinoma: evidence and evolving classification schemes. Clin Dermatol 2004; 22:189.

106. Person JR. An actinic keratosis is neither malignant nor premalignant: it is an initiated tumor. J Am Acad Dermatol 2003; 48:637.

107. Berhane T, Halliday GM, Cooke B, et al. Inflammation is associated with progression of actinic keratoses to squamous cell carcinomas in humans. Br J Dermatol 2002; 146:810.

108. Tanghetti E, Werschler P. Comparison of 5% 5-fluorouracil cream and 5% imiquimod cream in the management of actinic keratoses on the face and scalp. J Drugs Dermatol 2007; 6:144.

109. Wheeland RG. The pitfalls of treating all actinic keratoses as squamous cell carcinomas. Semin Cutan Med Surg 2005; 24:152.

110. Ehrig T, Cockerell C, Piacquadio D, et al. Actinic keratoses and the incidence of occult squamous cell carcinoma: a clinical-histopathologic correlation. Dermatol Surg 2006; 32:1261.

111. Alam M, Ratner D. Cutaneous squamous-cell carcinoma. N Engl J Med 2001; 344:975.

112. Ramos J, Villa J, Ruiz A, et al. UV dose determines key characteristics of nonmelanoma skin cancer. Cancer Epidemiol Biomarkers Prev 2004; 13:2006.

113. Adigun IA, Buhari MO, Ayorinde RO. Malignant skin tumor in Blacks: experience in a teaching hospital. West Afr J Med 2006; 25:276.

114. Parrish JA. Immunosuppression, skin cancer, and ultraviolet A radiation. N Engl J Med 2005; 353:2712.

115. Moloney FJ, Comber H, O'Lorcain P, et al. A population-based study of skin cancer incidence and prevalence in renal transplant recipients. Br J Dermatol 2006; 154:498.

116. Goyal JL, Rao VA, Srinivasan R, et al. Oculocutaneous manifestations in xeroderma pigmentosa. Br J Ophthalmol 1994; 78:295.

117. Edwards MJ, Hirsch RM, Broadwater JR, et al. Squamous cell carcinoma arising in previously burned or irradiated skin. Arch Surg 1989; 124:115.

118. Engler HS, Fernandez A, Bliven FE, et al. Cancer arising in scars of old burns and in chronic osteomyelitis, ulcers, and drainage sites. Surgery 1964; 55:654.

119. Mellemkjaer L, Holmich LR, Gridley G, et al. Risks for skin and other cancers up to 25 years after burn injuries. Epidemiology 2006; 17:668.

120. Veness MJ, Palme CE, Morgan GJ. High-risk cutaneous squamous cell carcinoma of the head and neck: results from 266 treated patients with metastatic lymph node disease. Cancer 2006; 106:2389.

121. Gupta R, Singh S, Hedau S, et al. Spindle cell carcinoma of head and neck: an immunohistochemical and molecular approach to its pathogenesis. J Clin Pathol 2007; 60:472.

122. Seike M, Ikeda M, Nakajima H, et al. Spindle cell squamous cell carcinoma showing continuous mesenchymal dedifferentiation in a single tumor. J Dermatol 2005; 32:813.

123. Eyden B, Banerjee SS. Spindle-cell squamous carcinoma exhibiting myofibroblastic differentiation. A study of two cases showing fibronexus junctions. Virchows Arch 2002; 440:36.

124. Sigel JE, Skacel M, Bergfeld WF, et al. The utility of cytokeratin 5/6 in the recognition of cutaneous spindle cell squamous cell carcinoma. J Cutan Pathol 2001; 28:520.

125. Takata T, Ito H, Ogawa I, et al. Spindle cell squamous carcinoma of the oral region. An immunohistochemical and ultrastructural study on the histogenesis and differential diagnosis with a clinicopathological analysis of six

cases. Virchows Arch A Pathol Anat Histopathol 1991; 419:177.

126. Suo Z, Holm R, Nesland JM. Squamous cell carcinomas, an immunohistochemical and ultrastructural study. Anticancer Res 1992; 12:2025.

127. Sprecher E. Genetic factors in the pathogenesis of UV-induced skin cancer1. Curr Probl Dermatol 2007; 35:28.

128. Grossman D, Leffell DJ. The molecular basis of nonmelanoma skin cancer: new understanding. Arch Dermatol 1997; 133:1263.

129. Lynch JM. Understanding Pseudoepitheliomatous Hyperplasia. Pathol Case Rev 2004; 9:36.

130. Marzano AV, Gasparini G, Caputo R. Cutaneous infection caused by Serratia marcescens. Cutis 2000; 66:461.

131. Gilaberte M, Bartralot R, Torres JM, et al. Cutaneous alternariosis in transplant recipients: clinicopathologic review of 9 cases. J Am Acad Dermatol 2005; 52:653.

132. Goel R, Wallace ML. Pseudoepitheliomatous hyperplasia secondary to cutaneous aspergillus. Am J Dermatopathol 2001; 23:224.

133. Scarisbrick JJ, Calonje E, Orchard G, et al. Pseudocarcinomatous change in lymphomatoid papulosis and primary cutaneous CD30+ lymphoma: a clinicopathologic and immunohistochemical study of 6 patients. J Am Acad Dermatol 2001; 44:239.

134. Courville P, Wechsler J, Thomine E, et al. Pseudoepitheliomatous hyperplasia in cutaneous T-cell lymphoma. A clinical, histopathological and immunohistochemical study with particular interest in epithelial growth factor expression. The French Study Group on Cutaneous Lymphoma. Br J Dermatol 1999; 140:421.

135. Kadin ME. Cutaneous Ki-1 lymphoma: pathology, immunology and clinical characteristics. Princess Takamatsu Symp 1987; 18:187.

136. Vucic M, Cupic H, Tomic K, et al. An unusual pattern of pseudoepitheliomatous hyperplasia associated with cutaneous primary melanoma: report of two cases with analysis of p53 and bcl-2 immunoreactivity. Acta Dermatovenerol Croat 2007; 15:72.

137. Meleti M, Mooi WJ, van der Waal I. Oral malignant melanoma associated with pseudoepitheliomatous hyperplasia. Report of a case. J Cutan Pathol 2006; 33:331.

138. Hanly AJ, Jorda M, Elgart GW. Cutaneous malignant melanoma associated with extensive pseudoepitheliomatous hyperplasia. Report of a case and discussion of the origin of pseudoepitheliomatous hyperplasia. J Cutan Pathol 2000; 27:153.

139. Dorji T, Cavazza A, Nappi O, et al. Spitz nevus of the tongue with pseudoepitheliomatous hyperplasia: report of three cases of a pseudomalignant condition. Am J Surg Pathol 2002; 26:774.

140. Johnston WH, Miller TA, Frileck SP. Atypical pseudoepitheliomatous hyperplasia and squamous cell carcinoma in chronic cutaneous sinuses and fistulas. Plast Reconstr Surg 1980; 66:395.

141. Czarnecki D, Staples M, Mar A, et al. Metastases from squamous cell carcinoma of the skin in southern Australia. Dermatology 1994; 189:52.

142. Palme CE, MacKay SG, Kalnins I, et al. The need for a better prognostic staging system in patients with metastatic cutaneous squamous cell carcinoma of the head and neck. Curr Opin Otolaryngol Head Neck Surg 2007; 15:103.

143. Neville JA, Welch E, Leffell DJ. Management of nonmelanoma skin cancer in 2007. Nat Clin Pract Oncol 2007; 4:462.

144. Bariani RL, Nahas FX, Barbosa MV, et al. Basal cell carcinoma: an updated epidemiological and therapeutically profile of an urban population. Acta Cir Bras 2006; 21:66.

145. Lear W, Dahlke E, Murray CA. Basal cell carcinoma: review of epidemiology, pathogenesis, and associated risk factors. J Cutan Med Surg 2007; 11:19.

146. Christenson LJ, Borrowman TA, Vachon CM, et al. Incidence of basal cell and squamous cell carcinomas in a population younger than 40 years. JAMA 2005; 294:681.

147. Ionescu DN, Arida M, Jukic DM. Metastatic basal cell carcinoma: four case reports, review of literature, and immunohistochemical evaluation. Arch Pathol Lab Med 2006; 130:45.

148. Abdulla FR, Feldman SR, Williford PM, et al. Tanning and skin cancer. Pediatr Dermatol 2005; 22:501.

149. Gallagher RP, Lee TK. Adverse effects of ultraviolet radiation: a brief review. Prog Biophys Mol Biol 2006; 92:119.

150. Almahroos M, Kurban AK. Ultraviolet carcinogenesis in nonmelanoma skin cancer part II: review and update on epidemiologic correlations. Skinmed 2004; 3:132.

151. Walker P, Hill D. Surgical treatment of basal cell carcinomas using standard postoperative histological assessment. Australas J Dermatol 2006; 47:1.

152. Wilkins K, Turner R, Dolev JC, et al. Cutaneous malignancy and human immunodeficiency virus disease. J Am Acad Dermatol 2006; 54:189.

153. Hassanpour SE, Kalantar-Hormozi A, Motamed S, et al. Basal cell carcinoma of scalp in patients with history of childhood therapeutic radiation: a retrospective study and comparison to nonirradiated patients. Ann Plast Surg 2006; 57:509.

154. Raasch BA, Buettner PG, Garbe C. Basal cell carcinoma: histological classification and body-site distribution. Br J Dermatol 2006; 155:401.

155. Paavilainen V, Aaltonen M, Tuominen J, et al. Histological characteristics of basal cell carcinoma of the eyelid. Ophthalmic Res 2007; 39:45.

156. Scrivener Y, Grosshans E, Cribier B. Variations of basal cell carcinomas according to gender, age, location and histopathological subtype. Br J Dermatol 2002; 147:41.

157. Askari SK, Schram SE, Wenner RA, et al. Evaluation of prospectively collected presenting signs/symptoms of biopsy-proven melanoma, basal cell carcinoma, squamous cell carcinoma, and seborrheic keratosis in an elderly male population. J Am Acad Dermatol 2007; 56:739.

158. Chen CC, Chen CL. Clinical and histopathologic findings of superficial basal cell carcinoma: A comparison with other basal cell carcinoma subtypes. J Chin Med Assoc 2006; 69:364.

159. Mathieu D, Fortin D. Intracranial invasion of a basal cell carcinoma of the scalp. Can J Neurol Sci 2005; 32:546.

160. Gufler H, Franke FE, Rau WS. High-resolution MRI of basal cell carcinomas of the face using a microscopy coil. AJR Am J Roentgenol 2007; 188:W480.

161. Smith JM, Irons GB. Metastatic basal cell carcinoma: review of the literature and report of three cases. Ann Plast Surg 1983; 11:551.

162. Farmer ER, Helwig EB. Metastatic basal cell carcinoma: a clinicopathologic study of seventeen cases. Cancer 1980; 46:748.

163. Bianchini R, Wolter M. Fatal outcome in a metatypical, giant, "horrifying" basal cell carcinoma. J Dermatol Surg Oncol 1987; 13:556.

164. Saladi RN, Singh F, Wei H, et al. Use of Ber-EP4 protein in recurrent metastatic basal cell carcinoma: a case report and review of the literature. Int J Dermatol 2004; 43:600.

165. Swanson PE, Fitzpatrick MM, Ritter JH, et al. Immunohistologic differential diagnosis of basal cell carcinoma, squamous cell carcinoma, and trichoepithelioma in small cutaneous biopsy specimens. J Cutan Pathol 1998; 25:153.

166. Morales-Ducret CR, van de Rijn M, LeBrun DP, et al. bcl-2 expression in primary malignancies of the skin. Arch Dermatol 1995; 131:909.

167. Stone DM, Hynes M, Armanini M, et al. The tumour-suppressor gene patched encodes a candidate receptor for Sonic hedgehog. Nature 1996; 384:129.

168. Kimonis VE, Mehta SG, Digiovanna JJ, et al. Radiological features in 82 patients with nevoid basal cell carcinoma (NBCC or Gorlin) syndrome. Genet Med 2004; 6:495.

169. Gorlin RJ. Nevoid basal cell carcinoma (Gorlin) syndrome. Genet Med 2004; 6:530.

170. Sellheyer K, Smoller BR. Dermatofibroma: upregulation of syndecan-1 expression in mesenchymal tissue. Am J Dermatopathol 2003; 25:392.

171. Takei Y, Fukushiro S, Ackerman AB. Criteria for histologic differentiation of desmoplastic trichoepithelioma (sclerosing epithelial hamartoma) from morphea-like basal-cell carcinoma. Am J Dermatopathol 1985; 7:207.

172. Rakha EA, El-Sayed ME, Green AR, et al. Breast carcinoma with basal differentiation: a proposal for pathology definition based on basal cytokeratin expression. Histopathology 2007; 50:434.

173. Jones C, Nonni AV, Fulford L, et al. CGH analysis of ductal carcinoma of the breast with basaloid/myoepithelial cell differentiation. Br J Cancer 2001; 85:422.

174. Kuijpers DI, Thissen MR, Neumann MH. Basal cell carcinoma: treatment options and prognosis, a scientific approach to a common malignancy. Am J Clin Dermatol 2002; 3:247.

175. Tillman DK Jr., Carroll MT. Topical imiquimod therapy for basal and squamous cell carcinomas: a clinical experience. Cutis 2007; 79:241.

176. Campbell RM, DiGiovanna JJ. Skin cancer chemoprevention with systemic retinoids: an adjunct in the management of selected high-risk patients. Dermatol Ther 2006; 19:306.

177. Costantino D, Lowe L, Brown DL. Basosquamous carcinoma-an under-recognized, high-risk cutaneous neoplasm: case study and review of the literature. J Plast Reconstr Aesthet Surg 2006; 59:424.

178. Sendur N, Karaman G, Dikicioglu E, et al. Cutaneous basosquamous carcinoma infiltrating cerebral tissue. J Eur Acad Dermatol Venereol 2004; 18:334.

179. Bowman PH, Ratz JL, Knoepp TG, et al. Basosquamous carcinoma. Dermatol Surg 2003; 29:830.

180. Jones MS, Helm KF, Maloney ME. The immunohistochemical characteristics of the basosquamous cell carcinoma. Dermatol Surg 1997; 23:181.

181. Goldstein DJ, Barr RJ, Santa Cruz DJ. Microcystic adnexal carcinoma: a distinct clinicopathologic entity. Cancer 1982; 50:566.

182. Gabillot-Carre M, Weill F, Mamelle G, et al. Microcystic adnexal carcinoma: report of seven cases including one with lung metastasis. Dermatology 2006; 212:221.

183. Ohta M, Hiramoto M, Ohtsuka H. Metastatic microcystic adnexal carcinoma: an autopsy case. Dermatol Surg 2004; 30:957.

184. Ban M, Sugie S, Kamiya H, et al. Microcystic adnexal carcinoma with lymph node metastasis. Dermatology 2003; 207:395.

185. Abbate M, Zeitouni NC, Seyler M, et al. Clinical course, risk factors, and treatment of microcystic adnexal carcinoma: a short series report. Dermatol Surg 2003; 29:1035.

186. Fischer S, Breuninger H, Metzler G, et al. Microcystic adnexal carcinoma: an often misdiagnosed, locally aggressive growing skin tumor. J Craniofac Surg 2005; 16:53.

187. Schwarze HP, Loche F, Lamant L, et al. Microcystic adnexal carcinoma induced by multiple radiation therapy. Int J Dermatol 2000; 39:369.

188. Antley CA, Carney M, Smoller BR. Microcystic adnexal carcinoma arising in the setting of previous radiation therapy. J Cutan Pathol 1999; 26:48.

189. Lei JY, Wang Y, Jaffe ES, et al. Microcystic adnexal carcinoma associated with primary immunodeficiency, recurrent diffuse herpes simplex virus infection, and cutaneous T-cell lymphoma. Am J Dermatopathol 2000; 22:524.

190. Carroll P, Goldstein GD, Brown CW Jr. Metastatic microcystic adnexal carcinoma in an immunocompromised patient. Dermatol Surg 2000; 26:531.

191. Chiller K, Passaro D, Scheuller M, et al. Microcystic adnexal carcinoma: forty-eight cases, their treatment, and their outcome. Arch Dermatol 2000; 136:1355.

192. Snow S, Madjar DD, Hardy S, et al. Microcystic adnexal carcinoma: report of 13 cases and review of the literature. Dermatol Surg 2001; 27:401.

193. Yavuzer R, Boyaci M, Sari A, et al. Microcystic adnexal carcinoma of the breast: a very rare breast skin tumor. Dermatol Surg 2002; 28:1092.

194. Buhl A, Landow S, Lee YC, et al. Microcystic adnexal carcinoma of the vulva. Gynecol Oncol 2001; 82:571.

195. Chi J, Jung YG, Rho YS, et al. Microcystic adnexal carcinoma of external auditory canal: report of a case. Otolaryngol Head Neck Surg 2002; 127:241.

196. Heenan PJ. Sebaceous differentiation in microcystic adnexal carcinoma. Am J Dermatopathol 1998; 20:537.

197. Wick MR, Cooper PH, Swanson PE, et al. Microcystic adnexal carcinoma. An immunohistochemical comparison with other cutaneous appendage tumors. Arch Dermatol 1990; 126:189.

198. Uchida N, Urano Y, Oura H, et al. Microcystic adnexal carcinoma. Case report with an immunohistochemical study. Dermatology 1993; 187:119.

199. Ongenae KC, Verhaegh ME, Vermeulen AH, et al. Microcystic adnexal carcinoma: an uncommon tumor with debatable origin. Dermatol Surg 2001; 27:979.

200. Kato N, Yasuoka A, Ueno H. Microcystic adnexal carcinoma: a case report with immunohistochemical and electron microscopical examinations. J Dermatol 1992; 19:51.

201. Eisen DB, Zloty D. Microcystic adnexal carcinoma involving a large portion of the face: when is surgery not reasonable? Dermatol Surg 2005; 31:1472.

202. Thomas CJ, Wood GC, Marks VJ. Mohs micrographic surgery in the treatment of rare aggressive cutaneous tumors: the Geisinger experience. Dermatol Surg 2007; 33:333.

203. Stein JM, Ormsby A, Esclamado R, et al. The effect of radiation therapy on microcystic adnexal carcinoma: a case report. Head Neck 2003; 25:251.

204. Reis JP, Tellechea O, Cunha MF, et al. Trichilemmal carcinoma: review of 8 cases. J Cutan Pathol 1993; 20:44.

205. Swanson PE, Marrogi AJ, Williams DJ, et al. Tricholemmal carcinoma: clinicopathologic study of 10 cases. J Cutan Pathol 1992; 19:100.

206. Boscaino A, Terracciano LM, Donofrio V, et al. Tricholemmal carcinoma: a study of seven cases. J Cutan Pathol 1992; 19:94.

207. Knoeller SM, Haag M, Adler CP, et al. Skeletal metastasis in tricholemmal carcinoma. Clin Orthop Relat Res 2004; 423:213–216.

208. Dekio S, Funaki M, Jidoi J, et al. Trichilemmal carcinoma on the thigh: report of a case. J Dermatol 1994; 21:494.

209. Garrett AB, Azmi FH, Ogburia KS. Trichilemmal carcinoma: a rare cutaneous malignancy: a report of two cases. Dermatol Surg 2004; 30:113.

210. Ikeda T, Tsuru K, Hayashi K, et al. Hypercalcemia of malignancy associated with trichilemmal carcinoma in burn scar. Acta Derm Venereol 2000; 80:396.

211. Ko T, Tada H, Hatoko M, et al. Trichilemmal carcinoma developing in a burn scar: a report of two cases. J Dermatol 1996; 23:463.

212. Wong TY, Suster S. Tricholemmal carcinoma. A clinicopathologic study of 13 cases. Am J Dermatopathol 1994; 16:463.

213. Kurokawa I, Senba Y, Nishimura K, et al. Cytokeratin expression in trichilemmal carcinoma suggests differentiation towards follicular infundibulum. In Vivo 2006; 20:583.

214. Jo JH, Ko HC, Jang HS, et al. Infiltrative trichilemmal carcinoma treated with 5% imiquimod cream. Dermatol Surg 2005; 31:973.

215. Toker C. Trabecular carcinoma of the skin. Arch Dermatol 1972; 105:107.

216. Garneski KM, Nghiem P. Merkel cell carcinoma adjuvant therapy: Current data support radiation but not chemotherapy. J Am Acad Dermatol 2007; 57:166–169.

217. Kanitakis J, Euvrard S, Chouvet B, et al. Merkel cell carcinoma in organ-transplant recipients: report of two cases with unusual histological features and literature review. J Cutan Pathol 2006; 33:686.

218. Gale KL, Milsom PB, de Beer J. Pr33 merkel cell carcinoma: report of 19 cases and review of the literature. ANZ J Surg 2007; 77(suppl 1):A68.

219. Snow SN, Larson PO, Hardy S, et al. Merkel cell carcinoma of the skin and mucosa: report of 12 cutaneous cases with 2 cases arising from the nasal mucosa. Dermatol Surg 2001; 27:165.

220. Barroeta JE, Farkas T. Merkel cell carcinoma and chronic lymphocytic leukemia (collision tumor) of the arm: a diagnosis by fine-needle aspiration biopsy. Diagn Cytopathol 2007; 35:293.

221. McLoone NM, McKenna K, Edgar D, et al. Merkel cell carcinoma in a patient with chronic sarcoidosis. Clin Exp Dermatol 2005; 30:580.

222. Lillis J, Ceilley RI, Nelson P. Merkel cell carcinoma in a patient with autoimmune hepatitis. J Drugs Dermatol 2005; 4:357.

223. Wirges ML, Saporito F, Smith J. Rapid growth of Merkel cell carcinoma after treatment with rituximab. J Drugs Dermatol 2006; 5:180.

224. Youker SR, Billingsley EM. Combined Merkel cell carcinoma and atypical fibroxanthoma. J Cutan Med Surg 2005; 9:6.

225. Walsh NM. Primary neuroendocrine (Merkel cell) carcinoma of the skin: morphologic diversity and implications thereof. Hum Pathol 2001; 32:680.

226. Huynh NT, Hunt MJ, Cachia AR, et al. Merkel cell carcinoma and multiple cutaneous squamous cell carcinomas in a patient with pityriasis rubra pilaris. Australas J Dermatol 2002; 43:48.

227. Gomez LG, DiMaio S, Silva EG, et al. Association between neuroendocrine (Merkel cell) carcinoma and squamous carcinoma of the skin. Am J Surg Pathol 1983; 7:171.

228. Rund CR, Fischer EG. Perinuclear dot-like cytokeratin 20 staining in small cell neuroendocrine carcinoma of the ovary (pulmonary-type). Appl Immunohistochem Mol Morphol 2006; 14:244.

229. Bobos M, Hytiroglou P, Kostopoulos I, et al. Immunohistochemical distinction between merkel cell carcinoma and small cell carcinoma of the lung. Am J Dermatopathol 2006; 28:99.

230. Nicholson SA, McDermott MB, Swanson PE, et al. CD99 and cytokeratin-20 in small-cell and basaloid tumors of the skin. Appl Immunohistochem Mol Morphol 2000; 8:37.

231. Kurokawa M, Nabeshima K, Akiyama Y, et al. CD56: a useful marker for diagnosing Merkel cell carcinoma. J Dermatol Sci 2003; 31:219.

232. Haneke E, Schulze HJ, Mahrle G. Immunohistochemical and immunoelectron microscopic demonstration of chromogranin A in formalin-fixed tissue of Merkel cell carcinoma. J Am Acad Dermatol 1993; 28:222.

233. Yang DT, Holden JA, Florell SR. CD117, CK20, TTF-1, and DNA topoisomerase II-alpha antigen expression in small cell tumors. J Cutan Pathol 2004; 31:254.

234. Sibley RK, Rosai J, Foucar E, et al. Neuroendocrine (Merkel cell) carcinoma of the skin. A histologic and ultrastructural study of two cases. Am J Surg Pathol 1980; 4:211.

235. van Muijen GN, Ruiter DJ, Warnaar SO. Intermediate filaments in Merkel cell tumors. Hum Pathol 1985; 16:590.

236. Leonard JH, Leonard P, Kearsley JH. Chromosomes 1, 11, and 13 are frequently involved in karyotypic abnormalities in metastatic Merkel cell carcinoma. Cancer Genet Cytogenet 1993; 67:65.

237. Gancberg D, Feoli F, Hamels J, et al. Trisomy 6 in Merkel cell carcinoma: a recurrent chromosomal aberration. Histopathology 2000; 37:445.

238. Senchenkov A, Barnes SA, Moran SL. Predictors of survival and recurrence in the surgical treatment of merkel cell carcinoma of the extremities. J Surg Oncol 2007; 95:229.

239. Ortin-Perez J, van Rijk MC, Valdes-Olmos RA, et al. Lymphatic mapping and sentinel node biopsy in Merkel's cell carcinoma. Eur J Surg Oncol 2007; 33:119.

240. Mojica P, Smith D, Ellenhorn JD. Adjuvant radiation therapy is associated with improved survival in Merkel cell carcinoma of the skin. J Clin Oncol 2007; 25:1043.

241. Yom SS, Rosenthal DI, El-Naggar AK, et al. Merkel cell carcinoma of the tongue and head and neck oral mucosal sites. Oral Surg Oral Med Oral Pathol Oral Radiol Endod 2006; 101:761.

242. Spitz S. Melanomas of childhood. Am J Pathol 1948; 24:591.

243. Weedon D, Little JH. Spindle and epithelioid cell nevi in children and adults. A review of 211 cases of the Spitz nevus. Cancer 1977; 40:217.

244. Binder SW, Asnong C, Paul E, et al. The histology and differential diagnosis of Spitz nevus. Semin Diagn Pathol 1993; 10:36.

245. Busam KJ, Barnhill RL. Pagetoid Spitz nevus. Intraepidermal Spitz tumor with prominent pagetoid spread. Am J Surg Pathol 1995; 19:1061.

246. Smith KJ, Barrett TL, Skelton HG 3rd, et al. Spindle cell and epithelioid cell nevi with atypia and metastasis (malignant Spitz nevus). Am J Surg Pathol 1989; 13:931.

247. Howat AJ, Variend S. Lymphatic invasion in Spitz nevi. Am J Surg Pathol 1985; 9:125.

248. Barnhill RL, Argenyi ZB, From L, et al. Atypical Spitz nevi/tumors: lack of consensus for diagnosis, discrimination from melanoma, and prediction of outcome. Hum Pathol 1999; 30:513.

249. Allen AC, Spitz S. Histogenesis and clinicopathologic correlation of nevi and malignant melanomas; current status. AMA Arch Derm Syphilol 1954; 69:150.

250. Kamino H, Flotte TJ, Misheloff E, et al. Eosinophilic globules in Spitz's nevi. New findings and a diagnostic sign. Am J Dermatopathol 1979; 1:319.

251. Barsky SH, Hannah JB. Extracellular hyaline bodies are basement membrane accumulations. Am J Clin Pathol 1987; 87:455.

252. Wesselmann U, Becker LR, Brocker EB, et al. Eosinophilic globules in spitz nevi: no evidence for apoptosis. Am J Dermatopathol 1998; 20:551.

253. Spatz A, Calonje E, Handfield-Jones S, Barnhill RL. Spitz tumors in children: a grading system for risk stratification. Arch Dermatol 1999; 135:282.

254. Kapur P, Selim MA, Roy LC, et al. Spitz nevi and atypical Spitz nevi/tumors: a histologic and immunohistochemical analysis. Mod Pathol 2005; 18:197.

255. Krengel S, Groteluschen F, Bartsch S, et al. Cadherin expression pattern in melanocytic tumors more likely depends on the melanocyte environment than on tumor cell progression. J Cutan Pathol 2004; 31:1.

256. Ribe A, McNutt NS. S100A6 protein expression is different in Spitz nevi and melanomas. Mod Pathol 2003; 16:505.

257. Bergman R, Azzam H, Sprecher E, et al. A comparative immunohistochemical study of MART-1 expression in Spitz nevi, ordinary melanocytic nevi, and malignant melanomas. J Am Acad Dermatol 2000; 42:496.

258. Evans MJ, Sanders DS, Grant JH, et al. Expression of Melan-A in Spitz, pigmented spindle cell nevi, and congenital nevi: comparative immunohistochemical study. Pediatr Dev Pathol 2000; 3:36.

259. Simonetti O, Lucarini G, Brancorsini D, et al. Immunohistochemical expression of vascular endothelial growth factor, matrix metalloproteinase 2, and matrix metalloproteinase 9 in cutaneous melanocytic lesions. Cancer 2002; 95:1963.

260. King MS, Porchia SJ, Hiatt KM. Differentiating spitzoid melanomas from Spitz nevi through CD99 expression. J Cutan Pathol 2007; 34:576.

261. Isabel Zhu Y, Fitzpatrick JE. Expression of c-kit (CD117) in Spitz nevus and malignant melanoma. J Cutan Pathol 2006; 33:33.

262. Stefanaki C, Stefanaki K, Antoniou C, et al. Cell cycle and apoptosis regulators in Spitz nevi: comparison with melanomas and common nevi. J Am Acad Dermatol 2007; 56:815.

263. Takata M, Saida T. Genetic alterations in melanocytic tumors. J Dermatol Sci 2006; 43:1.

264. Bogdan I, Burg G, Boni R. Spitz nevi display allelic deletions. Arch Dermatol 2001; 137:1417.

265. Mehregan AH, Mehregan DR, Broecker A. Epithelioid cell histiocytoma. A clinicopathologic and immunohistochemical study of eight cases. J Am Acad Dermatol 1992; 26:243.

266. Gelbard SN, Tripp JM, Marghoob AA, et al. Management of Spitz nevi: a survey of dermatologists in the United States. J Am Acad Dermatol 2002; 47:224.

267. Murphy ME, Boyer JD, Stashower ME, et al. The surgical management of Spitz nevi. Dermatol Surg 2002; 28:1065.

268. Casso EM, Grin-Jorgensen CM, Grant-Kels JM. Spitz nevi. J Am Acad Dermatol 1992; 27:901.

269. Lohmann CM, Coit DG, Brady MS, et al. Sentinel lymph node biopsy in patients with diagnostically controversial spitzoid melanocytic tumors. Am J Surg Pathol 2002; 26:47.

270. Patterson JW. Nevus cell aggregates in lymph nodes. Am J Clin Pathol 2004; 121:13.

271. Fontaine D, Parkhill W, Greer W, et al. Nevus cells in lymph nodes: an association with congenital cutaneous nevi. Am J Dermatopathol 2002; 24:1.

272. Curtin JA, Fridlyand J, Kageshita T, et al. Distinct sets of genetic alterations in melanoma. N Engl J Med 2005; 353:2135.

273. Whiteman DC, Stickley M, Watt P, et al. Anatomic site, sun exposure, and risk of cutaneous melanoma. J Clin Oncol 2006; 24:3172.

274. Kienstra MA, Padhya TA. Head and neck melanoma. Cancer Control 2005; 12:242.

275. Hoersch B, Leiter U, Garbe C. Is head and neck melanoma a distinct entity? A clinical registry-based comparative study in 5702 patients with melanoma. Br J Dermatol 2006; 155:771.

276. Leong SP, Accortt NA, Essner R, et al. Impact of sentinel node status and other risk factors on the clinical outcome of head and neck melanoma patients. Arch Otolaryngol Head Neck Surg 2006; 132:370.

277. Le Marchand L, Saltzman BS, Hankin JH, et al. Sun exposure, diet, and melanoma in Hawaii Caucasians. Am J Epidemiol 2006; 164:232.

278. Balch CM, Soong SJ, Gershenwald JE, et al. Prognostic factors analysis of 17,600 melanoma patients: validation of the American Joint Committee on Cancer melanoma staging system. J Clin Oncol 2001; 19:3622.

279. Zaballos P, Llambrich A, Puig S, et al. Dermoscopy is useful for the recognition of benign-malignant compound tumours. Br J Dermatol 2005; 153:653.

280. Massone C, Di Stefani A, Soyer HP. Dermoscopy for skin cancer detection. Curr Opin Oncol 2005; 17:147.

281. Braun RP, Rabinovitz HS, Oliviero M, et al. Dermoscopy of pigmented skin lesions. J Am Acad Dermatol 2005; 52:109.

282. Livestro DP, Muzikansky A, Kaine EM, et al. Biology of desmoplastic melanoma: a case-control comparison with other melanomas. J Clin Oncol 2005; 23:6739.

283. Hussussian CJ, Struewing JP, Goldstein AM, et al. Germline p16 mutations in familial melanoma. Nat Genet 1994; 8:15.

284. Kamb A, Shattuck-Eidens D, Eeles R, et al. Analysis of the p16 gene (CDKN2) as a candidate for the chromosome 9p melanoma susceptibility locus. Nat Genet 1994; 8:23.

285. Goldstein AM, Chidambaram A, Halpern A, et al. Rarity of CDK4 germline mutations in familial melanoma. Melanoma Res 2002; 12:51.

286. Stahl JM, Cheung M, Sharma A, et al. Loss of PTEN promotes tumor development in malignant melanoma. Cancer Res 2003; 63:2881.

287. You MJ, Castrillon DH, Bastian BC, et al. Genetic analysis of Pten and Ink4a/Arf interactions in the suppression of tumorigenesis in mice. Proc Natl Acad Sci U S A 2002; 99:1455.

288. Poynter JN, Elder JT, Fullen DR, et al. BRAF and NRAS mutations in melanoma and melanocytic nevi. Melanoma Res 2006; 16:267.

289. Deichmann M, Krahl D, Thome M, et al. The oncogenic B-raf V599E mutation occurs more frequently in melanomas at sun-protected body sites. Int J Oncol 2006; 29:139.

290. Curtin JA, Busam K, Pinkel D, et al. Somatic activation of KIT in distinct subtypes of melanoma. J Clin Oncol 2006; 24:4340.

291. Folpe AL, Cooper K. Best practices in diagnostic immunohistochemistry: pleomorphic cutaneous spindle cell tumors. Arch Pathol Lab Med 2007; 131:1517.

292. McKenna JK, Florell SR, Goldman GD, et al. Lentigo maligna/lentigo maligna melanoma: current state of diagnosis and treatment. Dermatol Surg 2006; 32:493.

293. Garbe C, Eigentler TK. Diagnosis and treatment of cutaneous melanoma: state of the art 2006. Melanoma Res 2007; 17:117.

294. Arora A, Lowe L, Su L, et al. Wide excision without radiation for desmoplastic melanoma. Cancer 2005; 104:1462.

295. MacNeill KN, Ghazarian D, McCready D, et al. Sentinel lymph node biopsy for cutaneous melanoma of the head and neck. Ann Surg Oncol 2005; 12:726.

296. Ugurel S, Hildenbrand R, Zimpfer A, et al. Lack of clinical efficacy of imatinib in metastatic melanoma. Br J Cancer 2005; 92:1398.

297. Wyman K, Atkins MB, Prieto V, et al. Multicenter Phase II trial of high-dose imatinib mesylate in metastatic melanoma: significant toxicity with no clinical efficacy. Cancer 2006; 106:2005.

298. Becker JC, Brocker EB, Schadendorf D, et al. Imatinib in melanoma: a selective treatment option based on KIT mutation status? J Clin Oncol 2007; 25:e9.

299. Antonescu CR, Busam KJ, Francone TD, et al. L576P KIT mutation in anal melanomas correlates with KIT protein expression and is sensitive to specific kinase inhibition. Int J Cancer 2007; 121:257.

300. Alexis JB, Martinez AE, Lutzky J. An immunohistochemical evaluation of c-kit (CD-117) expression in malignant melanoma, and results of imatinib mesylate (Gleevec) therapy in three patients. Melanoma Res 2005; 15:283.

301. Markovic SN, Erickson LA, Rao RD, et al. Malignant melanoma in the 21st century, part 2: staging, prognosis, and treatment. Mayo Clin Proc 2007; 82:490.

302. Neuber K, Eidam B. Expression of Fas ligand (CD95L) in primary malignant melanoma and melanoma metastases is associated with overall survival. Onkologie 2006; 29:361.

303. Coop CA, Schaefer SM, England RW. Extensive keloid formation and progression after each vaccination. Hum Vaccin 2007; 3:127.

304. Goel SK, Kuruvila M. Rare sequelae of herpes zoster in HIV positive patient. Indian J Dermatol Venereol Leprol 2002; 68:295.

305. Char F. Ehlers-Danlos syndrome. Birth Defects Orig Artic Ser 1971; 7:300.

306. Akintewe TA, Alabi GO. Scleroderma presenting with multiple keloids. Br Med J (Clin Res Ed) 1985; 291:448.

307. Layton AM, Yip J, Cunliffe WJ. A comparison of intralesional triamcinolone and cryosurgery in the treatment of acne keloids. Br J Dermatol 1994; 130:498.

308. Burk CJ, Aber C, Connelly EA. Ehlers-Danlos syndrome type IV: keloidal plaques of the lower extremities, amniotic band limb deformity, and a new mutation. J Am Acad Dermatol 2007; 56:S53.

309. Wang Z, Gao Z, Shi Y, et al. Inhibition of Smad3 expression decreases collagen synthesis in keloid disease fibroblasts. J Plast Reconstr Aesthet Surg 2007; 60:1193.

310. Berman B, Bieley HC. Adjunct therapies to surgical management of keloids. Dermatol Surg 1996; 22:126.

311. Onodera M, Ueno M, Ito O, et al. Factor XIIIa-positive dermal dendritic cells in keloids and hypertrophic and mature scars. Pathol Int 2007; 57:337.

312. Kikuchi K, Kadono T, Takehara K. Effects of various growth factors and histamine on cultured keloid fibroblasts. Dermatology 1995; 190:4.

313. Aiba S, Tagami H. Inverse correlation between CD34 expression and proline-4-hydroxylase immunoreactivity on spindle cells noted in hypertrophic scars and keloids. J Cutan Pathol 1997; 24:65.

314. Sato M. Upregulation of the Wnt/beta-catenin pathway induced by transforming growth factor-beta in hypertrophic scars and keloids. Acta Derm Venereol 2006; 86:300.

315. Ghazizadeh M. Essential role of IL-6 signaling pathway in keloid pathogenesis. J Nippon Med Sch 2007; 74:11.

316. Ghazizadeh M, Tosa M, Shimizu H, et al. Functional implications of the IL-6 signaling pathway in keloid pathogenesis. J Invest Dermatol 2007; 127:98.

317. Ong CT, Khoo YT, Tan EK, et al. Epithelial-mesenchymal interactions in keloid pathogenesis modulate vascular endothelial growth factor expression and secretion. J Pathol 2007; 211:95.

318. Chevray PM, Manson PN. Keloid scars are formed by polyclonal fibroblasts. Ann Plast Surg 2004; 52:605.

319. Sananto D, Noer S, Alsagaff JH. Gli-1 oncogene: the key to keloidogenesis? Plast Reconstr Surg 2007; 119:1146.

320. Murray JC, Pollack SV, Pinnell SR. Keloids: a review. J Am Acad Dermatol 1981; 4:461.

321. Selvaggi G, Boeckx W, De Wulf M, et al. Late results of burn wound scar after cerium nitrate-silver sulfadiazine and compressive therapy: scanning electron microscopy evaluation of a keloid scar. Plast Reconstr Surg 2007; 119:1965.

322. Ghazizadeh M, Miyata N, Sasaki Y, et al. Silver-stained nucleolar organizer regions in hypertrophic and keloid scars. Am J Dermatopathol 1997; 19:468.

323. Beer TW, Baldwin HC, Goddard JR, et al. Angiogenesis in pathological and surgical scars. Hum Pathol 1998; 29:1273.

324. Matsuoka LY, Uitto J, Wortsman J, et al. Ultrastructural characteristics of keloid fibroblasts. Am J Dermatopathol 1988; 10:505.

325. James WD, Besanceney CD, Odom RB. The ultrastructure of a keloid. J Am Acad Dermatol 1980; 3:50.

326. Bayat A, Arscott G, Ollier WE, et al. "Aggressive keloid": a severe variant of familial keloid scarring. J R Soc Med 2003; 96:554.

327. Marneros AG, Norris JE, Olsen BR, et al. Clinical genetics of familial keloids. Arch Dermatol 2001; 137:1429.

328. De Felice B, Ciarmiello LF, Mondola P, et al. Differential p63 and p53 expression in human keloid fibroblasts and hypertrophic scar fibroblasts. DNA Cell Biol 2007; 26:541.

329. Jagadeesan J, Bayat A. Transforming growth factor beta (TGFbeta) and keloid disease. Int J Surg 2007; 5:278.

330. Ishihara H, Yoshimoto H, Fujioka M, et al. Keloid fibroblasts resist ceramide-induced apoptosis by overexpression of insulin-like growth factor I receptor. J Invest Dermatol 2000; 115:1065.

331. Saed GM, Ladin D, Olson J, et al. Analysis of p53 gene mutations in keloids using polymerase chain reaction-based single-strand conformational polymorphism and DNA sequencing. Arch Dermatol 1998; 134:963.

332. Berman B, Villa A. Imiquimod 5% cream for keloid management. Dermatol Surg 2003; 29:1050.

333. Leventhal D, Furr M, Reiter D. Treatment of keloids and hypertrophic scars: a meta-analysis and review of the literature. Arch Facial Plast Surg 2006; 8:362.

334. Darzi MA, Chowdri NA, Kaul SK, et al. Evaluation of various methods of treating keloids and hypertrophic scars: a 10-year follow-up study. Br J Plast Surg 1992; 45:374.

335. Kauh YC, Rouda S, Mondragon G, et al. Major suppression of pro-alpha1(I) type I collagen gene expression in the dermis after keloid excision and immediate intra-wound injection of triamcinolone acetonide. J Am Acad Dermatol 1997; 37:586.

336. Jones K, Fuller CD, Luh JY, et al. Case report and summary of literature: giant perineal keloids treated with post-excisional radiotherapy. BMC Dermatol 2006; 6:7.

337. Klumpar DI, Murray JC, Anscher M. Keloids treated with excision followed by radiation therapy. J Am Acad Dermatol 1994; 31:225.

338. Kim A, DiCarlo J, Cohen C, et al. Are keloids really "gliloids"?: High-level expression of gli-1 oncogene in keloids. J Am Acad Dermatol 2001; 45:707.

339. O'Brien L, Pandit A. Silicon gel sheeting for preventing and treating hypertrophic and keloid scars. Cochrane Database Syst Rev 2006; 1:CD003826.

340. Sueki H, Whitaker D, Buchsbaum M, et al. Novel interactions between dermal dendrocytes and mast cells in human skin. Implications for hemostasis and matrix repair. Lab Invest 1993; 69:160.

341. McGibbon DH, Jones EW. Fibrous papule of the face (nose). Fibrosing nevocytic nevus. Am J Dermatopathol 1979; 1:345.

342. Cerio R, Rao BK, Spaull J, et al. An immunohistochemical study of fibrous papule of the nose: 25 cases. J Cutan Pathol 1989; 16:194.

343. Lee AN, Stein SL, Cohen LM. Clear cell fibrous papule with NKI/C3 expression: clinical and histologic features in six cases. Am J Dermatopathol 2005; 27:296.

344. Bansal C, Stewart D, Li A, et al. Histologic variants of fibrous papule. J Cutan Pathol 2005; 32:424.

345. Guitart J, Bergfeld WF, Tuthill RJ. Fibrous papule of the nose with granular cells: two cases. J Cutan Pathol 1991; 18:284.

346. Spiegel J, Nadji M, Penneys NS. Fibrous papule: an immunohistochemical study with an antibody to S-100 protein. J Am Acad Dermatol 1983; 9:360.

347. Shea CR, Salob S, Reed JA, et al. CD34-reactive fibrous papule of the nose. J Am Acad Dermatol 1996; 35:342.

348. Kimura S, Yamasaki Y. Ultrastructure of fibrous papule of the nose. J Dermatol 1983; 10:571.

349. Ragaz A, Berezowsky V. Fibrous papule of the face. A study of five cases by electron microscopy. Am J Dermatopathol 1979; 1:353.

350. Santa Cruz DJ, Prioleau PG. Fibrous papule of the face. An electron-microscopic study of two cases. Am J Dermatopathol 1979; 1:349.

351. Cerio R, Spaull J, Oliver GF, et al. A study of factor XIIIa and MAC 387 immunolabeling in normal and pathological skin. Am J Dermatopathol 1990; 12:221.

352. Enzinger F, Weiss S: Benign Fibrous Tissue Tumors: Nuchal Fibroma. St. Louis, MO: Mosby, 2001:284.

353. Michal M, Fetsch JF, Hes O, et al. Nuchal-type fibroma: a clinicopathologic study of 52 cases. Cancer 1999; 85:156.

354. Diwan AH, Graves ED, King JA, et al. Nuchal-type fibroma in two related patients with Gardner's syndrome. Am J Surg Pathol 2000; 24:1563.

355. Wehrli BM, Weiss SW, Yandow S, et al. Gardner-associated fibromas (GAF) in young patients: a distinct fibrous lesion that identifies unsuspected Gardner syndrome and risk for fibromatosis. Am J Surg Pathol 2001; 25:645.

356. Banney LA, Weedon D, Muir JB. Nuchal fibroma associated with scleredema, diabetes mellitus and organic solvent exposure. Australas J Dermatol 2000; 41:39.

357. Diwàn AH, Horenstein MG. Dermatofibrosarcoma protuberans association with nuchal-type fibroma. J Cutan Pathol 2004; 31:62.

358. Samadi DS, McLaughlin RB, Loevner LA, et al. Nuchal fibroma: a clinicopathological review. Ann Otol Rhinol Laryngol 2000; 109:52.

359. Balachandran K, Allen PW, MacCormac LB. Nuchal fibroma. A clinicopathological study of nine cases. Am J Surg Pathol 1995; 19:313.

360. Tsunemi Y, Saeki H, Tamaki K. Nuchal fibroma clearly visualized by computed tomography: a case report. Int J Dermatol 2005; 44:703.

361. Zamecnik M, Michal M. Nuchal-type fibroma is positive for CD34 and CD99. Am J Surg Pathol 2001; 25:970.

362. Laskin WB, Fetsch JF, Miettinen M. Nuchal fibrocartilaginous pseudotumor: a clinicopathologic study of five cases and review of the literature. Mod Pathol 1999; 12:663.

363. Yamamoto T, Katayama I, Nishioka K. Role of mast cells in dermatofibroma: recent viewpoints into the pathogenesis. Eur J Dermatol 2003; 13:419.

364. Yamamoto T, Sumi K, Yokozeki H, et al. Multiple cutaneous fibrous histiocytomas in association with systemic lupus erythematosus. J Dermatol 2005; 32:645.

365. Hui P, Glusac EJ, Sinard JH, et al. Clonal analysis of cutaneous fibrous histiocytoma (dermatofibroma). J Cutan Pathol 2002; 29:385.

366. Mentzel T, Kutzner H, Rutten A, et al. Benign fibrous histiocytoma (dermatofibroma) of the face: clinicopathologic and immunohistochemical study of 34 cases associated with an aggressive clinical course. Am J Dermatopathol 2001; 23:419.

367. Horenstein MG, Prieto VG, Nuckols JD, et al. Indeterminate fibrohistiocytic lesions of the skin: is there a spectrum between dermatofibroma and dermatofibrosarcoma protuberans? Am J Surg Pathol 2000; 24:996.

368. Rahbari H, Mehregan AH. Adnexal displacement and regression in association with histiocytoma (dermatofibroma). J Cutan Pathol 1985; 12:94.

369. Carstens HB, Schrodt GR. Ultrastructure of sclerosing hemangioma. Am J Pathol 1974; 77:377.

370. Goldblum JR, Tuthill RJ. CD34 and factor-XIIIa immunoreactivity in dermatofibrosarcoma protuberans and dermatofibroma. Am J Dermatopathol 1997; 19:147.

371. Calikoglu E, Augsburger E, Chavaz P, et al. CD44 and hyaluronate in the differential diagnosis of dermatofibroma and dermatofibrosarcoma protuberans. J Cutan Pathol 2003; 30:185.

372. Calikoglu E, Chavaz P, Saurat JH, et al. Decreased CD44 expression and stromal hyaluronate accumulation in myxoid dermatofibroma. Dermatology 2003; 207:104.

373. Katenkamp D, Stiller D. Cellular composition of the so-called dermatofibroma (histiocytoma cutis). Virchows Arch A Pathol Anat Histol 1975; 367:325.

374. Cerio R, Spaull J, Jones EW. Histiocytoma cutis: a tumour of dermal dendrocytes (dermal dendrocytoma). Br J Dermatol 1989; 120:197.

375. Nishio J, Iwasaki H, Ohjimi Y, et al. Overrepresentation of 17q22-qter and 22q13 in dermatofibrosarcoma protuberans but not in dermatofibroma: a comparative genomic hybridization study. Cancer Genet Cytogenet 2002; 132:102.

376. Riopel C, Musette P, Bodenant C, et al. Clear cell dermatofibroma: a case report with cytogenetic study. Ann Pathol 2004; 24:440.

377. Wang J, Morimitsu Y, Okamoto S, et al. COL1A1-PDGFB fusion transcripts in fibrosarcomatous areas of six dermatofibrosarcomas protuberans. J Mol Diagn 2000; 2:47.

378. Jha P, Moosavi C, Fanburg-Smith JC. Giant cell fibroblastoma: an update and addition of 86 new cases from the Armed Forces Institute of Pathology, in honor of Dr. Franz M. Enzinger. Ann Diagn Pathol 2007; 11:81.

379. Cin PD, Sciot R, de Wever I, et al. Cytogenetic and immunohistochemical evidence that giant cell fibroblastoma is related to dermatofibrosarcoma protuberans. Genes Chromosomes Cancer 1996; 15:73.

380. Maggoudi D, Vahtsevanos K, Psomaderis K, et al. Dermatofibrosarcoma protuberans of the face: report of 2 cases and an overview of the recent literature. J Oral Maxillofac Surg 2006; 64:140.

381. Gloster HM Jr. Dermatofibrosarcoma protuberans. J Am Acad Dermatol 1996; 35:355.

382. Parlette LE, Smith CK, Germain LM, et al. Accelerated growth of dermatofibrosarcoma protuberans during pregnancy. J Am Acad Dermatol 1999; 41:778.

383. Kransdorf MJ, Meis-Kindblom JM. Dermatofibrosarcoma protuberans: radiologic appearance. AJR Am J Roentgenol 1994; 163:391.

384. Torreggiani WC, Al-Ismail K, Munk PL, et al. Dermatofibrosarcoma protuberans: MR imaging features. AJR Am J Roentgenol 2002; 178:989.

385. Reimann JD, Fletcher CD. Myxoid dermatofibrosarcoma protuberans: a rare variant analyzed in a series of 23 cases. Am J Surg Pathol 2007; 31:1371.

386. Mendenhall WM, Zlotecki RA, Scarborough MT. Dermatofibrosarcoma protuberans. Cancer 2004; 101:2503.

387. Billings SD, Folpe AL. Cutaneous and subcutaneous fibrohistiocytic tumors of intermediate malignancy: an update. Am J Dermatopathol 2004; 26:141.

388. Abbott J, Oliveira A, nascimento A. The prognostic significance of fibrosarcomatous transformation in dermatofibrosarcoma protuberans. Am J Surg Pathol 2006; 30:436.

389. Goldblum JR, Reith JD, Weiss SW. Sarcomas arising in dermatofibrosarcoma protuberans: a reappraisal of biologic behavior in eighteen cases treated by wide local excision with extended clinical follow up. Am J Surg Pathol 2000; 24:1125.

390. Dominguez-Malagon H, Valdez-Carrillo Mdel C, Cano-Valdez AM. Dermatofibroma and dermatofibrosarcoma protuberans: a comparative ultrastructural study. Ultrastruct Pathol 2006; 30:283.

391. Patel KU, Szabo SS, Hernandez VS, et al. Dermatofibrosarcoma protuberans COL1A1-PDGFB fusion is identified in virtually all dermatofibrosarcoma protuberans cases when investigated by newly developed multiplex reverse transcription polymerase chain reaction and fluorescence in situ hybridization assays. Hum Pathol 2008; 39(2): 184–193.

392. Rubin BP, Schuetze SM, Eary JF, et al. Molecular targeting of platelet-derived growth factor B by imatinib mesylate in a patient with metastatic dermatofibrosarcoma protuberans. J Clin Oncol 2002; 20:3586.

393. Hisaoka M, Okamoto S, Morimitsu Y, et al. Dermatofibrosarcoma protuberans with fibrosarcomatous areas. Molecular abnormalities of the p53 pathway in fibrosarcomatous transformation of dermatofibrosarcoma protuberans. Virchows Arch 1998; 433:323.

394. Breuninger H, Sebastian G, Garbe C. Dermatofibrosarcoma protuberans—an update. J Dtsch Dermatol Ges 2004; 2:661.

395. Labonte S, Hanna W, Bandarchi-Chamkhaleh B. A study of CD117 expression in dermatofibrosarcoma protuberans and cellular dermatofibroma. J Cutan Pathol 2007; 34:857.

396. McArthur G. Molecularly targeted treatment for dermatofibrosarcoma protuberans. Semin Oncol 2004; 31:30.

397. Seavolt M, McCall M. Atypical fibroxanthoma: review of the literature and summary of 13 patients treated with mohs micrographic surgery. Dermatol Surg 2006; 32:435.

398. Kargi E, Gungor E, Verdi M, et al. Atypical fibroxanthoma and metastasis to the lung. Plast Reconstr Surg 2003; 111:1760.

399. Muenster MR, Hoang MP. Left facial mass in an elderly man. Metastasizing atypical fibroxanthoma of the skin. Arch Pathol Lab Med 2006; 130:735.

400. Cooper JZ, Newman SR, Scott GA, et al. Metastasizing atypical fibroxanthoma (cutaneous malignant histiocytoma): report of five cases. Dermatol Surg 2005; 31:221.

401. Mirza B, Weedon D. Atypical fibroxanthoma: a clinicopathological study of 89 cases. Australas J Dermatol 2005; 46:235.

402. Kaddu S, McMenamin ME, Fletcher CD. Atypical fibrous histiocytoma of the skin: clinicopathologic analysis of 59 cases with evidence of infrequent metastasis. Am J Surg Pathol 2002; 26:35.

403. Marrogi AJ, Dehner LP, Coffin CM, et al. Atypical fibrous histiocytoma of the skin and subcutis in childhood and adolescence. J Cutan Pathol 1992; 19:268.

404. Kovach BT, Sams HH, Stasko T. Multiple atypical fibroxanthomas in a cardiac transplant recipient. Dermatol Surg 2005; 31:467.

405. Hafner J, Kunzi W, Weinreich T. Malignant fibrous histiocytoma and atypical fibroxanthoma in renal transplant recipients. Dermatology 1999; 198:29.

406. Dilek FH, Akpolat N, Metin A, et al. Atypical fibroxanthoma of the skin and the lower lip in xeroderma pigmentosum. Br J Dermatol 2000; 143:618.

407. Youssef N, Vabres P, Buisson T, et al. Two unusual tumors in a patient with xeroderma pigmentosum:

408. Crowson AN, Carlson-Sweet K, Macinnis C, et al. Clear cell atypical fibroxanthoma: a clinicopathologic study. J Cutan Pathol 2002; 29:374.

409. Diaz-Cascajo C, Weyers W, Borghi S. Pigmented atypical fibroxanthoma: a tumor that may be easily mistaken for malignant melanoma. Am J Dermatopathol 2003; 25:1.

410. Rudisaile SN, Hurt MA, Santa Cruz DJ. Granular cell atypical fibroxanthoma. J Cutan Pathol 2005; 32:314.

411. Longacre TA, Smoller BR, Rouse RV. Atypical fibroxanthoma. Multiple immunohistologic profiles. Am J Surg Pathol 1993; 17:1199.

412. Monteagudo C, Calduch L, Navarro S, et al. CD99 immunoreactivity in atypical fibroxanthoma: a common feature of diagnostic value. Am J Clin Pathol 2002; 117:126.

413. Jensen K, Wilkinson B, Wines N, et al. Procollagen 1 expression in atypical fibroxanthoma and other tumors. J Cutan Pathol 2004; 31:57.

414. Bansal C, Sinkre P, Stewart D, et al. Two cases of cytokeratin positivity in atypical fibroxanthoma. J Clin Pathol 2007; 60:716.

415. Wilk M, Zelger BG, Nilles M, et al. The value of immunohistochemistry in atypical cutaneous fibrous histiocytoma. Am J Dermatopathol 2004; 26:367.

416. Barr RJ, Wuerker RB, Graham JH. Ultrastructure of atypical fibroxanthoma. Cancer 1977; 40:736.

417. Weedon D, Kerr JF. Atypical fibroxanthoma of skin: an electron microscope study. Pathology 1975; 7:173.

418. Worrell JT, Ansari MQ, Ansari SJ, et al. Atypical fibroxanthoma: DNA ploidy analysis of 14 cases with possible histogenetic implications. J Cutan Pathol 1993; 20:211.

419. Winkelmann RK, Peters MS. Atypical fibroxanthoma. A study with antibody to S-100 protein. Arch Dermatol 1985; 121:753.

420. Bansal C, Sinkre P, Stewart DT, et al. Two cases of cytokeratin positivity in atypical fibroxanthoma. J Clin Pathol 2007.

421. Chang J, Most D, Bresnick S, et al. Proliferative hemangiomas: analysis of cytokine gene expression and angiogenesis. Plast Reconstr Surg 1999; 103:1.

422. Marler JJ, Mulliken JB. Current management of hemangiomas and vascular malformations. Clin Plast Surg 2005; 32:99.

423. Garzon MC, Huang JT, Enjolras O, et al. Vascular malformations. Part II: associated syndromes. J Am Acad Dermatol 2007; 56:541.

424. Garzon MC, Huang JT, Enjolras O, et al. Vascular malformations: Part I. J Am Acad Dermatol 2007; 56:353.

425. Memeo M, Scardapane A, Stabile Ianora AA, Sabba C, Angelelli G. Hereditary haemorrhagic teleangiectasia: diagnostic imaging of visceral involvement. Curr Pharm Des 2006; 12:1227.

426. Smoller BR, Rosen S. Port-wine stains. A disease of altered neural modulation of blood vessels? Arch Dermatol 1986; 122:177.

427. North PE, Waner M, Mizeracki A, et al. GLUT1: a newly discovered immunohistochemical marker for juvenile hemangiomas. Hum Pathol 2000; 31:11.

428. Leon-Villapalos J, Wolfe K, Kangesu L. GLUT-1: an extra diagnostic tool to differentiate between haemangiomas and vascular malformations. Br J Plast Surg 2005; 58:348.

429. Tu J, Stoodley MA, Morgan MK, et al. Ultrastructural characteristics of hemorrhagic, nonhemorrhagic, and recurrent cavernous malformations. J Neurosurg 2005; 103:903.

430. Kanitakis J, Roger H, Soubrier M, et al. Cutaneous angiomas in POEMS syndrome. An ultrastructural and immunohistochemical study. Arch Dermatol 1988; 124:695.

431. Eerola I, Boon LM, Watanabe S, et al. Locus for susceptibility for familial capillary malformation ('port-wine stain') maps to 5q. Eur J Hum Genet 2002; 10:375.

432. Eerola I, Boon LM, Mulliken JB, et al. Capillary malformation-arteriovenous malformation, a new clinical and genetic disorder caused by RASA1 mutations. Am J Hum Genet 2003; 73:1240.

433. Brancati F, Valente EM, Tadini G, et al. Autosomal dominant hereditary benign telangiectasia maps to the CMC1 locus for capillary malformation on chromosome 5q14. J Med Genet 2003; 40:849.

434. Morris PN, Dunmore BJ, Tadros A, et al. Functional analysis of a mutant form of the receptor tyrosine kinase Tie2 causing venous malformations. J Mol Med 2005; 83:58.

435. Hashimoto T, Lam T, Boudreau NJ, et al. Abnormal balance in the angiopoietin-tie2 system in human brain arteriovenous malformations. Circ Res 2001; 89:111.

436. North PE, Waner M, Buckmiller L, et al. Vascular tumors of infancy and childhood: beyond capillary hemangioma. Cardiovasc Pathol 2006; 15:303.

437. McGill DJ, Mackay IR. Capillary vascular malformation response to increased ambient temperature is dependent upon anatomical location. Ann Plast Surg 2007; 58:193.

438. Ghosh A, Tibrewal SR, Thapa R. PHACES syndrome with congenital hypothyroidism. Indian Pediatr 2007; 44:144.

439. Hayashi Y, Ohi R, Tomita Y, et al. Bannayan-Zonana syndrome associated with lipomas, hemangiomas, and lymphangiomas. J Pediatr Surg 1992; 27:722.

440. Cheung DS, Warman ML, Mulliken JB. Hemangioma in twins. Ann Plast Surg 1997; 38:269.

441. Waner M, North PE, Scherer KA, et al. The nonrandom distribution of facial hemangiomas. Arch Dermatol 2003; 139:869.

442. Boye E, Yu Y, Paranya G, et al. Clonality and altered behavior of endothelial cells from hemangiomas. J Clin Invest 2001; 107:745.

443. Ritter MR, Dorrell MI, Edmonds J, et al. Insulin-like growth factor 2 and potential regulators of hemangioma growth and involution identified by large-scale expression analysis. Proc Natl Acad Sci U S A 2002; 99:7455.

444. Garzon M. Hemangiomas: update on classification, clinical presentation, and associated anomalies. Cutis 2000; 66:325.

445. Takahashi K, Mulliken JB, Kozakewich HP, et al. Cellular markers that distinguish the phases of hemangioma during infancy and childhood. J Clin Invest 1994; 93:2357.

446. Haggstrom AN, Drolet BA, Baselga E, et al. Prospective study of infantile hemangiomas: demographic, prenatal, and perinatal characteristics. J Pediatr 2007; 150:291.

447. Dubois J, Milot J, Jaeger BI, et al. Orbit and eyelid hemangiomas: is there a relationship between location and ocular problems? J Am Acad Dermatol 2006; 55:614.

448. Stigmar G, Crawford JS, Ward CM, et al. Ophthalmic sequelae of infantile hemangiomas of the eyelids and orbit. Am J Ophthalmol 1978; 85:806.

449. Dubois J, Garel L. Imaging and therapeutic approach of hemangiomas and vascular malformations in the pediatric age group. Pediatr Radiol 1999; 29:879.

450. Vilanova JC, Barcelo J, Smirniotopoulos JG, et al. Hemangioma from head to toe: MR imaging with pathologic correlation. Radiographics 2004; 24:367.

451. Sun ZJ, Zhao YF, Zhao JH. Mast cells in hemangioma: a double-edged sword. Med Hypotheses 2007; 68:805.

452. Tan ST, Velickovic M, Ruger BM, et al. Cellular and extracellular markers of hemangioma. Plast Reconstr Surg 2000; 106:529.

453. Domfeh AB, Fichera M, Hunt JL. Allelic loss of 3 different tumor suppressor gene loci in benign and malignant

454. endothelial tumors of the head and neck. Arch Pathol Lab Med 2006; 130:1184.

454. Smolinski KN, Yan AC. Hemangiomas of infancy: clinical and biological characteristics. Clin Pediatr (Phila) 2005; 44:747.

455. Vin-Christian K, McCalmont TH, Frieden IJ. Kaposiform hemangioendothelioma. An aggressive, locally invasive vascular tumor that can mimic hemangioma of infancy. Arch Dermatol 1997; 133:1573.

456. Hasan Q, Tan ST, Gush J, et al. Steroid therapy of a proliferating hemangioma: histochemical and molecular changes. Pediatrics 2000; 105:117.

457. Chen MT, Yeong EK, Horng SY. Intralesional corticosteroid therapy in proliferating head and neck hemangiomas: a review of 155 cases. J Pediatr Surg 2000; 35:420.

458. Chan YC. Current treatment practices in the management of cutaneous haemangioma. Expert Opin Pharmacother 2004; 5:1937.

459. Adams DM, Lucky AW. Cervicofacial vascular anomalies. I. Hemangiomas and other benign vascular tumors. Semin Pediatr Surg 2006; 15:124.

460. Zukerberg LR, Nickoloff BJ, Weiss SW. Kaposiform hemangioendothelioma of infancy and childhood. An aggressive neoplasm associated with Kasabach-Merritt syndrome and lymphangiomatosis. Am J Surg Pathol 1993; 17:321.

461. Mentzel T, Mazzoleni G, Dei Tos AP, et al. Kaposiform hemangioendothelioma in adults. Clinicopathologic and immunohistochemical analysis of three cases. Am J Clin Pathol 1997; 108:450.

462. Maguiness S, Guenther L. Kasabach-merritt syndrome. J Cutan Med Surg 2002; 6:335.

463. Lyons LL, North PE, Mac-Moune Lai F, et al. Kaposiform hemangioendothelioma: a study of 33 cases emphasizing its pathologic, immunophenotypic, and biologic uniqueness from juvenile hemangioma. Am J Surg Pathol 2004; 28:559.

464. Powell J. Update on hemangiomas and vascular malformations. Curr Opin Pediatr 1999; 11:457.

465. North PE, Waner M, Mizeracki A, et al. A unique microvascular phenotype shared by juvenile hemangiomas and human placenta. Arch Dermatol 2001; 137:559.

466. Beaubien ER, Ball NJ, Storwick GS. Kaposiform hemangioendothelioma: a locally aggressive vascular tumor. J Am Acad Dermatol 1998; 38:799.

467. Dubois J, Garel L, David M, et al. Vascular soft-tissue tumors in infancy: distinguishing features on Doppler sonography. AJR Am J Roentgenol 2002; 178:1541.

468. Sarkar M, Mulliken JB, Kozakewich HP, et al. Thrombocytopenic coagulopathy (Kasabach-Merritt phenomenon) is associated with Kaposiform hemangioendothelioma and not with common infantile hemangioma. Plast Reconstr Surg 1997; 100:1377.

469. Cheuk W, Wong KO, Wong CS, et al. Immunostaining for human herpesvirus 8 latent nuclear antigen-1 helps distinguish Kaposi sarcoma from its mimickers. Am J Clin Pathol 2004; 121:335.

470. Hu B, Lachman R, Phillips J, et al. Kasabach-Merritt syndrome-associated kaposiform hemangioendothelioma successfully treated with cyclophosphamide, vincristine, and actinomycin D. J Pediatr Hematol Oncol 1998; 20:567.

471. Wells GC, Whimster IW. Subcutaneous angiolymphoid hyperplasia with eosinophilia. Br J Dermatol 1969; 81:1.

472. Olsen TG, Helwig EB. Angiolymphoid hyperplasia with eosinophilia. A clinicopathologic study of 116 patients. J Am Acad Dermatol 1985; 12:781.

473. Reed RJ, Terazakis N. Subcutaneous angioblastic lymphoid hyperplasia with eosinophilia (Kimura's disease). Cancer 1972; 29:489.

474. Cornelius RS, Biddinger PW, Gluckman JL. Angiolymphoid hyperplasia with eosinophilia of the head and neck. AJNR Am J Neuroradiol 1995; 16:916.

475. Fetsch JF, Weiss SW. Observations concerning the pathogenesis of epithelioid hemangioma (angiolymphoid hyperplasia). Mod Pathol 1991; 4:449.

476. Fletcher CDM, Unni KK, Mertens F. Epithelioid Hemangioma. In World Health Organization Classification Of Tumours. Pathology and Genetics. Tumours of Soft Tissue and Bone. 2001; 159–160.

477. Sakamoto F, Hashimoto T, Takenouchi T, et al. Angiolymphoid hyperplasia with eosinophilia presenting multinucleated cells in histology: an ultrastructural study. J Cutan Pathol 1998; 25:322.

478. Mendlick MR, Nelson M, Pickering D, et al. Translocation t(1;3)(p36.3;q25) is a nonrandom aberration in epithelioid hemangioendothelioma. Am J Surg Pathol 2001; 25:684.

479. Kaur T, Sandhu K, Gupta S, et al. Treatment of angiolymphoid hyperplasia with eosinophilia with the carbon dioxide laser. J Dermatolog Treat 2004; 15:328.

480. Miller CJ, Ioffreda MD, Ammirati CT. Mohs micrographic surgery for angiolymphoid hyperplasia with eosinophilia. Dermatol Surg 2004; 30:1169.

481. Gupta G, Munro CS. Angiolymphoid hyperplasia with eosinophilia: successful treatment with pulsed dye laser using the double pulse technique. Br J Dermatol 2000; 143:214.

482. Shenefelt PD, Rinker M, Caradonna S. A case of angiolymphoid hyperplasia with eosinophilia treated with intralesional interferon alfa-2a. Arch Dermatol 2000; 136:837.

483. Redondo P, Del Olmo J, Idoate M. Angiolymphoid hyperplasia with eosinophilia successfully treated with imiquimod. Br J Dermatol 2004; 151:1110.

484. Satpathy A, Moss C, Raafat F, et al. Spontaneous regression of a rare tumour in a child: angiolymphoid hyperplasia with eosinophilia of the hand: case report and review of the literature. Br J Plast Surg 2005; 58:865.

485. Beral V, Peterman TA, Berkelman RL, et al. Kaposi's sarcoma among persons with AIDS: a sexually transmitted infection? Lancet 1990; 335:123.

486. Pica F, Volpi A. Transmission of human herpesvirus 8: an update. Curr Opin Infect Dis 2007; 20:152.

487. Martin JN, Ganem DE, Osmond DH, et al. Sexual transmission and the natural history of human herpesvirus 8 infection. N Engl J Med 1998; 338:948.

488. Regamey N, Tamm M, Wernli M, et al. Transmission of human herpesvirus 8 infection from renal-transplant donors to recipients. N Engl J Med 1998; 339:1358.

489. Hladik W, Dollard SC, Mermin J, et al. Transmission of human herpesvirus 8 by blood transfusion. N Engl J Med 2006; 355:1331.

490. Dukers NH, Rezza G. Human herpesvirus 8 epidemiology: what we do and do not know. AIDS 2003; 17:1717.

491. Whitby D, Marshall VA, Bagni RK, et al. Reactivation of Kaposi's sarcoma-associated herpesvirus by natural products from Kaposi's sarcoma endemic regions. Int J Cancer 2007; 120:321.

492. Yamamoto Y, Teruya K, Katano H, et al. Rapidly progressive human herpesvirus 8-associated solid anaplastic lymphoma in a patient with AIDS—associated Kaposi sarcoma. Leuk Lymphoma 2003; 44:1631.

493. Piette WW. The incidence of second malignancies in subsets of Kaposi's sarcoma. J Am Acad Dermatol 1987; 16:855.

494. Kato N, Harada M, Yamashiro K. Kaposi's sarcoma associated with lung cancer and immunosuppression. J Dermatol 1996; 23:564.

495. Franceschi S, Arniani S, Balzi D, et al. Survival of classic Kaposi's sarcoma and risk of second cancer. Br J Cancer 1996; 74:1812.

496. Hjalgrim H, Frisch M, Pukkala E, et al. Risk of second cancers in classical Kaposi's sarcoma. Int J Cancer 1997; 73:840.

497. Chen Z, Smith KJ, Skelton HG, et al. Telomerase activity in Kaposi's sarcoma, squamous cell carcinoma, and basal cell carcinoma. Exp Biol Med (Maywood) 2001; 226:753.

498. Casalone R, Albini A, Righi R, et al. Nonrandom chromosome changes in Kaposi sarcoma: cytogenetic and FISH results in a new cell line (KS-IMM) and literature review. Cancer Genet Cytogenet 2001; 124:16.

499. Judde JG, Lacoste V, Briere J, et al. Monoclonality or oligoclonality of human herpesvirus 8 terminal repeat sequences in Kaposi's sarcoma and other diseases. J Natl Cancer Inst 2000; 92:729.

500. Gill PS, Tsai YC, Rao AP, et al. Evidence for multiclonality in multicentric Kaposi's sarcoma. Proc Natl Acad Sci U S A 1998; 95:8257.

501. Davis DA, Scott DM. Lymphangioma-like Kaposi's sarcoma: etiology and literature review. J Am Acad Dermatol 2000; 43:123.

502. Smith KJ, Nelson A, Angritt P, et al. Kaposi's sarcoma in women: a clinicopathologic study. J Cutan Med Surg 1999; 3:132.

503. Falcone S, Murphy BJ, Weinfeld A. Gastric manifestations of AIDS: radiographic findings on upper gastrointestinal examination. Gastrointest Radiol 1991; 16:95.

504. Radin R. HIV infection: analysis in 259 consecutive patients with abnormal abdominal CT findings. Radiology 1995; 197:712.

505. Kao GF, Johnson FB, Sulica VI. The nature of hyaline (eosinophilic) globules and vascular slits of Kaposi's sarcoma. Am J Dermatopathol 1990; 12:256.

506. Senba M, Itakura H, Yamashita H, et al. Eosinophilic globules in Kaposi's sarcoma. A histochemical, immunohistochemical, and ultrastructural study. Acta Pathol Jpn 1986; 36:1327.

507. DeFatta RJ, Verret DJ, Adelson RT, et al. Kaposiform hemangioendothelioma: case report and literature review. Laryngoscope 2005; 115:1789.

508. Sironi M, Marchini R, Taccagni GL, et al. Juvenile cutaneous angiosarcoma following radiotherapy of a haemangioma. Pathologica 1988; 80:235.

509. Nanus DM, Kelsen D, Clark DG. Radiation-induced angiosarcoma. Cancer 1987; 60:777.

510. Del Mastro L, Garrone O, Guenzi M, et al. Angiosarcoma of the residual breast after conservative surgery and radiotherapy for primary carcinoma. Ann Oncol 1994; 5:163.

511. Mark RJ, Poen JC, Tran LM, et al. Angiosarcoma. A report of 67 patients and a review of the literature. Cancer 1996; 77:2400.

512. Schmid H, Zietz C. Human herpesvirus 8 and angiosarcoma: analysis of 40 cases and review of the literature. Pathology 2005; 37:284.

513. Hiatt KM, Nelson AM, Lichy JH, et al. Classic Kaposi Sarcoma (CKS) in the United States over the last two decades: A clinicopathologic and molecular study of 438 non-HIV related KS patients with comparison to HIV-related KS. Mod Pathol 2008; 21(5):572–582.

514. Zidan J, Robenstein W, Abzah A, et al. Treatment of Kaposi's sarcoma with vinblastine in patients with disseminated dermal disease. Isr Med Assoc J 2001; 3:251.

515. Cattelan AM, Trevenzoli M, Aversa SM. Recent advances in the treatment of AIDS-related Kaposi's sarcoma. Am J Clin Dermatol 2002; 3:451.

516. Aldenhoven M, Barlo NP, Sanders CJ. Therapeutic strategies for epidemic Kaposi's sarcoma. Int J STD AIDS 2006; 17:571.

517. Berman B, Perez OA, Zell D. Update on rosacea and anti-inflammatory-dose doxycycline. Drugs Today (Barc) 2007; 43:27.

518. Pu LL, Smith PD, Payne WG, et al. Overexpression of transforming growth factor beta-2 and its receptor in rhinophyma: an alternative mechanism of pathobiology. Ann Plast Surg 2000; 45:515.

519. Payne WG, Wang X, Walusimbi M, et al. Further evidence for the role of fibrosis in the pathobiology of rhinophyma. Ann Plast Surg 2002; 48:641.

520. Palleschi GM, Torchia D. Rosacea in a monozygotic twin. Australas J Dermatol 2007; 48:132.

521. Yazici AC, Tamer L, Ikizoglu G, et al. GSTM1 and GSTT1 null genotypes as possible heritable factors of rosacea. Photodermatol Photoimmunol Photomed 2006; 22:208.

522. Sapadin AN, Fleischmajer R. Tetracyclines: nonantibiotic properties and their clinical implications. J Am Acad Dermatol 2006; 54:258.

523. van Zuuren EJ, Gupta AK, Gover MD, et al. Systematic review of rosacea treatments. J Am Acad Dermatol 2007; 56:107.

524. Skala M, Delaney G, Towell V, et al. Rhinophyma treated with kilovoltage photons. Australas J Dermatol 2005; 46:88.

525. Payne WG, Ko F, Anspaugh S, et al. Down-regulating causes of fibrosis with tamoxifen: a possible cellular/molecular approach to treat rhinophyma. Ann Plast Surg 2006; 56:301.

526. Oelzner S, Elsner P. Bilateral chondrodermatitis nodularis chronica helicis on the free border of the helix in a woman. J Am Acad Dermatol 2003; 49:720.

527. Grigoryants V, Qureshi H, Patterson JW, et al. Pediatric chondrodermatitis nodularis helicis. J Craniofac Surg 2007; 18:228.

528. Rogers NE, Farris PK, Wang AR. Juvenile chondrodermatitis nodularis helicis: a case report and literature review. Pediatr Dermatol 2003; 20:488.

529. Magro CM, Frambach GE, Crowson AN. Chondrodermatitis nodularis helicis as a marker of internal disease [corrected] associated with microvascular injury. J Cutan Pathol 2005; 32:329.

530. Sasaki T, Nishizawa H, Sugita Y. Chondrodermatitis nodularis helicis in childhood dermatomyositis. Br J Dermatol 1999; 141:363.

531. Bottomley WW, Goodfield MD. Chondrodermatitis nodularis helicis occurring with systemic sclerosis–an underreported association? Clin Exp Dermatol 1994; 19:219.

532. Bard JW. Chondrodermatitis nodularis chronica helicis. Dermatologica 1981; 163:376.

533. Cribier B, Scrivener Y, Peltre B. Neural hyperplasia in chondrodermatitis nodularis chronica helicis. J Am Acad Dermatol 2006; 55:844.

534. Weedon D. Elastotic nodules of the ear. J Cutan Pathol 1981; 8:429.

535. Sinclair P. Excision technique for chondrodermatitis nodularis helicis. Australas J Dermatol 1996; 37:61.

536. de Ru JA, Lohuis PJ, Saleh HA, et al. Treatment of chondrodermatitis nodularis with removal of the underlying cartilage alone: retrospective analysis of experience in 37 lesions. J Laryngol Otol 2002; 116:677.

537. Hudson-Peacock MJ, Cox NH, Lawrence CM. The long-term results of cartilage removal alone for the treatment of chondrodermatitis nodularis. Br J Dermatol 1999; 141:703.

538. Moncrieff M, Sassoon EM. Effective treatment of chondrodermatitis nodularis chronica helicis using a conservative approach. Br J Dermatol 2004; 150:892.

539. Sanu A, Koppana R, Snow DG. Management of chondrodermatitis nodularis chronica helicis using a "doughnut pillow." J Laryngol Otol 2007; 121(11):1096–1098.

540. Kavanagh GM, Bradfield JW, Collins CM, et al. Weathering nodules of the ear: a clinicopathological study. Br J Dermatol 1996; 135:550.

541. Amichai B, Shiri J. Weathering nodules of the ear in a young woman. Br J Dermatol 1997; 137:659.

542. Hamilton KS, Johnson S, Smoller BR. The role of androgen receptors in the clinical course of nevus sebaceus of Jadassohn. Mod Pathol 2001; 14:539.

543. Terenzi V, Indrizzi E, Buonaccorsi S, et al. Nevus sebaceus of Jadassohn. J Craniofac Surg 2006; 17:1234.

544. Cribier B, Scrivener Y, Grosshans E. Tumors arising in nevus sebaceus: a study of 596 cases. J Am Acad Dermatol 2000; 42:263.

545. Diwan AH, Smith KJ, Brown R, et al. Mucoepidermoid carcinoma arising within nevus sebaceus of Jadassohn. J Cutan Pathol 2003; 30:652.

546. Dalle S, Skowron F, Balme B, et al. Apocrine carcinoma developed in nevus sebaceus of Jadassohn. Eur J Dermatol 2003; 13:487.

547. Miller CJ, Ioffreda MD, Billingsley EM. Sebaceous carcinoma, basal cell carcinoma, trichoadenoma, trichoblastoma, and syringocystadenoma papilliferum arising within a nevus sebaceus. Dermatol Surg 2004; 30:1546.

548. Premalata CS, Kumar RV, Malathi M, et al. Cutaneous leiomyosarcoma, trichoblastoma, and syringocystadenoma papilliferum arising from nevus sebaceus. Int J Dermatol 2007; 46:306.

549. Kazakov DV, Calonje E, Zelger B, et al. Sebaceous carcinoma arising in nevus sebaceus of Jadassohn: a clinicopathological study of five cases. Am J Dermatopathol 2007; 29:242.

550. Barth PG, Valk J, Kalsbeek GL, et al. Organoid nevus syndrome (linear nevus sebaceus of Jadassohn): clinical and radiological study of a case. Neuropadiatrie 1977; 8:418.

551. Munoz-Perez MA, Garcia-Hernandez MJ, Rios JJ, et al. Sebaceus naevi: a clinicopathologic study. J Eur Acad Dermatol Venereol 2002; 16:319.

552. Traboulsi EI, Zin A, Massicotte SJ, et al. Posterior scleral choristoma in the organoid nevus syndrome (linear nevus sebaceus of Jadassohn). Ophthalmology 1999; 106:2126.

553. Kaddu S, Schaeppi H, Kerl H, et al. Basaloid neoplasms in nevus sebaceus. J Cutan Pathol 2000; 27:327.

554. Hughes SM, Wilkerson AE, Winfield HL, et al. Familial nevus sebaceus in dizygotic male twins. J Am Acad Dermatol 2006; 54:S47.

555. Benedetto L, Sood U, Blumenthal N, et al. Familial nevus sebaceus. J Am Acad Dermatol 1990; 23:130.

556. Laino L, Steensel MA, Innocenzi D, et al. Familial occurrence of nevus sebaceus of Jadassohn: another case of paradominant inheritance? Eur J Dermatol 2001; 11:97.

557. Sahl WJ Jr. Familial nevus sebaceus of Jadassohn: occurrence in three generations. J Am Acad Dermatol 1990; 22:853.

24

Diseases of the Eye and Ocular Adnexa

Harry H. Brown

*Departments of Pathology and Ophthalmology, Harvey and Bernice Jones Eye Institute,
University of Arkansas for Medical Sciences, Little Rock, Arkansas, U.S.A.*

I. INTRODUCTION

The thought of pathological examination of ocular tissues to the general surgical pathologist may vary anywhere from apathy to annoyance to anathema, largely because the eye is a small and very complex organ. Its disease processes can be arcane, and accurate pathological diagnosis may require detailed clinical information, labor-intensive gross examination and histological techniques, and discriminating microscopic evaluation, all with a resultant low cost-benefit ratio (literally and figuratively). Many ocular pathological processes are visible to the ophthalmologist clinically by biomicroscopy (slit lamp) or ophthalmoscopy, or by special instrumentation such as optical coherence tomography (OCT) or ultrasound biomicroscopy, and at higher magnification than usually available to the general surgical pathologist. Thus, clinically apparent findings may go undetected or unrecognized at the gross bench. Likewise, with such refined techniques, pathological processes are also often accurately diagnosed clinically and treated, so that a pathological diagnosis may not be necessary or critical to patient therapy and treatment. Perhaps the most dramatic example, melanoma of the uveal tract, is one of the few malignancies treated without a pathological tissue diagnosis.

Nevertheless, an understanding of ocular diseases is necessary for optimal clinicopathological correlation and correct histopathological diagnosis. This chapter, therefore, will attempt to be a practical guide for the general surgical pathologist, dealing with the more common pathological specimens encountered. As such, it is organized not by specific tissue per se, but in addition by specimen type and procedure and the usual pathological processes for such procedures (i.e., the most common pathological entities the surgical pathologist might encounter when examining a specific specimen type). For instance, a corneal biopsy is almost always done to search for an infectious organism and virtually never for identifying a corneal dystrophy.

The scope of this chapter is also limited to only important or unique aspects of diseases that also occur at other sites. Many diseases of the eyelids and orbit that also occur in the skin and soft tissues elsewhere in the body are not described here, unless there are specific circumstances about their involvement of the ocular adnexa. The reader is referred to other chapters in this text for more detailed information about such entities. For more detailed and thorough investigation of specific ocular disease processes, a variety of resources are available (1–13).

II. EYELIDS

A. Anatomy

The anatomy of the eyelids is specialized primarily to provide protection to the eye in general and the cornea in particular. From without inward, the eyelids consist of the skin, subcutaneous tissue, orbicularis oculi muscle, tarsus (or tarsal plate) containing meibomian (sebaceous) glands, and conjunctiva (Fig. 1A, B). The skin of the eyelid is thin, with reduced epidermal thickness, diminished rete pegs, and more rarefied papillary and reticular dermis than in most other skin sites. Subcutaneous tissue likewise is extremely thin, if present at all, resulting in relatively close approximation of the orbicularis oculi skeletal muscle fibers to the skin, so that they are not infrequently present in skin biopsies or excisions of eyelid tissue. The tarsus gives structure and support to the eyelids and is better developed in the upper eyelid than the lower. It is composed of dense collagenous connective tissue (and not cartilage, as sometimes presumed), and surrounds the lobules of sebaceous glands, whose ducts open along the lid margin and whose secretions provide an evaporation retardant to the tear film. The palpebral conjunctiva lining the inner surface of the eyelids is very thin, with minimal stroma and tight adherence to the tarsus. The free edge of the eyelid, known as the lid margin, contains the cilia (eyelashes) and their associated sebaceous glands (glands of Zeis) and modified apocrine sweat glands (glands of Moll).

B. Specimen Handling

Eyelid skin specimens are handled in the same manner as dermatological specimens from other sites,

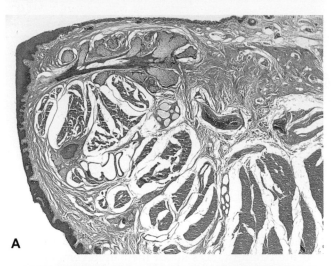

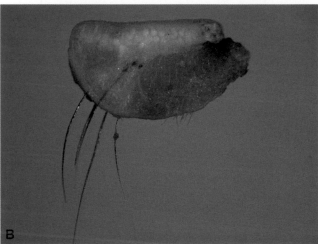

Figure 1 (**A**) Histological cross section of the eyelid, showing anatomical landmarks and relationships (H&E original magnification 25×). (**B**) Many of the eyelid structures may be visualized on magnified macroscopic examination of a cross section.

except for full-thickness eyelid wedge resections. These may be triangular or pentagonal in shape, with the lid margin (the free edge of the eyelid defining the palpebral fissure in vivo) at the base. The specimen can be oriented properly by determining whether the specimen is from the right or left side and upper or lower eyelid. The medial (or nasal), lateral (or temporal), and, if pentagonal, deep (superior if upper eyelid, inferior if lower eyelid) surgical margins should be inked, tangentially shaved (1-mm thick), and submitted to be embedded en face. The remaining central portion of the eyelid should then be serially sectioned perpendicular to the lid margin and submitted entirely, embedded in sequence and en face, so as to obtain histological full-thickness cross sections of the eyelid.

C. Diseases

Diseases that commonly affect the eyelids are generally the same that occur elsewhere on the body, and particularly, in the lower eyelid, are those that are prone to develop in sun-exposed sites. Those that result in common surgical pathology specimens include epidermal cyst, hidrocystoma, syringoma, acrochordon, squamous papilloma, verruca, molluscum contagiosum, melanocytic nevi, seborrheic keratosis, actinic keratosis, and basal cell carcinoma (14–18). These are all familiar entities to the general surgical pathologist and only rarely present challenges in diagnosis.

Basal Cell Carcinoma

Basal cell carcinoma is by far the most common malignant eyelid neoplasm, accounting for over 90% of malignancies, with squamous cell carcinoma, sebaceous carcinoma, and melanoma comprising the bulk of the remainder (19–21). They are more common on the sun-exposed lower eyelids than the relatively protected upper eyelids. Incidence increases with age, although occasionally young adults may be affected and consideration then given to the possibility of basal cell nevus syndrome (22,23). The typical clinical picture is one of a discrete, centrally ulcerated white-gray papule with telangiectatic rolled edges. Morpheaform or infiltrative basal cell carcinomas may be more white-yellow and indurated but lack discrete borders or significant elevation. Those that involve the medial canthal region have a propensity to invade deeply, recur more often, and require more extensive resection than at other periocular sites (24). Advanced tumors may cause extensive facial tissue destruction and grotesque cosmetic deformity; invasion of the eye, however, is quite rare (25).

Histopathological diagnosis of basal cell carcinoma relies on both tissue architecture and cellular morphology. Discrete, closely apposed nests of cohesive small epithelial cells with scant cytoplasm, displaying a palisading arrangement of nuclei at the peripheral margins of the nests, are the characteristic findings. Continuity with the basal layer of the epidermis is often present. Mitotic activity may be detected, but is neither atypical nor a prominent feature. The stroma surrounding individual nests is more densely fibrotic than normal dermis. Any of a number of patterns of differentiation may be observed, including keratotic, mucinous, and sebaceous. Cystic nests may result from accumulation of secretory products or cellular degeneration. The morpheaform or infiltrative basal cell carcinoma lacks the well-defined nesting pattern or differentiated features of the nodular type, and instead is identified by tongue-like trabecular cords of basaloid epithelial cells within a fibrotic stroma.

Immunohistochemistry is not necessary for the diagnosis of basal cell carcinoma in the vast majority of cases and is only used when other basaloid-appearing neoplasms such as Merkel cell carcinoma or adenoid cystic carcinoma are being considered.

Pathological specimens vary from incisional to excisional biopsy. More advanced cases may require full-thickness wedge resection of the eyelid. Mohs surgery is common for larger tumors and those involving the medial canthal region; otherwise, standard frozen section technique may be solicited for intraoperative assessment of the adequacy of excision (26). Exenteration is generally reserved for tumors deeply invasive into the orbit (27).

Squamous Cell Carcinoma

Squamous cell carcinoma of the eyelids accounts for 2% to 12% of all eyelid epithelial malignancies, and its incidence is increasing (28,29). In all respects, it is identical to its counterparts in other cutaneous sites and is described in detail elsewhere in this text. Most cases arise in a background of actinic keratosis. Generally, there is a low risk of invasion into the orbit and/or metastasis to regional lymph nodes (30,31). However, at least one study documented regional lymph node metastases in 24% of cases (31).

Sebaceous Tumefactions

Neoplasms of sebaceous differentiation are relatively prevalent in the eyelid in relation to their occurrence elsewhere because of the high number of sebaceous glands per unit area in the eyelid. In addition to the normal pilosebaceous structures of the skin, in the eyelid, there are also sebaceous glands associated with the eyelashes (glands of Zeis) and the sebaceous glands within the tarsal plates (meibomian glands), which are not associated with cilia but open directly onto the eyelid margin and produce an oily surface on the tear film to retard evaporation. Additional sebaceous glands are present as part of the pilosebaceous units in the caruncle, the fleshy nodule within the medial canthus. Any of these sebaceous glands may give rise to either reactive inflammatory (hordeolum or chalazion) and benign (sebaceous hyperplasia or adenoma) or malignant (sebaceous carcinoma) proliferations. Sebaceous carcinomas that arise in the glands of Zeis are more likely to be localized, discrete nodular neoplasms, while those in the meibomian glands may spread diffusely through the conjunctival epithelium and epidermis of the eyelid. This latter process may produce an indurated, red appearance, mimicking a chronic blepharoconjunctivitis and delaying the correct diagnosis for months to years (32–34). Sebaceous neoplasms, particularly adenomas, may be associated with the prior, concurrent, or subsequent development of visceral malignancies of the gastrointestinal tract (Muir–Torre syndrome, an autosomal dominant condition) (35,36). Sebaceous hyperplasia is often present as one feature of acne rosacea in older individuals. Histopathological classification of sebaceous proliferations is based on both architectural and cytomorphological features. Hyperplasia is a multilobular enlargement of histologically normal sebaceous lobules surrounding a dilated central pore. Sebaceous adenoma likewise is a well-differentiated proliferation of sebaceous

lobules, but without a normal architectural arrangement. Both show a single basaloid germinative cell layer at the periphery of the lobules, with rapid evolution to fully differentiated cells with microvesicular cytoplasm, low nuclear–cytoplasmic ratio, and small nuclei without significant nuclear pleomorphism or nucleoli. Mitotic figures are rare and, if present, are confined to the basal layers. Sebaceous cells may extend to the epidermis, but do not extend radially or intraepithelially. Sebaceous carcinoma is variable from well differentiated and similar to adenoma to poorly differentiated and difficult to identify as sebaceous at all. Such poorly differentiated cases may be confused with squamous cell carcinoma by the unwary. Sebaceous carcinoma is characterized by lobules of epithelial cells with high nuclear–cytoplasmic ratio, nuclear enlargement and hyperchromasia, mitotic activity including atypical mitotic figures, and comedo-type necrosis.

Reactive inflammatory processes.

Hordeolum. Hordeolum (stye) is a pustular, self-limited acute inflammation (microabscess) of the eyelid, relatively common in children. It may arise in the glands of Zeis and be present at or near the lid margin and be visible externally (external hordeolum) or, less commonly, in the meibomian glands and noted on eversion of the eyelid (internal hordeolum) (37). It is treated medically or rarely by incision and drainage, and thus does not come to the attention of the surgical pathologist.

Chalazion. Chalazion, in contrast, is a slowly developing, typically painless, subepithelial (and therefore flesh colored) nodule of either upper or lower eyelid that develops in both children and adults. It almost always arises from the meibomian glands and therefore is centered in the tarsus of the eyelid. Interruption in the flow of secretions in the meibomian gland ducts, often a result of chronic blepharitis, precipitates a release of the secretions into the surrounding tarsus and eyelid tissue, with an ensuing granulomatous inflammatory response.

Histopathologically, the granulomas consist of aggregates of epithelioid histiocytes, often centered about optically clear circular spaces corresponding to the foci formerly occupied by the lipid secretions, but now removed during tissue processing (Fig. 2A, B). When such spaces are present, the term "lipogranulomatous inflammation" is preferred; when not, infectious etiologies should be considered and appropriate histochemical stains for fungal and acid-fast bacilli employed. Multinucleated giant cells may be present, but in small numbers; presence of Touton giant cells is not a feature of chalazion. A surrounding admixture of lymphocytes and plasma cells is typical and may be prominent depending on the degree of evolution of the inflammatory reaction.

Rare cases of mycobacterial infection simulating lipogranulomatous inflammation have been described, in which the central clear spaces within the granulomas are rimmed by acute inflammatory cells, as opposed to the usual cuffing by epithelioid histiocytes (38). Again, histochemical stains for acid-fast organisms should be employed when this pattern of inflammation is encountered.

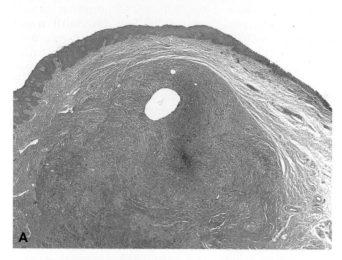

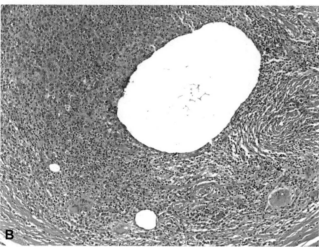

Figure 2 (**A**) Histological section of lipogranulomatous inflammation at the eyelid margin (chalazion) (H&E, original magnification 50×). (**B**) Higher power-demonstrating epithelioid histiocytes surrounding the central clear space and scattered multinucleated giant cells within the surrounding chronic inflammatory infiltrate (H&E, original magnification 200×).

The usual surgical procedure for chalazion is incision through the conjunctiva and curettage; thus, the pathological specimen consists of multiple minute fragments of irregularly shaped white-tan soft tissue, which should be filtered through a tea bag and submitted as such. Rarely, an excision of the nodule may be received, and more likely, in a recurrent case, where the clinical differential may include sebaceous or other neoplasms (39–41).

Sebaceous Hyperplasia. Proliferation of sebaceous glands is relatively common on the face, particularly the cheeks, in adults, presenting as one or more clustered small umbilicated soft yellow papules (42). They may follow chronic dermatitides or occur in the setting of acne rosacea. Only when they are clinically confused with other neoplasms such as basal cell carcinoma do they reach the surgical pathologist.

Histopathological features of sebaceous hyperplasia are a circumscribed, nodular expansion of enlarged sebaceous gland lobules surrounding a central duct. Basal germinative cells at the periphery rapidly develop cytoplasmic enlargement and microvesicular clearing as the cells produce their lipid secretory product. No cytological atypia or mitotic activity is present.

Sebaceous neoplasms.

Sebaceous Adenoma. Sebaceous adenoma is the most common type of sebaceous proliferation associated with Muir–Torre syndrome (sebaceous neoplasms, keratoacanthomas, and gastrointestinal malignancies) and, therefore when encountered, should elicit a comment in the surgical pathology report as to that possibility (36). Muir–Torre syndrome patients have been shown to harbor mutations in the DNA mismatch repair gene MSH2, or less commonly, MLH1 (43,44). Adenomas are rare in the eyelids, usually solitary, and differ from hyperplastic papules by being larger and lacking umbilication. When excised, they exhibit closely apposed lobules of sebaceous cells with slightly less orderly maturation from basal germinative cells at the periphery to mature sebocytes with abundant microvesicular cytoplasm centrally. Lobules are not arrayed around a central duct as in sebaceous hyperplasia. Mitotic activity is rare. Pagetoid intraepithelial infiltration by sebaceous cells is not a feature of sebaceous adenoma.

Sebaceous Carcinoma. While uncommon, as malignant neoplasms of the eyelid go (1–5%), sebaceous carcinoma (sebaceous cell carcinoma and sebaceous cell adenocarcinoma) is one of the most deadly, with five-year mortality rates as high as 25% (45). Improved survival has been documented in more recent series, with only 3% to 6% death rates (46,47).

Sebaceous carcinoma is more common in the upper eyelid than lower, but may involve both in a diffuse and/or multicentric fashion (46). Bilateral ocular involvement has not been reported. Women are twice as likely to be affected as men. Most cases develop in the sixth to seventh decade, although younger patients have been described, particularly those who have received radiation for retinoblastoma (48,49). The clinical appearance may vary from a discrete nodule, either deep or pedunculated, to a diffuse induration (Fig. 3A, B). The latter often defies diagnosis by posing ("masquerade syndrome") as a chronic blepharoconjunctivitis, and only when there is a lack of response to months, or even years, of topical medications is the possibility entertained and then confirmed by biopsy (32–34). The meibomian glands are the most common point of origin for sebaceous carcinoma, especially when the diffuse clinical presentation is manifest (46).

Histopathological examination of sebaceous carcinoma may vary from a lobular nesting pattern of well-differentiated cells showing clear-cut cytological sebaceous differentiation to poorly differentiated infiltrative cords and single cells without apparent cytoplasmic lipid (Fig. 4A, B). Comedo-type necrosis within lobules is another feature seen in sebaceous carcinoma (Fig. 4C). It is in the poorly differentiated

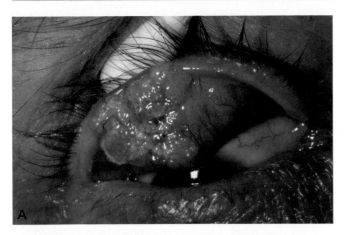

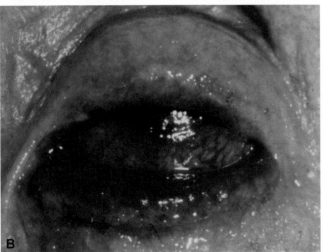

Figure 3 (**A**) Sebaceous carcinoma involving the upper eyelid palpebral conjunctiva as a multilobulated yellow mass with clinically discrete margins. (**B**) Sebaceous carcinoma masquerading as a chronic conjunctivitis, with diffuse indurated upper and lower eyelids and loss of cilia.

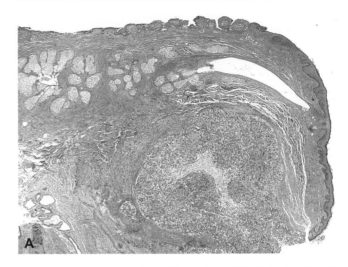

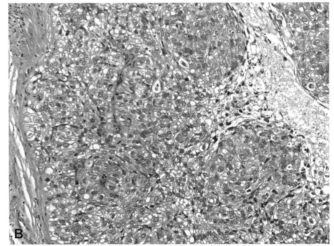

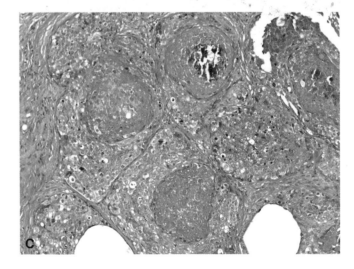

Figure 4 (**A**) Histological section of sebaceous carcinoma arising in the gland of Zeis, displacing the meibomian gland duct posteriorly (H&E, original magnification 50×). (**B**) Well-differentiated sebaceous carcinoma with microvesicular clearing of the cytoplasm due to intracytoplasmic lipid (H&E, original magnification 200×). (**C**) Comedonecrosis with calcification in a poorly differentiated sebaceous carcinoma (H&E, original magnification 200×).

tumors that diagnostic confusion arises, particularly with squamous and basal cell carcinomas. Sebaceous carcinoma may infiltrate the conjunctival and/or eyelid epithelium far afield, as a pagetoid pattern of single cells or small clusters of atypical cells (Fig. 5A). Such a pattern can create diagnostic confusion with an amelanotic malignant melanoma. Complete replacement of the surface epithelium may also occur and mimic squamous cell carcinoma in situ (Fig. 5B). Occasionally, there may be extensive intraepithelial involvement without an invasive component (50,51). In all these scenarios, the potential for histopathological misdiagnosis and subsequent inappropriate treatment and follow-up exists. A battery of histochemical and immunohistochemical stains may be necessary to determine the correct diagnosis (Table 1) (Fig. 5C) (52–56). In particular, a microvesicular intracytoplasmic pattern of epithelial membrane antigen (EMA) positivity is very helpful in diagnosis, but is rarely present in poorly differentiated cases.

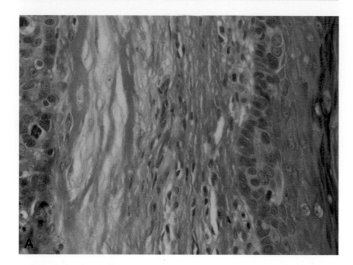
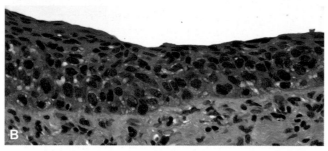
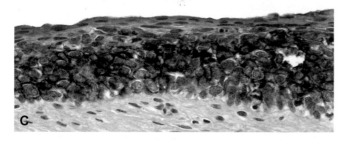

Figure 5 (**A**) Pagetoid involvement of the eyelid epidermis in sebaceous carcinoma. Note the identical cytomorphology with the invasive carcinoma at the bottom of the photomicrograph (H&E, original magnification 400×). (**B**) Intraepithelial sebaceous carcinoma with sheet-like, nearly complete effacement of the conjunctival epithelium. This histological pattern is easily confused with conjunctival intraepithelial neoplasia grade 3 (H&E, original magnification 400×). (**C**) Immunohistochemical stain berEP4 demonstrates strong positivity within the sebaceous carcinoma, but not in the compressed conjunctival epithelium at the surface (berEP4, original magnification 400×).

Table 1 Immunohistochemical Stains in The Differential Diagnosis of Malignant Epithelial Neoplasms of The Eyelid

Antibody	Sebaceous carcinoma	Basal cell carcinoma	Squamous cell carcinoma
AE1/AE3	+	+	+
EMA	+	−	Focal + to +
BRST-1	− to focal +	−	− to focal +
Cam 5.2	+	− to weak +	−

Accurate pathological diagnosis is important prognostically, since both basal and squamous cell carcinomas in the eyelids have a much lower rate of metastatic spread and overall mortality. Intraepithelial involvement as described above is an important factor in distinguishing well-differentiated sebaceous carcinoma from sebaceous adenoma, particularly when its radial extent exceeds the underlying lobular proliferation.

Histochemical stains to demonstrate intracytoplasmic lipid may be beneficial, but this requires frozen sections of tissue that has not been routinely processed and paraffin embedded. When given advance notice that sebaceous carcinoma is in the clinical differential, initial retention of a portion of the tissue is indicated. Formalin fixation does not remove the lipid, but maintaining the adherence of the tissue to the slide during the staining process can be challenging. Osmium staining of tissue processed for electron microscopy is another method of demonstrating intracytoplasmic lipid in questionable cases. As mentioned above, immunohistochemical panels may be helpful in differentiating poorly differentiated carcinomas of the eyelid and conjunctiva.

When the diagnosis of sebaceous carcinoma is confirmed, the usual course prior to definitive excision is to perform map biopsies of the palpebral, forniceal, and bulbar conjunctiva to determine the extent of intraepithelial involvement. Such biopsies are small and often difficult to interpret because of orientation problems and artifacts of handling, causing partial to complete loss of the epithelial surface. For these reasons and the additional artifacts produced by freezing, intraoperative consultations are not indicated for map biopsies. Frozen sections may be used at the time of definitive excision, however, again with the caveats listed above. In particular, distinction of conjunctival goblet cells as pagetoid tumor cells can be problematic.

Pathological parameters with prognostic implications, to be addressed in excision specimens, include tumor size, differentiation, intraepithelial spread, extension into the orbit, vascular, or lymphatic space invasion, and margin status. Overexpression of p53 has been correlated with clinically advanced cases (54).

Depending on the extent of invasive and intraepithelial involvement, management may vary from wide excision with cryotherapy at the margins to exenteration and regional lymph node sampling or dissection. Topical chemotherapy (mitomycin-C) may be beneficial for extensive or suspected pagetoid spread (57,58). Locally advanced disease with invasion into the orbit or the eye is rare. Recurrence rates vary but may be as high as 30%. Sebaceous carcinoma is metastatic to regional lymph nodes in up to 25% to 30% of cases; the incidence appears to be decreasing in more recent series, perhaps because of increased awareness, earlier detection, and more extensive mapping by ophthalmologists (46,47). Distant metastasis is uncommon. Visceral metastases typically involve the lung and liver, and less often the brain and bone (45).

Xanthelasma

Although only peripherally related to sebaceous tumefactions in that the cells of interest contain intracytoplasmic lipid, xanthelasma is a relatively common periocular condition and is described here because it is occasionally excised for cosmetic reasons. The yellow-tan plaques of xanthelasma cluster around the medial canthus bilaterally, involving both upper and lower eyelids (Fig. 6A) (59). They typically appear in middle age. Up to one-half of patients with xanthelasma will have an associated hyperlipidemia, usually hypercholesterolemia (59). Recurrences are relatively common following excision.

Histopathologically, xanthelasma are due to accumulations of lipid-laden histiocytes within the reticular dermis of the eyelid in a perivascular distribution (Fig. 6B). Occasional multinucleated histiocytes are present. No histological differences are apparent between patients with and without hyperlipidemia.

Treatment is for cosmesis only, and alternative therapies to excision include topical interferon alpha-2b, trichloroacetic acid, and laser ablation (59,60).

III. CONJUNCTIVA

A. Anatomy

The conjunctiva is the thin mucous membrane lining the inner surface of the eyelid and reflected onto the anterior epibulbar surface in the superior and inferior fornices. Thus, it can be subdivided into palpebral, forniceal, and epibulbar locations, each with differing histomorphology. The palpebral conjunctiva begins at the mucocutaneous junction along the eyelid margin and is tightly bound to the tarsal plate with only a thin, compressed stroma. The conjunctival epithelium is also thin and may show slight crypt-like invaginations into the stroma, known as pseudoglands of Henle. Accessory lacrimal glands are present subepithelially at the edge of the tarsus (glands of Wolfring) and in the fornix (glands of Krause). The fornix contains the highest density of goblet cells within the epithelium. The epibulbar conjunctival stroma, highly vascular within a loose collagenous background, again thins toward its termination at the corneoscleral limbus. A mild lymphoplasmacytic component is normally present.

B. Specimen Handling

Although diseases of the conjunctiva are relatively frequent in the clinical practice of ophthalmology, only few require surgical biopsy for diagnosis or excision for treatment. The most common specimens removed from the conjunctiva are papillomatous epithelial proliferations and pigmented lesions (61). Other processes that might come to the attention of the surgical pathologist are biopsies of granulomata in suspected sarcoidosis, lymphoproliferative disorders, amyloid deposits, and suspected autoimmune disease such as ocular cicatricial pemphigoid.

Biopsy and limited excision of conjunctiva are relatively easy and safe procedures, with minimal morbidity if the area removed is small. However, removal of significant portions of the conjunctiva risks the possibility of subsequent dry eye and scarring with symblepharon formation (adhesion of the eye to the eyelid), with resultant problems of ocular motility and eyelid restriction leading to corneal exposure.

Problems with conjunctival excisions from the surgical pathologist's perspective are mainly due to the handling and fixation of the specimen. The conjunctiva is rich in elastic fibers and tends to curl into a crinkled ball when excised, and if placed in formalin in that shape, it is for all intents and purposes impossible to evaluate margins of excision, or obtain properly oriented histological sections for

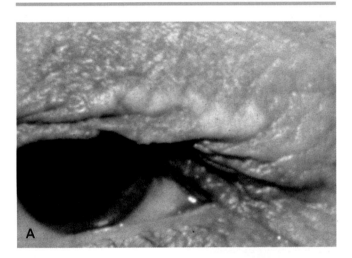

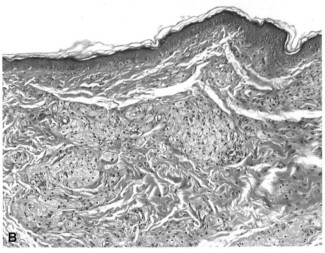

Figure 6 (A) Coalescing yellow nodules of xanthelasma involving the upper eyelid of a patient with dermatochalasis. (B) Histological section of xanthelasma, demonstrating clusters of lipid-laden histiocytes in a perivascular distribution within the dermis (H&E, original magnification 200×).

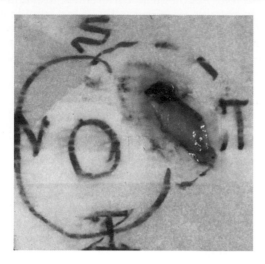

Figure 7 Intraoperative orientation of a conjunctival excision specimen from the left eye, demonstrating the optimal method for subsequent pathological examination.

examination and diagnosis. Ideally, conjunctival excisions should be laid flat, stromal side down on an absorbent paper, for 10 to 15 seconds, and then the specimen, adherent to the paper, placed in formalin, tissue side down. Once fixed, the tissue is then amenable to inking and sectioning. While on the paper, the specimen may also be oriented by the surgeon, by drawing a diagram as to the location on the eye, so that even more detailed information regarding margin status may be possible (Fig. 7). Small specimens (3–4 mm) may be submitted as received; larger specimens should be bisected or treated like a skin ellipse. Since the lesions commonly occur at the limbus, and the cornea is unlikely to be excised due to subsequent scarring, the limbal margin is usually the closest and most likely to be involved. If the specimen is received oriented, it should be sectioned such that the limbal margin is sampled. If peripheral corneal involvement is appreciated clinically, corneal epithelial debridement is often performed and submitted for cytological evaluation with or without cell block. If so, then the limbal tissue margin status becomes irrelevant.

Conjunctival specimens requiring special handling include those cases in which a lymphoproliferative process, a sebaceous neoplasm, or an autoimmune disorder such as ocular cicatricial pemphigoid is suspected. In these situations, the tissue should be submitted fresh so that ancillary studies such as flow cytometry for lymphoproliferative disorders and frozen sections for oil red O stains in sebaceous neoplasms or immunofluorescence in ocular cicatricial pemphigoid may be obtained. Optimal handling of these tissues therefore requires prior notification by the surgeon and timely handling by the surgical pathologist.

C. Diseases

Conjunctival Intraepithelial Neoplasia

Clinical features. Most cases of conjunctival intraepithelial neoplasia (CIN) arise within the interpalpebral fissure and are associated with solar elastosis of the conjunctival stroma, and it is presumed that sun exposure is causally related. Lesions usually arise at the nasal or temporal limbus and may spread both centripetally (onto the cornea) and centrifugally (Fig. 8A, B). They occur more commonly in middle-aged to elderly men with a significant history of sun exposure. CIN overlying solar elastosis is usually a discrete and circumscribed plaque-like thickening of the epithelium and is often keratinizing, resulting in the clinical appearance of leukoplakia. Some authors segregate this pattern of dysplasia from CIN, referring to these lesions instead as actinic keratosis (62). They also categorize the degree of dysplasia in these cases on nuclear features alone.

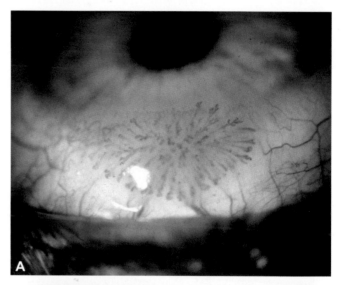

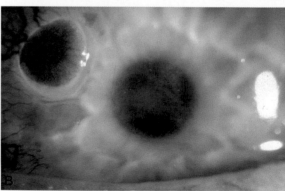

Figure 8 (A) Limbal module with papillomatous clinical features, which proved to be conjunctival intraepithelial neoplasia on pathological examination. Note the prominent vasculature of the papillary fronds. (B) Corneal intraepithelial neoplasia manifested by a diffuse frosting of the corneal epithelium, best seen in the pupillary zone. A disrcrete polypoid nodule with papillomatous features is present in the midperipheral cornea.

Nonkeratinizing CIN may be papillomatous and indistinguishable clinically from benign papillomas or ill-defined, thickened, gelatinous, gray discolorations of the conjunctiva and/or cornea. The latter clinical variant is not restricted to sun-exposed areas of the cornea and conjunctiva. Rare cases of corneal intraepithelial neoplasia without conjunctival involvement have been reported. Human papillomavirus (HPV) subtypes 16 and 18 have been identified by immunophenotyping and polymerase chain reaction (PCR) in some cases of CIN, although the correlation is not as strong as in the cervix, and the studies have been widely disparate in HPV detection, varying from 0% to 100% of cases (63–65).

CIN is graded using the same criteria as with cervical intraepithelial neoplasia: grade I (mild dysplasia; basal third of the epithelium involved); grade II (moderate dysplasia; up to two-thirds of epithelial thickness involved); and grade III (severe dysplasia/carcinoma in situ) (Fig. 9A, B). The WHO classification regards carcinoma in situ as a separate entity (66). The

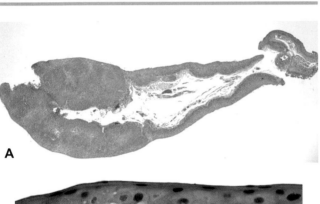

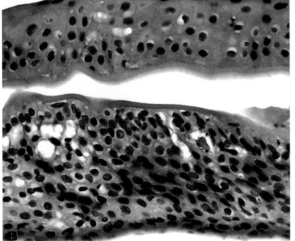

Figure 9 (A) Conjunctival intraepithelial neoplasia with marked acanthosis. The apparent papillomatous architecture in this case is an artifact of the tissue being folded upon itself (H&E, original magnification 20×). (B) Histological comparison of conjunctival epithelium with normal architecture and cytomorphology (*top*) with full-thickness dysplasia (*bottom*). Note the loss of maturation, nuclear hyperchromasia, and increased nucleus:cytoplasm ratio (H&E, original magnification 200×).

surgical pathologist should include in the report whether any associated solar damage and/or viral cytopathic effect is present. Of course, whatever the terminology used, the pathologist should make sure that the ophthalmologist understands his or her meaning so that no over- or undertreatment occurs.

Differential diagnosis. The chief histopathological differential diagnosis of CIN includes other intraepithelial proliferations that may result in partial to full thickness replacement of the epithelium. Principal among these mimickers, as mentioned before, is sebaceous carcinoma, which may simulate a chronic conjunctivitis and result in a long delay in diagnosis. Mitomycin C has been proposed as a treatment option for recurrent CIN, and specimens from patients who have received mitomycin topically may show significant cytologic atypia difficult to distinguish from CIN (67). However, the cytomorphologic changes associated with mitomycin are confined to the superficial layers of the conjunctival epithelium. Primary acquired melanosis (PAM) with atypia, when lacking pigment and replacing the conjunctival epithelium as a sheet of cells, may also mimic CIN. Conversely, rare cases of CIN containing melanin pigment have been reported, mimicking PAM with atypia. Immunohistochemical stains with cytokeratin (positive in CIN) and S-100 protein (positive in PAM) should be used in these situations to discriminate between the two.

Other than accurate histopathological diagnosis, the main responsibilities of the pathologist in examining conjunctival specimens with dysplasia are to (*i*) exclude an invasive squamous cell carcinoma and (*ii*) report the margin status, if possible. As to the former, such occurrences are uncommon except in HIV-positive individuals (68). Also, fortunately, when squamous cell carcinoma supervenes, it rarely results in regional lymph node metastasis or intraocular invasion. Locally more aggressive forms of carcinoma of the conjunctiva include spindle cell carcinoma and mucoepidermoid carcinoma, and, although rare, both should be considered in the differential diagnosis of invasive carcinoma of the conjunctiva (69–72). Mucoepidermoid carcinoma, in particular, may be subtle and easily mistaken for squamous cell carcinoma. Alternatively, the mucus-secreting component may not be present in the biopsy or initial excision and only becomes manifest in the recurrence or when intraocular invasion has supervened (72).

As to margin status, positive margins of CIN may portend an increased risk of recurrence (73,74). However, ophthalmologists typically use cryotherapy of the in vivo margins at the time of excision, so that reexcision for positive margins is not a standard procedure.

Melanoses and Melanocytic Proliferations

Melanotic and melanocytic processes of the conjunctiva are among the most difficult diagnostic dilemmas in ophthalmic pathology (Table 2). Even experts in the field do not agree on classification of lesions not clearly benign or malignant (75). Their appearance on

Table 2 Melanotic and Melanocytic Processes of the External Eye

1. Benign	Intraepithelial
a. Complexion-associated melanosis	
b. Ephelis	
c. Secondary melanosis	
i. Irritation (inflammation, exposure, etc.)	
ii. Systemic disease (Addison disease, Peutz-Jegher syndrome, etc.)	
d. Primary acquired melanosis without atypia	
e. Nevocellular nevus	
i. Junctional	
ii. Compound	Subepithelial
iii. Intrastromal	
f. Dendritic (blue/cellular blue) nevus	
g. Ocular/oculodermal melanocytosis (nevus of Ota)	
2. Premalignant	Intraepithelial
a. Primary acquired melanosis with atypia	
3. Malignant	Subepithelial
a. Melanoma	

otherwise pristine "whites of the eyes" may make the patient and clinician uneasy, no matter the age of the patient or the size of the lesion. In addition, terminology in the ophthalmic literature is often not well known or accepted by nonophthalmic pathologists (Fig. 10) (76). It is necessary for surgical pathologists to be conversant with the unique vocabulary understood by ophthalmologists in order to be able to communicate optimally with their clinical brethren. It is also incumbent upon both the clinician and pathologist to optimally obtain, preserve, and process the specimen. Biopsy specimens should be excised without excessive manipulation or crushing and oriented, fixed, inked, embedded, and sectioned, as

outlined previously. The conjunctival epithelium in cases of PAM may be friable and easily dislodged even after fixation, in which case, pathologic diagnosis may be impossible.

Congenital epibulbar melanocytic proliferations include nevocellular nevi, blue nevi (rare), and oculodermal melanocytosis (nevus of Ota) (77). Conjunctival nevi usually become apparent in childhood or adolescence, when pubertal hormonal changes cause increased pigmentation. They typically remain flat or plaque-like, even though, histologically, they evolve from junctional to intrastromal in the same fashion as nevi of the skin. Other similarities with cutaneous nevi include cellular pleomorphism and multinucleation. Conjunctival nevi often are associated with intrastromal invaginations and/or cysts lined by conjunctival epithelium (Fig. 11). This association is helpful both clinically and histologically as a feature usually associated with a benign melanocytic proliferation. Although evidence of a nevus may be present in up to 20% of conjunctival melanomas, a significant percentage of such cases also show features of PAM, and it is likely that PAM with atypia is the significant precursor lesion (78).

Oculodermal melanocytosis is characterized by diffuse, slate-gray discoloration of the episclera, sclera, and eyelid skin because of increased numbers of fusiform melanocytes in these tissues. Other features include melanocytic proliferation of the uveal tract, meninges of the optic nerve, and periosteum of the orbit. It is more common in Asians and African-Americans than in Caucasians, but the risk of developing melanoma is greater in whites. The majority of melanomas associated with oculodermal melanocytosis are not conjunctival but rather uveal, although rarely they may arise in the other areas of pigmentation (79). Pathologists are usually only consulted when malignant transformation is suspected.

Acquired melanosis refers to an area or areas of flat brown pigmentation of the conjunctiva. It occurs

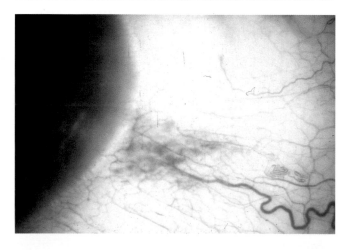

Figure 10 New-onset pigmentation of the perilimbal conjunctiva in an adult (primary acquired melanosis).

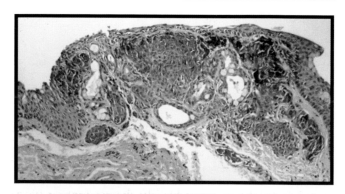

Figure 11 Histological section of a conjunctival nevus with both junctional and intrastromal components (compound nevus). Note the associated intrastromal epithelial microcysts lined by conjunctival epithelium, including goblet cells (H&E, original magnification 100×).

most commonly on the bulbar conjunctiva, plica semi-lunaris, and caruncle, but may also be present in non-sun-exposed areas of the conjunctiva. Pigmentation on the palpebral conjunctiva is unusual and an ominous finding. Acquired pigmentation may be either primary or secondary and either endogenous (chronic inflammatory disorders of the conjunctiva, Addison disease, etc.) or exogenous (e.g., topical epinephrine, silver solutions). Dark-skinned individuals are predisposed to complexion-associated melanosis, often including a circumferential ring at the limbus (80).

The term "primary acquired melanosis" has evolved to replace former monikers such as precancerous melanosis. PAM refers to a specific clinical scenario: the appearance of one or more flat ill-defined areas of brown pigment on the bulbar conjunctiva of one eye in a middle-aged Caucasian, without an identifiable antecedent cause (81). These areas of pigmentation may wax and wane and even disappear. The importance of PAM lies in the risk for development of malignant melanoma (hence, the former term "precancerous melanosis"); however, there is no conclusive clinical feature that predicts which patients will progress. The greater the extent of involvement of the conjunctiva, the greater is the risk for subsequent melanoma (82). Size greater than 6 mm and location other than at the limbus have been suggested as indications for biopsy; only histopathological examination can differentiate those lesions with atypia, at high risk (up to 90%) for subsequent melanoma, from those without atypia and essentially no risk to develop melanoma (78). Any lesion that clinically acquires depth is highly suspicious for development of melanoma.

PAM without atypia is defined as limitation of the melanocytes to the basal epithelial layer, without significant nuclear enlargement or hyperchromasia; some authors do not even require an increase in numbers of melanocytes to place pigmented lesions in this category (Fig. 12A).

Histopathological features in PAM are quite variable from patient to patient, from lesion to lesion, and even within a single lesion; therefore, multiple levels of sectioning should be performed. Atypia in PAM is based on melanocytic proliferation in which there is either cytological abnormality (epithelioid cell morphology, nuclear hyperchromasia, nucleoli) or architectural abnormality (pagetoid intraepithelial involvement, full thickness replacement) (Fig. 12B). Of the four criteria listed in Table 3, the latter two have the highest predictive value, with up to 90% of such cases subsequently developing melanoma (78). Immunohistochemical stains for melanocytes (S-100, HMB-45, MART-1, etc.) may be helpful to highlight equivocal cells, but do not address the question of atypia; proliferation markers thus far have shown variable results in reproducibly discriminating biopsies with atypia from those without (83–85).

In a more recent histopathological study, 29 cases of PAM with atypia were divided into low-risk and high-risk groups on the basis of morphological patterns as listed in Table 4 (86). The low-risk group had a 77% recurrence rate but only a 15% rate

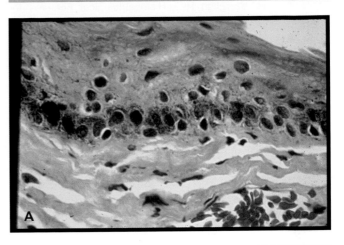

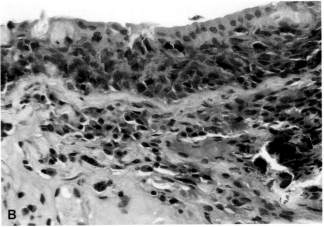

Figure 12 (A) Primary acquired melanosis without atypia, in this case showing only increased pigmentation of the basal epithelial cells without proliferation of the basally located melanocytes, identifiable by perinuclear clearing (artifactual) (H&E, original magnification 400×). (B) Primary acquired melanosis with atypia, in which cytologically atypical melanocytes are forming a solid sheet of cells beneath a monolayer of conjunctival epithelium containing goblet cells. Note the presence of melanophages within the stroma associated with a plasma cell infiltrate, not to be confused with invasive melanoma (H&E, original magnification 200×).

Table 3 Histopathological Criteria for Primary Acquired Melanosis with Atypia

Atypical feature	Development of invasive melanoma (%)
Basilar melanocytic hyperplasia with nuclear enlargement, hyperchromasia, +/− nucleoli and/or mitotic activity	22
Epithelioid cell morphology of melanocytes	75
Melanocytes singly or in clusters above the basal epithelium (pagetoid involvement)	90
Diffuse, near complete to complete replacement of epithelium by melanocytes	90

Table 4 Low Vs. High Risk Histopathological Features for Development of Melanoma in PAM with Atypia

Histopathological feature	PAM with atypia: without progression (%; $N = 13$)	PAM with atypia: progression to melanoma (%; $N = 16$)
Nucleus:cytoplasm ratio (N:C)		
High	100	0
Medium	0	81
Low	0	19
Nuclear hyperchromasia		
Present	100	50
Absent	0	50
Nucleoli		
Present	0	56
Absent	100	44
Nuclear size		
Small	55	6
Equal	45	75
Large	0	19
Architecture		
Lentiginous	100	37
Pagetoid	0	6
Mixed lentiginous and pagetoid	0	50

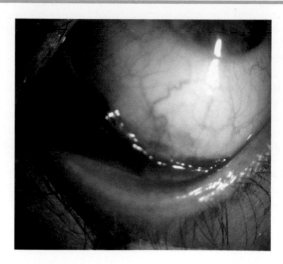

Figure 13 Malignant melanoma of the conjunctiva involving the inferior fornix and plica semilunaris. Note the associated bulbar conjunctival pigmentation indicative of preexisting primary acquired melanosis.

of invasive melanoma, while the high-risk group had a similar recurrence rate (63%) but a very high rate of invasive melanoma (94%).

There are a variety of caveats in the examination and diagnosis of conjunctival specimens for PAM:(78)

1. Misinterpretation of PAM as a junctional nevus in a middle-aged to elderly individual.
2. Overinterpretation of intraepithelial goblet cells containing melanin pigment for pagetoid involvement (i.e., PAM with atypia).
3. Overinterpretation of tangential sectioning of basal melanocytes for pagetoid involvement (i.e., PAM with atypia).
4. Misinterpretation of full-thickness replacement of the epithelium in PAM with atypia for CIN, grade III.
5. Misinterpretation of pagetoid intraepithelial involvement of PAM with atypia for pagetoid spread of sebaceous carcinoma.
6. Misinterpretation of melanophages in the stroma for invasive melanoma.
7. Misinterpretation of intraepithelial involvement in epithelial invaginations ("pseudoglands of Henle") for invasive melanoma.

If atypia is present, the lesion should be completely excised if possible. Cryotherapy of the base and margins is routinely performed in all cases where areas of pigmentation are not completely excised. If the lesion is extensive and resection is not feasible, mitomycin C has been used as an alternative therapy (87).

Malignant melanoma of the conjunctiva is a rare but potentially lethal neoplasm, with five-year mortality rates from 7% to 25% (Fig. 13) (88). Regional lymph node (preauricular, submandibular, and/or cervical neck) spread occurs in up to 40% of patients and usually, but not always, precedes visceral dissemination to the brain, lungs, and liver, most commonly (88). Tumor location other than at the limbus and positive margin status are the most important adverse prognostic factors for local recurrence and metastasis. Important pathological findings in resected specimens include tumor thickness, margin status, lymphovascular space involvement, mitotic activity, and presence of associated PAM. There is no consensus on discriminating values for the thickness of the melanoma: different studies have proposed thicknesses from 0.8 to 1.8 mm and even 4.0 mm as prognostic values, above which the likelihood of metastasis is significant (78,88). If the melanoma has invaded beyond the conjunctiva, either into the sclera or cornea, intraocularly, or into the eyelid or orbit, exenteration may be considered, although its effect on survival is debatable.

Dermoid

Limbal dermoid is a choristoma present at birth, most common at the inferotemporal aspect as a dome-shaped firm white-tan sessile nodule, up to 1.0 cm in diameter but usually 0.5 cm or less in diameter, straddling the limbus onto the peripheral cornea. It may be an isolated finding, but, especially when bilateral, represents one ocular manifestation of Goldenhar syndrome (preauricular skin appendage, eyelid coloboma, vertebral anomalies, hearing loss) (89).

Excision specimens demonstrate a nonkeratinizing stratified squamous epithelium that may or may not evidence goblet cells, overlying a dense collagenous stroma containing dermal pilosebaceous units. Occasionally, other elements such as bone, cartilage, and lacrimal gland are identified microscopically, and then the term "complex choristoma" is appropriate. These heterologous elements usually correspond to larger, more extensive growths, which may cover the cornea. Complex choristoma may be associated with linear nevus sebaceus of Jadassohn (cutaneous nevus sebaceus, cerebral atrophy with mental retardation and seizures) (90).

Another variation of dermoid occurs away from the limbus, in the superior temporal aspect of the conjunctiva toward the fornix, and may extend into the anterior orbit (91,92). In this type, a significant component of the mass is mature adipose tissue at its base, and therefore is termed "dermolipoma" (Fig. 14A, B). It also may represent one aspect of linear nevus sebaceus of Jadassohn. Adnexal structures are somewhat less likely to be present within the dermal layer on routine microscopic sections.

Dermoid if small is not treated; if it is large and causing complications such as corneal astigmatism or encroaching on the visual axis, it may be excised,

realizing the deep margin may be well within the sclera and result in thinning and possible ectasia. Surgical excision of dermolipoma likewise may cause interruption of drainage of the lacrimal gland and resultant dry eye symptoms.

IV. CORNEA

A. Anatomy

The cornea covers the anterior one-sixth of the eye circumference in adulthood, averaging 10.5 to 11.5 mm in diameter vertically and 0.5 to 1.0 mm more horizontally. Its stroma is continuous with the sclera at its periphery, known as the corneoscleral limbus, while its epithelium is continuous with the conjunctival epithelium at this same juncture. The cornea has an aspheric contour, steepest centrally, where it is also thinnest at around 0.5 mm. It is the principal refracting surface of the eye, and for optimal visual acuity, must be optically clear; thus, it is intricately ordered and avascular, and even minimal variations from normal may cause significant visual disability. The cornea is composed of five layers, from without inward, the corneal epithelium, Bowman layer, stroma, Descemet membrane, and the corneal endothelium (Fig. 15). The epithelium is a nonkeratinizing stratified squamous epithelium of five to seven layers centrally. Bowman layer is a uniform, acellular band of collagen 12 to 15 µm thick. The corneal stroma constitutes the bulk (90%) of the corneal thickness and

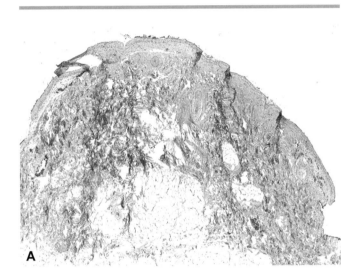

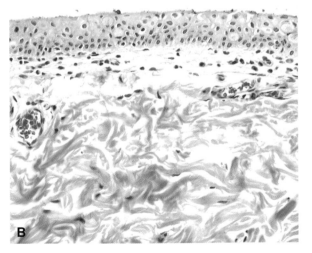

Figure 14 (**A**) Histological section of a conjunctival dermolipoma showing dermal adnexal pilar units and adipose tissue at the base (H&E, original magnification 50×). (**B**) The surface of the dermolipoma is lined by conjunctival epithelium containing occasional goblet cells. Note the subepithelial thick collagen bundles identical to that seen in the dermis of the skin (H&E, original magnification 400×).

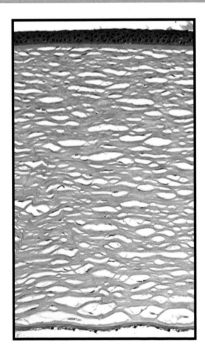

Figure 15 Histological cross section of normal cornea, demonstrating five layers visible on routine light microscopy. Note the artifactual clefts present between collagen lamellae within the stroma (H&E, original magnification 200×).

is composed of over 200 equally thick lamellae of collagen fibers, each fiber within a lamella running parallel to its mates. Keratocytes (stromal fibroblasts) are the only normal constituent cell within the stroma. Descemet membrane is the basement membrane of the corneal endothelium and increases in thickness with age, approaching the thickness of Bowman layer in late adulthood. The corneal endothelium is a monolayer of cuboidal cells lining the inner surface of the cornea, forming a hexagonal array when viewed en face. Periodic acid–Schiff (PAS) stain highlights not only Descemet membrane but also the paper-thin corneal epithelial basement membrane, not normally seen on routinely stained sections.

B. Specimen Handling

Corneal specimens generally come in two forms: round corneal buttons, 7 to 8 mm in diameter, and minute shaves or punch biopsies of corneal tissue, 1 to 2 mm in greatest dimension. Superficial keratectomy specimens are rare and may be variable in size and contour. Phototherapeutic keratectomy (PTK), i.e., ablation using an argon excimer laser, is becoming a more common alternative to surgical excision of diseases involving the anterior portions of the cornea (93). The handling and thought processes by the surgical pathologist for each type of specimen should be different; for example, biopsies are generally done for identification of a possible infectious organism, while corneal transplants are used to restore optical clarity to the visual axis.

Penetrating keratoplasty produces the most common surgical pathology specimens of the cornea. This procedure involves removal of the full thickness of the host cornea using a circular trephine and insertion of a donor cornea in its place. When the pathological process involves only the superficial cornea, a lamellar keratoplasty may be performed, with the anterior portion of the host cornea removed and the deep stroma, Descemet membrane, and the corneal endothelium remaining in situ. If only the surface of the cornea is involved, either a debridement of the epithelium or a superficial keratectomy may be the procedure of choice. Table 5 lists the possible surgical pathology corneal specimens and the most likely pathological conditions resulting therein.

Indications for corneal transplantation (i.e., penetrating keratoplasty) are variable worldwide: in the United States, failed prior grafts, Fuchs dystrophy,

pseudophakic or aphakic bullous keratopathy, and keratoconus and corneal scars account for the vast majority of pathological conditions, as shown in Table 6 (94–98).

Bullous Keratopathy

Introduction. Bullous keratopathy is the principal clinical manifestation of absorption of fluid into the cornea, which normally is dehydrated relative to its surroundings. This state is maintained by the corneal endothelial monolayer through the action of a Na^+/K^+-ATPase pump mechanism. Recent studies have identified aquaporin channels in the corneal endothelium, which may also aid in corneal dehydration (99). Functional (Fuchs dystrophy) or mechanical (intraocular surgery, graft rejection) damage to the endothelium allows aqueous fluid from the anterior chamber into the corneal stroma, and eventually to the corneal epithelium, where it may accumulate intracellularly and extracellularly, thus creating vesicles or bullae (Fig. 16). Rupture of bullae exposes nerve

Table 5 Corneal Specimen Types and Corresponding Pathological Processes

Procedure	Disease or condition
Epithelial debridement (cytological specimen)	Recurrent corneal erosion Corneal intraepithelial neoplasia Epithelial basement membrane dystrophy Band keratopathy (prior to chelation therapy)
Biopsy	Corneal ulcer
Superficial keratectomy	Pterygium Salzmann nodular degeneration Keloid
(Anterior) lamellar keratoplasty	Superficial stromal scar Anterior stromal dystrophy Band keratopathy
Penetrating keratoplasty	Pseudophakic bullous keratopathy Fuchs dystrophy Keratoconus Stromal scar Failed graft Stromal dystrophy
Posterior lamellar keratoplasty (DLEK; DSEK)	Pseudophakic bullous keratopathy Fuchs dystrophy

Table 6 Corneal Disorders Treated by Penetrating Keratoplasty (%)

	United States (Wills) 1996–2000 ($N = 1529$)	United States (Duke U.) 2000–2001 ($N = 374$)	Israel 1991–2000 ($N = 663$)	China 1994–2003 ($N = 229$)	Canada 1996–2004 ($N = 794$)
Failed graft	18	27	17	11	27
Fuchs dystrophy	15	24	2	0*	13
Pseudophakic or aphakic bullous keratopathy	27	17	12	12	25
Keratoconus	15	12	39	6	12
Scar	8	11	6	58	4
Other	17	12	24	13	19

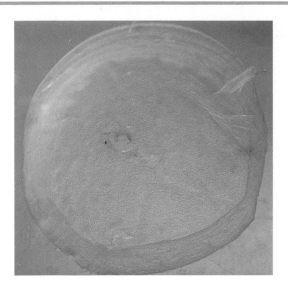

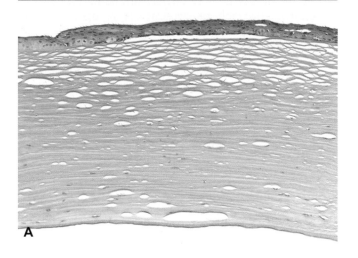

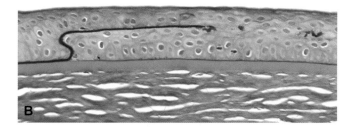

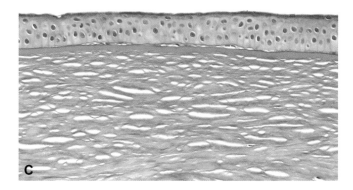

Figure 16 A penetrating keratoplasty specimen removed for bullous keratopathy. Note the microcystic pattern within the epithelial layer, which is artifactually disrupted paracentrally and thrown into folds at the upper right edge of the photograph.

endings, causing significant ocular pain, and disrupts the barrier function of the epithelium, potentiating possible microbial infection. The major causes of bullous keratopathy requiring penetrating keratoplasty are pseudophakia or aphakia, Fuchs dystrophy, and graft failure due to endothelial dysfunction or loss (100). The clinical features of each are described, followed by the common histopathological features, with exceptions as noted.

Pseudophakia.

Clinical Features. Pseudophakia refers to surgical extraction of a cataractous lens and insertion of an artificial replacement [intraocular lens (IOL) implant]; aphakia is cataract extraction without an IOL implant. The former is practically universal now, but has only been commonplace for the past 30 to 40 years. Recognition of the damage to the corneal endothelium during the procedure has led to advances in corneal protection, including smaller incisions, instillation of protective viscous gels into the anterior chamber prior to lens removal, and IOL placement, and more pliable implant materials. However, because of the attrition of endothelial cells (and their function) with aging and the large numbers of procedures performed, cataract extractions in the elderly still result in significant numbers of penetrating keratoplasty specimens with the clinical diagnosis of pseudophakic bullous keratopathy. Time of onset of bullous keratopathy from cataract surgery is variable from months to several years (101).

Pathology. Penetrating keratoplasty specimens of pseudophakic bullous keratopathy are often completely unremarkable on unaided gross examination; they typically are not vascularized and do not have discrete areas of scarring. Choosing a meridian for bisecting the cornea therefore is arbitrary. Care should be taken not to exert forceps' pressure on the cornea, particularly the endothelial (concave) surface.

Figure 17 (**A**) Bullous keratopathy in a patient with pseudophakia. Separation of the epithelium from Bowman layer is accompanied by degeneration of the basal epithelial cells. Note also the compaction and loss of artifactual clefts in the posterior stroma, and the absence of endothelial cells on the posterior surface (H&E, original magnification 100×). (**B**) PAS shows thickening and intraepithelial entrapment of the epithelial basement membrane (*left*), as compared with the normal thickness and basal location of the basement membrane (*right*) indicative of a resolved bulla. (PAS, original magnification 400×). (**C**) A thin degenerative pannus is characterized by fibroblast nuclei and collagen fibers separating the basal epithelium from Bowman layer (H&E, original magnification 400×).

When bisecting, the convex surface should be next to the cutting board.

The histopathological features of pseudophakic bullous keratopathy may be evident in all layers of the cornea, save Descemet membrane (Fig. 17A).

Subepithelial bullae may or may not be in the plane of sectioning, but where present show dome-shaped separation of the corneal epithelium from Bowman layer and degeneration of the basal epithelial cells, evidenced by loss of normal low columnar epithelial architecture, shrinkage of the cytoplasm, and pyknosis of the nuclei. Artifactual separation of the epithelium will not demonstrate alteration of the basal epithelial cell morphology. In the absence of bullae, the presence of thickened epithelial basement membrane on PAS stain, either in its normal subepithelial location or of reduplicated layers or scrolls of basement membrane present intraepithelially, are sequelae to previous episodes of epithelial separation (Fig. 17B). A thin fibrous (PAS-negative) membrane between the epithelium and Bowman layer is another indication of chronic bullous keratopathy and is known as a degenerative pannus (Fig. 17C). Stromal edema is characterized by a decrease or complete absence of clear spaces (clefts) between corneal stromal lamellae. These clefts are an artifact of tissue processing and normally are present relatively uniformly distributed throughout the stroma, histologically. Descemet membrane is normal in thickness and contour in pseudophakic and aphakic bullous keratopathy. The endothelial cells forming the monolayer lining the inner surface of the cornea are markedly decreased in numbers and, where present, are flattened and discontinuous. It is this lack of an intact endothelial monolayer that allows the normally dehydrated corneal stroma to imbibe fluid from the aqueous humor, which then traverses the stroma to form the subepithelial bullae.

Fuchs dystrophy.

Introduction. Corneal dystrophies are bilateral, localized, heritable diseases that vary in age of presentation, symptoms, and severity of visual disability. They may affect any layer of the cornea. Epithelial dystrophies typically cause pain without significant visual decrease, and if treated surgically, results in an epithelial debridement often best handled as a cytology specimen. Those affecting Bowman layer and the superficial corneal stroma may be treated by lamellar keratoplasty, in which, following nonpenetrating trephination, a cleavage plane is made within the corneal stroma, and the corneal button thus produced contains the corneal epithelium, Bowman layer, and anterior corneal stroma, leaving the posterior stroma, Descemet membrane, and endothelium intact. Stromal and endothelial dystrophies are the only ones treated by penetrating keratoplasty, and of these, Fuchs endothelial dystrophy is by far the most common.

Clinical Features. Fuchs dystrophy as yet has not been linked conclusively to a single specific chromosomal abnormality, although familial patterns of involvement with identified mutations have been described (102–105). Females are more often affected than males; onset of clinical signs and symptoms is rare before the sixth decade. Patients may complain of mildly decreased vision, a result of stromal edema, and pain from ruptured bullae. The diagnosis is made clinically by correlating the demographic findings and symptoms with the characteristic slit lamp biomicroscope appearance of corneal guttae (guttata),

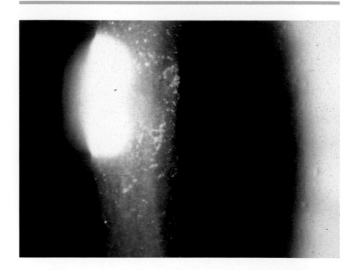

Figure 18 Slit lamp photograph of the irregular light reflections off the inner surface of the cornea in Fuchs dystrophy. Note also the drop-like pattern seen on retroillumination (*right side of photo*).

highlighted as "holes" or defects in the endothelial mosaic when viewed in specular reflection (Fig. 18). They are variable in numbers but invariably involve the central (axial) portion of the cornea. Those occurring at the periphery of the cornea and adjacent to Schwalbe ring and the trabecular meshwork are known as Hassall–Henle warts and are a universal finding in adults, without any clinical significance.

Pathology. Corneal guttae in keratoplasty specimens from patients with Fuchs dystrophy can be seen at the time of gross examination, with magnification and proper illumination, using a stereomicroscope; however, in the general surgical pathology practice, this is impractical (Fig. 19A, B). With the unaided eye, the corneal button is indistinguishable from that of a pseudophakic patient and should be handled in the same fashion.

The feature distinguishing Fuchs dystrophy from other causes of bullous keratopathy is the presence of guttae along the posterior surface of Descemet membrane. Histopathologically, guttae are mesa-topped discrete excrescences protruding posteriorly from an otherwise mildly to markedly thickened Descemet membrane (Fig. 20A). In some cases, the posterior surface of Descemet membrane is undulating, and the guttae are hidden within the substance of the membrane. PAS stain will invariably highlight these "buried" guttae as well as the surface guttae (Fig. 20B). Since the corneal button is usually taken from the central cornea, with a diameter of 7 to 8 mm, virtually any guttae present should be considered central and not to be confused with Hassall–Henle warts. The surviving endothelial cells become "trapped" in the valleys between guttae, and there is loss of a continuous endothelial monolayer. Another common histopathological finding of the endothelium in Fuchs dystrophy is melanin phagocytosis by remaining endothelial cells.

In virtually all other respects, the histopathological findings mirror those in pseudophakic bullous

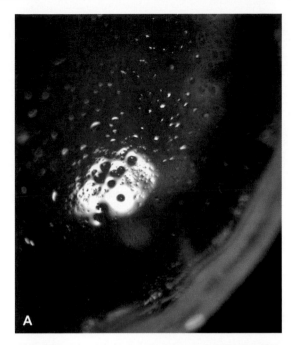

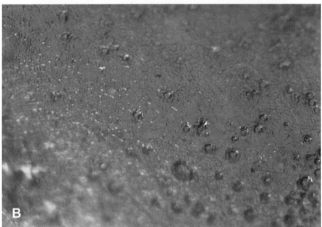

Figure 19 (**A**) Gross photograph of the penetrating keratoplasty specimen in Fuchs dystrophy, confirming the presence of corneal guttae as dark spots within the light reflex and light reflections elsewhere. (original magnification 3×).(**B**) Gross photograph of the endothelial mosaic showing drop-like excrescences interrupting the hexagonal array of endothelial cells. (original magnification 7×).

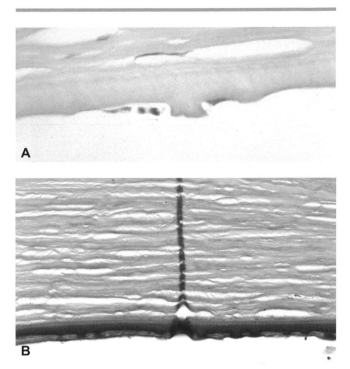

Figure 20 (**A**) Corneal gutta in histological sections appears as a mesa-like flat-topped protuberance on the inner surface of Descemet membrane, displacing the corneal endothelium (H&E, original magnification 400×). (**B**) In some cases of Fuchs dystrophy, the guttae are embedded within an abnormally and diffusely thick Descemet membrane, and are highlighted by PAS stain. (PAS, original magnification 400×).

keratopathy. It is not surprising, given the usual advanced patient age and relative frequency of cataract extraction in that age range, that specimens submitted as pseudophakic bullous keratopathy may also exhibit the guttae of Fuchs dystrophy and therefore be considered as comorbid conditions.

Apoptosis of corneal endothelium is increased in Fuchs dystrophy, and may be important in the pathogenesis of the disease (106). In a small subset of patients with a familial pattern of Fuchs dystrophy, mutations in COL8A2 gene on chromosome 1p have been identified, which may cause altered collagen formation (102,105).

Fuchs dystrophy may potentially recur in the donor cornea, although such an occurrence has yet to be proved (107). Because of the limited regenerative capacity of the corneal endothelium and the slow time course of the disease, it is more likely that the donor cornea came from an affected individual when guttae are seen in the graft subsequently.

Graft failure.

Introduction. Corneal transplants in general have a very high (>95%) initial rate of success (Fig. 21) (108). However, this percentage drops with time (as low as 50% at 5 years), so that graft failure is now rising as a reason for penetrating keratoplasty, even though many patients with failed grafts choose not to repeat the procedure (109). Graft failure may be due to effects of immunological rejection, nonimmunological factors, or both. Once a graft has failed, subsequent (repeat) graft survival rates are lower, attributable to additional factors such as the now-increased age of the patient, the increased likelihood of stromal neovascularization of the host cornea, and the development of glaucoma subsequent to the initial procedure (110). The pathological process precipitating the initial penetrating keratoplasty also affects the success of the graft: keratoconus patients and those with stromal dystrophies typically experience long periods of graft survival, while Fuchs dystrophy patients may fare relatively more poorly.

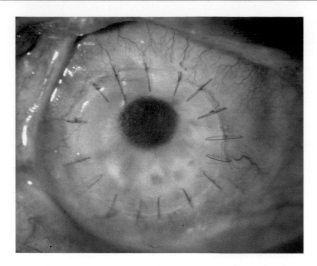

Figure 21 Failure of corneal grafts results in stromal edema as the corneal endothelium undergoes graft versus host rejection. Note the neovascularization of the graft at the donor-host interface, best seen at the 4:00 position in this slit lamp photograph.

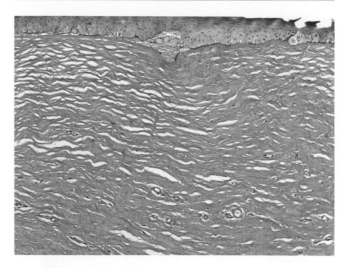

Figure 22 Neovascularization of the cornea, present both subepithelially and intrastromally in this photomicrograph, is important to document in penetrating keratoplasty specimens, as it is a major factor in primary and/or succeeding grafts failing (PAS, original magnification 400×).

Clinical Features. Repeat penetrating keratoplasty due to graft failure is usually performed as an end-stage treatment, and, as such, histopathological examination may not be reflective of the cause or causes of the failure. Immunologically mediated rejection and its immunosuppressive treatment, for instance, may render the pathological specimen devoid of a lymphocytic cell population. Supervening microbial keratitis may cause significant tissue destruction, in which case a search for possible organisms by histochemical stains is in order. In many cases the histopathological findings are either nonspecific or those of a bullous keratopathy. The most important histopathological finding to report is whether there is neovascularization present, since this is one of the major determinants as to survival of the new graft, and perhaps the only one detectable histologically (Fig. 22).

Pathology. A repeat penetrating keratoplasty specimen may be recognized by the retention of some radially arranged sutures at the periphery of the corneal button, or the scars left behind by sutures that have been removed. There is often partial to complete loss of transparency and a white-gray appearance to the cornea. Fine, usually radially arranged, arborizing blood vessels may be apparent. The cornea should be bisected perpendicular to the long axis of any areas of scarring or vascularization. On bisecting, the cornea is often slightly thickened because of edema.

Microscopically, as with the other etiologies, epithelial bullae may be present, characterized by separation of the epithelium from Bowman layer and degeneration of basal epithelial cells. In addition to the disruptions of Bowman layer at sites of suture tracks, a thin fibrous pannus may emanate from the stroma through these breaks onto the surface of

Bowman layer and extend radially for a short distance. Loss of artifactual clefts between stromal collagen lamellae correlates with the presence of stromal edema. Stromal neovascularization may be highlighted by PAS stain. Descemet membrane is usually unremarkable centrally, but is disrupted peripherally if a portion of the host cornea is also removed. A difference in thickness between the donor and host Descemet membranes is attributable to a difference in ages between the two, since Descemet membrane is generated (and therefore increases in thickness) throughout life. Endothelial cells are diminished in numbers and attenuated (flattened) in appearance. Although the endothelial cell loss may be due to immune-mediated rejection, by the time of regrafting no evidence of an inflammatory infiltrate remains. Occasionally, in other disease processes but particularly in repeat penetrating keratoplasty specimens, a thin retrocorneal fibrous membrane may be present, thought to arise from posterior migration of stromal keratocytes at the donor-host interface (Fig. 23) (111).

Another occurrence, unusual but important to note, is the absence of Descemet membrane and endothelium in the pathological specimen (112). This may be intentional, i.e., a lamellar keratoplasty, but that is a rare procedure and should be labeled as such, rather than a penetrating keratoplasty. If not, it may occur with either an initial or a repeat penetrating keratoplasty procedure and suggests that either the corneal trephine failed to penetrate Descemet membrane altogether or Descemet membrane detached from the trephined host cornea and remained in the eye on removal of the host cornea. In such instances, the donor graft inevitably fails, since the donor endothelium is not exposed to the anterior chamber and cannot function normally.

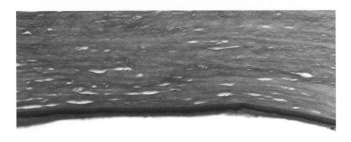

Figure 23 Formation of fibrous membranes on the inner surface of the graft may also cause failure. Such occurrences usually begin peripherally at the donor-host interface (H&E, original magnification 400×).

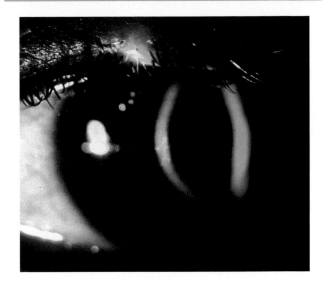

Figure 24 Keratoconus is an ectasia of the central cornea due to stromal thinning, and is recognized clinically by increased curvature of the cornea as seen in the slit beam of this slit lamp photograph.

Penetrating keratoplasty has been the standard treatment for bullous keratopathy, whatever the etiology, but newer techniques limited to replacement of the abnormal or absent endothelium only are currently being investigated. These include deep lamellar endothelial keratoplasty (DLEK) and Descemet stripping and (automated) endothelial keratoplasty (DSEK, DSAEK) (113,114). The possible advantages to these procedures include quicker visual recovery, better visual result, and increased resistance to trauma, since the host corneal stroma is retained, and the donor tissue is inserted through a small incision. Specimens from these procedures will, as the names imply, be limited to the tissue(s) removed, and will necessitate careful handling to ensure identification of the specimen within the specimen container, since it will be extremely thin and nearly transparent. Likewise, optimal microscopic sections will require embedding the specimen on edge and cutting multiple levels.

Keratoconus

Keratoconus is characterized by bilateral (but often asymmetric and metachronous) central corneal stromal thinning leading to conical ectasia (Fig. 24). It is more common in males and is usually diagnosed in the second or third decades of life. Most cases are sporadic, but in 5% to 25% of cases, a familial process with an apparent autosomal dominant pattern of inheritance may be discovered (115). Keratoconus has also been associated with Down, Marfan, and Turner syndromes. Symptoms begin with increased myopia and astigmatism because of steepening of the corneal curvature, followed by development of irregular astigmatism not correctable by spectacle lenses. Contact lenses will introduce a regular curvature for refraction but are often difficult to fit by the practitioner and poorly tolerated by the patient. Ultimately, penetrating keratoplasty is required to improve vision.

Several clues to the diagnosis are present at the time of gross examination of the corneal button. Not infrequently, the cornea will be folded on itself because of the central thinning. Some surgeons will

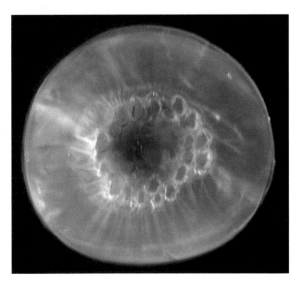

Figure 25 Gross photograph of a penetrating keratoplasty specimen for keratoconus. Note the midperipheral ring of pigment (Fleischer ring). The multiple paracentral circular epithelial defects are the result of cautery applied intraoperatively to reduce the curvature of the cornea.

apply cautery to the apex of the cone to flatten it prior to trephination so as to produce a more circular bed for the donor tissue, and the cautery marks are quite prominent when present (Fig. 25). A thin, faint brown arc may be visible on the anterior (convex) surface, known clinically as a Fleischer ring. There may be central stromal opacification if corneal scarring has occurred, such as a result of acute hydrops, when the stretched Descemet membrane ruptures. Vascularization of the cornea, however, is rare.

The cornea should be sectioned perpendicular to the pigment arc and either along or perpendicular to the corneal fold, if present. As with all corneal specimens, tissue sections should be embedded on edge to produce optimal histological cross sections of the cornea. Histologically, in addition to the central stromal thinning, one may see multiple minute discontinuities in Bowman layer, thought to be one of the earliest histological manifestations of the disease (Fig. 26A). The epithelium may be mildly acanthotic at the base of the cone and/or thinned at the apex, but is usually intact and otherwise unremarkable. Prussian blue stain will highlight focal intraepithelial positivity corresponding to Fleisher ring, most intense in the basal epithelium (Fig. 26B). The epithelial basement membrane is normal in thickness and location. If cautery was applied intraoperatively, its effects will be evident in loss of epithelium, Bowman layer, and even anterior corneal lamellae centrally and thermal injury to the epithelium and collagen at the edges of the burn. Descemet membrane and the endothelium are well preserved unless the patient had developed acute hydrops prior to penetrating keratoplasty, in which case, there will be a discontinuity and separation of the ends of Descemet membrane, with curling of the free ends toward the posterior stroma. Depending on the duration of time between rupture of Descemet and keratoplasty, endothelial cells will migrate to cover the denuded posterior stromal surface and ultimately begin to secrete a new basement membrane that may be highlighted by PAS stain.

Differential diagnosis. Keratoconus is not the only condition associated with central corneal thinning. Ectasia of the cornea may be an end result of *Herpes simplex* keratitis, healed corneal ulcer, and refractive surgical procedures [photorefractive keratectomy (PRK), laser in situ keratomileusis (LASIK)] (116). Ectatic herpetic corneas are usually vascularized and may continue to evidence a mononuclear inflammatory infiltrate. Healed ulcers will show absence of Bowman layer and loss of stromal lamellar architecture in the affected area. Post-LASIK corneas may most closely mimic keratoconus, but, if carefully examined, will demonstrate the peripheral break in Bowman layer and the apposition of the corneal flap to the deep corneal bed as a faint linear streak in the mid-stroma (Fig. 26C).

Stromal Dystrophy

Although these are rare surgical pathology specimens, stromal dystrophies have such unusual molecular and striking histopathological findings that they merit brief discussion. The three "classic" types with unique phenotypes and histopathological findings are granular dystrophy, lattice dystrophy, and macular dystrophy (117). Relatively recent molecular analysis has linked granular and lattice with two other variants, Avellino dystrophy and Reis–Buckler dystrophy (102,118). Granular and Reis–Buckler are characterized clinically by discrete punctate deposits: both

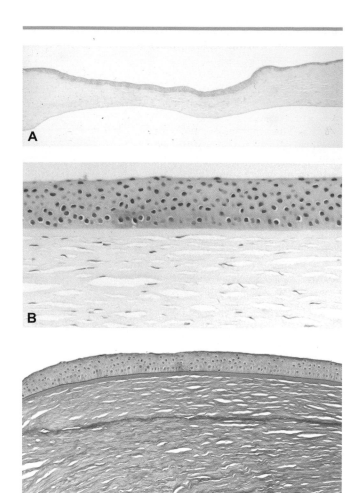

Figure 26 (**A**) Histological sections of keratoconus demonstrate reduced corneal thickness because of thinning of the stroma. The corneal stroma normally constitutes 90% of the entire corneal thickness (H&E, original magnification 100×). (**B**) The Fleischer ring visible clinically and in the pathological specimen is due to iron deposition within the corneal basal epithelium and can be highlighted by Prussian blue histochemical stain (Prussian blue, original magnification 400×). (**C**) Post-LASIK corneal ectasia may be differentiated from keratoconus when the interface between the corneal flap and the stromal bed is recognized, accentuated on periodic acid–Schiff histochemical stain in this photomicrograph (PAS, original magnification 400×).

superficial and deep in granular, only superficial in Reis–Bucklers. Lattice is so named for its crisscrossing linear deposits. Avellino combines elements of both granular and lattice. All have relatively clear cornea between the deposits. All also are autosomal dominant conditions in which significant visual disturbance may develop by middle age, leading to penetrating keratoplasty. Macular dystrophy, in contrast, is a diffuse clouding of the cornea without intervening clear spaces, is autosomal recessive, and causes more severe visual limitation at an earlier age, so that penetrating keratoplasty may be required by the third decade.

Histopathologically, the deposits of granular dystrophy are eosinophilic and a striking red on trichrome stain. They may be present in the basal epithelial layer, Bowman layer, and throughout the stroma. The stromal deposits seen in lattice dystrophy are more subtly eosinophilic and less well defined on hematoxylin- and eosin (H&E)-stained slides than those of granular dystrophy, but they are strongly orangeophilic on Congo red stain and exhibit the classic characteristics of amyloid under polarizing filters. Avellino dystrophy shows an admixture of both trichrome-positive stromal deposits with amyloid. Macular dystrophy is a localized mucopolysaccharidosis with strongly positive Alcian blue or colloidal iron deposits throughout the stroma, between collagen lamellae, and within stromal keratocytes. These and other useful histochemical stains in examining corneal specimens are listed in Table 7.

Molecular analysis has linked all but macular dystrophy to mutations of the transforming growth factor beta-induced gene (TGFB1) on chromosome 5q31, leading to aberrant protein folding of the gene protein pTGFB1 (initially termed "keratoepithelin") (119). Specific amino acid substitutions for arginines at positions 124 or 555 (e.g., Reis–Buckler: R124L substitution; granular R555W or R124S) lead to the different phenotypes noted above. Macular dystrophy has been linked to a mutation in CHST6 gene on chromosome 16, causing a decrease or absence of keratan sulfate (120). Excess production of other glycosaminoglycans as a cellular response likely contributes to the phenotypic picture. These stromal dystrophies may all eventually recur in the graft tissue.

C.   Corneal Biopsy

Biopsies of the cornea are generally only performed for attempts to uncover the etiology of unresolved corneal ulcers, i.e., those without a clear cause or unresponsive to topical therapy. Patients may be immunocompetent or immunocompromised, either locally due to topical corticosteroid therapy or systemically. Microbiological cultures have either been negative or not performed in cases suspected to be viral in etiology.

Ideally, biopsies should be taken at the edge of an ulcer rather than its base, where the tissue may be completely necrotic (121). It is obtained either by trephine (1.5–3.0 mm diameter) or with scalpel excision. The specimen may be divided by the surgeon in the operating room with portions submitted to both microbiology and surgical pathology. Therefore, the surgical pathological specimen size often is 1 mm in greatest dimension, or less, and requires care in locating and preserving the tissue at the gross bench and through tissue processing and embedding. As opposed to normally clear cornea, it is usually opaque white because of edema, inflammation, and/or necrosis, aiding in identification. Orientation of such a small specimen may be nearly impossible, but the tissue should be embedded on edge and multiple serial sections cut so that unstained slides will be available for histochemical and/or immunohistochemical stains without having to reface the block.

Histopathological examination of the tissue sections typically shows only necrotic corneal stroma, with or without inflammation. No other layers of the cornea may be identified because of sampling or orientation. The normal lamellar stromal architecture may or may not be recognizable. Types of microorganisms isolated from corneal specimens are listed in Table 8.

Acanthamoeba Keratitis

Acanthamoeba as an infectious disease of the cornea first came to attention in the 1970s in association with the use of contact lenses and/or hot tubs. In the United States, 85% of all cases of Acanthamoeba keratitis are seen in individuals who use contact lenses (1–2 new cases per million contact lens wearers per year) (122). Poor contact lens hygiene (use of or exposure to water containing the organism) is the main reason. The amoeba is free-living and can be isolated from all environments [air, water (both fresh and salt), and soil]. When conditions are not favorable, it becomes encysted and can remain so for extended

Table 7 Potentially Useful Histochemical Stains in Corneal Specimens

Histochemical stain	Pathologic process	Corneal location
Alcian blue, Colloidal iron	Macular dystrophy	Stroma
Congo red	Lattice dystrophy	Stroma
	Familial subepithelial amyloidosis (primary gelatinous droplike dystrophy)	Subepithelial
	Polymorphic amyloid degeneration	Stroma
Oil red O	Arcus senilis	Stroma
	Lipid keratopathy	Stroma
PAS	Epithelial basement membrane dystrophy	Epithelium
	Fuchs dystrophy	Descemet membrane
Prussian blue	Iron lines	Epithelium (basal)
	Hudson–Stahli line (age related)	
	Fleischer ring (base of cone in keratoconus)	
	Stocker line (advancing edge of pterygium)	
	Ferry line (edge of filtering bleb)	
	Hemosiderin (corneal bloodstaining)	Stroma
Rhodamine	Wilson disease	Descemet membrane
Trichrome	Granular dystrophy (deposits stain red)	Stroma
Von Kossa	Band keratopathy	Bowman layer

Table 8 Organisms Isolated in Infectious Keratitis

Type of infection
  Bacterial
    Gram-positive
      Staphylococcus epidermidis
      Staphylococcus aureus
      Streptococcus pneumoniae
      Streptococcus, groups D, G, or viridans
      Corynebacterium species
    Gram-negative
      Pseudomonas aeruginosa
      Haemophilus species
      Moraxella species
      Acinetobacter
      Proteus/Morganella species
      Serratia marcescens
      Neisseria species
    Acid-fast
      Mycobacterium species
    Viral
      Herpes simplex
      Adenovirus
      Herpes zoster
  Fungal
    Yeast
      Candida albicans
      Candida species other than *C.albicans*
    Filamentous
      Fusarium solani
      Aspergillus species
      Curvularia species
  Chlamydial
    Chlamydia trachomatis
      Serovars A-C: trachoma
      Serovars D-K: adult and neonatal inclusion conjunctivitis
  Parasitic
    Protozoa
      Acanthamoeba species
      Microsporidia species

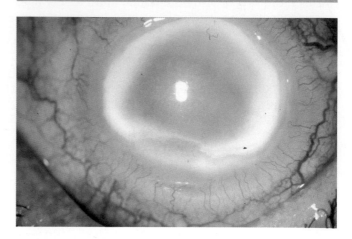

Figure 27 Acanthamoeba keratitis typically develops a ring-shaped corneal ulcer with stromal necrosis and may progress to corneal perforation.

periods before returning to an infective trophozoite form.

The classic clinical signs and symptoms are of ocular pain out of proportion to the clinical appearance of the eye, photophobia, and epiphora (increased tearing) (122,123). The early clinical picture may mimic a viral keratitis, but a ring-shaped corneal ulcer with surrounding stromal infiltrate supervenes in one to two months (Fig. 27). The corneal stroma may thin significantly or "melt," and may even perforate. A distinctive involvement of the radially arrayed corneal nerves may be present (radial keratoneuritis). Despite its virulent effects on the cornea, the organism only rarely infects intraocular tissues, although reactive intraocular inflammation is not uncommon (124).

The diagnosis of Acanthamoeba may be made in the microbiology laboratory by plating-affected corneal tissue onto a nonnutrient agar covered by a confluent growth of *Escherichia coli* at 90°F and observing the development of haphazard denuded tracks, as the amoeba have a moveable feast. Culture sensitivity, however, is poor, as low as 30% (122). Scanning confocal microscopy can identify both cysts and trophozoites in vivo and has been shown to be highly sensitive; it may in the future supplant the

need for culture, although now it is very limited in availability and involves considerable skill and expense (125).

Histopathological diagnosis may involve examination of a biopsy taken at the leading edge of the ulcer or infiltrate or of a penetrating keratoplasty specimen either in a severe corneal melt or for restoration of vision after quiescence due to successful medical therapy. The corneal tissue is usually necrotic because of action of proteases and cytokines, and viable inflammatory cells may be sparse or even absent (Fig. 28A). Acanthamoeba cysts are more easily recognized, since trophozoites may mimic stromal keratocytes or macrophages in size and form. Cysts are visible on routine H&E sections but can be highlighted by a number of histochemical stains including PAS, GMS, and trichrome (Fig. 28B). They appear as double-walled cysts, about 10 μm in diameter, with the outer wall undulating or scalloped. The trophozoite is slightly larger (10–25 μm), lacks a cyst wall, and contains within the cytoplasm a central nucleus with a prominent nucleolus. When compressed between stromal lamellae, the trophozoite is difficult to distinguish from a keratocyte or macrophage. PCR is possible as a diagnostic tool when biopsy specimens fail to yield positive results by culture or histopathology, but its utility is limited by expense and need for multiple screening primers (126).

Treatment with various antiamoebic (propamidine) and sometimes antifungal (miconazole) drugs in conjunction with disinfectant agents (PHMB, chlorhexidine) may be effective, particularly when prescribed early in the infectious process (122,123). However, even with resolution of the infection, penetrating keratoplasty may be required for improvement in vision. Identification of cysts in a penetrating keratoplasty specimen from a clinically quiescent patient does not necessarily put that patient at risk for recurrence, since it cannot be determined whether those cysts are nonviable remnants or only dormant.

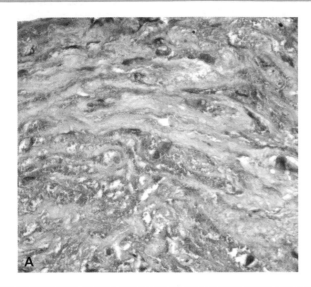

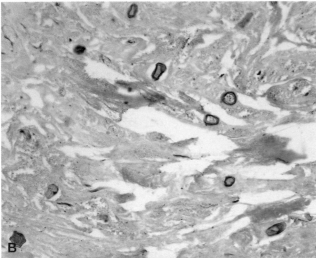

Figure 28 (**A**) Corneal biopsy specimen in suspected Acanthamoeba keratitis often show granular necrosis histologically; trophozooite forms of the amoeba are difficult to differentiate from stromal keratocytes or mononuclear histiocytes on histological examination (H&E, original magnification 400×). (**B**) Methenamine silver histochemical stain highlights the cyst forms of Acanthamoba, distinguished by their double wall and scalloped contour (Grocott methenamine silver, original magnification 400×).

Pterygium

Introduction. Pterygium and its little brother pinguecula are the result of solar damage (UVB rays) to the exposed portion of the ocular surface, i.e., within the interpalpebral fissure; only pterygium comes to the surgical pathologist, since it affects the cornea and therefore may impact visual acuity (Fig. 29). Pinguéculae are small, white-yellow nodules occurring on the conjunctival side of the corneal limbus, usually more evident nasally than temporally (Fig. 30). Pterygia are triangular growths of conjunctival tissue onto the surface of the cornea and are almost always based nasally.

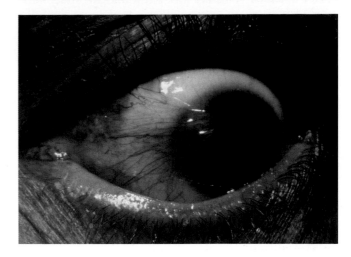

Figure 29 Pterygium is a wedge-shaped overgrowth of vascularized conjunctival tissue onto the cornea, most commonly seen at the nasal limbus.

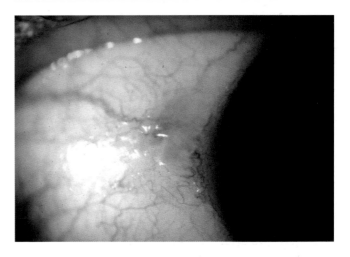

Figure 30 Pinguecula is a small (1–2 mm) yellow-white nodule at the limbus but without encroachment onto the cornea. Although more common nasally, they may occur temporally as well.

Clinical features. Pterygia occur in adults as winglike triangular overgrowths of vascularized conjunctival tissue onto the cornea, usually nasally. Those at sites other than the horizontal meridian are termed "atypical," or pseudopterygia. As with pinguecula, pterygium occurs in patients with significant sun exposure; incidence increases with age, and occurrence is more common in tropical zones than more temperate regions (127). Why there is progressive encroachment onto the cornea is not yet known. With advancement toward the central cornea, irregularity in corneal curvature may produce astigmatism, or the visual axis may be completely occluded by the overgrowth in advanced cases.

Pathology. Rarely do pathological specimens labeled pterygium appear even remotely as they did in vivo. Once excised, conjunctival tissue curls and folds upon itself and if placed in formalin in that state precludes orientation or optimal histological sectioning. If the surgeon carefully lays the specimen flat onto an absorbent paper prior to fixation, much more pathological and clinically relevant information may be gained.

Pterygium and pinguecula are histologically indistinguishable, unless there is evidence of corneal tissue microscopically. Both demonstrate solar elastosis of the subepithelial collagen identical to that seen in the dermis, with loss of eosinophilia, fragmentation, and clumping of collagen fibers (Fig. 31A, B). There is often congestion of the vasculature. A mild chronic inflammatory infiltrate may also be present within the affected stroma. The overlying epithelium may be variably atrophic, normal, or acanthotic; in a minority of cases, dysplastic features may be recognized as nuclear hyperchromasia, loss of maturation, and mitotic activity above the basal epithelium. The

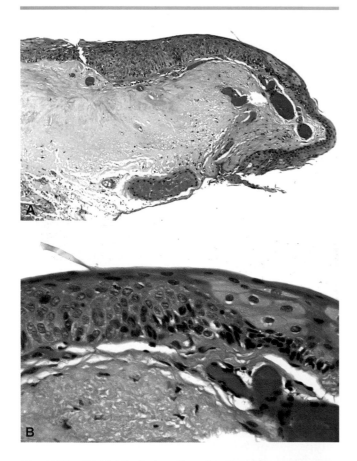

Figure 31 (**A**) Histological section of a pterygium is characterized by solar elastosis of the stromal collagen, identical in appearance to that of the dermis in actinically damaged skin (H&E, original magnification 100×). (**B**) The epithelium overlying a pinguecula or pterygium may demonstrate dysplastic features, as in this photomicrograph, ranging from mild to severe; development of squamous cell carcinoma, however, is rare (H&E, original magnification 400×).

growth of pterygium onto the cornea undermines or replaces the corneal epithelium, and there is destruction of Bowman layer beneath. If properly oriented, keratectomy specimens may demonstrate the corneal changes at the leading edge of the pterygium; however, more often than not, this is a serendipitous finding, since the excision specimens are rarely, if ever, received oriented and fixed in their in situ configuration.

Treatment. Pterygia that are actively growing, causing visual perturbations or restriction of movement or are suspicious for dysplasia, are excised by superficial keratectomy. Because of destruction of Bowman layer by the pterygium, and the incapacity of the cornea to regenerate it, a stromal scar at the site will inevitably result following excision. Clinical recurrence rates of 14% to 73% have been reported (128). Recurrences may require lamellar keratoplasty, and conjunctival flap or autograft; recurrent pterygia do not display the elastotic degeneration of the stroma, histologically.

V. GLAUCOMA

Another very common clinical entity for which surgical pathology specimens are extremely rare is glaucoma. Glaucoma, however, is not one but several disease processes linked by a common finding of characteristic visual field loss accompanied by an elevation in intraocular pressure. Intraocular pressure normally is maintained at 15 to 20 mm Hg through the balance of aqueous humor production and outflow. Production occurs by both active transport and passive diffusion in the ciliary processes. Aqueous humor circulates from the posterior chamber through the pupil into the anterior chamber, where it exits the eye via the aqueous outflow tract (trabecular meshwork into Schlemm canal and then into the systemic venous system (Fig. 32) (129). Glaucoma is subdivided according to the condition of the aqueous outflow tract: if the anterior chamber angle (where the outflow tract resides) appears unrestricted, the angle is considered "open" and the type of glaucoma, "open angle"; conversely, if the peripheral iris is physically blocking the outflow tract, then it is "closed angle" (or angle-closure) glaucoma. Either type may be primary or secondary. A third category of glaucoma is congenital glaucoma and is a result of abnormal anatomic development of the outflow tract. Primary open-angle glaucoma is one of the most common causes of visual disability in the United States, affecting 3% to 4% of the population older than 40 years, and is four to five times more common in African-Americans than Caucasians (130). Unfortunately, many patients with this insidious form of glaucoma are not diagnosed until significant visual loss has occurred, because of lack of symptoms. When medical management is inadequate in controlling intraocular pressure elevation, surgical procedures may result in specimens for the surgical pathologist. One of the more common surgical approaches is to excise a small portion of the posterior stromal lamellae of the peripheral cornea, a procedure

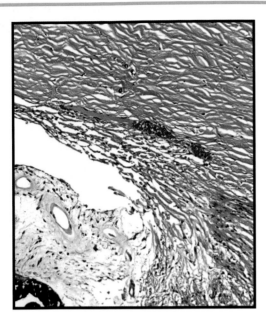

Figure 32 The juncture of the inner aspect of the peripheral cornea with the ciliary body and peripheral iris is termed the "anterior chamber angle" and is the principal site for egress of aqueous fluid from the eye. Specific structures include TM, SC, SS, CB, and I, and SR is not shown (at termination of Descemet membrane, only variably present in histological sections).

known as a trabeculectomy. The resultant pathological specimen is rarely more than 1 to 2 mm in greatest dimension, and in combination with the clarity of the cornea, may be difficult to find first at the dissecting table and second at the embedding center following tissue processing. Inking the specimen with Mercurochrome is helpful in identifying it through processing, yet not affecting the histological appearance. Although termed a "trabeculectomy," it is uncommon to find trabecular meshwork histologically; the typical specimen shows only the lamellar collagen of the corneal stroma, occasionally lined on one surface by Descemet membrane. Success or failure of the surgical procedure is not dependent on whether trabecular meshwork has actually been excised, so identifying trabecular meshwork histologically is not necessary. Perhaps this explains why these specimens are rarely submitted to the surgical pathologist if at all.

VI. LENS

A. Anatomy

The lens develops embryologically as a thickening (lens placode) and then infolding and sequestration (lens vesicle) of surface ectoderm. The fetal lens nucleus forms by elongation of the posterior lens epithelium lining its basement membrane, the lens capsule; these epithelial cells are not replaced so that the posterior lens capsule postnatally lacks an epithelial lining and remains stationary in thickness throughout life. Subsequent lens fibers forming the adult nucleus and lens cortex originate from lens epithelium at the equator of the lens where cell division and migration continue. In the adult, then, the anterior lens capsule is thicker than the posterior and is lined by lens epithelium; the lens cortex consists of acellular eosinophilic lamellae; the lens nucleus appears eosinophilic and homogeneous because of the longstanding compression of its fibers by each succeeding newly formed fiber at the lens equator.

B. Cataract

Cataract, i.e., opacification within the lens, may affect the lens nucleus, lens cortex, or the subcapsular zones at the anterior and posterior poles of the lens, either in isolation or in any combination. The most common forms in adults resulting in visual disability include nuclear sclerotic cataracts and posterior subcapsular cataracts (131). Both are associated with increasing age; posterior subcapsular cataracts in addition are common in diabetes and as a consequence of corticosteroid therapy.

Although removal of the lens is the most commonly performed intraocular surgical procedure in ophthalmology, it is not a standard surgical pathology specimen, and indeed, if submitted at all, is only for gross examination. Only in unusual cases is a cataract extraction examined histologically. Current surgical procedures typically remove only the lens nucleus intact, sonicating and/or aspirating the lens cortex piecemeal and leaving the lens capsule behind as a receptacle for placement of an IOL implant (Fig. 33). Often, a nuclear sclerotic cataract develops a brown translucency and is described clinically as a brunescent cataract. Histological examination of the lens nucleus cannot reliably distinguish a nuclear cataract from normal and therefore serves no essential purpose in patient care. Thus, lenses, when submitted to the surgical pathologist at all, are given only a gross examination and description.

It is in examination of enucleation or evisceration specimens that the cataractous changes of the lens cortex and subcapsular zones may be identified grossly and histologically. Cortical changes noted histologically include disruption of the lamellar architecture of lens fibers by fluid clefts and rounding up of lens fibers to form eosinophilic anuclear spheres (Morgagnian globules). The normal posterior lens capsule is normally devoid of lens epithelium, as mentioned above, with those cells having gone on to form the embryonic nucleus during fetal development. Posterior subcapsular cataract is identified histologically by migration of lens epithelium from the equator of the lens toward the posterior pole. This posterior migration may be either in the form of flattened nuclei along the lens capsule or large, pale cells with central nuclei ("bladder" cells of Wedl).

An increasingly common finding in enucleation specimens is the presence of an IOL implant status postcataract extraction. Currently, most lenses used

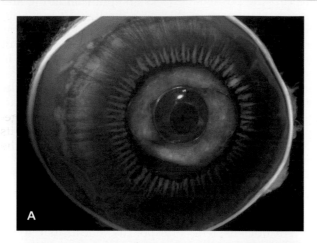

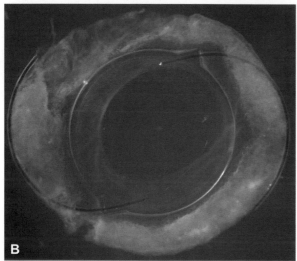

Figure 33 (**A**) Posterior chamber intraocular lens implant within the native capsular bag, as seen from behind after opening the eye coronally and preserving the anatomy of the anterior segment. (**B**) Surgical removal of a posterior chamber intraocular lens implant and the lens capsule, following traumatic dislocation. Note the secondary cataractous proliferation of the residual lens epithelium (Soemmerring ring). The central clear zone represents the anterior capsulotomy through which the native lens nucleus and cortex are removed and the implant inserted.

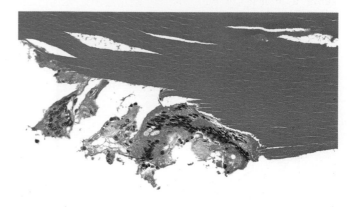

Figure 34 Multinucleated giant cells arrayed against frayed lens fibers in a phacoantigenic reaction after traumatic disruption of the lens capsule (H&E, original magnification 200×).

are placed into the residual lens capsule at the time of cataract extraction and, since the native lens is situated in the posterior chamber of the eye, are termed posterior chamber IOL implants. They are made of a number of substances including hard plastics like polymethylmethacrylate (PMMA) to flexible silicone. Depending on the polymer, the lens either dissolves in the solvents during tissue processing or does not adhere to the slide on sectioning, so that only an empty space signifying the location of the lens remains on histological examination. Suboptimal placement or subsequent dislocation of the lens may result in pathological injury to the iris and/or ciliary processes. Anterior chamber IOL implants are used much less frequently because of their higher

morbidity, particularly development of the UGH (uveitis, glaucoma, and hyphema) syndrome.

Rare forms of cataract include anterior subcapsular or anterior polar cataract, in which the lens epithelium undergoes apparent fibrous metaplasia, forming collagen fibers beneath the anterior lens capsule (132). In the fully developed form, lens epithelial cells from the equatorial edge migrate deep to the fibrous plaque and produce a new basement membrane, so that histologically from anterior to posterior one can identify anterior lens capsule (original), fibrous plaque, lens capsule (new), lens epithelium, and then lens cortex.

In cases where there has been traumatic disruption of the lens capsule, an inflammatory reaction may occur on exposure of the previously immune-privileged lens fibers, resulting in a zonal granulomatous inflammatory reaction replete with multinucleated giant cells (Fig. 34) (133). This condition was previously and inaccurately termed "phacoanaphylactic endophthalmitis"; the preferred nomenclature is phacoantigenic or lens-induced uveitis or endophthalmitis (134). Leakage of denatured, soluble lens protein through an intact lens capsule in a hypermature cataract (complete liquefaction of the lens cortex) may lead to one form of secondary open-angle glaucoma known as phacolytic glaucoma. Histologically, macrophages with pale cytoplasm align along the anterior chamber angle and in the trabecular meshwork in enucleation specimens of such cases.

VII. INTRAOCULAR CONDITIONS

A. Enucleation

Introduction

Eyes are removed for a variety of reasons; by far the most common one given on a surgical pathology requisition form is some permutation of "blind,

Table 9 Indications for Enucleation (Mayo Clinic 1999–2000)

Reason for enucleation	%
Tumor	48
End-stage glaucoma	13
Phthisis (or atrophia) bulbi	12
Recent trauma	11
Chronic retinal detachment	9
Infection or inflammation	7

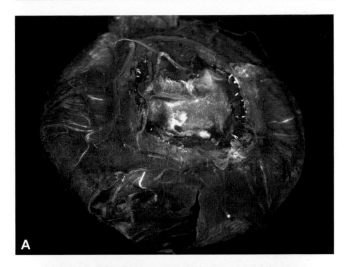

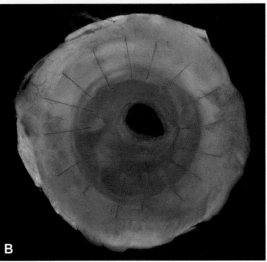

painful eye." This of course gives no clue to the surgical pathologist as to what to look for or expect when examining the specimen. Sometimes the enucleating surgeon is an oculoplastics expert, only recruited to do the procedure and has no more detailed patient history to offer, and trying to track down the clinical information is difficult, time consuming, and, unfortunately, often fruitless. Thus, it is up to the surgical pathologist to attempt to discover the root cause leading to removal of the eye. The reasons and percentages for removal of the eye vary according to the institution or practice. The experience at the Mayo clinic from 1990 to 2000 is shown in Table 9 (135). It is heavily weighted toward tumors because of its wide referral base; trauma and phthisis bulbi are the most common reasons at most institutions.

In the author's experience, there are four main categorizations for enucleation specimens: those that are end-stage degenerations of a variety of disease processes, often termed, clinically, "phthisis bulbi"; those with a history or external evidence of penetrating trauma, such as open or sutured lacerations; those with fulminant intraocular, usually suppurative, inflammation (endophthalmitis or panophthalmitis); and those harboring an intraocular mass. Limited excisions of portions of the eye, such as iridocyclectomy, may be performed by specialists in ocular oncology, but, rarely, if they ever come to the attention of the general surgical pathologist. Removal of the cornea and the entire intraocular contents, leaving the sclera and its extraocular muscle attachments, is termed an "evisceration," and is sometimes performed for an improved cosmetic result postoperatively because of the continued actions of the extraocular muscles (Fig. 35A, B) (136).

Specimen Handling

Eyes removed surgically should be fixed in 10% neutral buffered formalin for 24 to 48 hours prior to opening. Injection of formalin intraocularly is neither necessary nor indicated. If fresh tissue of an intraocular neoplasm is needed for special studies (e.g., flow cytometry or cytogenetics), a small (2–3 mm) block of tissue may be removed through a scleral opening, and the eye then placed in fixative as above. Once properly fixed, the eye may be washed in running tap water for 15 to 30 minutes and then placed in 50% ethanol to resurrect natural coloring and allow for detailed gross examination without noxious fumes. Ideally, a stereoscopic dissecting microscope is available for both external and internal ocular examination, because

Figure 35 (**A**) Gross appearance of an intact evisceration specimen with the cornea removed. The external surface of the specimen corresponds to the external aspect of the choroid, i.e., that side next to the sclera in situ. (**B**) The cornea and rim of scleral tissue removed from the front of the evisceration specimen, in this case, demonstrating a perforating corneal ulcer in the donor tissue of a penetrating keratoplasty.

many ocular pathological conditions are on the order of millimeters in dimensions and will go unrecognized to the unaided or untrained eye. To accurately assess and localize intraocular processes, the eye must be oriented properly by identification of certain external anatomic landmarks (Fig. 36). The horizontal meridian of the eye is identified by finding the long posterior ciliary arteries, two in number, which enter the sclera just medially and laterally to the optic nerve and travel obliquely forward through the sclera toward the equator of the globe. Their paths are visible as red-purple streaks through the white sclera, defining the horizontal plane of the eye (long posterior ciliary nerves accompany the arteries). Identification of the insertions of the oblique muscles confirms the laterality of the eye. The superior oblique muscle,

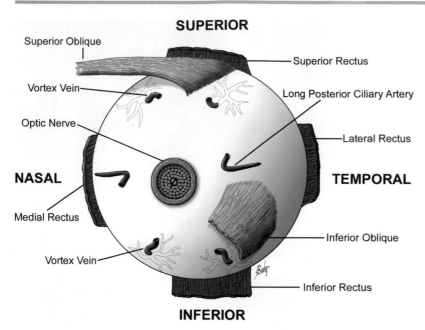

Figure 36 Drawing of the posterior aspect of the eye. Locating the paired long posterior ciliary arteries identifies the horizontal plane of the eye. The oblique muscle insertions are useful in determining laterality of the eye: the superior oblique is tendinous and inserts in the superior temporal quadrant, while the inferior oblique is muscular and inserts temporal to the optic nerve near the horizontal plane. The four vortex veins exit the eye slightly posterior to the equator in roughly the oblique meridians. *Source*: From Ref. 226.

having changed direction by passing through the cartilaginous trochlea attached to the superomedial wall of the orbit, is a white, fibrous tendon inserting posterolaterally into the sclera in the superior to superotemporal quadrant of the eye, posterior to the equator. The inferior oblique muscle has almost no tendinous component and therefore is beefy red-tan right up to its insertion point just temporal to the optic nerve. Once properly oriented, detailed external examination of the cornea, conjunctiva, and episclera can be undertaken under stereoscopic magnification. Transillumination of the eye using a small but bright light source will highlight defects in light transmission such as pigmented masses or areas of hemorrhage, and guides the pathologist in the correct plane of sectioning. If the optic nerve is more than 2 mm in length, it should be cross-sectioned 1 mm behind the globe and examined macroscopically for evidence of atrophy, demyelination, meningeal hemorrhage, or masses. The usual plane of section for opening the eye is horizontal, beginning posteriorly just above the optic nerve and progressing forward, using the long posterior ciliary arteries as guides. Once the back of the lens is encountered, the blade should be continued around it rather than through it, since in adults, the lens is very hard and attempting to cut through it may easily displace it and disrupt the anatomy of the anterior segment. The ideal plane of section will pass through the superior edge of the pupil. After completion of the section, the inferior calotte (cup) containing the optic nerve head, macula, and lens may be viewed under magnification. By placing the calotte back in 50% ethanol, light reflections from the vitreous surface are eliminated, resulting in far superior stereomacroscopic examination. The superior calotte is then examined in the same fashion. If deep cassettes and embedding molds are available, the inferior calotte

may be processed as is; if not, a second cut parallel to the first, just inferior to the optic nerve, is made [often called the "P-O" section (pupil-optic nerve)]. This may be accomplished by placing the inferior calotte upside down in the cassette and using the upper edge of the cassette as a cutting guide. Secondary planes of section and additional blocks may be necessary to examine pathological processes that would not be included in the P-O section. Special conditions that may alter this routine method would be (i) presence of an intraocular tumor, in which the plane should bisect the mass (located by transillumination) in order to determine maximum tumor height; (ii) a penetrating wound (surgical or traumatic), in which the plane of section should be perpendicular to the laceration; and (iii) presence of an IOL implant, in which the eye should be opened in a coronal plane at the equator of the eye, so as not to disrupt the implant or its environs. An artificial lens should be suspected whenever the pupil appears black on external examination, because the native lens will opacify somewhat yellow to gray-white with fixation and therefore visible behind the iris. Obviously, when the pupil is not visible externally, such as with opacification of the cornea or accumulation of cells within the anterior chamber, this determination is not possible. When opened coronally, orientation of the resulting anterior and posterior calottes may be maintained by placing a meridional streak of ink straddling the equator at the superior (12:00) position of the eye prior to sectioning. Once gross examination is complete, secondary planes of section of both calottes are necessary to obtain microscopic sections of the anterior and posterior segments. The posterior calotte is sectioned horizontally, beginning at the equator and progressing posteriorly while viewing the optic nerve head and macula, while the anterior calotte is sectioned vertically from back to front, perpendicular to the corneoscleral limbal incision for the cataract extraction, but avoiding the IOL implant. Prosthetic devices such as artificial lenses and extrascleral buckles do not need to be removed prior to tissue processing. Even when resistant to dissolution in the alcohols and organic solvents of tissue processing, they in general do not adhere to the glass slides and thus are not present microscopically.

Phthisis Bulbi

Clinical features. Phthisis bulbi literally means "shrunken eye" and is the end result of a variety of ocular conditions and disease processes, usually because of longstanding chronic inflammation, retinal detachment, or other degenerative processes. Depending on the initial insult, any of a wide variety of histological findings within the eye may be discovered (137).

Pathology. On external examination, the eye is small (<22-mm maximum diameter) and squared when viewed from the front, each side corresponding to a rectus muscle insertion (Fig. 37A, B). This results from ocular hypotension (intraocular pressure <5–6 mm Hg) allowing for greater tractional effect on the softened eye by the four rectus muscles. The cornea likewise may be reduced in size and is often opacified and/or vascularized. The anterior chamber angle may evidence peripheral anterior synechiae (adhesions between the iris root and the trabecular meshwork).

Deposition of calcium may be present, beginning as a fine basophilic stippling in Bowman layer and progressing to plaques of calcium in it and the anterior stroma (Fig. 38A, B). This condition is known as band keratopathy because of its clinical appearance as a horizontal white strip within the interpalpebral fissure. There may also be corneal pannus (fibrous or fibrovascular tissue between the epithelium and Bowman layer) or stromal scarring (destruction of normal lamellar architecture) and/or vascularization. A retrocorneal fibrous membrane may be present emanating from a disruption of Descemet membrane, or more extensive fibrous proliferation may completely obliterate the anterior chamber and extend posteriorly through the pupil (fibrous ingrowth). Migration of corneal endothelium posteriorly to blanket the surfaces of the anterior chamber angle and anterior iris may also occur, a condition termed "endothelialization" or "descemetization" because of the resultant basement membrane material deposited by the aberrantly situated endothelium. Often there is a mild chronic inflammatory infiltrate within the uvea (iris, ciliary body, and/or choroid). The lens, if present, is usually cataractous and often calcified. Fibrovascular proliferation within the posterior chamber may encompass the lens anteriorly and be adherent to a funnel-shaped, tractionally detached retina (Fig. 39). Depending on the age of the detachment, the retina will show degenerative changes and gliosis of one or more layers (Fig. 40). Macrocystic changes are common in longstanding cases. An exudative form of retinal detachment may be present in

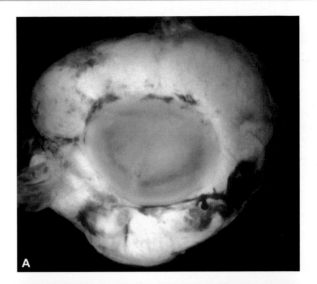

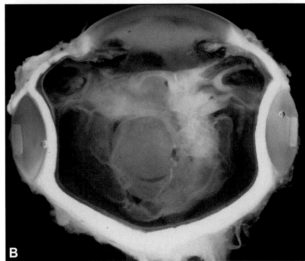

Figure 37 (**A**) Phthisis bulbi: a small, squared eye with opacification of the cornea and/or anterior chamber on external examination. (**B**) Same eye in cross section, showing an encircling equatorial scleral buckle, with a complete retinal detachment and macrocystic degeneration, fibrous obliteration of the posterior chamber, and absence of the lens.

other instances, in which bullous detachment of the retina overlies proteinaceous eosinophilic subretinal fluid containing innumerable cholesterol crystals (strikingly iridescent on gross examination) and phagocytic histiocytes containing PAS-positive intracytoplasmic material. This histological pattern is known as a Coats-type response for its similarity to a childhood form of unilateral exudative retinal detachment due to abnormally permeable retinal vessels. Membranes, variably composed of fibrovascular tissue, glial tissue, and retinal pigment epithelial-derived cells, may occur both preretinally and subretinally. Rarely, there is massive gliosis of the retina with complete effacement of the normal architecture sufficient to produce a mass effect (138).

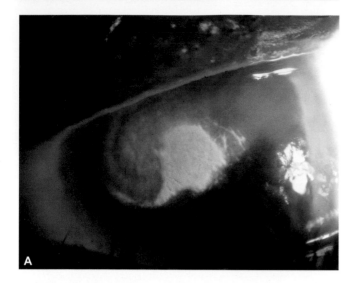

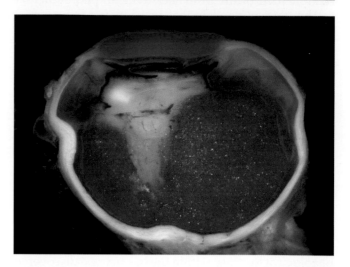

Figure 39 Tractional forces of a posterior chamber cyclitic membrane have caused centripetal displacement of the ciliary body and a funnel-shaped retinal detachment. Iridescent cholesterol crystals are present within the proteinaceous subretinal fluid. Note the presence of a posterior chamber intraocular lens implant on the anterior aspect of the cyclitic membrane.

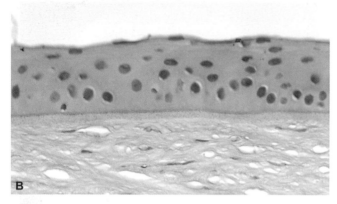

Figure 38 (A) Band keratopathy is characterized by an interpalpebral horizontal white opacification of the superficial cornea on slit lamp examination and is a relatively common development in chronically inflamed or degenerated eyes. (B) Histological evidence of band keratopathy begins as shown in this photomicrograph, with a fine basophilic stippling at the level of the epithelial basement membrane and Bowman layer. It may progress in advanced cases to thick calcific plaques in Bowman layer and the anterior stroma (H&E, original magnification 400×).

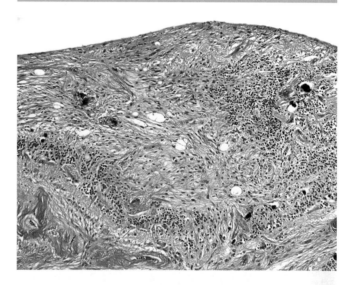

Figure 40 Gliosis of the inner retina with disruption of the retinal microanatomy. Scattered calcospherites are present as well (H&E, original magnification 100×).

Clues to the underlying etiology responsible for the retinal damage may be found in some cases. Microaneurysms within the inner nuclear layer are most often a sign of diabetic retinopathy, particularly when combined with preretinal neovascularization at the optic nerve head or elsewhere on the retinal surface (Fig. 41A). Other signs of diabetes include iris neovascularization, lacy vacuolization of the iris pigment epithelium, thickened basement membrane of ciliary and choroidal capillary networks, and evidence of panretinal photocoagulation (Fig. 41B, C). Diffuse atrophy of the nerve fiber layer and disappearance of the ganglion cells, in concert with a deeply excavated optic nerve head, indicate chronic open-angle glaucoma as the culprit (Fig. 42A–C). Atrophy of the entire inner retina to the level of the outer portion of the inner nuclear layer is the characteristic histopathological appearance of a prior central retinal artery occlusion, while retention of the retinal layers but significant deposition of hemosiderin in a perivascular distribution suggests a prior central retinal vein occlusion.

The retinal pigment epithelium (RPE) may be replaced by bone (thought to be due to metaplasia of the RPE), forming a thin shell within the eye or as a nodular mass (Fig. 43A, B) (139). Drusen, dome-shaped to plaque-like excrescences on the inner aspect of Bruch membrane are common and may become

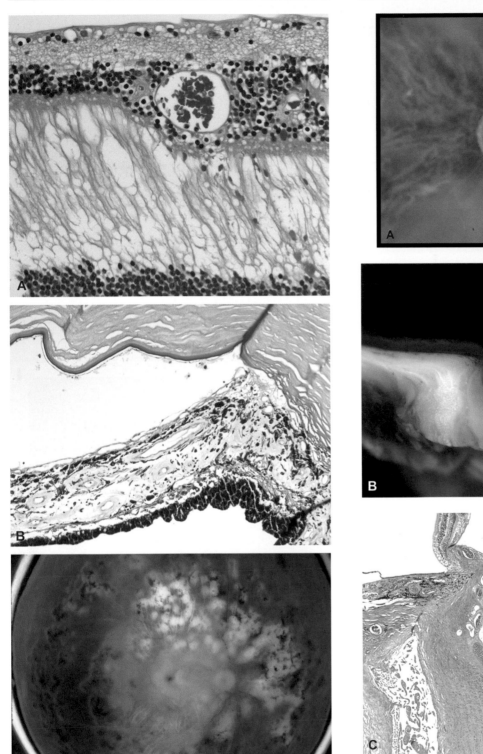

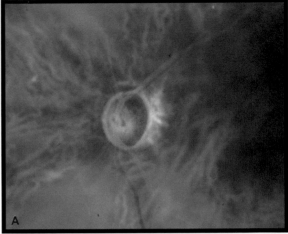

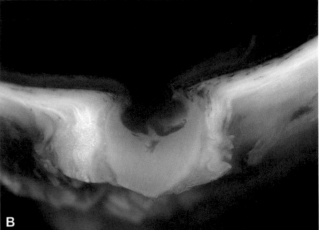

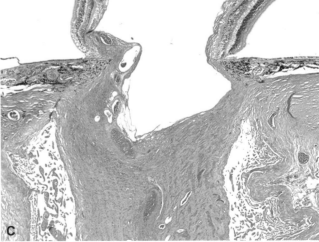

Figure 41 (**A**) Histological appearance of a retinal microaneurysm within the deep capillary plexus in the inner nuclear layer, in a patient with proliferative diabetic retinopathy status, postpanretinal photocoagulation (H&E, original magnification 400×). (**B**) Neovascularization of the surface of the iris (rubeosis iridis) in the same patient, with involvement of the anterior chamber angle causing peripheral anterior synechia (neovascular glaucoma) (H&E, original magnification 200×). (**C**) Gross appearance of panretinal photocoagulation healed scars. Note that the macula is usually not treated.

Figure 42 (**A**) Advanced chronic open-angle glaucoma causes loss of axonal tissue forming the optic nerve, resulting in a deeply excavated appearance on gross examination. Note the visibility of the lamina cribrosa in the base of the cup, most pronounced superiorly. (**B**) Cross section through the optic nerve head demonstrates the characteristic "beanpot" shape with undermined edges at the disc margin. (**C**) Histological correlate to the gross appearance, with undermining of the margins of the optic nerve head imparting a beanpot appearance on cross section.

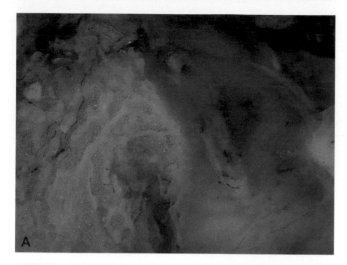

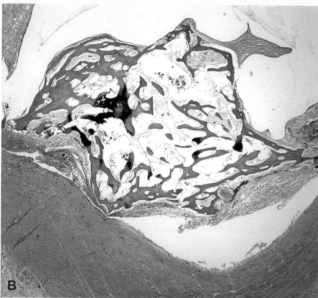

Figure 43 (**A**) Osseous metaplasia of the retinal pigment epithelium (RPE) forming a tumoral mass on gross examination of the eye. Note the bony trabeculae and intervening yellow lipid globules of marrow adipose tissue in the left half of the field. (**B**) Histological correlation with the gross appearance. Such a degree of bone formation may necessitate decalcifying the eye even before attempting to open it for gross examination (H&E, original magnification 20×).

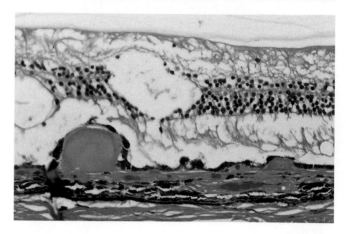

Figure 44 Histological section of drusen, eosinophilic deposits on Bruch membrane, elevating the retinal pigment epithelium. In this case the drusen are peripheral and the overlying retinal contains typical cystoid spaces in the outer plexiform layer, an almost universal finding in adults.

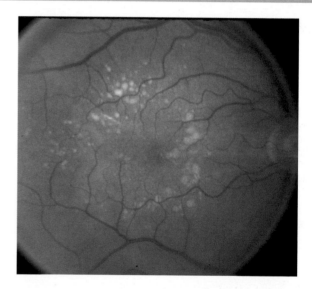

Figure 45 Fundus photograph of drusen in the macula, the so-called dry form of ARMD. Only about 10% of cases will develop the "wet" or neovascular form of ARMD with its attendant's severe visual loss. *Abbreviation*: ARMD, age-related macular degeneration.

calcified (Fig. 44). Those occurring beneath the macula, in association with thickened and calcified Bruch membrane, are characteristic of the atrophic or so-called dry form of age-related macular degeneration (Fig. 45) (140). Subretinal neovascular membranes arising from the choroidal circulation form breaks through in the brittle Bruch membrane in 8% to 10% of cases, the "wet" form of age-related macular degeneration. Hemorrhage from this neovascular tissue and subsequent organization in the subretinal space results in a disciform scar with significant central visual loss due to overlying retinal photoreceptor

degeneration (Fig. 46A, B). The sclera posteriorly is thickened, and with shrinkage of the eye, often irregular in contour. The optic nerve is shrunken from demyelinaton and neural tissue atrophy, with expansion of the meningeal space and wrinkling of the dura mater (Fig. 47).

Trauma. Eyes enucleated as a result of traumatic injury often manifest evidence of a penetrating wound (Fig. 48). An attempt at primary repair (i.e., embedded sutures) may or may not be evident. The globe in

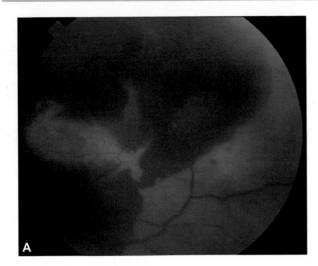

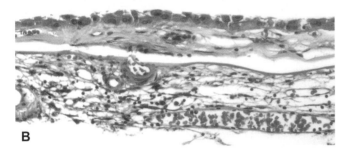

Figure 46 (**A**) Fundus photograph of subretinal hemorrhage in the macula as a result of subretinal neovascularization in ARMD. (**B**) Histological section of a subretinal neovascular membrane elevating the retinal pigment epithelium. Note the break in Bruch membrane through which a capillary from the choroid is penetrating. Subretinal neovascular membranes are also referred to as CNV since the choroid is the source of the new vessel proliferation (H&E, original magnification 400×). *Abbreviations*: ARMD, age-related macular degeneration; CNV, choroidal neovascularization.

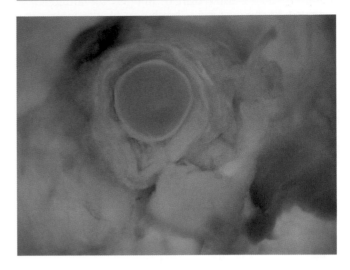

Figure 47 Gross examination of a cross section of the optic nerve immediately behind the eye showing complete demyelination of the nerve; with neuronal tissue loss, the meningeal space becomes wider and the dura becomes somewhat wrinkled.

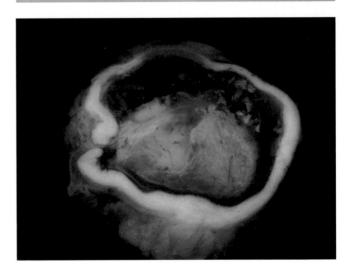

Figure 48 Phthisical eye, following penetrating trauma. In addition to the internal disorganization, there is a full-thickness defect of the sclera equatorially. The wound was not visible externally because of the epibulbar reparative granulation tissue and fibrosis.

general and wound in particular should be accurately described and measured for medicolegal purposes. Transillumination of the eye should be attempted but is usually noncontributory because of filling of the globe with hemorrhage. The plane of section for opening the eye is determined by the orientation of the wound; ideally, the plane of section should be anterior-posterior and perpendicular to the linear wound. If the wound is meridional, necessitating opening the eye in a coronal plane, secondary sectioning to examine anterior and posterior segments will be required. Coronal sectioning of the eye is also recommended when an IOL implant is present in order to expose the implant and its relationship to the lens capsule without artifactual disruption.

Severe trauma to the eye may be either blunt or penetrating, depending on the nature and force of the injurious agent. Ocular trauma is a common process, at least in urban settings. Many cases involve blunt force injury in young males because of assault and may result in serious damage to one or both eyes. Sometimes the visual complications of blunt trauma develop months to years following the insult (141). Penetrating injuries may be intentional but are often accidental, and while the majority are due to a foreign object, occasionally ruptured globes result from blunt trauma.

Sympathetic ophthalmia. Sympathetic ophthalmia is a rare but potentially vision-threatening granulomatous inflammatory complication involving both eyes, following penetrating injury to one eye (142). A putative, as yet unidentified, antigen (or antigens) is exposed to the systemic circulation by the injury and elicits a T-cell-mediated response (143). It is postulated that if the damaged ("exciting") eye is removed within two weeks of injury or onset of inflammation, the immune response is abrogated and the fellow ("sympathizing") eye may be spared. However, cases have occurred within time spans as short as five days following injury. Despite its rare occurrence, it may be the most important reason for pathological examination of an eye enucleated for penetrating trauma.

Clinical features of sympathetic ophthalmia include the usual features of uveitis: keratic precipitates on the corneal endothelium, perilimbal congestion termed "ciliary flush," cells and flare in the aqueous humor, posterior synechiae (adhesions between iris and lens), cells in the vitreous, retinal vascular sheathing, and yellow subretinal infiltrates (corresponding to Dalen-Fuchs nodules, see below). If the inflammation is severe, an exudative retinal detachment may supervene and obscure visualization of the subretinal infiltrates.

The sine qua non histopathological feature of sympathetic ophthalmia is the presence of nonnecrotizing granulomatous inflammation within the choroid, classically sparing the choriocapillaris (Fig. 49). This sparing is not universal, but is cited as the main histopathological distinguishing sympathetic ophthalmia from another type of granulomatous choroiditis, Vogt-Koyanagi-Harada syndrome (VKH), a disease with which sympathetic ophthalmia shares many clinical features as well. Other granulomatous inflammatory processes must also be considered in the histopathological differential diagnosis, including mycobacterial and fungal infections, sarcoidosis, and phacoantigenic endophthalmitis, as mentioned previously. The inflammation in sympathetic ophthalmia is usually diffuse, although occasionally discrete granulomas are present.

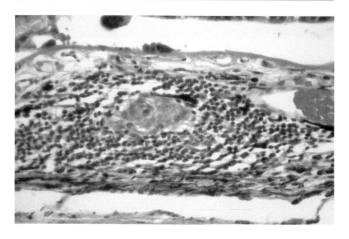

Figure 49 Discrete minute granuloma in the choroid, with a surrounding lymphoplasmacytic infiltrate. In sympathetic ophthalmia, the inflammation may spare the choriocapillaris, as demonstrated here (H&E, original magnification 200×).

Epithelioid histiocytes and occasionally multinucleate giant cells exhibiting melanin pigment phagocytosis are present within the granulomatous areas. Macrophage-rich subretinal pigment epithelial inflammatory cell aggregates (Dalen-Fuchs nodules) are also characteristic, but not pathognomonic, of sympathetic ophthalmia. Presence of eosinophils as a component of the uveal inflammation is thought by some to be the earliest histopathological finding in sympathetic ophthalmia, and eosinophils are more prevalent in severe cases and those without prior corticosteroid therapy. The lymphocytes present are predominantly T cells.

Treatment of sympathetic ophthalmia consists of aggressive corticosteroid therapy at the earliest sign of uveitis. Severe or refractory cases may require more potent immunosuppressive agents such as cyclosporine A (143).

Common pathological findings attributable to trauma include hyphema (hemorrhage into the anterior chamber) with bloodstaining of the cornea, angle recession, Vossius ring, glaukomflecken, vitreous hemorrhage, retinal detachment with intraretinal hemorrhage, necrosis, and full-thickness disruption and hemorrhagic ciliochoroidal detachment.

One potential complication of hyphema, bloodstaining of the cornea, occurs in less than 10% of all traumatic hyphemas, but is present in a significantly higher percentage of severe ("8-ball") hyphemas (Fig. 50A) (144). The etiology of corneal bloodstaining is thought to be due to sustained elevation of intraocular pressure. Corneal endothelial dysfunction or loss, however, may predispose to bloodstaining at normal intraocular pressure levels. The cornea becomes diffusely yellow-tan to brown, more intensely centrally. The opacification may last for years, and clears gradually from the periphery toward the visual axis. Histopathologically, corneal bloodstaining is characterized by innumerable minute red hemoglobin fragments, greater centrally than peripherally, which may involve the cornea transmurally (Fig. 50B). Descemet membrane and Bowman layer are relatively spared, however. With time, keratocytes, and possibly macrophages, phagocytose the hemoglobin. Hemosiderin deposits then appear in greatest concentraton in the posterior stroma, centrally. Keratocyte necrosis is a common sequela.

Angle recession is a tear in the anterior face of the ciliary body, between the insertion of the iris root and the ciliary attachment to the scleral spur (Fig. 51A, B). It is seen most commonly after blunt trauma to the eye (145). With the anterior-posterior compressive force of a blow, the eye expands at the equator, stretching the ciliary body. The resulting tear causes the plane of the iris to move posteriorly (recessed), making the anterior chamber deeper. Glaucoma may be a long-term complication of angle recession, often not manifest until many years after the injury. It is believed that the trabecular meshwork may be subclinically damaged at the time of injury, and with time, scarring causes decreased aqueous outflow and thus elevated intraocular pressure.

Another manifestation of an anterior-posterior compressive blow is a Vossius ring, an imprinting of

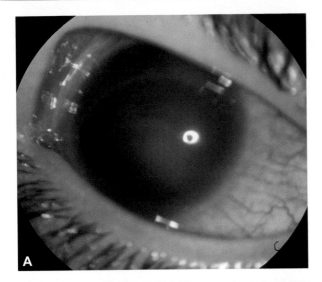

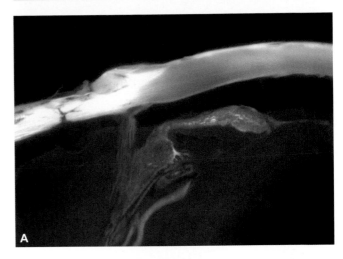

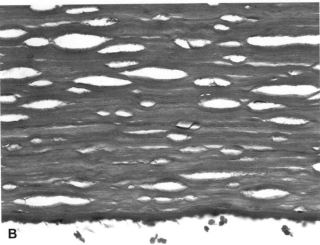

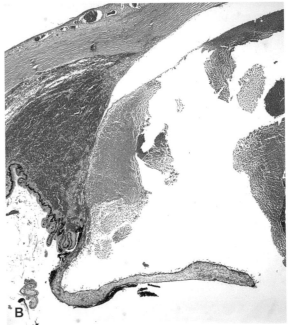

Figure 50 (**A**) Photograph of a so-called 8-ball hyphema in a patient following blunt trauma. (**B**) Histological section of the cornea shows minute erythrocyte fragments within the corneal stroma, most evident along the edges of artifactual clefts between collagen lamellae. Descemet membrane is typically spared. With time, the fragments clear, beginning peripherally at the limbus and proceeding centrally (H&E, original magnification 400×).

Figure 51 (**A**) Gross photograph of an enucleation specimen with angle recession and severe intraocular hemorrhage as a result of blunt trauma. Note the V-shaped cleft in the anterior face of the ciliary body. The ciliary body is also hemorrhagically detached, with only its remaining attachment at the scleral spur. (**B**) Histological section of angle recession with marked posterior displacement of the iris. Note the diffuse hemorrhage within the ciliary body and the presence of blood in the anterior chamber (hyphema) (H&E, original magnification 20×).

melanin pigment from the iris pigment epithelium onto the anterior lens capsule (Fig. 52). An identical appearance may be seen in postmortem eyes, but in that situation, it is far more likely a result of autolysis and not a pathological finding.

Glaukomflecken are minute, ill-defined, white subcapsular opacities in the lens in association with acute elevations in intraocular pressure, as with acute angle closure glaucoma. They correspond histopathologically to foci of lens epithelial necrosis, and clinically they may either disappear or persist after the pressure is normalized.

Traumatic retinal detachment is a common sequela of penetrating trauma, and may result in permanent visual loss even if repaired. Because of

their high metabolic demand, and because they are supplied by the choriocapillaris and not the retinal circulation, retinal photoreceptors begin to degenerate quickly in retinal detachment. On histopathological examination, this is seen as loss of outer segments and blunting of inner segments, progressing to complete loss of both outer and inner segments and dropout of nuclei in the outer nuclear layer (Fig. 53). Clues to identify artifactual detachment of the retina as a function of fixation and processing include the

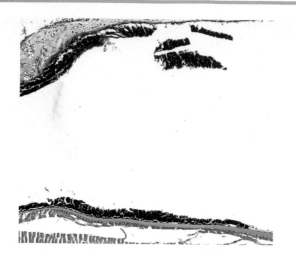

Figure 52 Vossius ring manifested as dislocation of iris pigment epithelium onto the anterior lens capsule. In surgically enucleated eyes, this histological appearance is likely a pathological finding resulting from blunt trauma; in postmortem eyes, it is usually an autolytic artifact (H&E, original magnification 100×).

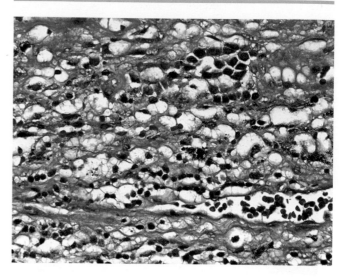

Figure 54 Cluster of hematopoietic precursors within the choroid in a case of penetrating ocular injury and enucleation within days. Note the extravascular location and size differential in comparison to lymphocytes in the lower portion of the field (H&E, original magnification 400×).

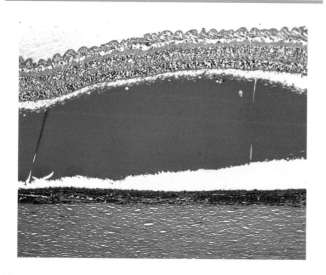

Figure 53 Histological section of a retinal detachment, with proteinaceous eosinophilic subretinal fluid occupying the subretinal space. Note, in addition, the degeneration of photoreceptor outer and inner segments of the retina (H&E, original magnification 40×).

effusions separating the two layers occur not infrequently when the eye is entered. It is a dreaded complication of intraocular surgery, for the massive filling of the suprachoroidal space will cause expulsion of the intraocular tissues if not checked.

An interesting incidental finding often seen in traumatically injured eyes is the presence of foci of extramedullary hematopoiesis within the choroid (Fig. 54) (146). It is not thought to be marrow embolism but rather recruitment of progenitor cells with subsequent proliferation.

VIII. UVEA

A. Anatomy

The uveal tract is from anterior to posterior, composed of the iris, ciliary body, and choroid. It is the predominant vascular layer of the eye. Posteriorly, it separates the sclera externally from the retina internally, and anteriorly, it divides the anterior chamber from the posterior chamber. The iris from anterior to posterior is composed of the stroma, a loose fibrovascular tissue with dendritic melanocytes and the smooth muscle fibers of the sphincter pupillae surrounding its free edge at the pupillary margin, and a double layer of pigment epithelium posteriorly. The dilator pupillae smooth muscle fibers are inconspicuous wisps immediately anterior to the pigment epithelium. Vessels within the stroma have a surrounding distinct acellular zone, or cuff, to allow for changes in tortuosity during changes in pupillary diameter, and this cuff is helpful in identifying iris tissue in cases of ruptured globe with possible extrusion of intraocular contents.

absence of any fluid or proteinaceous material in the subretinal space, preservation of photoreceptor outer and inner segments, and adherence of melanin pigment granules to the photoreceptor outer segments.

Hemorrhagic detachment of the choroid is also a common complication of penetrating trauma. The choroid is bound to the sclera only at the optic nerve head and at the vortex veins, so that hemorrhages and

The iris is connected at its periphery to the anterior face of the ciliary body, known as the iris root. The ciliary body is a roughly triangular-shaped structure with its base the anterior face, its hypotenuse the border abutting the sclera, and its apex directed posteriorly. It is subdivided into the pars plicata, or that portion anteriorly containing the ciliary processes, and the pars plana, or flat portion, posteriorly. The free surface of the ciliary body is lined by a continuation of the double layer of epithelium, but in contrast to the iris, only the outermost layer is pigmented; the layer lining the free surface is nonpigmented. The smooth muscle fibers of the ciliary muscle form the bulk of the triangular cross-sectional area, separated by fibrous tissue containing variable numbers of uveal melanocytes. At the ora serrata, the double layer of ciliary epithelium is continuous with the retina: the nonpigmented layer with the neurosensory retina and the pigmented layer with the RPE. The tapered stroma of the ciliary body is continuous with the choroid, which extends posteriorly to the edge of the optic nerve head. The choroid is composed of arteriovenous vascular tissue with graduated caliber from the choriocapillaris as the monolayer capillary network immediately external to Bruch membrane (on which the RPE rests internally) to larger vessels at its border with the sclera.

B. Specimen Handling

Examination of uveal tissue in isolation is almost nonexistent; the usual scenarios in which that might occur are for identification of extruded intraocular tissue in a surgical exploration of a ruptured globe, or of an incidental (and minute) biopsy of an unusual iris appearance during a cataract extraction or glaucoma procedure. The clues given above in the anatomy of the iris and ciliary body are helpful in the former; the latter is usually for a pigmented macule or small nodule and may be insufficient or inconclusive diagnostically. However, the iris is the easiest intraocular tissue to observe and obtain for pathological examination. Lesions of the iris are amenable to fine needle aspiration, biopsy, and excision, with retention of visual function.

Iridocyclectomy for an iris or ciliary body mass is possible, but again is almost nonexistent outside of a specialized academic setting. Therefore, this discussion pertains to diseases of the uvea for which enucleation is performed; most commonly, these are uveal malignant melanoma and serious inflammatory conditions.

Handling an enucleated eye specimen removed for an intraocular tumor requires careful gross inspection and handling by the pathologist. Unless there is some mitigating circumstance, the eye should fix in 10% neutral buffered formalin for 24 to 48 hours (preferably 48 hours) prior to opening. Only if unfixed tumor tissue is required for ancillary tests should the eye wall be incised before adequate fixation. If necessary, a small hinged flap or window through the sclera overlying the tumor can be made and a cube of uveal tissue removed prior to placing the whole eye in formalin. Obviously, the surgical pathologist must locate the intraocular tumor beforehand to attempt this, and without clinical information, the only recourse is transillumination of the eye as described below. This flap or window technique is challenging but preferable to making a larger incision into the vitreous cavity, which will cause the eye to collapse and possibly contaminate the epibulbar surface with malignant cells.

On gross examination, in addition to the usual external measurements of the eye in three dimensions, cornea and optic nerve, the scleral surface of the eye should be carefully inspected for evidence of abnormal pigmentation or masses. The eye is then transilluminated by using a point source of light placed against the eye from behind, while in a darkened room. Pigmented tumors will block light transmission (as will hemorrhage); the technique is less sensitive for amelanotic masses. The outlines of the transillumination defect can be marked with ink on the scleral surface, so that the plane of section can be chosen to bisect the tumor. The four vortex veins (Fig. 36) must be identified, since they are the most common sites of egress of intraocular melanoma; the vortex vein(s) within or nearest to the tumor should be identified, inspected, and superficially shaved off the sclera and submitted separately before opening the eye. Any areas of scleral pigmentation are suspect and should be included in histological sections, either separately or as part of the main specimen. Although rare for uveal melanomas, optic nerve invasion is possible and a 1-mm thick cross section of the optic nerve surgical margin should be shaved and submitted en face. Once the eye is opened in an anterior-posterior plane determined by the tumor location, the maximum basal dimension and tumor height on the cut surface are recorded. The specific uveal tissues involved, shape of growth, degree and homogeneity of pigmentation, presence or absence of hemorrhage and/or necrosis, and associated pathological processes (retinal detachment, cataract, etc.) should be included in the gross description (Fig. 55). A second cut parallel to the initial plane, 3-mm thick to include the optic nerve, is submitted; the remaining tissue may be sectioned and submitted as necessary, usually parallel to but occasionally perpendicular to the original plane, to document any additional findings of prognostic significance, such as intrascleral extension.

Tissue processing of whole eye specimens benefits from gentle, prolonged dehydration and clearing, but in practical terms, for busy general surgical pathology practices, special processing times may not be feasible. Histological sections are routinely cut at 5 µm; multiple levels of sectioning may be necessary to fulfill all the criteria for pathological staging. PAS stain is beneficial in determining the presence and type of so-called matrix-rich microcirculation architecture within the melanoma. Immunohistochemical stains to confirm the melanocytic nature of the tumor are rarely required.

Clinical Findings

Malignant melanoma is the most common primary intraocular malignancy in adults, with a prevalence of

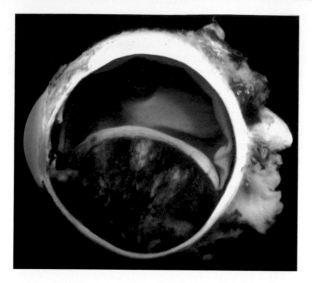

Figure 55 Malignant melanoma of the choroid on cut surface displaying variegated pigmentation, a dome-shaped configuration, and involvement of the ciliary body anteriorly. Tumor height and basal dimension are important parameters and are easily obtained if the tumor is bisected.

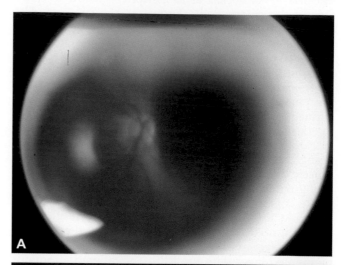

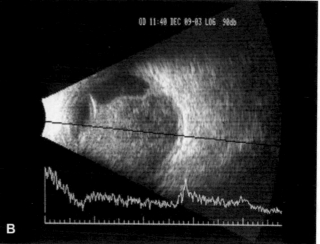

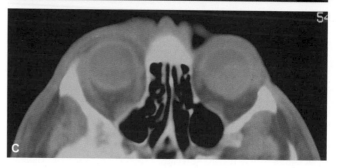

Figure 56 (**A**) Fundoscopic appearance of the same tumor prior to enucleation, showing a smooth-surfaced brown elevated mass obscuring the macula and encroaching upon the optic nerve head. (**B**) Ultrasound examination prior to enucleation showed a large mass with low internal reflectivity, consistent with the diagnosis of uveal melanoma. (**C**) CT scan confirms the ultrasound findings, and in addition suggests the possibility of extraocular extension posteriorly. This was confirmed at the time of enucleation.

one per six to seven million per year in the United States. Affected patients typically present in the fifth to sixth decades; men outnumber women slightly. Presenting symptoms of visual field loss and decreased vision pertain to the retinal detachment caused by the tumor (Fig. 56A). Small tumors may be asymptomatic and discovered only on routine fundoscopy. Helpful ancillary studies include ultrasound, particularly A-scan, which demonstrates low echogenicity within the mass, and imaging studies to potentially identify extraocular extension (Fig. 56B, C).

Tumoral processes of the iris are readily identified by the patient and therefore are usually detected early in development (Fig. 57). Personal photographs may be useful to date the onset and progression of the process. Even minute growth of an iris tumor can be documented by serial slit lamp photography. Depending on the clinical appearance, growth characteristics, patient age, systemic status, and concomitant ocular findings, the ophthalmologist can then form a specific differential diagnostic list of iris masses (147). Table 10 outlines some of the more common possibilities.

Pathology

The uveal tract of the eye normally contains throughout its stroma dendritic melanocytes of neural crest origin, not to be confused with the melanin-containing pigment epithelium lining the uveal tract of neuroepithelial origin. It is the uveal dendritic melanocyte that gives rise to intraocular melanoma, either from a preexisting nevus or de novo. Most uveal melanomas are centered at or posterior to the equator, and therefore, the choroid is the predominant uveal tissue

involved. Typically, choroidal melanoma grows centripetally toward the center of the eye as a dome-shaped mass, and may assume a mushroom or collarbutton shape if rupture through Bruch membrane

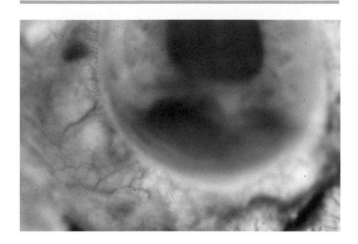

Figure 57 Malignant melanoma involving the inferior iris and ciliary body. Perilimbal pigmentation at the 8:00 position proved to be extraocular extension of the melanoma.

Table 10 Iris Tumefactions

Iris tumefaction	Clinical characteristic(s)
Juvenile xanthogranuloma	Yellow-pink to gray nodule in infant/, resolves with time/corticosteroids, may cause spontaneous hyphema
Brushfield spot	Down syndrome; 10–20 per eye, white-yellow, fluffy
Lisch nodule	Neurofibromatosis type 1; multiple iris nevi
Nevus/melanocytoma	Brown, flat to mildly elevated, minimal distortion of iris landmarks; congenital/childhood onset, stationary to slow growth
Melanoma	May be localized or diffuse ("ring"), white ("tapioca") to brown-black, growth into anterior chamber angle, and/or ciliary body; adults (wide range)
Metastasis	Gelatinous to solid, white-gray to brown; may mimic primary melanoma; adults
Peripheral nerve sheath tumor	Rare, both schwannoma, neurofibroma reported
Leiomyoma	Rare
Sarcoid	Multiple small white nodules at pupillary margin (Koeppe nodule) or elsewhere (Busacca nodule), adult onset, often with posterior chorioretinitis

occurs. Occasionally it grows diffusely, following the contour of the normal choroid and with only minimal elevation. Since the ciliary body is an annular structure three-dimensionally, diffuse melanoma of the ciliary body is termed "ring melanoma." Likewise, melanoma of the iris may be diffuse or may appear as multiple amelanotic tan-white nodules, so-called tapioca melanoma. Choroidal melanoma is clinically categorized by size for prognosis and treatment purposes, as shown in Table 11.

Histopathological examination of uveal melanoma begins with the determination of cell type, as

Table 11 Size Classification of Melanoma of The Posterior Uvea

Category	Basal diameter	Height
Small	<10 mm	<3mm
Medium	>10 and <15 mm and/or	>3 and <10 mm
Large	>15 mm and/or	>10 mm

Table 12 Cytomorphology of Melanoma of The Posterior Uvea

	Spindle cell	Epithelioid cell
Nucleus	Elliptical	Round
	Dispersed chromatin	Coarse, vesicular chromatin
	+/− longitudinal central streak	
Nucleolus	Punctate, basophilic, central	Large, eosinophilic, central
Cytoplasm	Eosinophilic to melanotic	Eosinophilic to melanotic
Cytoplasmic border	Ill defined	Well defined
	Syncytial arrangement of cells	+/− cytoplasmic retraction from surrounding cells

described in Table 12 (148). A spindle cell with an elongated elliptical nucleus containing a punctate central nucleolus corresponds to a spindle B cell of the original Callender classification. A spindle A cell is characterized by a longitudinal groove in the nucleus that lacks a nucleolus. Epithelioid cells are round to polygonal with discrete cell membranes, ample eosinophilic cytoplasm with or without melanin pigment, and round to oval nuclei containing a conspicuous central nucleolus (Fig. 58). Current dogma considers a tumor composed entirely of

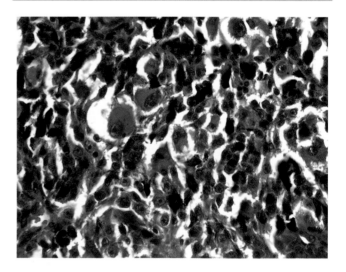

Figure 58 Histological section of malignant melanoma of the choroid, predominantly epithelioid cell type. Note the large cell size with prominent eosinophilic cytoplasm, round to oval nuclei with large central nucleoli and discrete cell borders. However, there is significant variation in cell size and morphology.

spindle A cells to be benign, i.e., a choroidal nevus, so that to diagnose a spindle cell melanoma one must identify at least some spindle B cells (148). The current classification therefore includes either spindle cell nevus or spindle cell melanoma. Unfortunately, not all tumor cells fit nicely into either spindle A, B, or epithelioid categories; rather, cells appear as if on a continuum from spindle at one end to epithelioid at the other. This obviously creates problems in classification and in interobserver variability. It may also explain why the majority of cases are classified as mixed type (spindle and epithelioid cells). There is no clear consensus among ophthalmic pathologists as to how many epithelioid cells must be identified to consider a tumor mixed, also giving rise to interobserver disagreement (149). A rare uveal melanoma will be completely necrotic, so that determination of cell type is impossible. Despite these shortcomings, classification based on cell type has clinical prognostic significance: patients with spindle cell melanomas have 15-year survival rates on the order of 60%; those with nonspindle (mixed or epithelioid) tumors have 15-year survival rates on the order of 40% (150).

Melanomas of the iris are categorized as to cell type in the same fashion as posterior melanomas: spindle cell, epithelioid cell, and mixed spindle, and epithelioid. Spindle cell type is present in slightly over half, epithelioid cell type is rare (2–4%), and mixed cell type makes up the remainder. In contrast, only 20% of diffuse iris melanomas are spindle cell type, with over two-thirds mixed cell type (151).

In addition to cell type and presence of necrosis, mitotic activity should be quantified per 40 high-power field examinations. Mitotic activity in most cases is low. Presence of tumor-infiltrating lymphocytes (>100 per 20 high-power fields) may also have prognostic significance, although it is inverse to that of cutaneous melanomas; lymphocytic infiltrate within a choroidal melanoma is an adverse prognostic factor (152). Studies have shown an inverse correlation between nucleolar size and variability and long-term survival, but such measurements are labor intensive and were performed using sophisticated image-analyzing methodology (153,154). Specific examples of so-called matrix-rich microcirculation patterns [particularly, closed loops, networks (three closed loops, back-to-back), arcs, and parallel arrays with cross-linking] have been positively correlated with death from metastasis (Fig. 59) (155–157). Determination of such patterns may be enhanced by examining PAS-stained sections. Interestingly, such patterns have been reported to be visible in vivo with confocal indocyanine green angiography. Immunohistochemical proliferation markers may also be useful in predicting biological behavior, although results have varied (158). Presence of intrascleral or extrascleral extension should be noted when present, and if present, whether there is intraluminal vortex vein involvement (Fig. 60). Extraocular extension of a uveal melanoma is reported to occur in up to 17% of cases; most are either microscopic or, if grossly apparent, small (<5-mm maximum dimension) (159). Finally, tumor-associated coexisting pathological processes

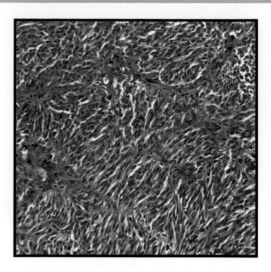

Figure 59 Matrix-rich microcirculation patterns of arcs and loops in uveal melanoma, particularly when there are closed loops in back-to-back configuration, convey an increased risk of death due to disease.

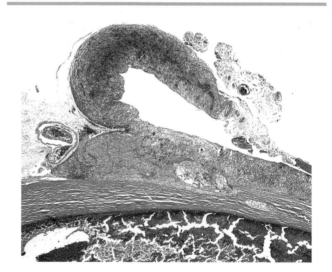

Figure 60 Extraocular extension of choroidal melanoma along and within a vortex vein, the usual method of egress. Note the intraluminal tumor thrombus at the left edge of the field (H&E, original magnification 20×).

should be documented, such as retinal detachment, cataract, and angle closure. Checklists have been published to facilitate reporting of pathological examination of melanomas and other intraocular tumors (160).

The main histopathological differential diagnosis of uveal melanoma is melanocytoma, also called magnocellular nevus. This tumor typically involves the optic nerve head, but, rarely, may form masses in the choroid or ciliary body (161–163). It is a uniformly heavily pigmented jet-black tumor that may show foci of necrosis and/or extraocular extension, features normally worrisome for malignancy. Rare reports have described ciliary body melanocytoma extending through emissarial channels into the episclera, resulting in a dumbbell-shaped mass (162). Necrosis may cause release of melanin pigment into the aqueous humor, leading to accumulation in the aqueous outflow tract and a subsequent elevated intraocular pressure (so-called melanomalytic glaucoma). Histopathological examination of melanocytoma shows cells so uniformly heavily pigmented that cell shape and nuclear features are obscured. Bleaching the sections is necessary to allow the polygonal cells of melanocytoma with their benign nuclear features (round to oval nuclei, dispersed chromatin, inconspicuous to absent nucleolus) and low nuclear:cytoplasmic ratio to be appreciated.

Treatment of melanoma is varied. Small tumors may first be followed to document growth, since the clinical differential diagnosis for these tumors is a choroidal nevus. Medium-size tumors may either be enucleated or treated with brachytherapy (I-125 plaque); survival rates do not significantly differ between these options (164). Other primary or adjunctive treatment options such as helium ion radiation and transpupillary thermoplasty are possible for small- or medium-size tumors. Large tumors require enucleation; preoperative radiation has shown no benefit (165).

Local excision or alternative treatment modality failures followed by enucleation may show treatment effects, reportedly even including a change in the cell type of the melanoma. Melanomas of the uveal tract disseminate hematogenously and not by lymphatics; usual sites of metastatic disease are the liver, lungs, and bone (166). In the Collaborative Ocular Melanoma Study (COMS), results for tumors treated by either (125) I brachytherapy or enucleation were as follows: 5-, 10-, and 12-year rates of death due to metastatic melanoma were 10%, 18%, and 21%, respectively, in the former, and 11%, 17%, and 17%, respectively, in the latter (164). Older patient age and larger maximum basal tumor diameter were the most important predictors of death due to metastatic melanoma. Melanomas of the iris are exceedingly uncommon, representing only 3% of melanomas involving the uveal tract (167). They also differ in having a much better prognosis, with metastatic and mortality rates in the 2–5% range. Age at diagnosis is in the fifth decade, approximately 10 years earlier than posterior uveal melanomas. Most (>85%) iris melanomas are centered below the horizontal plane of the iris; in 10%, the growth is diffuse throughout all quadrants. Localized melanomas of the iris average 6 mm (range 1–17 mm) in greatest basal dimension and 2 mm (range 1–4 mm) in height. In an ophthalmic oncology referral practice, iris nevi outnumber melanomas by 5:1 (147).

Diffuse iris melanomas represent about 10% of all iris melanomas (151). They manifest as heterochromia iridis, and affected patients typically have more symptomatology than those with localized tumors because of extensive anterior chamber angle involvement (with elevated intraocular pressure), cataract, and uveitis. They are not amenable to local resection,

requiring either enucleation or radiation therapy for treatment. Perhaps because of delayed diagnosis and/or higher incidence of epithelioid cells in diffuse iris melanomas as compared with localized tumors, diffuse iris melanomas have higher rates of metastasis (10–15%) than their discrete counterparts (168). Prognostic factors for increased risk of metastasis include: older age at diagnosis, elevated intraocular pressure, tumor involvement of the iris root (+/− angle involvement), and extraocular extension of melanoma.

Metastatic melanoma has been reported to involve the choroid, but such occurrences are extremely rare in comparison with primary uveal melanoma. Metastatic melanoma (as with other types of metastases) is less likely to assume the characteristic dome or mushroom shapes of primary choroidal melanoma, but rather to be a relatively flat, discoid tumor. Histopathologically, metastatic melanoma cells are often more anaplastic and mitotically active than their primary counterparts.

IX. RETINA

A. Anatomy

The retina is composed of 10 layers, with the innermost 9 considered the neurosensory retina and the 10th, the RPE. This distinction is clinically important, since a potential space exists between the neurosensory retina and RPE because of embryonic development. It is in this space that fluid or blood may accumulate, causing an exudative (or serous) retinal detachment. To reiterate, a retinal detachment refers to a separation between the neurosensory retina and the RPE.

The nine layers of the neurosensory retina, from inward out, are (*i*) internal limiting membrane (a true PAS-positive basement membrane); (*ii*) nerve fiber layer (formed by the axons of the ganglion cells); (*iii*) ganglion cell layer; (*iv*) inner plexiform layer (an anuclear synaptic zone); (*v*) inner nuclear layer (nuclei of bipolar, amacrine, horizontal, and Muller cells); (*vi*) outer plexiform layer (watershed zone between retinal and choroidal circulations); (*vii*) outer nuclear layer (nuclei of rod and cone photoreceptors); (*viii*) external limiting layer (not a true membrane, appears as such on routine H&E stains but actually a result of terminal bar junctions between adjacent cells, and (*ix*) photoreceptors (rod and cone inner and outer segments (Fig. 61). The retinal pigment epithelium is a monolayer of cuboidal cells, attached to Bruch membrane on their basal aspect.

Topographically, the retina is divided into zones: peripapillary refers to the zone immediately surrounding the optic nerve head; the macula is that retina temporal to the optic nerve, bounded by the superior and inferior temporal vascular arcades, and centered about the fovea (fovea centralis). As mentioned before, the retina terminates peripherally at the ora serrata, so named because of the scalloped appearance, most pronounced on the nasal side, of the juncture between the neurosensory retina and the pars plana.

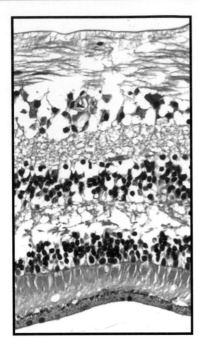

Figure 61 Histological cross section of the retina (H&E, original magnification 200×).

B. Specimen Handling

As before with the uvea, retinal tissue in isolation is almost never a surgical pathology specimen. Fragments of retina may occasionally be identified in biopsy specimens received from explorations of ruptured globes, easily recognized as such when the lamellar architecture of both nuclear and plexiform layers are present, but difficult to distinguish from lymphocytes when only nuclear layer fragments are present. Surgical repair of macular holes during vitrectomy involves incising the internal limiting membrane and peeling a premacular glial membrane adherent to the internal limiting membrane from the inner surface of the retina. These specimens are exceedingly hard to find in the specimen container, since the minute, ultrathin membrane is cellophane-like and may be transparent. Fortunately, indocyanine green is used to aid in visualizing the membrane intraoperatively and staining the excised membrane. However, it leaches out in formalin, so the specimen should be examined and submitted as soon as it is received. As with minute corneal biopsies, a drop of Mercurochrome applied to the membrane will improve tremendously the chances of recovering it after tissue processing. PAS stain is used to identify the internal limiting membrane within the specimen.

C. Retinoblastoma

Much has been discovered in the past two decades regarding the pathogenesis of retinoblastoma, heralded by the discovery within tumor cells of a mutation on chromosome 13q14, the localization of the mutation to the retinoblastoma gene (RB1), the recognition that the normal gene product (pRB1) acts as a tumor suppressor, and that the mutation results in an aberrant gene product incapable of regulating cell proliferation (169).

With the recognition that both alleles of chromosome 13 must be affected for tumors to develop, Knudson's "two-hit" hypothesis was borne out (170).

Clinical Features

Retinoblastoma is the most common malignant intraocular tumor in children, with approximately 250 to 300 new cases each year in the United States. It comprises about 4% of all pediatric malignancies (171). The usual age at presentation is less than 5 years, and the mean is 18 to 24 months in the United States. Children with the germ line mutation are often diagnosed by the age of one year, and usually develop multifocal disease in one eye and/or bilateral disease. Onset in utero or later in childhood or even in adulthood has been documented, but is rare. No sex or ethnic predilection is apparent. Discovery of the tumor is heralded by the development of cosmetic problems often first noticed by the parents (172). The pupil of the affected eye may have an abnormal appearance (white pupil, or leukocoria) or loss of the red reflex within the pupil may be seen in photographs of the infant or child (Fig. 62). Loss of vision may cause the eye to deviate (strabismus), usually inward toward the nose (esotropia). Rarely the tumor will be diffuse within the eye and simulate an endophthalmitis. Only in advanced cases with extraocular extension will there be proptosis. Demonstration of calcification within the tumor, a common occurrence,

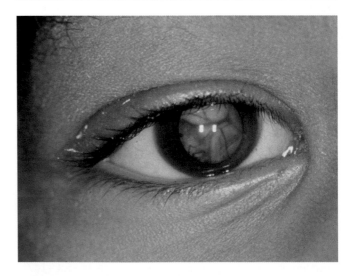

Figure 62 Abnormal pupillary reflex in a young child is highly suspicious for retinoblastoma. In this case, however, the exudative retinal detachment of Coats disease caused the abnormal pupillary appearance. Among other causes of leukocoria are cataract, persistent hyperplastic primary vitreous, and intraocular inflammatory processes such as toxocariasis.

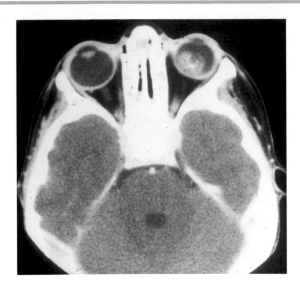

Figure 63 CT scan demonstrating calcification within an intraocular mass in a child, strongly suggestive of retinoblastoma.

is a helpful radiographic finding in differentiating clinical mimics such as Coats disease or causes of retinal detachment from retinoblastoma (Fig. 63).

Pathology

Eyes enucleated for the clinical diagnosis of retinoblastoma must be handled with special care for a number of reasons. Fresh tissue may be requested (or obtained by the surgeon prior to receipt by the pathologist) for molecular genetic analysis or chemotherapy sensitivity studies. This obviously requires opening the globe prior to fixation. As anyone who has attempted this knows, loss of intraocular pressure causes the eye to collapse, and release of vitreous fluid makes for a slippery external surface. More importantly, retinoblastoma is frequently friable and necrotic, and contamination of the external surface of the eye is almost de rigeur when opened in the fresh state. If possible, a small superficial incision through the sclera into the base of the tumor without violating the vitreous is preferable to a complete cross section of the eye.

It is incumbent upon the surgical pathologist to remove any surgical margins from the dissecting field prior to opening the eye. In the case of retinoblastoma, this means the optic nerve margin, since invasion of the optic nerve is the usual mode of egress. The optic nerve surgical margin should be inked and then shaved and embedded en face, producing a cross section for microscopic examination. If opening the eye in the fresh state is not requested, it should be fixed routinely for 24 to 48 hours and then handled as above. Transillumination prior to opening may or may not be beneficial in determining the location of the tumor and the plane of sectioning. If not otherwise indicated, the usual horizontal plane is taken. In addition to the separately submitted optic nerve surgical margin, histological sections of the eye must include

multiple levels through the optic nerve head in order to evaluate for tumor invasion microscopically.

Once opened, the tumor location and growth pattern should be evaluated. Exophytic growth displaces the adjacent normal retina away from the eye wall and therefore causes retinal detachment (Fig. 64A). Endophytic growth of the tumor does not produce this effect. However, the tumor may exhibit a mixture of both endo- and exophytic patterns. Multifocality and vitreous seeding by the tumor should be described, but may be difficult to differentiate from artifactual contamination because of tumor friability and the mucoid "sticky" nature of the vitreous gel. Again, due to the presence of tumor necrosis, the gross appearance may be a variegated gray-white. Presence or absence of involvement of the optic nerve head should be documented. Absence of a discrete mass

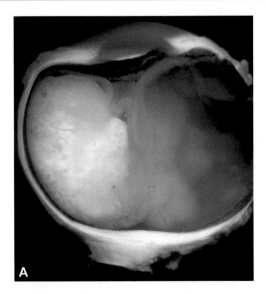

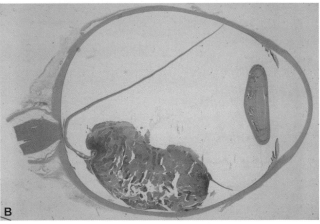

Figure 64 (**A**) Gross appearance of an exophytic retinoblastoma, demonstrating a variegated gray-white cut surface and complete retinal detachment. (**B**) Photomicrograph of an enucleation specimen of retinoblastoma. The variegated appearance grossly corresponds to the interlacing areas of viable (hematoxyphilic) and nonviable (eosinophilic) tumor cells (H&E, original magnification 1.5×).

but a rather diffuse whitening and thickening of the retina with cells in the vitreous, posterior, and anterior chambers is characteristic of the diffuse form of the tumor. Layering of retinoblastoma cells in the anterior chamber is termed "pseudohypopyon," since it resembles clinically the accumulation of acute inflammatory cells in the anterior chamber in uveitis or endophthalmitis. Retinocytoma, the clinically benign variant, has been described as having a more translucent gray quality, with pigmentary changes and calcification at its periphery.

Microscopically, retinoblastoma belongs to the class of small blue round cell tumors of childhood, and undifferentiated retinoblastoma might be difficult to distinguish from intraocular metastases of other round cell tumors, except for their usual location in the uveal tract and not the retina (Fig. 64B). Tumors may appear at any location in the retina and may appear to arise from any nuclear layer, although differentiation of tumor cells attempts to recapitulate photoreceptor cell development. Differentiation within retinoblastoma is identified by rosette formation, i.e., a circular arrangement of cell nuclei. Homer Wright rosette is the least-specific type, being seen in other neuroectodermal tumors such as medulloblastoma, neuroblastoma, and the Ewing sarcoma/PNET spectrum. It is characterized by a tangle of neurofibrillary material within the center of the rosette. Flexner–Wintersteiner rosette has an optically empty center to the rosette, with an accentuation of the cell borders rimming the space because of terminal bar formations between adjacent cells (Fig. 65). This feature is similar to that seen in the normal external limiting membrane of the retina, and Flexner–Wintersteiner rosette is therefore more specific, although not pathognomonic, for retinoblastoma. The most differentiated form of rosette is the fleurette, which, in addition to the terminal bar formation, shows abortive attempts at photoreceptor development as nubbins of eosinophilic

buds protruding into the lumen of the rosette. Retinocytoma, as might be expected of a benign counterpart to retinoblastoma, consists of cytologically and architecturally well-differentiated cells without mitotic activity or necrosis.

Other typical findings in retinoblastoma include the presence of geographical areas of necrosis surrounding islands of viable tumor cells clustered around a central vessel (pseudorosette). Because of the rapid proliferation of tumor cells, those reaching a critical distance from their vascular supply die; this distance (slightly over 0.1 mm) from the central vessel is relatively constant, so that the pseudorosettes are somewhat uniform in diameter. Also because of rapid cell turnover, DNA from necrotic cells often coats basement membranes within the eye, imparting a basophilic linear hue to tumor vessels, the internal limiting membrane of the adjacent retina and the lens capsule. Calcification occurs within necrotic areas as variably fine to coarse granules. In up to one-third of cases, neovascularization of the anterior iris surface may develop.

Immunohistochemical stains are virtually never needed for diagnostic purposes; as might be expected, retinoblastomas have shown neuron-specific enolase and synaptophysin positivity.

Various histopathological parameters have been correlated with disease-free survival; those with statistical significance for poor reduced survival are optic nerve involvement at the surgical margin (50–85% mortality rate at 5 years) and extrascleral involvement (13–69% mortality rate) (173). In addition, massive choroidal invasion and/or involvement of the retrolaminar optic nerve, (beyond the lamina cribrosa of the sclera) but not at the surgical margin, portend an increased risk of orbital recurrence and/or metastasis. Once past the lamina cribrosa, the tumor may gain access to the subarachnoid space and spread via the cerebrospinal fluid.

In addition to intracranial dissemination, retinoblastoma may metastasize hematogenously to the lungs, liver and bone, most commonly (171).

Finally, children with germ line mutations in RB1 are at risk for a variety of nonocular malignancies such as pinealoblastoma (so-called trilateral retinoblastoma), osteosarcoma, and other soft tissue tumors, melanoma, leukemia, and carcinomas of squamous and sebaceous origin. Risk of development of a second malignancy increases approximately 1% per year following diagnosis (174).

Treatment

Most cases of retinoblastoma are unilateral and without evidence of metastasis at the time of diagnosis, and are highly curable (>95%) with enucleation alone (175). For unilateral tumors with favorable clinical parameters (Table 13), cryotherapy or thermotherapy, with or without chemoreduction, or plaque radiotherapy may be employed so as to hopefully retain the eye and vision without reducing patient survival. In bilateral cases, the eye harboring the more advanced tumor is often enucleated; chemoreduction is the main line of defense, however.

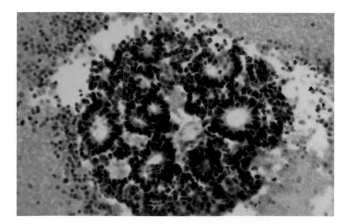

Figure 65 Numerous Flexner–Wintersteiner rosettes are present in a tumor pseudorosette. Note the central vessel and uniform distance of viable tumor from the center, with an abrupt transition to tumor necrosis once the critical distance from the metabolic supply is reached (H&E, original magnification 200×).

Table 13 International Classification Scheme of Retinoblastoma (2003)

Group	Features
A	Tumor ≤3 mm in greatest basal dimension or thickness
B	Tumor >3 mm in greatest dimension OR macular or peripapillary location OR with clear subretinal fluid ≤3 mm from tumor margin
C	Tumor with focal seeding (subretinal and/or vitreous) ≤3 mm from tumor
D	Tumor with diffuse seeding (subretinal and/or vitreous) >3mm from tumor
E	Tumor size >50% of ocular volume *or* neovascular glaucoma *or* opaque media due to hemorrhage *or* invasion into optic nerve, choroid, sclera, anterior chamber, or orbit

processes may involve the orbit, requiring pathological assessment for proper patient care. The incidence of benign versus malignant conditions evolves with age, with most childhood diseases being benign (e.g., dermoid cyst, lymphangioma, optic nerve glioma) and only few malignant (rhabdomyosarcoma), while in adults malignant processes assume a significant proportion (lymphoma, contiguous spread of adnexal or sinus neoplasms, metastatic neoplasms). Tables 14 and 15 list several of the more common entities, which may come within the purview of the surgical pathologist. It should be apparent that such a cosmetically disfiguring procedure as an exenteration is reserved only for conditions in which the potential for improvement in survival exists.

X. ORBIT

A. Introduction

As stated at the outset, because of the large overlap with identical diseases and tumors discussed elsewhere in this text, only those with unique or important aspects regarding their orbital involvement will be addressed in this section. A wide variety of tumoral

B. Anatomy

The orbit is the conical- to pear-shaped space, approximately 30 cc in volume, surrounded, except at its base, by portions of seven bones. At the base, the orbital septum, a fibrous fascia, connects the orbital rim to the tarsi of the upper and lower eyelids and separates the orbital tissues from those of the eyelid. The bulk of the orbital space is occupied by the eye

Table 14 Potential Primary Orbital Surgical Specimens

Type of process	Tissue	Benign process	Procedure	Malignant neoplasm	Procedure
Primary	Lacrimal gland	Pleomorphic adenoma	Excision	Adenoid cystic carcinoma	Excision or exenteration
		Dacryoadenitis (e.g., sarcoid)	Biopsy	Malignant lymphoma	Biopsy
	Soft tissues	Thyroid orbitopathy	None or biopsy	Malignant lymphoma	Biopsy
		Idiopathic orbital inflammation (pseudotumor)	None or biopsy	Rhabdomyo-sarcoma	Biopsy
		Dermoid cyst/Epidermal cyst	Excision		
		Venous malformation (cavernous hemangioma)	Excision		
	Bone	Langerhans cell histiocytosis	Biopsy or curettage		
	Optic nerve	Meningioma	None or Excision	Malignant meningioma	Excision or exenteration
		Juvenile pilocytic astrocytoma	None or excision	Glioblastoma multiforme	Biopsy or excision

Table 15 Secondary Processes Involving The Orbit

Type	Primary site	Disease process	Surgical procedure
Secondary	Intraocular	Malignant melanoma	Enucleation or exenteration
		Retinoblastoma	Enucleation or exenteration
	Ocular adnexae		
	Conjunctiva	Malignant melanoma	Exenteration
		Squamous cell carcinoma	Exenteration
		Mucoepidermoid carcinoma	
	Eyelid/periocular skin	Basal cell carcinoma	Exenteration
		Squamous cell carcinoma	Exenteration
		Sebaceous carcinoma	Exenteration
		Malignant melanoma	Exenteration
	Paranasal sinus	Mucocele	Excision
		Invasive zygomycosis	Debridement, possible exenteration
		Squamous cell carcinoma	Exenteration
	Metastatic	Breast carcinoma	Biopsy
		Lung carcinoma	Biopsy
		Prostatic adenocarcinoma	Biopsy

and surrounding adipose tissue. Specialized structures in the orbit include the optic nerve, 2.5 to 3.0 cm in length, six extraocular muscles (four recti: superior, medial, inferior, and lateral; two oblique: superior and inferior), the levator palpebrae superioris muscle, and the lacrimal gland in the superior temporal aspect. The lacrimal gland is actually not entirely within the orbit; it is subdivided into the larger orbital and smaller palpebral lobes by the aponeurosis of the levator palpebrae superioris.

Any mass effect within the tissues of the orbit will displace the eye forward (proptosis or exophthalmos). Proptosis may be axial, if the mass effect is directly behind the globe and within the space bounded by the four rectus muscles (intraconal, as in optic nerve neoplasms), or nonaxial, if the mass effect is extraconal (i.e., lacrimal gland neoplasms displace the eye down and nasally). Important associations with surrounding structures include the paranasal sinuses (ethmoid and sphenoid medially, frontal superiorly, and maxillary inferiorly), the cavernous sinus posteriorly, and the lacrimal sac and nasolacrimal duct anteriorly at the inferior nasal aspect.

C.   Specimen Handling

Specimens from the orbit come to the surgical pathologist in three shapes and sizes: incisional biopsies on the order of millimeters to one centimeter; excisions of discrete masses, usually greater than one centimeter; and exenterations, in which either partial or complete removal of the orbital contents, including the eye if present, is removed. Exenterations may be either lid sparing or lid encompassing. Biopsies and excisions are handled as with soft tissues anywhere else in the body; excisions should be inked prior to sectioning, in case margin status is important for patient management. Exenteration specimens should be oriented prior to dissection and any palpable or visible mass lesion measured and described in relation to its anatomic location. Helpful clues to orientation include the horizontal plane of the palpebral fissure, identification of the caruncle, which is the fleshy mound of tissue in the medial canthus between the eyelids, the more developed and slightly larger superior tarsus (and eyelashes) in the upper eyelid as compared with the lower, and, in lid-sparing procedures, the slight nasal displacement of the pupil within the iris. If the location of the tumor is not discerned by clinical history, previous biopsy, or gross inspection, palpation will usually suffice to identify the abnormally firm focus. Once identified, the skin and soft tissue margins should be inked, although, in complete exenterations, positive soft tissue margins indicate tumor abuts the bone, and, if the bony wall is visually unremarkable intraoperatively, no further treatment is indicated. Rarely, if there is bone destruction by the neoplasm, fragments or portions of bone may be present as part of the exenteration specimen (Fig. 66A). The deep (apical) margin containing the surgical transection of the optic nerve should be shaved and submitted en face; remaining margins may be taken perpendicular

to the outer surface, in a meridional (anterior-posterior) plane from the outside in to, but not necessarily including, the eye. The eye is exceedingly rarely involved by an infiltrating neoplasm and only in those cases is it necessary to document scleral and/or corneal invasion. Three sections of tumor should suffice for pathological diagnosis. The remainder of the orbital tissues may be sampled in the major and minor meridians in the same fashion. Proper orientation of the specimen can be confirmed grossly and microscopically by finding the lacrimal gland in the section taken from the superior temporal quadrant. Once the orbital tissues have been sampled, the eye may be removed and handled as an enucleation specimen. If histological capabilities exist for oversize blocks and glass slides, complete cross sections of the entire specimen may be submitted to include the tumor in relation to the eye and eyelids, but this is beyond the scope of most surgical pathology practices (Fig. 66B).

D.   Malformations

Dermoid Cyst

Dermoid cysts are thought to arise from surface ectoderm embryologically entrapped within suture lines of adjoining bones, for there is usually a bony defect overlying their location. They typically become manifest in childhood in the superior temporal or superior medial quadrants of the orbit and expand slowly with age (176). Rupture of the cyst wall may result in an inflammatory clinical picture. When excised in toto, they appear as egg-shaped, white-tan, thin-walled cysts, and on sectioning, exude a creamy to flaky white contents in which hair may be evident. Histological sections show the cyst lining to be keratinizing stratified squamous epithelium, beneath which are pilosebaceous units in a loose collagenous stroma. A brisk foreign body granulomatous response ensues if the cyst contents are released into the surrounding tissues, which may destroy the epidermal lining entirely; the pathological diagnosis then rests on identification of hair and/or keratin within the granulomatous reaction.

Venous Malformation (Cavernous Hemangioma)

Cavernous hemangioma, now generally considered to be a venous malformation, is one of the more common surgical pathology specimens from the orbit (177,178). It is a slowly expanding, ovoid, circumscribed mass and thus is rarely detected before adulthood. It may be either intraconal or extraconal in the posterior orbit. Because of the slow velocity of blood through its anastomosing channels, thrombosis is common. Venous malformation is excised when either vision or cosmesis is compromised, and can be isolated and removed without bleeding complications. On gross examination, the red-purple mass has a mildly knobby surface and may appear thinly encapsulated. When sectioned, the spongy appearance with closely packed thin-walled vascular spaces containing blood is characteristic (Fig. 67A). Histological sections

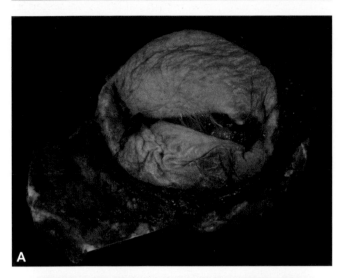

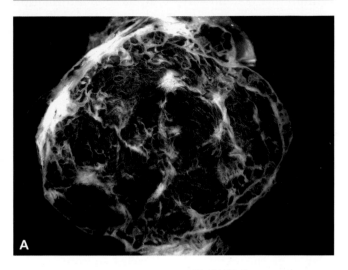

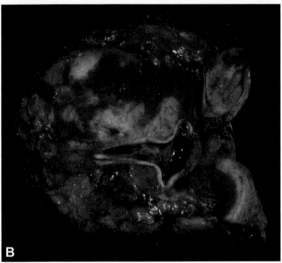

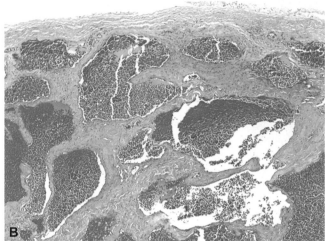

Figure 66 (**A**) Exenteration specimen, including a portion of the maxilla and inferior lateral orbital rim, in a patient with a large malignant melanoma of the orbit. (**B**) A vertical cross section of the exenteration specimen shows a hemorrhagic, variegated tan-brown mass filling the orbit and collapsing the eye. On microscopic examination, a small intraocular focus in an otherwise necrotic eye indicated that the process began as an intraocular uveal melanoma, with massive extraocular extension.

Figure 67 (**A**) Gross appearance of the cut surface of a venous malformation as a circumscribed lobular mass with a thin white fibrous surface and interconnecting white septa outlining congested, cystic vascular spaces. (**B**) Histological section of venous malformation showing congested dilated vascular channels lined by flattened endothelium and containing smooth muscle elements within the variably thick septa (H&E, original magnification 100×).

demonstrate endothelial-lined spaces containing smooth muscle elements within the fibrous septa (Fig. 67B). Foci of thrombosis with granulation tissue may mimic the capillary proliferation pattern seen in juvenile hemangioma.

Lymphatic Malformation (Lymphangioma)

Although the presence of lymphatics within the orbit has been debated, current evidence suggests that they do exist at least in the vicinity of the lacrimal gland and the dura of the optic nerve (179,180). Malformation of lymphatic channels in the orbit usually becomes manifest in childhood as proptosis because

of ill-defined cystic masses on imaging studies (181). It may enlarge rapidly, simulating rhabdomyosarcoma, if hemorrhage into the channels occurs. Its appearance at the time of surgery has been likened to a "chocolate cyst." In addition to its worrisome growth, it may compress the optic nerve, causing visual loss, necessitating prompt surgical intervention. Removal may be incomplete because of its infiltrative nature and involvement of vital structures.

Microscopic examination reveals variably sized cystic spaces lined by flattened endothelium and containing proteinaceous fluid or erythrocytes. The walls surrounding the channels contain fibrous tissue and lymphoid aggregates, sometimes with follicle formation. Smooth muscle is usually lacking.

Immunohistochemically, lymphatic malformation endothelial cells may be highlighted by D2-40 antibody, supporting the lymphatic nature of the malformation (182).

Inflammation

Graves orbitopathy is the most common cause of proptosis, both bilateral and unilateral, in adults. It rarely comes to the attention of the surgical pathologist, however, because it is diagnosed serologically and by radiographic studies and treated medically by radioactive ablation of the thyroid. CT or MR imaging shows a characteristic fusiform expansion of the extraocular muscles but sparing of their tendons. The medial rectus is the most commonly involved, but typically more than one muscle is affected. Only when there is sufficient mass effect from inflammation and edema of the extraocular muscles to compromise vision by compressing the optic nerve is surgical management indicated in the active phase of the disease. If a biopsy were to be performed, histologically, it would demonstrate interstitial edema and a B-cell predominant lymphocytic infiltrate. Decompression of the orbit by medial orbitotomy with herniation of the orbital tissues into the ethmoid sinus may result in a specimen from the paranasal sinus, totally unrelated to the orbital disease process. When an extraocular muscle is submitted for examination, often the surgical procedure is for strabismus because of end-stage fibrotic and fat replacement of muscle fibers, causing restriction of eye movement.

Idiopathic. Idiopathic orbital inflammation is the preferred term for what is often referred to as orbital pseudotumor (183,184). The clinical picture is one of a relatively acute onset of unilateral proptosis with conjunctival injection and pain on eye movement. Typically, adults are affected, although it can occur in younger age groups. On imaging studies, an ill-defined mass lesion may involve one or more tissues of the orbit; if a single tissue only is affected, then it is appropriate to use the specific term instead of the more general ''orbital'' inflammation, e.g., inflammation confined to an extraocular muscle is myositis and lacrimal gland dacryoadenitis. Biopsies performed in the active stages of the disease show tissue infiltration by a scattered polymorphous inflammatory infiltrate, predominantly lymphoplasmacytic, but with minor populations of eosinophils and neutrophils. Granulomatous inflammation is not typical, although it has been described; if present, histochemical stains for microorganisms are indicated. Likewise, vasculitis within the tissue is rare in idiopathic orbital inflammation and should raise the suspicion for a systemic vasculitis such as Wegener granulomatosis. Most cases are diagnosed on clinical grounds, and biopsies are generally reserved for cases unresponsive to the usual corticosteroid therapy regimen. Fibrosis then dominates the histological pattern, with only a sparse inflammatory component; some regard this sclerosing pattern of idiopathic orbital inflammation as a distinct entity unrelated to the more acute process described above (Fig. 68) (185).

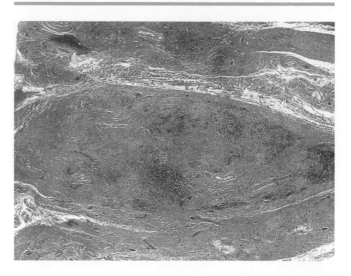

Figure 68 Histological pattern of idiopathic orbital inflammation at low power, showing a patchwork of lymphoplasmacytic infiltrates in a densely sclerotic background (H&E, original magnification 50×).

This pattern may be associated with other immunologically mediated fibrosing conditions such as retroperitoneal and mediastinal fibrosis, Riedel thyroiditis, and sclerosing cholangitis (186). In severe cases, the fibrosis may cause complete restriction of ocular motility, the so-called frozen orbit. Immunosuppressive and radiation therapy may have some efficacy in ameliorating the process.

XI. LACRIMAL GLAND

The lacrimal gland is composed of serous acini aggregated in lobules, separated by thin fibrovascular septa, draining via multiple ducts into the superior lateral fornix of the conjunctiva. Only occasional lymphocytes and plasma cells, singly and in small aggregates, are normally present. Mass effect within the lacrimal gland may be a result of inflammation (dacryoadenitis), duct obstruction (dacryops), and cellular proliferations. Involvement by certain inflammatory processes such as sarcoidosis may be bilateral. The most common benign epithelial neoplasm is pleomorphic adenoma; other varieties include oncocytoma and monomorphic adenoma (187). Interestingly, only one case of Warthin tumor has been described (188). Of the primary malignancies of the orbit in adults, many will likely involve or originate in the region of the lacrimal gland. Adenoid cystic carcinoma is the most common epithelial malignancy of the lacrimal gland. Because of its propensity for perineural invasion, adenoid cystic carcinoma is not often completely eradicated by exenteration; local resection with adjuvant therapy may be as efficacious in local control and survival (189). The malignant component of malignant mixed tumor (carcinoma ex pleomorphic adenoma) is usually either a poorly differentiated adenocarcinoma or adenoid cystic carcinoma. Primary epithelial malignancies other than these, while documented, are rare. Tumors primarily involving salivary glands are described elsewhere in the text and not elaborated upon here.

A. Lymphoproliferative Processes

Of the nonepithelial tumoral expansions of the lacrimal gland, lymphoproliferative processes are by far the most common and certain to cross the examining table of a general pathologist. They may arise elsewhere within the orbit or in the conjunctiva and less commonly in the eyelid; this discussion includes all periocular sites. They may be unilateral or bilateral. Most cases of orbital and conjunctival proliferations are localized disease processes, while eyelid involvement has a high association with systemic disease (190). Suspected lymphoproliferative disorders of the periocular region require forewarning to the surgical pathologist by the surgeon, since fresh tissue is usually necessary for ancillary studies to provide the most accurate and precise histopathological diagnosis. It is therefore incumbent upon the ophthalmologist to alert the pathologist to the possibility that the specimen represents a lymphoproliferative process, and incumbent upon the pathologist to handle the tissue appropriately and in a timely fashion. Unfortunately, the amount of tissue excised is often insufficient in amount and quality to allow for all possible ancillary studies. The pathologist is then required to prioritize specimen allocation in order to achieve the maximal diagnostic potential of the tissue. The following list is one approach to handling and distribution of suspected lymphoid tissue received fresh:

1. Touch preparation of freshly cut surface, fixed immediately in 95% ethanol and stained with H&E.
2. Intraoperative microscopic examination:
    a. If a lymphoid cell population is identified, submit as follows (in order of importance):
        (i). Place a section in zinc formalin for histopathological examination;
        (ii). Send a portion to flow cytometry for a lymphoma workup;
        (iii). Submit a portion to cytogenetics for chromosomal analysis; and
        (iv). Snap-freeze a portion and hold for possible molecular studies (B-cell/T-cell gene rearrangement).
    b. If either only a few or no lymphoid cells are identified, discuss with the surgeon regarding obtaining additional tissue or performing frozen section intraoperative consultation on the existing specimen:
        (i). If the clinical suspicion of a lymphoproliferative disorder remains high, additional biopsy material is recommended, repeating steps 1 and 2.
        (ii). If a frozen section is warranted, freeze a thin cross section of the tissue, examine, and report.

(iii). If no frozen section is requested, fix the tissue in 10% neutral buffered formalin and process routinely.

Fine needle aspiration is not routinely performed for orbital and/or conjunctival neoplasms at most institutions, but is a possible method of obtaining material for screening diagnosis (191,192). If a lymphoproliferative process is identified, and enough material for flow cytometry obtained, an incisional biopsy may not be necessary prior to systemic workup. For accurate lymphoma classification, however, histopathological morphological diagnosis is required (193).

B. Clinical Findings

Ocular adnexal lymphoproliferative disorders run the gamut from benign reactive hyperplasias to high-grade malignant lymphomas. They typically present in the fifth to seventh decades, although conjunctival lymphoid hyperplasias are not uncommon in children. Women are afflicted more often than men. The most common site of involvement is the orbit, usually superior temporal in the lacrimal gland, and patients present with proptosis, often with inferior displacement. Molding of the mass to the contour of the eye is a characteristic feature on imaging studies (Fig. 69A) (194). If the mass is sufficient to restrict extraocular muscle movement, there may be diplopia (double vision) and/or ptosis (drooping of the eyelid). Lymphoproliferative disorders involving the conjunctiva appear as pink "salmon-patch" elevations of the conjunctiva, usually in the bulbar conjunctiva or fornices (Fig. 69B) (195). Histopathological diagnosis of lymphoproliferative disorders is relatively straightforward at the benign and malignant extremes, but can be difficult, if not impossible, to categorize in the intermediate, often indeterminate, gray zone (196). Since there are no lymph nodes in the orbit, the anatomical landmarks of nodal architecture (and their effacement) are of no help in diagnosis. Features favoring a benign diagnosis include: the presence of reactive lymphoid follicles, with normal follicular architecture; a zonal polymorphous infiltrate of both T- and B-cell lymphocytes and plasma cells; and a lack of overt malignant nuclear features. Partial or diffuse involvement and/or replacement of normal lacrimal gland parenchyma by a relatively monomorphous population of small to intermediate lymphocytes is more consistent with a neoplastic lymphoid proliferation (Fig. 70A). However, malignant lymphomas may evolve from presumably preexisting reactive proliferations, and partial effacement of a reactive architectural pattern by lymphoma must be kept in mind. Small, relatively well-differentiated lymphocytes are the most common cell population in orbital lymphoproliferative processes and therefore are difficult to classify as malignant on cytomorphological characteristics alone (Fig. 70B). Immunophenotyping is a key adjunct, especially in problematic cases, and may be accomplished by flow cytometry and/or immunohistochemistry. Gene rearrangement studies are usually reserved for

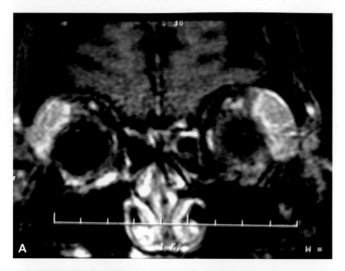

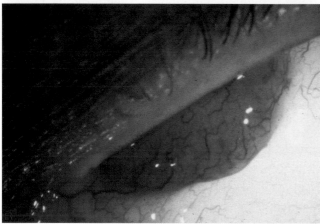

Figure 69 (**A**) Bilateral superior temporal masses, as seen on MR scan, are highly suspicious for a lymphoproliferative process. Note that the masses conform to the globes, rather than indenting or invading them. (**B**) Conjunctival involvement appears as a fleshy, salmon-pink mass.

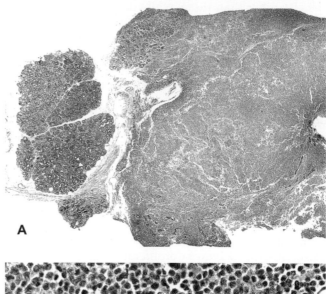

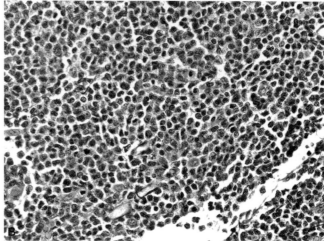

Figure 70 (**A**) Partial effacement of the lacrimal gland by a diffuse lymphoproliferative process (H&E, original magnification 25×). (**B**) At high power, lymphocytes are small with irregular nuclear contours. Immunophenotypying demonstrated typical pattern of mantle cell lymphoma (CD5+, CD20+, FMC7+, cyclin D1+, CD10-, CD23-) (H&E, original magnification 400×).

cases deemed inconclusive by histopathological and immunophenotypic analysis and may be beyond the scope of a general surgical pathology practice, requiring consultation with a reference laboratory.

C.   Extranodal Marginal Zone B-Cell Lymphoma

Extranodal marginal zone B-cell lymphoma (MALT lymphoma) is the most common type of lymphoma to involve the orbit, and may or may not arise in or involve the lacrimal gland (Table 16) (197). MALT lymphoma may demonstrate either partial or diffuse involvement and/or replacement of normal lacrimal gland parenchyma by a relatively monomorphous population of small to intermediate lymphocytes (Fig. 70A). Nuclei show membrane irregularities, vesicular to coarse chromatin, and small nucleoli. Another general characteristic of MALT lymphoma is the monocytoid morphology of neoplastic lymphocytes.

Infiltration of residual ductal elements by neoplastic lymphocytes (lymphoepithelial lesions), typical of MALT lymphoma in salivary gland, is uncommon in the lacrimal gland. As alluded to above, residual follicular architecture may be present.

MALT lymphomas are associated with an indolent course, and, particularly, if localized to the orbit as they often are, have an excellent prognosis with radiation therapy (198).

Treatment

Treatment of ocular adnexal lymphoproliferative disorders is radiation, if localized (stage IE), and radiation plus chemotherapy, if systemic. Radiation dosages range from 15 to 20 Gy for hyperplasia/atypical hyperplasia/indeterminate to 30 to 35 Gy for lymphoma (198,199). Corticosteroid therapy may

Table 16 Incidence of Malignant Lymphoma Subtypes in the Orbit

Malignant lymphoma subtypes	Percentage of orbital cases
Extranodal marginal zone (MALT lymphoma)	64
Follicle center	10
Grade I	1
Grade II	9
Diffuse large B cell	9
Plasmacytoma	6
Lymphoplasmacytic-immunocytoma	5
T cell	3
Mantle cell	2

be attempted first for benign hyperplasia. Radiation treatment morbidity may include dry eye, radiation retinopathy, and cataract, particularly at higher dosages (199).

Certain controversies have flared in the past two decades regarding lymphoproliferative processes in the orbit because of apparent inconsistencies between clinical presentation and behavior, clinical behavior and pathological diagnosis, pathological diagnosis and immunophenotype, and immunophenotype and molecular analysis. For instance, initial dogma was that bilaterality was a marker for systemic disease, and eyelid and orbital involvement were more likely to disseminate than conjunctival disease (194). Larger, more recent studies are divided as to the validity of those conclusions (190,200). Previous authors questioned the relevance of pathological diagnosis, stating that there was no significant difference in development of systemic disease between orbital reactive and/or atypical hyperplasias and frank orbital malignant lymphomas (201). More recent experience indicates that reactive processes are not at risk for systemic involvement, and that the risk is minor for low-grade lymphomas (7% dissemination, median follow-up 44 months) (196). Finally, initial studies showed that the development of systemic disease was not different between proliferations demonstrating monoclonality versus those that did not (194). More recent evidence shows that there is a significant correlation between documentation of monoclonality (either by immunophenotype or by gene rearrangement) and (*i*) dissemination at the time of diagnosis, (*ii*) persistence of disease at follow-up, and (*iii*) lymphoma-related death (196).

Although the vast majority of ocular adnexal and orbital lymphomas are of B-cell lineage, rare cases of T-cell lymphoma and Hodgkin lymphoma have been documented (202,203).

XII. OPTIC NERVE

A. Neoplasms

Optic Glioma

Optic nerve glioma (juvenile pilocytic astrocytoma) is the most common primary tumor of the optic nerve and accounts for about 1% of all intracranial tumors.

The majority occur in the first decade of life, with a median age of 6.5 years and a mean age of 11 (204). Those occurring in children are almost invariably benign; indeed, some have regarded them as astrocytic hamartomas, particularly when associated with neurofibromatosis type 1 (NF1). This association is relatively common; i.e., anywhere from 10% to 70% of patients with optic nerve glioma will have NF1, and from 10% to 30% of patients with NF1 will develop optic glioma (205). Most optic nerve gliomas, however, are sporadic, and females are preferentially affected. The tumors are almost always unilateral. Gliomas occurring in adults are much more likely to behave in a malignant fashion (206).

Symptomatology results from compression or atrophy of axons within the affected segment of the nerve, causing visual decrease or complete loss. The mass effect of the tumor may produce an axial proptosis, sometimes with a downward displacement. Loss of vision may secondarily cause a strabismus. Fundoscopic examination may show the effects of venous compression, with optic disc edema, venous stasis retinopathy or the full-blown "strawberry sundae" pattern of retinal hemorrhage in central retinal vein occlusion. Opticociliary shunts may develop between the retinal and choroidal circulations at the optic disc. Radiographic imaging classically demonstrates a fusiform enlargement of the affected portion of the optic nerve, sometimes with rather clear demarcation from the unaffected portion. The optic canal may be widened but does not necessarily correlate with intracranial involvement; rather it may be a result of arachnoid hyperplasia, which not uncommonly accompanies the tumor. Invasion beyond the confines of the dura is not a feature of glioma of childhood.

Pathology. The prototypical gross appearance of optic glioma is one of a fusiform, uniform expansion of the optic nerve, well beyond its normal 3-mm diameter on cross section. The external aspect is smooth and white, as the dura is intact surrounding the glioma. The white-gray cut surface may contain gray, myxoid, or gelatinous foci and/or areas of hemorrhage.

The histopathological appearance on low power shows dilation of the normal fascicular arrangement of axons surrounded by fibrovascular septa. The fascicles are only mildly hypercellular as compared with normal, with spindle nuclei and bland chromatin and abundant pale eosinophilic neurofibrillary cytoplasmic processes. Mitotic activity, if detected, is sparse. Coarse eosinophilic Rosenthal fibers may be abundant within the neurofibrillary background. A microcystic pattern is not uncommon in areas. The meninges surrounding the affected portion of the nerve may show meningeal hyperplasia, further expanding the diameter of the nerve (Fig. 71A, B).

Treatment. Optic nerve glioma of childhood has a natural course of self-limited slow growth; rarely, it may even demonstrate spontaneous regression (207–209). Most cases are carefully followed if the vision and radiographic appearance are stable. Only rarely is surgical excision indicated for cosmetic improvement or if intracranial involvement with

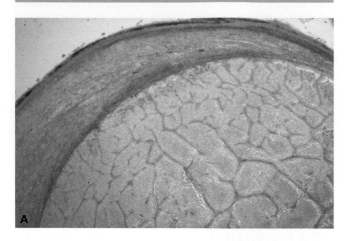

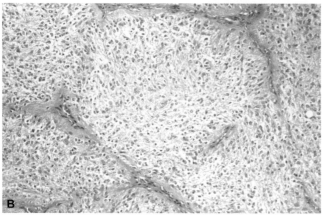

Figure 71 (**A**) Low-power photomicrograph of an optic nerve glioma, showing variable enlargement of the fascicular arrangement of the normal nerve, without significant hypercellularity. Note the expansion of the meninges, due to meningeal hyperplasia and not extrapial extension of the glioma (H&E, original magnification 25×). (**B**) At higher power, there is some degree of hypercellularity within individual fascicles, but without nuclear enlargement, hyperchromasia, pleomorphism, or mitotic activity (H&E, original magnification 100×).

contralateral vision loss develops. When surgery is performed, only the affected portion of the nerve is excised; the eye remains in place. Radiation and chemotherapy as therapeutic alternatives have had questionable results. Astrocytic optic nerve tumor in adulthood, in contrast, is a frankly malignant neoplasm both in clinical behavior and in histopathological appearance (i.e., glioblastoma multiforme) (206,210). Most patients rapidly evolve from unilateral to bilateral visual loss and die within one year of onset; again, radiation and chemotherapy have not appreciably improved survival rates or duration for this rare neoplasm.

Meningioma

Meningioma of the ocular adnexa most commonly involves the intraorbital or intracanalicular optic nerve, either as a primary site or secondarily from an adjacent intracranial location such as the sphenoid

wing or tuberculum sella (211). In rare cases, orbital meningioma arises without apparent connection to either the optic nerve or intracranially and is thought to originate from ectopic congenital meningothelial rests. It typically manifests in middle-aged females as a slowly progressive decrease in visual acuity and color desaturation, with only mild (2–5 mm) axial proptosis; a significant number of patients are asymptomatic, however (212). Occurrences in adult males and children are uncommon. Bilateral involvement seems to preferentially affect adolescents. Ocular funduscopic examination, depending on the location and extent of the tumor, may show an optic disc that is variably normal, elevated, or atrophic. Opticociliary shunt vessels, papillary vessels that shunt retinal venous drainage to the choroidal circulation, develop in up to one-third of cases. Radiographic studies demonstrate a tubular expansion of the optic nerve, often with a bulbous dilatation at the orbital apex. Calcification is often detected.

Pathology. Gross examination of a resected optic nerve meningioma recapitulates the radiographic appearance. On cut surface, the optic nerve itself may either be compressed by the surrounding meningothelial proliferation or infiltrated and partially to completely effaced. The tumor may be confined by the dura, but often invades through into the surrounding perioptic soft tissues. On microscopic examination, the tumor displays the typical syncytial whorling to streaming pattern of meningothelial cells with round to oval uniform nuclei, dispersed chromatin, and occasional intranuclear cytoplasmic invaginations. Atypical features (nuclear pleomorphism, increased mitotic activity, necrosis and "sheeting") are rare. Psammoma bodies are usually infrequent. The histopathological diagnosis is usually straightforward; rarely, the syncytial arrangement may simulate a nonnecrotizing granulomatous inflammation or the fibrous subtype a solitary fibrous tumor/hemangiopericytoma.

Treatment. The natural evolution of optic nerve meningioma is one of slow, inexorable visual decline, which may take years to cause significant impairment (213). Aggressive behavior is rare. Thus, surgical intervention is almost never necessary for tumors confined to the orbit; radiation in fractionated doses or stereotactic radiosurgery may be used if clinically indicated (214). If an intracranial component threatens vital structures or the opposite optic nerve via the optic chiasm, an intracranial surgical procedure may be performed, but the intraorbital component is not disturbed.

XIII.   SOFT TISSUE

Although fibrous histiocytoma historically has been ranked as the most common mesenchymal tumor of the orbit in adults, it is an uncommon pathological diagnosis in the current lexicon. Some cases now would undoubtedly be classified in the solitary fibrous tumor–hemangiopericytoma spectrum of spindle cell neoplasms. The clinical, radiographic, and gross and microscopic pathological findings of these and other soft tissue neoplasms such as peripheral nerve sheath tumors do not differ from those occurring in sites other than the orbit, and are further described elsewhere in the text.

A. Rhabdomyosarcoma

Rhabdomyosarcoma is the most common malignant orbital neoplasm in childhood, usually presenting as a rapidly enlarging mass in a child in the latter part of the first decade (215). Although they may arise from pluripotential cells in any quadrant of the orbit, the most common location is superior nasal, thus displacing the eye forward, inferiorly and temporally. The rapid enlargement necessitates prompt diagnosis and treatment, which now is a largely successful combination of chemotherapy and radiation (216). Therefore, a biopsy is all that is now done surgically, which may tax the ability of the surgical pathologist to accurately distinguish the neoplasm from the other small round blue cell tumors of childhood.

The most common subtype of rhabdomyosarcoma in the orbit is embryonal, in which sheets of undifferentiated hyperchromatic small cells with minimal cytoplasm and high mitotic activity efface the normal orbital tissues. Alveolar rhabdomyosarcoma is less common, occurs in a slightly older age group, and is more likely to involve the inferior rather than the superior orbit (217). The dyscohesive nature of the neoplastic cells in the central foci of nests of tumor, the architecture for which the subtype is named, is not always apparent, but by FISH or cytogenetic evaluation the characteristic 2:13 translocation may be identified and allow proper categorization.

XIV. SECONDARY/METASTATIC NEOPLASMS

Secondary malignancies, either direct spread from the eyelid or contiguous paranasal sinuses or metastatic from distant sites, increase in incidence with increasing age. In these cases, clinical information and/or prior pathological material may be available to guide the pathologist in gross dissection and microscopical diagnosis. Since the most common paranasal sinus malignancy is squamous cell carcinoma, it follows that squamous cell carcinoma of the orbit is high on the list of possibilities when examining an orbital exenteration, particularly if no ancillary clinical information is available. Of the cutaneous primaries of the eyelids, basal cell carcinoma is far and away the most common; of those that invade the orbit, medial canthal location and infiltrative histopathological growth pattern are characteristic. Metastases to the orbit are nearly always carcinomas; in men, a lung primary is the most common, while in women breast carcinomas predominate (218). Paradoxically, rare metastases (particularly scirrhous breast carcinomas) may cause enophthalmos (retraction of the eye into the orbit) rather than proptosis, as might be expected from a tumoral process. Occasionally, the metastasis is the presenting sign of the malignancy; most often, in these cases, an occult lung primary is discovered on systemic examination.

Melanomas involving the orbit may be either primary or secondary (219). Of the primary melanomas reported, a large majority have been associated with some preexisting form of oculodermal melanocytosis or cellular blue nevus (220,221). Secondary involvement of the orbit from a primary uveal melanoma is far and away the most common type of orbital melanoma (222). Extraocular extension of a uveal melanoma is reported to occur in up to 17% of cases; most are either microscopic or, if grossly apparent, small (<5-mm maximum dimension) (159,223). Extraocular extension of a primary intraocular malignancy, so sufficiently advanced as to present as a large orbital mass, is extremely unusual in developed countries today, but must be entertained at the time of gross dissection and microscopic examination. Obvious distortion of the eye or discontinuity in the eye wall on sectioning should raise one's suspicions. Secondary orbital involvement by melanoma due to contiguous spread from a conjunctival or eyelid melanoma is also possible. Exenteration for an ocular adnexal malignant melanoma, while beneficial in local control, has not shown any improvement in patient survival (222). Melanoma metastatic from distant sites may involve the orbit; of the cases reported, most originate as cutaneous melanomas and account for from 6% to 16% of all orbital metastases (224). Rarely, orbital metastasis from a uveal melanoma of the contralateral eye may occur (225).

REFERENCES

1. Albert DM, Miller JW, Azar DT, et al. Albert & Jakobiec's Principles and Practice of Ophthalmology. Ophthalmic Pathology, 3rd ed. Section 13. Philadelphia: WB Saunders, 2008.
2. Garner A, Klintworth GK. Pathobiology of Ocular Disease. A Dynamic Approach, 3rd ed. New York: Informa Healthcare 2008.
3. Garrity JA. Henderson's Orbital Tumors. 4th ed. Philadelphia: Lippincott Williams & Wilkins, 2007.
4. Yanoff M, Fine BS. Ocular Pathology. 5th ed. Philadelphia: CV Mosby, 2002.
5. Lee WR. Ophthalmic Histopathology. New York : Springer-Verlag, 2002.
6. Shields JA. Atlas of Orbital Tumors. Philadelphia: Lippincott Williams & Wilkins, 1999.
7. Shields JA, Shields CL. Atlas of Eyelid and Conjunctival Tumors. Philadelphia, PA: Lippincott Williams & Wilkins, 1999.
8. Shields JA, Shields CL. Atlas of Intraocular tumors. Philadelphia: Lippincott Williams & Wilkins, 1999.
9. Apple DJ, Rabb MF. Ocular Pathology: Clinical Applications and Self-Assessment. 5th ed. St. Louis, MO: CV Mosby, 1998.
10. Tasman W, Jaeger EA, eds. Duane's Clinical Ophthalmology, vol. 1–5. Philadelphia: Lippincott Williams & Wilkins, 1998.
11. Sassani JW, ed. Ophthalmic Pathology with Clinical Correlations. Philadelphia: Lippincott-Raven, 1997.
12. Spencer WH, ed. Ophthalmic Pathology: An Atlas and Textbook. 4th ed. vol. 1–4. Philadelphia: WB Saunders, 1996.
13. McLean IW, Burnier MN, Zimmerman LE, et al. Tumors of the Eye and Ocular Adnexa, Atlas of Tumor Pathology,

3rd Series Fascicle 12. Washington DC: Armed Forces Institute of Pathology, 1995.

14. Plowman PN. Eyelid tumours. Orbit 2007; 26:207–213.

15. Chi MJ, Baek SH. Clinical analysis of benign eyelid and conjunctival tumors. Ophthalmologica 2006; 220:43–51.

16. Mencia-Gutierrez E, Gutierrez-Diaz E, Redondo-Marcos I, et al. Cutaneous horns of the eyelid: a clinicopathological study of 48 cases. J Cutan Pathol 2004; 31:539–543.

17. Ozdal PC, Callejo SA, Codere F, et al. Benign ocular adnexal tumours of apocrine, eccrine or hair follicle origin. Can J Ophthalmol 2003; 38:357–363.

18. Deokule S, Child V, tarin S, et al. Diagnostic accuracy of benign eyelid skin lesions in the minor operation theatre. Orbit 2003; 22:235–238.

19. Prabhakaran VC, Gupta A, Huilgol SC, et al. Basal cell carcinoma of the eyelids. Compr Ophthalmol Update 2007; 8:1–14.

20. Allali J, D'Hermies F, Renard G. Basal cell carcinomas of the eyelids. Ophthalmologica 2005; 219:57–71.

21. Margo CE, Waltz K. Basal cell carcinoma of the eyelid and periocular skin. Surv Ophthalmol 1993; 38:169–192.

22. Taylor SF, Cook AE, Leatherbarrow B. Review of patients with basal cell nevus syndrome. Ophthal Plast Reconstr Surg 2006; 22:259–265.

23. Honavar HG, Shields JA, Shields CL, et al. Basal cell carcinoma of the eyelid associated with Gorlin-Goltz syndrome. Ophthalmology 2001; 108:1115–1123.

24. Leibovitch I, McNab A, Sullivan T, et al. Orbital invasion by periocular basal cell carcinoma. Ophthalmology 2005; 112:717–723.

25. Aldred WV, Ramirez VG, Nicholson DH. Intraocular invasion by basal cell carcinoma of the lid. Arch Ophthalmol 1980; 98:1821–1822.

26. Nemet AY, Deckel Y, Martin PA, et al. Management of periocular basal and squamous cell carcinoma: a series of 485 cases. Am J Ophthalmol 2006; 142:293–297.

27. Tyers AG. Orbital exenteration for invasive skin tumours. Eye 2006; 20:1165–1170.

28. Limawararut V, Leibovitch I, Sullivan T, et al. Periocular squamous cell carcinoma. Clin Experiment Ophthalmol 2007; 35:174–185.

29. Lin HY, Cheng CY, Hsu WM, et al. Incidence of eyelid cancers in Taiwan: a 21-year review. Ophthalmology 2006; 113:2101–2107.

30. Donaldson MJ, Sullivan TJ, Whitehead KJ, et al. Squamous cell carcinoma of the eyelids. Br J Ophthalmol 2002; 86:1161–1165.

31. Faustina M, Diba R, Ahmadi MA, et al. Patterns of regional and distant metastasis in patients with eyelid and periocular squamous cell carcinoma. Ophthalmology 2004; 111:1930–1932.

32. Shields JA, Demirci H, Marr BP, et al. Sebaceous carcinoma of the ocular region: a review. Surv Ophthalmol 2005; 50:103–122.

33. Kass LG, Hornblass A. Sebaceous carcinoma of the ocular adnexa. Surv Ophthalmol 1989; 33:477–490.

34. Brownstein S, Codere F, Jackson WB. Masquerade syndrome. Ophthalmology 1980; 87:259–262.

35. Singh AD, Mudhar HS, Bhola R, et al. Sebaceous adenoma of the eyelid in Muir-Torre syndrome. Arch Ophthalmol 2005; 123:562–565.

36. Rishi K, Font RL. Sebaceous gland tumors of the eyelids and conjunctiva in the Muir-Torre syndrome. A clinicopathologic study of five cases and literature review. Ophthal Plast Reconstr Surg 2004; 20:31–36.

37. Wald ER. Periorbital and orbital infections. Pediatr Rev 2004; 25:312–320.

38. Gonzales-Fernandez F, Kaltreider SA. Orbital lipogranulomatous inflammation harboring *Mycobacterium abscessus*. Ophthal Plast Reconstr Surg 2001; 17:374–380.

39. Rawlings NG, Brownstein S, Jordan DR. Merkel cell carcinoma masquerading as a chalazion. Can J Ophthalmol 2007; 42:469–470.

40. Ramlee N, Ramli N, Tajudin LS. Pleomorphic adenoma in the palpebral lobe of the lacrimal gland misdiagnosed as chalazion. Orbit 2007; 26:137–139.

41. Tailor R, Inkster C, Hanson I, et al. Metastatic renal cell carcinoma presenting as a chalazion. Eye 2007; 21: 564–565.

42. Prioleau G, Santa Cruz DJ. Sebaceous gland neoplasia. J Cutan Pathol 1984; 11:396–414.

43. Honchel R, Halling KC, Schaid DJ, et al. Microsatellite instability in Muir-Torre syndrome. Cancer Res 1994; 54:1159–1163.

44. Mathiak M, Rutten A, Mangold E, et al. Loss of DNA mismatch repair proteins in skin tumors from patients with Muir-Torre Syndrome and MSH2 or MLH1 germline mutations: establishment of immunohistochemical analysis as a screening test. Am J Surg Pathol 2002; 26:338–343.

45. Rao NA, Hidayat AA, McLean IW, et al. Sebaceous carcinomas of the ocular adnexa: A clinicopathologic study of 104 cases, with five-year follow-up. Hum Pathol 1982; 13:113–122.

46. Shields JA, Demirci H, Marr BP, et al. Sebaceous carcinoma of the eyelids: personal experience with 60 cases. Ophthalmology 2004; 111:2151–2157.

47. Muqit MM, Roberts F, Lee WR, et al. Improved survival rates in sebaceous carcinoma of the eyelid. Eye 2004; 18:49–53.

48. Kivela T, Asko-Seljavaara S, Pihkala U, et al. Sebaceous carcinoma of the eyelid associated with retinoblastoma. Ophthalmology 2001; 108:1124–1128.

49. Rundle P, Shields JA, Shields CL, et al. Sebaceous gland carcinoma of the eyelid seventeen years after irradiation for bilateral retinoblastoma. Eye 1999; 13(pt 1):109–110.

50. Leibovitch I, Selva D, Huilgol S, et al. Intraepithelial sebaceous carcinoma of the eyelid misdiagnosed as Bowen's disease. J Cutan Pathol 2006; 33:303–308.

51. Margo CE, Grossniklaus HE. Intraepithelial sebaceous neoplasia without underlying invasive carcinoma. Surv Ophthalmol 1995; 39:293–301.

52. Sinard JH. Immunohistochemical distinction of ocular sebaceous carcinoma from basal cell and squamous cell carcinoma. Arch Ophthalmol 1999; 117:776–783.

53. Johnson JS, Lee JA, Cotton DW, et al. Dimorphic immunohistochemical staining in ocular sebaceous neoplasms: a useful diagnostic aid. Eye 1999; 13(pt 1):104–108.

54. Cabral ES, Auerbach A, Killian JK, et al. Distinction of benign sebaceous proliferations from sebacecous carcinomas by immunohistochemistry. Am J Dermatopathol 2006; 28:465–471.

55. Fan YS, Carr RA, Sanders DS, et al. Characteristic Ber-EP4 and EMA expression in sebaceoma is immunohistochemically distinct from basal cell carcinoma. Histopathology 2007; 51:80–86.

56. Kodama T, Hayasaka S, Setogawa T. Immunohistochemical localization of epidermal growth factor receptor and epithelial antigen in tumors of the human conjunctiva, eyelid, lacrimal gland, and orbit. Graefes Arch Clin Exp Ophthalmol 1995; 233:672–676.

57. Tumuluri K, Kourt G, Martin P. Mitomycin C in sebaceous gland carcinoma with pagetoid spread. Br J Ophthalmol 2004; 88:718–719.

58. Shields CL, Naseripour M, Shields JA, et al. Topical mitomycin-C for pagetoid invasion of the conjunctiva by eyelid sebaceous gland carcinoma. Ophthalmology 2002; 109:2129–2133.

59. Rohrich RJ, Janis JE, Pownell PH. Xanthelasma palpebrarum: a review and current management principles. Plast Reconstr Surg 2002; 110:1310–1314.

60. Doi H, Ogawa Y. A new operative method for treatment of xanthelasma or xanthoma palpebrarum: microsurgical inverted peeling. Plast Reconstr Surg 1998; 102:1171–1174.
61. Shields CL, Demirci H, Karatza E. Clinical survey of 1643 melanocytic and nonmelanocytic conjunctival tumors. Ophthalmology 2004; 111:1747–1754.
62. Mauriello JA Jr., Napolitano J, McLean I. Actinic keratosis and dysplasia of the conjunctiva: a clinicopathological study of 45 cases. Can J Ophthalmol 1995; 30:312–316.
63. Scott IU, Karp CL, Nuovo GJ. Human papillomavirus 16 and 18 expression in conjunctival intraepithelial neoplasia. Ophthalmology 2002; 109:542–547.
64. Eng H-L, Lin T-M, Chen S-Y, et al. Failure to detect human papillomavirus DNA in malignant epithelial neoplasms of conjunctiva by polymerase chain reaction. Am J Clin Pathol 2002; 117:429–436.
65. Tulvatana W, Bhattarakosol P, Sansopha L, et al. Risk factors for conjunctival squamous cell neoplasia: a matched case-control study. Br J Ophthalmol 2003; 87: 396–398.
66. Campbell RJ. Histological typing of tumours of the eye and its adnexa. 2nd ed. World Health Organization, International Histological Classification of Tumors Springer-Verlag, Berlin, 1998:12.
67. Salomao DR, Mathers WD, Sutphin JE, et al. Cytologic changes in the conjunctiva mimicking malignancy after topical mitomycin C chemotherapy. Ophthalmology 1999; 106:1756–1761.
68. Pe'er J. Ocular surface squamous neoplasia. Ophthalmol Clin North Am 2005; 18:1–13.
69. Slusker-Shternfeld I, Syed NA, Sires BA. Invasive spindle cell carcinoma of the conjunctiva. Arch Ophthalmol 1997; 115:288–289.
70. Cervantes G, Rodriguez AA Jr., Leal AG. Squamous cell carcinoma of the conjunctiva: clinicopathological features in 287 cases. Can J Ophthalmol 2002; 37:14–19.
71. Carrau RL, Stillman E, Canaan RE. Mucoepidermoid carcinoma of the conjunctiva. Ophthal Plast Reconstr Surg 1994; 10:163–168.
72. Hwang IP, Jordan DR, Brownstein S, et al. Mucoepidermoid carcinoma of the conjunctiva: a series of three cases. Ophthalmology 2002; 107:801–805.
73. Lee GA, Hirst LW. Ocular surface squamous neoplasia. Surv Ophthalmol 1995; 39:429–450.
74. Doganay S, Er H, Tasar A, et al. Surgical excision, cryotherapy, autolimbal transplantation and mitomycin-C in treatment of conjunctival-corneal intraepithelial neoplasia. Int Ophthalmol 2005; 26:53–57.
75. Grossniklaus HE, Margo CE, Solomon AR. Indeterminate melanocytic proliferations of the conjunctiva. Trans Am Ophthalmol Soc 1999; 97:157–168.
76. Ackerman AB, Sood R, Koenig M. Primary acquired melanosis of the conjunctiva is melanoma in situ. Mod Pathol 1991; 4:253–263.
77. Shields CL, Shields JA. Tumors of the conjunctiva and cornea. Surv Ophthalmol 2004; 49:3–24.
78. Jakobiec FA, Folberg R, Iwamoto T. Clinicopathologic characteristics of premalignant and malignant melanocytic lesions of the conjunctiva. Ophthalmology 1989; 96:147–166.
79. Patel BC, Egan CA, Lucius RW, et al. Cutaneous malignant melanoma and oculodermal melanocytosis (nevus of Ota): report of a case and review of the literature. J Am Acad Dermatol 1998; 38:862–865.
80. McLean IW. Differential diagnosis of the conjunctival melanoses. Ann Diagn Pathol 1998; 2:264–270.
81. Rodriguez-Sains RS. Pigmented conjunctival neoplasms. Orbit 2002; 21:231–238.
82. Shields JA, Shields CL, Mashayekhi A, et al. Primary acquired melanosis of the conjunctiva: risks for progression to melanoma in 311 eyes. The 2006 Lorenz E. Zimmerman Lecture. Ophthalmology 2008; 115:511–519.
83. Sharara NA, Alexander RA, Luther PJ, et al. Differential immunoreactivity of melanocytic lesions of the conjunctiva. Histopathology 2001; 39:426–431.
84. Pache M, Glatz-Krieger K, Sauter G, et al. Expression of sex hormone receptors and cell cycle proteins in melanocytic lesions of the ocular conjunctiva. Graefes Arch Clin Exp Ophthalmol 2006; 244:113–117.
85. Chowers I, Livni N, Solomon A, et al. MIB-1 and PC-10 immunostaining for the assessment of proliferative activity in primary acquired melanosis without and with atypia. Br J Ophthalmol 1998; 82:1316–1319.
86. Sugiura M, Colby KA, Mihm MC Jr., et al. Low-risk and high-risk histologic features in conjunctival primary acquired melanosis with atypia: clinicopathologic analysis of 29 cases. Am J Surg Pathol 2007; 31:185–192.
87. Chalasani R, Giblin M, Conway RM. Role of topical chemotherapy for primary acquired melanosis and malignant melanoma of the conjunctiva and cornea: review of the evidence and recommendations for treatment. Clin Exp Ophthalmol 2006; 34:708–714.
88. Shields CL. Conjunctival melanoma: risk factors for recurrence, exenteration, metastasis, and death in 150 consecutive patients. Trans Am Ophthalmol Soc 2000; 98:471–492.
89. Tasse C, Majewski F, Bohringer S, et al. A family with autosomal dominant oculo-auriculo-vertebral spectrum. Clin Dysmorphol 2007; 16:1–7.
90. Pushker N, Mehta M, Bajaj MS, et al. Atypical oculo-orbital complex choristoma in organoid nevus syndrome. J Pediatr Ophthalmol Strabismus 2006; 43:119–122.
91. Shields CL, Shields JA. Conjunctival tumors in children. Curr Opin Ophthalmol 2007; 18:351–360.
92. Punia RS, Nanda A, Mohan H, et al. Clinicopathological study of dermolipoma—a report of four cases. Indian J Pathol Microbiol 2006; 49:605–607.
93. Ayres BD, Rapuano CJ. Excimer laser phototherapeutic keratectomy. Ocul Surf 2006; 4:196–206.
94. Cosar CB, Sridhar MS, Cohen EJ, et al. Indications for penetrating keratoplasty and associated procedures, 1996–2000. Cornea 2002; 21:148–151.
95. Dorrepaal SJ, Cao KY, Slomovic AR. Indications for penetrating keratoplasty in a tertiary referral centre in Canada, 1996–2004. Can J Ophthalmol 2007; 42:244–250.
96. Zhang C, Xu J. Indications for penetrating keratoplasty in East China, 1994–2003. Graefes Arch Clin Exp Ophthalmol 2005; 243:1005–1009.
97. Kang PC, Klintworth GK, Kim T, et al. Trends in the indications for penetrating keratoplasty, 1980-2001. Cornea 2005; 24:801–803.
98. Yahalom C, Mechoulam H, Solomon A, et al. Forty years of changing indications in penetrating keratoplasty in Israel. Cornea 2005; 24:256–258.
99. Macnamara E, Sams GW, Smith K, et al. Aquaporin-1 expression is decreased in human and mouse corneal endothelial dysfunction. Mol Vis 2004; 10:51–56.
100. Thompson RW Jr., Price MO, Bowers PJ, et al. Long-term graft survival after penetrating keratoplasty. Ophthalmology 2003; 110:1396–1402.
101. Morrison LK, Waltman SR. Management of pseudophakic bullous keratopathy. Ophthalmic Surg 1989; 20:205–210.
102. Klintworth GK. The molecular genetics of the corneal dystrophies—current status. Front Biosci 2003; 8:687–713.
103. Sundin OH, Broman KW, Chang HH, et al. A common locus for late-onset Fuchs corneal dystrophy maps to 18q21.2–q21.32. Invest Ophthalmol Vis Sci 2006; 47: 3919–3926.
104. Sundin OH, Jun AS, Broman KW, et al. Linkage of late-onset Fuchs corneal dystrophy to a novel locus at 13pTel-13q12.13. Invest Ophthalmol Vis Sci 2006; 47:140–145.

105. Gottsch JD, Sundin OH, Liu SH, et al. Inheritance of a novel COL8A2 mutation defines a distinct early-onset subtype of fuchs corneal dystrophy. Invest Ophthalmol Vis Sci 2005; 46:1934–1939.

106. Borderie VM, Baudrimont M, Vallee A, et al. Corneal endothelial cell apoptosis in patients with Fuchs dystrophy. Invest Ophthalmol Vis Sci 2000; 41:2501–2505.

107. Christopoulos V, Garner A. Emergence of cornea guttata in donor tissue: a causee of late graft failure. Eye 1993; 7 (pt 6):772–774.

108. Teenan DW, Sim KT, Hawksworth NR. Outcomes of corneal transplantation: a corneal surgeon vs the general ophthalmologist. Eye 2003; 17:727–730.

109. Price MO, Thompson RW Jr., Price FW Jr.Risk factors for various causes of failure in initial corneal grafts. Arch Ophthalmol 2003; 121:1087–1092.

110. Sit M, Weisbrod DJ, Naor J, et al. Corneal graft outcome study. Cornea 2001; 20:129–133.

111. Kremer I, Rapuano CJ, Cohen EJ, et al. Retrocorneal fibrous membranes in failed corneal grafts. Am J Ophthalmol 1993; 115:478–483.

112. Pieramici D, Green WR, Stark WJ. Stripping of Descemet's membrane: a clinicopathologic correlation. Ophthalmic Surg 1994; 25:226–231.

113. Price MO, Price FW. Descemet's stripping endothelial keratoplasty. Curr Opin Ophthalmol 2007; 18:290–294.

114. Covert DJ, Koenig SB. Descemet stripping and automated endothelial keratoplasty (DSAEK) in eyes with failed penetrating keratoplasty. Cornea 2007; 26:692–696.

115. Edwards M, McGhee CN, Dean S. The genetics of keratoconus. Clin Experiment Ophthalmol 2001; 29:345–351.

116. Randleman JB. Post-laser in-situ keratomileusis ectasia: current understanding and future directions. Curr Opin Ophthalmol 2006; 17:406–412.

117. Santos LN, Fernandes BF, de Moura LR, et al. Histopathologic study of corneal stromal dystrophies: a 10-year experience. Cornea 2007; 26:1027–1031.

118. Klintworth GK. Advances in the molecular genetics of corneal dystrophies. Am J Ophthalmol 1999; 128:747–754.

119. Yoo SY, Kim TI, Lee SY, et al. Development of a DNA chip for the diagnosis of the most common corneal dystrophies caused by mutations in the betaigh3 gene. Br J Ophthalmol 2007; 91:722–727.

120. Liu NP, Smith CF, Bowling BL, et al. Macular corneal dystrophy types I and II are caused by distinct mutations in the CHST6 gene in Iceland. Mol Vis 2006; 12:1148–1152.

121. Leibowitz HM, Villazon S. Corneal Procedures. In: Leibowitz HM, Waring GO III, eds. Corneal Disorders: clinical diagnosis and management. 2nd ed. Philadelphia: WB Saunders, 1998:982–983.

122. Illingworth CD, Cook SD. *Acanthamoeba* keratitis. Surv Ophthalmol 1998; 42:493–508.

123. Kumar R, Lloyd D. Recent advances in the treatment of *Acanthamoeba* keratitis. Clin Infect Dis 2002; 35:434–441. (Epub 2002, Jul 16).

124. Moshari A, McLean IW, Dodds MT, et al. Chorioretinitis after keratitis caused by *Acanthamoeba*. Ophthalmology 2001; 108:2232–2236.

125. Matsumoto Y, Dogru M, Sato EA, et al. The application of in vivo confocal scanning laser microscopy in the management of Acanthamoeba keratitis. Mol Vis 2007; 13:1319–1326.

126. Year H, Zamfir O, Bourcier T, et al. Comparison of PCR, microscopic examination and culture for the early diagnosis and characterization of Acanthamoeba isolates from ocular infections. Eur J Clin Microbiol Infect Dis 2007; 26:221–224.

127. Di Girolamo N, Chui J, Coroneo MT, et al. Pathogenesis of pterygia: role of cytokines, growth factors, and matrix metalloproteinases. Prog Retin Eye Res 2004; 23:195–228.

128. Ang LP, Chua JL, Tan DT. Current concepts and techniques in pterygium treatment. Curr Opin Ophthalmol 2007; 18:308–313.

129. Kardon RH, Weingeist TA. Chapter 43: Anatomy of the ciliary body and outflow pathways. In: Tasman W, Jaeger EA, eds. Duane's Clinical Ophthalmology, vol 3. Philadelphia: JB Lippincott, 1994:1–26.

130. Racette L, Wilson MR, Zangwill LM, et al. Primary open-angle glaucoma in blacks: a review. Surv Ophthalmol 2003; 48:295–313.

131. Eagle RC, Spencer WH. Lens. In: Spencer WH, ed. Ophthalmic Pathology: An Atlas and Textbook. 4th ed. Philadelphia: WB Saunders, 1996:372–437.

132. Klintworth GK, Garner A. The causes, types and morphology of cataracts. In: Garner A, Klintworth GK, eds. Pathobiology of Ocular Disease. A dynamic approach. 2nd ed. New York: Marcel Dekker, 1994:481–532.

133. Thach AB, Marak GE JR, McLean IW, et al. Phacoanaphylactic endophthalmitis: a clinicopathologic review. Int Ophthalmol Clin 1991; 15:271–279.

134. Khalil MK, Lorenzetti DW. Lens-induced inflammations. Can J Ophthalmol 1986; 21:96–102.

135. Kitzmann AS, Weaver AL, Lohse CM, et al. Clinicopathologic correlations in 646 consecutive surgical eye specimens, 1990-2000. Am J Clin Pathol 2003; 119:594–601.

136. Chaudhry IA, AlKuraya HS, Shamsi FA, et al. Current indications and resultant complications of evisceration. Ophthalmic Epidemiol 2007; 14:93–97.

137. Saeed MU, Chang BY, Khandwala M, et al. Twenty year review of histopathological findings in enucleated/eviscerated eyes. J Clin Pathol 2006; 59:153–155.

138. Gelisken F, Inhoffen W, Rohrbach JM, et al. Massive retinal gliosis: a late complication of retinal detachment surgery. Graefes Arch Clin Exp Ophthalmol 2004; 242:255–258.

139. Yoon YD, Aaberg TM Sr, Wojno TH, et al. Osseous metaplasia in proliferative vitreoretinopathy. Am J Ophthalmol 1998; 125:558–559.

140. Curcio CA, Medeiros NF, Millican CL. The Alabama age-related macular degeneration grading system for donor eyes. Invest Ophthalmol Vis Sci 1998; 39:1085–1096.

141. Girkin CA, McGwin G Jr., Long C, et al. Glaucoma after ocular contusion: a cohort study of the United States Eye Injury Registry. J Glaucoma 2005; 14:470–473.

142. Gurdal C, Erdener U, Irkec M, et al. Incidence of sympathetic ophthalmia after penetrating eye injury and choice of treatment. Ocul Immunol Inflamm 2002; 10:223–227.

143. Damico FM, Kiss S, Young LH. Sympathetic ophthalmia. Semin Ophthalmol 2005; 20:191–197.

144. Fraser C, Liew S, Fitzsimmons R, et al. Spontaneous resolution of corneal blood staining. Clin Experiment Ophthalmol 2006; 34:279–280.

145. Tumbocon JA, Latina MA. Angle recession glaucoma. Int Ophthalmol Clin 2002; 42:69–78.

146. Mudhar HS, Ford AL, Ebrahimi KB, et al. Intraocular choroidal extramedullary haematopoiesis. Histopathology 2005; 46:694–696.

147. Shields JA. Sanborn GE. Augsburger JJ. The differential diagnosis of malignant melanoma of the iris: a clinical study of 200 patients. Ophthalmology 1983; 90:716–720.

148. McLean IW, Foster WD, Zimmerman LE, et al. Modifications of Callender's classification of uveal melanoma at the Armed Forces Institute of Pathology. Am J Ophthalmol 1983; 96:502–509.

149. Seddon JM, Polivogianis L, Hsieh CC, et al. Death from uveal melanoma. Number of epithelioid cells and inverse

SD of nucleolar area as prognostic factors. Arch Ophthalmol 1987; 105:801–806.

150. Isager P, Ehlers N, Overgaard J. Prognostic factors for survival after enucleation for choroidal and ciliary body melanomas. Acta Ophthalmol Scand 2004; 82:517–525.

151. Demirci H, Shields CL, Shields JA, et al. Diffuse iris melanoma: a report of 25 cases. Ophthalmology 2002; 109:1553–1560.

152. Niederkorn JY, Wang S. Immunology of intraocular tumors. Ocul Immunol Inflamm 2005; 13:105–110.

153. Coleman K, Baak JP, van Diest PJ, et al. Prognostic value of morphometric features and the callender classification in uveal melanomas. Ophthalmology 1996; 103:1634–1641.

154. Moshari A, McLean IW. Uveal melanoma: mean of the longest nucleoli measured on silver-stained sections. Invest Ophthalmol Vis Sci 2001; 42:1160–1163.

155. Al-Jamal RT, Makitie T, Kivela T. Nucleolar diameter and microvascular factors as independent predictors of mortality from malignant melanoma of the choroid and ciliary body. Invest Ophthalmol Vis Sci 2003; 44:2381–2389.

156. Kivela T, Makitie T, Al-Jamal RT, et al. Microvascular loops and networks in uveal melanoma. Can J Ophthalmol 2004; 39:409–421.

157. Folberg R, Maniotis AJ. Vasculogenic mimicry. APMIS 2004; 112:508–525.

158. Al-Jamal RT, Kivela T. KI-67 immunopositivity in choroidal and ciliary body melanoma with respect to nucleolar diameter and other prognostic factors. Curr Eye Res 2006; 31:57–67.

159. Blanco G. Diagnosis and treatment of orbital invasion in uveal melanoma. Can J Ophthalmol 2004; 39:388–396.

160. Folberg R, Salomao D, Grossniklaus HE, et al. Recommendations for the reporting of tissues removed as part of the surgical treatment of common malignancies of the eye and its adnexa. The Association of Directors of Anatomic and Surgical Pathology. Hum Pathol 2003; 34:114–118.

161. Shields JA, Eagle RC Jr., Shields CL, et al. Progressive growth of an iris melanocytoma in a child. Am J Ophthalmol 2002; 133:287–289.

162. Rummelt V, Naumann GOH, Folberg R, et al. Surgical management of melanocytoma of the ciliary body with extrascleral extension. Am J Ophthalmol 1994; 117: 169–176.

163. Cialdini AP, Sahel JA, Jalkh AE, et al. Malignant transformation of an iris melanocytoma. Graefes Arch Clin Exp Ophthalmol 1989; 227:348–354.

164. Collaborative Ocular Melanoma Study Group. The COMS randomized trial of iodine 125 brachytherapy for choroidal melanoma: V. Twelve-year mortality rates and prognostic factor: COMS report No. 28. Arch Ophthalmol 2006; 124:1684–1693.

165. Hawkins BS, Collaborative Ocular Melanoma Study Group. The Collaborative Ocular Melanoma Study (COMS) randomized trial of pre-enucleation radiation of large choroidal melanoma: IV. Ten-year mortality findings and prognostic factors. COMS report No. 24. Am J Ophthalmol 2004; 138:936–951.

166. Collaborative Ocular Melanoma Study Group. Assessment of metastatic disease status at death in 435 patients with large choroidal melanoma in the Collaborative Ocular Melanoma Study (COMS): COMS report No. 15. Arch Ophthalmol 2001; 119:670–676.

167. Yap-Veloso MIR, Simmons RB, Simmons RJ. Iris melanomas: diagnosis and management. Int Ophthalmol Clin 1997; 37:87–100.

168. Shields CL, Shields JA, Materin M, et al. Iris melanoma: risk factors for metastasis in 169 consecutive patients. Ophthalmology 2001; 108:172–178.

169. MacPherson D, Dyer MA. Retinoblastoma: from the two-hit hypothesis to targeted chemotherapy. Cancer Res 2007; 67:7547–7550.

170. Knudson AG Jr, Hethcote H, Brown B. Mutation and childhood cancer: a probabilistic model for the incidence of retinoblastoma. Proc Natl Acad Sci U. S. A. 1975; 72: 5116–5120.

171. Balmer A, Zografos L, Munier F. Diagnosis and current management of retinoblastoma. Oncogene 2006; 25: 5341–5349.

172. Shields CL, Shields JA. Basic understanding of current classification and management of retinoblastoma. Curr Opin Ophthalmol 2006; 17:228–234.

173. Khelfaoui F, Validire P, Auperin A, et al. Histopathologic risk factors in retinoblastoma: a retrospective study of 172 patients treated in a single institution. Cancer 1996; 77:1206–1213.

174. Shields CL, Mashayekhi A, Au AK, et al. The international classification of retinoblastoma predicts chemoreduction success. Ophthalmology 2006; 113:2276–2280.

175. Rodriguez-Galindo C, Chantada GL, Haik BG, et al. Treatment of retinoblastoma: current status and future perspectives. Curr Treat Options Neurol 2007; 9:294–307.

176. Ahuja R, Azar NF. Orbital dermoids in children. Semin Ophthalmol 2006; 21:207–211.

177. McNab A. Orbital vascular anatomy and vascular lesions. Orbit 2003; 22:77–79.

178. Rootman J. Vascular malformations of the orbit: hemodynamic concepts. Orbit 2003; 22:103–120.

179. Dickinson AJ, Gausas RF. Orbital lymphatics: do they exist? Eye 2006; 20:1145–1148.

180. Gausas RF, Daly T, Fogt F. D2-40 expression demonstrates lymphatic vessel characteristics in the dural portion of the optic nerve sheath. Ophthal Plast Reconstr Surg 2007; 23:32–36.

181. Bilaniuk LT. Vascular lesions of the orbit in children. Neuroimaging Clin N Am 2005; 15:107–120.

182. Fukunaga M. Expression of D2-40 in lymphatic endothelium of normal tissues and in vascular tumours. Histopathol 2005; 46:396–402.

183. Gordon LK. Orbital inflammatory disease: a diagnostic and therapeutic challenge. Eye 2006; 20:1196–1206.

184. Lutt JR, Lim LL, Phal PM, et al. Orbital inflammatory disease. Semin Arthritis Rheum 2007; 2008; 37(4):207–222. (Epub 2007, Sep 4).

185. Hsuan JD, Selva D, McNab AA, et al. Idiopathic sclerosing orbital inflammation. Arch Ophthalmol 2006; 124: 1244–1250.

186. Kyhn M, Herning M, Prause JU, et al. Orbital involvement in multifocal fibrosclerosis. Acta Ophthalmol Scand 2004; 82(3 pt 1):323–324.

187. Calle CA, Castillo IG, Eagle RC, et al. Oncocytoma of the lacrimal gland: case report and review of the literature. Orbit 2006; 25:243–247.

188. Bonavolonta G, Tranfa F, Staibano S, et al. Warthin tumor of the lacrimal gland. Am J Ophthalmol 1997; 124:857–858.

189. Perez DF, Pires FR, Almeida OP, et al. Epithelial lacrimal gland tumors: a clinicopathological study of 18 cases. Otolaryngol Head Neck Surg 2006; 134:321–325.

190. Coupland SE, Hummel M, Stein H. Ocular adnexal lymphomas: five case presentations and a review of the literature. Surv Ophthalmol 2002; 47:470–490.

191. Laucirica R, Font RL. Cytologic evaluation of lymphoproliferative lesions of the orbit/ocular adnexa: an analysis of 46 cases. Diagn Cytopathol 1996; 15:241–245.

192. Nassar DL, Raab SS, Silverman JF, et al. Fine-needle aspiration for the diagnosis of orbital hematolymphoid lesions. Diagn Cytopathol 2000; 23:314–317.

193. Plaisier MB, Sie-Go DM, Berendschot TT, et al. Ocular adnexal lymphoma classified using the WHO classification: not only histology and stage, but also gender is a predictor of outcome. Orbit 2007; 26:83–88.

194. Weber AL, Jakobiec FA, Sabates NR. Lymphoproliferative disease of the orbit. Neuroimaging Clin N Am 1996; 6: 93–111.

195. Shields CL, Shields JA, Carvalho C, et al. Conjunctival lymphoid tumors: clinical analysis of 117 cases and relationship to systemic lymphoma. Ophthalmology 2001; 108:979–984.

196. Coupland SE, Krause L, Delecluse H-J, et al. Lymphoproliferative lesions of the ocular adnexa: analysis of 117 cases. Ophthalmology 1998; 105:1430–1441.

197. Ruiz A, Reischl U, Swerdlow SH, et al. Extranodal marginal zone B-cell lymphomas of the ocular adnexa: multiparameter analysis of 34 cases including interphase molecular cytogenetics and PCR for Chlamydia psittaci. Am J Surg Pathol 2007; 31:792–802.

198. Lee S, Chang OS, Kim GE, et al. Role of radiotherapy for primary orbital lymphoma. Am J Clin Oncol 2002; 25:261–265.

199. Stafford SL, Kozelsky TF, Garrity JA, et al. Orbital lymphoma: radiotherapy outcome and complications. Radiother Oncol 2001; 59:139–144.

200. Johnson TE, Tse DT, Byren GE, et al. Ocular-adnexal lymphoid tumors: a clinicopathologic and molecular genetic study of 77 patients. Ophthal Plast Reconstr Surg 1999; 15:171–179.

201. Polito E, Leccisotti A. Prognosis of orbital lymphoid hyperplasia. Graefes Arch Clin Exp Ophthalmol 1996; 234:150–154.

202. Coupland SE, Foss H-D, Assaf C, et al. T-cell and T/natural killer-cell lymphomas involving the ocular and ocular adnexal tissues. Ophthalmology 1999; 106: 2109–2120.

203. Sahjpaul R, Elisevich K, Allen L. Hodgkin's disease of the orbit with intracranial extension. Ophthalmic Surg Lasers 1996; 27:239–242.

204. Jahraus CD, Tarbell NJ. Optic pathway gliomas. Pediatr Blood Cancer 2006; 46:586–596.

205. Listernick R, Ferner RF, Liu GT, et al. Optic pathway gliomas in neurofibromatosis-1: controversies and recommendations. Ann Neurol 2007; 61:189–198.

206. Hartel PH, Rosen C, Larzo C, et al. Malignant optic nerve glioma (glioblastoma multiforme): a case report and literature review. W V Med J 2006; 102:29–31.

207. Astrup J. Natural history and clinical management of optic pathway glioma. Br J Neurosurg 2003; 17: 327–335.

208. Piccirilli M, Lenzi J, Delfinis C, et al. Spontaneous regression of optic pathways gliomas in three patients with neurofibromatosis type I and critical review of the literature. Childs Nerv Syst 2006; 22:1332–1337.

209. Ahn Y, Cho B-K, Kim S-K, et al. Optic pathway glioma: outcome and prognostic factors in a surgical series. Childs Nerv Syst 2006; 22:1136–1142.

210. Wabbels B, Demmler A, Seitz J, et al. Unilateral adult malignant optic nerve glioma. Graefes Arch Clin Exp Ophthalmol 2004; 242:741–748.

211. Moster ML. Detection and treatment of optic nerve sheath meningioma. Curr Neurol Neurosci Rep 2005; 5:367–375.

212. Saeed P, Rootman J, Nugent RA, et al. Optic nerve sheath meningiomas. Ophthalmology 2003; 110:2019–2030.

213. Miller NR. New concepts in the diagnosis and management of optic nerve sheath meningioma. J Neuroophthalmol 2006; 26:200–208.

214. Andrews DW, Faroozan R, Yang BP, et al. Fractionated stereotactic radiotherapy for the treatment of optic nerve sheath meningiomas: preliminary observations of 33 optic nerves in 30 patients with historical comparison to observation with or without prior surgery. Neurosurgery 2002; 51:890–902; (discussion 903-904).

215. Shields CL, Shields JA, Honavar SG, et al. Clinical spectrum of primary ophthalmic rhabdomyosarcoma. Ophthalmology 2001; 108:2284–2292.

216. Shields JA, Shields CL. Rhabdomyosarcoma: review for the ophthalmologist. Surv Ophthalmol 2003; 48:39–57.

217. Seregard S. Management of alveolar rhabdomyosarcoma of the orbit. Acta Ophthalmol Scand 2002; 80:660–664.

218. Amemiya T, Hayashida H, Dake Y. Metastatic orbital tumors in Japan: a review of the literature. Ophthalmic Epidemiol 2002; 9:35–47.

219. Shields JA, Shields CL. Orbital malignant melanoma: the 2002 Sean B. Murphy lecture. Ophthal Plast Reconstr Surg 2003; 19:262–269.

220. Tellado M, Specht CS, McLean IW, et al. Primary orbital melanoma. Ophthalmology 1996; 103:929–932.

221. Gunduz K, Shields JA, Shields CL, et al. Periorbital cellular blue nevus leading to orbitopalpebral and intracranial melanoma. Ophthalmology 1998; 105:2046–2050.

222. Liarikos S, Rapidis A, Roumeliotis A, et al. Secondary orbital melanomas: analysis of 15 cases. J Craniomaxillofac Surg 2000; 28:148–152.

223. Seregard S, Kock E. Prognostic indicators following enucleation for posterior uveal melanoma: a multivariate analysis of long-term survival with minimized loss to follow-up. Acta Ophthalmol Scand 1995; 73:340–344.

224. Shields JA, Shields CL, Brotman HK, et al. Cancer metastatic to the orbit: the 2000 Robert M. Curtis lecture. Ophthal Plast Reconstr Surg 2001; 17:346–354.

225. Shields JA, Perez N, Shields CL, et al. Orbital melanoma metastatic from contralateral choroid: management by complete surgical resection. Ophthalmic Surg Lasers 2002; 33:416–420.

226. Hogan MJ, Alvarado JA, Weddell JE. Histology of the Human Eye: An Atlas and Textbook. Philadelphia: WB Saunders, 1971.

25

Infectious Diseases of the Head and Neck

Panna Mahadevia and Margaret Brandwein-Gensler
Department of Pathology, Albert Einstein College of Medicine,
Montefiore Medical Center—Moses Division, Bronx, New York, U.S.A.

To understand infectious disease, one has to understand people, and how they live.

The strange and exotic become pedestrian when they show up on your doorstep. A disease may be extraordinarily rare in one era yet become commonplace one decade later. Epidemics, population shifts, and immigration patterns profoundly affect the spectrum of infectious disease we see. What a cat carries on its paws, how the Chinese prepare their fish, how households in Northern Africa store their grains, are all details which, because of the "smallness" of our world, ultimately affect what we see under our microscopes.

I. COMMON CLINICAL ENTITIES

A. Bacterial Sinusitis

Acute Sinusitis

Clinical. Bacterial sinusitis is a common entity. It may follow severe upper respiratory viral infection or develop because of underlying anatomic predisposition (e.g., poor sinus aeration and drainage). Patients complain of sudden onset of symptoms like headache, fever, nasal discharge, pain, and swelling over the affected sinuses. Radiologically, sinus opacification or an air-fluid level is seen. Untreated sinusitis may progress to serious sequelae such as orbital cellulitis, meningitis, epidural or subdural or intracranial abscess, or cavernous sinus thrombosis.

Etiology. In nonimmunocompromised individuals, acute bacterial sinusitis is usually caused by *Streptococcus pneumonia* or *Hemophilus influenza*, transmitted via ororespiratory droplets. Introduction of the 7-valent pneumococcal vaccine in children has shifted the causative agents for acute sinusitis for both children and adults; Brook and colleagues demonstrated decreasing culture recovery of *S. pneumonia* and increasing recovery of *H. influenza* (1,2). *Pseudomonas aeruginosa* and *Staphylococcus aureus* are recovered from AIDS patients with bacterial sinusitis; these bacteria rarely cause non-nosocomial sinusitis in immunocompetent hosts (3,4).

Treatment. The treatment goals are to eradicate the infection and improve drainage and aeration of the sinus. Sinus puncture and irrigation will allow for culture recovery with drug sensitivity evaluation and relief of symptoms. Endoscopic sinus surgery can also address drainage impairments. Topical spray and oral vasoconstrictors are also used to further aid sinus drainage. Amoxicillin, clarithromycin, and azithromycin are the recommended first-line antimicrobials; they cover *S. pneumoniae, H. influenzae, Moraxella catarrhalis*, and anaerobic bacteria.

Chronic Sinusitis

Clinical. Adult chronic sinusitis is associated with impaired sinus aeration, drainage, or allergies. Patients complain of facial pain, headache, thick nasal drainage, nasal obstruction, decreased smell, and bad breath. Fever does not occur in chronic sinusitis. Acute exacerbation of chronic sinusitis (AECS) is heralded by worsening of symptoms or development of new symptoms.

Etiology. Chronic sinusitis and AECS are more often associated with anaerobic bacteria (*Peptostreptococcus* sp., *Fusobacterium* sp., and *Propionibacterium acnes*), emphasizing the importance of normal sinus aeration (5).

Complications of Chronic Sinusitis

Complications include polyp or mucocele formation. The loose lamina propria of the Schneiderian mucosa is easily distended by repeated bouts of inflammation to form polyps. The term mucocele is applied to two different pathological conditions: the blockage of a sinus osteum and the blockage of a minor salivary duct. When an osteum is blocked, the sinus can slowly become distended by an expanding mucocele or mucopyocele. These mucoceles most often occur in sinuses with dependent drainage, such as the frontal sinus; the ethmoid and sphenoid sinuses are less often involved. Their slow expansion may result in bone remodeling, significant skull deformity, and globe displacement.

A mucous retention cyst is the result of a significant blockage of a minor salivary duct and is also essentially a mucocele. It usually presents radiologically as an asymptomatic smooth mucous-filled cyst on the antral floor. Unlike the mucocele developing from a blocked osteum, a mucous retention cyst does not have the same potential to expand and remodel bone.

Differential diagnosis. The clinical differential diagnosis of chronic sinusitis includes Wegener's granulomatous (WG) and Churg-Strauss syndrome. Chronic sinusitis in younger patients should bring to mind immotile cilia syndrome and Kartagener's syndrome (immotile cilia, bronchiectasis, and situs inversus). Ultrastructural examination of shed respiratory cells is useful in confirming abnormal cilia morphology. Brush biopsies submitted in gluteraldehyde can be used for visualizing the ultrastructure of ciliated cells.

Sinonasal polyposis is rare in children and should prompt an investigation for cystic fibrosis (CF). Up to 50% of all patients with CF have nasal polyposis. A study of nasal polyposis in 27 children and adolescents found 36% of them to have CF (6). Histologically, polyps in CF are generally not inflamed and lack the eosinophils and thickened basement membrane of allergic polyps. CF polyps contain predominantly acid mucin, which stains blue on alcian blue stain and purple-blue on periodic acid–Schiff stain (7).

Treatment. Chronic sinusitis requires at least three to four weeks of antimicrobial therapy, ideally guided by culture results. Amoxiciliin-clavulanate, second-generation cephalosporins, and erythromycin-sulfasoxazole are recommended first-line antibiotics. Other individualized supportive therapies include steroids, decongestants, nasal irrigations, mucolytic agents, antihistamines, and antiallergic immunotherapies. Patients should be supported with smoking cessation programs. Patients who are refractory to medical therapy or have evidence of anatomic obstruction may undergo endoscopic sinus surgery.

B. Tonsillitis, Tonsillar Hyperplasia, and Peritonsillar Abscess

Tonsillitis

Clinical. Acute tonsillitis causes extreme pharyngeal pain radiating to the ears, muffled voice, and swelling of regional lymph nodes. The tonsils are enlarged, reddened with a purulent yellow or white exudate. Chronic obstructive tonsillitis represents massive tonsillar hypertrophy ("kissing tonsils"), which causes chronic upper airway obstruction, obstructive sleep apnea, and significant school absences. The airway obstruction may be so severe as to lead to growth retardation and cor pulmonale as a result of chronic hypoxia.

Etiology. *Streptococcus* is the most commonly isolated causative agent. Rare cases of acute necrotizing *Clostridium difficile* tonsillitis and gonococcus tonsillitis have been reported (8,9). Adenoviruses, parainfluenza virus, herpes simplex virus (HSV), and Epstein-Barr virus (EBV) may cause "bacterial culture negative" tonsillitis. Infectious mononucleosis (IM) tonsillitis reveals a "dirty" gray membrane.

Histopathology. Most tonsillectomy specimens show lymphoid hyperplasia, *Actinomyces* colonies, and acutely inflamed keratinous debris (keratin plugs) within the tonsillar crypts. Bacterial colonies, intramucosal neutrophils, and tonsillar fibrosis are seen in chronic tonsillitis and may be quite pronounced. Post-IM tonsillectomy specimens can reveal atypical lymphoid infiltrate and Reed-Sternberg-like cells within tonsillar sinusoids. Eliciting a clinical history of recent IM will avoid a misdiagnosis of Hodgkin's disease (HD).

Treatment. Tonsillectomy is recommended for patients with three or more episodes of tonsillitis per year despite adequate medical therapy. Tonsillectomy and/or adenoidectomy are indicated for chronic mouth breathing, as this may distort facial growth (adenoid facies), chronic airway obstruction and sleep apnea, persistent foul taste or bad breath, peritonsillar abscess unresponsive to medical therapy and drainage, recurrent acute otitis media (AOM), or chronic serous otitis media (SOM).

Tonsillar Hyperplasia

Actinomyces are commonly seen in tonsillectomy specimens and has been suggested as a cause of tonsillar hypertrophy (10). Toh and colleagues (11) studied 834 tonsillectomy specimens and found a significant association between *Actinomyces* and sleep apnea, as compared with a clinical history of chronic tonsillitis. On the other hand, no dose-related association was found between *Actinomyces* and tonsillar size. The lack of association between *Actinomyces* and chronic tonsillitis may reflect previous antibiotic treatment. It is presently unresolved as to whether exposure to *Actinomyces* toxins is responsible for inducing tonsillar hyperplasia.

Peritonsillar Abscess

Clinical. Purulent recurrent tonsillitis may "point" superiorly and posteriorly filling the parapharyngeal space with pus and resulting in a peritonsillar abscess ("quincy"). Patients with peritonsillar abscess have trismus, pain, and a muffled ("hot potato") voice. Examination reveals a fluctuant mass distorting the lateral soft palate and tonsillar fossa. If untreated, severe quincy may result in upper airway obstruction.

Etiology. Cultures are usually polymicrobial, *Streptococcus pyogenes*, *Prevotella* sp., and *Peptostreptococcus* sp. are most commonly found.

Treatment. Treatment involves draining the abscess and antibiotic therapy. Fine needle aspiration of the abscess allows for culture and drug sensitivity determination. Penicillin is the first-line antimicrobial of choice; clindamycin or second- or third-generation cephalosporins can cover β-lactamase producing penicillin-resistant organisms.

Lemeire's Disease

Lemiere's disease represents a rare aggressive oropharyngeal infection. It is caused by *Fusobacterium necrophorum*, a gram-negative obligate anaerobe, which is part of the normal oral flora; infection with this organism became extremely rare after the advent of antibiotics. More recently, an increased incidence has been reported from the Children's Hospital of Wisconsin (12). This may be due to changes in the treatment patterns for pharyngitis with a marked reduction in the use of oral antibiotics for children and increased use of second- and third-generation cephalosporins, which are inactive against *Fusobacterium*. The initial symptoms in Lemeire's disease include pharyngitis, cervical pain, and swelling. Peritonsillar abscesses may then form. The illness progresses to bacteremia, septic thrombophlebitis, and thrombocytopenia.

The author (MBG) has examined autopsy tissue from a young woman with Lemierre's syndrome; the pharynx revealed diffuse necrosis, thrombosis, and hemorrhage with little inflammatory response.

Treatment. Treatment includes intravenous β-lactamase-resistant antibiotics such as ticarcillin-clavulanate, ampicillin-sulbactam, metronidozole, or clindamycin plus surgical drainage or debridement of necrotic tissue.

C. Otitis Externa

Otitis Externa

Clinical. Otitis externa ("Swimmer's ear," "hot-weather ear" "jungle rot") is an infection of the external auditory canal (EAC) involving cutaneous tissues but not extending to the underlying cartilage or bone. Patients complain of itching, purulent discharge, and ear fullness or pressure. The EAC contains flaky, keratinous debris, which may be blackened. An unusual progression of otitis externa to form a calcified mycetoma has been described (13).

Etiology. S. aureus is the most commonly isolated organism. *P. aeruginosa* is also commonly isolated, especially in warmer climates or with aquatic environments (14). In warmer climates, the EAC may also become colonized with fungus, commonly *Aspergillus* and *Candida* (15). *Aspergillus niger* colonization is responsible for the blackened debris.

The differential diagnosis of keratinous flakes from the EAC includes cholesteatoma (epidermal inclusion cyst) and well-differentiated squamous carcinoma. The latter might be easily overlooked both clinically and histologically, as it may not come to mind. Squamous carcinoma of the EAC is very rare but often masquerades as a "draining ear." Therefore, keratinous flakes on biopsy should prompt the pathologist to order deeper sections, or at least consider the possibility of a well-differentiated squamous carcinoma. Biopsies of chronic otitis externa should routinely include a Gomori methenamine silver stain. Fruiting heads, pigmented conidia of *A. niger*, and birefringent calcium oxalate crystals (associated with *Aspergillus* infection) can be observed (16).

Treatment. Mycotic otitis externa is responsive to local debridement and topical antifungal solutions. Bacterial otitis externa, if unresponsive to topical solutions (a combination of neomycin, polymyxin B, and hydroxycortisone), will require oral antibiotics.

Malignant Otitis Externa

Clinical. "Malignant" or necrotizing external otitis (MEO) is an aggressive, spreading infection that causes deep soft tissue necrosis of the external ear, temporal bone osteomyelitis, cranial nerve deficits, and septicemia (17,18). It is seen most often in elderly diabetics; but can also occur in immunodeficient patients (e.g., HIV, malnutrition, malignancy) and children (19–21). Patients present with severe otalgia and otorrhea usually unresponsive to topical antibiotics. If untreated, MEO may progress to invasive mastoiditis, cranial nerve invasion, brain abscess, and death (19,21). The diagnosis is established correlating clinical, laboratory, and radiological findings. The erythrocyte sedimentation rate is markedly increased, although nonspecific. Tissue diagnosis is usually not required.

Etiology. P. aeruginosa is most commonly isolated, less often *S. aureus*, *Proteus mirabilis*, or *Aspergillus*. A rare case due to Malassezia has also been reported (22). An iatrogenic component has been appreciated; in a case control study, 86% of patients with MEO had prior ear irrigations, usually for cerumen impactions, as compared with 15% of matched controls (18).

Treatment. Six to eight weeks of oral antipseudomonal quinolones, especially ciprofloxacin, has replaced previous protocols of intravenous antimicrobials and has also obviated the need for surgical deridement (18).

D. Otitis Media

Acute Otitis Media

Clinical. AOM is a common disease of childhood. Patients present with sudden onset of fever and ear pain, usually preceding a viral upper airway infection. Minimal clinical criteria for diagnosis of AOM include limited tympanic membrane (TM) mobility on pneumatic otoscopy, TM erythema, and fluid behind the TM. The TM may bulge, or perforate, in which case otorrhea develops.

Etiology. Children are susceptible to developing AOM because of the straight, horizontal position of the Eustachian tube during childhood. The Eustachian tube takes on a vertical and kinked position as the base of skull and maxilla grow. Bacterial pathogens gain access into the middle ear space directly through influx from the pharynx. *S. pneumoniae*, *H. influenza*, and *Moraxella* sp. are the most common causative bacteria. A significant reduction in the incidence of childhood AOM of 6% has been observed after the introduction of the heptavalent pneumococcal vaccine (23).

Treatment. To reduce overdiagnosis and overtreatment of AOM, which can lead to the emergence of resistant bacterial strains, children between six months and two years should receive antibiotics only if the diagnosis is certain (acute onset, middle ear effusion, and middle ear inflammation) or if there is a fever greater than 39°C. Infants younger than six months can receive antibiotics even if the diagnosis is uncertain. For children older than two years, antibiotics should be prescribed if the diagnosis is certain and there is a fever greater than 39°C.

Serous Otitis Media (Otitis Media with Effusion)

SOM describes a collection of fluid within the middle ear, which may develop de novo or result from recurrent AOM. Patients are usually asymptomatic and found to have conductive hearing loss. The TM is dull or opaque with limited mobility; it can bulge or appear retracted. A fluid level and bubbles may be seen behind the TM. "Glue ear" (chronic catarrhal otitis media) refers to mucin filling the middle ear with a retracted, immobile TM.

Chronic pediatric SOM can result in conductive hearing loss and may impede speech development. In adults, SOM, especially unilateral SOM, is uncommon and should prompt an investigation to rule out nasopharyngeal neoplasia, which might compress the torus tubaris, thus interfering with middle ear aeration.

Treatment. SOM may resolve spontaneously. Antihistamines and decongestants had been the mainstay of medical therapy, but meta-analysis confirms their ineffectiveness (24). SOM persisting over 12 weeks should be drained (myringotomy), and middle ear ventilation is reestablished by tympanostomy tube placement. Adenoidectomy may also be indicated.

Chronic Suppurative Otitis Media

Clinical. Chronic suppurative otitis media (CSOM) is defined as chronic otorrhea and a perforated TM. It may occur in a wide patient age range. Patients present with malodorous otorrhea. Granulation tissue and debris may fill the external canal, and the TM is perforated. Sequelae of CSOM include chronic quiescent mastoiditis, acute purulent mastoiditis, or cholesteatoma, which may erode and destroy the middle ear space. Meningitis, lateral sinus thrombosis, and intracranial abscess formation are uncommon and serious complications (25). CSOM can heal by fibrosis and sclerosis (tympanosclerosis, fibroosseus sclerosis of the ossicles), resulting in a "frozen" (immobile) middle ear.

Etiology. P. aeruginosa is most common pathogen associated with CSOM, followed by S. aureus, K. pneumoniae, and Proteus sp.

Treatment. The treatment goals for CSOM are eradication of infection, aural toilet, and control of granulation tissue. Topical aminoglycosides and fluoroquinolones (ciprofloxacin, tobramycin, piperacillin) can cover CSOM pathogens; however, aminoglycosides have known vestibular and cochlear toxicities. Removal of debris either by aural irrigation or micromanipulation allows for greater efficacy of topical antimicrobials. Persistent infection can stimulate growth of granulation tissue, which in turn impedes penetration of topical antimicrobials. Tympanoplasty or tympanomastoidectomy may be necessary to control granulation tissue, remove secondary cholesteotoma, and restore conductive hearing. Resolved CSOM can be treated by myringoplasty to repair the TM defect.

Histopathology. Middle ear pathology specimens may be seen as the result of treatment of CSOM and/or chronic mastoiditis. The mucosa of? the middle ear is normally lined by a simple epithelium. Chronic infection may induce goblet cell metaplasia and hyperplasia, which is especially prominent in glue ear. Minor salivary glands are not normally present in the middle ear. Chronic otitis media will result in mucin-filled gland-like structures in the submucosa, acute and chronic inflammatory infiltrate, and fibrosis. Mastoid bone will reveal reactive bony remodeling, new bone growth, and acute and/or chronic inflammatory infiltrate. A cholesteatoma is histologically identical to an epidermal inclusion cyst; one sees a squamous lining and abundant flaky keratin.

II. SPECIFIC BACTERIAL AND MYCOBACTERIAL DISEASES

A. Syphilis

Syphilis is a sexually transmitted infection caused by *Treponema pallidum* (treponema—Greek: turning thread, palidum—Latin: pale), a long (5–20 μm) slender spirochete, which rotates along its long axis and may "creep" and "crawl" along solid surfaces. Primary and secondary syphilis have the proclivity to affect skin and mucosa. Tertiary syphilis has a predisposition for the central nervous and cardiovascular systems.

Epidemiology and Historical Perspective

Syphilis was known as "the great pox" (in distinction to smallpox), as a terrible pandemic swept through Europe and Asia in the 15th century. It was also called "Italian Disease" (probably by the French) and "French Disease" (probably by the Italian). Theories on its origin abound: one is that syphilis was brought to Spain from the West Indies by Columbus' crew. Another theory holds that *T. pallidum* is a mutated form of *Treponema pertenue,* which is related to *T. pallidum* and endemic to Africa. Syphilis is contracted through sexual relations and blood transfusions. By contrast, *T. pertenue* is transmitted through nonvenereal direct contact.

The rate of reported syphilis dropped precipitously in the 1940's, with the development of penicillin; it became possible for the first time to cure infection and halt its further spread. The reported case rate in the United States for 1977 was 10.4/100,000, a decrease of 99% from 1940! Changing patterns in sexual behavior and prostitution led to some resurgence, the reported rate peaked at 20.3 cases/100,000 in 1990. The general trend since 1991 is an overall decline in the reported

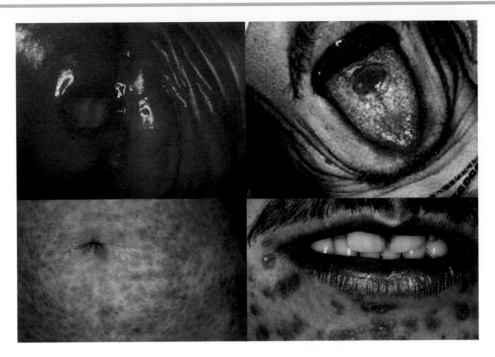

Figure 1 Syphilis: primary and secondary lesions. Upper left panel: This silvery gray penile erosion is a manifestation of primary syphilis. Upper right panel: Oral chancres can occur on the dorsal tongue; this ulcerated lesion has a purple base and irregular raised border. Lower left panel: Generalized macular/papular rash of secondary syphilis. Lower right panel: Coalescing macular/papular lesions facial lesions of secondary syphilis. *Source:* From http://www.clinical-virology.org/gallery/images/non_viral/PRIMARY_SYPHILIS-1.jpg (upper left panel), http://www.gettestedchicago.com/services.asp?service=What+does+syphilis+look+like%3F, accessed Jan 2008 (upper right panel), and http://www.clinical-virology.org (lower left and right panel).

case rate, which was around 3 cases/100,000 in 2005. For 2004, the highest reported rates per 100,000 were in Louisiana (7.4), Maryland (6.9), Georgia (6.3), New Mexico (4.4), Florida (4.3), and New York (3.8); the incidences were highest among men aged 35 to 39 (12.4/100,00) and women aged 20 to 24 (3/100,000). The rates among African-Americans are six times greater than among non-Hispanic white Americans (26–28).

Clinical. Syphilis may be clinically divided into three distinct phases: primary, secondary, and tertiary; it is worth remembering that primary and secondary syphilis can potentially escape medical attention.

Primary Syphilis—Oral Manifestations

Primary syphilis develops one week to three months after initial exposure; a characteristic chancre develops at the site of infection. While chancres are obvious on the penis, they may easily escape awareness on the cervix, which explains the generally lower reported rates for women. Intraoral chancres can develop after oral sex; the lips are most commonly affected, followed by tongue, and tonsil. Fiumara has pointed out that tonsillar chancres have a tendency to occur on the left tonsil, rather than the right, correlating with right-handedness. (29).

Cutaneous chancres are typically, painless, hard, raised lesions, which develop shallow ulcerations with sharp raised borders. Mucosal primary chancres can appear as silvery gray erosions, granulation tissue, or nonspecific deep ulcers with a red/brown or purple base and irregular raised border (30–32) (Fig. 1). Chancres can last three to seven weeks and spontaneously heal with minimal scarring, ("cigarette paper thin" and semitranslucent), thus enabling individuals to avoid seeking medical attention.

The natural history of primary syphilis is altered in HIV-seropositive patients. Chancres can be more numerous, last longer, or persist, rather than spontaneously resolve. Chancres may rapidly progress to the destructive gummatous stage, which is seen in tertiary syphilis (see below) (28).

Secondary Syphilis—Head and Neck Manifestations

Secondary syphilis results from systemic dissemination and becomes manifest weeks to months after primary infection; individuals develop fever and generalized macular/papular rash. The rash affects scalp, eyebrows, and beard hair follicles causing a patchy "moth-eaten" alopecia (alopecia syphilitica). Macular/papular lesions coalesce in warm moist areas to form hyperplastic lesions, condyloma lata, which have a proclivity for anogenital and intertriginous areas, and the ears and nasolabial folds of the face. Condyloma lata do not reflect the initial site of inoculation but like chancres, they are also infectious. Generalized lymphadenopathy occurs with a predisposition for periarticular sites (i.e., epitrochlear and inguinal lymph nodes).

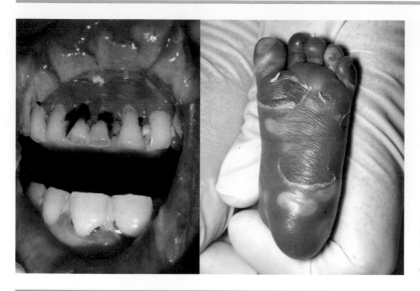

Figure 2 Left panel: Silvery gray mucous patches of secondary syphilis. Right panel: Desquamating rash in early congenital syphilis. *Source*: From http://www.adhb.govt.nz/newborn/TeachingResources/Dermatology/InfectiveLesions.htm, accessed Jan 2008.

At least 30% of patients with secondary syphilis develop various oral manifestations. Patients may present with pharyngitis or tonsillitis (33). They can develop condyloma lata, "mucous patches," or maculopapular lesions, all of which are infectious. Mucous patches are raised, flat, macerated lesions, with a thin grayish membrane (34) (Fig. 2). Rarely, ulcerative nodular lesions develop in secondary syphilis (35), referred to as lues malignum.

Untreated secondary syphilis will lapse into latency. One quarter of patients may experience recurrent mucocutaneous symptoms during the first year, which may last up to four years. About one-third of untreated patients will progress to develop tertiary syphilis (see below).

Otosyphilis

Otosyphilis was a common complication of syphilis in the preantibiotic era. Although now rare, its incidence is rising in HIV-seropositive individuals. It is usually seen in the secondary stage, but may also occur in primary and tertiary stages and congenital syphilis. Syphilitic involvement of the cochlea, vestibule, and labyrinth results in fluctuating sensorineural hearing loss, tinnitus, vertigo, and nystagmus (36,37). The diagnosis of otosyphilis is established by positive serology (see below) in patients with cochlear-vestibular symptoms after exclusion of other causes.

Tertiary Syphilis

Tertiary syphilis manifests years to decades after primary infection in about one-third of untreated patients. The notorious Tuskeegee study was conducted by the U.S. Public Health Service between 1932 and 1972 on 399 African-American males with late-stage infection with the murky goal of studying the progression of untreated tertiary syphilis. These men were misled into believing that they were receiving treatment for "bad blood," but effective therapy for syphilis (in 1945, penicillin became the drug of choice) was withheld (38).

Tertiary syphilis most commonly affects the cardiovascular and central nervous systems. Cardiovascular syphilis results in a coronary artery vasculitis and aortitis, which may cause aneurysmal dilatation. The aortic intima becomes contracted and scarred, resulting in a characteristic "pebbled" or "tree bark" appearance.

Neurosyphilis causes chronic meningitis with lymphoplasmacytic endarteritis. The brain and nerves may be directly infected, causing neural loss, cranial nerve deficits (e.g., eight nerve deafness, vestibular symptoms), sensorimotor loss (tabes dorsalis, taboparesis), progressive dementia, and psychiatric disorders.

Tertiary Syphilis—Head and Neck Manifestations

Gummas are painless raised ulcerative masses, which can rapidly enlarge becoming necrotic and destructive. They are noninfectious, can occur anywhere, but are most often seen in the liver. In the head and neck, gummas most commonly involve the palate but can also develop in the sinonasal tract, larynx, temporal bones, and ossicles. Sinonasal gummas may clinically present with chronic sinusitis and radiographic evidence of destruction; thus mimicking sinonasal fungal disease or Wegener's granulomatosis (WG).

Atrophic glossitis (luetic glossitis) is another manifestation of tertiary syphilis. The tongue appears smooth, atrophic, or wrinkled and shrunken. It is the result of obliterative vasculitis, muscular atrophy, and fibrosis. A fourfold increase in risk of developing carcinoma has been noted in luetic glossitis (32). A 1949 report on 330 patients with tongue carcinoma demonstrated positive syphilis serology in 22% of them (39). This association was probably potentiated by the carcinogenic effects of prepenicillin therapies (arsenic and heavy metals) (32). The rate of syphilis serology in patients with tongue cancer is now much lower, 8% in a report from 1995 (40).

Mandibular resorption is another manifestation of tertiary syphilis, described in 6 of 68 patients with oral tertiary syphilis (41), which may lead to spontaneous fracture.

Congenital Syphilis

Congenital syphilis results from maternal infection up to two years prior to pregnancy. The rate of congenital syphilis is declining in developed countries; the case rate for the United States in 2005 was 8/100,000 live births (42). But worldwide, more than 1 million pregnancies are impacted by syphilis annually, resulting in stillbirths, low-weight or premature births, and congenital syphilis. Africa is especially plagued by lack of access to health care and lack of widespread maternal screening (43,44).

Treponema crosses the placenta in early pregnancy, but symptomatic fetal infection begins at the fourth gestational month, when immunocompetence develops, suggesting that much of the pathobiology of congenital syphilis depends on the host reaction, rather than direct effect of *Treponema*. Congenital syphilis may be divided into early and late congenital syphilis. Early congenital syphilis is diagnosed within the first two years, usually between three and eight weeks of life, when babies develop mucocutaneous condyloma lata and extensive erythematous and desquamating rash (Fig. 2). Late congenital syphilis may be diagnosed after the first two years until the third decade of life, overlapping in age with acquired syphilis. It may present with interstitial keratitis, neurosyphilis, gummas, and bony lesions.

Congenital Syphilis—Head and Neck Manifestations

Osteomyelitis and osteochondritis are features of early and late congenital syphilis causing temporal bone osteomyelitis, vomer collapse (saddle nose deformity), and anterior tibial saber shin deformity. The latter results from periosteitis inducing bony overgrowth. Teeth are small, abnormally notched, and unusually shaped (Hutchinson's incisors and "mulberry" molars). A study of 271 patients with congenital syphilis revealed the following head and neck manifestations: frontal bossing of Parrot (86%) (Fig. 3), shortened maxilla with concave midface (84%), high arched palate (76.4%), saddle nose deformity (73%), mulberry molars (65%), sternoclavicular thickening (Higoumenakis' sign) (39%), mandibular protuberance (26%), rhagades (circumfrential wrinkles of perioral skin, 19%), and Hutchinson's triad, which consists of notched incisors (63%), ocular interstitial keratitis (9%), and VIII nerve deafness (3%) (45).

Histopathology

Primary syphilis. A nonspecific lymphoplasmacytic infiltrate characterizes all stages and is most dense in the primary chancre. The overlying epidermis is thin and eventually ulcerates. Lymphoplasmacytic vasculitis with a "coat sleeve"-like arrangement, endothelial proliferation (obliterative endarteritis), and lymphoplasmacytic neuritis can be seen.

The Steiner modification of Warthin–Starry or Dieterle stains will reveal the spirochetes especially around vessels, but they may be localized in the epidermis (or squamous mucosa) or in dermis or

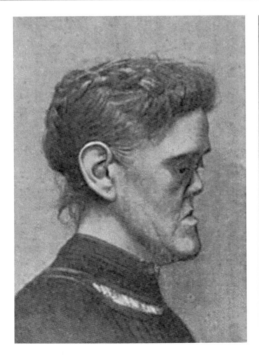 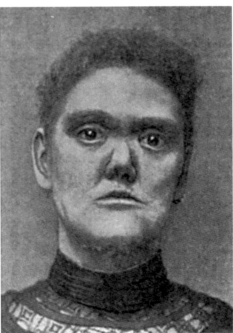

Figure 3 Parrot's frontal bossing. Untreated congenital syphilis leads to a progressive osteitis, resulting in frontal bossing and saddle-nose deformity. *Source*: From http://www.gutenberg.org.

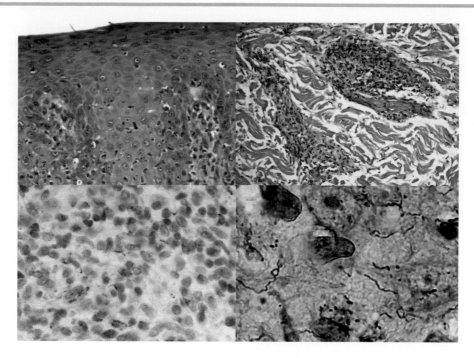

Figure 4 Secondary syphilis. Upper left panel: Epidermis with spongiotic changes and neutrophilic infiltrate (hematoxylin and eosin). Upper right panel: Para-adnexal chronic inflammatory infiltrate. Lower left panel: Numerous spirochetes are demonstrated by immunohistochemistry. Lower right panel: Dieterle staining demonstrates numerous elongated coiled spirochetes clustering at sites of neutrophilic infiltrates. *Source*: Courtesy of Dr. A Weber, Zurich, Switzerland (upper left panel).

submucosa. Intracellular spirochetes may be found within endothelial cells and histiocytes (46).

Secondary syphilis. Dense lymphoplasmacytic infiltrates are seen. Granulomatous reaction with Langerhan's multinucleated giant cells and epithelioid histiocytes are a late finding. Plasma cells may be sparse or absent. Spirochetes may be seen in the secondary lesions predominantly around vessels (Fig. 4). Endovascular proliferation is variable and more likely present in older lesions. Condyloma lata consists of epithelial hyperplasia with elongated rete pegs, dense lymphoplasmacytic infiltrate with perivascular cuffing of plasma cells. Lymph nodes reveal noncaseating granulomata, perivascular cuffing of plasmacytes, and capsular fibrosis.

Tertiary syphilis. The gummas of late, secondary, and tertiary syphilis reveal necrosis, granulomas, multinucleated Langerhan's type giant cells and obliterative endarteritis. Spirochetes may be rarely observed in gummas by special stains.

Congenital syphilis. Congenital syphilis may have the histological features seen in all stages and spirochetes can be identified by the usual techniques. Bone findings include osteochondritis, periostitis, osteomyelitis, and osteonecrosis. Granulation tissue causes generalized osteoclastic resorption.

Demonstrating Spirochetes

Historically, the classic "dark field" study involves searching for motile spirochetes by examining chancre transudate suspended in saline (Fig. 5). This can only

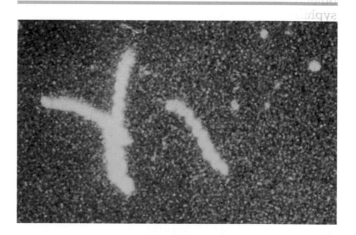

Figure 5 *Treponema pallidum.* Darkfield examination for motile *Treponema pallidum* spirochetes requires the use of chancre transudate suspended in saline. *Source*: Courtesy of Dr. Nasser Said-Al-Naief, Birmingham, Alabama, U.S.A.

be performed on fresh, undried transudate, and there is the potential for confusion with commensal spirochetes such as *Treponema microdentium*. Immunohistochemistry (IHC) with commercial polyclonal antibodies is more sensitive than silver stain and can be used on paraffin-embedded tissue (47). Polymerase chain reaction (PCR) may be helpful for tissues that are negative by immunohistochemical studies;

sensitivity is dependent on primer design or selection of region to amplify. (47).

Serological Identification

Serology is a diagnostic cornerstone for syphilis. In the United States, VDRL (venereal disease research laboratory) and RPR (rapid plasma reagin) remain the first-line indirect screening tests. Positive results are confirmed by fluorescent treponemal antibody absorption test (FTA-ABS), which is more specific. In the FTA-ABS, serum antibodies are combined with *T. pallidum*; antibody-antigen complexes are detected by the addition of fluorescent human anti-IgG immunoglobulin.

VDRL titers can be used to moniter treatment effect. Most patients become nonreactive to VDRL and RPR tests after adequate therapy, but some remain persistently positive (serofast). The FTA-ABS test usually remains positive for life but may become nonreactive in patients with tertiary syphilis. False-negative VDRL tests may be seen in early primary, late latent, and late syphilis. False-positive VDRL can occur with systemic lupus erythematosis, pregnancy (1–2%), malaria, IM, rheumatoid arthritis, polyarteritis nodosum, viral infection, mycoplasma pneumoniae, and Chlamydia. The FTA-ABS can be positive in nonsyphilitic spirochete infections (endemic syphilis, yaws, pinta, bejel).

Differential Diagnosis

The diagnosis of syphilis should be considered in any mucosal lesion with a plasmacytic infiltrate. On the other hand, one should remember that the lesions of syphilis may also be poor in plasma cells. Necrotizing granulomata should also prompt consideration of late syphilis.

Yaws. Yaws, (framboesia tropica) is a nonvenereal infection by *T. pallidum pertenue* seen in children and young adults primarily in nongenital, unclothed areas. Yaws is endemic in Central and West Africa, Southeast Asia, Central and South America, and the Caribbean. The initial lesion in yaws is an exophytic, pruritic, infectious, facial ulcer, which expands and fuses with smaller satellite lesions. The primary lesion regresses and scars. In secondary yaws, there are nonspecific constitutional symptoms, multiple, diffuse mucocutaneous lesions, periostitis, and osteitis. Tertiary yaws is characterized by subcutaneous and osseous gummas and neurological disease (48).

Bejel. *T. pallidum endemecium* is endemic to the Middle East and southern Sahara and infects mostly children. Primary bejel is characterized by multiple small papules and ulcers. In secondary bejel, children develop oropharyngeal ulcerated mucous patches, cutaneous condyloma lata, and osteitis/periosteitis. Tertiary bejel is marked by gummas of the upper airways and bones.

Pinta. *T. pallidum carateum* is endemic to Mexico and South America and causes a relatively mild cutaneous infection. It is seen in young adults. The primary cutaneous lesion is an expanding, coalescing macular/papule usually on the lower limbs. Secondary pinta is characterized by an eruption of erythematous scaling papules (pintids) that coalesce into psoriaform plaques. In tertiary pinta, hyperpigmented and hypopigmented cutaneous lesions develop.

Histologically, the spirochetes of endemic syphilis tend to be more epidermotrophic than *T. pallidum* and produce less endothelial proliferation (48). Clinicopathological correlation is necessary; serological tests cannot distinguish between endemic syphilis and venereal syphilis. PCR-based studies can distinguish between *T. pallidum pallidum, T. pallidum pertenue, T. pallidum endemecium,* and *T. pallidum carateum.*

Treatment. Penicillin G is the drug of choice for all stages of syphilis. The Jarisch-Herxheimer reaction is an acute febrile reaction that can develop within 24 hours of initiating treatment for syphilis.

B. Gonorrhea

A sexually transmitted infection caused by *Neisseria gonorrhea*, a gram-negative nonmotile diplococcus. It is the second-most common sexually transmitted disease (STD) in the United States after Chlamydia. Its virulence is due to pili formation, which impedes phagocytosis and aids in bacterial adherence. Infections by *N. gonorrhea* are primarily localized in the genitourinary tract and oral cavity; occasionally systemic manefestations can develop.

Transmission and Epidemiology

Gonorrhea ("flow of seed") is an STD caused by *N. gonorrhea* (gonococcus). Nonsexual mucosal/digital contact or mucosal contact with fomites (towels, sheets) may also transmit the bacteria, although they are susceptible to drying and sunlight. Notably, it can be transmitted manually to mucosal surfaces in children; therefore pediatric gonococcal infection does not necessarily indicate child abuse. Gonococcal infection may be transmitted to neonates during vaginal birth delivery causing gonococcal conjunctivitis, which may progress to scarring and blindness (gonococcal ophthalmia neonatorum). This has led to the widespread administration of conjunctival silver nitrate prophylaxis to newborns.

Gonorrhea is *much* more prevalent in the United States than syphilis. A peak of 300 cases/100,000 occurred in the World War II–era. Reported incidences declined between 1950 and 1960, and sharply increased again in the late 1960s, corresponding to "the sexual revolution" and the Vietnam War. Because of educational, screening, and surveillance programs for STDs, which include evaluation and treatment of sexual partners, infection rates have steadily decreased from 1975 through 1997, with a plateau in recent years. Over 330,000 cases were reported in 2005, 115.6 cases/100,000 (49); it has been estimated that only about half of all cases are reported. Geographically, the distribution is similar to that for syphilis: the Southern United States has the highest rates, namely Mississippi (272), Louisiana (211), Alabama (207), South Carolina (203), Ohio (182), and Georgia (179), per 100,000 (50).

Clinical. Primary *N. gonorrhea* infection after genitourinary contact is asymptomatic in 80% of women, thereby escaping detection. In contrast, more than 90% of men infected in the same way develop symptoms. Oropharyngeal contact after fellatio frequently leads to symptoms in both men and women within one week of exposure; patients may develop oropharyngeal mucosal erythema, purulent, exudative and ulcerative tonsillitis and pharyngitis, and cervical lymphadenopathy (8,51).

Urogenital symptoms (purulent drainage, burning itching—"the clap") occur within days of exposure and do not abate if untreated; thus men with gonorrhea are more likely to receive medical attention; in contrast, the symptoms of primary syphilis abate if untreated, and infection can easily escape notice. Anal infection can lead to painful and purulent proctitis. In women, pelvic inflammatory disease from untreated gonorrhea infection leads to infertility. Systemic dissemination leads to fever, polyarthralgias, and disseminated rash. The rash may be vesicular/pustular, purpuric, or form hemorrhagic bullae (52). Gonococcemia may also lead to cholecystitis and hepatitis (Fitz-Hugh-Curtis syndrome) and septic arthritis.

Histopathology.   The pathologist may encounter gonorrhea as an incidental finding in tonsillectomy specimens. *Neisseria* other than *gonococcus* may be present in the pharynx or tonsils, but do not cause tonsillitis and are generally not observed histologically. In *gonococcus* tonsillitis, intracellular diplococci may be observed on Brown and Brenn or methylene blue stain in the submucosa (53). Intracellular organisms may also be occasionally observed in chlamydial tonsillitis, another STD. If skin is biopsied during gonococcemia, one sees fibrin deposition, leukocytoclastic reaction, and hemorrhage; gram-negative diplococci are seen only rarely.

Other diagnostics.   The diagnosis of gonorrhea is primarily established by culture (Thayer Martin media with an enhanced CO_2 concentration). DNA detection methods (PCR and non-PCR-based) and enzyme immunoassays (EIAs) can be used on swab specimens. Reliance *solely* on nonculture techniques to establish the diagnosis is discouraged as it does not allow for monitoring of gonococcal isolate drug susceptibilities.

Treatment.   Fluoroquinolone-resistant gonorrhea is widespread in the United States, with increasing prevalence. Current CDC treatment recommendations are IM ceftriaxone or oral cefixime; coinfection with chlamydial should be ruled out for all patients with STD (54).

C. Rhinoscleroma

A chronic, progressive, disfiguring upper aerodigestive tract infection caused by *Klebsiella rhinoscleromatis* (Type III Klebsiella), a gram-negative bacillus of low infectivity:

Background and Epidemiology

The term rhinoscleroma was minted in the late 19th century by Ferdinand Von Hebra and his son-in-law Moritz Kohn (aka Kaposi) to describe patients presenting with hard ("sclero") noses ("rhino"); it was

assumed to be an indolent malignant process (55). Mikulicz demonstrated that this disease was inflammatory, not neoplastic (56); *K. rhinoscleromatis*, the causative bacterium, was identified in 1882 (57). Interestingly, aniline dye workers were noted to have an increased prevalence of rhinoscleroma in San Salvador in the late 19th century. The dye was derived from *Indigofera tinctoria*, a legume associated with *Bacillus indigogenous*; Quevedo concluded that this was identical to von Frisch's bacillus (58). Rhinoscleroma is endemic at tropical latitudes, (Central America, Chili, Central Africa), subtropical latitudes (India, Indonesia, Egypt, Algeria, Morroco), and temperate latitudes (Eastern and Central Europe, Russian republics) (59,60). Mayan art is thought to depict nasal deformities consistent of rhinoscleroma (58,61), which would indicate that the disease predated colonization of the "New World" (Fig. 6).

K. rhinoscleromatis is a noncommensural organism of low infectivity; transmission between humans is assumed to occur only after prolonged exposure. Increased incidence among family members and household contacts has been reported, but this still remains controversial (58–60,62). A genetic predisposition has

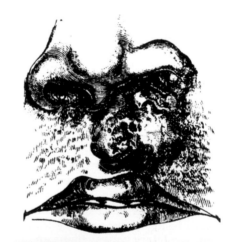

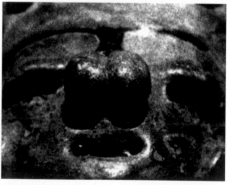

Figure 6   Rhinoscleroma. Upper panel: Original illustration from Von Hebra and Kaposi's report of a patient with a slow-growing, hard, nasal cavity mass. Lower panel: Aztec statue from El Salvador with a deformed nose thought to represent rhinoscleroma (59).

been demonstrated; histocompatiblity leukocyte antigen (HLA) haplotype DQA1*03011-DQB1*0301 significantly increases susceptibility to rhinoscleroma (63). Rhinoscleroma has been referred to as the "disease of the great unwashed" (58). Social conditions may vary but poor hygiene and crowded environments are a common thread. In one mountainous endemic site in Indonesia, many families sleep together in large, poorly ventilated houses, huddled together with their dogs and domestic fowls for warmth (59,60).

Clinical. Rhinoscleroma affects the entire upper aerodigestive tract, most commonly the sinonasal cavity (95–100%) and pharynx (50%) (61,64). Laryngotracheal involvement occurs in 15% to 80% of cases but is rarely seen without sinonasal disease (65). The term "scleroma" has been advocated to emphasize that infection is not limited to the nasal cavity (66); this nosology never gained popularity for fear of confusion with systemic sclerosis or scleroderma (61).

Initial catarrhal phase. Disease usually presents in the second and third decades of life, with a female predominance (61). The natural course evolves through three clinicopathological stages. The initial phase is the "rhinitic/catarrhal" stage; mucosa is red, atrophic with foul purulent discharge and crusting. The clinical differential diagnosis in this early stage includes infection with *Klebsiella ozena.*

Second proliferative phase. The second phase, the florid proliferative granulomatous stage, occurs months to years later. Nasal obstruction and epistaxis is common. Patients commonly present with polypoid masses protruding through the external nares. The inflammatory masses may distort the midface soft tissues, resulting in a "rhinoceros-like" appearance. Clinical remissions and relapses are frequent. The clinical differential diagnosis during this phase includes leprosy and syphilis. Laryngotracheobronchial and intracranial extension can occur during this stage. Other infections may be superimposed, resulting in significant morbidity and mortality (62).

Third sclerotic phase. The final sclerotic stage is characterized by fibrosis and inflammation, culminating in disfigurement, stenosis, and loss of function.

Immunological considerations. The histological resemblance of rhinoscleroma to lepromatous leprosy (LL) and atypical mycobacteriosis mirrors immunological similarities with respect to defective T-lymphocyte response. The foamy histiocytes in these three processes fail to transform into epithelioid histiocytes, which have more efficient bactericidal capacities. In LL and rhinoscleroma, the T helper and suppresser cells are scattered throughout the inflammatory infiltrate, without the purposeful segregation seen in granulomas. By contrast, the granulomas of tuberculoid leprosy (TL) or sarcoid reveal T suppresser cells rimming the periphery of granulomas and T helper cells percolating within them (67). The absolute T-cell counts in patients with rhinoscleroma are altered, with decreased T helper cells and increased T suppresser cells (68). Intrinsic alterations in cell-mediated immunity, perhaps directly caused by *K. rhinoscleromatis*, account for disease chronicity. Rhinoscleroma has been reported in AIDS, but to date

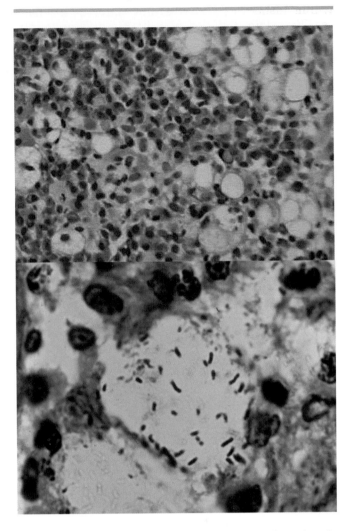

Figure 7 Rhinoscleroma. Upper panel: Hematoxylin and eosin stain reveals a lymphoplasmacytic infiltrate and foamy histiocytes or Mikulicz cells. Lower panel: Intrahistiocytic bacilli are seen best on Warthin–Starry stain.

the mucocutaneous infections do not greatly differ from the cases occurring in the usual hosts, except for one case presenting with gingival ulcers (69).

Histopathology. Dense, acute, and chronic inflammation with characteristic foamy macrophages (Mikulicz cells) is seen (Fig. 7). Mikulicz cells are large tissue histiocytes with numerous vacuoles containing viable and nonviable bacilli. They are sparse in the initial catarrhal and final sclerotic stages and most abundant in the second florid proliferative granulomatous stage. Multinucleated Mikulicz cells, plasma cells, and Russell bodies are also abundant in this stage (70). This phase is referred to as the "granulomatous" stage; however true granulomas are never seen.

The infection may involve regional lymph nodes. A Rosai Dorfman disease–like reaction has been reported in a patient with rhinoscleroma involving a periparotid lymph node (71).

Special stains (periodic acid–Schiff, Warthin–Starry, and Hotchiss Mc Manus) will reveal the bacilli within histiocytes (72). Warthin–Starry is the most sensitive stain. IHC for type III *Klebsiella* antigen is also specific (72).

Other diagnostics. Tissue cultures for *K. rhinoscleromatis* may be positive only in 50% of cases, and are more likely to be positive in the florid proliferative granulomatous stage.

Differential diagnosis. The differential diagnoses include atypical mycobacterial infection, LL, and syphilis. Atypical mycobacterial infection appears as a histiocytic infiltrate, rather than a granulomatous reaction; it can be ruled out by a Ziehl-Neelsen stain. LL also appears as a diffuse histiocytic infiltrate (Virchow cells) and can be ruled out by Fite–Farraco stain. When a lymphoplasmacytic infiltrate dominates, the diagnosis of syphilis should be considered. The overlying respiratory mucosa may demonstrate squamous metaplasia with significant hyperplasia mimicking a carcinomatous process.

Treatment. Treatment involves surgical debridement and prolonged antibiotic therapy. Antibiotics such as streptomycin, doxycycline, tetracycline, rifampin, second- and third-generation cephalosporins, sulfonamides, clofazimine, ciprofloxacin, and ofloxacin have demonstrated effectiveness (61,62,64,73). Nasal washes with topical antibiotics such as acriflavine 2% or rifampin have been used. Long-term follow-up is necessary as relapses are common. Education in elementary hygiene is essential in reducing the incidence in endemic areas.

D. Actinomycoses

This is an infection with the anaerobic gram-positive filamentous bacterium *Actinomyces israelli*, which may cause draining cervicofacial infection, and occasionally pulmonary, gastrointestinal, or disseminated infections.

Background

The cause of bovine "lumpy-jaw" was identified by Harz in 1877 and named *Actinomyces bovis* (Actinomyces: "strahlen-pilz" or "ray-fungus") (74). *Actinomyces israelii* is a commensural organism present around teeth, especially carious teeth, in tonsillar crypts, saliva, and in dental plaque. It is classified as a filamentous bacteria, rather than a fungus because (*i*) it reproduces by fission rather than sporulation (as do perfect fungi) or filamentous budding (as do imperfect fungi) and (*ii*) the presence of muramic acid in cell walls, and the absence of mitochondria, both features of bacteria (75).

Clinical Presentation

Actinomyces is a contributing agent of gingivitis and caries (76). *Actinomyces* has limited infectious potential in most individuals; antecedent trauma (poor dentition and dental extraction, previous irradiation) or debilitation (immunosuppression, diabetes, malignancy) are necessary predisposing factors for invasive infection. Actinomyces most commonly manifests as cervicofacial infection; it may also cause infection of the

thoracic and abdominal and pelvic cavities (77). Cervicofacial abscesses develop secondary to periapical infection. Characteristically, cervicofacial actinomycosis produces a firm, slow-growing, and painless mass, which ultimately develops multiple fistulae that drain pale yellow "sulfur granules" (Fig. 8). The fistulae can be quite long, tunneling into soft tissues of the back and chest. In the absence of draining fistulae, this presentation may mimic neoplasia. There may also be an acute clinical presentation with fever and tenderness, also lacking fistulae (78,79). Pneumonia may develop in debilitated patients after aspiration of oral actinomycosis. Pulmonary infection can also progress to form communicating sinus tracts to the vertebrae, sternum, ribs, pericardium, and chest wall. Abdominal actinomycosis can develop after appendiceal abscess or a bowel perforation. Lower abdominal infections may also drain into the inguinal area or through the

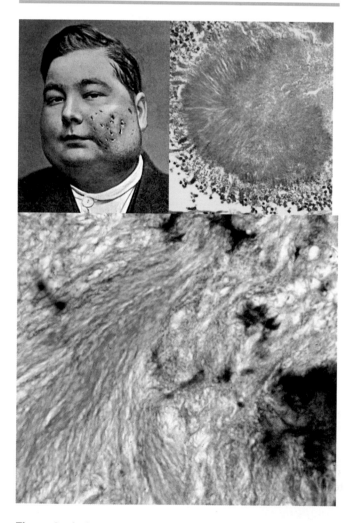

Figure 8 Actinomycosis. Upper left panel: Cervicofacial actinomycosis of the maxilla causing multiple draining fistulae. Upper right panel: Colonies of actinomycosis (sulfur granules) within pharyngeal tonsil. Lower panel: Fine strands of bacilli are appreciated on periodic acid–Schiff stain. *Source*: From www.gutenberg.org/files (upper left panel).

abdominal wall. Bacteremia may develop, usually in the immunosuppressed (80).

Rarely, *Actinomyces* may cause sinonasal, oral, laryngeal, or hypopharyngeal infection (81–87). Many patients have no obvious predisposing conditions; in these cases some proceeding microtrauma is hypothesized. Actinomycoses of the thyroid has been reported, either as extension of cervicofacial infection or as an isolated infection (88). In patients with AIDS, sinonasal and lingual actinomycosis have been reported (89–91).

Etiology

A. israelli is the most common isolate; *A. naeslundii*, *A. pyogenes*, *A. denticolens*, *A. odontolyticus*, and other subspecies can also cause infection. Actinomycosis is invariably part of a polymicrobial infection, including other bacteria, which magnify the pathogenic potential of Actinomycoses; these include *Actinobacillus actinomycetemcomitans*, followed by *Peptostreptococcus*, *Prevotella*, *Fusobacterium*, *Bacteroides*, *Staphylococcus* and *Streptococcus* species, and Enterobacteriaceae.

Histopathology

Actinomyces colonies appear as blue clumps on hematoxylin and eosin; the filamentous hyphae fan out in a ray-like manner. Gram-positive slender branching bacilli are seen on Brown and Brenn stain; the bacilli stain black or gray on Gomori methanamine silver. The bacillary filaments have club-shaped or "beaded" ends and may mimic fungi in their tendency to branch. However, their very narrow width (~0.5 µm) is beyond the range of fungal hyphal diameters. In disseminated disease, there is lesser tendency for the organisms to form the "sulfur granule" clumps. Actinomyces are not acid-fast and do not stain with Ziehl-Neelsen, although occasionally they may be weakly acid-fast. This can help distinguish *Actinomyces* from *Nocardia*; the latter filamentous bacteria do not stain well with hematoxylin and eosin stain but do stain well with a modified Ziehl-Neelsen. The distinction between these two filamentous bacteria is important as their sensitivities to antibiotic differ: penicillin is the drug of choice for *Actinomyces*, while *Nocardia* is unresponsive to penicillin and can be treated with sulfa drugs.

The diagnosis of actinomycosis is confirmed by anaerobic culture. Many reported cases lack confirmatory cultures, due to the absence of anaerobic conditions, or overgrowth of other bacteria and the failure to recognize *Actinomyces* as a pathogen and perform appropriate subcultures. Antimicrobial susceptibility testing is not necessary in the management of actinomycosis because of their predictable response to antibiotics.

Treatment

High-dose penicillin is the cornerstone of therapy. The risk developing penicillin resistance appears to be minimal. Lack of a clinical response to penicillin usually indicates the presence of resistant companion bacteria, which may require antimicrobial modification (i.e., additional agents that are active against these companion bacteria).

E. Mycobacteria and Atypical Mycobacteria

Mycobacterium tuberculosis—*M. tuberculosis* (MTB) is a strict aerobic bacillus (1.0–4.0 µm long); its multilayered cell membrane is composed of complex lipids and waxes and is responsible for its characteristic staining and immunogenic properties. Once stained, it is resistant to decolorization by acid alcohol, and hence is "acid-fast." MTB is the cause of cavitary pneumonia and progressive disseminated systemic infection.

Epidemiology and Background

TB was so named because of its tendency to form "tubercles" or softened nodules of infection. Koch identified the organism in 1882 (Koch's bacillus). TB is long recognized as being associated with crowded conditions and poor sanitary and nutritional status. MTB is spread through inhalation of aerosolized droplets; ingestion of *M. bovis* and probably MTB can also cause infection; however mucosal breaks are probably required (92). Rarely, MTB is transmitted by trauma (tuberculosis verrucosa cutis or Laennec's prosector's warts) (93).

The early 1990s was marked by disease resurgence in the United States caused by (*i*) immigration patterns, (*ii*) reactivation of disease in the elderly, and (*iii*) the AIDS pandemic. In 1993, over 25,000 cases were reported (10/100,000), which represented a 14% increase over 1985 rates, an incidence nadir since the inception of national reporting in 1953 (53/100,000). The disease incidence has been steadily declining since 1993; 14,097 cases (4.8/100,000) were reported in 2005 (94). Fifty-five percent of all TB cases occur in foreign-born persons; their case rate is more than eight times greater than that of U.S.-born persons. The most commonly affected patients are from Mexico, the Philippines, Vietnam, India, and China.

F. Clinical Stages: Primary TB

Primary TB is usually a subclinical pulmonary infection in the upper lobes, where the oxygen tension is highest (Simon's focus). The pulmonary infection and draining lymph nodes (Ghon complex) heal as calcified granulomas. Latent bacilli remain in these foci and are capable of reactivation. Primary infections become inactivated, but patients are at lifelong risk for developing active disease. Less commonly, primary pulmonary infection progresses to symptomatic pulmonary disease (progressive primary infection); children and young adults are most susceptible.

G. Reactivation of TB

Disease reactivation develops many years after primary exposure and is referred to as progressive secondary infection or (endogenous) reinfection TB. ("Reinfection tuberculosis" is a misnomer as it implies an exogenous source.) Patients present with fever, weight loss, and pulmonary symptoms such as bloody sputum. Cavitary TB develops and can spread systemically (also referred to as "miliary TB") favoring kidneys, adrenals, bone marrow, spleen, ovaries, testes, meninges, and bones; however, extrapulmonary TB is actually uncommon during secondary infection. In a review of patients with TB from Boston City Hospital during the years 1968 to 1977, it was estimated that 4.5% of all cases of TB (over 1500 in total) had extrapulmonary manifestations (95).

H. MTB in the Head and Neck

Head and neck involvement in TB is relatively rare and thought to result from direct contact with expectorated sputum as well as hematogenous/lymphatic spread. A retrospective analysis of 1315 TB patients revealed that 128 patients (9.7%) had head and neck involvement (96). Cervical TB lymphadenitis (scrofula) represents the most common head and neck presentation (83–95%) (96–98). Other head and neck sites that can be affected include salivary glands, larynx, oral cavity, pharynx, eyes, ears, skin, thyroid, sinonasal tract, nasopharynx, and retropharyngeal space (96–98). Sinonasal TB may be associated with extension into the underlying bone, resulting in a destructive radiographic appearing mimicking neoplasia (99).

I. Primary Sinonasal Tract TB

In rare cases, nasopharyngeal and sinonasal TB can present as a primary upper airway infection (100–105). This is presumably the direct result of inhalation, however chest X rays alone are an insensitive method for excluding pulmonary involvement; patients with positive sputum may have "negative" radiographs. Nasopharyngeal and sinonasal TB may clinically and histologically mimic WG. This distinction is of grave consequence, as administering steroids and immunosuppressive agents as indicated for active WG may result in miliary progression of unrecognized TB.

J. Mucocutaneous TB—Lupus vulgaris

Lupus vulgaris (LV) is the term for mucocutaneous secondary TB, which is usually caused by hematogenous or lymphatic spread. The term "lupus" (wolf) was generalized to describe all facial lesions with "ragged ulceration" in which disease had an "animal-like" ability to devour flesh. Virchow believed the term lupus originated in the Middle Ages. In the reign of the Stuart (1371–1390), deaths due to "cancer and wolf" were tabulated together. These lesions were also called "noli me tangere" (Don't meddle with me) as they became "enraged by the Application of even the mildest Medicament" (Daniel Turner 1731) (106).

LV is commonly associated with cervical lymphadenitis or upper airway mucosal disease (107). The face is the most common site for LV, especially the nose and cheeks. LV presents as soft brown papules with a characteristic "apple jelly" appearance reminiscent of "a bruise or a decayed spot on an apple" (106). The lesions of secondary TB may also become hypertrophic (lupus verrucosus) or ulcerative (lupus necrogenica). LV is usually seen in patients with strong immune responses (strong reactors to PPD or purified protein derivative); hypersensitivity to acid fast bacilli probably enhances the destructive nature of these lesions which heal with dense and deforming scars.

Orofacial TB, (tuberculosis cutis orofacialis) is a result of autoinoculation from infectious sputum in patients with active pulmonary disease. The anterior and lateral tongue, palate, and lips are affected by extremely painful, small, yellow-red nodules, which ulcerate.

K. Laryngeal TB

Historically, laryngeal TB ("laryngeal phthisis"—phthisis: to dry up) was one of the most common laryngeal diseases of the preantibiotic era. Eighty years ago Sir St. Clair Thompson wrote, "There is no specific disease of the larynx as common as tuberculosis" (107). An autopsy study from the 1940s revealed that almost 40% of patients dying from TB had laryngeal infection (108). Interestingly, 88% of patients with laryngeal infection also had gastrointestinal TB, presumably a result of swallowed infectious sputum (108). In that era, laryngeal TB was accompanied by the stigmata of cavitary pulmonary disease, highly infectious sputum, and progression to end-stage miliary infection with poor prognosis.

Currently, laryngeal TB is quite rare and seen in 1% of infected patients (109–111). Instead of presenting with major constitutional symptoms (fever, weight loss, night sweats, fatigue, and hemoptysis), patients present with hoarseness, cough, hemoptysis, and dysphagia. The mode of spread is still through expectorated sputum. While the association with cavitary pulmonary disease is uncommon; most patients with laryngeal TB also have infectious sputum, still favoring direct pulmonary spread rather than hematogenous seeding.

The lesions of laryngeal TB have also changed. Ulcerative, granulomatous lesions of the posterior larynx were common in the preantibiotic era and probably related to the clinical practice of encouraging patients to lie supine for most of their illness (112). Currently, laryngeal TB can affect any site in the larynx. They are commonly unilateral (113). Lesions may be hypertrophic, polypoid, exophytic, nodular, or ulcerated, clinically mimicking carcinoma (114). Seventy percent of lesions affect the anterior two-thirds of the vocal cords, similar to the distribution of most vocal cord carcinomas (115).

Histopathology

Patients with normal immunity will produce necrotizing granulomatous reactions with epithelioid histiocytes, giant cells, and lymphoplasmacytic infiltrate (Fig. 9). The diagnosis of TB is made with

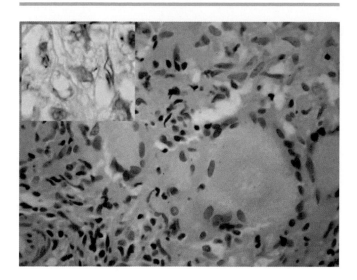

Figure 9 Tuberculosis. Epithelioid granulomata with Langerhans' multinucleated cells. Inset: Acid-fast stain reveals characteristic bacilli.

Ziehl-Neelsen stain and patience. In relatively healthy patients, one might have to search, and examine step sections, to find a solitary "red snapper." The acid-fast bacilli do not stain with hematoxylin and eosin stain or Gram stain.

LV reveals ulceration with adjacent hyperplasia and hyperkeratosis. Epithelioid granulomas with giant cells and chronic inflammation suggest a diagnosis of TB, but other pathogens (fungal, treponemal) need be ruled out. Necrosis is usually minimal in LV, and acid-fast bacilli may be rare.

Serological Testing

The tuberculin skin test (Mantoux test, PPD, or purified protein derivative) is the traditional screening test for latent primary TB infection; a positive tuberculin skin test initiates a course of therapy to eradicate latent infection. PPD is of limited use for those previously immunized with bacilli Calmette-Guerin (BCG) and the immunosuppressed. Newer serological tests assess the response of antigen-specific memory T cells to MTB, specifically interferon-γ (IFN-γ) in response to previously encountered mycobacterial proteins ESAT-6 (early secretory antigenic target protein 6) and CFP-10 (culture filtrate protein 10) (116). T-SPOT-TB and QuantiFERON-TB Gold are two enzyme-linked immunoassay kits available to assess latent MTB infection.

Culture and PCR Identification

Treatment for suspected cases of TB must be instituted prior to culture confirmation, as MTB does not exhibit detectable growth for weeks. The PCR assay can be performed on body fluids such as sputum. It provides rapid diagnosis, can distinguish between MTB and MOTT species (mycobacteria other than TB), and

detect partially treated culture-negative MTB. On the other hand, PCR assays do not necessarily reflect active infection nor can assess drug sensitivity.

Diagnostic Tests for Paraffin-Embedded Tissues

PCR for MTB can also be performed on formalin-fixed paraffin-embedded tissues, with greater sensitivity than the standard Ziehl-Neelsen stain (117,118). In-situ hybridization with species-specific probes can also be performed on pathology specimens (119).

Treatment. Initial four-drug therapy is recommended with either daily drug regimens or directly observed intermittent therapy; the latter regimen has the advantage of increased compliance. The recommended drugs for a six-month course of therapy are isoniazid, rifampin, pyrazinamide, and ethambutol. Ethambutol may be dropped if the culture drug sensitivities return favorable results. If symptoms resolve in the initial two months, and sputum smear becomes negative for AFB, then pyrazinamide may also be dropped. HIV-seropositive patients require extended treatment protocols. Multidrug-resistant TB requires the addition of an anti-TB aminoglycoside, a fluoroquinolone, and cycloserine, ethionamide, or amino salicylic acid.

MOTT (Mycobacteria other than *M. tuberculosis*)
This is a large group of acid-fast bacilli, only some of which are human pathogens. Pathogenic MOTT cause localized infection (subcutaneous, lymphadenitis) in immunocompetant individuals, serious pneumonias in patients with underlying pulmonary disease, and fulminant disseminated disease in AIDS victims.

Background. Mycobacteria other than *M. tuberculosis*, referred to as "MOTT" (mycobacteria other than TB) or as atypical, anonymous, or nontuberculous mycobacteria, are present in water, milk, (especially unpastuerized milk), dust, soil, and birds (*Mycobacterium avium*). Infection is transmitted as a result of environmental exposures, not human-to-human transmission. Nail salons and hot tubs are potential current sources of water-borne MOTT (120,121). The Runyon classification system, described in the 1950s, is based on the growth and pigment characteristics of MOTT. Runyon group I are photochromogens: cultures produce bright yellow pigment upon exposure to light. Group II are scotochromogens: cultures produce bright orange pigment when grown either in dark or light conditions. Group III fail to produce pigment under any condition and are called nonphotochromogens. Group IV MOTT represent rapid growers, forming visible cultures within days rather than weeks. This classification allows for preliminary identification of the more common MOTT (122).

Of historical interest, cervical lymphadenitis was also called scrofula, or "the King's scrofula," "the King's Evil" or "the King's touch." From the reign of Clovis the First of France in the fifth century, until 18th century England (Queen Anne), and 19th century France (Charles the Tenth), reigning monarchs, by divine right, could cure scrofula by a touch and the pronouncement "The King touches thee and God heals thee." These cures evolved into elaborate galas with feasting and distribution of gold pieces, "touch pieces," which were kept as lifetime mementos (123,124).

Clinical. There are four common presentations for MOTT: (*i*) cervical lymphadenitis (e.g., *M. scrofulaeum, M. kansasii*), (*ii*) ulcerative granulomatous skin disease (*M. ulcerans, M. murinium, M. intermedium, M. fortuitum*), (*iii*) pneumonia in patients with underlying pulmonary disease such as emphysema, e.g., *M. kansasii,* and (*iv*) serious pneumonias and generalized infections in patients with AIDS [e.g., *M. avium-intracellulare* (MAI)]. MOTT does not cause pulmonary infection in immunocompetant hosts or in normal lungs.

Mycobacterial Cervical Lymphadenitis

Primary cervical TB lymphadenitis is thought to be the result of infection through disruptions in tonsillar mucosa. Mycobacterial cervical lymphadenitis occurs over a wide age range, usually in immunocompetant individuals. Patients are generally afebrile with enlarged erythematous upper cervical lymph nodes. Involvement of submental, preauricular, middle, or lower cervical chain is much less common (125,126). Lymph nodes may form cutaneous fistulas to the neck or face. *M. scrofulaceum, M. kansasii,* and MAI are most commonly recovered.

Histopathology. Histologically, mycobacterial lymphadenitis is similar to MTB disease; granulomas with multinucleated giant cells, abscess formation with marked necrosis, and variable amounts of acid-fast bacilli are seen. Histologically, the actual bacilli of MTB and MOTT are indistinguishable. MOTT infections in AIDS patients differ from that of normal hosts in that they lack well-formed granulomas. Typically, disseminated infections are seen in any organ as sheets of foamy macrophages with innumerable acid-fast bacilli. A rare tissue reaction has been described in lymph nodes and skin of patients with AIDS in which fibroblasts act as "facultative histiocytes" phagocytosing acid-fast bacilli. This results in a spindled "pseudosarcomatous" type of tissue reaction termed "*Mycobacterium avium-intracellulare*" pseudotumor or (more correctly) "Spindled Nontuberculous Mycobacteriosis" (SNM) (127–129). These lesions resemble fibrohistiocytic tumors or nodular sclerosis type HD. This underscore the importance of examining Ziehl-Neelsen stains in practically every AIDS patient (Fig. 10).

Treatment. MOTT is less sensitive to standard anti-MTB drugs. Macrolides, such as clarithromycin and azithromycin, have greater activity against MOTT than standard anti-MTB drugs alone. However for cervical lymphadenitis, resection is the treatment of choice over antimicrobial therapy. This was demonstrated in a recent prospective randomized control study of 100 children with confirmed non-TB mycobacterial treated either with surgical excision or clarithromycin and rifabutin (130). Mycobacterial cervical lymphadenitis may also be caused by *M. tuberculosis* and *M. bovis.* The distinction between MOTT and MTB relies on cultures, or PCR techniques, which has

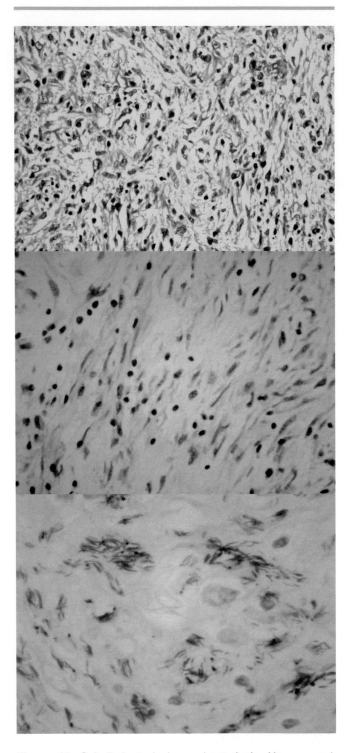

Figure 10 Spindled atypical mycobacteriosis. Upper panel: Cervical lymph node with fascicles of bland spindle cells mixed with sparse mononuclear cells. (hematoxylin and eosin). Middle panel: Inflammatory cells and foamy histiocytes are scarce, and no necrosis is present. An infectious process might easily by overlooked in this setting. Lower panel: Innumerable acid-fast bacilli within fibroblastic cells. (Ziehl–Neelsen)

important epidemiological and treatment repercussions. One-third to one-half of patients with mycobacterial lymphadenitis have radiographic evidence of pulmonary disease, indicating that mycobacterial cervical lymphadenitis can be the presenting symptom of pulmonary MTB disease (123,124,131). These patients then require the recommended full anti-MTB therapy (see above) to eradicate the pulmonary focus. In the latter instance it has been postulated that the primary pulmonary infection gives rise to cervical infection via drainage to mediastinum lymph nodes and subsequently inferior deep cervical lymph nodes or from the pleura to axillary lymph nodes to inferior deep cervical lymph nodes.

L.   Leprosy – Hansen's Disease

Hansen's disease is a contagious, chronic, progressive granulomatous disease caused by *Mycobacterium leprae* (Hansen's bacillus) involving skin, mucosa, and peripheral nerves.

Epidemiology and Background

Biblical writings, which date back 3000 years, describe leprosy (tzara'as) as depressed, hypopigmented lesions containing white hairs (Leviticus 13:1–46). Leprosy is seen mostly in tropical climates and in rural areas. In 2002, 763,917 new cases were reported worldwide, 90% of which were in Brazil, Madagascar, Mozambique, Tanzania, and Nepal (132). For that same year, 133 new cases were diagnosed in the United States; 108 of them were immigrants and refugees living in California, Florida, Hawaii, Louisiana, Texas, Puerto Rico, and New York City (133). The incidence of leprosy in native-born Americans is very low, 11 cases in total for 2002, 8 of which were from Texas (130,134); almost half of all native-born Americans who develop leprosy are Hispanic (134).

Leprosy is generally a disease of low infectivity transmitted by prolonged exposure through nasal secretions or injured skin. Nasal secretions contain high concentrations of bacilli, while the amount of bacilli in skin lesions is variable. Other modes of transmission have also been proposed, such as breast milk, mosquitoes, and bedbugs; however their significance in the overall transmission of leprosy is unknown. Transmission of infection closely relates to the immune status of the infected individual.

Immunological Considerations

The Ridley Joplin criteria classify patients into the following five immunological categories on the basis of cutaneous, histological, and peripheral nerve findings: tuberculoid tuberculoid (TT), borderline tuberculoid (BT), borderline borderline (BB), borderline lepromatous (BL), and lepromatous leprosy (LL) (135). TT represents the most robust immune response with the fewest number of bacilli. LL represents the opposite immunological pole, patients are anergic to the lepromin test (purified suspension of killed *M. leprae*), and lesions contain abundant bacilli. The rate of infection is higher for household contact with infected individuals, especially those with LL, indicating the importance of exposure dose. One significant feature of the Ridley Joplin grading system is that the polar groups (TL and LL) are relatively

"stable" and do not shift immunological responses, whereas patients with borderline lesions (BT, BB, BL) may either upgrade or downgrade their immune responses.

Clinical

M. leprae survives better at cooler temperatures closer to 30°C. Hence it affects skin, peripheral nerves, and upper airway mucosa, rather than viscera. Patients present with cutaneous hypopigmented or hyperpigmented hypesthetic macular lesions (Fig. 11). The early lesions may also be tender, erythematous, and indurated (erythema nodosum leprosum) and ultimately ulcerate (136). Neural involvement is common to all forms of leprosy and results in pain and muscle atrophy. Sensory loss ultimately leads to repeated mechanical trauma and secondary infections. The classical signs of leprous nerve involvement include claw hand, foot drop, lagophthalmos, and anesthesia.

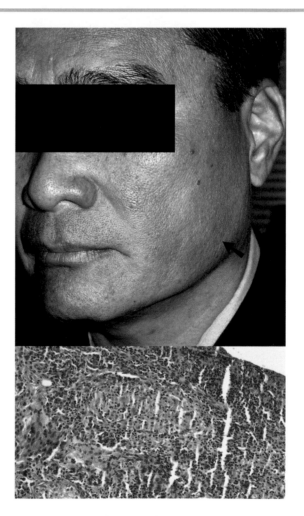

Figure 11   Tuberculoid leprosy. Upper panel: Borderline tuberculoid leprosy presenting as a subtle, red-brown, partially anesthetic plaque on the left face; its inferior border (*arrow*) is sharply demarcated, which is characteristic of tuberculoid leprosy. Lower panel: Periadnexal non-necrotizing granuloma. *Source*: Courtesy of Dr. Brian Thomas, Bronx, New York, U.S.A.

Lepromatous Leprosy—Head and Neck Manifestations

LL usually begins with nonspecific symptoms of chronic mucopurulent rhinitis; the mucus contains copious mycobacteria. The diagnosis is not suspected prior to the development of skin lesions. The earlobes and nose become enlarged and infiltrated. The widespread symmetrical facial lesions progressive coarsen facial features (leonine facies). Late sinonasal lesions are nodular, ulcerative and may ultimately lead to nasal collapse. LL is also associated with mycobacillemia and involvement of liver, spleen, and bone marrow.

Laryngeal involvement usually follows nasal disease, and can be common, (137,138) especially in LL and advanced cases (139). The epiglottis is most often involved and appears thickened and irregular. Vocal cord paralysis may develop because of recurrent laryngeal nerve involvement. Oral manifestations usually appear in 20% to 60% of cases. Lesions are usually located on the hard palate, uvula, ventral tongue, lips, and gums. The anterior maxilla may be destroyed with loss of teeth.

Histopathology. TL reveals epithelioid granulomas and relatively few organisms, which are seen only on Fite–Faraco or modified Fite stains. Nerves are cuffed by lymphocytes or granulomas, or may contain free acid-fast bacilli. LL reveals diffuse histiocytic infiltrate incapable of undergoing "epithelioid" transformation and granuloma formation (Fig. 12). These foamy histiocytes (lepra cells, Virchow cells) may be "stuffed" with abundant mycobacilli (globi) and remain uncleared by the host. Free bacilli are abundant within nerves. BT, BB, and borderline leprosy will demonstrate a mixture of ill-formed granulomas and foamy histiocytes.

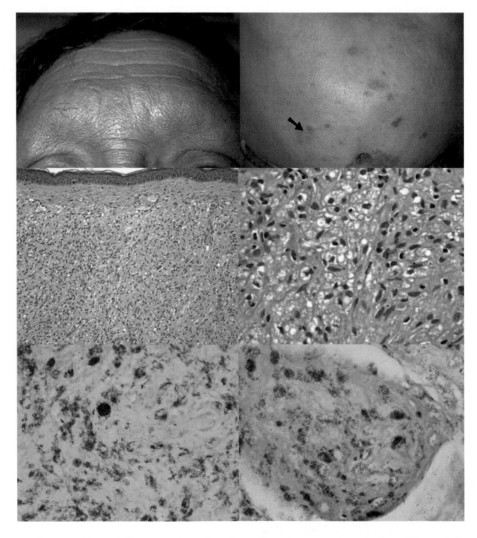

Figure 12 Lepromatous leprosy. Upper left panel: Complete loss of eyebrows and eyelashes. Upper right panel: Erythematous hyperpigmented patches and a hypopigmented patch (*arrow*). Middle left panel: Diffuse dermal infiltrate of histiocytes without granuloma formation. Middle left right panel: Vacuolated mononuclear histiocytes or lepra cells admixed with occasional small lymphocytes (hematoxylin-eosin). Lower left panel: Fite stain demonstrating innumerable acid-fast bacilli throughout the dermis. Lower right panel: Numerous acid-fast bacilli, *Mycobacterium leprae*, in nerve (Fite stain). *Source*: From Ref. 130 and courtesy of Dr. Mary Schwartz, Houston, Texas, U.S.A.

The diagnosis of leprosy is more difficult to determine early in the disease course when mycobacilli may be sparse and granulomas are not fully developed. Mycobacteria may be sparsely present or absent histologically in TL. In a biopsy study of 30 cases of laryngeal leprosy, only 7 revealed histological evidence of bacilli, most often, as expected, in those cases with foamy cells (138).

The histoid form leprosy (140) is seen in late leprosy and is characterized by spindle-shaped histiocytes forming dermatofibroma-like tumors; an analogous lesion is the SNM (see above).

Differential diagnosis. The differential diagnosis includes MTB, atypical mycobacteria, systemic lupus erythematosis, sarcoidosis, leishmaniasis and mycosis fungiodes. Clinical suspicion and histopathological findings secure the diagnosis. Perineural cuffing by lymphocytes, granulomas, or free organisms are important diagnostic features of leprosy, and not seen with MTB infections. Free mycobacilli and mycobacilli-laden foamy histiocytes are present even in biopsies of "normal" skin; limited inflammatory reaction is pathognomonic for LL. The Fite–Faraco stain is specific for *M. leprae*, and is not known to stain other mycobacteria.

Culture and PCR identification. *M. leprae* does not grow in culture. It can be inoculated into mouse foot pads and into nine-banded armadillos (who have a lower body temperature) where it grows very slowly, dividing at a rate once in 12 to 14 days. PCR detection is extremely sensitive and especially helpful in establishing the diagnosis in paucibacillary Hansen's disease (130). It can be applied to formalin-fixed paraffin-embedded specimens. PCR testing cannot distinguish between live and dead bacilli and therefore cannot assess treatment effect. Serological antibody tests to antiphenolic glycolipid 1 titers or slit-skin smears correlate with bacterial load and can be used to monitor response to therapy.

Treatment. Dapsone, rifampin, and clofazimine are commonly used. However prolonged treatment is required, which is expensive and associated with adverse side effects.

M. Cat Scratch Disease

Regional lymphadenitis is usually caused by *Bartonelli henselae*, a rickettsial-like gram-negative bacterium, which is introduced via skin breaks.

Clinical

Cat scratch disease (CSD) is a disease of the immunocompetent; children and young adults are most often affected (griffes de chat (141)). An erythematous lesion develops within 3 to 10 days at the site of a cat scratch, lick, or bite. It progresses through vesicular and papular stages spontaneously resolving within one to three weeks. The cat appears healthy throughout this time. CSD then comes to medical attention up to seven weeks later with painful regional lymphadenopathy, most commonly affecting axillary and cervical lymph nodes (142). In the head and neck, preauricular and submandibular lymph nodes may be involved (143). Not all patients will recall an incident with a cat, therefore the diagnosis of CSD might escape consideration.

Lymphadenopathy has been reported in more than 80% of patients and may persist longer than six months in 20% of cases. CSD may also be accompanied by fever, headache, myalgias, and secondary skin rashes (erythema nodosum erythema annulare, erythema multiforme, thrombocytopenic purpura). Rarely, 1% to 2% of patients can develop severe systemic infection such as encephalitis, osteomyelitis, hepatitis, and pleuritis (144). Atypical manifestations occur in 5% of patients and include Parinaud's oculoglandular syndrome, characterized by conjunctival granulomas, nonsuppurative conjunctivitis, and preauricular lymphadenopathy (142,145).

Etiology

Most cases are caused by *B. henselae*, (previously referred to as "*Rochalimaea henselae*") a rickettsial-like gram-negative bacterium (146). Rarely *Afipia felis* is recovered (147,148). These organisms are obligate intracellular organisms associated with soil picked up on cat paws and thus transmitted to humans (146,149).

Histopathology

Early CSD may reveal only nonspecific lymphoid hyperplasia and sinus histiocytosis. Epithelioid granulomas coalesce to form necrotizing microabscesses with polymorphonuclear cells and fibrin. The necrotic areas are rimmed with pallisading epithelioid histiocytes and lymphocytes (Fig. 13). The finding of stellate necrosis is neither sensitive nor specific for CSD. The bacilli stain with Warthin–Starry and are weakly positive with Brown and Hopp stain; they are seen within capillaries and macrophages. In practice, they

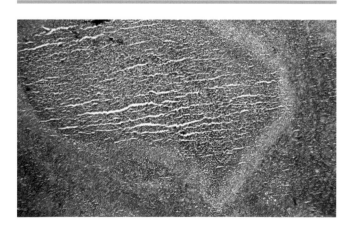

Figure 13 Cat scratch disease (CSD). Stellate necrosis rimmed with epithelioid histiocytes and lymphocytes should raise the possibility of CSD, however these findings are neither sensitive nor specific. Look for bacilli within capillaries and macrophages by Warthin–Starry stain; in practice, they are very difficult to find. (hematoxylin and eosin)

may be very difficult to identify. Skin biopsies from the primary lesions of CSD reveal epithelial hyperplasia, histiocytic, and inflammatory infiltrate, which progresses to form the same necrotic pallisading granulomas.

Serology and PCR

Serum antibody studies are the cornerstone of diagnosis; on occasion they have demonstrated that patients with CSD are coinfected with both *B. henselae* and *A. felinis* (147). PCR assays can be applied to archival pathology specimens with greater sensitivity and specificity than Warthin–Starry stain and IHC (147,150).

Treatment

Treatment of CSD is mostly supportive for mild to moderate disease manifestations. Patients with severe symptoms may require antibiotics, but there are no standardized regimens. Erythromycin, azithromycin, ciprofloxacin, gentamycin, rifamicin, and trimetoprim/sulfomethoxazole are thought to be effective (142). Surgery is indicated for CSD only to confirm the diagnosis. Needle aspiration of a suppurative lymph node may relieve local pain. Incision and drainage is to be avoided, as this may result in cutaneous fistula formation.

Bacillary Angiomatosis

Clinical presentation. Bacillary Angiomatosis (BA) is characterized by mucocutaneous vascular lesions and constitutional symptoms (fever, chills, and headache). In addition to mucocutaneous sites, BA can affect the liver, spleen, bone, brain, lungs, lymph nodes, and heart (151–154). Patients present with single or multiple cutaneous papules or nodules, 0.5 to 4.0 cm in size, which may be red, violet, friable, tender, and ulcerated. Mucocutaneous lesions can affect the face, extremities, scrotum, nasal cavity, oral cavity, and pharynx (155,156). Deeper subcutaneous nodules resembling cellulitis may develop and erode underlying bone. The mucocutaneous lesions may resemble Kaposi's sarcoma (KS) or verruga peruana (VP), the chronic cutaneous manifestation of infection with *Bartonella bacilliformis* (the agent of Carrion's disease or Oroyo fever).

Histopathology. The diagnosis of BA is based on correlating characteristic clinical and histopathological findings. There is a lobular proliferation of capillaries with plump protuberant "tombstone"-like epithelioid endothelial cells. The endothelial cells have vesicular, hyperchromatic, and pleomorphic nuclei. Necrotic cellular debris and atypical mitotic figures are seen mimicking malignancy. Neutrophils are diffuse and tend to aggregate around eosinophilic granular material that corresponds to masses of slender bacilli, which can be seen on Warthin–Starry stain; the bacilli stain variably with Steiner and Brown and Brenn stains and are morphologically similar to the bacilli of CSD.

Etiology. Infection may be acquired through exposure to cats, soil, or waste. *Bartonella henselae*

(formally *R. hensleae*) and *Rickettsia quintana* (Trench fever) have been isolated from BA (152,157). Host immune response is pivotal to the manifestation of infection. Exposure to the same bacteria will cause CSD (see above), which is localized to lymph nodes in immunocompetent hosts, or systemic long-term infections in immunocompromised individuals (HIV patients, organ transplant recipients) (158).

Differential diagnosis. The differential diagnosis of BA includes pyogenic granuloma and KS. Pyogenic granuloma lacks cytological pleomorphism and clusters of bacilli. KS is composed of spindled cells producing slit-like spaces, hyaline globules (which stain with periodic acid–Schiff, phosphotungstic acid hematoxylin, and trichrome) and the presence of HHV-8 (Human herpesvirus 8) are pathognomonic for KS. KS also lacks nuclear debris, lobular configuration, and bacilli.

Interestingly, BA resembles VP caused by *B. bacilliformis*, which is related to *A. felis* and *R. henselae* (159). VP is the result of an angioblastic response to *Bartonella* infection, with plump, atypical epithelioid endothelial cells. VP can regress as the lesion becomes progressively infiltrated by lymphocytes. VP has a number of different patterns, which may also mimic neoplasia: the spindled pattern of VP may be indistinguishable from KS and the epithelioid pattern of VP mimics carcinoma or other epithelioid neoplasms (159). The correct diagnosis of VP lies in recognizing the infectious nature of these lesions, and the clinical history (patients are from endemic areas in South America, such as Peru). Intracellular clumps of *Bartonella* bacilli (Rocha-Lima bodies) are best visualized on Giemsa stain. Warthin–Starry stain is negative for *B. bacilliformis*, which can distinguish it from *B. henselae*/BA, which does stain with Warthin–Starry.

Culture, PCR, and serological identification. Routine culture methods are inadequate for isolation of the causative bacilli, as they are fastidious and slow growing. The use of enriched medium, cell lyses centrifugation, and prolonged incubation are recommended. Serological tests may not reliably distinguish between *Bartonella quintana* and *R. henselae*. Cross-reactivity with Chlamydia has also been reported. PCR can be used on clinical specimens to confirm the diagnosis (157).

Treatment. Erythromycin is the first drug of choice for BA; doxycycline is also effective for patients who tolerate erythromycin poorly. Serious infections require a third-generation cephalosporin or aminoglycoside to prevent septicemia (160).

III. FUNGAL DISEASES

A. Sinonasal Fungal Disease

General Aspects

There are four clinicopathological classifications of sinonasal mycotic disease: (*i*) acute invasive fulminant infection, (*ii*) chronic invasive infection, (*iii*) noninvasive mycotic colonization ("fungus ball" or mycetoma), and (*iv*) allergic fungal sinusitis (AFS) (Table 1).

Table 1 Classification of Sinonasal Fungal Disease

Invasive	Acute fulminant invasive
	Chronic granulomatous
	Chronic invasive
Noninvasive	Fungus ball or mycetoma
	Allergic fungal sinusitis

It is important for the pathologist to have sound understanding of the differences between these entities. These different diseases can be caused by various fungi, but *Aspergillus* is by far the most commonly isolated agent of all types of sinonasal fungal disease (161,162). The term "aspergilloma" is to be avoided, as it has been applied in the context of different disease entities. Noninvasive forms of fungal sinusitis are much more prevalent than invasive fungal disease.

The term "invasive fungal sinusitis" refers to the presence of tissue invasion, which may vary in degree. This cannot be reliably determined radiographically; mycetomas and AFS may form inflammatory expansile masses with bony erosion, mimicking an invasive phenomenon. Invasive fungal sinusitis can be subclassified as either acute or chronic. Chronic invasive fungal sinusitis can be further classified as chronic granulomatous sinusitis, which is seen most often in endemic regions, and chronic invasive fungal sinusitis, which can be seen in diabetic patients.

Fungal hyphae may be sparse in AFS or may be confined to vessels in early invasive sinusitis. Importantly, pathology reporting should distinguish whether hyphae are present within mucin, or within tissue, as this has therapeutic implications. Fungal hyphae may be impossible to classify without culture confirmation. On the other hand, pathological correlation is necessary to distinguish clinical infection from laboratory contamination.

Aspergillosis

Aspergillosis is a disease caused by *Aspergillus*, (a member of the family *Moniliaceae*, class *Hyphomycetes*, phylum Deuteromycota), which has septated thin branching hyphae and forms petallike "fruiting heads" bearing pigmented conidia during sexual reproduction.

Historical background. *Aspergillus* derives its name from the Latin "aspergere," meaning "to pour." The fungus was so named by Micheli, a priest, who noted that the conidial heads resembled the Catholic Church's aspergillum, or holy water font (Fig. 14) (163). As an etymological aside, "aspersions" is derived from "aspergillum"; during the rite of Asperges, the sprinkling of holy water, a particular individual may have been deemed to require more sprinkling than others, thereby having aspersions cast on him.

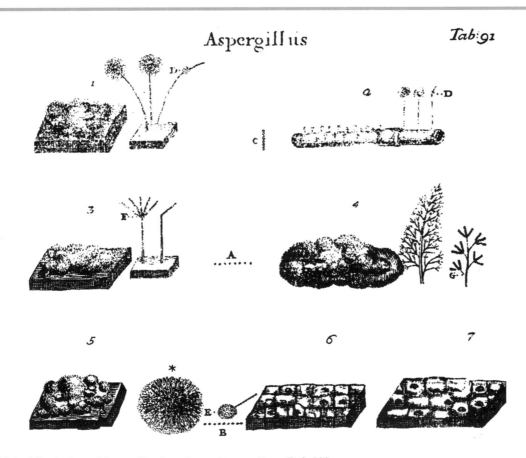

Figure 14 Original illustration of Aspergillus in culture. *Source*: From Ref. 163.

Aspergillus is abundant in soil, decaying organic matter (fallen leaves, compost heaps), and stored grains (164). *Aspergillus flavus* is the most prevalent environmental species, but climatic differences influence species prevalence (165). Indoor airborne *Aspergillus* concentrations are usually greater than outdoor concentrations. *Aspergillus* is one of the most common indoor isolates from areas affected by hurricanes Katrina and Rita (166), and is a common isolate from hospital patient care areas (167). Aspergillus is transmitted by inhalation of airborne spores. Historically, clusters of fatal infections were associated with hospital renovations, specifically exposure to fireproofing materials (168).

Acute Fulminant Aspergillus Sinusitis

Clinical presentation. Acute fulminant invasive aspergillosis occurs most often in granulopenic patients with hematological malignancies; it can also develop in AIDS patients (169), transplant recipients, and occasionally in immunocompetent patients (170). Presenting complaints include fever, headache, nasal discharge, sinus pain, and periorbital and maxillary swelling (171). Initially, nasal and palatal mucosa appear pale and ischemic and then become blackened and gangrenous (Fig. 15). *Aspergillus*' ability for vascular invasion is potentiated by production of elastase and proteases (172). Needless to say, tremendous morbidity and high mortality rates are associated with fulminant invasive *Aspergillus* sinusitis. The

infection spreads through vessels and nerves and can extend intracranial; the orbital nerve can become involved with ensuing blindness.

Histopathology. Invasive aspergillosis is a necrotizing infection; the degree of accompanying inflammation varies with the patient's state of immunity. Granulocytopenic patients have minimal inflammation. The hyphae invade tissue diffusely in all directions. Fungal vascular invasion results in mycotic vascular thrombosis and zones of coagulative necrosis with cellular debris. *Aspergillus* hyphae are thin (2–5 μm), septated, with acutely angled (45°) branching. The hyphae appear "stiff," with less bending than other fungi (Fig. 16). The hyphae may also appear fragmented, swollen, and degenerated. Hyphae can be seen on hematoxylin and eosin stain, thus it is possible to diagnose invasive aspergillosis on frozen section intraoperative consultation (173). Gomori methanamine silver will stain the hyphae and accentuate

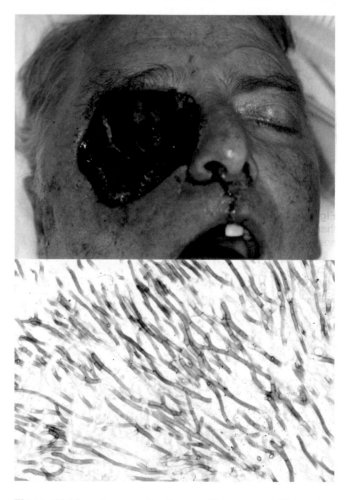

Figure 16 Invasive mycotic disease. Upper panel: This unfortunate person required aggressive debridement for invasive mycotic sinusitis. Lower panel: Invasive Aspergillosis—The thin septated hyphae are relatively stiff and parallel hyphae walls; 45° branching angles are frequent. Inflammatory reaction is not present (Gomori methenamine silver). *Source*: Courtesy of Dr. William Lawson, Mount Sinai, New York.

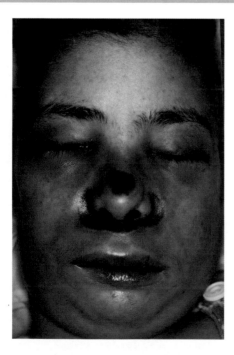

Figure 15 Invasive fungal sinusitis. Periorbital and facial edema, vascular congestion, and thrombotic hemmorrhage of the soft tissues herald invasive mycotic sinusitis. The course of untreated cases is swift and fulminant. *Source*: Courtesy of Dr. William Lawson, Mount Sinai, New York, U.S.A.

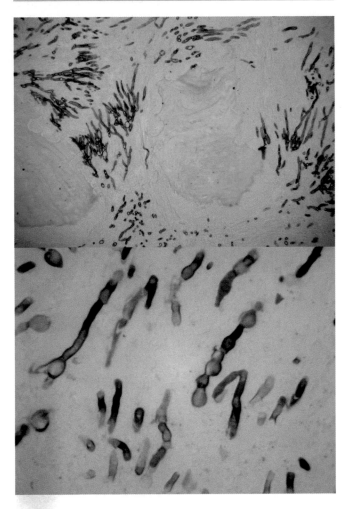

Figure 17 Invasive mycotic disease. Upper panel: Fungi other than *Aspergillus* can also cause invasive infection in the immunosuppressed patient. Lower panel: Septated branching hyphae with intercalated swellings. This was identified as a Penicillium on mycology culture.

Chronic Invasive/Chronic Granulomatous Aspergillus Sinusitis

Background and etiology. Chronic granulomatous *Aspergillus* sinusitis is a disease of immunocompent hosts usually seen in highly endemic areas, such as Sudan, Saudi Arabia, or India (165,176,177). It has rarely been reported in the United States (178) and in African-Americans (179). The disease is almost exclusively associated with *A. flavus* and probably caused by prolonged exposure to large doses of fungus. *Aspergillus* has been recovered from straw roofs, earthen floors, bedding, and grains stored within homes (176). The dusty air of summer sandstorms further disseminates the fungal spores and encourages their growth. Furthermore, asymptomatic nasal colonization with *Aspergillus* has been demonstrated in endemic regions.

The term "chronic invasive fungal sinusitis" describes fungal sinonasal infection with documented tissue invasion but no granulomatous reaction. While this may overlap with endemic fungal sinusitis, chronic invasive fungal sinusitis also describes a subset of patients with nonneutropenic immunosuppression, usually uncontrolled diabetes or chronic renal failure. It is usually associated with *Aspergillus* or *Mucorales* infection.

Clinical presentation. Patients complain of nasal obstruction, discharge, and pain. Proptosis is a common finding. Imaging studies usually reveal an inflammatory process involving multiple paranasal sinuses, with bony erosion and remodeling. Frequently, the process can extend beyond the sinuses to involve the brain, cavernous sinus, and orbit.

Histopathology.

Chronic Granulomatous Fungal Sinusitis. Chronic granulomatous *Aspergillus* sinusitis is characterized by nonnecrotizing and necrotizing granulomas, extensive fibrinoid necrosis, foreign body and Langerhan's type multinucleated giant cells, and eosinophil microabscesses (Fig. 18). Vasculitis, vascular proliferation, and perivascular fibrosis are seen;

septations. There is no "pinching" at septations points, unlike the pseudoseptation of *Candida* (Fig. 17).

Serology. Serum *Aspergillus* galactomannan is not reliable in establishing the initial diagnosis of sinonasal aspergillosis (174). However, once the diagnosis has been established, *Aspergillus* galactomannan levels may be followed in immunosuppressed patients to assess treatment efficacy.

Treatment. If invasive aspergillosis is suspected, rapid intervention is indicated. Tissue examination establishes the diagnosis. Infected tissue is bloodless due to vascular thrombosis; debridement is necessary as this tissue is not susceptible to systemic agents. Systemic antifungal therapy is always indicated; voriconazole is the first drug of choice. Direct sinonasal instillation of amphotericin B has also been recommended (175). If feasible, immunosuppression in transplant recipients should be reduced or neutropenia should be addressed with growth factors.

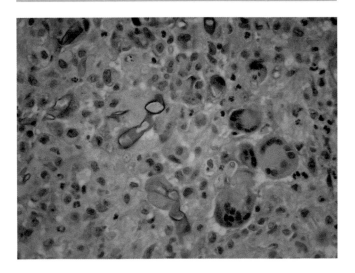

Figure 18 Chronic granulomatous fungal sinusitis can be seen in individuals from endemic regions.

these vascular changes are attributed to *A. flavus* aflatoxins (165,176). Branching septated fungal hyphal are abundant; they may also appear swollen and degenerated. Fungal tissue invasion is seen, but vascular invasion is absent.

Chronic Invasive Fungal Sinusitis. An exuberant granulomatous reaction is not seen in chronic invasive fungal sinusitis; a strong acute and chronic inflammatory response is present. By definition, fungal tissue invasion is seen, which distinguishes this process from a mycetoma or a pronounced AFS. One might see some granuloma formation and vascular invasion.

Treatment. Most patients respond to surgical debridement. However, there is a significant recurrence rate, which may be improved with antifungal therapy (165).

Fungus Ball/Mycetoma

Background and etiology. Fungus ball/mycetoma represents fungal reproduction within a sinus cavity; this is the only context in sinonasal fungal disease in which fungal sexual reproduction might be seen. *Aspergillus fumigatus* and *A. flavus* are most commonly isolated from mycetomas (180,181). A history of previous endodontic treatment is common among patients with fungus balls (181,182). Endodontic procedures are thought to contribute to the formation of antral fungus balls. Progressive loss of the fungistatic effect of eugenol, one component of the endodontic sealer, allows for the zinc oxide, another sealer component, to promote *Aspergillus* spore germination (182). Anecdotally, *Aspergillus* fungus balls have been attributed to smoking marijuana (183). Marijuana samples contain viable *Aspergillus* spores, which easily pass through the filterless marihuana cigarettes (184).

Clinical presentation. Patients may complain of nasal obstruction, discharge, and sinus pain, but not proptosis. Some patients are totally asymptomatic and come to attention with an incidental radiographic paranasal sinus finding. Radiological findings include sinus opacification, calcifications, and bony remodeling. Single sinuses are more commonly involved than multiple sinuses, most often the maxillary antrum, followed by sphenoid, ethmoid, and frontal sinuses (182,183).

Histopathology. The size of the fungus ball, and the extent of associated inflammation, can greatly vary. Some mycetomas are merely microscopic and found in the context of an acute and chronic sinusitis (Fig. 19). Others can produce a significant inflammatory mass, with a centrifugal pattern of abundant hyphae and acute and chronic inflammatory debris (Fig. 20). The matted dense conglomeration of hyphae is refractile on hematoxylin and eosin and stains with Gomori methanamine silver. The hyphae remain separate from the Schneiderian mucosa; tissue invasion, vascular invasion, and granulomas are not seen.

"Fruiting heads" (conidial heads) are a striking finding and allow for differentiation between *Aspergillus* species (Fig. 21). Sterigmata arise from the conidiophores and bear secondary sterigmata, or phialides (vaselike structures), which bud off chains of

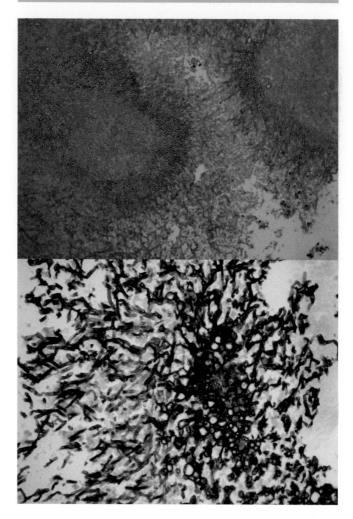

Figure 19 Fungus ball (mycetoma). Upper panel: A mass of refractile hyphae can be seen on hematoxylin and eosin. Lower panel: Pleomorphic septated hyphae (Gomori methanamine silver).

pigmented conidia for a daisy petallike effect. The color of the conidia will distinguish species: they are brown/black for *A. niger* (niger—Lat. black), yellow/green for *A. flavus* (flavus—Lat. yellow), and green for *A. fumigatus* (fumigatus—Lat. Smoky—descriptive of the "smoky plumes of conidia," which rise from the cultures). Examination of paraffin-embedded tissue morphology of the "fruiting heads" is not as detailed as lactophenol blue culture preparations, but may still allow for speciation. Fontana-Masson melanin stain can be positive for *A. niger*, highlighting the fruiting heads, but not *A. flavus* or *A. fumigatus* (185). Calcium oxalate crystals are characteristic of *A. niger*, and occasionally seen with *A. flavus*. They may be seen as radiating clusters of birerefringent crystals, which stain strongly with Alizarin red S (pH 7); silver nitrate-rubeanic acid with 5% acetic acid pretreatment specifically detects oxalate (186). The calcium depositions can become quite dense and organized.

PCR techniques. *Aspergillus* fungus balls can be specifically identified by their fruiting heads; it is

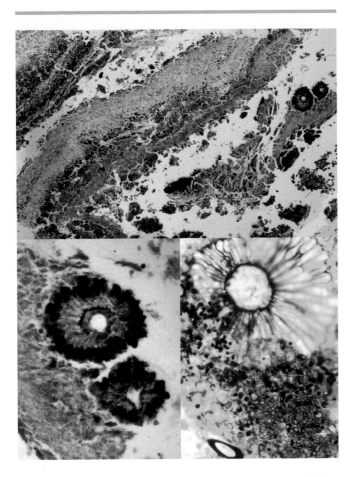

Figure 20 Aspergillus niger mycetoma. Upper panel: Low power reveals layers of conidia, hyphae, and inflammatory debris (hemantoxylin and eosin). Lower left: Fruiting heads—Note how the brown/black pigmentation is obvious on hematoxylin and eosin stain. Lower right: Fruiting head (Gomori methanamine silver).

usually not possible to identify the causative fungi for non-*Aspergillus* fungus balls in pathology specimens. PCR and in situ hybridization have been applied to paraffin-embedded specimens and can identify and speciate the causative fungi (185,187). This may be of epidemiological interest, but has no therapeutic implications.

Treatment. Most patients remain recurrence-free after conservative curettage (functional endoscopic sinus surgery, FESS). Some otolaryngologists recommend irrigation with saline or iodine solutions. No additional antimycotic therapy is indicated (182).

Allergic Fungal Sinusitis (Eosinophilic Mucin Rhinosinusitis)

Background and etiology. Katzenstein first described this entity in a group of patients with allergic symptoms; their sinonasal contents were histologically similar to that seen in allergic bronchopulmonary aspergillosis (188). AFS is also referred to as eosinophilic sinusitis with allergic mucin, chronic hyperplastic eosinophilic sinusitis, and eosinophilic

mucin rhinosinusitis (EMRS). It has an incidence of 6% to 9% of all the hyperplastic sinus disease requiring surgery (189). Importantly, the role of fungi in this process is actually still speculative. Many cases are associated with *A. fumigatus, A. flavus,* or the demateaceous fungi; but given their environmental ubiquity, fungi may be incidental to the process. The fungal hypothesis holds that susceptible individuals develop extreme eosinophil-driven hypersensitivity reactions to the ubiquitous fungi, and that an immune T_H2-like lymphocyte-mediated response to fungal antigens is responsible for the process. T_H2 cells regulate IgE production and allergic inflammatory response. Proof of this hypothesis would require demonstration that the sinonasal T_H lymphocytes are *specifically activated* in response to the colonizing fungi, but those data do not exist (190). Presently, although fungal hyphae are present within AFS, their role in initiating or promoting this disease remains circumstantial.

Fungal hyphae are not always found within allergic mucin. Is AFS a different entity from eosinophilic sinusitis with allergic mucin but without fungi or part of the same disease spectrum? This latter entity has also been referred to as "AFS-like syndrome" or "eosinophilic mucin rhinosinusitis." EMRS may be a distinct entity from AFS. Ferguson reviewed the literature and her own accrued experience and compared the clinicopathological features of 431 patients with AFS with 69 patients with EMRS (191). Mean patient age was significantly younger for AFS than EMRS (31 vs. 48). Asthma, aspirin sensitivity, and bilateral disease were significantly more common in EMRS than AFS (93% vs. 41%, 54% vs. 13%, and 100% vs. 54%, respectively). Pathologically, allergic sinusitis with more abundant and thick allergic mucin is more likely to contain fungal hyphae (192). These clinicopathological distinctions support the view that AFS and EMRS may be different entities.

Clinical presentation. Patients with AFS have a history of allergic sinusitis, nasal polyposis, and possibly allergic asthma (193,194). Visual changes and facial distortion may be present because of an enlarging inflammatory mass (Fig. 22). Radiographically, a heterogeneous inflammatory soft tissue mass and associated sinonasal polyposis can be seen; bony destruction and remodeling may also be present. Ferromagnetic elements in associated with the fungi result in a serpiginous pattern of increased attenuation on CT examination. Serum eosinophilia, elevated IgE, cutaneous sensitivity to fungal antigens, and the presence of fungal-specific serum precipitins all support the diagnosis of allergic mycotic sinusitis.

Histopathology. At low power, allergic mucin contains red and blue onion skin–like laminations, which are composed of debris, degenerated epithelial cells, degranulating eosinophils, and polymorphonuclear leukocytes (Fig. 22). The Schneiderian mucosa is infiltrated by eosinophils. Charcot–Leyden crystals are present within the allergic mucin; they are pink/orange hexagonal, bipyramidal, needlelike, nonpolarizable crystals, which result from eosinophil degranulation. The presence of Charcot–Leyden defines

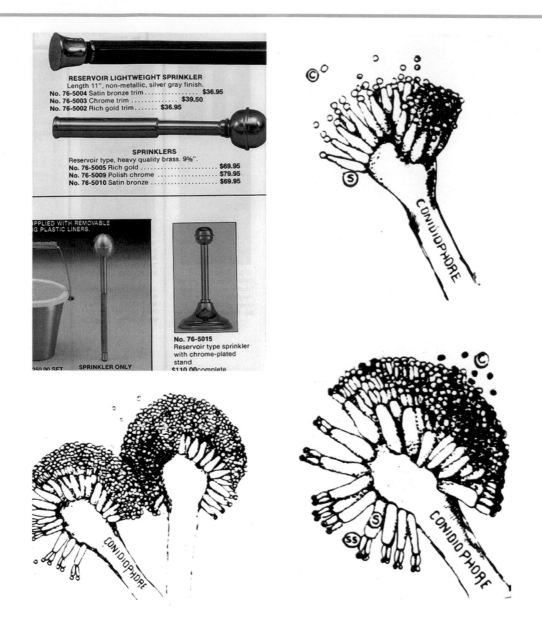

Figure 21 The fruiting heads of *Aspergillus*. The structure of the conidiophores, sterigmata, and the color of the conidia, are distinguishing features of *Aspergillus* subtypes. This level of detail is not seen on histology, but on microscopy of the culture. Upper right: *Aspergillus fumigatus* has primary sterigmata (S) bearing conidia (C). Lower left: *Aspergillus flavus* condiophores may or may not bear secondary sterigmata bearing conidia (C). Lower right: A niger has paired secondary sterigmata (SS) bearing conidia (C).

allergic mucin. Hyphae are sparse and noninvasive; if present, they are usually seen only after a Gomori methanamine silver stain. The greater the amount and thickness of the allergic mucin, the more likely hyphae will be found. Tissue artifact such as folds can mimic hyphae; artifactual "hyphae" are usually slightly out of the plane of focus and usually parallel to the ripples of mucin, whereas true hyphae are in the plane of focus (Fig. 23).

Treatment. FESS will accomplish removal of the inspisated allergic mucin and improved sinus aeration and drainage. Patients experience initial dramatic relief of symptoms; however disease recidivism is common and usually some additional form of therapy is required, including specific fungal and nonfungal immunotherapy, systemic or local corticosteroids, and antifungal antimicrobial therapies (193–195).

Mucormycosis and Entomophthoromycosis

Mucormycosis and Entomophthoromycosis are diseases caused by *Mucorales* and *Entomophthorales*, members of the fungal class *Zygomycetes*. These primitive fungi have wide, pleomorphic hyphae; Mucorales are nonseptate and branching, *Entomophthorales* have few branch points, and may have septations.

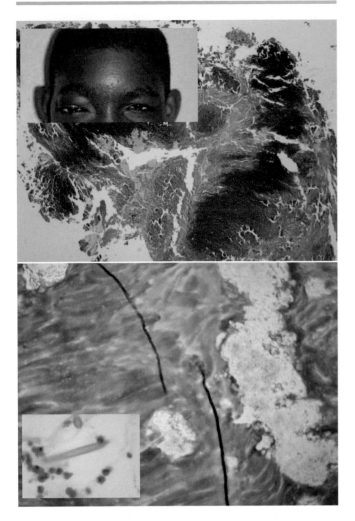

Figure 22 Allergic fungal sinusistis. Upper panel: "Ripples" of eosinophils alternating with mucous hint at allergic fungal disease. The denser, and more abundant the allergic mucin, the greater the likelihood fungal hyphae will be identified (hematoxylin and eosin). Upper inset: Proptosis due to long-standing allergic fungal sinusitis. Lower panel: Few hyphal fragments can be found. Exact identification of these fragments in tissue sections may be impossible (Gomori methanamine silver). Lower inset: Charcot–Leyden crystals—thick and thin needlelike non-polarizable crystals (hematoxylin and eosin).

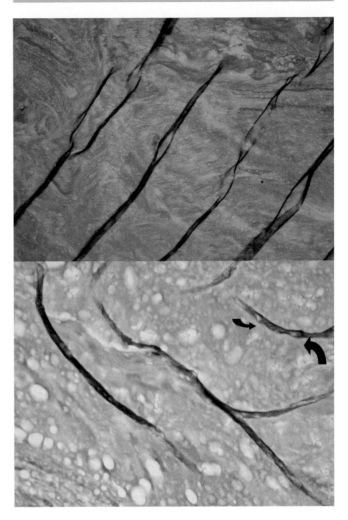

Figure 23 Recognizing hyphae. Upper panel: Artifact such as folds can mimic hyphae; artifactual "hyphae" are usually slightly out of the plane of focus and are parallel to the ripples of mucin (Gomori methanamine silver). Lower panel: True hyphae, seen here, are in the plane of focus and are of variable length. Here we see branching hyphae with globose swellings (*arrows*) (Gomori methanamine silver).

Mucorales

Background and etiology. Mucorales can be found in decaying fruit, especially with high sugar content, vegetables, soil, old bread, and manure. Spices, herbal teas, and birdseed have been found to harbor *Rhizopus* and *Absidia*, (members of family *Mucoracea*, order *Mucorales*) (196). *Rhizopus, Rhizomucor,* and *Absidia* are the most common human pathogens of mucormycosis and are transmitted by inhalation; *Rhizopus* accounts for 90% of cases of rhinocerebral mucormycosis (Fig. 24). Rarely, mucormycosis can be caused by other genera such as *Suksenaea, Apophysomyces, Cunninhamella, Cokermyces,* and *Syncephalastrum spp.*

Mucormycosis is thought to be 10- to 50-fold less common than *Aspergillus* or *Candida* infections; an estimated 500 cases per year are seen in the United States (197). Infection can usually be classified as either rhinocerebral, pulmonary, gastrointestinal, cutaneous, or disseminated. The incidence of mucormycosis has been rising in some settings such as transplant centers (197). Nosocomial infection has been associated with Elastoplast® bandages (198–200). In one report, two patients developed rhinocerebral zygomycosis after receiving steroids from the same physician, and the infection source was traced to the central air-conditioning filter in that office building (201). An outbreak of gastric mucormycosis caused by *Rhizopus microsporus* has been associated with contaminated wooden tongue depressors, which were used to prepare oral medications administered by nasogastric tube (202).

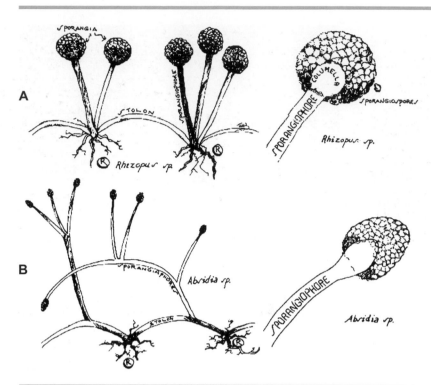

Figure 24 Two examples of sporangiophore morphology. Rhyzopus: Clusters of rhizoids arise directly—opposite groups of sporagiophores. Stolons connect one nodal point to the next. The columella extends into the globose sporangium like a "finger in a balloon." Absidia: Freely branching sporangiophores arise on stolons between the nodal points of rhizoids (R). The columella extends into the piriform sporangium.

Rhizopus elaborates ketone reductase; it favors the acidic, high glucose environment of uncontrolled diabetics who are most susceptible to this infection (197,203–205). Mucor hyphae invade vessels and form endovascular thrombi causing tissue necrosis. Diabetic microangiopathy further potentiates local ischemia and increases susceptibility to infection. The low pH of necrotic tissue provides fertile media for fungal growth and also impairs polymorphonuclear leukocyte function. Mucormycosis has also been associated with immunodeficient/granulocytopenic conditions such as acute leukemia, disseminated cancer, corticosteroids therapy, and prolonged immunosuppressive therapy, conditions of chronic metabolic acidosis such as renal disease and extensive burns and also deferoxamine therapy (197,205,206,208–211). *Rhizopus* requires free iron for rapid growth; it utilizes the iron chelator deferoxamine as siderophore to scavenge serum iron. Patients with myelodysplasia may have iron overload from transfusions; they are also at risk for mucormycosis. Patients with systemic acidosis (diabetics, renal failure) have elevated serum iron because of the disruption in the iron-binding capacity of transferrin in an acidic environment; this also potentiates the risk for developing mucormycosis (197).

Clinical presentation. Mucormycosis of the head and neck is predominantly manifested as invasive rhinocerebral infection presenting with symptoms of sinusitis and periorbital cellulitis: eye or facial pain, numbness, nasal obstruction, bloody nasal discharge, blurry vision, and soft tissue swelling. Diabetics can present with sudden blindness due to optic nerve invasion (205,207). Granulocytopenic patients may develop rapid fulminant infection, while diabetics

can develop a more chronic invasive infection with a longer prodrome. Palatal and sinonasal mucosa initially appear normal, then become progressively erythematous, violaceous, then black and necrotic. The black necrotic intranasal or palatal eschar is highly suggestive of mucormycosis; it is seen in 40% of patients (205). Intraorbital or intracranial extension is a common and feared complication.

AIDS patients rarely develop mucormycosis, as their polymorphonuclear cell function is intact; when they do develop this infection, it is usually in the context of other associated risk factors such as diabetes or lymphoma (174,211). Mucormycosis has been occasionally documented in nondiabetic, nonimmunosuppressed patients; it has been suggested that chronic rhinosinusitis may be a predisposing factor for these individuals (212). Mucormycosis can rarely manifest as a sinus fungus ball (213,214).

Histopathology. The diagnosis is confirmed by tissue examination. Mucorales have broad hyphae (7–20 μm) with "floppy" twisting and folding. *Mucorales* hyphae have been likened to empty bent-cellophane tubes; they are basophilic on hematoxylin and eosin stain (Fig. 25). The outer hyphal walls are slightly refractile, with uneven thickness. Septations are absent or erratic, but hyphal folding may mimic septations. Hyphal branching forms variable angles ranging from 45° to 90° due to the general "floppiness" of the hyphae.

Vascular invasion and thrombotic infarction are characteristic of acute fulminant rhinocerebral mucormycosis. Surrounding tissue will reveal hemorrhage and necrosis. Fungal nerve invasion can occur and extend into the central nervous system (CNS). The

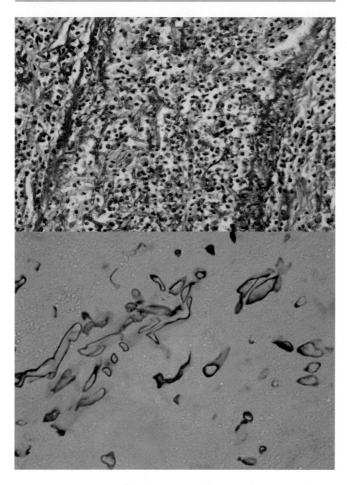

Figure 25 Mucormycosis. Upper panel: Wide pleomorphic branching hyphae are seen intravascularly on hematoxylin and eosin stain. Lower panel: Gomori methanamine silver stain reveals invasive, wide hyphae with sparse septations.

inflammation may contain rare multinucleated foreign body giant cells with ingested hyphal fragments. The round large sporangium of *Zygomycetes* is rarely observed within tissue sections (215,216). Mucormyces sporangia appear as simple large round conidiophores, and collapsed umbrella- or parachute-like conidiophores, filled with conidia.

A case of fatal culture confirmed *Saksenea vasoformis* invasive rhinocerebral zygomycoses has been described (217). At autopsy, the broad hyphae evoked a granulomatous inflammation.

Serology. No reliable serological PCR test exists and cultures may be negative; therefore empiric therapy is indicated before the diagnosis is established.

Treatment. The goals of treatment are: (*i*) debridement or resection of infected tissues, (*ii*) administration of systemic antifungal therapy, and (*iii*) correction of underlying hyperglycemia or neutropenia. Debridement or resection is necessary, as the avascular necrotic tissue cannot be penetrated by systemic antifungal agents. Amphotericin B is the first drug of choice.

Entomopthorales

Background and epidemiology. The *Entomophthorales* derive their name from the Greek word "entomon," meaning insect, reflecting their original identification as insect pathogens or parasites (219). Human pathogens in this order include *Basidiobolus ranarum*, *Conidiobolus coronatus*, and less commonly *Conidiobolus incongruous* (219). Entomophthorales have been isolated from plants, insects, and feces of frogs, lizards, and turtles (220–222). *Basidiobolus* has been isolated from the gastrointestinal tract of various reptiles and amphibians along the Southern Florida coast (220). Entomophthorales may cause chronic granulomatous rhinoentomophthoromycosis in immunocompetant hosts from tropical regions such as Central and West Africa, India, Caribbean Islands, and South America (223–225). Rhinoentomophthoromycosis in native-born Americans is uncommon (226).

Clinical course. Basidiobolomycoses predominantly manifest as subcutaneous infections; gastrointestinal infections are less common. Chronic invasive sinusitis is rarely caused by *Basidiobolus* (226). In contrast, conidiobolomycosis most commonly causes chronic invasive facial rhinocerebral infections. It begins with submucosal nasal expansile swelling and progresses to cause erosion, destruction, and deformity of the nasal and labial soft tissues (226–230). The rhinoceros-like mid-face expansion is similar to that which may be seen in advanced cases of rhinoscleroma (Fig. 26).

Histopathology. Chronic invasive rhinoentomophthoromycosis are granulomatous infections with foreign body giant cell reaction. Tissue invasion can be seen, but angioinvasion is not part of the disease process. *Basidiobolus* and *Conidiobolus* have septated pleomorphic wide thin-walled hyphae (4–10 μm) with less branching than the *Mucorales*. A Splendore–Hoeppli phenomenon is characteristic and is seen as a bright fringe-like, halo-like, or threadlike eosinophilic precipitate around fungal hyphae. This reaction is not specific for the *Entomophthorales*, and can also be seen with other organisms such as *Sporothrix*, and *Schistosoma* (Fig. 27).

Serology. Enzyme-linked immunosorbent assays (ELISAs) and immunodiffusion antibody assays to *Basidiobolus* and *Conidiobolus* have been developed but are not widely available (219,222).

Treatment. Itraconazole and potassium iodide are reasonable first-line antifungal choices (222,230).

Pseudoallescheriasis

Pseudoallescheriasis is a infection with *Pseudoallescheria boydii* (also historically referred to as *Allescheria boydii*, *Petriellidium boydii*, *Pseudallescheria sheari*, *and Monosporium apiospermum*), a fungus with thin, septated branching hyphae, intercalated swellings, and pear-shaped macroconidia.

Background and etiology. *P. boydii* is a ubiquitous filamentous fungus present in soil, decaying vegetation, polluted freshwater, sewage, swamps, waterlogged pastures, coastal tidelands, and livestock manure (231,232). *P. boydii* is a teleomorph (perfect

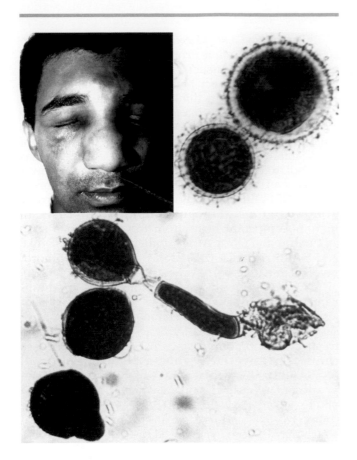

Figure 26 Rhinofacial Entomopthoromycosis: *Conidiobolus coronatus.* Upper left panel: Rhinoceros-like distension of nose. Upper right panel: Resting villose sporangiola. Lower panel: Globose primary sporangiola developing from sporangiophores. Note "beaks" (or basal papillae), which are the former points of attachment to the sporangiophores. The sporangiola discharge the spores. *Source*: Courtesy of Dr. Carlos da Silva Lacaz, Sao Paulo, Brazil.

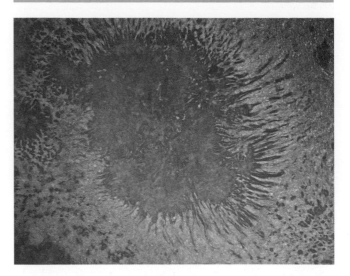

Figure 27 Splendore–Hoeppli phenomenon. Characteristic and is seen as a bright fringe-like, halo-like, or threadlike eosinophilic precipitate around fungal hyphae.

or sexual fungus); the genus *Scedosporium* represents the corresponding imperfect (anamorph, asexual) form with two pathogenic species: *Scedosporium apiospermum and Scedosporium prolificans*. Distinction between the perfect and imperfect forms can be accomplished only by studying the clinical isolates. *P. boydii* is an uncommon infectious agent with low pathogenicity in immunocompetent hosts; infection with *Scedosporium* is much rarer. Infection is acquired by inhalation or soft tissue trauma.

Clinical presentation. The vast majority of *P. boydii* infections present as posttraumatic subcutaneous mycetomas ("Madura foot") (233). *P. boydii* pneumonia can occur after freshwater aspiration in near-drowning incidents. Nosocomial pulmonary colonization can be seen in patients with underlying pulmonary disease (e.g., CF) or immunosuppression (231,234). *P. boydii* can cause deep systemic infection after trauma or surgery, usually in immunosuppressed individuals (AIDS, leukemia, organ transplant, diabetes, steroid therapy); this may manifest

as osteomyelitis, septic arthritis, myocarditis, endocarditis, and CNS infection (235).

In the head and neck, *P. boydii* may cause sinusitis in both immunocompromised and immunocompetent patients (236–243). Bates recently compiled 26 cases of *P. boydii* sinusitis from the literature (236). Immunosuppressed patients with *P. boydii* sinusitis were more likely to demonstrate tissue invasion and develop fatal infection. *P. boydii* has also been involved in parotitis and otomycosis (244).

Histopathology. Both *Pseudallescheria* and *Scedosporium* form acutely branching, slender, septated hyphae with parallel cell walls. Tissue invasion and vascular invasion may be seen. Unless conidia are present, *Pseudallescheria/Scedosporium* cannot reliably be distinguished from *Aspergillus*. Hyphal intercalary swellings (intercalary chlamydoconidia) and abundant large, irregularly shaped ovoid and pear-shaped chlamydoconidia (15–20 µm) (Greek: chlamydo—cloak or envelope) are specific for *Pseudallescheria/Scedosporium*. Chlamydoconidia are asexually produced spores that can be formed in tissues by both *Pseudallescheria* and *Scedosporium* under appropriate conditions. They are unicellular, round to pyriform, and gold to brown colored. Characteristic tissue chlamydoconidia plus thin septated hyphae allow for the preliminary histological diagnosis of pseudallescheriasis.

Pseudallescheria is distinguished from *Scedosporium* by examining the cultured isolate. When cultured on appropriate media (cornmeal agar or potato dextrose agar), *P. boydii* should form the organs of sexual reproduction, cleistothecia, which are golden to dark brown fruiting bodies (completely closed ascocarps). Clinical isolates that do not demonstrate a sexual state are designated *Scedosporium* spp.

Treatment. *Pseudallescheria* and *Scedosporium* are resistant to amphotericin B; voriconazole is an appropriate first-line drug (245).

Phaeohyphomycosis

Subcutaneous or deep tissue fungal infection caused by the family of pigmented saprophytic fungi (family Dematiaceae, phylum Deuteromycota). In the head and neck, the demateaceous fungi are associated with noninvasive and invasive sinonasal fungal disease.

Background and etiology. The demateaceous fungi (black molds) are distributed worldwide and found in soil, wood, plants, and water. This group contains over 60 genera of human pathogens including *Alternaria, Curvularia, Bipolaris, Cladosporium, Exserohilum, Exophiala,* and *Wangiella.* One feature common to the demateaceous fungi is the presence of melanin in the cell wall, which enhances fungal virulence by scavenging free radicals and hypochlorite produced by phagocytic cells during their oxidative burst (246).

Typically, demateaceous fungi are of low virulence. Localized, subcutaneous infection (chromomycoses) may occur in immunocompetent individuals after penetrating injury. Invasive infection may occur in immunocompromised patients (AIDS, bone marrow or solid organ transplants, diabetes, chronic granulomatous disease, renal failure with peritoneal dialysis and steroids), especially those with indwelling catheters (247). A nosocomial outbreak of demateaceous fungemia was traced to a deionized water source used in the preparation of a prevenipuncture skin disinfectant (248).

Clinical features. Subcutaneous phaeohyphomycosis usually appear as erythematous nodules or plaques. Noncutaneous phaeohyphomycosis may present as sinusitis, bronchopneumonia, CNS infection, ocular disease, prosthetic valve endocarditis, arthritis, osteomyelitis, fungemia, endocarditis, peritonitis, and gastrointestinal disease. The demateaceous fungi can precipitate allergic sinusitis (see below) and asthma. The presence of *Alternaria* in the drip pan unit of an air conditioner was associated with the development of asthma, which was reversed after the allergen was removed (249).

The spectrum of demateaceous paranasal sinus disease includes acute fulminant sinusitis, chronic invasive sinusitis, and AFS (Fig. 28). Previous intranasal steroids (250,251) and aquatic exposure (250,252) have been associated with demateaceous sinus disease. Of interest, one patient with presumed phaeohyphomycosis sinusitis had come into close physical contact with a patient with *Drechslera osteomyelitis,* suggesting rare person-to-person contagion (253).

The gross appearance of material encountered during surgery has been described as "muddy," "cheesy," "hamburger-like," "greasy," "sticky," "putty-like," "fecal-like," and "peanut butter–like."

Histopathology. The inflammatory response is composed of lymphocytes, eosinophils, and plasma cells; occasionally a granulomatous reaction is present. In demateaceous allergic sinusitis, allergic mucin can be seen, with sparse hyphae. Tissue invasion by demateaceous fungi may occur in immunocompromised patients. Demateaceous fungal hyphae are pleomorphic and irregular, and they are wider than *Aspergillus* and thinner than *Zygomycetes.* Their distinctive brown

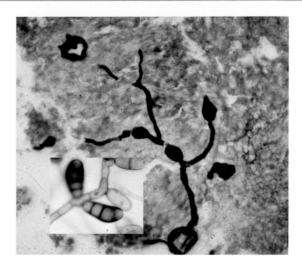

Figure 28 Allergic fungal sinusitis. These thin septated hyphal fragments reveal occasional tear-shaped macroconidia, reminiscent of Curvularia. Cultures confirmed Curvularia (Gomori methenamine silver). Inset: Macroconidia of Curvularia in culture.

pigment may be seen in unstained and hematoxylin and eosin-stained slides. Fontana Masson can stain the demateaceous fungi, although longer staining times may be required (246). The fungi do not sporulate during infections; therefore the distinctions in conidial morphology and conidial germination are seen only in laboratory cultures preparations (Figs. 29, 30).

Treatment. Noninvasive demateaceous sinus disease may be treated by FESS; adjuvant therapy such as intranasal steroids and immunotherapy are recommended for AFS. Fulminant-invasive demateaceous sinus infection requires rapid intervention with surgical debridement and systemic antifungal therapy; itraconazole and voriconazole are first-line drugs of choice (246).

Bipolaris and Exserohilum

Infections previously classified as *Drechslera* are grouped as *Bipolaris* (254). *Bipolaris/Drechslera* and *Exserohilum* have taxonomic similarities on the basis of spore morphology and patterns of germination. *Bipolaris* and *Exserohilum* can cause the full spectrum of invasive and noninvasive fungal sinus disease in both immunocompetent and immunocompromised individuals (255–261).

Culture morphology will reveal that the conidiophores, which directly bear conidia, are geniculate (genu—knee), with a zigzag, or "bent-knee" appearance. The "genu" is a site of conidial attachment (254). The site of germ tube formation in the germinating macroconidia is useful in discriminating these fungi. *Bipolaris* macroconidia are fusoid and germinate from the terminal ends (polar germination, hence bipolar). *Exserohilum* macroconidia may be quite long and usually have polar germination, but may have amphigenous

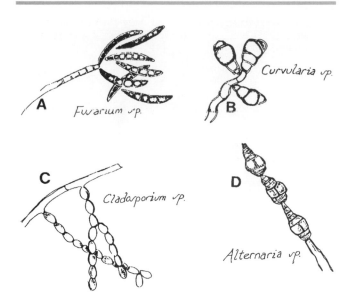

Figure 29 Demateaceous fungi: Conidial morphology. (**A**) Long, slightly curved banana-shaped tapered macroconidia of *Fusarium sp.* (**B**). *Curvularia sp.* macroconidia are straight to slightly curved., with three to four septae, depending on species. (**C**) *Cladosporium sp.* with branching chain of smooth conidia. (**D**) *Alternaria sp.* produces conidial chains with rounded ends and pointed apices. Horizontal septations alternate with vertical ones.

germination. They are distinguished by the "bent" terminal germ tubes, which emerge from the lateral side of the terminal cell. Their conidial hilum (point of attachment with the conidiophore) has a pronounced distinctive protrusion.

Curvularia

Curvularia can cause the full spectrum of invasive and noninvasive fungal sinus disease in both immunocompetent and immunocompromised individuals (262–265). Hyphal fragments may be regular and septated or pleomorphic and pigmented. Acutely

branching, thin, septated hyphae have been illustrated, with pleomorphism reminiscent of, but thinner than, Mucorales. The macroconidia of *Curvularia lunata* have three septa and four cells. They can be distinguished from *Bipolaris* and *Exserohilum* as follows: in the mature macroconidia, the second cell from the tip (opposite the hilar attachment) has a thicker darker wall. This second cell swells, causing the characteristic bend (curve) of the genera.

Alternaria

Alternaria is a saprophyte present in various vegetables and grains (266). It produces a mycotoxin fatal to laboratory animals at high doses (267). Alternaria causes AFS and invasive sinus infection in both immunosuppressed and immunocompetent individuals (268–273). One patient pitched hay in Florida for many years, which suggests long-term exposure to *Alternaria* (271). *Alternaria* was the leading cultured pathogen causing AFS (24.3%) in a series of 37 patients from the Mayo clinic (273). A number of healthy patients have been reported with chronic allergic sinusitis that progressed to chronic invasive infection with fistulae formation of the hard palate (269–271).

Histologically, a granulomatous reaction with hyphal fragments within foreign body giant cells can be seen. The hyphae have "parallel" walls (i.e., nonpleomorphic) and are septated with rare branching. A beaded appearance of hyphal fragments is observed reflecting *Alternaria's* ability to produce conidial chains (sympodial growth). The macroconidia are pointed at one end and rounded at the other end. The septations are seen to alternate horizontally and longitudinally (hence *Alternaria*). The sympodial growth of the macroconidia can be likened to a chain of hand grenades.

Cladosporium

Cladosporium is one of the most common fungi isolated from nasal mucus of healthy volunteers (274). It has been implicated as a trigger of AFS (275), and is a rare cause of invasive fungal sinusitis (276,277). Cladosporium hyphae are pigmented, relatively thin, with

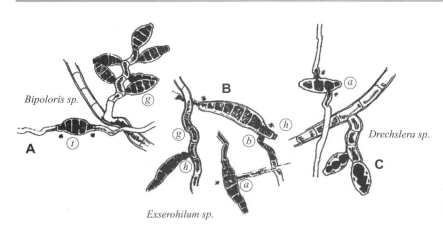

Exserohilum sp.

Figure 30 Demateaceous fungi: Conidial morphology. The macroconidial morphology and patterns of germination (*) aid in distinguishing among the demateaceous fungi. Note the geniculate conidiophore (*g*). (**A**) *Bipolaris sp.* macroconidia in general have three to five septations and germinate from terminal ends. (*t*). (**B**) *Exserohilum sp.* with long macroconidia. The conidial hilum (*h*) has a pronounced protrusion. Polar germinations have a "bend" (*b*) and may emerge from the lateral side of the terminal cell. Amphigenous germination also may be seen. (**C**) *Drechslera sp.* macroconidia are cylindrical, without a prominent hilum and have amphigenous germination (*a*). *Drechslera biseptata* has two to three septae.

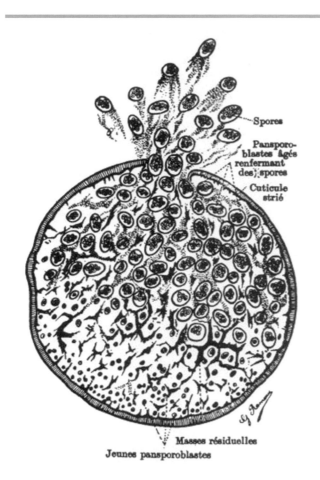

Figure 31 Rhinosporidiosis. Release of spores from mature spherule. *Source*: From Ref. 278.

frequent branching. The conidia of *Cladosporium* are nonseptated, and thus distinguished from the macroconidia of other demateaceous fungi. The conidia grow in long delicate chains, as does *Alternaria* macroconidia, but the morphology of these two fungal conidia are sufficiently distinctive.

Hyalohyphomycosis

Hyalohyphomycosis is an infection by Hyphomycetes (family Moniliaceae, phylum Deuteromycota) fungi, which are glassy (hyaline), uncolored, or lightly colored in culture. Candida is a hyphomycete, a commensural organism and a pathogen. Other saprophytic fungi such as Fusarium are opportunistic human pathogens.

Fusarium. Fusarium is a pathogen of flowers, fruits, vegetables, and grains, widely dispersed in the environment. It produces potent mycotoxin (T2 and others), which contaminate cereals and grains. Fusariosis occurs most often among compromised hosts (bone marrow and solid organ transplant recipients, burn patients, neutropenic patients, diabetics) (279–281). *Fusarium* may be an uncommon cause of invasive sinonasal infection (276,282,283). Fusarium hyphae are

uniform, 2 to 7 μm wide, and septated, with acutely angled branching, similar to *Aspergillus*. However, *Fusarium* has twisted and ribbonlike hyphae with constrictions at hyphal branch points, distinguishing it from *Aspergillus* and *Zygomycetes*. *Fusarium* produced colorless microconidia and characteristic macroconidia. The latter have four to six cells, with tapering at either end; they resemble septated bananas.

Candidiasis. Candidiasis is an infection by *Candida albicans*, a common commensural imperfect fungus with yeast forms (2–4 μm), which forms pseudohyphae.

Candida will be discussed in more detail in section III.B.1 Candida is a rare cause of sinusitis and invasive sinonasal disease in cancer patients, AIDS patients, and immunocompetant patients (284–286).

Sporotrichosis

This is an uncommon infection in the United States caused by *Sporothrix schenkii*, a dimorphic fungus, which appears in tissue as small budding yeasts, with typical elongated cigar or football-shaped forms up to 10 μm in diameter.

Background and etiology. Sporotrichosis is most often seen in tropical and subtropical regions. It is caused by *S. schenkii*, which is ubiquitous with a worldwide distribution. *S. schenkii* has been isolated from soil, wood, plant thorns, and grains and is commonly recovered from cats, rodents, and armadillos (287). Sporotrichosis is usually acquired after inoculation from environmental sources (thorns, splinters, sphagnum moss, or infected grasses) or zoonotic transmission (bites by animals or birds, insect stings). Occupations such as horticulture, gardening, beekeeping, carpentry, agriculture, animal husbandry, and veterinary practice have been associated with Sporotrichosis (287,288).

Clinical. Sporotrichosis most commonly presents as cutaneous and subcutaneous infection, which can extend to regional lymph nodes; the extremities are most often involved. In the head and neck, facial skin is the most common site of involvement (8%) (288). The oral mucosa may be involved (0.3%) either as the primary disease manifestation or in the setting of systemic infection (289). Sinonasal and laryngeal sporotrichosis have been reported, albeit very rarely (290–294).

Histology. The inflammatory response is usually granulomatous and can be necrotizing. Epithelial hyperplasia may be present. Yeast-like fungal elements are very commonly observed in confirmed cases of sporotrichosis (89%) (288). *S. schenkii* yeasts are globose, cigar-, or spindle-shaped, approximately 10 μm in length. They are not visible on hematoxylin and eosin–stained sections but can be seen on periodic acid–Schiff or Gomori methanamine silver stain. Single budding with a narrow isthmus can be seen, similar to *Cryptococcus* budding. Production of short hyphae within infected tissue has been occasionally observed (295,296). These hyphae aggregate around hair follicles or in the lower dermis are nonseptate and infrequently branch. "Asteroid"-like bodies may be seen in immunocompetent hosts (Splendore–Hoeppli

Table 2 Comparative Histomorphology of Fungal Yeast Forms

Organism	Size (microns)	Shape	Staining characteristics
Blastomyces	6–15	Round to oval, wide-necked budding protoplasmic retraction	GMS: + (positive) entire organism PAS: + capsule Mucin: weak or negative
Coccicidiodomyces	80	Round endospores 2–5 μm	H&E: entire organism Mucin: − (negative)
Cryptococcus	4–10	Round to oval, thin-necked budding	H&E: only nucleus PAS/DPAS: + capsule Mucin: + strong GMS: + entire organism
Histoplasma	2–5	Round, thin-necked budding	H&E: intranuclear, Prominent retraction halo GMS: + entire organism
Myospherulosis	Up to 120	Cysts, no budding	H&E: "battered" RBCs Hgb: +, GMS/iron: − Mucicarmine/PAS: −
Paracoccidioidomyces	4–20	Round to oval, "ship's wheel" budding	H&E: retraction artifact GMS, PAS: entire organism+
Pneumocystis	4–7	"boat" shaped	H&E: only nuclei GMS: + entire organism
Sporothrix	to 10	Football shaped, thin-necked budding	Splendore–Hoeppli GMS: + entire organism
Torulopsis	to 5	Round, oval, thin necked	H&E, PAS, GMS: + entire organism
Rhinosporidium	to 300 round	2–5 endospores	PAS/DPAS: + Mucin capsule GMS: capsule and endospores +

Abbreviations: H&E, hematoxylin and eosin; GMS, Gomori methenamine silver; PAS, periodic acid–Schiff; D-PAS, digested periodic acid–Schiff.

phenomenon), which appear as eosinophilic needle-like rays emanating from the fungal spores. These asteroid bodies are usually seen within microabscesses (297).

The differential diagnosis includes *Cryptococcus neoformans*; collapsed *Cryptococcal* yeasts can have a cigar-shaped silhouette. One reliable point of distinction is the thick double-walled mucinophilic polysaccharide capsule of *Cryptococcus*, which is not seen in *Sporothrix*. The differential diagnosis of also includes *Candida glabrata* and *Blastomyces dermatitidis* can also be included in the differential diagnosis (see below). Table 2 summarizes the comparative features of tissue fungal yeast forms.

Culture and skin testing. Confirmation is obtained by culture identification. The sporotrichin skin test may be useful. Serological testing for sporotrichosis is available, but of variable sensitivity and specificity.

Treatment. Itraconazole is the drug of choice, with high cure rates and less toxicity than is seen with amphotericin B. Saturated solution of potassium iodide is also effective and cheap (287).

Cryptococcosis

This is infection by *C. neoformans*, round to oval yeasts, 4 to 10 μm, with narrow-necked budding and a thick mucinophilic capsule that is usually self-limited and localized in immunocompetant individuals, and disseminated and potentially fatal in immunosuppressed individuals.

Cryptococcus is an extremely rare cause of sinusitis; cryptococcal pansinusitis has been reported in an AIDS patient with cryptococcal meningitis (298). It is also a rare cause of sinusitis in immunocompetent patients (299,300). Cryptococcosis will be discussed in detail in section III.B.5 in the context of laryngeal infections.

Blastomycosis

This is infection caused by *Blastomyces dermatitides*, spherical dimorphous yeast, 6 to 15 μm, which forms single broad-necked budding structures.

B. dermatitides may be a cause of sinusitis, usually concomitant with pulmonary disease (301,302).

Rhinosporidiosis

This is infection by *Rhinosporidium seeberi*—a mesomycetozoea, a new class phylogenetically at the animal-fungal divergence in the evolutionary tree. *Rhinosporidium* forms very large spherules (300 μm) containing hundreds of endospores (Fig. 32) (278).

Background and epidemiology. *R. seeberi* is present worldwide, and is endemic to India, Sri Lanka, Malaysia, Brazil, and Argentina. In the United States, cases have been reported from the rural south and west (303–305). Mucosal trauma (e.g., by digital contamination, dust storms) is considered necessary in establishing infection. For example, the proclivity of rhinosporidiosis to affect the lower nasal septum was thought to be due to digital trauma. For Muslims, "the habit of removing the last drops of urine following micturition by cleaning the penile meatus with a stone may have predisposed them to contamination causing (urethral) infection" (306). Men and animals bathing together in stagnant waters have been associated with many cases (307).

The nature of etiological agent of Rhinosporidiosis has long been elusive (308) (Fig. 31). Originally it was considered a fungus, and more recently, blue-green algae. However, recent molecular genetic investigations have lead to the reclassification of Rhinosporidium as a Mesomycetozoea, a novel clade that is phylogenetically at the animal-fungal divergence in the evolutionary tree (309,310).

Clinical presentation. Patients infected with rhinosporidiosis generally are healthy. Rhinosporidium most commonly infects the conjunctiva and nasal cavity, causing friable lobulated red-pink polyps. Other upper respiratory sites, such as larynx, and genitourinary sites, may also be involved. (307). Nasal and urethral infections have a male predominance; a female predominance is seen in conjunctival infections. Subcutaneous infections as well as disseminated rhinosporidiosis are rare (306,311,312). One patient with disseminated disease was a grave digger and street sweeper, suggesting soil-related inoculation (311).

Histopathology. Rhinosporidiosis is invariably accompanied by an intense acute inflammatory and lymphoplasmacytic infiltrate. The cysts (spherules or sporangia) are numerous, round, large (300 μm), and thick walled (Fig. 32). The cyst wall is birefringent, and stains with hematoxylin and eosin, Gomori methanamine silver, digested-periodic acid–Schiff, and mucicarmine. The largest, most mature cysts are closest to the mucosal surface. Hundreds to thousands of small (2–9 μm) spores (endospores) are seen within mature cysts. The spores are initially uninuclear, but mature to form clusters of 12 to 16 "naked nuclei" (endospores or sporozoites). Mitotic figures are infrequently observed within these spores (313). The cysts extrude the "spore morulas" into the surrounding tissue from a pore. In cases of disseminated rhinosporidiosis, single spores may be present in body fluids such as urine (Fig. 33).

The differential diagnosis includes *Coccidioides immitis*. In fact, Seeber initially believed that *Rhinosporidium* was related to *C. immitis*; but its spherules are not as large (60 μm); its walls are not as thick, birefringent, or mucinophilic; and its endospores are not as numerous.

Treatment. Rhinosporidiosis is treated by surgical removal. Anecdotally, dapsone treatment has also been reported (314).

Myospherulosis

An inflammatory, noninfectious condition caused by exogenous or endogenous lipids that react with erythrocytes to form "spherules" - the histological hallmark of this condition.

Background. Myospherulosis is a condition resulting from the interaction of erythrocytes with petroleum, lanolin, or traumatized adipose tissue (315–317). It was originally described as the development of painful soft tissue masses in Africans (315). Histologically, this condition was marked by a "Swiss cheese" pattern of cysts with "bags of spherules" likened to bags of marbles, hence the name

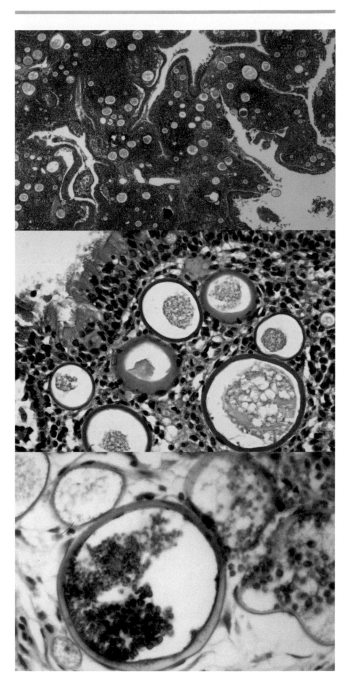

Figure 32 Rhinosporidiosis. Upper panel: Multiple spherules and intense lymphoplasmacytic reaction. Middle panel: The spherules can be as large as 300 μm. Lower panel: Note the thick wall of the mature spherules, which are filled with innumerable spores, approximately 6 to 7 μm in size.

myospherulosis or intramuscular spherules. It was postulated that injection of foreign material for scarification may have contributed to this process. Subsequently, other patients were reported with persistent sinusitis, pain, and swelling after Caldwell-Luc maxillotomy; the use of petroleum-based tetracycline impregnated packing was a common feature in these cases (316).

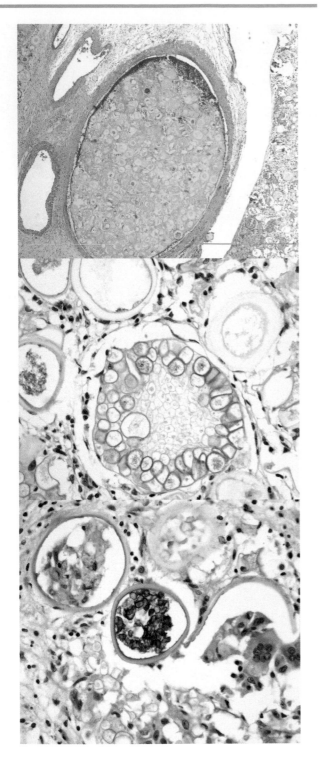

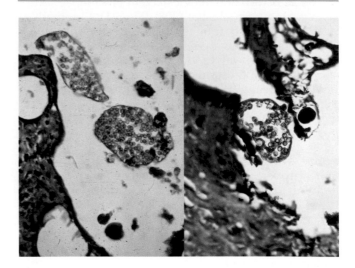

Figure 34 Myospherulosis. Left panel: "Encapsulated" erythrocytes mimic fungi or prototheca, hematoxylin and eosin stain. Right panel: Hemoglobin stain confirms their true nature. *Source*: Courtesy of Dr. Juan Rosai.

Figure 33 Disseminated, fatal rhinosporiodiosis in a grave digger. Upper panel: Low-power view of endovascular embolus of rhinosporodiosis. Middle and lower panel: Higher power views of spherules in different states of maturation (hematoxylin and eosin). *Source*: Courtesy of Dr. HM Sian, Singapore.

Etiology. The spherules were originally thought to be fungi, algae, or pollen. Rosai demonstrated that these puzzling spherules were actually red blood cells (RBCs) (317). The use of lipid-based sinus packing (bacitracin-zinc, hydrocortisone, and neomycin-polymyxin ointment) is associated with development of sinonasal myospherulosis (318). Other causes of myospherulosis include infection, such as coexistent mycetoma (319) and traumatic fat necrosis. Rarely, sinonasal myospherulosis may occur spontaneously (320).

Histology. The characteristic appearance is of numerous pseudocysts with a Swiss cheese appearance. Within these spaces, large (100 μm) saclike structures ("parent bodies") are present delineated by thin, nonrefractile membranes. These sacs contain numerous spherules; 5 to 7 μm in size, their appearance are likened to "bags of marbles." The spherules are brown, misshapen erythrocytes. Okajima's hemoglobin stain confirms their nature as erythrocytes. Gomori methanamine silver, iron stain, and periodic acid–Schiff stains are negative (Fig. 34).

Differential diagnosis. Failure to recognize the noninfectious nature of myospherulosis may lead to unwarranted therapy. The spherules may mimic *Coccidioidomyces* and *Rhinosporidium*. The saccule membranes of myospherulosis are approximately 1 μm in thickness, not like the thicker, double-walled, birefringent capsules of *Coccidioidomyces* and *Rhinosporidium*, which both stain with Gomori methanamine silver. Negative periodic acid–Schiff stain rules out cellulose (chitin) and inhaled pollen.

Treatment and clinical implications. The development of myospherulosis requires surgical debridement to establish the diagnosis and treat the condition. Patients developing myo spherulosis following sinonasal surgery are more likely to develop sinonasal adhesions requiring revision surgery. It is reasonable to avoid lipid-based ointments after sinus surgery, and opt for water-soluble antibiotic lubricants (318).

B. Oral and Laryngeal Fungal Disease

Candidiasis

Clinical. Oral candidiasis (OC) (thrush) can be classified as either primary or secondary; the latter can be due to a number of common or rare immunodeficiency conditions (Table 3). Primary OC usually affects adults who often have some predisposing condition such as diabetes, dentures, decreased saliva due to radiation or Sjogren's syndrome or use of steroid inhalants or tobacco (321,322) (Fig. 35). Newborn thrush is common in the first months of life and related to perinatal exposure or concomitant diaper rash. Childhood thrush can be seen with chronic use of steroid inhalants for asthma.

The chief complaints for oral thrush are burning and pain; the most commonly affected sites are buccal commissure, buccal mucosa, palate, and tongue. Examination reveals mucosal ulceration and pseudomembrane with a white creamy or milk curd–like exudate. Stripping the membrane leaves a raw bleeding surface.

Laryngeal candidiasis may be due to local factors, such as steroid inhalants (323) or prior radiation, or caused by systemic immunosuppression such as neutropenia or AIDS (324–327). Patients with laryngeal candidiasis present with hoarseness, dysphagia, and odynophagia.

Chronic hyperplastic candidiasis refers to an intraoral leukoplakia caused by superficially invasive *Candida* infection. It may appear either homogeneous or nodular (speckled erythroleukoplakia) and is seen most on the buccal mucosa, followed by palate, and tongue. Nodular lesions can cause soreness or discomfort, whereas homogenous lesions are usually asymptomatic (321). They are often seen together with other Candida lesions such as angular cheilitis, denture stomatitis, or median rhomboid glossitis.

Histopathology. The infected mucosa is usually acutely inflamed, but sometimes inflammation is minimal. Candida pseudohyphae can be seen with either

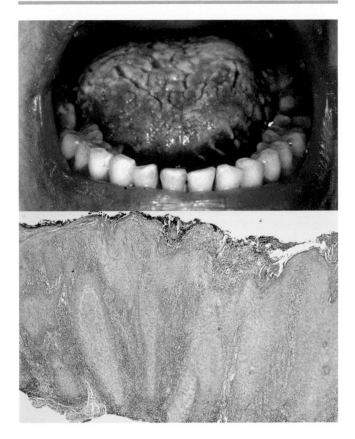

Figure 35 Oral Candida. Upper panel: Thick curd-like exudate in a leukemic patient. Lower panel: Chronic hyperplastic Candidiasis (hematoxylin and eosin stain). The presence of hyperplasia, and inflammation, should prompt the ordering of fungal special stains. However, oral Candida may also be associated with minimal inflammation. Therefore we recommend that pathologists be liberal in ordering fungal stains. *Source*: Courtesy of Dr. Marie Ramer DDS, Mount Sinai, New York, U.S.A.

Table 3 Classification of Oral Candidosis

Primary oral candidosis	Secondary oral candidosis
The "Primary Triad"	Familial chronic mucocutaneous candidosis
Pseudomembranous (acute)	Diffuse chronic mucocutaneous candidosis
Erythematous (acute and chronic)	Candidosis endocrinopathy syndrome
Hyperplastic (chronic)	Familial mucocutaneous candidosis
Plaque-like	Severe combined immunedeficiency
Nodular/speckled	DiGeorge syndrome
Other candida-associated lesions	Chronic granulomatous disease
Denture stomatitis	AIDS
Angular cheilitis	
Median rhomboid glossitis	
Linear gingival erythema	

Source: From Ref. 321.

periodic acid–Schiff or Gomori methanamine silver stains superficially invading mucosa (Fig. 36). Candida invasion always stops short of penetrating the junction between the parakeratotic layer and the stratum spinosum. The pseudohyphae are thin, regular, and "pinched" at the point of pseudoseptation. True branching is not seen. Small, oval, globose yeast cells are abundant, imparting a "spaghetti and meatballs" appearance.

Chronic hyperplastic candidiasis. The squamous mucosa is hyperplastic; homogenous leukoplakia may be either orthokeratotic or parakeratotic (Fig. 35). Nodular leukoplakia may demonstrate variable mucosal thickness; parakeratosis is common. Acute inflammation and microabscesses are seen. Epithelial dysplasia is generally absent in homogenous leukoplakia and is more common in nodular leukoplakias. In some cases, hyphae can be quite sparse and seen after a considerable search.

Mechanism. What are the mechanisms that allow this very common commensural organism to become an invasive pathogen? *C. albicans* and

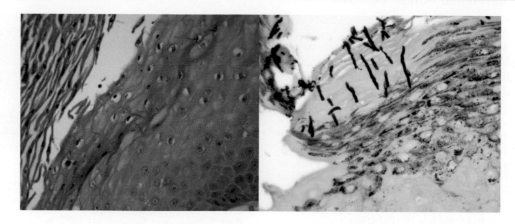

Figure 36 Oral Candida (high power). Left panel: Superficially invasive oral Candida (hematoxylin and eosin stain). Right panel: *Candida pseudohyphae*, Gomori methanamine silver stain.

C. glabrata are capable of a phenomenon known as "switching," which allows them to alter phenotype and other factors, thus evading host immune mechanisms. Switching may augment *Candida's* ability for adhesion and superficial invasion. *C. glabrata* has a greater ability to adhere to denture surfaces than *C. albicans* (328). Candida proteinases function optimally at acidic pH and are further responsible for virulence (321). The mechanism predisposing some diabetics to develop OC is not clear; however increased glucose concentration in saliva and continuous denture wearing are probably important contributing factors (329).

Treatment. Predisposing conditions should be addressed, i.e., smoking, poor denture hygiene, sleeping with dentures. Topical fluconozole is the first-line treatment of OC. The treatment for Candida laryngitis is standard systemic antifungal therapy (amphotericin B). Chronic hyperplastic candidiasis may be conservatively treated by laser excision.

Coccidioidomycosis

This is infection by *Coccidioides,* yeasts that produce large spherules (80 μm) filled with endospores 2 to 5 μm. Infection may be subclinical, cause minor flu-like symptoms, or result in serious pneumonia and disseminated disease.

Background and epidemiology. *C. immitis* is endemic in the Southwestern United States (southern Texas, New Mexico, Arizona, and California) and in Northern Mexico as well as Central America (Guatemala and Honduras) and South America (Venezuela and Argentina) (330). An estimated 150,000 cases of coccidioidomycosis (San Joaquin Valley fever or valley fever, desert rheumatism, the bumps) occur in the United States annually; approximately 60% of cases occur in Arizona (331). In endemic areas, it is said to be as common as chicken pox (332). About 20% of annually reported cases are diagnosed outside endemic areas, thus widening the relevancy of this organism (333).

Coccidioides endospores are released into the environment and germinate to form hyphae, which bear barrel-shaped, infectious arthrospores. Cool, moist weather and alkaline soil (which inhibits competing organisms) are conditions favoring germination. There is seasonal variation in the rate of skin-test conversion; the higher rate of infection is seen at the end of summer (333).

Professions involved in soil disrupting activities in endemic areas (e.g., archeological, construction, or agricultural workers) increase risk of infection (Fig. 37). Point source epidemics have been related to archeological digs; especially Native American sites in the western United States, even outside recognized endemic regions. Sifting of dirt during archeological activities can result in particularly high exposure risk (333–336). On another note, there are over 350,000 individuals in the United States military stationed in endemic areas, and the infection rate has been increasing in this population. Thus coccidioidomycosis is also an emerging threat to the health and readiness of our military personnel (337).

Coccidioides is extraordinarily infectious: 10 arthroconidia will cause infection in animals (338). Handling laboratory Petri dishes and glassware have caused disease. Direct human-to-human transmission usually does not occur; endospores are not infectious but must first germinate to yield the infectious arthrospores. Several hospital staff has developed infections after removing a plaster cast from a patient with an osteomyelitis caused by *Coccidioides* (339). It was postulated that the dressing under the cast had supported the growth of the mycelial phase, which bore infectious arthrospores. Infectious arthrospores have also been exported by the shipping of Indian artifacts wrapped in a dusty packing materials (340) and agricultural products (341) and have also been found in San Joaquin Valley cotton (342).

Clinical course. Infection manifestation can range from subclinical to disseminated and lethal, depending on the dose exposure and host factors such as immune status, nationality, and pregnancy.

illness or self-limited pneumonia. Persistent lung infection may result in cavitary lesions.

Disseminated infection. Disseminated disease develops in about 0.5% of individuals. African Americans and Filipinos are 175 and 10 times more likely to develop disseminated disease, respectively, than Caucasians, probably due to differences in cell-mediated immunity (344). Immunocompromise (HIV infection, diabetes), late trimester pregnancy, and age extremes (very young and elderly) are conditions associated with greater rates of clinical infection and disseminated disease. Disseminated infection can involve meninges, bones, joints, soft tissues, and skin (345). Skin lesions commonly affect the face and form papules, pustules, or suppurative, necrotic, granulomatous, verrucous, or nodular lesions. AIDS patients may have initial presentations indistinguishable from the immunocompetent, e.g., pulmonary infiltrates or erythematous skin lesions. Alternatively, they may present with disseminated coccidioidomycosis and involvement of atypical sites such as lymph node, liver, or brain (346,347). Disseminated or extrapulmonary coccidioidomycosis is an AIDS-defining illness.

Laryngeal coccidioidomycosis and other head and neck manifestations. Laryngotracheal coccidioidomycosis may occur with or without concurrent pulmonary disease (348,349). Patients present with hoarseness and stridor and may progress to upper airway obstruction. The larynx and trachea have edematous, erythematous polypoid type tissue. Other head and neck sites include skin and subcutis of the scalp and neck, lymph nodes, tonsil, retropharynx, and tongue (333,350). Temporal bone involvement can result in otitis media, ossicular destruction, mastoiditis, facial nerve paralysis, and subperiosteal abscess formation (345).

Etiology. C. immitis is the major disease pathogen and found mainly in the central valley of California. More recently, C. posadasii, another pathogen, has been identified; it is found mainly in Nevada, Utah, Texas, New Mexico, Arizona, Northern Mexico, and in endemic areas of South America (351).

Histopathology. Coccidioidomyces evokes granulomatous reaction with foreign body–type giant cells; inflammation may be accompanied by tissue eosinophilia (Spendore–Hoeppli phenomenon) (Fig. b37). The fungal spherules are large, ranging from 30 to 80 μm. The spherule capsule is thick and the internal and external limits give it a double-walled appearance, but it is not as thick or bilaminated as is Rhinosporidium. The capsule is best stained by Gomori methanamine silver stain, but it can also be seen on hematoxylin and eosin, Giemsa and Papanicolau stains. Spherules containing endospores are diagnostic; occasionally mycelia may be present at the periphery of pulmonary cavitary lesions or skin lesions (352). C. immitis and C. posadasii are indistinguishable, but this is of no clinical significance as they have identical susceptibilities to antifungal agents (351).

When Coccidioidomyces endospores (2–5 μm) are released from spherules, they may be confused with other yeasts mimicking *Histoplasma, Cryptococcus,* or *Candida*. Small immature spherules may mimic

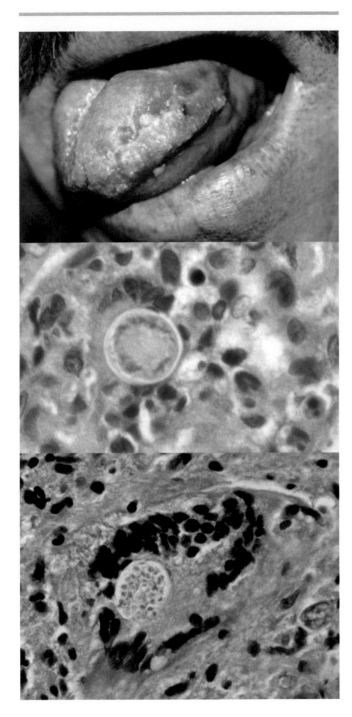

Figure 37 Coccidioidomycosis. Upper panel: Mexican farm worker with ulcerating tongue lesion (350). Middle and Lower panels: Granulomatous reaction with multinucleated giant cells containing large thick-walled spherules. Coccidioidomyces ranges in size up to 80 μm; the refractile cell wall ranges from 2 to 4 μm (hematoxylin and eosin stain). *Source*: Courtesy of Dr. Raphael Rodriquez (upper panel).

About 60% of infected individuals are asymptomatic, 25% develop arthralgias, fever, and rash (343). Skin lesions vary from maculo-papular eruption to erythema multiforme. Pulmonary disease can develop in 40% of individuals and may manifest as a flu-like

Blastomyces. The differential diagnosis includes *Rhinosporidium,* which has larger spherules (350 μm). The capsule of *Rhinosporidium* stains with mucicarmine stain, while that of *Coccidioidomyces* does not.

Serological identification and PCR. Acute serum antibodies and a newly converted skin reaction to coccidioidin antigen may be helpful diagnostic adjuncts. The serological diagnosis of coccidioidomycosis is confirmed by detecting IgM and IgG antibodies directed against the organism. False-negative tests can occur early in the infection and in anergic patients with disseminated disease. Serological testing by multiple modalities (enzyme-linked immunoassay, immunodiffusion, complement fixation) is recommended for immunocompromised patients with suspected coccidioidomycosis (343). Nested PCR assays have been developed, which can confirm the presence of *Coccidioidomyces* in formalin-fixed paraffin-embedded tissues (351,353).

Treatment. Patients with uncomplicated primary coccidioidomycosis may be observed; there are no prospective randomized clinical trials to address the issue as to whether these patients might benefit from oral azole therapy (354). African-Americans, Filipinos, HIV/AIDS patients, and diabetics warrant more aggressive treatment with fluconozole, as they are at risk for disseminated infection. Amphotericin B is the drug of choice for third-trimester pregnant women, as they are also at-risk for disseminated infection. Patients with more advanced disease require either IV amphotericin or high-dose azole therapy with or without intrathecal amphotericin (354).

Paracoccidioidomycosis

This is an infection by *Paracoccidioides brasiliensis,* a dimorphic fungus. The yeasts are spherical, 4 to 20 μm in diameter, with multiple budding daughter yeasts producing the characteristic "Ship's wheel" pattern. *P. brasiliensis* is found in soil and plants and is endemic to rural subtropical regions of Central and South America.

Background and epidemiology. Paracoccidioidomycosis (South American Blastomycosis, Lutz disease, Lutz-Splendore-Almeida disease) is endemic to rural regions of Mexico, Brazil, Columbia, Venezuela, Uruguay, and Argentina. It is predominantly seen in adult males living in endemic regions or having visited these areas (355). Seventy percent of infected individuals have some agricultural exposure. Infection occurs much less frequently in women; estrogen has a protective role inhibiting the transition of conidia into yeasts, a critical step in disease pathogenesis (356). The incidence of paracoccidioidomycosis among Brazilian AIDS patients is generally low, probably due to widespread trimethoprim sulfamethoxazole prophylaxis for *Pneumocystis carinii,* which also arrests progression of *P. brasiliensis* (356).

Paracoccidioidomycosis is acquired by aspiration. Oral infection is also thought to be acquired in the act of teeth cleaning with infected wood fragments (357,358) and further potentiated by alcohol and smoking exposure. There is no evidence of human-to-human transmission.

Clinical course. Clinical manifestations can range from subclinical infections to clinically apparent infections in immunocompetent and immunosuppressed patients (359). Pulmonary involvement is common. Reactivation of quiescent disease is the main mechanism of chronic infection. *Paracoccidioides* has a predilection of facial skin and upper airway mucosa; often oral infection is the initial and main disease manifestation. The oral lesions are typically erythematous, granular, and hyperplastic, speckled with pinpoint hemorrhages resulting in a "mulberry-like" (framboesiform) surface referred to as "moriforme stomatitis" (360–362) (Fig. 38). The lips can become thickened and firm. Bone infection is uncommon; juvenile oral infection can destroy alveolar bone causing tooth loss. Palatal perforation is also a rare presentation (363). Cervical adenopathy may be due to oral infection, or secondary to pulmonary infection. Hematogenous dissemination can result in serious and potentially fatal CNS or systemic infection.

Histopathology. Infection is characterized by suppurative granulomas with multinucleated giant cells containing round yeasts, 2 to 10 μm, and up to 30 μm in diameter. They have bilaminated refractile walls 0.2 to 1 μm thick; ultrastructurally these walls have an inner electron lucent layer and an external electron dense layer. Multiple budding daughter yeasts are characteristic and diagnostic; they may virtually rim the mother yeast capsule mimicking the spokes on a mariner's wheel (Fig. 38). This is best observed on Gomori methanamine silver and periodic acid–Schiff stains. The small, newly released daughter spores may be confused with other small yeasts such as *Histoplasma.* Single budding yeasts forms are also present, mimicking *Blastomyces,* which is the main differential diagnosis, hence the synonym South American *Blastomyces. Paracoccidioides* may be birefringent, polarizing with a Maltese cross appearance, which is not specific for *Paracoccidioides.*

Serological identification and PCR. *P. brasiliensis* produces a 43 kDa glycoprotein, gp-43, during the infectious yeast phase. This antigen, and corresponding antibodies, can be detected in serum, urine, and cerebral spinal fluid by complement fixation, immunodiffusion, and ELISA techniques. PCR can be used to detect *P. brasiliensis* in archival pathology specimens (364).

Treatment. Itraconazole is the drug of choice. Ketoconazole is also effective, but itraconazole is preferred because of less toxicity (365). Fluconozole can be used for CNS disease.

Blastomycosis

This is an infection caused by *B. dermatitides,* spherical dimorphous yeast, 6 to 15 μm, which forms single broad-necked budding structures. The hyphal form is *Ajellomyces dermatitidis.*

Epidemiology. *B. dermatitidis* (North American Blastomycosis, Gilchrist's disease, Chicago disease) is endemic in the Ohio and Mississippi River basins

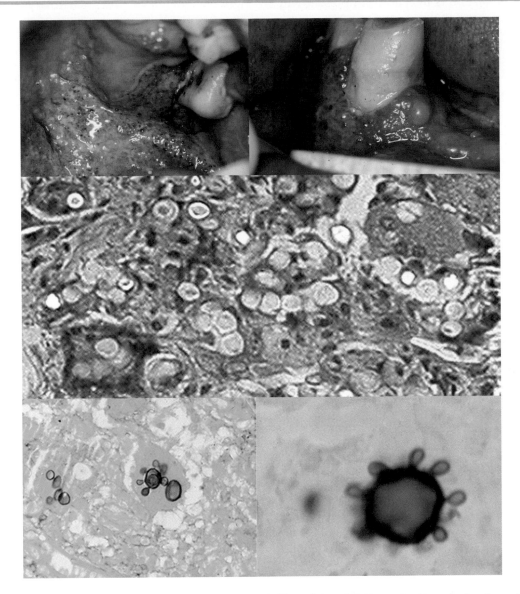

Figure 38 Paracoccidioidomycosis (South American blastomycosis). Upper left and right panels: Granular "mulberry-like" (framboesi-form) lesions of oral paracoccidioidomycosis. Center panel: Granulomatous reaction with refractile intracellular yeasts. Lower left and right panels: Grocott silver stains demonstrate the characteristic multiple budding yeasts (Mariner's wheel formation). *Source*: Courtesy of Dr. Ameida of Piracicaba, Brazil (gingival cases), Courtesy of Drs Sposto, Onofre, and Navarro, Sao Paulo, Brazil (palatal case), and http://www.saber.ula.ve/tropical/index.html.es, Accessed January 2008 (Grocott silver stains).

and around the Great Lakes. Blastomycosis is not a nationally notifiable disease and so its epidemiological patterns are not well characterized. Because of major epidemics in Wisconsin, Illinois, and Mississippi, this disease is reportable in these states (366–369). North American blastomycosis is not confined to North America and has also been detected in South America, India, and Africa. Canine blastomycosis follows the same geographic distribution as human disease, which is due to similar outdoor exposures and not interspecies transmission (370,371). Point sources for Blastomycosis usually involve woodsy and watery environments, rotting wood, and construction sites; however historically it has been

difficult to isolate *Blastomyces* from soil specimens after point source infections. Recently, PCR-based studies comparing patient isolates and soil samples have elucidated that not all isolated environmental strains are pathogens, whereas other strains are more rarely detected in soil but have a greater association with clinical infection (372).

Clinical. Blastomyces usually causes infection after inhalation; the majority of patients are immunocompetent. There are three different disease manifestations: infections may be asymptomatic, acute, or chronic and insidious. Asymptomatic infection will resolve spontaneously. Patients with acute pneumonia present with fever, productive cough, and myalgias.

Those with more insidious infection can present with anorexia, weight loss, malaise, and chronic cough, mimicking TB or malignancy; thus blastomycosis can often evade clinical suspicion. Hematogenous systemic dissemination is common in these cases. Extrapulmonary presentation implies primary lung infection. Another mode of infection is traumatic inoculation, although this is rare (373). Disseminated blastomycosis should be ruled out whenever there is presentation with dermal disease.

Head and neck manifestations of blastomycosis. In a report of 102 patients with blastomycosis, 41% had pulmonary disease and 45% had skin lesions (374). (Fig. 39). Twenty-three patients had lesions involving the head and neck, most of which were cutaneous

lesions (70%). Five patients had laryngeal lesions and two had nasal lesions. Cervical adenopathy has been reported in 55 to 10% of cases (375). Skin lesions appear as papules, pustules, or subcutaneous nodules that ultimately ulcerate. The borders are serpiginous with numerous crusting microabscesses or may have verrucous-like appearance (376). In the larynx, blastomycosis appears as erythematous or white masses with irregular borders that may impair vocal cord mobility—an appearance that can be identical to carcinoma. In fact, a number of unfortunate "laryngeal carcinomas" have been reported that actually represented cases of blastomycosis (377–379). Deep laryngeal fissures or laryngocutaneous fistulas may form. Oral lesions may present as warty lesions, or as

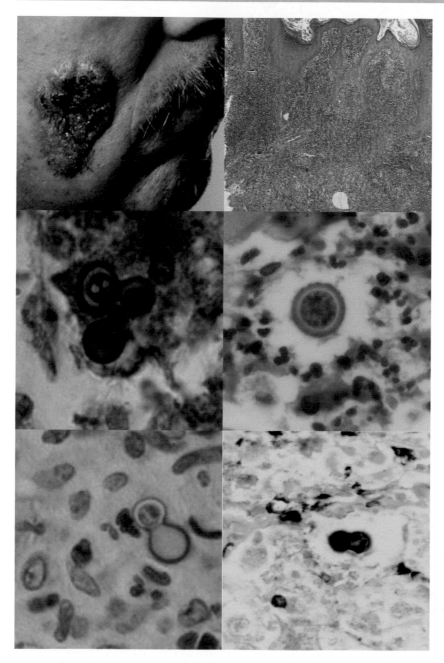

Figure 39 Blastomycosis. Upper: Blastomycotic infection causes verrucoid inflammatory lesions. Note the characteristic space between the thick outer wall and the protoplasm, and the dumbbell-shaped, broad-neck budding. The wall will stain with periodic acid–Schiff but weakly or not at all with mucin stain. Lower right: Gomori methanamine silver stain.

severe, draining periodontal disease, or as draining sinuses mimicking actinomycosis (380).

Immunocompromised patients (diabetics or those receiving corticosteroids or cytological cancer therapy) are more likely to develop disseminated disease (375). Blastomycosis is rare in HIV-infected individuals (381).

Histopathology. *Blastomyces* can induce a hyperplastic, hyperkeratotic verrucoid response, mimicking seborrhea keratosis, squamous carcinoma or verrucous carcinoma (VC). Acute and chronic granulomatous reaction with necrosis is seen. The organisms are round, 6 to 15 μm wide, with very distinctive thick refractile cell walls, and characteristic broad based budding (Fig. 39). This broad budding imparts a "dumbbell" or lollipop-shaped appearance. Another characteristic feature for *Blastomyces* is the retraction artifact between the cell wall and the protoplasm. Special stains are helpful but the organisms can be seen in routine hematoxylin and eosin and Papanicolau stains. Periodic acid–Schiff and Gomori methanamine silver will stain the cell wall. *Blastomyces* will stain weakly or be nonreactive with the mucicarmine stain.

The primary diagnosis can be established by identifying the yeasts either in tissue, sputum, or pus. Culture identification can take between 5 and 30 days.

Differential diagnosis. The morphological differential diagnosis includes *Cryptococcus* and *Paracoccidioides*. *Cryptococcus* will also stain strongly with periodic acid–Schiff and Gomori methanamine silver. Unlike *Blastomyces*, *Cryptococcus* will react strongly with the mucicarmine stain. *Paracoccidioides* can be much larger than *Blastomyces* and forms multiple budding structures.

Serological identification. An EIA for antibodies to the A antigen of *B. dermatitidis* is a sensitive and rapid test available through reference laboratories.

Treatment. Amphotericin B and itraconazole are the current drugs of choice. High-dose amphotericin is recommended for severe pulmonary or extrapulmonary infection, whereas itraconazole can be used for mild to moderate pulmonary infection.

Cryptococcosis

This is an infection by *C. neoformans*, round to oval yeasts, 4 to 10 μm, with narrow-necked budding and a thick mucinophilic capsule that is usually self-limited and localized in immunocompetent individuals, and disseminated and potentially fatal in immunosuppressed individuals.

Background. *C. neoformans* is ubiquitous yeast with worldwide distribution that is usually acquired through inhalation of environmental sources; pigeon guano represents the most important disease vector. Pigeons have unusual nesting habits; unlike other birds, they do not rid their nests of excreta. The nests become progressively transformed into a "plaster-like mass of dried fecal material" (382). Pigeon guano is a realized ecological niche for *Cryptococcus*, which is able to undergo sexual reproduction in this setting; its hyphal sexual form is

Filobasidiella neoformans (383). Pet birds have also been a rare source of infection in the United States (384).

Clinical presentation. Cryptococcosis manifests as a self-limited, subclinical, or subacute pulmonary infection in immunocompetent hosts. Individuals with AIDS or organ transplants comprise the usual immunosuppressed hosts; infection is likely due to reactivation of latent infection, rather than new exposure. They can develop disseminated disease involving lungs and CNS and present with fever, malaise, cough, headache and altered mental status. Other involved sites include spinal cord, lymph nodes, spleen, bone marrow, liver, kidney, adrenal, and thyroid glands (385–387).

Head and neck manifestations of cryptococcosis. In the head and neck, the larynx and oral cavity can be involved; lesions may be "warty" or ulcerating (387–389). Laryngeal cryptococcosis can occur as an isolated lesion or in the setting of pulmonary infection. Patients with laryngeal infection may be immunocompetent, or have locally altered immunity (e.g., steroid inhalants), or have systemic immunosuppression.

Immune reconstitution syndrome. AIDS patients with CD4 counts lower than 100/mL are predisposed to disseminated infection. After 1996, HAART (highly active antiretroviral therapy) has resulted in a decreased incidence of cryptococcosis from 6% to 12% to 3%. However, immune reconstitution with HAART may result in an intense symptomatic inflammatory response. Immune reconstitution syndrome (IRIS) occurs in 10% to 25% of HIV patients who receive HAART, which mirrors rising CD4 cell counts. IRIS is typically associated with infections (opportunistic and other infections) and malignancies such as KS. IRIS linked with Cryptococcal infection has been associated with the development of lymphadenitis and CNS manifestations such as meningitis.

Histopathology. Cryptococcosis is diagnosed by histopathology or cytology. Granulomatous inflammation with foreign body–type giant cells and intracellular and extracellular organisms are seen in immunocompetent patients. In immunosuppressed patients, the inflammatory reaction may be limited (390). The yeasts are not readily stained by hematoxylin and eosin, though the stain may accentuate their nuclei (Fig. 40). Gomori methanamine silver will stain the organisms, while mucicarmine and digested periodic acid–Schiff stain will accentuate the polysaccharide capsule. Uncollapsed round yeasts are 6 to 7 μm but may be as large as 20 μm. Single budding yeasts with narrow necks are seen. Collapsed yeasts take on a "boatlike" or sickle-type shape, similar to *Pneumocystis*. Capsule-deficient *Cryptococcus*, seen in AIDS, may be difficult to identify, as they do not stain with mucicarmine (391,392). Fontana Masson stain will be helpful in this setting (393). India ink preparation and latex agglutination tests are used to identify organisms and capsular polysaccharide antigens, respectively, in body fluids such as CSF. EIAs are available for serum antibodies to *Cryptococcus* capsular polysaccharide and are valuable in the detection of meningitis. The diagnosis should be confirmed by culture, however lack of growth does not rule out infection.

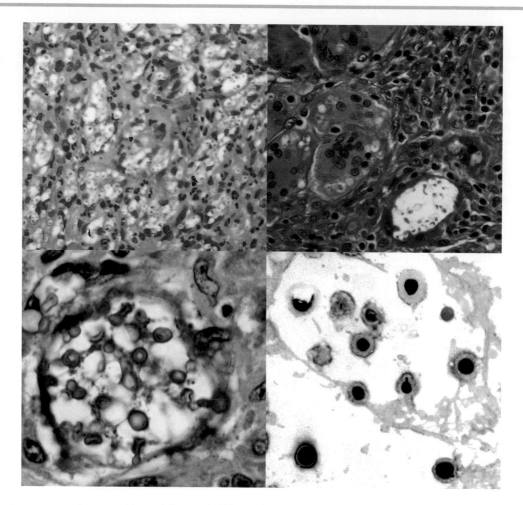

Figure 40 Cryptococcus neoformans. Upper left panel: Primary laryngeal cryptococcus in an 80-year-old gentleman on low-dose steroids. The clearing effect around the intracellular organisms can be appreciated on low power. Upper right panel: Primary laryngeal Cryptococcosis in a nonimmunosuppressed woman. Multinucleated giant cells containing small yeast forms. Lower left panel: Mucicarmine stain accentuates the inner and outer limits of the polysaccharide capsule. Lower right panel: Gomori methenamine silver stain densely stains the entire organism, leaving a negative impression of the capsule. Occasional narrow-necked budding is seen. *Source*: Courtesy of Dr. Leslie Smallman, Birmingham, England (upper right panel).

Differential diagnosis. The differential diagnosis includes *Sporothrix, Pneumocystis, Blastomyces, Histoplasma,* and *C. glabrata. Blastomyces, Histoplasma,* and *Cryptococcus* all have a polysaccharide cell wall that stains with digested periodic acid–Schiff. *Blastomyces* can be distinguished from *Cryptococcus* by its wider budding isthmus, its protoplasmic retraction artifact, and lack of strong reaction with the mucicarmine stain (see III.B.5). The other organisms can be distinguished from *Cryptococcus* on the basis of their size and shape. *Histoplasma capsulatum,* is smaller and intracellular; *S. schenkii,* has the football shaped yeasts in addition to the rounded forms; *P. carinii* is approximately the same size as *Cryptococcus* but does not vary in size as the latter does, and budding forms are not evident with *Pneumocystis* (Table 2).

Treatment. Pulmonary cryptococcosis in the immunocompetent host does not require therapy. Intravenous amphotericin B is used to treat disseminated and meningeal infections. AIDS patients with

CD4 counts less than 100/mL may require lifelong oral fluconozole to suppress *Cryptococcus.*

Histoplasmosis

This is an infection by *H. capsulatum*, a small spherical to oval yeast, 2 to 5 μm, usually intracellular, within histiocytes.

Historical perspective. Histoplasmosis (Darling's disease) was elucidated in the early 20th century by Samuel Darling, a pathologist working in Panama, who discovered intrahistiocytic organisms he dubbed "Histoplasma." The term "Capsulatum" was derived from the "refractile rim" observed around the organisms (394).

The European starling (*Sturnus vulgaris linnaeus*) is the major vector of histoplasmosis and was introduced to North America during the design of Central Park in New York City in the late 19th century. One of the intentions was to fill the park with all the birds mentioned in Shakespeare's writings. A murmuration of 60 starlings was released in Central Park in 1890. In 1895, it was noted: "They seemed to have left the park and have established themselves in various favorable places in the upper part of the city . . . (Such as) . . . the roof of the Museum of Natural History and at other points. . . . as they have already endured our most severe winters, we may doubtless regard the species as thoroughly naturalized . . . " (395,396). Since then, the starlings successfully and rapidly multiplied to become one of the most numerous birds in North America. This tremendous ecological success has been attributed to the adaptation of a southwest migratory pattern and the ability of starlings to oust other birds out of their roosts. Thus the lines:

> I'll have a starling shall be taught to speak
> Nothing but "Mortimer," and give it to him (397)

were indirectly responsible for countless cases of disease, ruined crops, and downed airplanes in the United States.

Epidemiology and background. Histoplasmosis is common to North and Central America, and is also endemic to Europe, Russia, and the Far East (398,399). In the United States, it is endemic in the Mississippi and Ohio River Valleys in the Midwest. It can be isolated from starling roosts, bat caves, pigeon's excrement, and chicken coops. Exposure occurs via aerosolized bird or bat droppings and contaminated soil and fertilizers. Starling congregations are especially risky, as these gregarious birds amass by the thousands in a Hitchcock-like fashion, and the accumulation of their droppings can become especially dense, necessitating public health decontamination measures (399,400). Point source epidemics have been traced to construction sites associated with bird roosts (401).

Clinical course. Most individuals with normal immunity exposed to small doses of *Histoplasma* develop subclinical pulmonary infection; a massive inhaled dose can lead to acute pneumonia. Persons with emphysema can develop chronic cavitating pulmonary infection and sclerosing mediastinitis. Disseminated systemic infections occur in the elderly, AIDS patients, or those immunosuppressed by chemotherapy or hematological malignancy. It can occur after primary infection; reactivation of latent infection is a less frequent mechanism (402). Patients with disseminated infection present with fever, septicemia, weakness, anorexia, weight loss, pneumonia, hepatic or renal failure, CNS infection, or mucocutaneous lesions (402,403). The cutaneous lesions have a predilection for the face; they can appear as plaques, crusted papules, or nodules. *Histoplasma* has greater dermatotropism for HIV-infected individuals; dermal lesions are three times more common than mucosal lesions (404). Disseminated and extrapulmonary histoplasmosis is included in the criteria for AIDS.

Head and neck manifestations of histoplasmosis. Both immunocompetent and immunosuppressed individuals may develop infection of the gingiva, tongue, palate, and larynx (Fig. 41). Patients with oral histoplasmosis present with pharyngitis, tonsillitis, cervical lymphadenopathy; lesions are extremely painful,

indurated, ulcerating, or verrucoid and can erode bone (405–413). Exophytic lesions may mimic carcinoma. Ulcerating lesions occur around the nose and mouth (414). Oropharyngeal infection usually occurs with active pulmonary histoplasmosis but can also develop in the absence of detectable lung disease (412). Additionally, oropharyngeal histoplasmosis may serve as the sentinel of disseminated infection.

Mucocutaneous histoplasmosis may develop soon after initiation of HAART in some HIV-infected individuals as part of the IRIS syndrome. The introduction of HAART paradoxically worsens clinical response to some infections despite improvement of the immunological status (404).

Etiology. Two varieties of *Histoplasma* are pathogenic to humans: H. *capsulatum var capsulatum* and H. *capsulatum var duboisi*. The latter is seen in Africa. *Histoplasma* is a dimorphic fungus; its hyphal form is *Emmonsiella capsulatum*. The microconidal/spores of E. *capsulatum* are infectious. They form yeasts at 37°C in vitro or in vivo. *Histoplasma* survives and replicates within the phagosomes of host histiocytes.

Immunological considerations. Primary infection is largely self-limited in immunocompetent individuals because of the development of T-cell-mediated immunity and macrophage fungistatic activity. Active infection is the result of disrupted host-pathogen balance (415).

Histopathology. *Histoplasma* is seen as "intracellular and extracellular petite hematoxylinophilic bodies each surrounded by a small halo" (416) (Fig. 41). Careful observation reveals an intracellular nucleus. Granulomatous reaction may be present; the overlying mucosa can be hyperplastic. The three characteristic morphological features of *Histoplasma*, the intrahistiocytic location, the "halo" effect around each organism, and its nuclei, are best observed in hematoxylin and eosin–stained sections. The halo or "capsule" does not stain and is actually an artifact of tissue embedding. The organism does stain with Gomori methanamine silver stain, but high background makes it unsuitable for evaluation of these small organisms. Periodic acid–Schiff will stain the organisms with less background. Solitary and multiple thin-necked budding may be seen. A touch preparation can be superior in revealing the fine morphology of *Histoplasma*, and if possible, should always be an adjunct to tissue biopsy.

Differential diagnosis. The differential diagnosis includes other small intracellular organisms such as *Leishmania tropica*, and *L mexicana complex*, which may also cause mucocutaneous lesions [Oriental sore, "Old World" sore (*L tropica*) and espundia, "New World" sore (*L mexicana/braziliensis*)]. *Trypanosome cruzi* is another small intracellular protozoan pathogen that may be the cause of mucocutaneous lesions in addition to systemic disease. The distinction between *Histoplasma* and these protozoa is particularly important in cases of disseminated infection as the treatments differ (antifungal agents versus antiprotozoan agents).

Leishmania and *Trypanosome* are within the same size range as *Histoplasma* (2–4 μm) but lack the prominent clear halo of *Histoplasma*. *Leishmania* and

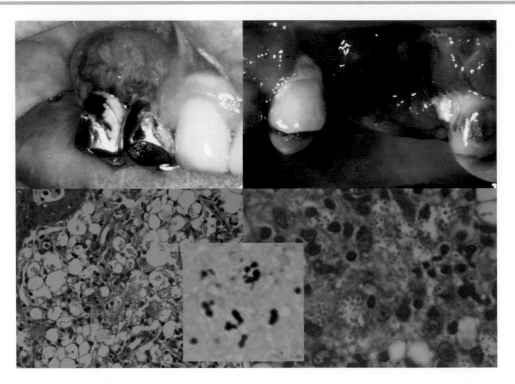

Figure 41   Histoplasmosis. Upper left panel: Granulomatous inflammatory lesion of premolar gingivae in a 75-year-old man with active pulmonary histoplasmosis. Upper right panel: Granulomatous inflammatory palatal mass. Lower left panel: Submucosal histiocytic infiltrate containing "petite" organisms. Lower right panel: Small intrahistiocytic organisms surrounded by a halo with faint, darker nuclei (hematoxylin and eosin). Inset: Gomori methanamine silver stain highlights the thin-necked budding. This budding pattern is similar to that seen with Cryptococcus. However, Histoplasma is much smaller (2–4 μm) than Cryptococcus (>6 μm). *Source*: Courtesy of Dr. Charles Cobb, DDS, Missouri, U.S.A. (upper left panel).

Trypanosome can be seen in hematoxylin and eosin and reticulin stains. *Histoplasma* is a round organism; *Leishmania* and *T. cruzi* have a "diaper pin" shape. *Histoplasma* will stain with Gomori methanamine silver stain; *Trypanosome* and *Leishmania* will not. Both *Trypanosome* and *Leishmania* have intracellular kinetoplasts adjacent to round nuclei. The kinetoplasts are impossible to visualize on paraffin-embedded tissue slide, but may be seen on Giemsa stained touch preparations.

The differential diagnosis in AIDS patients includes *P. carinii* and *Penicilicium marneffei*. Both of these organisms appear as rounded yeast forms with intracellular nuclei visible on hematoxylin and eosin stain. *P. carinii* is not intracellular, is slightly larger than *H. capsulatum* (4–6 μm vs. 2–5 μm), lacks the clear halo, and is "boat-shaped." *P. marneffei* has been rarely reported in patients with AIDS (417). It is a biphasic fungus and is also intracellular. *P. marneffei* lacks a clear halo, and septated hyphal forms may be seen.

Culture, serological identification, and PCR.   Fungal cultures provide the strongest evidence for identification, but they can be negative in up to 20% of patients with disseminated infection and 50% of chronic infections, and require up to four weeks for growth. Serological antibody tests are possible in up to 90% of patients, but only two to six weeks after exposure. Immunosuppressed individuals may not develop elevated antibodies. On the other hand, serum titers may be elevated from previous exposure but not indicative of active infection. During active infection, *Histoplasma* antigens are released and may be detected in body fluids: blood, urine, cerebral spinal fluid, and bronchial alveolar lavage. Antigen detection using antibodies to *Histoplasma*-specific polysaccharides provides a rapid and accurate method for establishing the diagnosis of histoplasmosis early in the disease (418). Antigen detection sensitivity is greater in the urine than serum; detection in cerebral spinal fluid is positive in only 50% of *Histoplasma* meningitis. The titers can be used to measure response to therapy. Lastly, there are commercially available PCR and DNA probe kits for detection of *Histoplasma*.

Treatment.   Itraconazole is the drug of choice for mild to moderate infections; fluconozole is a second-line agent. Posaconazole is also effective and used in patients who do not respond, or cannot tolerate, other antifungal drugs.

IV.   VIRAL DISEASE

A.   HIV, Related Infections, and Tumors

Human Immunodeficiency Virus

A ribonucleic acid (RNA) retrovirus, lentivirus subfamily, approximately 10 kb (kilo-base pair) long, capable of selectively binding CD4 cells, namely

T-helper/inducer lymphocytes, via its GP-120 envelope protein. The enveloped virions are 120 to 160 nm, with a characteristic central bar-shaped core nucleiod 60 to 100 nm. HIV integrates randomly into the host genome; viral replication involves production of a double-stranded DNA intermediate provirus via reverse transcriptase (RT).

Background and epidemiology. HIV infection is transmitted by semen, blood and blood products, breast milk, and placental circulation. HIV-1 is the primary causative virus of the acquired immunodeficiency syndrome (AIDS). HIV-2 was isolated in West Africa; its prevalence in the United States is extremely low. AIDS originated in Central Africa; sera from Ugandan children collected in the early 1970s revealed a high prevalence of antibodies to HTLV-III (HIV) (419). AIDS (slim disease) was seen in Zaire since the late 1970s (420,421). It is thought that either HIV had mutated from other T-lymphotrophic retroviruses or moved from nonsusceptible to susceptible populations. A related virus, Simian T lymphocyte virus-III (STLV-III), is naturally present among African primates; some, like the African green monkey, remain healthy, while others, (Macaques, rhesus monkeys) develop immunodeficiency (422,423). Healthy West Africans have been found to harbor a retrovirus (human T lymphocyte virus-IV or HTLV-IV) distinct from the HIV (HTLV-III) but similar to STLV-III (424). HIV may then represent a mutation from a natural simian or human reservoir.

The rise of AIDS in Central Africa is in no way coincidental to the massive small pox vaccination in Africa in the late 1960s and 1970s. One possibility is iatrogenic infection through contaminated needles (ped-o-jet lancets) employed in the vaccination campaigns because of unavailability of disposable needles (425,426). Another possibility is that of viral interactions with vaccinia-activated latent HIV (427).

In Central and West Africa, (Zaire, Uganda, Rwanda, Burundi, Senegal) HIV was transmitted through promiscuity and contact with prostitutes (426–429). HIV spread to Haiti and then the United States via tourist/immigrant contacts with prostitutes. AIDS first appeared in the United States among homosexuals and Haitian immigrants in two major cities with large homosexual populations: namely New York City and San Francisco (430). It was initially termed the "gay-related immunedeficiency syndrome." The *San Francisco Chronicle* newspaper published the "seven deadly symptoms" associated with the disease: (*i*) persistent fever for more than four or five days, (*ii*) unexplained weight loss of 10 to 20 pounds in a few months, (*iii*) general aches and pains similar to an acute viral syndrome for over 10 days. (*iv*) sore or swollen lymph glands for over a week. (*v*) appearance of blue or purplish skin spots (KS). (*vi*) persistent or worsening herpes sores for over five weeks. and (*vii*) loss of sensorimotor ability or defects in mental or neural function (431). These are the features characteristics of HIV infection. During that era, promiscuity among segments of the homosexual community reached gargantuan proportions, with possible *pro annum* sexual contacts

numbering in the hundreds (432). Like a fatal "chain letter," intravenous drug abuse and blood donations widened the circle of vulnerability to include intravenous drug abusers, hemophiliacs, and other recipients of infected blood and blood products.

In the United States, the incidence of new cases and related deaths continued to increase until the mid-1990, when the use of HAART became widespread. As of 2003, more than 1 million persons in the United States are living with HIV/AIDS; approximately 40,000 new cases of HIV infection and 16,000 to 17,000 AIDS-related deaths occur annually (433). Transmission is greatest among the male-to-male sexual contact group (434). Globally, an estimated 38 million people (range 35–42 million) are living with HIV/AIDS. The devastating impact of this disease, with respect to suffering, mortality, disruption to families, local economies, and infrastructure is greatest in Sub-Saharan and South Africa, where 25 million (range 23.1–27.9 million) are living with HIV/AIDS (435).

The HIV virion and genome. HIV (HTLV-III, human T lymphotrophic virus) is an RNA retrovirus, which gains access into host cells by binding CD4 receptors, chemokine coreceptors (CXCR4, CCR5), and other cell surface proteins (431,436). A feature common to all retroviruses is their ability to integrate into the host genome and hijack cellular transcriptional machinery for its own expression and replication. The virion is composed of two copies of positive single-stranded RNA encoding nine genes. Each RNA strand is tightly bound to nucleocapsid proteins, p7, and the enzymes necessary for replication (RT, proteases, ribonucleases, integrase). The viral RNA is enclosed in a capsid of p24, which is surrounded by a matrix of p17, which in turn is surrounded by the viral envelope composed of a phospholipid bilayer procured from the host membrane during virion budding. The viral envelope is embedded with host proteins and studded with about 70 copies of a complex HIV protein (Env) consisting of a stem of gp41 capped by three molecules of gp120. This glycoprotein complex enables the virus to attach and fuse with target cells initiating infection (437).

HIV genome is flanked by 640-nucleotide long terminal repeat (LTR) sequences, which ultimately control viral activity by initiating transcription by RNA polymerase II (RNAPII). TAR (Trans Activating Responsive Element) is an important element within the LTR, which projects away from the rest of the genome in a hairpin configuration. After HIV-1 integration, the provirus becomes organized into nucleosomes, and basal viral transcriptional activity is very low. The hairpin portion prevents full viral transcription and only a small number of RNA transcripts are produced, which includes tat (transactivator of transcription) protein (438). Tat is very important to activation and replication of integrated HIV. Tat recruits the TATA-binding protein, transcription factor IIB, and positive transcription and elongation factor b, (PTEF-b) to the promoter region to form an active preinitiation complex (PIC). Cyclin-dependent kinase 9 and cyclin-T become part of this complex, hyperphosphorylating and activating RNAPII. RNAPII transcribes the TAR in the LTR (439,440). Once a threshold is reached, an explosive positive feedback loop occurs for further *tat* upregulation. Newly synthesized tat protein returns to the nucleus and exerts its transactivating function, destabilizing the nucleosome, triggering chromatin remodeling, eliminating the hairpin RNA structure, and resulting in transcription of integrated HIV. Other newly synthesized tat is secreted and taken up by other HIV-infected cells further amplifying viral activation, and also taken up by noninfected cells, impacting cellular processes.

Extracellular tat has cytokine-like activities, upregulating interleukin (IL)-2 and IL-2 receptor, which enhances the spread of HIV among T cells, IL-4, IL-4 receptor, and IL-6, which may promote tumorigenesis of B-cells, and IL-8, and IL-10 (440). At physiological concentrations, tat upregulates Bcl-2, which may protect infected cells from apoptosis. Intracellular tat also promotes cellular proliferation; *tat* transgenic mice develop skins tumors, KS-like lesions, and hepatocellular carcinomas (441,442). *Tat* may contribute to genomic instability by interfering with DNA repair machinery (443).

The internal segment of the HIV genome contains *gag* (encoding structural core proteins), *pol* (encoding RT, protease, and integrase), and *env* genes (encoding envelope glycoproteins). These three genes are uniformly present in all retroviruses and are necessary for viral replication. The six accessory genes are *REV, VIF, NEF, VPR, VPU,* and *TAT,* the latter of which is described above. They are called accessory genes as they are not necessary for viral replication in some in vitro systems, but they are important in disease pathogenesis (444).

Rev (regulator of expression of virion) encodes a protein, which allows HIV mRNA with a Rev response element (RRE) to be exported from the nucleus to the cytoplasm and avoid splicing. When rev is absent, host RNA splicing machinery quickly splices HIV mRNA so that only the smaller, regulatory proteins are produced; in the presence of rev, HIV mRNA is exported from the nucleus before splicing, so that HIV RNA genome and structural proteins can also be produced (445). Vif (viral infectivity factor) is essential for HIV replication in lymphocytes and macrophages, but not in most cell lines. It appears that vif promotes efficient RT after virion entry (444).

Nef is a versatile protein with multiple activities. Nef is necessary for the development of high viral load. Australian patients infected with *nef*-defective derivative of HIV had low-level replication and significant delay in the progression to AIDS (446). Nef has three distinct activities: (*i*) it mediates T-cell activation, (*ii*) it increases intracellular trafficking of surface receptors, and (*iii*) it stimulates infectivity of virions after infection. *Nef* downregulates CD4 by triggering endocytosis of the HIV-CD4 complex. This acts as an immigration quota, limiting the influx of HIV into the cells, which allows for viral replication and prevents the cytotoxic effect caused by large numbers of virus or provirus; excess CD4 also inhibits virion budding. *Nef* downregulates class I major histocompatibility complex accomplishing immune evasion. It increases

viral infectiousness by playing a role in the uncoating of the viral core after fusion (444).

Vpr (viral protein R) is involved in regulating nuclear import of the HIV-1 preintegration complex, and is required for virus replication in nondividing cells such as macrophages. *Vpr* induces cell cycle arrest and apoptosis in proliferating cells, which can result in immune dysfunction (447). HIV-2 contains Vpr and a related protein Vpx (viral protein X). Two functions of Vpr in HIV-1 are divided between Vpr and Vpx in HIV-2; HIV-2 Vpr protein induces cell cycle arrest and Vpx protein is required for nuclear import. Finally, *Vpu* (viral protein U) enhances the release of assembled virions. The relatively compact genome of HIV accommodates these multiple gene regions by utilizing overlapping reading frames and posttranscriptional splicing modifications.

HIV tropism. HIV binds with T4 cell (T helper/inducer cells) and monocytes, macrophages, CNS glial cells, astrocytes, and neurons. Infected monocytes can secondarily infect mucosal and gastrointestinal epithelial cells. HIV-1 entry is mediated through the interaction of HIV gp120 and the target cell CD4 receptors plus chemokine coreceptors (CXCR4, CCR5). HIV strains are classified as either syncytium inducing (SI) or nonsyncitial inducing (N-SI). The SI strain preferentially infects T cells (T-tropic) via CXCR4 and is associated with more rapid disease progression. T-tropic isolates replicate in both CD4 T cells and macrophages. The N-SI strain (macrophage or M-tropic) preferentially infects macrophages rather than T cells using the β-chemokine receptor CCR5 for entry. HIVs that use only the CCR5 receptor are termed R5, HIVs that use CXCR4 are termed X4 and those that use both are X4R5. Macrophages appear to be the first cells infected by HIV and a reservoir for viral persistence and transmission. In tonsils and adenoids of HIV-infected patients, macrophages fuse into multinucleated giant cells that produce huge amounts of viruses.

Primary infection and latency. HIV viremia follows infection, peaking at about six weeks and becoming undetectable after about eight weeks. Antibody seroconversion is detectable after week six, and peaks at approximately eight to ten weeks. A vigorous cytotoxic T-cell response immediately follows infection, specifically targeting envelope proteins and internal proteins (*gag* and *nef*). This response selects against viral replication and is a selection pressure toward early integration. The pressure toward integration and latency allows HIV to effectively elude the host immune system while it is still intact. After seroconversion, proviral integration is followed by viral latency. During latency, T4 cell counts and immune function are normal and HIV may be not detectable at all.

The mechanism for HIV latency has not been elucidated but could relate to DNA methylation or direct activity of the host cellular products on the integrated HIV genome (448). Latency may last up to a decade or longer. Differences in viral replication are demonstrated throughout the course of infection. HIV isolated in early infection replicates more slowly and at a lower level compared with HIV recovered after progression to AIDS. This represents mutation from R5 N-SI type virus to an X4 SI virus, which is associated with increased destruction of CD4 lymphocytes. Replication can lead to the emergence of up to 10 mutations *per* replication cycle; can give rise to highly cytopathic strains and viruses that can infect other tissues, such as the brain, the bowel, and the kidney (448).

HIV/AIDS

Tables 4–6 summarize the criteria for HIV infection, the CD4 lymphocyte categories that are used to guide clinical and therapeutic management of HIV-infected individuals, and the clinical categories for HIV/AIDS, respectively. Primary HIV infection may be entirely asymptomatic, but more than half of infected patients present with fever, malaise, myalgias, diarrhea, pharyngitis, macular erythematous rash, lymphadenopathy, splenomegaly, and/or weight loss. The acute illness occurs three to six weeks after primary exposure and may last up to two weeks; milder symptoms may persist for months.

Clinical manifestations commonly involve the head and neck. Mucosal ulcerations can accompany acute HIV seroconversion; they are probably the direct result of HIV infection (chancre of HIV). These lesions are multiple, painful, small (0.3–1.5 cm) discreet ulcers, which have been reported on the palate, esophagus, anus, and penis and relate to sexual activity (449).

The advent of HAART has dramatically shifted the infectious manifestations for HIV-seropositive patients. Opportunistic infections are rare for early stage patients with CD4 counts greater than 500 cells/mm^3. Intermediate stage patients with CD4 counts between 500 and 200 cells/mm^3 may manifest some early signs of HIV infection. AIDS (advanced stage infection) is diagnosed with counts less than 200 cells/mm^3. Opportunistic infections occur in this CD4 count range, especially with counts below 50 cells/mm^3.

OC, oral hairy leukoplakia (OHL), KS, non-Hodgkin's lymphoma (NHL), and necrotizing ulcerative gingivitis/periodontitis are strongly associated with HIV; these conditions may be present in up to

Table 4 Criteria for HIV Infection for Adolescents and Adults

1. Repeatedly reactive screening tests positive for HIV antibody (e.g., enzyme immunoassay) with specific antibody confirmed Western blot or immunofluorescence assay
2. Direct identification of virus in host tissues by virus isolation
3. HIV antigen detection
4. Positive result on any other highly specific licensed test for HIV

Table 5 CD+4 Lymphocytes Categories: Used to Guide Clinical and Therapeutic Actions in the Management of HIV-Infected Adolescents and Adults

Category 1: Greater or equal to 500 cells/mL	Early stage, opportunistic infections rare
Category 2: Between 200–499 cells/mL	Intermediate stage, early signs of HIV infection
Category 3: Less than 200 cells/mL	Advanced stage, opportunistic infections occur in this range

Table 6 Clinical Categories of HIV Infection

Category A: ([formerly referred to as pre -ARC (AIDS-related complex) or pre-AIDS)], excludes conditions of categories B and C
Asymptomatic HIV infection
Persistent generalized lymphadenopathy
Acute (primary) HIV infection with accompanying illness or history of acute HIV infection

Category B: (formerly referred to as ARC), HIV seropositivity plus at least one of the following
Bacillary angiomatosis
Oral candidiasis
Vulvovaginal candidiasis, poorly responsive to therapy
Fever or diarrhea (>1 month duration)
Hairy leukoplakia
Herpes zoster, two or more episodes or more than one dermatome
Idiopathic thrombocytopenic purpura
Listeriosis
Pelvic inflammatory disease
Peripheral neuropathy

Category C: AIDS = HIV seropositivity plus at least one of the following,
CD +4 lymphocytes less than 200 cells/mL
Candidiasis of bronchi, trachea, lungs, or esophagus
Invasive uterine cervical carcinoma
Coccidioidomycosis, disseminated or extrapulmonary
Cryptococcosis, extrapulmonary
Cryptosporidiosis, chronic intestinal (>1 month)
CMV retinitis, or disease other than liver, spleen or lymph nodes
Encephalopathy, HIV related
Herpes simplex virus, chronic ulcerations (>1 month) or bronchitis, pneumonitis, esophagitis
Histoplasmosis, disseminated or extrapulmonary
Isosporiasis, chronic intestinal (>1 month)
Kaposi's sarcoma
Lymphoma: Burkitt's, immunoblastic, or primary brain
Mycobacterium avium complex, or M kansasii, disseminated or extrapulmonary
Mycobacterium tuberculosis, pulmonary or extrapulmonary
Mycobacterium, other or unidentified species, disseminated or extrapulmonary
Pneumocystic carinii pneumonia
Pneumonia, recurrent, bacterial or viral
Progressive multifocal leukoencephalopathy
Salmonella septicemia, recurrent
Toxoplasmosis of brain
Wasting syndrome due to HIV

50% of seropositive patients and up to 80% of AIDS patients. Painful HSV lesions may be present, and reactivation of herpes zoster may be seen. With the advent of HAART, the prevalence of OC, OHL, and HIV-associated periodontal disease has decreased in adults, but the prevalence of KS remains unchanged. The incidence of HPV-associated (human papillomavirus) oral lesions and HIV-related salivary gland disease has increased (450).

Persistent generalized adenopathy (PGA) is a common presenting symptom of AIDS. Lymph nodes early in the course of AIDS reveal reactive follicular hyperplasia and follicular lysis: an influx of mantle cells and polymorphonuclear cells into germinal centers with their architectural disruption. Multinucleated giant cells and monocytoid B cells (somewhat larger than B cells with abundant pale cytoplasm and vesicular nuclei) can be seen in sinusoids. As the disease progresses, the number of follicles decrease, and a "washed out" paucicellularity develops. Terminal lymph nodes may have a virtual absence of lymphocytes; one sees only macrophages, fibroblasts, and granulocytes.

Treatment. The introduction of HAART is responsible for a dramatic drop in AIDS mortality, from 29.4/1000 person-years in 1994 to 8.8/100 person-years in 1997 (451). Unfortunately, on a global level, only a small proportion of seropositive patients have access to HAART. Three classes of drugs are used to treat HIV infection: RT inhibitors, protease inhibitors (PI), and fusion inhibitors. RT inhibitors interfere with reverse transcription; there are two types of RT inhibitors: nucleoside/nucleotide RT inhibitors, which incorporate nucleoside/nucleotide analogues into the HIV DNA that bind competitively blocking replication. The main options for dual nucleoside/nucleotide analogue inhibitors are tenofovir/emtricitabine, zidovudine/lamivudine, and abacavir/lamivudine, which are given in fixed-dose combinations. Nonnucleoside RT inhibitors (nevirapine, delavirdine, efavirenz) bind to RT. PIs (saquinavir-HGC, ritonavir, indinavir, nelfinavir) interfere with the protease enzyme, which is necessary for virion production. Fusion inhibitors (enfuvirtide) interfere with the ability of HIV virions to fuse with the cellular membrane, thereby blocking entry into host cells. HIV mutations are common events, and different strains can emerge throughout the course of the disease that could be resistant to antiretroviral drugs. Therefore, treatment strategy involves combinations of antiretroviral drugs (HAART). Antiretroviral drugs from at least two different classes are given at one time; this has been demonstrated to effectively suppress HIV.

Recommendations are that treatment should be offered to persons with <350 CD4 T cells/mm^3 or plasma HIV RNA levels of >55,000 copies/mL. The recommendation to treat asymptomatic patients should be based on the willingness and readiness of the person to begin therapy, the degree of existing immunodeficiency as determined by the CD4 T-cell count, the risk for disease progression as determined by the CD4 T-cell count and level of plasma HIV RNA, the potential benefits and risks of initiating therapy in an asymptomatic person, and the likelihood of adherence to the prescribed treatment regimen (452).

Pneumocystosis

This is an infection by *P. carinii* (*Pneumocystis jirovecii*), a small (4–7 μm) fungus that primarily causes pneumonia in immunosuppressed patients. Extrapulmonary pneumocystosis is very uncommon and usually affects immunosuppressed individuals. Extrapulmonary pneumocystosis in HIV-seropositive individuals has a predisposition for the ear.

Background and etiology. Pneumocystis was first identified in 1909 by Carlos Chagas, and believed to be a new trypanosomal organism; Antonio Carinii identified the organism in rat lungs in 1910 (453). In the 1950s, sporadic outbreaks of interstitial plasma cell pneumonia occurred among premature and malnourished children in post–World War II Central and Eastern Europe. In 1952, Vanek and Jirovec reported the association of pulmonary *P. carinii* in malnourished infants with interstitial plasma cell pneumonia (454). Genomic studies of ribosomal RNA confirm that *Pneumocystis* is more closely related to fungi than protozoa (455). There is stringent host specificity; *P. carinii* f. sp. *hominus* can only infect humans; humans cannot become infected from an animal reservoir. The nomenclature has recently been changed and *P. carinii* f. sp. *Hominus* has been renamed *Pneumocystis jironvecci*.

The high seroprevalence of antibodies to *Pneumocystis* in young children led to the assumption that *P. carinii* infection results from reactivation of latent infection. However, *P. carinii* is not ubiquitous, and epidemic-like clusters of *Pneumocystis* pneumonia (PCP) have been reported; both facts suggest that infection can also be newly acquired (454). *Pneumocystis* is transmitted from human-to-human; immunocompetent individuals can become transient asymptomatic carriers. Health care workers in contact with AIDS patients with PCP may become transiently colonized with *Pneumocystis*, in turn transmitting infection to other immunocompromised patients (456,457). *P. carinii* f. sp. *hominus* can be recovered from nasopharyngeal and oral samples from individuals in direct contact with patients with PCP, (456,457) but larger studies demonstrate the overall rarity of asymptomatic upper airway colonization in healthy individuals (458,459).

Head and neck manifestations of pneumocystis. Extrapulmonary pneumocystosis is extremely uncommon and usually develops in immunosuppressed patients. Ng and colleagues reviewed 16 non-AIDS patients with extrapulmonary pneumocystosis: 13 were immunosuppressed, 11 of them had concurrent PCP (454). Extrapulmonary pneumocystosis was limited to the hilar or tracheal lymph nodes in five patients. Widespread infection developed in the remaining eight patients, involving two or more sites (i.e., spleen, thymus, lumens of blood vessels, liver, bone marrow, adrenals, brain, kidneys, gastrointestinal tract, heart, liver, thyroid, pericardium, and hard palate).

Extrapulmonary pneumocystosis in HIV-seropositive individuals is more likely to occur in those receiving aerosolized pentamidine PCP prophylaxis, as these antifungal agents are not systemically absorbed. Ng and colleagues noted that HIV-associated extrapulmonary pneumocystosis was clinically distinct from the non-HIV-infected group. Seropositive individuals tended to have infection restricted to the ear or eye with a better prognosis; limited infection to the eye or ear was not observed in any seronegative immunosuppressed individuals. Otic pneumocystosis may present as otitis externa, EAC polyps, middle ear infections, or subcutaneous nodules (460–466). Otic infection is thought to result from *Pneumocystis* colonizing the nasopharynx and ascending the Eustachian tube.

Three cases of pneumocystosis apparently restricted to the thyroid have also been reported. All were diagnosed with AIDS, and only one received aerosolized pentamidine prophylaxis (456).

Histopathology. Extrapulmonary pneumocystosis reveals the same foamy frothy granular exudate seen in pulmonary infection, without much inflammatory response. Faint basophilic nuclei of *Pneumocystis* may be seen on hematoxylin and eosin stain. Gomori methanamine silver stain can reveal fungal cysts which are partially collapsed, "cup-shaped" or boat-shaped generally the size of erythrocytes (Fig. 42). Monoclonal immunohistochemical antibodies to *Pneumocystis* are commercially available and can be especially helpful in confirming the diagnosis, particularly in extrapulmonary sites.

Treatment. Patients with aural pneumocystosis can respond well to oral antifungal therapy (trimethoprim/sulfamethoxazole) (461). Systemic trimethoprim/sulfamethoxazole is necessary for PCP and may be necessary for extrapulmonary visceral infection (454).

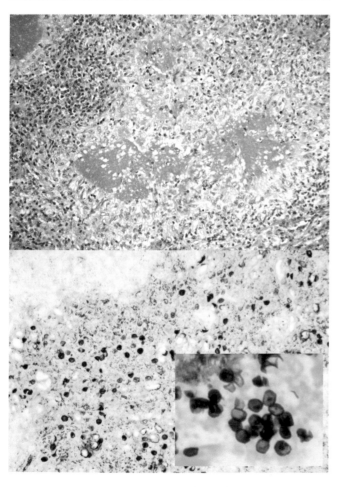

Figure 42 Pneumocystosis. Upper panel: An unusual granulomatous reaction with *Pneumocystis carinii* (hematoxylin and eosin). Lower panel: Gomori methanamine silver stains reveal pleomorphic yeast forms; collapsed "navicular" shapes can be seen. Nuclei can also be seen within the organisms as "dots."

Kaposi's Sarcoma and HHV-8

Background and epidemiology. KS is a multicentric, angioproliferative disorder characterized by proliferating spindle cells, inflammation, and neoangiogenesis (467). KS is classified into four forms: (*i*) classic KS, (*ii*) endemic or African KS, (*iii*) iatrogenic KS, which develops in HIV-seronegative immunosuppressed patients, and lastly (*iv*) epidemic or HIV-KS. Classic KS occurs in elderly Mediterranean or Eastern European men, 50 to 70 years (468). Up to one-third of classic KS patients may develop secondary malignancies, often NHL. Endemic or African KS is seen in HIV-seronegative African boys and men (469). Iatrogenic KS most commonly develops in renal or other solid organ transplant recipients (470). HIV-KS is the most common HIV-associated neoplasm; the risk of HIV-KS is highest among male homosexuals as compared with other HIV-seropositive groups.

HHV-8 DNA can be identified in all forms of KS. HHV-8 [Kaposi-Sarcoma associated Herpesvirus (KSHV)] is also associated with primary effusion lymphoma and multicentric Castleman's disease (467,471,472). There is a solid causative relationship between HHV-8 and KS. HHV-8 seroconversion in HIV-seropositive individuals is found to precede the development of HIV-KS. The presence of HHV-8 DNA in peripheral blood mononuclear cells in HHV-8/HIV-seropositive homosexual men is predictive for the development of KS; between 30% and 50% of these men will develop HIV-KS within 10 years of seroconversion (473,474). Yet HHV-8 alone is not sufficient for the promotion of KS, and not all dual HHV-8/HIV-seropositive individuals will develop HIV-KS.

The prevalence of HHV-8 exposure varies geographically and is highest in regions where classic and endemic KS are common. HHV-8 seroprevalence is high in southern Italy (23%), Zambia (40%), Uganda (50%), and as high as 87% in Botswana and 89% in Tanzania (475–479). By contrast, the seroprevalence of HHV-8 in United States blood donors is very low (5.2%) (480). The mode of transmission of HHV-8 is not entirely clear. HHV-8 seroconversion is directly proportional to the number of previous sexual partners. However the detection rates of HHV-8 in semen from dual HHV-8/HIV-seropositive men is variable (481). While HHV-8 DNA can be detected in blood peripheral mononuclear cells, HHV-8 is not readily transmitted through blood products. There is little evidence for HHV-8 acquisition among transfusion recipients even in countries found retrospectively to have significant HHV-8 seroprevalence in blood donors (482). HHV-8 DNA in patients with HIV-KS is more often detected in saliva, as compared with other body fluids, with higher concentrations (481,483). Thus oral secretions may represent a significant mode of transmission and could also explain the predilection of HIV-KS for the oral cavity.

Clinical. Classic KS manifests as soft red nodules on the lower limbs, and less commonly, on upper limbs. Lesions may be multicentric and coalescent, but rarely exceed 2 cm in size. Classic KS may uncommonly affect the head and neck; 8% involve facial skin or eyelids, nose, and ears, and only 2% affect the mucosa (conjunctiva, palate, tongue, gingiva, and tonsil) (484–486). By contrast, HIV-KS commonly affects cutaneous head and neck sites (32%) and mucosal surfaces [palate, gingiva, buccal mucosa, dorsal tongue, larynx, trachea, paranasal sinuses (19%)] (467,484,487–489).

KS evolves through three stages: patch, plaque, and nodular. The patch stage, which is the earliest stage, is characterized by single or multiple, flat, bruise-like, blue, purple, red macules. Multiple individual lesions may become confluent. The plaque stage represents the progression of patches to form elevated plaques. The nodular stage is characterized by raised, spongy lesions and exophytic masses, which can become fixed as they invade underlying tissue.

Histopathology. Patch KS appears as proliferating irregular, jagged, thin-walled "vascular spaces" lined by plump endothelial cells and surrounded by inflammation. Slit-like vessels are present around preexisting blood vessels and skin adnexal, and between collagen fibers. The patch stage may resemble granulation tissue. Extravasated RBCs and hemosiderin may be present.

Plaque KS has a more prominent spindle cell component than the patch KS. The proliferating spindle cells are admixed with slit-like blood vessels; extravasated RBCs and hemosiderin may be present. Eosinophilic globules or "red bodies" are seen in plaque KS. They are usually smaller than erythrocytes and highly sensitive and specific for KS. They stain with phosphotungstic acid hematoxylin, periodic acid–Schiff, and trichrome stains.

Nodular KS appears as interlacing bundles of long, plump, pleomorphic spindle cells, slit-like blood vessels, and extravasated RBCs. Mitotic figures are easily recognized. The degree of vascular space formation correlates with tumor differentiation. Well-differentiated tumors produce dilated ectatic spaces, angiosarcomatous anastomotic spaces, which are likened to blood-filled mazes and "glomeruloid" formations, which are loose "skein-like" clusters of capillaries resembling glomeruli. Poorly differentiated KS contains packed spindle cells with or without slit-like or cleft-like spaces. Erythrocytes are usually abundant within the slit-like spaces and hemosiderin deposition is also present. However, areas of KS may be depleted of erythrocytes, focally mimicking other sarcomas. KS may frequently metastasize to lymph nodes, and early metastases may be confined to subcapsular sinusoids.

KS is reactive for HHV-8, vimentin, CD31, CD34, and variably expresses Factor VIII by IHC.

Treatment. Treatment choices are based on symptoms, location and extent of the lesion, and the general medical condition of the patient. Superficial skin KS can be treated with local resection or cryosurgery. Small intraoral KS interfering with function may be resected or debulked. Alternatively, intralesional injection of vinblastine and 3% sodium tetradecyl sulfate is another option; one double-blind randomized control study demonstrated some efficacy with this approach (490).

Laryngeal KS requires immediate therapy, as it may rapidly progress to cause airway obstruction. Radiotherapy, laser debulking, or intralesional vinblastine may provide regression or palliation.

Iatrogenic KS may regress spontaneously with reduction of immunosuppression; persistent iatrogenic KS may be treated by chemotherapy. Likewise, systemic chemotherapy is recommended for other forms of aggressive or widespread KS. Chemotherapeutic agents such as vincristine, vinblastine, adriamycin, doxorubicin, bleomycin, INF-α, alitretinoin, and pegylated liposomal doxorubicin have been used to treat KS. There has also been a recent interest in treating KS with thalidomide.

AIDS-Related Parotid Cysts

This is a bilateral parotid enlargement caused by intraglandular lymphoid infiltrate and hyperplasia of intraparotid/periparotid lymph nodes, resulting in cystic dilatation of salivary ducts. AIDS-related parotid cysts (ARPC) is a manifestation of diffuse infiltrative lymphocytosis syndrome (DILS), defined as persistent CD8 lymphocytosis and lymphoid infiltrate in various organs, in association with HIV infection.

Background and etiology. AIDS patients may develop cystic and solid parotid tumors referred to as "AIDS-related parotid cysts," or ARPC (491–499). ARPC is a manifestation of DILS, which is characterized by salivary and lacrimal swelling, sicca syndrome, and persistent circulating and visceral infiltrate of CD-8 cells. There are superficial similarities and some major distinctions between ARPC and Sjogren's syndrome (Table 7) (500). Patients with ARPC lack serum autoantibodies but have autoimmune Sjogren's type symptoms (xerostomia and xerophthalmia, and arthritic pain) (491,492,496,497). They may have severe sialadenitis on lip biopsies, on par with that seen in Sjogren's disease (501,502). The infiltrate of DLIS is

Table 7 Comparison Between Diffuse Infiltrative Lymphocytosis Syndrome (DILS) and Sjogren's Syndrome

Variable	Sjogren's syndrome	DILS
Sicca syndrome	Present	present
Glandular manifestations	Moderate parotid enlargement	Moderate to severe parotid enlargement
Extraglandular manifestations	Mainly pulmonary, gastrointestinal, renal, and neurological involvement	Mainly musculoskeletal, pulmonary, gastrointestinal, and neurological involvement
Infiltrating lymphocytes	CD4	CD8
Autoantibodies	High frequency of RA factor, ANA, anti-Ro/SSA and anti-LaSSB Ro (rarely)	Low frequency of RA factor, ANA, anti-Ro (rarely)
HLA associations	B8, DR2, DR3, and DR4	B45, B49, B50, DR11(DR5) and DRw6

Source: From Ref. 500.

predominantly CD8 lymphocytes, whereas CD4 cells are prevalent in SS. EBV has been associated with both Sjogren's syndrome and DLIS; HIV has been detected in minor salivary ductal epithelium of patients with DILS (501,502). Persistent generalized AIDS lymphadenopathy involving periparotid/intraparotid lymph nodes adds another pathogenetic overlay to ARPC. The hyperplastic lymph nodes cause obstruction and cystification of intranodal salivary ducts (503).

Clinical. Patients typically present with painless enlarging parotid masses. Imaging studies reveal that these masses are usually multiple and bilateral. Patients may also complain of rheumatological symptoms such as arthralgias, lower back pain, fibromylagia, bursitis, tendonitis, and osteoarthritis (500).

Histopathology. ARPC comprises cystic dilatation of intranodal parotid ducts. The lymph nodes are reactive, usually with florid follicular hyperplasia and follicle lysis. A lymphoid infiltrate typically extends into the parotid parenchyma in a periductal manner (503). Lymphoepithelial islands are seen. There is histological overlap between ARPC and benign lymphoepithelial lesion (BLEL). BLEL tends to be more solid than ARPC, with a greater degree of acinar atrophy. Multinucleated giant cells with peripherally located nuclei are more often seen in ARPC, but are occasionally seen in BLEL.

Treatment. Patients with ARPC complain of cosmetic deformity. ARPC may regress spontaneously or after initiation of HAART (504). Cysts may be aspirated; doxycycline sclerotherapy can limit their growth or allow for regression.

AIDS-Related Nasopharyngeal Lesions

This is an adenoidal hypertrophy in AIDS patients relating to generalized persistent lymphadenopathy.

Adenoidal enlargement is a common, incidental imaging finding for HIV-seropositive patients (505,506). These patients may also be symptomatic and present with middle ear effusions, nasal obstruction, nasal congestion, pharyngitis, and lymphadenopathy (507,508).

Histopathology. The adenoidal hyperplasia is accompanied by follicular hyperplasia and follicular lysis. The latter finding appears as an influx of lymphocytes into follicles with fragmentation of germinal centers. Involuted follicles are also seen. The paracortical and interfollicular zones are expanded with immunoblasts and plasma cells. Multinucleated giant cells are seen and their nuclei are usually peripherally located but are occasionally located centrally. They are seen in early stage of HIV infection and absent from advanced stage disease (508).

The Herpesvirus family. Herpes comes from the Greek *"herpein"* meaning –"to creep,"as herpesviruses cause chronic/latent/recurrent infections. The Herpesvirus family is characterized by double-stranded DNA core surrounded by capsid proteins and ensheathed in an envelope. Herpesviruses pathogens include: Cytomegalovirus (CMV), Epstein-Barr virus (EBV), herpes simplex virus (HSV), and Varicella

Zoster virus (VZV). (Varicella zoster, the agent of chickenpox and herpes zoster, will not be included in the following discussions.)

B. Cytomegalovirus

CMV is a large herpesvirus (180 nm diameter) trophic for endothelial cells, B and T cells, mononuclear cells, neurons, and salivary gland. Symptomatic systemic infection can affect the retina, lungs, kidneys, gastrointestinal tract, and brain. CMV-infected cells are characteristically enlarged ("mega") with large eosinophilic intranuclear and amphophilic cytoplasmic inclusions.

Epidemiology

In the United States, between 50% and 80% of adults become infected with CMV by the age of 40. CMV is ubiquitous, and is more widespread in developing countries and areas with lower socioeconomic conditions. It is transmitted through sexual intercourse, saliva, blood, and breast milk. CMV is inactivated by heat, soap, detergent, and disinfectant and therefore is not transmitted by household contact (509). Latency follows infection; CMV latency does not involve a change in the pattern of viral transcription, rather CD8 cytotoxic T-cell suppression of CMV replication. Viral shedding ceases with latency, but can persist in children with congenital CMV infection, as well those with HIV seropositivity. CMV reactivation can develop, and is more likely to occur in the immunosuppressed. There are many different CMV strains with strain-specific mutations encoding for gB, an envelope protein and immune target. Strain-specific immunity, therefore, does not offer cross-protection. Up to 20% of immunocompetent individuals are infected with multiple CMV strains; the infection rate for multiple CMV strains is higher in HIV-seropositive individuals.

CMV is one of the most common of all congenital infections; approximately 30,000 to 40,000 infants are born annually with congenital CMV infection, and approximately 8000 of them have serious disabilities (510). In the United States, about 1% to 4% of women develop primary CMV infection during pregnancy. Maternal CMV infection is usually clinically silent; 5% of women develop mononucleosis-type symptoms (CMV disease). Vertical transmission occurs in 30% to 40% of primary maternal CMV infections, either transplacentally, during vaginal delivery, or by nursing. The risk of vertical transmission after CMV reactivation during pregnancy is much lower, around 1% to 3% (509).

Clinical Course: Congenital CMV

The earlier the intrauterine infection, the greater the impact seen. Infection during full-term delivery or nursing has no neurodevelopmental sequelae. About 10% to 15% of congenital CMV infections are symptomatic (509). Symptomatic congenital infections are associated with significant rates of disease mortality (30%); cognitive impairment (50–80%); sensorineural hearing loss (30–60%); visual impairment (20–35%);

and neuro-developmental, behavioral, and neuromuscular disorders (30–60%). Infants can demonstrate intrauterine growth retardation, hepatosplenomegaly, microcephaly, and cerebral calcifications; seizures, visual deficits, and hearing loss are common (511). One-third of children with symptomatic congenital CMV infection, however, have normal developmental outcomes. Conversely, some babies with asymptomatic congenital CMV infection do go on to develop deficits.

Clinical Course: CMV Infection in Organ Transplant Recipients

CMV infection is a major cause of morbidity and mortality in solid organ and bone marrow transplant recipients. Risk for active CMV infection is greatest for CMV naïve recipients of organs from CMV-seropositive donors. HLA donor/recipient disparities further increase the risk for posttransplant CMV infection.

The effects of CMV infection in transplant recipients can be classified as either direct or indirect. Infection is defined as a significant rise in CMV-specific serum antibodies. CMV disease is marked by fever, malaise, myalgias, and headache (512). Direct effects of CMV disease include pneumonitis, enterocolitis, nephritis, hepatitis, and encephalitis. Indirect effects of posttransplant CMV infection include allograph injury and rejection, increased cardiovascular complications, and more rarely, posttransplant lymphoproliferative disorder (PTLD). The risk of acute allograph rejection increases 60% with posttransplant CMV viremia and 150% with CMV disease (513). Chronic allograph rejection, myocardial infarction, heart failure, and cardiac arrhythmias are further sequelae of posttransplant CMV infection.

Clinical Course: CMV in AIDS

CMV was formerly one of the most important opportunistic pathogens for AIDS patients before the introduction of HAART; in this era of HAART, the incidence of CMV disease has greatly decreased. However, CMV still has a significant impact on the progression to AIDS. Patients seropositive for both HIV and CMV are 2.5 times more likely to progress to AIDS and death than HIV-seropositive/CMV-seronegative individuals (514). Plasma CMV viremia is a stronger predictor for CMV disease and death than CD4 cell counts or plasma HIV RNA concentration (514). CMV disease typically occurs when latent virus reactivates in AIDS patients with CD4 cell counts below 100 cells/mm^3 or when HAART fails to reconstitute normal CMV-specific immune responses.

CMV retinitis is the most common clinical manifestation, accounting for 85% of all CMV disease in AIDS patients. However, its incidence has dramatically dropped from 17.1/100 to 5.6/100 patient-years with the institution of HAART (512). Paradoxically, CMV retinitis is replaced by immune reconstitution uveitis, a serious complication of HAART, which also leads to blindness. Immune reconstitution uveitis develops in a substantial proportional of AIDS patients with CMV retinitis receiving HAART (515).

It is characterized by posterior chamber inflammation, macular and disc edema, neovascularization, cataracts, and epiretinal membrane formation. The intraocular inflammatory cells include CMV-specific cytotoxic T cells and increased CMV-specific Th2 cells (516). Other systemic manifestations of CMV disease in AIDS patients include gastrointestinal ulcerations (15%), pneumonia, and encephalitis, the latter of which now accounts for less than 1% of CMV disease in this group (666).

Clinical Course: CMV in the Head and Neck

Upper respiratory tract CMV disease was uncommon in AIDS patients in the pre-HAART era; currently it is even rarer. CMV disease can cause oropharyngeal, nasal, nasopharyngeal, and laryngotracheal ulcerations in patients with active AIDS (518–524). The ulcers are "well-punched out" without peripheral indurations (Fig. 43). Vasculitis due to CMV endothelial infection

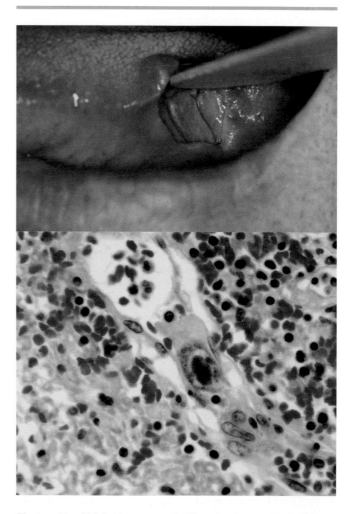

Figure 43 CMV. Upper panel: Sharply demarcated ulcer of lateral tongue. Lower panel: Endothelial cytomegalic cell with intranuclear amphophilic inclusions, peri-inclusion halo, and fine eosinophilic cytoplasmic inclusions (hematoxylin and eosin). *Source*: Courtesy of Dr. David A Evans, Sacramento, California, U.S.A. (upper panel).

appears to be an underlying disease mechanism. Ulcers are self-limiting and usually resolve with gancyclovir. CMV prophylaxis for organ recipients has rendered ulcerative CMV upper airway disease rare for this group too (525).

A vocal cord paralysis (without mucosal ulceration) has been reported secondary to laryngeal neuritis; CMV inclusions within the recurrent laryngeal nerve were demonstrated at autopsy (526). CMV parotitis has been reported; fine needle aspirate revealed the characteristic and diagnostic cytomegalic cells (527). Overall, CMV does not commonly cause symptomatic parotid disease and is not involved in the pathogenesis of ARPC (528).

Pathogenesis. CMV infects endothelial cells; detached circulating cytomegalic endothelial cells can serve as a vehicle, along with circulating infected polymorphonuclear cells and monocytes, for further disease dissemination (529). CMV also infects epithelial cells, renal tubules, and salivary ducts. In the brain, CMV infects all cellular components, including neuronal, glial, monocytic, and endothelial cells.

Viral synergy plays a crucial role in the downward spiral of immune function; CMV synergistically interacts with HIV to potentiate immunosuppression by a number of mechanisms. One such mechanism involves transactivation of viral activating factors. CMV produces transactivating proteins, which activate HIV LTR regions, thereby upregulating viral transcription and promoting active HIV replication. Specifically, CMV immediate-early region-2 protein can transactivate HIV LTR (530). Alternatively, CMV can induce cytokines that activate HIV-latent provirus through signal transduction (531). If CMV and HIV are coinfectants of the same cell, then HIV can form pseudotypes with an expanded tropism for cells with CMV receptors (532). In turn, upregulated HIV replication potentiates the reactivation of latent CMV infection, furthering the vicious cycle. H9 lymphoblastoid cell lines coinfected with HIV-1 and CMV demonstrate enhanced transcription CMV late region antigens as well as enhanced HIV replication (533).

CMV directly impairs cell-mediated immunity through a variety of mechanisms; infected monocytes have decreased antigen-presenting functions and downregulated IL-1 production (534). Marked decrease in IL-1 may contribute to the depressed lymphocyte responses. CMV can directly suppress null killer cell function and inhibit mitogen-induced T-cell proliferation (535). CMV has been demonstrated to have long-lasting influence on peripheral total lymphocyte counts; total CD8 T-cell counts are twice as high in older (>60 years) CMV-seropositive individuals as compared to CMV-seronegative cohorts (536). A relative inflation of CMV-specific CD8 T cells has been demonstrated in healthy elderly CMV-seropositive individuals (537). It has been postulated that the magnitude of CMV-specific CD8 clonal expansion occurs at the expense of a more generalized immune repertoire, thus contributing to aging immune senescence. Likewise, a relative expansion of CMV-specific CD8 T cells has been demonstrated in the immunosuppressed (538). Therefore

CMV can directly compromise immune function by overutilization of limited CD8 T-cell resources.

Histopathology. Cytomegalic-infected endothelial cells can be seen adjacent to ulceration. The classic cytomegalic cell has a large pink intranuclear inclusion, surrounded by a clear halo, and, less commonly, an amphophilic cytoplasmic inclusion (Fig. 43). The combination of intranuclear and intracyoplasmic inclusions is seen only in the lytic replicative phase, which occurs in a minority of infected cells. Infected cells produce a large amount of immediate early antigens (IEAs) and early antigens (EAs), which can be detected by IHC prior to replication and formation of classic CMV inclusions. In early infections, IHC for EA is therefore more sensitive than in situ hybridization for CMV genome.

Serology. Seroconversion can be reliably diagnosed by observed elevation of CMV IgG. Elevated serum CMV IgM suggests recent or ongoing infection. CMV DNA can be detected by PCR of whole blood, plasma, amniotic fluid, fetal cord blood, and cerebral spinal fluid.

Treatment. Currently, there is no available treatment for primary maternal infection during pregnancy. Polymerase inhibitors (Ganciclovir, Cidofovir, Foscarnet) and translation inhibitors (Fomivirsen) can be administered to immunosuppressed patients with CMV infection; these drugs are known animal teratogens and are not recommended during pregnancy. Ganciclovir is the recommended first drug of choice, and foscarnet should be reserved for ganciclovir-resistant CMV.

Control of CMV infection in organ recipients has resulted in significant reduction in rates of CMV disease and organ rejection. CMV-seronegative organ recipients benefit from valacyclovir prophylaxis with respect to lower acute rejection rates; however, this may be due to direct effects of the antiviral medication as most episodes of acute graft rejection occur prior to detection of CMV viremia (512).

C. Epstein-Barr Virus

This is an enveloped icosahedral herpesvirus with 173 kb double-stranded linear DNA, with a diameter of 110 to 120 nm. Epstein-Barr virus (EBV or HHV-4) is strongly tropic for B cells, epithelium, and T cells.

Overview and Pathobiology

The Epstein-Barr virus (EBV or HHV-4) is a member of the HHVs family and is ubiquitous throughout humanity. Most adults worldwide have antibodies to EBV. Subclinical seroconversion usually occurs at a young age under poorer socioeconomic conditions. In higher socioeconomic conditions, seroconversion occurs in teenagers and young adults and is associated with the clinical syndrome of IM.

The greatest relevance of EBV is as a promoter of malignancy. The development of an EBV vaccine would represent, in effect, a formidable anticancer campaign (539,540). Many carcinomas, lymphomas, and other lymphoproliferative disorders have

Table 8 Diseases Associated with EBV

Primary infection	Infectious mononucleosis
	EBV-associated hemophagocytic syndrome
	Gianotti-Crosti syndrome
Chronic infection and lymphoproliferative disorders	Lymphoproliferative disorders in immunocompromised hosts
	Duncan disease—X-linked recessive lymphoproliferative disorder
	Hemophagocytic lymphohistiocytosis
	Severe chronic active EBV infection
	Hypersensitivity to mosquito bites
	Hydroa vacciniforme
Lymphomas and leukemias	Burkitt's lymphoma
	Lymphoma in immunocompromised hosts
	Pyothorax-associated lymphoma
	Primary effusion lymphoma (coinfection with HHV-8)
	Methotrexate-associated lymphoma
	Lymphomatoid granulomatosis
	Sinonasal NK/T cell lymphoma
	Aggressive NK/T cell lymphoma/ leukemia
	Chronic NK cell leukemia
	Hodgkin's lymphoma
	Angioimmunoblastic T cell lymphoma
Carcinomas	Nasopharyngeal carcinoma
	Gastric carcinoma
	Okinawa oral squamous cell carcinoma
	Malignant lymphoepithelial carcinoma salivary glands
Other epithelial lesions	Oral hairy leukoplakia
Sarcomas	Leiomyosarcoma

well-established associations with EBV. Table 8 summarizes clinical conditions currently associated with EBV infection, many of which are beyond the scope of this chapter. How does a single virus induce such a wide range of neoplasia? The answer lies within host genetic and immunological factors as well as in various environmental factors, which promote the array of EBV-associated pathology.

EBV strains. EBV is genetically diverse, with a number of immunologically distinct genotypes (541–545). Geographic and host genetic predispositions appear to be the basis for the seroepidemiological findings. There are biological differences between EBV genotypes: genotype A (EBV-1) has a proclivity for B cells and transforms them into immortalized lymphocytoblastoid (LCB) cell lines with greater efficiency than genotype B, while genotype B (EBV-2) has increased lytic ability. However, there is generally no association between different genotypes inducing different pathologies; tumor genotype distribution tends to follow geographical prevalence. Overall, genotype A is the most commonly encountered, and is prevalent in nasopharyngeal carcinomas (NPC) from patients in Asia, Europe, and the United States. Genotype B (Jijoye virus) has been found predominantly in Central Africa and New Guinea, but still is less common than genotype A in these regions; it is

uncommon in NPC. Genotype C is prevalent in NPC from patients in Southern China. Genotype D is common in the United States, Africa, and Korea. Genotype F is commonly seen in NPC in patients from Southern China and Taiwan and is rare outside China. Multistrain coinfections can develop in both immunocompetant and immunocompromised patients (544–547).

Establishing latent infection—The lymphoid compartment. EBV is transmitted through saliva. After primary pharyngeal infection, EBV gains entry into mucosal-associated B cells by binding the viral glycoprotein gp350/220 (BLLF-1) with the CD-21 antigen (complement component receptor C3D, CR2). EBV infects resting memory B cells and successfully establishes latent infection in this compartment by ultimately escaping immunosurveillance. Latent infection is oncologically benign to both host and virus, as none of the latent proteins expressed drive cell growth.

Upon entry into B cells, EBV expresses EBV nuclear antigens (EBNAs) and latent membrane proteins (LMPs), which induce B cells to become activated proliferating lymphoblasts. The blasts migrate to the germinal centers, while the viral program shifts to coordinate LMP1 and LMP2 expression. LMP1 and LMP2 activate B cells in a ligand-independent manner, promoting latent infection by mimicking an antigen activated B-cell primary response without the necessity for normal external signaling by antigen-specific T helper cells. Thus EBV uses subterfuge rather than replication to promote latency; activated B cells amplify viral genome as they proliferate. Some of these activated B cells exit the cell cycle and persist as infected memory cells that do not elicit a cytotoxic T-cell response. Most B cells end-differentiate into plasma cells that are permissive for lytic viral replication (548,549).

Three latency profiles have been identified: only EBERs (see below) and EBNA1 are expressed in latency I; this profile is seen in Burkett's lymphoma (BL). In latency II, EBERs, EBNA1, LMP1, and LMP2 are expressed; this profile is seen in hairy leukoplakia and NPC. All of the latency proteins and EBERs are expressed in the latency III program, which is seen in immunosuppression-associated lymphoproliferations and in IM.

Establishing latent infection—The epithelial compartment. The upper airway epithelium predominantly serves as an important compartment for viral replication, amplification, and shedding. EBV is capable of infecting, replicating, and persisting in oropharyngeal and nasopharyngeal epithelium (550–556). Productive lytic lingual infection in HIV-seronegative individuals is rare (557). In vitro study demonstrates that cell-to-cell EBV infection may occur through apical CR2-like membrane receptors, whereas cell-free virion infection may occur at the basolateral cell membrane, and is mediated by integrins (554). In vivo study reveals that intraepithelial monocytes, rather than latently infected B cells, may be directly responsible for establishing infection in stratified oral epithelium (555). Latently infected memory B cells can become activated in immunosuppressed individuals, behaving like normal memory B cells in secondary response and transmitting EBV to submucosal monocytes. In turn, monocytes/macrophages transmucosally migrate, transmitting virus to differentiated epithelium in the stratum spinosum. Differential expression of EBV membrane glycoproteins impacts viral cellular tropism. EBV virions produced by B cells have a greater affinity for epithelium; they have low levels of membrane glycoprotein gp42, thus promoting efficient binding of membrane glycoprotein gHgLR onto epithelial cells. In contrast, virions produced within epithelium have greater efficiency in infecting B cells; they have high gp42 levels that bind HLA class II receptors on B cells (556).

Clonal infection. Latent EBV exists as a circular, nonintegrated episome. Particularities in episomal size allow for the determination of infection clonality. The terminal repeat (TR) sequences are 500-bp fragments, 4 to 12 copies of which normally flank each terminus of the viral genome; TR sequences facilitate circular episome formation. The number of TR sequences, and accordingly the total size of the episome, varies in increments of 500 bp. If tissues contain polyclonal populations of EBV-infected cells, digestion and Southern blot will reveal TR fragments of varying sizes with a "ladder" effect. A clonal expansion of EBV-infected tumor cells will reveal a dominant single band for the TR by Southern blot after restriction enzyme digestion. By extension, EBV viral clonality suggests that the tumor is a clonal expansion derived from a single EBV-infected cell. EBV integration, in addition to clonal episomes, can be detected in NPC, although it is not a necessary event (558).

EBV proteins: EBNA. EBNA are transcribed during early infection. EBNA1 is important in the establishment and maintenance of latent infection. EBNA1 tethers the origin of replication for the multicopy plasmid form of the viral genome (ori-p), enabling EBV to segregate with the host genome during mitoses and be transmitted to daughter cells of activated B cells (559,560). EBNA2 is a transactivating protein necessary for B-cell immortalization; EBNA2 transactivates cellular (CD21, CD23, C-FGR, c-MYC) and viral promoters (LMP1 promoter) through the Notch1 signal transduction pathway (561). EBNA leader protein (EBNA-LP) is a coactivator that reinforces the transactivating properties of EBNA2. EBNA3A, 3B, 3C are proteins that act as transcriptional regulators, with repressing and activating properties. EBNA3C recruits the human histone deacetylase to its targets (562). This can account for the silencing properties of EBNA3C, as histone deacetylation globally represses transcription. The removal of acetyl groups alters histone conformation, allowing them to wrap more tightly around the DNA, interfering with transcription.

EBV-encoded small RNAS. EBV-encoded small RNAs (EBER 1 and 2) are untranslated; nonpolyadenylated RNA sequences abundantly produced in latently infected nonreplicating cells, approximately 10^5 copies/cell. The functions of EBER1 and EBER2 remain elusive. It is likely that they act through binding to and modifying the properties of host cellular proteins. EBER is known to bind to at least three proteins: the La antigen; ribosomal protein L22 (EAP); and the INF-inducible, double-stranded RNA-activated protein kinase (PKR) (563,564). In vitro study reveals that high EBER expression in epithelial cell lines has transforming properties (565).

EBV proteins: LMP. As mentioned, the coordinated expression of LMP1 and LMP2 establishes latent EBV infection in memory B cells. LMP1 functions as a ligand-independent activated membrane receptor causing permanent activation of several signal transduction cascades, including NFkB and the c-jun N-terminal kinase (JNK)/AP-1 pathways (566,567). The C-terminal activating regions (CTAR1) of LMP1 interact with the TRAF [tumor necrosis factor (TNF) receptor-associated factors] family of proteins (568). Thus LMP1 acts as a constitutively activated member of the TNF receptor family and activates nuclear NFkB, a transcription factor, thereby initiating cell proliferation. LMP2A is also a membrane protein; its intracytoplasmic tail contains an immunoreceptor tyrosine-based activation motif (ITAM). Binding tyrosine kinases to phosphorylated LMP2A-ITAM suppresses the activating signal normally generated by the B-cell receptor (569).

LMP has been shown to have transforming properties for both epithelial and lymphoid cells. Transfected epithelial cells with upregulated LMP show decreased maturation, reduced cytokeratin expression, decreased desmosomal junctions, and features of transformation (loss of contact inhibition, anchorage-independent growth) (570–573). LMP1 has been shown to inhibit p53-mediated apoptosis in epithelial cells (574,575).

EBV protein: ZEBRA. Heterologous DNA (hetDNA) is a rearranged, inverted EBV DNA segment that contains BZLF1, a gene that triggers the transition from viral latency to productive lytic infection (576). BZLF1 encodes for ZEBRA (also known as Zta or EB-1), a DNA-binding transcriptional transactivator of EBV genes normally silenced during latent infection. The BZLF1 promoter region contains ZEBRA response elements (ZRE), whereby ZEBRA can amplify its own production. The BZLF1 promoter also has phorbol acetate (TPA) response elements (TRE), through which phorbol esters can disrupt latency. ZEBRA protein stimulates the production of Rta, an EBV protein encoded by BRLF1, and then ZEBRA and Rta synergistically activate transcription of a subset of early lytic cycle genes that encode proteins necessary for lytic EBV replication (577). ZEBRA binds to the origin of lytic cycle replication (oriLyt) and recruits other viral proteins essential for lytic replication.

It was originally suspected that ZEBRA could function as an oncoprotein, as it was demonstrated to bind tumor suppressor wild-type (WT) p53, but not the mutated p53 protein (578). However, the impact of ZEBRA on p53 function remains controversial; opposing effects on p53 transcriptional function has been found in different cell types. In some cell lines, BZLF1 potentiates p53 function and inhibits cell cycle progression (579). It has been speculated that BZLF1-induced activation of p53 function may enhance the efficiency of lytic EBV replication (580).

Infectious Mononucleosis

Clinical course. Primary EBV exposure during childhood is usually subclinical. IM can develop in one-third to one-half of individuals exposed to EBV after adolescence (581). The incidence of IM in the United States is estimated at 45/100,000 patients (582). Patients experience a nonspecific prodrome of headache, malaise, and fatigue for three to five days, followed by palatal petechiae, pharyngitis, tonsillitis, cervical adenopathy, abdominal pain, and fever (583). The pharyngitis/tonsillitis may be ulcerative, and in extreme cases causes upper airway obstruction. There is generalized lymphadenopathy including posterior cervical nodes and hepatosplenomegaly. Occasionally cardiac, respiratory, or renal complications occur. CNS involvement (meningitis, encephalitis, transverse myelitis, neuritis) can develop; these patients usually do not manifest the more typical features of pharyngitis and lymphadenopathy (583). Multiple cranial nerve palsies may occur (584).

IM is rarely fatal; deaths have resulted from splenic rupture, respiratory tract obstruction, hepatitis, hemophagocytosis, and encephalitis. Uncomplicated IM can resolve within three to four weeks; occasional patients are symptomatic for months, but IM rarely lasts longer than four months. The diagnosis of chronic fatigue syndrome (CFS) should be considered for patients remaining symptomatic after six months.

Children with IM tend to be less symptomatic with shorter illnesses than young adults, or have subclinical illnesses. Viral dose and the maturity of host immune system are thought to account for the differences between the pediatric and adolescent disease courses.

Pathogenesis. Replicating EBV is highly immunogenic, inducing a robust cytotoxic T-cell response. The characteristic peripheral lymphocytosis of IM represents an antigen-specific clonal expansion of CD8 T cells (583). High levels of circulating cytokines (TNF-α and IFN-γ) contribute to the systemic manifestations of IM. Acute IM resolves as the infected B cells are eliminated, but a residual pool of latently infected memory B cells remains. Some B cells will reenter the productive lytic phase as plasma cells; this is especially true for individuals who normally shed EBV in their saliva. However, the overall immune balance is maintained by cytotoxic T-cell surveillance of these reactivated plasma cells.

Histopathology. Lymph node biopsies or tonsillectomies are usually not performed for clinically typical cases of IM. Occasionally, one can see tonsillectomies from patients with recent IM. Reed-Sternberg-like cells and atypical lymphocytic infiltrate may be observed in these specimens, and one should be careful not to over diagnose HD. Interestingly, HD rarely involves the tonsil.

Lymph nodes in IM are generally partially effaced with follicular hyperplasia. The paracortical region is distended with proliferating immunoblasts, nuclear debris, and tingible body macrophages as well

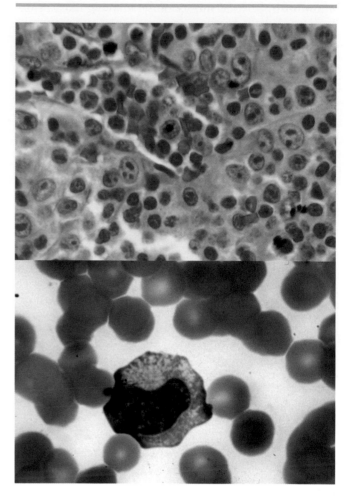

Figure 44 Infectious mononucleosis. Upper panel: This lymph node reveals proliferating immunoblasts in the paracortical region and atypical lymphocytes with irregular nuclear contours, coarse chromatin pattern, and multiple nucleoli. Lower panel: Downey cells represent atypical cytotoxic T-cells.

as Reed-Sternberg-like cells (Fig. 44). The immunoblasts may proliferate to the point of forming sheets, mimicking immunoblastic lymphoma.

Serology. Peripheral lymphocytosis is diagnostic for IM, with atypical T-cell lymphocytes or Downey cells. The "monospot" test (also called the heterophil test, Paul-Bunnell IgM test) screens for two or more non-Forssman IgM heterophil antibodies, which cross-react with glycolipids (Forssman antigens) found on RBCs from sheep or horses, but not other species. Patient serum is mixed with two different antigen suspensions: guinea pig kidney antigen will absorb Forssmann antibodies, which are nonspecific for IM, while the second antigen suspension, beef RBC stroma, will remove IgM (including EBV IgM) and serves as the negative control. The patient serum is then mixed with horse RBC. Serum from patients with IM adsorbed with guinea pig kidney will agglutinate the horse RBCs, whereas little or no RBC agglutination is seen with serum first adsorbed with beef stroma. The sensitivity of the monospot test is up to 90% by week 3 or 4.

If the monospot is negative, then specific antibody tests can be performed: IgG to EA and EBNA, and IgM and IgG to viral capsid antigen (VCA). VCA-IgM rises first and disappears after about four weeks. VCA-IgG peaks at weeks 2 to 4 and then persists for life at low levels. Rising VCA titers indicate reactivation of latent infection. Early antigen-diffuse (EA-D) IgG also rises early in the acute illness and disappears within three to six months. EBNA1 IgG rises after the second month and remains elevated throughout life.

Treatment. There is no specific treatment for IM; supportive treatment may be necessary to relieve symptoms. A short course of corticosteroids may be administered to relieve upper airway swelling.

Severe Chronic Active EBV Infection

Severe chronic active EBV (SCAEBV) infection is defined as persistently high EBV DNA in monocytes and plasma plus high titers of EBV antibodies; SCAEBV is seen most commonly in Japan (585–587). Patients with SCAEBV can develop pancytopenia, interstitial pneumonia, uveitis, and hepatitis. Some patients develop oligoclonal or monoclonal proliferations, which can culminate in either T-cell, NK-cell, or B-cell lymphomas. The prognosis of SCAEBV is very poor, with a mortality that approaches 50%. Patients usually die of lymphoma, haemophagocytic syndrome, or fulminant hepatitis.

Patients with SCAEBV may have congenital or acquired defective cytotoxic T-cell responses to EBV and also demonstrate evidence of infected activated Th1 and Th2 cells. This defective cytotoxic T-cell response may allow EBV to survive in NK or T cells as well as in B cells and contributes to the development of the disease.

EBV-Lymphoproliferative Disorders

Aids-related lymphomas. AIDS-related lymphomas (ARLs) are mostly of B-cell origin and contain clonal EBV. The predominant ARL is diffuse large B-cell type, often arising in the CNS. The associated EBV gene expression pattern resembles PTLD, suggesting a similar EBV-driven proliferative process that eventually leads to lymphoma. BL is a less commonly encountered type of ARL and resembles sporadic BL; only 30% to 40% of AIDS-related BL are associated with EBV (588). Chronic antigenic stimulation and HIV-induced B-cell proliferation contribute to the pathogenesis of ARL.

Posttransplant lymphoproliferative disorder. PTLD is a complication in transplant recipients treated with immunosuppressive drugs; the majority are EBV associated B-cell proliferations. In solid-organ transplant PTLD, the EBV is of host origin; in bone marrow transplant PTLD, the EBV is generally of donor origin (589). Frequently, PTLD is associated with primary EBV exposure; therefore testing donor and recipient EBV serostatus can assess risk for PTLD. The early PTLD process represents a polyclonal expansion of EBV-infected B cells that may spontaneously regress with reduction of immunosuppressive therapy or infusion of EBV-reactive cytotoxic T cells. PTLD can progress to a polymorphic B-cell proliferation with emerging malignant clones or develop into diffuse large B-cell lymphoma.

Ataxia-telangectasia. Ataxia-telangiectasia (AT) is characterized by cerebellar ataxia, telangiectasias, and susceptibility to infections and malignancies. This autosomal recessive syndrome is associated with mutations in AT-mutated (ATM) gene on chromosome 11q22–23, which encodes ATM protein kinase. ATM protein kinase is critical in activating p53 and promoting apoptosis in response to DNA double-strand breaks. Loss of ATM in AT patients renders them more sensitive to mutagens. AT patients also demonstrate deficiencies of EBV-specific immunosurveillance. Thus AT patients have an increased incidence of EBV-lymphoproliferative disorders (EBV-LPD) (590).

Wiskott-aldrich syndrome. Wiskott-Aldrich syndrome (WAS) is characterized by severe eczema, thrombocytopenia, and immunodeficiency. This X-linked recessive syndrome is associated with mutations in the WAS protein (WASP) gene located on chromosome Xp11.22–11.23. WASP is present only in hematopoietic cells and regulates actin polymerization; it is involved in actin cytoskeletal–based signal transduction pathways, filopod formation, and immune synapse formation (591). Most patients with WAS have defects in both cellular and humoral immunity. Lymphocytes and platelets from WAS patients show cytoskeletal abnormalities, and T cells show diminished proliferative response to stimulation through the T-cell receptor-CD3 complex. Defective immune synapse formation contributes to the immunodeficiency with loss of normal engagement between T-cell receptors and antigen-presenting cells (592). The combined immune defects render WAS patients vulnerable to EBV-LPD (590,593).

X-linked lymphoproliferative syndrome. Primary EBV infection usually progresses to a fatal illness for patients with X-linked lymphoproliferative syndrome (XLP, Duncan's disease, fatal mononucleosis). XLP is related to mutations in the signaling lymphocyte activation molecule (SLAM)-associated protein (SAP) gene on chromosome Xq25. SLAM is a self-ligand membrane protein on B and T cells that initiates signal transduction pathways; T-cell SAP binds to SLAM as a negative regulator. EBV immune response is generally over reactive because of nonfunctional SAP protein. EBV-CTL activity is diminished and the inhibition of NK cell function allows for the survival of EBV-transformed B cells. Individuals with XLP are usually asymptomatic until their first exposure to EBV. Primary infection generally causes severe or fatal IM associated with fulminant hepatitis and/or haemophagocytic syndrome. Long-term survivors often develop hypo- or agammaglobulinemia and/or malignant lymphoma (588,590).

Burkitt's lymphoma. BL is a high-grade lymphoma composed of small uncleaved lymphocytes. BL can be classified as endemic, sporadic, or AIDS related. Endemic BL is seen in African children, with a predilection for craniofacial bones and a strong association (>95%) with EBV (594). A massive prospective screening of about 42,000 Ugandan children was performed in the 1970s. Thirty-one children among this group developed BL, mostly in the mandible, maxilla, and orbit. Children with significantly elevated VCA antibodies had a thirty-fold excess risk of developing BL (594).

Sporadic BL is histologically identical to endemic BL, but represents a different disease entity. Sporadic BL is rare and uncommonly associated with EBV (15% of cases). It occurs in older patients; disease is most often intrabdominal (595). AIDS-related BL, as mentioned above, is similar to sporadic BL; only 305 to 40% of AIDS-related BL are associated with EBV (588). Rearrangement of the c-MYC proto-oncogene is a hallmark of all BL; over 80% of BL cases have a translocation of the c-MYC oncogene at q24, chromosome 8, most often to the Ig-heavy chain regions on chromosome 14 [t(8;14)(q24.1;q32)], or chromosome 2 (κ light chains) or chromosome 22 (λ light chains).

The "BL belt" is characterized by holoendemic malaria, poverty, and malnutrition. There is a significant association between malarial infection and the development of BL, but the relationship between these diseases is not well understood. Malarial infection is known to impair T helper cell function (596), which could allow for loss of EBV-specific immunosurveillance.

Indigenous plants in the "BL belt" promote BL; *Euphorbia tiruncalli* and other *Euphorbia sp.* are known to reactivate latent EBV infection through BZLF1 phorbol acetate (TPA) response elements. Extracts of *Euphorbia* have been shown to induce translocations in infected cord blood B cells and to reactivate lytic infection in Raji cells (597,598). *Euphorbia* plants are often used as oral medications for relief of headaches, sore throats, diarrhea, and wounds. For example, *Euphorbia tirucalli* leaves are boiled and ingested or the branches are roasted and chewed. The tendency for oral exposure is thought to promote the tumorigesis specifically in the jaws (599).

Hodgkin's disease. Indirect evidence has long supported an association between EBV and HD. Rising EBV antibody titers could be detected prior to the development of HD, and occasional cases of IM progressing to HD have been documented. Strong evidence for the pathogenic role of EBV comes from in situ studies (600). Up to 50% of cases of HD in the United States are associated with EBV (601,602). However, EBV-positive HD is even more common in underdeveloped countries, especially in children younger than 10 years (603–606). Three mechanistic models for HD have been proposed: HD of childhood (mixed cellularity, EBV+), HD of young adults (nodular sclerosis, EBV–), and HD of older adults (mixed cellularity, EBV+) (607). EBV is present in nearly 100% of AIDS-related HD (608).

Nasopharyngeal Carcinoma

NPC represents a malignancy with significant and distinct viral, geographic, racial, and ethnic associations.

EBV has been well established as a promoter of NPC. IgG and IgA antibodies to VCA and EA are commonly elevated among patients with NPC, and antibody titers have been demonstrated to rise prior to the discovery of carcinoma (609,610). NPC is endemic to Southern China, especially the Kwangtung province, and also the Kiangsu, Fukien, Taiwan, and Chekiang provinces (611). Elevated incidences are also found in Southeast Asia, Tunisia, Algeria, Morocco, Uganda, Kenya, New Guinea, Papua, Greenland, and the Arctic (612–616). In 2002, approximately 80,000 new cases were diagnosed worldwide; the estimated number of mortalities exceeded 50,000 (616). Migration of high- or intermediate-risk persons to lower-risk countries will not ameliorate this risk; southern Chinese living in Singapore, Malaysia, and Japan have rates of NPC comparable with natives of southern China. The incidence of NPC among Chinese living in the United States is about half of that observed in southern China, but remains 10 to 20 times higher than the incidence among U.S. whites and blacks (616). The incidence of NPC in North African immigrants and their offspring living in Israel is higher than in native Israelis. Familial aggregation of NPC is well documented; familial case clustering is the result of genetic susceptibility and the accumulation of environmental exposures. There is a 4- to 10-fold excess risk among first-degree relatives with NPC (614,617–619).

NPC and salted fish. Boat-dwelling fishermen and their families, known as Tankas, consume more salted fish and have a significantly higher incidence of NPC as compared with land dwellers. Ho first suggested the relationship between Cantonese salted fish intake and carcinogenesis in 1971. Salted fish is a cheap dietary staple in Southern China where the NPC incidence is 50/100,000, but is not a dietary staple in Northern China where the incidence of NPC is much lower (1/100,000) (611).

Traditionally, fish is salted rather than cooked, since fuel is much more expensive than the sea salt. Salted fish is commonly the first solid food given to weaned babies. Retrospective case-control study revealed that weekly ingestion of salted fish during childhood conferred 40 times excess relative risk (RR) in developing NPC. Salted Cantonese-type fish contains mutagenic nitrosamines and induces nasal and other tumors in rats (620–623). The source of nitrates in salted fish is related to the manner of fish preparation. Nitrates are present in the sea salt used to prepare the fish. Rather than gut and clean the fish after being caught, fish are salted whole and ungutted undergoing partial putrification (referred to as "soft meat"). Nitrate-reducing bacteria are responsible for the nitrate production (624,625).

NPC and smoke exposure. Cigarette smoking increases the risk for developing NPC by two- to sixfold, in a dose-related fashion (626–631). Prolonged exposure to indoor smoke is also an implicated promoter. The incidence of NPC in central Africa is greatest in the southern mountainous regions where cooking is performed indoors because of the cold climate. Smoke is a constant indoor companion for it is not vented through chimneys but escapes slowly and passively through thatched grass roofs. Specimens of soot taken from the interior of huts of patients with NPC contain significant amounts of carcinogenic aromatic hydrocarbons (612,632).

NPC and phorbol esters. Folk medicines and herbal drugs derived from native plants in Southern China and the central African BL belt also have carcinogenic effects. *Euphorbiaceae* and *Thymelaeaceae* are two families of trees, shrubs and bushes common to tropical and subtropical areas and have been used in the production of traditional herbal medicines. Case-control studies have demonstrated two- to fourfold excess risk of NPC in association with use of traditional medicines (628,633).

Examples of *Euphorbiaceae* and *Thymelaeaceae* include *Euphorbia lathyris, Croton tiglium, Croton megalocarpus, Croton macrostachyus, Jatropha curcas*, and *Aleurites fordii*; these plants contain diterpene esters (such as phorbol esters), which cause reactivation of EBV in latently infected Raji cells (634–636). Croton oil contains 12-0-tetradecanoyl-phorbol-13-acetate (TPA) and is a classic example of a tumor initiator. Tung oil is derived from *A. fordii*, and 85% of the world's tung oil is produced in Southern China. Tung oil is ubiquitous as a waterproofing agent, in wood polish, and in bases for oil paints, varnishes, and inks. Inhalation of pollen and contaminated soil dust can also exert a promoting effect; soil extracts from around *A. fordii* (tung oil trees) can reactivate latent EBV in Raji cells (635).

NPC and EBV. NPC is histologically classified as either keratinizing or nonkeratinizing, replacing the former WHO I/II/III classification schema (637). Nonkeratinizing NPC comprises 75% to 99% of all NPCs; nonkeratinizing NPC is further subclassified as either undifferentiated or differentiated. EBV is present in the majority of nonkeratinizing NPCs. In addition to the serological associations between EBV and NPC presented above, EBV clonality within NPC and precursor lesions provides irrefutable evidence for a causal relationship (638–640). In contrast, patients with keratinizing NPC generally do not have elevated EBV titers, and EBV in situ hybridization studies are negative (641,642).

EBV viral load can be used as a biomarker for prognostication and disease monitoring. Serum EBV DNA concentrations directly correlate with stage at diagnosis; they have been demonstrated to fall within hours of initial surgical therapy. If EBV DNA persists after surgery, then recurrence is likely. Overall, serum viral load is better than EBV antibodies titers with respect to prediction and detection of disease relapse (643–647).

Undifferentiated Salivary Carcinoma (Eskimo Tumor)

Undifferentiated salivary lymphoepithelial carcinoma is an uncommon malignancy with a predilection for Greenland Eskimos (Inuit's), Aleutians, and Chinese (648). These tumors are frequently associated with EBV; viral clonality and elevated serum antibodies have been demonstrated (649–653). Sporadic salivary lymphoepithelial carcinomas are rarer than the endemic form and their association with EBV is variable. Interestingly, two EBV positive salivary lymphoepithelial carcinomas have been associated with autoimmune syndromes (654). One unusual sporadic salivary lymphoepithelial carcinoma demonstrated transition to a low-grade myoepithelial component; both epithelial and myoepithelial components were positive for EBV (655).

Oral Hairy Leukoplakia

This is a hyperplastic oral lesion, usually on the lateral tongue, caused by productive EBV infection. It is usually seen in immunosuppressed patients; it is considered a marker for the progression to AIDS in HIV-seropositive individuals.

Background. The two most common oral AIDS lesions seen in the post-HAART era are OHL and OC. OHL was first described in AIDS patients (656,657) but can also be encountered in other immunosuppressed groups, and is occasionally seen in immunocompetent individuals (658–661). Subclinical OHL appears to be rare. In a screening study of 90 diabetic persons, 90 pregnant women, and 30 healthy controls, subclinical OHL was detected by cytology in only one (diabetic) subject (662).

Clinical presentation. OHL presents as a white plaque on the lateral tongue with ill-defined borders, and a raised, corrugated, or "hairy"-like appearance. It can also develop on other areas of the tongue or in the oral cavity (663) (Fig. 45).

OHL and the risk of progression to aids. OHL is considered a risk marker for the progression to AIDS. The presence of OHL has been significantly associated with high HIV viral loads (>3000 copies/ul), oral Candida, lack of HAART therapy, and the presence of antifungal therapy (664,665).

Histopathology. OHL is composed of hyperplastic, hyperparakeratotic squamous epithelium with "hair-like" keratin projections forming an irregular

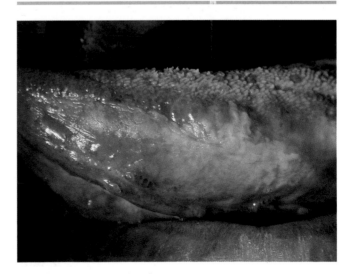

Figure 45 Hairy leukoplakia. Leukoplakic corrugated appearance of lesions on lateral tongue border. *Source*: Courtesy of Dr. Marie Ramer DDS, Mount Sinai, New York, U.S.A.

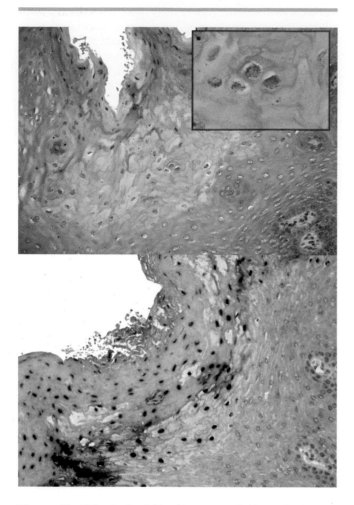

Figure 46 Hairy leukoplakia. Upper panel: Hyperplastic and hyperkeratotic lingual mucosa with a "spiky" surface. Inset: Nuclear chromatin condensed at the nuclear membrane results in a "string-of-beads"-like appearance. Intranuclear viral inclusions are present (hematoxylin and eosin). Lower panel: ISH for Epstein-Barr virus. *Source*: Courtesy of Dr. Adham Fahmy, Mount Sinai, New York.

ridged surface (Fig. 46). Characteristic intranuclear Cowdry A–type "ground-glass" inclusions can be seen in the upper stratum spinosum. Surrounding the intranuclear inclusions are "beads" of marginalized chromatin. Intracellular edema is seen. These cytological changes are sensitive indicators for EBV infection. Candida super infection may be present, but should not obfuscate the diagnosis.

Differential diagnosis. OHL is different from "hairy tongue"; the latter is a symmetrical lesion of the dorsal midline tongue. Hairy tongue may develop secondary to radiation, smoking, or antibiotic administration, which would alter normal bacterial flora; often its development is idiopathic. Histologically, hairy tongue is hyperkeratotic, but not hyperplastic, with abundant bacterial colonies. Intranuclear inclusions and koilocytic change are not seen.

Pathobiology of EBV infection in HL. OHL is characterized by high copy number of EBV in the

replicative phase; there is also evidence for latent epithelial infection (666,667). For each patient, multiple different EBV strains can be detected within the epithelial compartment (668,669). EBV-infected epithelium has the densest localization in the stratum spinosum (670–674). This leads to the hypothesis that the superficial tongue is directly and repeatedly infected by exposure to saliva (666).

EBV infection of the epithelial compartment may be established either by cell-to-cell transfer (cell transfer infection) or as a result of direct viral uptake by epithelial cells. Cell transfer is a much more efficient process than direct viral infection and is important in the promotion of lingual EBV infection. Cell transfer infection may be mediated by intraepithelial monocytes, Langerhan's cells (dendritic cells), or B cells (555,676,677). Cell transfer EBV infection mediated by B cells is likely important in Waldeyer's ring. In OLH, however, the process is probably not mediated by B –cells, as they are not a common intraepithelial component (667,675). It is likely that monocytes/ Langerhan's cells promote lingual EBV infection (555,675).

Marked tropism of cell transfer infection for differentiated stratified epithelium has been demonstrated (555,676,677), consistent with the finding of preferential localization of lytic and latent infection to the stratum spinosum. On the other hand, direct viral infection of epithelium is another possible mechanism, although less efficient. Cell-free virion infection can occur at the basolateral aspect of the cell membrane, and is mediated by integrins (554). This is consistent with the finding of EBV within the basal reserve layer of OHL by in situ PCR (678).

Treatment. Treatment options for patients with symptomatic OHL include surgery, systemic antiviral therapy, and topical treatment. Topical therapy is the first treatment of choice; podophylin resin/acyclovir cream has been demonstrated to completely resolve lesions (663). Surgery can provide relief from the symptoms of burning sensations, but does not prevent the development of new lesions. Systemic antiviral therapy is associated with adverse side effects (nausea, vomiting, diarrhea), and new lesions can reappear after the drug is discontinued.

Sinonasal NK/T-Cell Lymphoma

Sinonasal lymphomas can be classified as either NK/ T-cell or B-cell type; each group has unique geographic, etiological, and clinicopathological features. EBV is strongly associated with sinonasal NK/T-cell lymphomas; this phenotype is more common in Asian countries (Japan, China, Hong Kong, Indonesia) and Central and South America (679–685). Clonal EBV has been demonstrated within the neoplastic cells. The B-cell phenotype is rare in Asian patients with sinonasal lymphomas, and these tumors are invariably EBV-negative (686).

"Western" sinonasal lymphomas are more likely to have the EBV-negative B-cell phenotype (686,687). EBV-positive NK/T-cell phenotype sinonasal lymphomas are less common in Western populations; when seen, they often occur in patients of Asian or Hispanic descent (688). EBV is involved in the pathogenesis of upper aerodigestive tract B-cell lymphomas in the context of HIV-associated lymphomas or EBV-associated lymphoproliferative disease.

D. Herpes Simplex Virus

This is a double-stranded DNA (150 kb) herpesvirus that is trophic for epithelium and nerve ganglia. HSV-1 and HSV-2 are ubiquitously distributed worldwide. HSV-1 affects the upper airway; both HSV-1 and HSV-2 cause genital infections. HSV infection may also result in recurrent episodic or disseminated disease.

Epidemiology

HSV-1 is a ubiquitous virus; in less-developed countries, seroconversion happens during childhood or adolescence. It is transmitted by contact with infectious saliva, and can also be sexually transmitted. In more-developed countries, or middle- or upper-socioeconomic strata, seroconversion can take place between the 3rd and 4th decades of life. The U.S. seroprevalence for HSV-1 for the period of 1999 to 2004 was 57.7% (95% CI, 55.9–59.5%), which represents a significant decrease from the seroprevalence of 62% (95% CI, 59.6–64.6%) for the period of 1988 to 1994 (689).

HSV-2 is usually transmitted sexually. The U.S. seroprevalence for HSV-2 for the period of 1999 to 2004 was 17% (95% CI, 15.8–18.3%), representing a significant decrease from the seroprevalence of 21% (95% CI, 19.1–23.1%) for the period of 1988 to 1994 (689). Seroprevalence is higher in African-Americans than Caucasians, and females have slightly higher seroprevalence than males.

Clinical Course

Primary HSV-1 exposure/infection. Primary exposure to HSV-1 during childhood usually results in subclinical seroconversion. The incubation period ranges from 2 to 12 days, and is commonly four days long; it is followed by viral shedding into the saliva, which can last for 7 to 10 days, but may persist as long as 23 days (690). Intermittent HSV shedding in saliva can persist in up to 75% of asymptomatic individuals, and is a significant source of viral transmission (691–693).

Symptomatic primary oropharyngeal infection is characterized by a prodrome of fever, headache, and myalgias, followed by severe gingivostomatitis. The gums are red, swollen, and friable. Painful vesicles erupt on the inner lip, anterior gingiva, and oral mucosa (Fig. 47). Tiny vesicles may appear around the nose. The lesions heal within two weeks. Rarely, primary gingivostomatitis can progress to herpetic encephalitis, which is commonly fatal. Both symptomatic and subclinical primary infection result in latent HSV infection of sensory ganglion nuclei. The trigeminal ganglion is the primary site for HSV-1 latency.

HSV-1 can also be sexually transmitted and is an increasing cause for genital herpes. Genital HSV-1

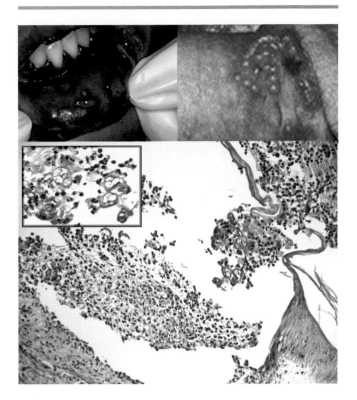

Figure 47 Herpes simplex. Upper left panel: Primary symptomatic HSV-1 infection. Vesicles on the inner lip, most are ulcerated and covered with a grayish slough. Upper right panel: Crops of penile vesicles in HSV-2 infection. Lower panel: Intraepithelial vesicle formation with acute inflammatory exudate. Inset: Large infected cells with pale "cleared out" nuclei (hematoxylin and eosin). Source: http://www.clinical-virology.org (upper left and right panels).

infections are less severe and less prone to recurrence than genital HSV-2 infections (690).

Reactivation of HSV-1. Reactivation (recrudescence) of latent infection occurs in up to half of infected individuals. It can be stimulated by emotional factors; hormonal changes; excess of sunlight, fever, trauma, and dental procedures. Reactivation results in viral replication within nerve ganglia; the virus then translocates anterograde to the dermatome. The patient experiences tingling and pain and then develops clusters of coalescing vesicles. The vesicles ulcerate and crust within 72 to 96 hours. Immunocompetent individuals tend to have mucocutaneous labial lesions, (herpes labialis) but not intraoral lesions. By contrast, AIDS patients with reactivated HSV-1 infection develop a wider distribution of oral lesions that persist longer (694). Mucocutaneous herpes lasting more than one month was an original defining AIDS criterion prior to serological testing, and remains a diagnostic criterion (Table 6).

Reactivation of HSV is one of the causes for Bell's palsy (695–697), in addition to Lyme's disease and VZV.

Herpetic whitlow. Herpetic whitlow refers to intensely painful pustules and vesicles that develop on the fingertips; they are caused by inoculation from oral or genital HSV lesions. Whitlow was an occupational hazard of hospital personnel and dentists in the era prior to universal precautions. Whitlow can be seen in thumb-sucking children, individuals with a history of oral or genital herpes, and immunocompromised patients.

Primary HSV-2 exposure/infection. HSV-2 is associated with genital herpes and is usually sexually transmitted. The majority of HSV-2 seroconversion is asymptomatic (698). HSV-1 antibodies protect against HSV-1 genital infection but not HSV-2 infection; the presence of HSV-1 antibodies reduces the severity of HSV-2 disease (690).

Symptomatic primary HSV-2 infection is associated with fever, malaise, and lymphadenopathy. Men develop painful penile vesicles, dysuria, and penile discharge (Fig. 47). Women develop vulvar and cervical lesions, and experience vulvar pain, and dysuria. Although uncommon, HSV-2 can also cause oral ulcerations.

Reactivation of HSV-2. The major morbidity of HSV-2 infection is the high rate of reactivation. In one study, 90% of patients experienced symptomatic recurrence within the first 12 months; 38% had 6 recurrences and 20% had more than 10 recurrences in the first year (699). In general, subclinical and symptomatic reactivated infections are more common with HSV-2 than HSV-1. Recurrent HSV-2 infection is preceded by a prodrome of tenderness, pain, and burning at the site of eruption; the symptoms are more severe in women than in men. Women develop painful genital vesicles that heal within 8 to 10 days. Men develop penile vesicles. Asymptomatic HSV-2 reactivation has also been associated with HSV-2 oral shedding, implying a more generalized systemic process (700).

Disseminated HSV infection. Disseminated HSV infection can develop in pregnant women, immunosuppressed individuals, including transplant recipients, cancer patients, and rarely in immunocompetent individuals; disseminated infection progresses rapidly to cause encephalitis, hepatitis, multiorgan failure, and death (701–704). Localized HSV lymphadenitis and tonsillitis have been rarely reported (705–709).

Neonatal HSV infection. Symptomatic or asymptomatic pregnant women shedding HSV can infect their babies; pregnant women with primary genital HSV infection have the highest risk of neonatal transmission (710). The majority of HSV-infected infants are born to asymptomatic mothers; babies can develop encephalitis, keratoconjunctivitis, and hepatitis. The unfortunate sequelae of TORCH (Toxoplasmosis, Other Agents, Rubella, CMV, and Herpes Simplex) neonatal infections include mental retardation, microencephaly, microphthalmia, and blindness.

Pathobiology of HSV—lytic infection. HSV binds to epidermal, mucosal, and neuronal cells by attaching to heparin sulfate proteoglycan receptors via gB and gC viral glycoproteins; binding of gD to membrane receptors triggers fusion of the viral envelope with the cell membrane (711). The HSV capsid is transported to the nuclear pores. The genome is released intranuclearly, it circularizes and transcription commences.

Several viral talents enable HSV to achieve productive infection: it subterfuges host RNAPII for viral transcription (712), and it causes degradation of most cellular synthetic processes (713). The latter process is efficiently accomplished by "virion host shut-off protein" (VHS or UL41) (714).

HSV encodes three sets of genes: alpha, or immediate early genes; beta, or early delayed genes; and gamma, or late expressed genes. α-Trans-inducing factor (α-TIF or virion protein 16) is a viral tegument protein that induces transcription of immediate early proteins (715). Five IEAs are expressed 2two to four hours after infection, which regulate viral gene expression. "Infected cell polypeptides": ICP0, ICP4, and ICP27 are consecutively expressed α-gene products, which regulate expression of beta and gamma genes (716).

Late (χ) genes are transcribed seven hours after infection and encode for membrane glycoproteins; however, some χ genes (encoding gB and gD) are expressed early. Transcription of both β and χ genes are dependent on the trans-activator ICP4 (717). (Interestingly, in the recurrent theme of viral-viral interactions, ICP4 is able to transactivate promoter regions in HPV16 early regions and HIV LTR) (718,719).

HSV plasmids are produced in a "rolling circle" mechanism within the host nucleus, yielding concatemers that are cleaved, and packaged, into awaiting preformed capsids. Virion envelopes are derived from host nuclear membrane; the host nuclear membranes develop thick reduplicated patches, which contain viral glycoproteins. Virions travel through the cytoplasm to egress via cytoplasmic vesicles.

HSV latency. After primary infection, HSV is transported retrograde in type C neuronal axons to the ganglia, where it establishes latency (720). Infectious virions or viral proteins are not detected, enabling latent infection to evade immunosurveillance. ICP0 protein is encoded by the HSV-1 α0 gene (also referred to as "alpha zero" or IE110) and is a candidate gene regulator of reactivation (715). During latency, latency-associated transcript (LAT), a viral RNA transcript, inhibits HSV-1 α0 expression by an antisense microRNA mechanism (721). LAT transcripts also block apoptotic pathways, downregulating TGF-β1 and SMAD3 and inhibiting caspases (722,723). Inhibition of host apoptosis is an important survival mechanism enabling viruses to perpetuate latency.

HSV interference with cell-mediated immunity. One of the mechanisms by which HSV interferes with cell-mediated immunity is through the inhibition of antigen presentation. ICP47 is produced during the second hour of keratinocyte infection. ICP47 binds and inactivates cellular peptide transporter proteins, (TAP, transporter-associated with antigen presentation), thereby interfering with the transport of viral peptides and their presentation to HLA class I molecules within the endoplasmic reticulum (720). Thus HSV-infected cells lack membrane HLA class I molecules and elude cytotoxic T-cell detection. Becker proposed an interesting hypothesis regarding the evolutionary role of pain in HSV's ability to evade immune detection and gain access to sensory neurons

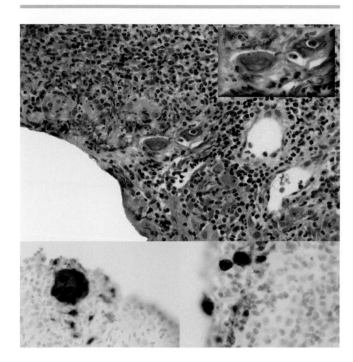

Figure 48 Herpes simplex. Upper panel: An oral ulceration due to HSV infection. Inset: Characteristic nuclear molding is seen in these multinucleated cells (hematoxylin and eosin). Lower panel: Immunohistochemistry for HSV-1.

(720). The CGRP neuropeptide (calcitonin gene–related peptide) is released by type C axons in the skin and mucosa and is responsible for the sensation of pain. CGRP also suppresses the antigen presenting function of Langerhan's cells. The hypothesis states that HSV evolved to infect skin and mucosa using pain to inactivate Langerhan's cells and downstream antigen-presenting activities. Furthermore, HSV infects immature dendritic cells (Langerhan's precursor cells), thereby gaining access to type C neurons.

Histopathology. The hallmark of HSV infection is intramucosal/intraepithelial vesicle formation (Fig. 47). Infected nuclei are enlarged, with homogeneous basophilic or clear ground-glass inclusions and peripheral chromatin beading. These nuclei are present in the basal and parabasal layers of early lesions and extend throughout the epithelium in later lesions. Multinucleated syncytial cells can be seen with intranuclear and cytoplasmic inclusions (Fig. 48). The multiple nuclei "mold" with each other, rather than overlap one another.

HSV infection of solid organs results in zones of necrosis. Ghost cells with intranuclear inclusions, and multinucleated syncytial cells, can be observed at the periphery of the necrosis.

The differential diagnosis includes EBV infection; the nuclear chromatin can marginate, causing a beaded appearance for both HSV and EBV infections. EBV infection is not associated with vesicle formation or necrosis. Measles infection results in multinucleated syncytial giant cells; these nuclei appear crowded and overlapping, with prominent eosinophilic nuclear and cytoplasmic inclusions.

IHC for HSV antibodies will be helpful in confirming the diagnosis; intranuclear immunostaining should be seen.

Treatment. Antiviral drugs targeting viral DNA synthesis are effective against HSV; these drugs inhibit virus replication and may shorten the duration of symptoms; they do not eradicate HSV. Acyclovir is the drug of choice for initial and recurrent genital HSV; mucocutaneous HSV, HSV encephalitis, and suppressive HSV therapy. Oral acyclovir can be effective in suppressing herpes labialis in immunocompromised patients with frequently recurrent infections. Famciclovir and valacyclovir can be administered for recurrent genital HSV.

E. HPV

This is a large group of small double-stranded DNA epitheliotrophic viruses with 8000 bp. The viral capsid is 20-sided icosahedral structure composed of 72 capsomeres. In the head and neck, HPV is the causative agent for laryngeal papillomas, sinonasal papillomas, and a subset of squamous cell carcinomas (SCCs).

Overview: Transmission and Pathobiology of HPV

The warts of the horned cottontail rabbit are known to regress spontaneously, even after malignant transformation (Fig. 49). Pedestrian skin warts, condylomata, and laryngeal papillomas, likewise share the mercurial quality of "here today, gone tomorrow"; they are impacted by hormonal, immunological, psychological, and other factors yet unknown. Papillomavirus is both a ubiquitous and mysterious foe of humanity, causing warts of little consequence and benign and malignant diseases of significant morbidity and mortality.

Transmission of HPV. It is well established that urogenital and upper airway HPV infections can be transmitted by sexual activity. Patients with HPV-positive oropharyngeal SCC are likely to have antibodies to HPV16 L1, a validated measure of lifetime sexual exposure (724,725). Upper airway infection can also occur by vertical maternal fetal transmission, either through direct exposure during vaginal delivery or intrauterine exposure (desquamated cells within amniotic fluid or transplacental). Lastly, transmission can occur through routine household contact (sharing eating utensils) and autoinoculation.

A recent literature meta-analysis examined the HPV recovery rates from neonatal oral and/or genital samples taken at the time of delivery (726). The authors found that the pooled transmission rate from mother to child was 18% for vaginal deliveries and 8% for Cesarean sections. For babies born to HPV-positive mothers, the pooled RR of neonatal exposure is 4.8 (95% CI, 2.1–10.9). The data, however, did not support the recommendation of Cesarean section for all HPV-positive mothers. Interesting, some neonates with positive samples had HPV-negative mothers raising the issue of other exposure sources such as equipment or personnel (727).

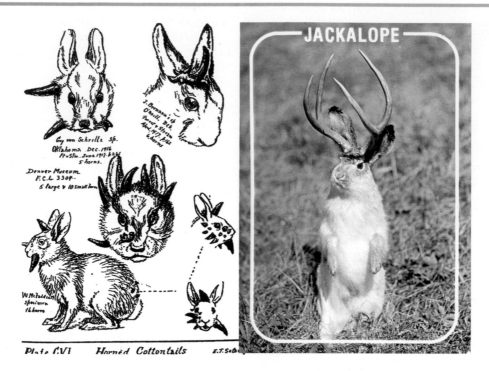

Figure 49 Left panel: The Shope virus was originally isolated from the keratinous growths of "horned" cottontail rabbits in the West. Right panel: The "jackalope" of barroom fame, may have been inspired by sightings of these horned cottontails.

The pertinent question is, "How often does neonatal exposure result in clinical infection?" Prospective longitudinal studies indicate that HPV recovery rates in oral and/or genital samples from exposed neonates fluctuate with time and are probably influenced by maternal anti-HPV antibody transmission through breast milk (728). Studies in preschool children further support the transient nature of subclinical oral HPV infections as well as the acquisition of new infection from household members or other children (729).

Juvenile onset laryngeal papillomatosis (JOLP) is the result of vertical maternal fetal transmission. JOLP is extremely rare in the overall population (4.3/ 100,000 children), in contrast to the high prevalence of HPV. The most frequent manifestation of genital HPV is cervical dysplasia; genital condylomas are less common by one or two orders of magnitude. The presence of genital condylomata during pregnancy put babies at risk for developing JOLP; 68% of patients with laryngeal papillomas surveyed confirmed maternal histories of condylomata (730). JOLP has been estimated to occur in 7 of every 1000 infants born to mothers with genital condylomata during pregnancy; the RR of developing JOLP in this setting was 231 (95% CI, 135–396) (731). Interestingly, the next generation does not appear to be affected; children born to parents with recurrent respiratory papillomatosis (RRP) were not affected with laryngeal papillomas (732). We will see below that oropharyngeal HPV infection is an important mechanism of head and neck SCC carcinogenesis. Could neonatal/childhood

HPV acquisition also contribute to oropharyngeal carcinogenesis? This may be so, as HPV infection has been detected in tonsillectomy specimens of asymptomatic children, including high-risk (HR)-HPV (733–735).

Pathobiology of HPV. Papillomavirus was first extensively studied in cotton-tailed rabbits by Richard Shope (736). There are numerous mammalian species-specific forms of PV. The HPV genome is roughly one-twentieth the size of herpesvirus genome, with a fraction of encoded proteins compared with herpesvirus. Yet HPV has tremendous genotypic diversity; over 100 different human types are known. A viral type is defined as having 50% or more unique genomic sequences when compared with other known types. HPV types have been classified into HR, representing HPV 16,18,31,33,35 and low-risk (LR), representing HPV 6,11,13,32,34,40,42,44,53,55,63.

Some HPV types have well-established associations with various entities. HPV2 and HPV4 cause cutaneous and oral verruca and HPV1 and HPV2 cause plantar warts. HPV7 is associated with "Butcher's warts." HPV5 and HPV8 are associated with epidermodysplasia verruciformis; an uncommon autosomal recessive disorder characterized by multiple, flat warts with a propensity for malignant transformation. HPV13 is usually found in Heck's disease, an intraoral form of flat condylomas. HPV6 and HPV11 are commonly associated with benign condylomas and exophytic papillomas of the anogenital region and upper aerodigestive tract. HPV16, 18, and occasionally 31, 33, and 35 are associated with uterine cervical dysplasia and neoplasia, VC, and oropharyngeal carcinomas. Occasionally multiple viral types can be present within a lesion; rarely LR-HPV alone can be identified within cancers.

The life cycle of HPV is tightly regulated by the state of differentiation of the host epithelium. There are three modes of HPV DNA replication. Initial HPV infection targets basal and parabasal cells; some mucosal/epidermal abrasion is necessary to establish infection here. During initial basal cell infection, HPV produces between 50 and 100 episomes per cell. The second mode represents low-level replication in the basal cells, which serve as the reservoir for the duration of infection. During this phase the HPV genome replicates once per S phase. The third phase is called vegetative DNA replication. Virion production can occur only in more the terminally differentiated keratinizing ("permissive") cells of the stratum spinosum and stratum granulosum.

The HPV genome is divided into E (early) and L (late) regions: the early regions promote viral replication and regulate viral functions, while the late regions are necessary for virion production (737,738). The E1 and E2 proteins are replication factors; E1 protein has helicase activity and promotes HPV DNA strand separation ahead of the replication complex. E2 protein recruits host polymerases and accessory proteins to coordinate viral transcription and replication. E2 protein also functions as transcriptional activator of E6 and E7 at low concentrations and suppresses transcription of these genes at high concentrations. The E4 protein facilitates cellular maturation and nonlytic HPV release.

HR-HPV genome contains two important promoters, the early promoter (known as p97 for HPV16 and HPV31 and p105 for HPV18) initiates transcription upstream of the E6 open reading frame (ORF). The late promoter, p742, is located in the E7 ORF; it is activated during the vegetative replication phase of HPV.

HR-HPV E6 protein has an affinity to bind host WT p53 protein as part of a complex with ubiquitin ligase, thus abrogating the proapoptotic tumor-suppressor pathway. HR-HPV E7 protein has an affinity to bind pRB (retinoblastoma protein), thus deregulating cell-cycle progression to S phase. Normally, cells migrating from the basal reserve layer cease to enter the mitotic cycle, but HR-HPV E7 is responsible for reentry of infected cells into the cell cycle despite their upward migration. The mechanisms by which HPV promotes carcinogenesis will be further discussed at the end of this section.

The upstream regulatory region (URR), also referred to as "long control region," or LCR, is a noncoding region located between the L1 and E6 regions. The 5' segment of URR contains transcription termination signals and a nuclear matrix attachment region (which organizes the attachment of viral DNA to nucleosomes), the central region contains epithelial-specific enhancer regions, which promote HPV-type specific tissue tropism, and the 3' segment contains the replication origin and E6 promoter (739).

L1 and L2 regions encode capsid proteins; they are expressed only during productive infection. The L1 protein (major capsid protein) is able to self-assemble into virus-like particles inducing a host immune response. The HPV vaccine Gardasil is composed of HPV 6/11/16/18 L1 proteins.

Heck's Disease (Focal Epithelial Hyperplasia, Multifocal Papillomavirus Epithelial Hyperplasia)

Clinical presentation. Focal epithelial hyperplasia (FEH), or Heck's disease, has a strong genetic predisposition, and is seen among American Navajo Indians, South American Indians, Greenlandic, Alaskan, and Canadian Eskimos, and Laplanders; it is extremely rare among Caucasians (740–743). It is usually diagnosed within the first two decades of life.

The lesions are soft, pale, sharply circumscribed, and elevated, round to oval, papular or plaque like, either red, pink, gray, or white (Fig. 50). They have a smooth pearly surface and "disappear" when the mucosa is stretched. They may be single, but often are multiple and clustered; in extreme cases the confluent lesions result in a "cobblestone" mucosa. For this reason, the term "multifocal papillomavirus epithelial hyperplasia" has been suggested as a replacement for "FEH" (744). There is a predilection for the lower lip, buccal mucosa, tongue, and commissure.

Etiology. HPV13 is usually detected within the lesions (741,742); HPV32 is detected less frequently (742,745). Transmission occurs via routine household contact; it is common for siblings to be affected (743).

Histology. Lesions are characterized by hyperkeratosis, parakeratosis, hyperplasia, acanthosis, and elongated anastamosing rete pegs. The horizontal outgrowth of the distal rete pegs has been likened to a "bronze age ax" (Fig. 50). Squamous metaplasia and hyperplasia may be present in underlying minor salivary ducts. Typical koilocytes can be seen. A characteristic finding is "mitosoid" nuclear degeneration; the nuclei are enlarged with clumped chromatin mimicking mitotic figures.

Treatment. The lesions may regress spontaneously. Persistent lesions can be treated with CO_2 laser excision and INF (topical or systemic) (746,747).

Condylomata, Papillomata, Verruca, Bowenoid Papulomatosis

Clinical presentation. Condylomata accuminatum, squamous (or exophytic) papillomata, verruca, and Bowenoid papulomatosis (BP) are all HPV-related lesions; each has a characteristically distinct histological appearance. They may be seen in both immunocompetent and HIV-seropositive individuals. Since the institution of HAART therapy (1996 and onward) the incidence of HPV oral mucosal lesions has been *increasing* (748).

These lesions can occur in the oral cavity, especially the labial mucosa, tongue, buccal mucosa, and floor of mouth. They can be single or multiple, sessile or pedunculated, and variably sized. They are soft, white/gray, with a papillary, "pebbly," spiky surface or cauliflower-like (749,750).

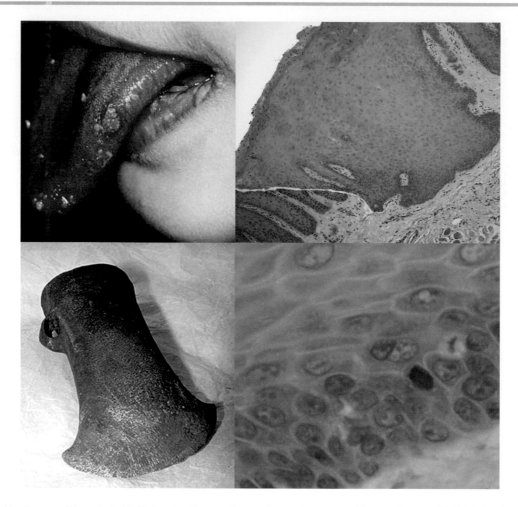

Figure 50 Heck's disease. Upper left: Multiple raised, smooth papules on tongue and lips on 4-year-old child. (746). Upper right: The silhouette of the broadened and hyperplastic epithelium has been likened to a "Bronze age axe." Lower left: "Bronze age axe." Lower right: Brick-shaped "mitosoid" body.

Bowenoid papulosis deserves specific mention; the term "Bowenoid" was coined to distinguish it from Bowen's disease (BD), also known as erythroplasia of Queyrat. BD describes a solitary erythematous macule of the genital skin, which histologically corresponds to carcinoma-in situ (CIS). As would be expected, BD can progress to invasive SCC. In distinction, the term "Bowenoid papulomatosis" was originally coined to describe lesions that resembled BD histologically (CIS), but clinically differed in their appearance (single or multiple *raised* lesions) and biological potential (cured by excision). Mucosal BP can occur in the oral cavity, and may be seen in immunosuppressed patients as well as immunocompetent individuals (751,752). The reader should be aware that a spectrum of HPV-related oral dysplastic lesions exists, including "koilocytic dysplasia" and "dysplastic warts."

Etiology. Squamous papillomas and condylomas are associated with LR-HPV. HR-HPV can also be detected in oral condylomata from immunocompetent and HIV-seropositive patients (753). BP has been

associated with HPV16/18 as well as other HR-HPV (751,752). More unusual HPV types may be associated with oral lesions in AIDS patients, such as HPV7, which is usually associated with "Butcher's" warts, and HPV32, which is occasionally associated with Heck's disease (754). Verrucas are associated with HPV2 and HPV4 (755–757).

Histology. Condylomas and papillomas are characterized by papillary proliferations of acanthotic and parakeratotic squamous epithelium. Papillomas tend to be more exophytic with well-defined fibrovascular stalks, whereas condylomata are more sessile, broad based, with extension of the proliferating epithelium into underlying minor salivary ducts. Condylomas may have thin elongated rete pegs pointing toward the center of the lesion, a feature lacking in papillomas. Koilocytes, defined by condensed "raisin-shaped" nuclei, or binucleated or multinucleated cells, plus perinuclear halos, may be seen in either entity.

Verrucas are hyperplastic, hyperkeratotic lesions with an exophytic serrated surface contour. Serrated spires are produced by pointed mounds of parakeratosis. A pronounced granular layer is present, even in mucosal verruca, and is generally not present in condylomas and papillomas. The rete pegs of verruca are also elongated and relatively thin, pointing toward the lesion's center.

The CIS of BP histologically differs from conventional CIS. The histological elements of BD include dyskeratotic cells, multinucleated cells, apoptotic fragments, atypical mitotic figures, and mitosoid bodies scattered throughout the mucosa; it may or may not have a full thickness distribution. Hyperkeratosis is usually present with a variable degree of verrucoid hyperplasia.

Treatment. All of these lesions can be treated by conservative excision, laser ablation, cryotherapy, or topical podophylin. Injected or topical INF has also been used to treat BP. Immunosuppressed patients are more likely than immunocompetent patients to develop recurrent lesions. BP usually follows an indolent course and may occasionally regress. However, BP can recur after excision and occasionally can progress to invasive carcinoma.

Laryngeal Papilloma

Juvenile onset laryngeal papillomatosis.
Clinical Presentation. The initial presentation of JOLP may be within the first few months after birth up to the second decade of life, with no gender predominance. (758). Hoarseness and weak cry are common presentations. Laryngoscopy reveals papillomas, which can be single or multiple and virtually carpeting the endolarynx.

Clinical Course. Multiple recurrences (RRP) are a common and serious consequence of this disease. Progression to RRP can be predicted by initial presentation with multiple lesions at four years of age or younger (759). A grimmer outcome is the extension of papillomas into the trachea, bronchi, and lungs, which can develop in 9% of individuals (758). Previous tracheostomy put children at risk for this complication. RRP can resolve at puberty, but may also persist into adulthood. Malignant change can occur in RRP, either with the acquisition of HR-HPV or in concert with external promoters such as irradiation, and cigarette smoking (760–763).

Etiology. An infectious etiology for laryngeal papillomas was suspected by Ullman in 1923; he was able to produce papilloma-like growths on his arm and that of his assistant after injection of cell-free tissue extracts derived from a laryngeal papilloma from a child (764). LR-HPV causes laryngeal papillomas; HPV11 is associated with more aggressive clinical course than HPV6 (758). HPV remains in the surrounding laryngeal mucosa and is the source of disease recurrence (765).

HPV may evade immune recognition by down-regulating class I MHC cell surface expression via decreased TAP-1 levels. TAP proteins facilitate the entry of viral peptides into the rough endoplasmic reticulum, making them available to be complexed with MHC-I molecules. There is a statistically significant correlation between decreased TAP-1 expression

in tissues and disease recurrence (766,767). We have seen the identical mechanism of immune evasion by HSV.

Adult onset laryngeal papillomas.
Clinical Presentation. JOLP and adult onset laryngeal papillomas (AOLPs) are considered the same disease; they are both caused by HPV infection and have the potential to develop multiple recurrences. Yet striking epidemiological and clinical distinctions remain between the two entities. AOLPs occur after the second decade of life, with a strong male predominance; laryngeal infection may be sexually transmitted (768). Patients who present with single lesions are less likely to develop RRP (769).

Treatment. Microlaryngoscopy with laser excision is the therapeutic mainstay. The goals of surgery are symptomatic relief and airway maintenance. It may be necessary to leave behind papilloma in the regions of the anterior commissure and posterior cricoid to avoid laryngeal scarring. INF-α therapy is associated with decreased disease severity for RRP, however therapy cessation results in relapse, and prolonged drug use is associated with significant side effects. Intralesional injections with cidofovir have been used for both JOLP and AOLP (770,771). Cidofovir is a cytosine nucleoside analogue of deoxycytidine monophosphate; its metabolite becomes incorporated into the viral DNA and acts as a competitive inhibitor to viral DNA polymerase. HPV lacks its own DNA polymerase and hijacks the host polymerase for replication. Therefore the mechanism by which cidofovir impacts HPV is unclear. Lastly, vaccination trials for RRP patients using immune modulating heat shock protein linked to HPV6/11 proteins are under development (772).

Verrucous Carcinoma And Verrucous Hyperplasia

VC—historical perspective. VC is a clinicopathologically distinct well-differentiated variant of SCC, which is "cytologically benign yet clinically aggressive." It was brought to the attention of pathologists by Ackerman in 1948 (773). Rudolf Virchow and Heinrich Waldeyer had become unfortunately well acquainted with VC during the autopsy of Prince Frederick III of Germany. He died with of a long-standing, indolent, and unrecognized laryngeal VC that ultimately progressed to develop squamous carcinoma (774). Virchow had examined many biopsies from Prince Frederick's laryngeal tumor and pronounced them benign due to the lack of infiltration and pleomorphism.

Clinical presentation. VC presents as a slow growing gray/white firm warty tumor with a cauliflower-like surface and sharply demarcated margins. A male predominance is seen with VC (775). There is also an association with cigarettes and chewing tobacco for oral VC. The oral cavity is a common site for VC, usually on the buccal mucosa or gingiva; the larynx is a less common site.

Etiology. Similarities of VC to the "Buschke-Lowenstein" giant condylomas fueled interest in the association of VC and HPV. HPV (mostly HPV18) has been detected in 20% to 100% of patients with oral, labial, or laryngeal VC (776–781).

Histology. Superficial biopsies are notorious for revealing only dense hyperkeratosis and parakeratosis without any dysplasia. The diagnosis of VC relies on identifying broad, hyperplastic, pushing, and club-shaped rete pegs; these regions also contain minimum anaplasia. Pathologists and surgeons should always bear in mind the possibility of a "hybrid tumor," i.e., the spontaneous or postradiation occurrence of both a VC and a squamous carcinoma. Many sections must be examined to rule out this possibility; cervical lymph node dissection is not indicated unless a hybrid component is identified.

Verrucous Hyperplasia

Clinical. Verrucous hyperplasia (VH) (proliferative VH) is a precursor lesion for both VC and squamous carcinoma. It may be a single lesion or multiple confluent lesions. They may appear as flat leukoplakia, or as warty papillations, or may be clinically indistinguishable from VC. The site distribution for 66 cases of VH in order of decreasing frequency is gingiva, buccal mucosa, tongue, floor of mouth, lip, and palate (782).

Etiology. HPV has been detected in 29% of cases by PCR (783).

Histology. VH shares many features with VC, yet falls short of the diagnostic criteria for VC. VH is seen as epithelial hyperplasia, hyperkeratosis, with hyperplastic and anastamosing rete pegs (784,785). Keratin-filled clefts punctuate the epithelium, and papillation formation may be seen. However, the pushing and burrowing nature of the club-shaped rete pegs, which define VC, are not seen in VH. Cytological atypia is not prominent.

Treatment. VH is persistent and irreversible; excisional biopsies are often accompanied by multiple recurrences. Extensive multifocal disease can be an especially frustrating problem, as radiotherapy, chemotherapy, and retinoids appear to have no impact on the ultimate course of this disease. Topical 5-aminolevulinic acid-mediated photodynamic therapy (786) and resection with adjuvant immune modulation (787) are newer treatment modalities that hold promise.

Inverting Papilloma

This gray/white firm polypoid tumor arises predominantly in the area of the middle meatus and may fill the nasal cavity and maxillary sinus. A possible infectious etiology has been suggested for almost 25 years ago by Kusiak and Hudson, who fortuitously found small (40–50 nm) crystalline-like intranuclear viral particles by electron microscopy (788).

Table 9 summarizes 33 genotype-based investigations published as English peer-reviewed full manuscripts between 1987 and 2006, studying HPV in IP (789–821). Table 10 represents the pooled analysis from our review studies by methodology (822). A wide range of detection rates are seen for studies using ISH techniques (0–79%), and PCR, either with type-specific probes (0–77%) or consensus probes

(2–67%). Interestingly, as detection thresholds have decreased, and the number of published reports using PCR-based techniques has increased, we see no increase in the overall range of HPV detection rates. Weighted estimates revealed similar detection rates across methods, 26.8% (95% CI, 16.4–37.2%) by ISH, 25.2% (95% CI, 14.7–35.6%) by consensus PCR, and 23.6% (95% CI, 12.2–35.0%) by type-specific PCR.

Interestingly, the HPV detection rate significantly increases in dysplastic IP and SCC-ex-IP with increasing ratio of HR- to LR-HPV types (Table 11). Dysplasia in IP results from either primary infection or secondary coinfection with HR-HPV. Progression to malignancy requires additional steps such as loss of tumor suppressor genes and viral integration. From a pragmatic viewpoint, the detection of HPV within IP has prognostic implications with regard to recurrence and malignant potential.

HPV and Head and Neck Squamous Cell Carcinoma

HPV and oropharyngeal SCC. Site-specific upper aerodigestive tract studies demonstrate a significant and strong association with HPV16 infection and oropharyngeal cancer, especially those of the palatine tonsil. Table 12 (724,725,823–843) summarizes 23 studies of oropharyngeal SCC published from 2000 to 2007; the HPV detection rates range from 13% to 82%. HPV-associated oropharyngeal SCC tend to have basaloid-type histology. A number of studies demonstrate a significant association between "never smoking" status, oropharyngeal SCC, and HPV infection, as compared to patients classified as smokers (823,825,827,829,835,837).

Serum HPV16 antibodies are predictive for oropharyngeal SCC; HPV16 exposure for this group is related to sexual activities. Furniss and colleagues demonstrated that HPV16 seropositivity is associated with more than 10 oral sex partners and more than 12 sexual partners; they found a fourfold increased RR for developing oropharyngeal SCC, even when adjusted for smoking (724). DeSouza and colleagues found that more than 26 vaginal sex partners and more than 6 oral sex partners/lifetime increased the RR for developing oropharyngeal SCC by 4.2 and 8.6, respectively (839).

A number of studies demonstrate an improved prognosis for patients with HPV-positive SCC (724,823,825,826,838,844). Furniss reported improved survival for patients with HPV-positive oropharyngeal SCC, as compared with the HPV-negative group, on Cox regression analysis (Hazard ratios of 0.4 and 0.5 for serum and tumor evidence of HPV, respectively) (724). Weinberger and colleagues demonstrated a dramatic increase in the association with improved outcome when patients were stratified according to HPV viral load and p16 status, as compared with HPV status alone. High copy number (median 46 copies/cell) plus high p16 expression associated with significant improvement in OS at five years (75%) compared with HPV-negative cases (15%) and low copy number median (3.6 copies/cell) plus low p16 expression (13%), (Hazard ratio 5.26) (838).

Table 9 Detection Methodology for HPV in Inverted Papillomas

Author	Year	Target	Method[a]	HPV types	Positive cases/subjects (%)*	Median age	M:F	Comments
Respler	1987	DNA	SB	11	+1/2 (50%)	12.5	1:1	
Syrjanen	1987	DNA	ISH	6/11/16/18	5/14 HPV11 (36%) 1/14 HPV16 (7%) 4/14 HPV11 and 16 (29%)	58	2:1	4 coinfections 1 recurrence
Brandsma	1987	DNA	SB, ISH	2, 6/11, 16/18	+2/9 HPV11 (22% by SB) +1/6 HPV6 (17% by ISH)	NA		+1 HPV11 (ISH) probably exophytic papilloma
Weber	1988	DNA	ISH	6b, 11	+16/21 (76%)	45	2.5:1	+1 case with SCC, +3 cases with "atypia"
Brandwein	1989	RNA	ISH	6/11, 16/18	+3/7 (43%) HPV6/11 +2/7 (29%) HPV16/18	60	6:1	+3 cases with dysplasia, +1 case with SCC
Siivonen	1989	DNA	ISH	6/11, 16	+8/21 (38%) HPV11 +8/21 (38%) HPV16	56	3.2:1	+3 cases with SCC, 3 cases with coinfection
Ishibashi	1990	DNA	SB	6/11, 16/18	+1/7 (14%) HPV6	61	1.3:1	
Bryan	1990	DNA	PCR	6/11	+10/13 (77%) HPV6/11			
Judd	1991	DNA	ISH, PCR	6/11, 16/18, 33	0/9 HPV+	67	1:1.3	
Furuta	1991	DNA	ISH, PCR, DB	6/11, 16/18	+3/26 (12%) HPV11 (DB and ISH) +1/26 (4%) HPV16 (DB and ISH)	NA		+1 case by DB and ISH with SCC, 1 additional IP with SCC, + HPV16 by PCR
Sarkar	1992	DNA	ISH, PCR	6b/11, 16/18	0/24 HPV+			
McLachlin	1992	DNA	ISH, PCR	6/11, 16/18, 31/33/35	+3/17 (18%) HPV6/11 +1/17 (6%) HPV16	57	14:1	+1 case with dysplasia, +1 HPV16 case with SCC
Kashima	1992	DNA	PCR	6/11, 16/18	+7/29 (24%) HPV6/11	NA		+1 case with dysplasia, +2 cases with SCC
Wu	1993	RNA	ISH, PCR, SB	57b	+12/15 (80%) HPV57b	NA		
Tang	1994	DNA	ISH	6/11, 16/18, 31/33/35	0/26	NA		
Buchwald	1995	DNA	ISH, PCR	6/11, 16/18, 31/33/35, 45, 51, 52 consensus L1 (MY09/MY11)	+4/57 HPV6/11 (7%) +1/57 HPV18 (2%)	NA		+2 cases with SCC
Beck	1995	DNA	PCR	6/11, 16/18, 31/33, 35, 57 consensus L1, MY09/MY11, E6 (WD72, WD76, WD66, WD67, WD154)	+18/39 (46%) HPV6/11 +5/39 (13%) HPV16/18	59 mean	2.6:1	+5 with dysplasia, +10 with SCC
MacDonald	1995	DNA	PCR	6/11, 16/18	+8/20 (40%) HPV6/11 +1/20 (5%) HPV16	NA		+1 case with SCC
Gaffey	1996	DNA, RNA	ISH	6/11, 16/18, 31/33, 35, 42–45, 51, 52, 56	+1/20 (5%) HPV16 +1/20 (5%) HPV11	NA		+1 HPV11 case with SCC
Shen	1996	DNA	PCR	6/11, 16/18 consensus L1, MY09/MY11	+17/46 (37%) HPV6/11 +1/46 (2%) HPV16	NA		Includes +1/6 with SCC (HPV16)
Ogura	1996	DNA	PCR	2a, 5b, 6b, 11, 16/18, 57, 58	+2/9 (22%) HPV16 +1/9 (11%) HPV57	51	1.4:1	

(Continued)

Table 9 Detection Methodology for HPV in Inverted Papillomas (Continued)

Author	Year	Target	Method[a]	HPV types	Positive cases/subjects (%)*	Median age	M:F	Comments
Caruana	1997	DNA	PCR	6b, 11, 16/18, 31/33 consensus L1, MY09/MY11	+2/19 (11%) HPV6b/11 +7/19 (37%) HPV16	64	1.6:1	+4/8 cases with dysplasia −2/4 cases with SCC
Bernauer	1997	DNA	PCR	6/11, 16/18 consensus L1, MY09/MY11	+7/22 (33%) consensus primers +1/22 (5%) HPV18	53	2.5:1	+2/2 cases with SCC, one of which was HPV18
Hwang	1998	DNA	PCR	6/11, 16/18, 33	+3/42 (7%) HPV6/11+2/42 (5%) HPV16	NA		+1 case with dysplasia +2 cases with SCC
Mirza	1998	DNA	ISH	6/11, 16/18	+5/28 (18%) HPV6/11 +2/28 (7%) HPV16/18	NA		+1 case with dysplasia +1 case with SCC +1 case with low-risk/high-risk coinfection
Kassim	1998	DNA	PCR	16	4/10 (40%) HPV16	49	All male	
Saegusa	1999	DNA	PCR	16/18	+6/28 (36%) HPV16/18	NA		
Weiner	1999	DNA	PCR	6b/11, 16/18 consensus L1, MY09/MY11, GP5+/GP6+	+3/83 (4%) HPV11 +2/83 (3%) HPV16 +1/83 (1%) HPV18	NA		Includes +1/7 with SCC, 6 SCC arose in IP, 1 arose in an oncocytic papilloma, derivation of one positive case not specified
Kraft	2001	DNA	ISH, PCR	6/11, 16/18, 31/33/51 consensus L1, MY09/MY11	+1/29 (3%) HPV11	NA		
Fischer	2005	DNA	PCR	consensus L1, CP66F, CP69F	+4/6 (67%) HPV+	NA		Sequencing in +3 cases: homology with HPV 21/34/56/60/66/80
McKay	2005	DNA	PCR	6/11, 16/18, 31/33, 35, 45, 52, consensus L1, MY09/MY11	+1/14 (7%) HPV11+2/14 (14%) HPV18	NA		HPV integration present in 4 cases with severe dysplasia or SCC
Katori	2006	DNA	ISH		+12/29 (41%) HPV6/11 +9/29 (31%) HPV16/18	52 mean	1.9:1	+5 cases with severe dysplasia and +4 cases with SCC. No mention of coinfection, we assume there was none.
Hoffman	2006	DNA	PCR	6/11, 16, consensus L1/L2, MY09/MY11	+3/26 (12%) HPV6/11 +2/26 (8%) other IP with consensus primers	61	1.9:1	

[a]ISH, in situ hybridization; PCR, polymerase chain reaction; SB, southern blot; SCC, squamous cell carcinoma.

Table 10 HPV Detection Rates in Inverted Papaillomas—By Method

	In situ hybridization	Type specific PCR	PCR consensus
Number of studies	15	10	11
Total case examined	328	210	349
Detection range	0–79%	0–77%	2–67%
Weighted prevalence[a]	26.8% (95%CI 16.4–37.2)	23.6% (95%CI 12.2–35.0)	25.2% (95%CI 14.7–35.6)
Pooled (crude) prevalence	26% (84/328)	22% (46/210)	23% (80/349)

[a]Weighted prevalence estimated by random-effects inverse-variance with continuity correction.
Source: From Ref. 822.

Table 11 Association of HPV in benign versus dysplastic versus malignant IP

Diagnosis	Overall HPV		HPV6/11 positive cases/total		HPV16/18 positive cases/total	
	Pos/total	Weighted prevalence (95%CI)[a]	Pos/total	Pooled prevalence (range)	Pos/total	Pooled prevalence (range)
IP, no dysplasia or low-grade dysplasia	129/597	22.3% (15.9–28.6)	102/597	17.1% (0–76.9%)	21/597	3.5% (0–33.3%)
IP with moderate to severe dysplasia	32/54	55.8% (30.5–81.0)	17/54	31.5% (0–66.7%)	15/54	27.8 (0–100%)
IP with SCC	34/65	55.1% (37.0–73.2)	9/65[b]	13.8% (0–100%)	22/65[b]	33.8 (0–100%)

[a]Weighted prevalence estimated by random-effects inverse-variance with continuity correction.
[b]One additional carcinoma was coinfected with 6/11 and 16/18, and the remaining HPV in a carcinoma was untyped.
Source: From Ref. 822.

One hypothesis states that the HPV + WT p53 tumor phenotype is more radiosensitive, as some apoptotic promoting p53 function remains (724). However, this improved survival may not be related solely to radiosensitivity. Licitra and colleagues reported on patients with oropharyngeal SCC treated by primary surgery +/− adjuvant radiotherapy (836). A 61% reduction in five-year mortality rate for HPV-positive patients was seen, when adjusted for adjuvant radiotherapy; this would argue against radiosensitivity as the sole explanation for these differences. It is known that integrated HPV E6 and E7 are immunogenic; another hypothesis is that an increased host immunogenic response also contributes to improved survival.

HPV in oral and laryngeal SCC. HPV does contribute to the carcinogenesis of a subset of oral cavity and laryngeal SCC; overall HPV is less frequently associated with both of these cancers than with oropharyngeal SCC. Table 13 (724,725,823,826–830, 832–835,837,840–843,845–850) summarizes 23 studies published from 2000 to 2007 examining HPV in oral cavity SCC; the HR-HPV detection rates range from 0% to 83%. Studies comparing the HPV status in patients with oral versus oropharyngeal SCC (725,823,826,828,830,833,835,837) plus those studies that also include a normal patient control group (724,827,829,832,834,840,843), almost consistently demonstrate a greater frequency of HPV with oropharyngeal SCC as compared with oral SCC. Only the study by Nemes (837) showed a converse relationship.

HPV detection in laryngeal carcinomas is summarized in Table 14, which includes 16 studies published from 2000 to 2007; the HPV detection rates range from 0% to 52% (724,823,826–828,830,834,839, 843,851–858). Overall, the HPV detection rates in laryngeal SCC are lower than those seen with oral

cavity and oropharyngeal SCC. HPV16 is most frequently demonstrated. Dual infection with LR and HR-HPV types can be seen. Rarely, a laryngeal SCC, not associated with papillomatosis, may harbor only a LR-HPV viral type (857). Szladek studied 25 laryngeal SCC and demonstrated HPV in 12 cases. In addition, the TTV ubiquitous transfusion transmissible virus, genotype 1TTV was present in 11 cases; HPV and geneotype 1-TTV coinfection was significantly associated with decreased time to tumor progression (p < 0.001) by univariate analysis (858).

Mechanisms of HPV-induced carcinogenesis: E6. The immortalization of HPV16- and HPV18-transfected cell lines is dependent on E6 and E7 transcription (859,860). HPV E6 protein binds with p53 tumor suppressor protein, enhancing its degradation by the ubiquitin-proteasome system (861–863). E6 first binds to the E6-associated protein (E6-AP), an E3-ubiquitin-protein-ligase. The E6/E6-AP complex binds to p53, resulting in p53 ubiquitinization and subsequent proteasomal degradation (863). Normally, E6-AP plays a minor role in p53 degradation. Mutated p53 is an extremely common event in carcinogenesis, abrogating the protective post-DNA damage pathways of growth arrest and apoptosis. Functional p53 inactivation has a similar impact, leading to cell cycle dysregulation and promoting chromosomal instability. In contrast, LR-HPV E6 is not able to induce p53 degradation in vitro (864).

E6 has additional oncogenic activities independent of p53 protein; HR E6 proteins can bind numerous other cellular proteins, promoting their degradation in both E6-AP dependent and E6-AP independent pathways (865). One such example is the binding of E6 to PDZ-domain containing proteins; PDZ domains are protein-protein recognition sites; PDZ-domain-containing proteins are involved in a

Table 12 HPV Detection Rates in Patients with Oropharyngeal Squamous Cell Carcinoma

Author	Year	Country	Serum Ab	Method, target	Pos	Total	%	Comments
Gillison	2000	United States		PCR, MY09/MY11	34	60	57	Most HPV 16. HPV more likely in nonsmokers (7/8) than smokers (27/51)
Mellin	2000	Sweden		PCR, GP5/GP6	26	60	43	More women in HPV+ group
Schwartz	2001	United States		PCR type specific 6,11,16,18 E6	18	44	41	HPV more common in never smokers 14/42 than ever smokers
Mork	2001	Scandinavia	yes	PCR, GP5/GP6, E1	9	18	50[t]	
Ringstrom	2002	United States		PCR, MY09/MY11	15	29	52	All HPV16
Dahlstrom	2003	United States	yes		41	70	59	HPV16 more common in never smokers (24/35) than ever smokers (17/35) Serum HPV16 L1 Ab predictive for oropharyngeal SCC, OR 59.53 (95% CI: 5.71-620-2)
El-Mofty	2003	United States		PCR, SPF10	10	11	91	All tonsil HPV16,
Herrero	2003	Multiple	yes	PCR, GP5/GP6	26	142	18[t]	Serum HPV16 E6 or E7Ab predictive for oropharyngeal SCC, OR = 9.2 (95% CI: 4.8-17.7)
Begum	2005	United States		ISH, HPV16	37	45	82	
El-Mofty	2005	United States		PCR SPF10	12	20	60	HPV 16
Hansson	2005	Sweden		PCR, MY09/MY11, GP5/GP6	21	46	46[o]	HR-HPV DNA in oral mouthwash samples predictive for oropharyngeal SCC, OR = 230 (44-1200) on multivariate regression analysis
Ibieta	2005	Mexico		PCR, MY09/M11, GP5/GP6	4	9	44	Most HPV16, no tonsillar SCC included, only retromolar trigone
Koppikar	2005	India		PCR, MY09/MY11	2	6	33	Most were HPV16, but 14% were multiple HPV infections, (including HPV18, 8, 38)
Kreimer	2005	Multiple	yes	PCR, GP5/GP6	25	141	18[s]	Serum HPV VLP Ab plus high tumor viral load predictive for oropharyngeal SCC, OR 12.0 (95% CI 5.2-27.5)
Tachezy	2005	Czech		PCR, GP5/GP6	32	56	57	HPV more common in never smokers (7/7) than ever smokers 28/61
Licitra	2006	Italy		PCR HPV16, HPV18	17	90	19	All HPV16, 2 SCC integrated only, remaining both episomal and integrated
Nemes	2006	Hungary		PCR, MY09/MY11,	1	8	13	Most HPV16, most integrated HPV more common in never smokers (7/18) than ever smokers 26/61
Weinberger	2006	United States		qPCR HPV16 E6	48	79	61	
DeSouza	2007	United States		ISH, HPV16, PCR, MY09/MY11	72	100	72	
Furniss	2007	United States	yes	PCR, SPF1A, SPF2B	116	288	40.3[s]	High HPV16 L1 serum Ab titer predictive for oropharyngeal SCC, OR = 30.3 (95% CI 12.4-73.6)
Pintos	2007	Canada	yes	PCR, MY09/MY11	9	17	53[s]	Serum HPV16 VLP predictive for oropharyngeal SCC, OR = 27.68 (95% CI 7.5 – 102.2) by crude analysis
Smith	2007	United States	yes	PCR, MY09/MY11	35	62	56[s]	Serum HPV16 E6/E7Ab predictive for oropharyngeal SCC, OR = 72.8 (95% CI 16.0–330),
Schlecht	2007	United States		PCR, MY09/MY11	7	17	41	Most HPV16

Abbreviations: OR, Overall risk; Ab, serum antibodies; ISH, in-situ hybridization; PCR, polymerase chain reaction; HR, high-risk; s, seropositivity results; t, tumor results; o, oral mouthwash results; VLP, viral like particles; CI, confidence intervals.

variety of cell signaling and adhesion pathways. E6-mediated degradation of PDZ-domain-containing proteins, such as the Scribble protein, which in necessary for establishing cell polarity (866), may promote the loss of squamous polarity that is common to HPV-induced dysplasia and neoplasia. E6 can also function as a transcription promoter. E6, in concert with Myc,

upregulates TERT transcription, which increases telomerase activity and thereby suppresses normal cell senescence (867).

Mechanisms of HPV-induced carcinogenesis: E7. The E7 protein forms complexes with retinoblastoma proteins (p105[RB], p130, p107) and releases E2F transcription factors (867–869). Active Rb is

Table 13 HPV Detection Rates in Patients with Squamous Cell Carcinoma of the Oral Cavity

Author	Year	Country	Method, target	Pos	Total	%
Gillison	2000	United States	PCR, MY09/MY11	10	84	12
Mork	2001	Scandinavia	Serum Ab, HPV16, PCR, GP5/GP6, E1	4	59	7[t]
Ringstrom	2002	United States	PCR, MY09/MY11	2	41	5
Chen	2002	Taiwan	In-situ PCR	24	29	83
El-Mofty	2003	United States	PCR, SPF10	0	15	0
Herrero	2003	Multiple	Serum Ab, PCR, GP5/GP6	30	766	4[t]
Dahlstrom	2003	United States	Serum Ab, HPV16	8	50	16[s]
Correnti	2004	Venezuela	PCR, MY09/MY11	8	16	50
Zhang	2004	China	PCR HPV16/18, E6 type specific primers	54	73	74
Begum	2005	United States	HPV16, ISH	0	61	0
Kreimer	2005	Multiple	Serum Ab, PCR, GP5/GP6,	28	764	4[s]
Hansson	2005	Sweden	PCR, MY09/MY11, GP5/GP6	15	85	18
Tachezy	2005	Czech	PCR, GP5/GP6	3	12	25
Koppikar	2005	India	PCR, MY09/MY11	28	83	34
Ibieta	2005	Mexico	PCR, MY09/M11, GP5/GP6	16	36	44
Boy	2006	South Africa	PCR, HPV, 16 E1, HPV18	7	59	12
Nemes	2006	Hungary	PCR, MY09/MY11	31	68	46
Pintos	2007	Canada	Serum Ab, PCR, MY09/MY11	5	49	10[s]
Furniss	2007	United States	Serum Ab, PCR, SPF1A, SPF2B	28	190	15[s]
Sugiyama	2007	Japan	PCR, HPV16, E7	24	66	36
Balderas-Loaeza	2007	Mexico	PCR, MY09/MY11, GP5/GP6	26	62	42
Smith	2007	United States	Serum Ab, PCR, MY09/MY11	59	142	42[s]
Schlecht	2007	United States	PCR, MY09/MY11	0	7	0

Note: s, reflects seropositivity results.

Table 14 HPV Detection Rates in Patients with Laryngeal Squamous Cell Carcinoma

Author	Year	Country	Method, target	Pos	Total	%	Comments
Brito	2000	Brazil	ISH	4	45	9	
Gillison	2000	United States	PCR, MY09/MY11	16	86	19	
Venuti	2000	Italy	PCR, MY09/MY11	13	25	52	HPV16, HPV45, HPV6, integration, only HPV16-positive tumors transcriptionally active
Mork	2001	Scandinavia	Serum Ab PCR GP5/GP6 E1	1	32	3	
Almadori	2001	Italy	PCR, MY09/MY11	15	42	36	HPV16, HPV18, HPV33
Ringstrom	2002	United States	PCR, MY09/MY11	1	10	10	HPV16
El-Mofty	2003	United States	PCR, SPF10	2	7	29	HPV16, HPV31
Dahlstrom	2003	United States	Serum Ab, HPV 16	5	14	36	
Begum	2005	United States	HPV16, ISH	0	54	0	
Koppikar	2005	India	PCR, MY09/MY11	0	2	0	
Torrente	2005	Chile	PCR, MY09/MY11	10	31	32	3 were integrated HPV16, 2 were HPV58, 1 each HPV39, 45, 51, 59, 66, 69
Szladek	2005	Hungary	PCR, MY09/MY11	12	25	48	Both low-risk (8) and high-risk (4) HPV found in SCC, same prevalence as control group. Genotype 1TTV found in 11/25
Olivera	2006	Brazil	PCR, GP5/GP6	41	110	37	HPV16, HPV18
Manjarrez	2006	Mexico	In situ PCR L1C1L1C2	4	16	25	2 cases LR and HR, 1 case HR, 1 case LR only
Koskinen	2007	Scandinavia	PCR, MY09/MY11 GP5/GP6, SPF10	3	69	4	
DeSouza	2007	United States	ISH, HPV16, PCR, MY09/MY11	4	16	25	
Furniss	2007	United States	Serum Ab, PCR SPF1A, SPF2B	14	45	31	

hypophosphorylated; it binds transcription factors such as E2F, repressing cell-cycle progression. HR E7 binds hypophosphorylated Rb, thereby releasing E2F and promoting transcription of genes involved in DNA synthesis and cell-cycle progression. Similar to the mechanism of HR E6, HR E7 Rb binding results in ubiquitin-mediated proteolysis (870). E7 from LR papillomavirus (e.g., cottontail rabbit papillomavirus) has less Rb-binding-affinity (871); the transforming capacity of LR-E7 is greatly reduced compared with that of HR-E7 (872).

The HPV+/p53 WT tumor phenotype. The data supports two distinct pathways for upper aerodigestive tract carcinogenesis. Nonvirally mediated carcinogenesis, which is most often promoted by smoking, is the result of accumulation of multiple genetic hits, including p53 mutations, and/or multiple genomic losses, including loss of heterozygosity (LOH) at 17p13, resulting in loss of p53 function, and LOH 9p21, and causing loss of tumor suppressor gene INK4a, which encodes p16 protein. The HPV16-mediated pathway is more often associated with WT p53 and elevated p16 protein; p16 can serve as a surrogate marker for HPV infection.

Transcriptionally silent HPV in head and neck squamous cell carcinomas (HNSCCs) are considered as incidental passengers. Braakhuis compared patterns of LOH for HPV + transcriptionally active HNSCC, versus HPV-negative HNSCC, versus HPV+ but transcriptionally silent HNSCC. All transcriptionally active HPV + HNSCC had WT p53, and a significantly lower rate of LOH for 3p, 9p, and 17p than HPV-negative HNSCC. HPV + transcriptionally silent HNSCC had LOH patterns similar to the HPV-negative tumors (873).

HPV integration. In general, HPV integration is a rare phenomenon, but malignant transformation is thought to rapidly progress after integration. Carcinomas can harbor both episomal and integrated HPV, and integration is not a necessary event (874). When integration does occur, the E6 and E7 regions are invariably integrated into the host genome. Different regions, such as L1 or E2, can be lost upon integration. The E2 ORF is a 48-kd DNA-binding protein with regulatory and suppressive activities on the p97/p105 gene promoter for HPV16/18. The loss of E2 regulatory activity over E6/E7 leads to E6/E7 overexpression.

F.   Molluscum Contagiosum

This is a contagious skin papular lesions caused by a large double-stranded DNA poxvirus, 300 nm in diameter, with a "brick-shaped" virion and a dumbbell-shaped nucleioid core. This virus is tropic for skin and rarely for mucosa.

Background

Molluscum contagiosum (MC) is transmitted by direct contact and by fomites. It has a worldwide distribution and is seen in conditions of crowding and poor hygiene; it may also be sexually transmitted.

Clinical course. MCs are small, discrete, flesh-colored, pearly papules, 2 to 6 mm, with characteristic small central umbilicated depressions or crusting (Fig. 51). Cheesy keratinous infectious material can be expressed from the central depression. Sexually transmitted lesions are often located in the genitalia, lower abdomen, and inner thighs. In children, MC is usually transmitted by direct contact or fomites

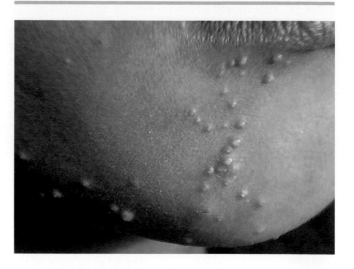

Figure 51   Molluscum contagiosum 1.Cluster of small, pearly papules with characteristic umbilicated central compression. *Source*: http://www.clinical-virology.org.

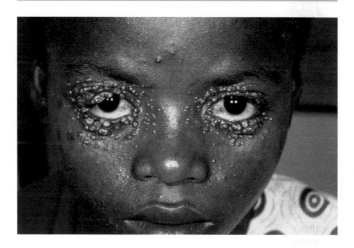

Figure 52   Molluscum contagiosum 2. Patients with HIV/AIDS can have extensive, multiple lesions. *Source*: Photo courtesy of Ben Naafs and http://www.cehjournal.org/extra/53_05_01.html, accessed January 2008.

(clothing, toys) (875). Childhood MC usually occurs on the limbs, neck, and occasionally face and eyelids (876). Lesions are usually asymptomatic and nonpruritic but can become symptomatic after rupture or secondary bacterial infection.

Immunosuppressed hosts (AIDS patients, renal transplant recipients, patients on steroids, etc.) may develop multiple lesions, which can become large and confluent (877). MC in AIDS patients tends to occur on the facial skin and eyelids (Fig. 52). Low CD4 cell counts have been associated with widespread facial MC, which serves as a marker for severe AIDS. Rarely, MC in immunosuppressed hosts can affect mucosal surfaces (878).

G. Measles

Measles (rubeola) is an acute childhood illness caused by an RNA paramyxovirus (120–250 nm) with a lipoprotein envelope, which contains F (fusion) proteins and H (hemagglutinin) proteins.

Clinical Course

Measles is uncommon in the United States, thanks to the live attenuated measles virus (MV) vaccine, but may still occur among nonimmunized children, as witnessed by an epidemic in the 1990s (882). In developing countries with poor nutrition and immunity, fatal infection can be common (883). Measles is highly contagious and transmitted by ororespiratory secretions. After an incubation period (10–12 days) children develop high fever, conjunctivitis, photophobia, lymphadenopathy, and small intraoral erythematous vesicles and ulcers (Koplick's spots), usually on the lower buccal mucosa (Fig. 54). A generalized skin rash follows, beginning on the face, and spreading to the trunk and extremities (Fig. 55). The rash usually resolves within 10 days. Measles is infectious from the onset of the prodromal symptoms until day 4 of the rash.

Pneumonia (interstitial giant cell pneumonia) and acute encephalitis are serious immediate complications of measles; they occur, although rarely, in normal patients. Subacute sclerosing panencephalitis (SSPE) is a rare, progressive, fatal, late sequel to measles characterized by mental deterioration and motor abnormalities. SSPE is detectable 5 to 10 years after primary measles and is the result of defective, nonreplicative MV persistence in the brain. Immunosuppressed patients are likely to develop serious sequelae after infection. Their rashes may be atypical and last longer, possibly obscuring the clinical

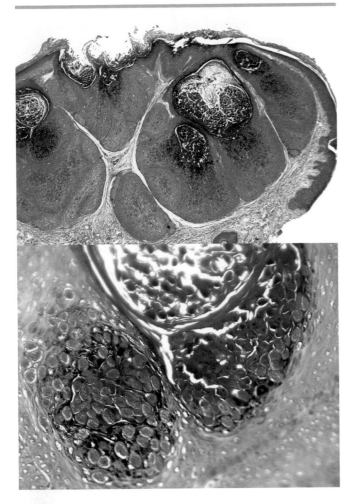

Figure 53 Molluscum contagiosum. Upper panel: Molluscum papules are composed of cup-shaped epithelial hyperplasia filled with transformed enlarged infected keratinocytes distended with Henderson–Paterson viral inclusions, or molluscum bodies. Lower panel: Keratinocytes distorted by pink granular cytoplasmic inclusions. Mature pox bodies (Henderson–Patterson bodies) are dense, basophilic "packettes" of assembled virions (hematoxylin and eosin).

Histopathology. MC is characterized by cup-shaped epithelial hyperplasia, the center of which is filled with transformed enlarged infected keratinocytes distended with Henderson-Paterson viral inclusions, or molluscum bodies (879,880) (Fig. 53). These molluscum bodies appear as granular, eosinophilic, cytoplasmic inclusions in the lower epithelium. As they mature in the upper epithelium, the molluscum bodies usurp the entire cell; they are dense, compact, homogeneous, and basophilic. The molluscum bodies contain infectious replicating virions.

Treatment. MC is a self-limiting disease; the lesions involute within six to nine months. However lesions may be treated by curettage or cryosurgery. Oral cimetidine can be an alternative to local therapies; however, facial MC is less responsive to oral cimetidine than lesions at other sites (881).

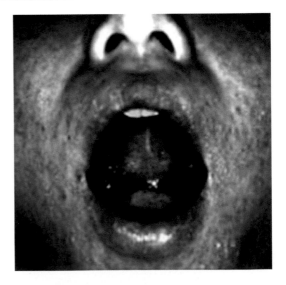

Figure 54 Measles. Intraoral ulcers (Koplick's spots) and erythematous facial rash. *Source*: http://www.clinical-virology.org.

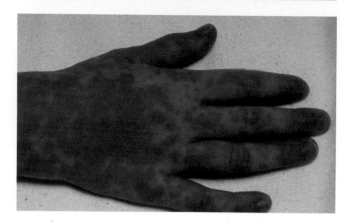

Figure 55 Measles. Measles rash spreads from the face and trunk to the extremities.

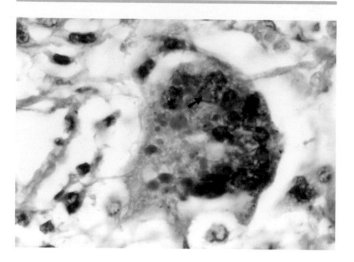

Figure 56 Measles. Multinucleated giant cells with intranuclear (Cowdry A) (*arrow*) and intracytoplasmic eosinophilic inclusions (hematoxylin and eosin).

diagnosis. Postvaccination fatal disseminated infection may rarely develop in immunosuppressed children (884).

There is mounting evidence that measles infection is involved in the pathogenesis of otosclerosis, the most common cause of acquired hearing loss (885). The combination of decreased serum antimeasles IgG and conductive hearing loss is highly specific and sensitive for the diagnosis of otosclerosis. MV-like nucleocapsid structures are present in osteoblasts of otosclerosis, and measles antigens and RNA are detected in active otosclerosis. Detectable perilymph antimeasles IgG and decreased serum antimeasles IgG are found in patients with otosclerosis. The incidence of otosclerosis has decreased with the introduction of the measles vaccine (885). MV is also implicated in the complex pathogenesis of Paget's disease of bone. MV nucleocapsid mRNA and protein have been demonstrated in osteoclasts from Paget's disease, and in vitro models demonstrate that transfection with MV nucleocapsid gene results in the formation Pagetoid bone (886).

Histopathology

Historically, characteristic Warthin–Finkeldey (WF) cells were observed in tonsillectomy specimens of children who developed measles (887,888). These syncytial giant cells are of T-cell origin; they contain numerous nuclei, up to 100 per cell, which have a crowded, "bunch of grapes" appearance (Fig. 56). Both nuclear and cytoplasmic eosinophilic inclusions are seen, distinguishing WF cells from other multinucleated giant cells (Table 15).

WF cells can be seen in the stratum corneum, tonsils, as well as in other organs, most notably lungs, in disseminated infection. Skin biopsies also reveal focal parakeratosis and necrosis high in the epidermis near the granular layer. Cytology of nasal and lacrimal secretions, as well as sputum and urine, may also reveal WF cells. The histological diagnosis of measles can be confirmed by commercially available antibodies.

HSV also results in formation of multinucleated syncytial giant cells; their nuclear inclusions are

Table 15 Histological Comparison of Selected Viral Infections

Virus	MNSGC	Intranuclear inclusions	Cytoplasmic inclusions	Site
Herpes simplex	Yes	Cleared out, steel-gray, glassy, nuclear molding	Rare	Epithelium, LN, other
Measles (*Warthin-Finkeldey*)	Yes	Eosinophilic, nuclear crowding (bunch of grapes)	Eosinophilic	Epithelium, lungs, other
HIV	WS-like cells	No	No	In LN
EBV	No	Beaded, marginated chromatin, amphophilic	No	Tongue mucosa, RS-like cells in LN and tonsils
CMV (*Cowdry inclusions*)	No	Large, basophilic amphophilic	Large	Endothelium, lungs, other
HPV (*koilocytes*)	No	Brick- or raisin-shaped nuclei	No	Epithelium
Molluscum contagiosum (*Henderson-Patterson*)	No	No	Initially pink granular inclusions, become dense and basophilic	Skin

Abbreviations: MNSGC, multinucleated syncytial giant cells; LN, lymph node; WS-like, Warthin-Finkeldey-like; RS-like, Reed Sternberg-like.

"cleared out" or amphophilic, not frankly eosinophilic, and they lacks eosinophilic cytoplasmic inclusions. WF-like cells can also be seen in reactive lymph nodes and lymph nodes of patients with AIDS, Hodgkin's lymphoma and NHL, and reactive lymph nodes (889). In these cases, the prominent eosinophilic intranuclear and intracytoplasmic inclusions are lacking.

H. Mumps

Mumps is a highly contagious, self-limiting illness caused by an RNA paramyxovirus (150–250 nm). Characteristically, it affects salivary glands as well as other glandular organs.

Clinical

Mumps (epidemic parotitis) is an acute illness of children and young adults transmitted by ororespiratory secretions. It is uncommon in the United States due to immunization programs. The Jeryl Lynn vaccine substrain, which is used in the United States as a monovalent vaccine or as part of the combined MMR (measles mumps rubella) vaccine has an efficacy of up to 95% after two immunizations, with no complications; vaccine efficacy decreases during outbreak conditions (890,891).

Infection is characterized by a prodrome of fever, headache, malaise, and nausea, followed by acute, painful parotid swelling. In most cases, there is initial unilateral involvement with subsequent infection of the other gland. The involved gland has a characteristic boggy consistency. Subacute infection can develop in one-third to one-half of individuals. Saliva remains infectious for up to six weeks (892). Other salivary glands, lacrimal glands, and thyroid may also be involved (893). Presternal edema (Gillis sign), facial edema including eyelids and neck, dyspnea, and supraglottic edema have been reported (894,895).

Disseminated infection is more likely to occur in adults, causing abdominal pain, hepatosplenomegaly, pancreatitis, lymphadenopathy, deafness, myocarditis, polyarthritis, and meningitis/encephalitis. Orchitis and epidydimitis, followed by atrophy, can develop in up to one-third of postpubescent males. Mastitis develops in approximately 15% of women (896). Generally, mumps is self-limiting, even after sequelae such as meningitis and encephalitis, and usually resolves without morbidity.

Histopathology

Mumps infection is rarely observed by histopathology. Infected tissue reveals hemorrhage, necrosis, edema, and a dense lymphoplasmacytic infiltrate permeating periductal and periacinar tissue. Vacuolation and necrosis of the acini and ducts can be seen (892,897). Viral inclusions are not seen.

The diagnosis is best confirmed by serum isoamylase fractions and serum IgM mumps titers. Real-time PCR assays have been developed, which allow for earlier detection of infection, with greater sensitivity, and can be applied to oral specimens, urine, and cerebral spinal fluid (898).

V. PROTOZOAN

A. Toxoplasmosis

Toxoplasmosis is caused by *Toxoplasma gondii*, one of the most common of all mammalian protozoan parasites. The usual route of human infection is through the ingestion of oocysts from poorly cooked or raw meats of secondary hosts or food and water contaminated by fecal oocysts. Infection is usually asymptomatic or mild, but the repercussions of congenital infection or systemic infection in the immunosuppressed are severe or fatal.

Background and Epidemiology

Toxoplasma (toxon = arc, plasma = form) is an obligate intracellular parasite initially isolated at the turn of the century in gondis, Tunisian rodents (899). Domestic cats and small rodents are major natural reservoirs for these protozoa. The potentially infectious oocysts (10–12 μm) are formed in the intestinal epithelium of the animal reservoir. Stray cats and household cats can pass huge numbers of oocysts in their feces. The excreted oocysts pass unsporulated and thus are noninfectious; they require oxygen for sporulation. Feces may remain infectious for up to one year (900), and during this time become dispersed by houseflies or roaches. Oocysts are sensitive to boiling water, but survive drying, freezing, and disinfectants.

Toxoplasmosis can be transmitted to humans by ingestion of food or water contaminated by fecal oocysts or by eating undercooked or raw meat of secondary hosts (901). Oocytes have been isolated in soil from yards populated by cats; children playing in infected soil or sandboxes or gardeners working in infected soil are at risk for infection (902). Herbivores (cows, lambs, pigs) grazing in infected soil can become secondary hosts; ingestion of raw or barely cooked meat (e.g., steak Tartar, Kibbe, or fondue Bourguignome) from secondary hosts is another vector for infection. Transmission from blood or organ transplantation is rare.

Clinical course. Ingested sporulated oocytes release tachyzoites (trophozoites), which invade and infect cells. The tachyzoites divide to form cysts (10–100 μm) filled with thousands of organisms. These cysts may remain latent in host tissue and serve as potential reservoirs for reactivation or chronic infection. Infection is usually asymptomatic or mild in immunocompetent hosts. Lymphadenopathy, fever, myalgias, anorexia, headache, sore throat, and rash are uncommon symptoms. Posterior cervical lymph nodes are the most commonly involved nodes; periparotid and submandibular lymph nodes and the tonsils can also be involved (903).

Immunocompetent hosts may rarely develop necrotizing infections such as retinitis, encephalitis myocarditis, hepatitis, and pneumonitis. In an epidemic stemming from infected water in British

Columbia, of 100 people diagnosed with acute infection, 51 developed lymphadenopathy and 20 developed retinitis (904).

AIDS toxoplasmosis is most commonly thought to result from reactivation of previous infection. For immunosuppressed individuals, the most serious infectious sequelae include encephalitis, myocarditis, pneumonitis, and hepatitis. Toxoplasma encephalitis is the most frequent cause of intracerebral mass lesions in AIDS.

Toxoplasmosis in pregnant women can seriously impact the fetus. The risk of fetal loss is greatest during first trimester infection; the risk of severe congenital infection is greatest with third trimester infection. A cohort of 339 women from France who contracted toxoplasmosis during pregnancy was studied; the overall risk of fetal infection was 7.4% (905). Transplacental transmission may result in severe intracranial infections causing microcephaly, hydrocephaly, cerebral calcifications, chorioretinitis, mental retardation, blindness, and seizure disorders.

Histopathology. Lymph nodes reveal irregular clusters of eosinophilic epithelioid histiocytes surrounding and percolating into germinal centers (Fig. 57). The constellation of microgranulomas (collections with fewer than 25 epithelioid cells), follicular hyperplasia, and lack of either Langerhan's or foreign body giant cells, is highly specific for toxoplasmosis (906). Nuclear debris, tingible body macrophages, paracortical hyperplasia, and monocytoid B cells in interfollicular and sinusoidal areas are also seen. Nonnecrotic macrogranulomas (collections with > 25 but < 50 epithelioid cells) may be seen but are relatively sparse (< 3/slide). Microgranulomas within germinal centers are also considered to specific for toxoplasmosis (906).

Tachyzoites, especially extracellular tachyzoites, are hardly perceptible on hematoxylin and eosin stain

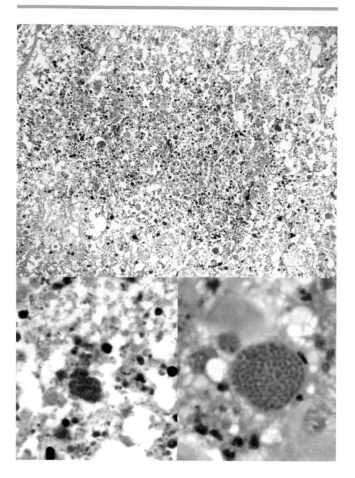

Figure 58 Toxoplasmosis. Upper panel: Intracerebral toxoplasmosis with necrosis and abscess formation. Lower left and right panels: Intracerebral cysts of trophozoites (hematoxylin and eosin).

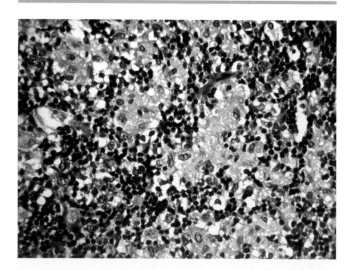

Figure 57 Toxoplasmosis. Clusters of epithelioid histiocytes can be seen in interfollicular regions. Trophozoites are very difficult to visualize on lymph node sections (hematoxylin and eosin).

but might be observed with Giemsa staining. They are 6 × 2 μm, "banana-shaped" or "crescent-shaped," with a nucleus. The encysted forms of *T. gondii* are more easily visualized; mature oocysts (12 μm in diameter) contain eight infective sporozoites. They can be seen on hematoxylin and eosin in CNS infections (Fig. 58), but are rarely present in lymph nodes. Histologically, chronic toxoplasmosis tonsillitis is similar to lymphadenitis (907). Disseminated infections reveal necrosis, intracellular and extracellular tachyzoites, and encysted tachyzoites.

IHC, PCR, and serology. IHC and PCR can be performed on formalin-fixed paraffin-embedded tissue to enhance detection sensitivity and specificity (Fig. 59).

The Sabin Feldman Dye test, developed in 1948, was a mainstay of serological diagnosis for detection of IgG antibodies. In the presence of serum IgG antibodies and complement, the live tachyzoiites lose their affinity for methylene blue dye. The dye test is highly sensitive and specific, but cannot detect IgM, which would be most important in congenital infection. ELISA testing is currently the most widely used serum test, and assays are available for IgM and IgG.

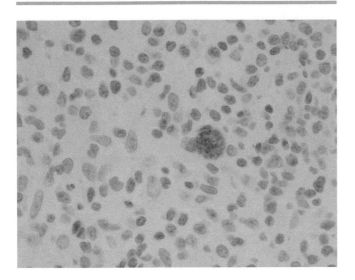

Figure 59 Immunohistochemistry for toxoplasmosis.

IgM antibody titers rise within the first week after infection.

Direct detection methods should be used for fetal infections and infections of the immunosuppressed. PCR can be performed on amniotic fluid and blood or body fluids from HIV-seropositive patients.

Treatment. Toxoplasmosis is usually self-limited. Treatment is required for severe or persistent symptoms or for immunocompromised patients. The therapy of choice is a combination of pyrimethamine and sulfodiazine or rovamycin. Importantly, these drugs are active against tachyzoites but not cysts; hence lifelong drug maintenance is necessary for immunocompromised patients. Azithromycin has been found to have some effect on the tissue cysts phase (908).

B. Trichinosis

This is a protozoan infection by *Trichinella* transmitted through ingestion of infected meat. After the initial gastrointestinal phase, *Trichinella* encysts in skeletal muscle causing muscular symptoms.

Background and Etiology

Ingestion of inadequately cooked or stored infected meat, usually pork, will result in transmission of *Trichinella*. Conversely, cooking meat to a minimum of 60°C for 30 minutes per pound or deep-freezing for at least three weeks at −15°C will kill the parasites. The federal prohibition against feeding raw-meat garbage to hogs and commercial or home freezing of pork has greatly decreased the incidence of trichinosis in the United States. Between 1997 and 2001, an average of 12 cases of trichinosis were reported annually (909). By contrast, over 10,000 cases of human trichinosis were reported between 1995 and 1997 worldwide, and it's been estimated that as many as 11 million people

may be infected. Romania, Argentina, Croatia, Lithuania, and Yugoslavia have the highest infection rates (910). Meats other than pig that can also cause trichinosis include bear, horse, walrus, dog, cat, wallaby, and kangaroo (911,912).

Most cases of trichinosis follow infection with *Trichinella spiralis*, however infections with *Trichinella nativa, Trichinella britovi, Trichinella murrelli, Trichinella nelsoni, and Trichinella pseudospiralis* have also been described (911,913). After ingestion of infected meat, which contains the encysted larvae, the immature worms are released in the stomach and superficially invade small intestinal mucosa. They develop through four larval stages, mature, mate, and lay eggs on the second day. By day 6, the female worms deposit motile, immature larvae, which enter the systemic circulation via intestinal lymphatics and venules. These larvae become encysted within host skeletal muscle. The parasite alters the skeletal intracellular environment and may remain viable for years (914). *Trichinella* especially favors muscles with a rich blood supply, such as the extraoccular and intrinsic laryngeal muscles, diaphragm, deltoid, and gastrocnemius muscles.

Clinical Course

Most cases follow a self-limited course; severity depends on the size of the inoculum. Early symptoms include fever, nausea, vomiting, headache, fatigue, and diarrhea. These symptoms correspond to the intestinal invasion phase. After the first week, symptoms correspond to larval migration into muscle (muscle phase): they include symmetrical periorbital or facial edema, myositis, blurry vision, and peripheral eosinophilia. Eye movement and swallowing may be extremely painful. In a recent study of *T. britovi* infection, muscle weakness and restricted motion of the upper extremities were common symptoms; no objective arthritis or muscle weakness were present (915). The profound diffuse weakness might suggest myositis or myasthenia gravis (916).

Blindness can result from retinal invasion by migrating larvae. Parasite invasion into the lungs, heart, and CNS may be seen in rare serious cases, and fatalities are rare (914).

Histopathology

The deltoid and gastrocnemius muscles are recommended sites for diagnostic muscle biopsies. The larvae appear as tightly coiled worms within an intramuscular double-walled capsule (Fig. 60). If the larvae are missed on muscle biopsy due to sampling error, nonspecific myositis may be seen. *Trichinella* may be an incidental finding in the sternocleidomastoid muscle of radical neck dissections or in laryngectomy specimens (usually for carcinoma) (917). Calcified cysts denote remote infection. When the larvae migrate elsewhere, such as to the myocardium and CNS, they do not become encysted.

T. pseudospiralis and *Trichinella paupae* do not become encysted within human muscle (910). Aside from this, and size differences, all species and

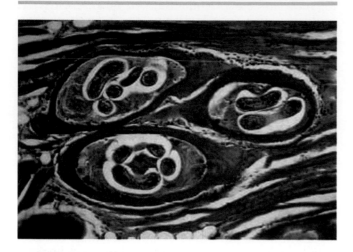

Figure 60 Trichinosis. Encysted larvae within skeletal muscle (hematoxylin and eosin). *Source*: From http://www.humanillnesses. com/original/T-Ty/Trichinosis.html

genotypes of *Trichinella* are morphologically indistinguishable at all developmental stages (918).

Serology

Laboratory findings include elevated transaminases, muscle creatinine kinase, peripheral eosinophilia, and anti-*Trichinella* antibodies. ELISA tests are highly reliable in detecting the specific antibody as early as in the first week of infection. Other tests include complement fixation, indirect fluorescent antibody, and the bentonite flocculation test, which becomes positive during the third week and may remain positive for one year (919).

Treatment

Administration of anthelmintics (mebendazole, albendazole, thiabendazole) at the intestinal invasion stage (within the first 3 days of infection) can prevent the muscular invasion phase (914). If tissue invasion does occur, then therapy is aimed at minimizing damage; antipyretics, analgesics, and prednisone (50 mg/day) are administered.

VI. UNKNOWN ETIOLOGY

A. Malakoplakia

This is a tumor-like inflammatory process characterized by a histiocytic infiltrate with intracellular "targetoid" calcified concretions termed "Michaelis–Gutmann" (MG) bodies. It is probably the result of an acquired monocyte bactericidal defect in the face of a chronic bacterial infection.

Background and Etiology

Malakoplakia (from the Greek "malacos" meaning soft, and "plakia" meaning places) is a chronic inflammatory response to certain bacteria in the setting of defective macrophage host response. It is an acquired macrophage defect localized to an organ site and promoted by a specific bacterial host interaction. Low-level cyclic guanosine monophosphate (c-GMP) is associated with abnormal lysosomal function (decreased bactericidal activity and poor lysosomal granule release) (920). There is a propensity for malakoplakia to occur in individuals with underlying immunosuppressive conditions (AIDS, transplantation, hematopoietic malignancies, etc.), or who have other concurrent chronic infections such as TB. A literature review of 153 cases of malakoplakia (in the pre-AIDS era) revealed that 40% of patients had some underlying immunosuppressive condition (921). It is possible that malakoplakia results from an overwhelmed phagocytic system challenged with chronic bacterial infection with particular antigenic properties. Different bacteria have been associated within malakoplakia, most often *Escherichia coli*, *Klebsiella*, and *Rhodococcus equi* (922,923).

Clinical Course

Malakoplakia most commonly develops in the urinary bladder, kidneys, and less commonly in the genital tract. It may also affect the skin, bone, lungs, and gastrointestinal tract. In the head and neck, it affects the parotid, temporal bone, ear, thyroid, ocular adnexae, tongue, tonsil, sinonasal tract, larynx, and soft tissues of the neck (924–933). Submucosal malakoplakia appears as multiple yellow tumor-like nodules or masses; malakoplakia of the head and neck is rarely observed as mucosal plaques. Massive nasopharyngeal malakoplakia has been described (926).

Histopathology

The stage of the disease process is reflected in the histology (926,934,935). The early disease phase (prediagnostic malakoplakia) is characterized by an infiltrate of plasma cells and epithelioid histiocytes (Von Hansemann cells) within an edematous stroma. In the classic or granulomatous phase, MG bodies, giant histiocytes, and abundant lymphocytes are seen. The late fibrotic phase is characterized by abundant collagen and numerous fibroblasts surrounding scattered MG bodies and histiocytes.

MG bodies are calcified lamellar bodies, 5 to 10 μm, with a targetoid or "owl's eye" appearance; they are composed of calcium and phosphorus, (in the form of hydroxyapatite), iron, and bacterial wall glycolipids (lipid A) (Fig. 61). MG bodies react with periodic acid–Schiff, Von Kossa, Prussian blue, and alizarin red, consistent with polysaccharide, calcium, and iron, respectively. MG bodies are gram-negative and may react with Gomori methanamine silver stain. Clumps of intrahistiocytic and extracellular gram-negative coccobaccilli may be seen on Brown and Brenn stain.

Ultrastructurally, MG bodies are phagolysosomes, which form laminated calcified concretions. Whorls of membrane segments are present in the phagolysosomes. Bacteria are present, partially

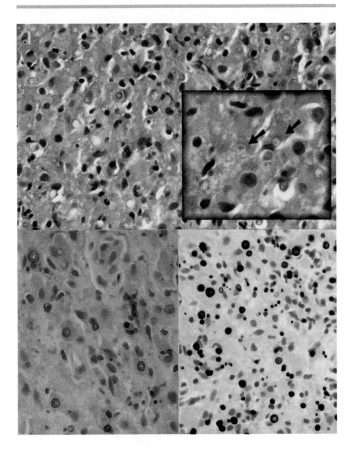

Figure 61 Malakoplakia Upper panel and inset: Targetoid intracellular Michaelis–Gutman (MG) bodies (hematoxylin and eosin). Lower left panel: MG bodies on Prussian blue iron stain. Lower right panel: MG bodies on Von Kossa calcium stain. *Source*: Courtesy of Dr. Maomi Li, Montefiore, Bronx, New York, U.S.A.

degraded or intact, leaving little doubt as to their involvement in the formation of malakoplakia (927). MG bodies are S-100-negative.

The differential diagnosis of malakoplakia includes other infections, which have a prominent histiocytic infiltrate (LL, atypical mycobacterial infection, Whipple's disease, rhinoscleroma, and histoplasmosis) as well as entities such as inflammatory myofibroblastic tumor and granular cell tumor. Special stains (Ziehl-Neelsen, Fite, periodic acid–Schiff, digested-periodic acid–Schiff, Warthin–Starry, and Gomori methanamine silver) are indicated to rule out the above organisms. This is especially true in early cases of malakoplakia (prediagnostic malakoplakia) where MG bodies are rare or scarce.

Treatment

The lesions are usually debrided or excised by diagnostic/palliative purposes. Successful resolution has been reported with long-term antibiotics such as trimethoprim sulfamethoxazole, quinolones, penicillins, and clofaimines. Vitamin C and the cholinergic agonist bethanechol chloride have been used to

increase c-GMP levels. Conversely, steroids can stabilize lysosomal membranes and can worsen malakoplakia.

B. Sarcoid

This is a multisystem disorder of uncertain etiology. The diagnosis is established by clinicoradiological correlation in the presence of the histopathological findings of characteristic granulomas, which are typically nonnecrotizing. The disease is usually self-limiting.

Predispositions for Sarcoidosis

The incidences of sarcoidosis are highest in Scandinavia, United Kingdom, and the United States. It is 10 times more common among African-Americans than whites with an incidence of 35–38/100,000 among African-Americans (936). Generally, there is an inverse relationship between susceptibility to MTB and sarcoidosis; it is virtually nonexistent among ethnic groups with high susceptibility to MTB such as the Eskimos, Indians, and Chinese. There is a known familial association for sarcoidosis; the ACCESS study (a case-control etiologic study of sarcoidosis) demonstrated a fivefold increase in RR for family members (937). HLA class I haplotype HLA-B8 is associated with susceptibility to sarcoidosis. For class II HLA genes, the HLA-DRB1*1101 allele is significantly associated with sarcoidosis in both blacks and whites; HLA-DRB1-F47 and HLA-DRB1*1501 were significantly associated with sarcoidosis in whites (936).

Clinical

Sarcoidosis is most often diagnosed between the second and fourth decades of life. Many patients are totally asymptomatic and diagnosed after an incidental chest X ray reveals the typical findings of hilar lymphadenopathy and a diffuse pulmonary reticular pattern. A screening program in Denmark estimated that asymptomatic sarcoidosis was four times more prevalent than symptomatic cases; a Swedish autopsy study suggested that the incidence of subclinical cases was even greater (938,939).

Patients may present with nonspecific symptoms such as fever, malaise, and weight loss. The more typical symptomatic presentation includes lymphadenopathy, hepatosplenomegaly and pulmonary, arthritic, and ocular symptoms. Lofgren's syndrome refers to the acute manifestation of sarcoidosis: erythema nodosum, hilar lymphadenopathy fever, and polyarthritis. It is more common in white women. Most symptomatic patients follow a self-limiting course as the disease "burns out" within two years. Fewer individuals will progress to severe pulmonary fibrosis and renal involvement. Mortality due to sarcoidosis is rare (940).

In the head and neck, sarcoidosis typically involves the anterior or posterior cervical lymph nodes. Extranodal head and neck manifestations can

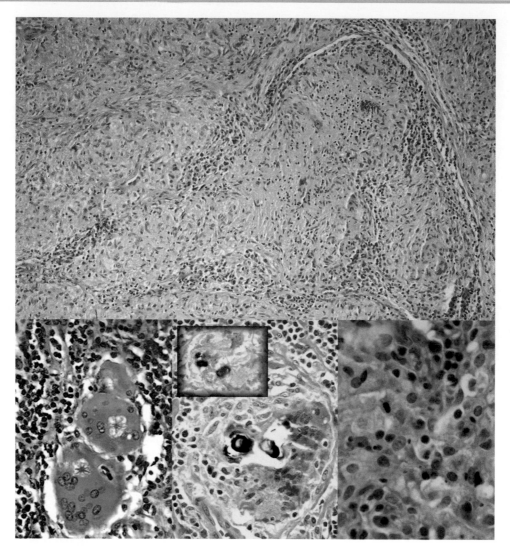

Figure 62 Sarcoid (hematoxylin and eosin except where noted). Upper panel: Low power view of hyalinized noncaseating granulomas, typical for sarcoid. Lower left panel: Asteroid bodies. Lower center panel: Calcified, lamellated, Schauman concretions. Inset: Alizarin red stain for calcium. Lower right panel: Pigmented ovoid intrahistiocytic Hamazaki–Wesenberg inclusions. *Source*: Courtesy of Dr. Martha Warnock, San Francisco, California, U.S.A. (lower left panel).

be seen in 38% of sarcoid patients (940). The eye is most common head and neck extranodal site involved by sarcoidosis, followed by parotid and lacrimal glands involvement, and upper respiratory tract submucosa (940–942). Heerfordt's syndrome (uveoparotid fever) is a rare, acute presentation of sarcoidosis with a self-limiting course. Patients present with fever, parotid and lacrimal gland swelling, and uveitis (inflammation of the interior eye); cranial nerve palsies may also develop.

Causes

Sarcoidosis is viewed as a disease that develops in genetically susceptible individuals and is triggered by exposure to sensitizing antigens, resulting in an exaggerated immune response. Both infectious agents and noninfectious antigens have been suspected as being responsible for triggering the disease. There are obvious histological similarities between sarcoid and mycobacterial granulomas, and occasionally mycobacteria are found within sarcoid granulomas. The recovery of cell-wall-deficient mycobacterial forms from sarcoidosis patients has bolstered the association (943). A recent meta-analysis of published PCR-based studies has concluded that there is a significant association between sarcoidosis and MTB as well as atypical mycobacteria. However, the association with cell-wall deficient mycobacteria has been refuted (944) and the PCR-based associations are not uniformly accepted. Other infectious agents that have been queried as possible triggers have included *P. acnes* (945) and *Borrelia burgdorferi* (946). Possible noninfectious environmental triggers include beryllium, aluminum, zirconium, titanium, pine pollen, peanut dust, and clay ingestion.

Histopathology

The granulomas of sarcoidosis are characteristically uniform, small, compact, nonconfluent, and nonnecrotic; they are composed of epithelioid histiocytes with multinucleated giant cells, rimmed by T-suppressor cells and contain interspersed T-helper cells. Up to one-third of specimens from sarcoid patients may contain some degree of central necrosis (947). Over time, the granulomas heal by fibrosis, commencing at the periphery and progressing inward.

Sarcoid granulomas can contain typical inclusions: asteroid bodies, Schaumann bodies, and Hamazaki-Wesenberg inclusions; however, these inclusions are neither sensitive nor specific (Fig. 62). Asteroid bodies are star-like crystalline inclusions seen within multinucleated giant cells. Schaumann described calcified laminated concretions within multinucleated giant cells (948,949). Hamasaki-Wesenberg inclusions are seen within histiocytes, unrelated to granulomas, and are round, (coccoid), oval, or rod-shaped golden brown inclusions, 3 to 15 μm; they stain with Ziehl-Neelsen stain, and the intensified Kinyoun stain. They can be relatively large, mimicking yeasts (950,951).

Other Diagnostics

The Kviem test relies on the specific hypersensitivity that sarcoid patients have to the "sarcoid antigen." It involves subcutaneous injection of heat-sterilized tissue homogenates from tissue (spleen or liver) involved by sarcoid. The injection site is biopsied four to six weeks later. A positive Kviem test reveals sarcoid granulomas at the injection site. The sensitivity of the Kviem test varies with disease activity: up to almost 90% of patients recently diagnosed with subacute cases may have positive Kviem tests, while patients with chronic or inactive sarcoid may have low or nonexistent rates of reaction to the Kviem test. On the other hand, false positivity with the Kviem test is rare (947), as seen in MTB or leukemia (952).

Angiotensin-converting enzyme (ACE) converts angiotensin I to angiotensin II. Its main tissue sources are foamy histiocytes and epithelioid histiocytes. Elevated serum ACE can be seen in sarcoidosis, especially patients with active pulmonary disease, and may be helpful in clinically establishing the diagnosis. ACE is not elevated in inactive sarcoidosis. The overall false-positive rate for serum ACE is 2% to 4%; it may be elevated in diabetes, Gaucher's disease, hyperthyroidism, chronic renal disease, liver disease, leprosy, silicosis, berylliosis, amyloidosis, MTB or MAI infection, and asbestosis (952)

Differential Diagnosis

Sarcoid granulomas are not entirely specific for sarcoid. Ziehl-Neelson stains should always be performed to rule out mycobacteria. Sarcoid-like granulomas can be observed with rheumatoid arthritis (953) and have also been seen as a reaction to various malignancies (954–956).

Treatment

Corticosteroids remain the cornerstone of therapy but other regimens using cytotoxic agents (methotrexate, azathioprine, cyclophasphamide), antimicrobials (choroquine, hydrochloroquine, minocycline), and cytokine modulators (pentoxifyline, thalidomide, Infliximab) have emerged (957). This latter class of drugs targets TNF-α released by pulmonary macrophages.

VII. ACKNOWLEDGMENT

We would like to thank Jonathan Neuman for proofreading this work.

REFERENCES

1. Brook I, Foote A, Hausfeld JN. Frequency of recovery of pathogens causing acute maxillary sinusitis in adults before and after introduction of vacciniation of children with the 7-valent pneumococcal vaccine. J Med Microbiol 2006; 55:943–946.
2. Brook I, Gober AE. Frequency of recovery of pathogens from the nasopharynx of children with acute maxillary sinusitis before and after the introduction of vaccination with the 7-valent pneumococcal vaccine. Int J Pediatr Otorhinolaryngol 2007; 71:575–579.
3. Hern JD, Ghufoor K, Jayaraj SM, et al. ENT manifestations of Pseudomonas aeruginosa infection in HIV and AIDS. Int J Clin Pract 1998; 52:141–144.
4. Gurney TA, Lee KC, Murr AH. Contemporary issues in rhinosinusitis and HIV infection. Curr Opin Otolaryngol Head Neck Surg 2003; 11:45–48.
5. Brook I. Bacteriology of chronic sinusitis and acute exacerbation of chronic sinusitis. Arch Otolaryngol Head Neck Surg 2006; 132:1099–1101.
6. Triglia JM, Bellus JF. Nasal polyposis in children. Diagnostic and therapeutic problems. Ann Pediatr Paris 1992; 39: 473–477.
7. Oppenheimer EH, Rosenstein BJ. Differential pathology of nasal polyps in cystic fibrosis and atopy. Lab Invest 1979; 40:445–449.
8. Balmelli C, Ganthard HF. Gonococcal tonsillar infection—a case report and literature review. Infection 2003; 31: 362–365.
9. Gerber JE. Acute necrotizing bacterial tonsillitis with Clostridium perfringens. Am J Forensic Med Pathol 2001; 22:177–179.
10. Bhargava D, Bhusnurmath B, Sundaram KR, et al. Tonsillar actinomycosis: a clinicopathological study. Acta Trop 2001; 80:163–168.
11. Toh ST, Yuen HW, Goh YH. Actinomycetes colonization of tonsils: a comparative study between patients with and without recurrent tonsillitis. J Laryngol Otol 2007; 121:775–778.
12. Ramirez S, Hild TG, Rudolph CN, et al. Increased diagnosis of Lemierre syndrome and other Fusobacterium necrophorum infections at a Children's Hospital. Pediatrics 2003; 112:380–385.
13. Hoshino T, Matsumoto M. Otomycosis: subdermal growth in calcified mass. Eur Arch Otorhinolaryngol 2006; 263:875–888.

14. Dibb WL. Microbial aetiology of otitis externa. J of Infect 1991; 22:233–239.

15. Vennewald I, Schonlebe J, Klemm E. Mycological and histological investigations in humans with middle ear infections. Mycoses 2003; 46:12–18.

16. Landry MM, Parkins CW. Calcium oxalate crystal deposition in necrotizing otomycosis caused by *Aspergillus niger*. Modern Pathol 1993; 6:493–496.

17. Chandler JR. Malignant external otitis. Laryngoscope 1968; 78:1257–1293.

18. Grandis JR, Branstetter BF, Yu VL. The changing face of malignant (necrotizing) external otitis: clinical, radiological, and anatomic correlations. Lancet: Infect Dis 2004; 4:34–39.

19. Rees BD, Luntz M, Telischi FF, et al. Necrotizing external otitis in patients with AIDS. Laryngoscope 1997; 107: 456–460.

20. Nir D, Nir T, Danino J, et al. Malignant external otitis in an infant. J Laryngol Otol 1990; 104:488–490.

21. Sreepada GS, Kwartler JA. Skull base osteomyelitis secondary to malignant external otitis. Curr Opin Otolaryngol Head Neck Surg 2003; 11:316–323.

22. Chai FC, Auret K, Christiansen K, et al. Malignant otitis externa caused by Malassezia sympodialis. Head Neck 2000; 22:87–89.

23. Eskola J, Kilpi T, Palmu A, et al. Efficacy of a pneumococcal conjugate vaccine against acute otitis media. N Engl J Med 2001; 344:403–409.

24. Griffin GH, Flynn C, Bailey RE, et al. Antihistamines and/or decongestant for otitis media with effusion (OME) in children. Cochrane database Syst Rev 2006; 4:CD003423.

25. Dubey SP, Larawin V. Complications of chronic suppurative otitis media and their management. Laryngoscope 2007; 117:264–267.

26. Centers for Disease control and Prevention (CDC). Available at: www.cdc.gov/std/stats/figures/fig26.htm. Accessed July 2007.

27. Centers for Disease control and Prevention (CDC). Available at: www.cdc.gov/std/stats04/syphilis.htm. Accessed July 2007.

28. Golden MR, Marra CM, Holmes KK. Update on syphilis: resurgence of an old problem. JAMA 2003; 290:1510–1514.

29. Fiumara NJ, Walker EA. Primary syphilis of the tonsil. Arch Otolaryngol 1982; 108:43–44.

30. Leao JC, Gueiros LA, Porter SR. Oral manifestations of syphilis. Clinics 2006; 61:161–166.

31. Bruce AJ, Rogers RS. Oral manifestations of sexually transmitted diseases. Clin Dermatol 2004; 22:520–527.

32. Little JW. Syphilis: an update. Oral Surg Oral Med Oral Pathol Oral Radiol Endod 2005; 100:3–9.

33. Hamlyn E, Marriott D, Gallagher RM. Secondary syphilis presenting as tonsillitis in three patients. J Laryngol Otol 2006; 120:602–604.

34. Zawar V, Chuh A, Gugle A. Oral lesions of syphilis: an isolated, rare manifestation. Dermatol Online J 2005; 11:46.

35. Yuen HW, Luke KS, Yeoh KH. An unusual presentation of secondary syphilis in otolaryngology. Otolaryngol Head Neck Surg 2001; 125:277–229.

36. Song JJ, Lee HM, Chae SW, et al. Bilateral otosyphilis in a patient with HIV infection. Eur Arch Otorhinolaryngol 2005; 262:972–974.

37. Klemm E, Wollina U. Otosyphilis: report on six cases. J Eur Acad Dermatol Venereol 2004; 18:429–434.

38. Centers for Disease control and Prevention (CDC). Available at: www.cdc.gov.mill1.sjlibrary.org/nchstp/od/tuskegee/time.htm. Accessed July 2007.

39. Gibbel MI, Cross JH, Ariel IM. Cancer of the tongue. A review of 330 cases. Cancer 1949; 2:411–423.

40. Dickenson AJ, Currie WJR, Avery BS. Screening for syphilis in patients with carcinoma of the tongue. Brit J Oral Maxillofacial Surg 1995; 33:319–320.

41. Meyer I, Shklar G: The oral manifestations of acquired syphillis. Oral Surg Oral Med Oral Pathol 1967; 23:45–57.

42. Centers for Disease control and Prevention (CDC). Available at: www.cdc.gov/std/stats/syphilis.htm. Accessed July 2007.

43. Gurlek A, Alaybeyoglu NY, Demir CY, et al. The continuing scourge of congenital syphilis in 21st century: a case report. Int J Pediatr Otorhinolaryngol 2005; 69: 1117–1121.

44. Saloojee H, Velaphi S, Goga Y, et al. The prevention and management of congenital syphilis: ans overview and recommendations. Bull of the WHO 2004; 82:424–429.

45. Fiumara NJ, Lessell S. Manifestations of late congenital syphilis. An analysis of 271 patients. Arch Dermatol 1970; 12:78–83.

46. Barrett AW, Villarroel Dorrego M, Hodgson TA, et al. The histopathology of syphilis of the oral mucosa. J Oral Pathol Med 2004; 33:286–291.

47. Behrhof W, Springer E, Brauninger W, et al. PCR testing for Treponema pallidum in paraffin-embedded skin biopsies: test design and impact on the diagnosis of syphilis. J Clin Pathol 2007; 61(3):390–395.

48. Farnsworth N, Rosen T. Endemic treponematosis: review and update. Clin Dermatol 2006; 24:181–190.

49. Centers for Disease control and Prevention (CDC). Available at: www.cdc.gov/std/stats/Tables/Table1.htm. Accessed July 2007.

50. Centers for Disease control and Prevention (CDC). Available at: www.cdc.gov/std/stats/Tables/Table12.htm. Accessed July 2007.

51. Little JW. Gonorrhea. Update. Oral Surg Oral Med Oral Pathol Oral Radiol Endodontol 2006; 101:137–143.

52. Ackerman AB: Hemorrhagic bullae in gonococcemia. New Engl J Med 1970; 282:793–794.

53. Veien NK, From E, Kvorning SA. Microscopy of tonsillar smears and sections in tonsillar gonorrhoea. Acta Otolaryngol 1976; 82:451–454.

54. Centers for Disease control and Prevention (CDC). Available at: www.cdc.gov/std/treatment/2006/updated-regimens.htm. Accessed July 2007.

55. Von Hebra F, Kohn M. Ueber ein eigenthumliches Neubebilde an der Nase. Wiener Med Wochenschrift 1870; 20:1–5.

56. Mikulicz J. Ueber das Rhinosclerom (Hebra). Archiv fur Klinische Chirurgie 1876; 20:485–533.

57. Von Frisch A. Zur Aetiologie des Rhinscleroms. Wien Med Wochenschr 1882; 32:96–97.

58. Quevedo J. Scleroma in Guatemala, with a study of the disease based on the experience of 108 cases. Ann Otol Rhinol Laryngol 1945; 58:613–645.

59. Muzyka MM, Gubina KM. Problems of the epidemiology of scleroma. I Geographical distribution of scleroma. J Hyg Epidemiol Microbiol Immunol 1971; 15:233–242.

60. Muzyka MM, Gubina KM. Problems of the epidemiology of scleroma. II. Some aspects of the problem of endemic focus formation. J Hyg Epidemiol Microbiol Immunol 1972; 16:8–18.

61. Hart CA, Rao SK. Rhinoscleroma. J Med Microbiol 2000; 49:395–396.

62. Vozmediano JMF, Hita JCA, Cabrerizo AG. Rhinoscleroma in three siblings. Ped Dermatol 2004; 21:134–138.

63. Sanchez-Marin LA, Bross-Soriano D, Arrieta J, et al. Association of HLA-DQA1*03011-DQB1*0301 haplotype with the development of respiratory scleroma. Otolaryngol Head Neck Surg 2007; 136:481–483.

64. Maguina C, Cortez-Escalante J, Osores-Plenge F, et al. Rhinoscleroma: Eight Peruvian Cases. Rev Inst Med Trop S Paulo 2006; 48:295–299.

65. Iyengar P, Laughlin S, Keshavjee S, et al. Rhinoscleroma of the larynx. Histopathol 2005; 47:225–226.

66. Andraca R, Edson RS, Kern EB. Rhinoscleroma: A growing concern in the United States? Mayo Clin Proc 1993; 68:1151–1157.

67. Modlin RL, Hofman FM, Meyers PR, et al. In-situ demonstration of T-cell subsets in granulomatous inflammation: leprosy, rhinoscleroma and sarcoidosis. Clin Exp Immunol 1983; 51:430–438.

68. Berron P, Berron R, Ortiz-Ortiz L. Alterations in the T-lymphocyte subpopulation in patients with rhinoscleroma. J Clin Microbiol 1988; 26:1031–1033.

69. Paul C, Pialoux G, Dupont B, et al. Infection due to *Klebsiella rhinoscleromatis* in two patients infected with HIV. Clin Infect Dis 1993; 16:441–442.

70. Abaikhail A, Satti MB, Uthman MAE, et al. Rhinoscleroma: a clinicopathological study from the Gulf region. Sing Med J 2007; 48:148–151.

71. Kasper HU, Hegenbarth V, Buhtz P. Rhinoscleroma associated with Rosai-Dorfman reaction of regional lymph nodes. Pathoil Internat 2004; 54:101–104.

72. Meyers PR, Shum TK, Becker TS, et al. Scleroma (Rhinoscleroma). A histologic immunohistochemical study with bacterial correlates. Arch Pathol Lab Med 1983; 107: 377–383.

73. Bhargava D, Date A. Pathology in focus: Palatal presentation of scleroma. J Laryngol Otol 2001; 115:679–680.

74. Bostroem (1891) in: Peabody JW, Seabury JH: Actinomycosis and Nocardiosis. J Chron Dis 1957, 5:374–400.

75. Rippon JW. Medical Mycology. The Pathogenic Fungi and the Pathogenic Actinomyces. 3rd Ed. Philadelphia, PA: WB Saunders1988:15.

76. Bennhoff DF. Actinomycosis: diagnostic and therapeutic considerations and a review of 32 cases. Laryngoscope 1984; 94:1198–1217.

77. Brandenburg JH, Finch WW, Kirkham WR. Actinomycosis of the larynx and pharynx. Ann Otol Rhinol Laryngol 1978; 86:739–742.

78. Balatsouras DG, Kaberos AK, Eliopoulis PN, et al. Cervicofacial actinomycosis presenting as acute upper respiratory tract. J Laryngol Otol 1994; 108:801–803.

79. Gaffney RJ, Walsh MA. Cervicofacial actinomycosis: an unusual cause of submandibular swelling. J Laryngol Otol 1993; 107:1169–1170.

80. Cone LA, Leung MM, Hirschberg J. Actinomyces odontolyticus bacteremia. Emerging Infect Dis 2003; 9: 1629–1632.

81. Thomas R, Kameswaran M, Ahmed S, et al. Actinomycosis of the vallecula: report of a case and review of the literature. J Laryngol Otol 1995; 109:154–156.

82. Artesi L, Gorini E, Lecce S, et al. Laryngeal actinomycosis. Otolaryngol Head Neck Surg 2006; 135:161–162.

83. Syed MA, Ayshford CA, Uppal HS, et al. Actinomycosis of the post-cricoid space: an unusal cause of dysphagia. J Laryngol Otol 2001; 115:428–429.

84. Atespare A, Keskin G, Ercin C, et al. Actinomycosis of the tongue, a diagnostic dilemma. J Laryngol Otol 2006; 120: 681–683.

85. Belmont M, Behar PM, Wax MK. Atypical presentations of actinomycosis. Head Neck 1999; 21:264–268.

86. Baliga S, Shenoy S, Wilson G, et al. An unusual case of actinomycosis. Ear Nose Throat J 2002; 81:44–55.

87. Ozcan C, Talas D, Gorur K, et al. Actinomycosis of the middle turbinate: an unusual cause of nasal obstruction. Eur Arch Otorhinolaryngol 2005; 262:412–415.

88. Yiotakis J, Tzounakos P, Manolopoulous L, et al. Actinomycosis of the thyroid gland masquerading as a neoplasm. J Laryngol Otol 1997; 111:172–174.

89. Kingdom TT, Tami TA. Actinomycosis of the nasal septum in a patient infected with HIV. Otolaryngol Head Neck Surg 1994; 111:130–133.

90. Watkins KV, Richmond AS, Langstein IM. Nonhealing extraction site due to *Actinomyces naeslundii* in patient with AIDS. Oral Surg Oral Med Oral Pathol 1991; 71: 675–677.

91. Vazquez AM, Marti C, Renaga I, et al. Actinomycosis of the tongue associated with HIV infection: Case report. J Oral Maxillofac Surg 1997; 65:579–581.

92. Belal A. Latent tuberculosis in tonsils and adenoids. J Laryngol Otol 1951; 65:414–425.

93. Golden RL. Sir William Osler and the anatomic tubercle. J Am Acad Dermatol 1987; 16:1071–1074.

94. Centers for Disease control and Prevention (CDC). Available at: www.cdc.gov/tb/surv/surv2005/PDF/TBSurvFullReport.pdf. Accessed August 2007.

95. Alvarez S, Mc Cabe W. Extrapulmonary tuberculosis revisited: A review of experience at Boston City and other hospitals. Medicine 1984; 63:25–55.

96. Menon K, Bem C, Gouldesbrough D, et al. A clinical review of 128 cases of head and neck tuberculosis presenting over a 10-year period in Bradford, UK. J Laryngol Otol 2007; 121:362–368.

97. Al-Serhani AM. Mycobacterial infection of the head and neck: Presentation and diagnosis. Laryngoscope 2001; 111:2012–2016.

98. Nalini B, Vinayak S. Tuberculosis in ear, nose, and throat practice: its presentation and diagnosis. Am J Otolaryngol 2006; 27:39–45.

99. Jang YJ, Jung SW, Koo TW, et al. Sinonasal tuberculosis associated with osteomyelitis of the ethmoid bone and cervical lymphadenopathy. J Laryngol Otol 2001; 115: 736–739.

100. Messervy M. Primary tuberculoma of the nose with presenting symptoms and lesions resembling a malignant granuloma. J Laryngol Otol 1971; 85:177–184.

101. Batra K, Chaudhary N, Motwani G, et al. An unusual case of primary nasal tuberculosis with epistaxis and epilepsy. Ear Nose Throat J 2002; 81:842–844.

102. Chopra RK, Kerner MM, Calcaterra TC. Primary nasopharyngeal tuberculosis: a case report and review of this rare entity. Otolaryngol Head Neck Surg 1994; 111: 820–823.

103. Harrison NK, Knight RK. Tuberculosis of the nasopharynx misdiagnosed as Wegener's granulomatosis. Thorax 1986; 41:219–222.

104. Waldron J, Van Hasselt CA, Skinner DW et al. Tuberculosis of the nasopharynx: clinicopathological features. Clin Otolaryngol 1992; 17:57–59.

105. Bath AP, O'Flynn P, Gibbin KP. Nasopharyngeal tuberculosis. J Laryngol Otol 1992; 106:1079–1080.

106. Russell B. The history of lupus vulgaris: its recognition, nature, treatment and prevention. Proc Royal Soc Med 1954; 48:127–138.

107. Thompson, Sir St. Clair. Tuberculosis of the Larynx: Ten Years Experience in a Sanatorium. London: HMSO, 1924.

108. Auerbach O. Laryngeal tuberculosis. Arch Otolaryngol 1946; 44:191–201.

109. Lim JY, Kim KM, Choi EC, et al. Current clinical propensity of laryngeal tuberculosis: review of 60 cases. Eur Arch Otorhinolaryngol 2006; 263:838–842.

110. Sutbeyaz Y, Ucuncu H, Karasen RM, et al. The association of secondary tonsillar and laryngeal tuberculosis: a case report and literature review. Auris Nasus Larynx 2000; 27:371–374.

111. Coscaron BE, Santa Cruz RS, Serradilla Lopez JM. Tuberculous epiglottitis, an atypical form of laryngeal tuberculosis. Presentation of a case and review of literature. An Otorrinolaryngol Ibero Am 2005; 32:55–63.

112. Dworetsky JP, Risch OC. Laryngeal tuberculosis: A study of 500 cases of pulmonary tuberculosis with a resume based on 28 years of experience. Ann Otol Rhinol Laryngol 1941; 50:745–757.

113. Bailey CM, Windle-Taylor PC. Tuberculosis laryngitis: a series of 37 patients. Laryngoscope 1981; 91:93–100.

114. Pino Rivero V, Marcos Garcia M, Gonzales Palomino A, et al. Laryngeal tuberculosis masquerading as carcinoma. Report of one case and literature review. An Otorrinolaryngol Ibero Am 2005; 32:47–53.

115. Thaller SR, Gross JF, Pilch BZ, et al. Laryngeal tuberculosis as manifested in the decades 1963–1983. Laryngoscope 1987; 97:848–850.

116. Richeldi L. An update on the diagnosis of tuberculosis infection. Am J Respir Crit Care Med 2006; 174:736–742.

117. Hillemann D, Galle J, Vollmer E, et al. Real-time PCR assay for improved detection of Mycobacterium tuberculosis complex in paraffin-embedded tissues. Int J Tuberc Lung Dis 2006; 10:340–342.

118. Park DY, Kim JY, Choi KU, et al. Comparison of polymerase chain reaction with histopathologic features for diagnosis of tuberculosis in formalin-fixed, paraffin-embedded histologic specimens. Arch Pathol Lab Med 2003; 127:326–330.

119. Zerbi P, Schonau A, Bonetto S, et al. Amplified *in-situ* hybridization with peptide nucleic acid probes for differentiation of Mycobacterium tuberculosis complex and nontuberculous Mycobacterium species on formalin-fixed, paraffin-embedded archival biopsy and autopsy samples. Am J Clin Pathol 2001; 16:770–775.

120. Vulgia DJ, Jang Y, Zizek C, et al. Mycobacteria in nail salon whirlpool footbaths, California. Emerging Infect Dis 2005; 11:616–618.

121. Edson RS, Terrell CL, Brutinel WM, et al. *Mycobacterium intermedium* granulomatous dermatitis from hot tub exposure. Emerging Infect Dis 2006; 12:821–822.

122. Runyon EH. Anonymous mycobacteria in pulmonary disease. Med Clin North Am 1959; 43:273–290.

123. German JL, Black TC, Chapman JS. TB of superficial lymph nodes. Dis Chest 1956; 30:326–337.

124. Kent D. Tuberculosis lymphadenitis: not a localized disease process. Am J Med Sci 1967; 254:866–874.

125. Saitz EW. Cervical lymphadenitis caused by atypical mycobacteria. Ped Clin No Am 1981; 28:823–839.

126. Stewart MG, Starke JR, Coker NJ. Nontuberculous mycobacterial infections of the head and neck. Arch Otolaryngol Head Neck Surg 1994; 120:873–876.

127. Brandwein M, Choi HS, Strauchen J, et al. Spindled nontuberculous mycobacteriosis in AIDS mimicking neoplasia. Evidence of dual histiocytic and fibroblast-like characteristics of spindle cells. Virchow Arch A 1990; 416:281–286.

128. Umlas J, Federman M, Crawford C, et al. Spindle cell pseudotumor due to *Mycobacterial avium-intracellulare* in AIDS patients. Am J Surg Pathol 1991; 15:1181–1187.

129. Chen KTK. Mycobacterial spindle cell pseudotumor of lymph nodes. Am J Surg Pathol 1992; 16:276–281.

130. Anderson H, Stryjewska B, Boyanton BL, et al. Hansen disease in the United States in the 21st century: a review of the literature. Arch Pathol Lab Med 2007; 131:982–986.

131. Lindeboom JA, Kuijper EJ, Bruijnesteijn ES, et al. Surgical excision versus antibiotic treatment for nontuberculous mycobacterial cervicofacial lymphadenitis in children: A multicenter, randomized, controlled trial. Clin Infect Dis 2007; 44:1057–1064.

132. Centers for Disease control and Prevention (CDC). Available at: www.cdc.gov/ncidod/dbmd/diseaseinfo/hansens_t.htm. Accessed July 2007.

133. Pfeifer LA. A Summary of Hansen's Disease in the United States-2002. Baton Rouge, LA: National Hansen's Disease Programs, 2003.

134. Taylor JP, Vitek I, Enriquez V, et al. A continuing focus of Hansen's disease in Texas. Am J Trop Med Hyg 1999; 60:449–452.

135. Ridley DS, Jopling WH. Classification of leprosy according to immunity - a five group system. Int J Lepr 1965; 34:255–273.

136. Kustner EC, Cruz MP, Dansis CP, et al. Lepromatous leprosy: A review and case report. Med Oral Patol Oral Cir Bucal 2006; 11:E474–E478.

137. Soni NK. Leprosy of the larynx. J Laryngol Otol 1992; 106:518–520.

138. Gupta JC, Gandagule VN, Nigam JP, et al. A clinicopathological study of laryngeal lesions in 30 cases of leprosy. Lepr India 1980; 52:557–565.

139. Yoshie Y. Clinical and histopathological studies on leprosy of the larynx. Int J Leprosy 1955; 24:352–353.

140. Wade HW. The histoid variety of lepromatous leprosy. In J Leprosy 1963; 31:129–141.

141. Debre R, Lamet M, Jammet ML, et al. La maladie des griffes de chat. Bull et Mem de la Soc Med des Hosp de Paris 1950; 66:76–79.

142. Ridder GJ, Boedeker CC, Technau-Ihling K, et al. Cat-scratch disease: otolaryngologic manifestations and management. Otolaryngol Head Neck Surg 2005; 132:353–358.

143. McEwan J, Basha S, Rogers S, et al. An unusual presentation of cat-scratch disease. J Laryngol Otol 2001; 115: 826–828.

144. Margileth AM, Wear DJ, English CK. Systemic cat scratch disease: Report of 23 patients with prolonged or recurrent severe bacterial infection. J Infect Dis 1987; 155:390–402.

145. Regnery R, Tappero J. Unraveling mysteries associated with cat-scratch disease, bacillary angiomatosis and related syndromes. Emerging Infect Dis 1995; 1:16–21.

146. O'Connor SP, Dorsch M, Stiegerwalt AG, et al. 16 S rRNA sequences of *Bartonella bacilliformis* and cat scratch disease bacillus reveal phylogenetic relationships with the alpha-2 subgroup of the class *Proteobacteria*. J Clin Microbiol 1991; 29:2144–2150.

147. Giladi M, Avidor B, Kletter Y, et al. Cat scratch disease: The rare role of Afipia felis. J Clin Microbiol 1998; 36: 2499–2502.

148. English CK, Wear DJ, Margileth AM, et al. Cat-Scratch Disease. Isolation and culture of the bacterial agent. JAMA 1988; 259:1347–1352.

149. Birkess KA, George VG, White EH, et al. Intracellular growth of *Afipia felis*, a putative etiologic agent of Cat scratch Disease. Infect and Immun 1992; 60:2281–2287.

150. Qian X, Jin L, Hayden RT, et al. Diagnosis of cat-scratch disease with *Bartonella henselae* infection in formalin-fixed paraffin-embedded tissues by two different PCR assays. Diagn Mol Pathol 2005; 14:146–151.

151. Leboit PE, Egbert BM, Stoler MH, et al. Epithelioid haemangioma-like vascular proliferation in AIDS: Manifestation of cat scratch disease bacillus infection? Lancet 1988; 1:960–963.

152. Koehler JE, LeBoit PE, Egbert BM, et al. Cutaneous vascular lesions and disseminated cat-scratch disease in AIDS patients and AIDS-related complex. Ann Intern Med 1988; 109:449–455.

153. Kemper CA, Lombard CM, Deresinski SC, et al. Visceral bacillary epithelioid angiomatosis: possible manifestations of disseminated cat scratch disease in the immunocompromised host: a report of two cases. Am J Med 1990; 89:216–222.

154. LeBoit PE, Berger TG, Egbert BM, et al. Bacillary angiomatosis. The histopathology and differential diagnosis of a pseudoneoplastic infection in patients with HIV disease. Am J Surg Pathol 1989; 13:909–920.

155. Lopez de Blanc S, Samuelli R, Femopase F, et al. Bacillary angiomatosis affecting the oral cavity. Report of two cases and review. J Oral Pathol Med 2000; 29:91–96.

156. Vickery CL, Dempewolf S, Porubsky ES, et al. Bacillary angiomatosis presenting as a nasal mass with epistaxis. Otolaryngol Head Neck Surg 1996; 114:443–446.

157. Sala M, Font B, Sanfeliu I, et al. Bacillary Angiomatosis caused by *Bartonella quintana*. Ann N Y Acad Sci 2005; 1063:3302–307.

158. Resto-Ruiz S, Burgess A, Anderson BE. The role of the host immune response in pathogenesis of *Bartonella henselae*. DNA and cell biology 2003; 22:431–440.

159. Arias-Stella J, Lieberman PH, Garcia-Caceres U, et al. Verruga Peruana mimicking malignant neoplasms. Am J Dermatopathol 1987; 9:279–291.

160. Schwartz RA and Lambert WC. Bacillary Angiomatosis. Available at: http://www.emedicine.com/derm/topic44.htm#section~Treatment. Accessed September 2007.

161. Stamberger H, Jakes R, Beaufort F. Aspergillosis of the paranasal sinuses. X-ray diagnosis, histopathology and clinical aspects. Ann Otol Rhinol Laryngol 1984; 93:251–256.

162. Taxy JB. Paranasal fungal sinusitis: contributions of histopathology to diagnosis: a report of 60 cases and literature review. Am J Surg Pathol 2006; 30:713–720.

163. Micheli PA. Nova plantarum genera juxta Tournefortii methodum disposita Florence, 1729, pp. 212–213.

164. Magan N, Aldred D. Post-harvest control strategies: minimizing mycotoxins in the food chain. Int J Food Microbiol 2007; 119:131–139 (epub 2007 Jul 31).

165. Hedayati MT, Pasqualotto AC, Warn PA, et al. Aspergillus flavus: human pathogen, allergen, and mycotoxin producer. Microbiology 2007; 153:1677–1692.

166. Rao CY, Riggs MA, Chew GL, et al. Characterization of airborne molds, endotoxins, and glucans in homes in New Orleans after Hurricanes Katrina and Rita. Appl Environ Microbiol 2007; 73:1630–1634.

167. Falvey DG, Streifel AJ. Ten-year air sample analysis of Aspergillus prevalence in a university hospital. J Hosp Infect 2007; 67:35–41.

168. Aisner J, Schimpff SC, Bennett JE, et al. *Aspergillus* infections in cancer patients. Association with fireproofing materials in a new hospital. JAMA 1976; 235:411–412.

169. Hunt SM, Miyamoto C, Cornelius RS, et al. Invasive fungal sinusitis in the acquired immunodeficiency syndrome. Otolaryngol Clin North America 2000; 33:335–347.

170. Siddiqui AA, Shah AA, Basher SH. Craniocerebral aspergillosis of sinonasal origin in immunocompetent patients: clinical spectrum and outcome in 25 cases. Neurosurg 2004; 55:602–611.

171. Risk SS, Kraus DH, Gerresheim G, et al. Aggressive combination treatment for invasive fungal sinusitis in immuno-compromised patients. Ear Nose Throat J 2000; 79:278–285.

172. Rhodes JC, Bode RB, McCuan-Kirsch CM: Elastase production in clinical isolates of *Aspergillus*. Diagn Microbio Infect Dis 1988; 10:165–170.

173. Ghadiali MT, Deckard NA, Farooq U, et al. Frozen section biopsy analysis for acute invasive fungal rhinosinusitis. Otolaryngol Head Neck Surg 2007; 136:714–719.

174. Kostamo K, Richardson M, Eerola E, et al. Negative impact of Aspergillus galactomannan and DNA detection in the diagnosis of fungal rhinosinusitis. J Med Microbiol 2007; 56:1322–1327.

175. Vener C, Carrabba M, Fracchiolla NS, et al. Invasive fungal sinusitis: an effective combined treatment in five

176. Sandison AT, Gentiles JC, Davidson CM, et al. Aspergilloma of paranasal sinuses and orbit in northern Sudanese. Sabouraudia 1967; 6:57–69.

177. Veress B, Malik OA, El Tayeb AA, et al. Further observations on the primary paranasal *Aspergillus* granuloma in the Sudan. A morphological study of 46 cases. Am J Trop Med Hyg 1973; 22:765–772.

178. Busaba NY, Colden DG, Faquin WC, et al. Chronic invasive fungal sinusitis: a report of two atypical cases. Ear Nose Throat J 2002; 81:462–466.

179. Currens J, Hutcheson PS, Slavin RG, et al. Primary paranasal Aspergillus granuloma: case report and review of the literature. Am J Rhinol 2002; 16:165–168.

180. Ferreiro JA, Carlson BA, Cody T. Paranasal sinus fungus balls. Head Neck 1997; 19:481–486.

181. Klossek JM, Serrano E, Peloquin L, et al. Functional endoscopic sinus surgery and 109 mycetomas of paranasal sinuses. Laryngoscope 1997; 107:112–117.

182. Grosjean P, Weber T. Fungus balls of the paranasal sinuses: a review. Eur Arch Otorhinolaryngol 2007; 264: 461–470.

183. Schwartz IS. Marijuana and fungal infection. Am J Clin Pathol 1985; 84:256.

184. Kagen SL. Aspergillus: An inhalable contaminant of marihuana. N Engl J Med 1981; 304:483–484.

185. Perez-Jaffe LA, Lanza DC, Loevner LA, et al. In-situ hybridization for Aspergillus and Penicillium in allergic fungal sinusitis: a rapid means of speciating fungal pathogens in tissues. Laryngoscope 1997; 107:233–240.

186. Kurreon F, Green GH, Rowles SL. Localized deposition of calcium oxalate around a pulmonary *Aspergillus niger* fungus ball. Am J Clin Pathol 1975; 64:556–563.

187. Willinger B, Obradovic A, Selitsch B, et al. Detection and identification of fungi from fungus balls of the maxillary sinus by molecular techniques. J Clin Microbiol 2003; 41: 581–585.

188. Katzenstein AL, Sale SR, Greenberger PA. Pathologic findings in allergic *Aspergillus* sinusitis: a newly recognized form of sinusitis. Am J Surg Pathol 1983; 7:439–443.

189. Schubert MS. Allergic fungal sinusitis. Clin Rev Allergy Immunol 2006; 30:205–216.

190. Borish L, Rosenwasser L, Steinke JW. Fungi in chronic hyperplastic eosinophilic sinusitis: reasonable doubt. Clin Rev Allergy Immunol 2006; 30:195–204.

191. Ferguson BJ. Eosinophilic mucin rhinosinusitis: a distinct clinicopathologic entity. Laryngoscope 2000; 110:799–813.

192. Lara JF, Gomez JD. Allergic mucin with and without fungus. Arch Pathol Lab Med 2001; 125:1442–1447.

193. Willard CC, Eusterman VD, Massengil PL. Allergic fungal sinusitis: report of 3 cases and review of the literature. Oral Surg Oral Med Oral Pathol 2003; 96:550–560.

194. Marple B, Newcomber M, Schwade N, et al. Natural history of allergic fungal rhinosinusitis: A 4 to 10 year follow-up. Otolaryngol Head Neck 2002; 127:361–366.

195. Kuhn FA, Swain R. Allergic fungal sinusitis: diagnosis and treatment. Curr Opin Otolaryngol Head Neck Surg 2002; 11:1–5.

196. Tansey MR. Efficient isolation of thermophilic and thermotolerant mucoralean fungi. Mycopathologia 1984; 85: 31–42.

197. Spellberg B, Edwards J, Ibrahim A. Novel perspectives on mucormycosis: pathophysiology, presentation, and management. Clin Microbiol Rev 2005; 18:556–569.

198. Gartenberg G, Bottone EJ, Keusch GT, et al. Hospital-acquired mucormycosis (*Rhizopus rhizopodiformius*) of skin and subcutaneous tissue: epidemiology, mycology, and treatment. N Engl J Med 1978; 299:1115–1118.

haematological patients. Leuk Lymphoma 2007; 48: 1577–1586.

199. Keys TF, Haldorson RN, Rhodes KII, et al. Nosocomial outbreak of *Rhizopus* infections associated with Elastoplast wound dressings–Minnesota. MMWR 1978; 27:33–34.

200. Bottone EJ, Weitzman I, Hanna BA. Rhizopus rhizopodiformis: emerging etiological agent of mucormycosis. J Clin Microbiol 1979; 9:530–537.

201. England AC, Weinstein M, Ellner JJ, et al. Two cases of rhinocerebral zygomycosis (mucormycosis) with common epidemiologic and environmental features. Am Rev Respir Dis 1981; 124:497–498.

202. Maravã-Poma E, Rodrãguez-Tudela JL, de Jalãn JG, et al. Outbreak of gastric mucormycosis associated with the use of wooden tongue depressors in critically ill patients. Intensive Care Med 2004; 30:724–728.

203. Auluck A. Maxillary necrosis by mucormycosis. a case report and literature review. Med Oral Patol Oral Cir Bucal 2007; 12(5):E360–E364.

204. Kyrmizakis DE, Doxas PG, Hajiioannou JK, et al. Palate ulcer due to mucormycosis. J Laryngol Otol 2002; 116:146–147.

205. Munir N, Jones NS. Rhinocerebral mucormycosis with orbital and intracranial extension: a case report and review of optimum management. J Laryngol Otol 2007; 121:192–195.

206. Hilal AA, Taj-Aldeen SJ, Mirghani AH. Rhinoorbital mucormycosis secondary to Rhizopus oryzae: a case report and literature review. Ear Nose Throat J 2004; 83:556, 558–560, 562.

207. Margo CE, Linden C, Strickland-Marmol LB, et al. Rhinocerebral mucormycosis with perineural spread. Ophthal Plast Reconstr Surg 2007; 23:326–327.

208. Ladurner R, Brandacher G, Steurer W, et al. Lessons to be learned from a complicated case of rhino-cerebral mucormycosis in a renal allograft recipient. Transpl Int 2003; 16:885–889.

209. Kara IO, Tasova Y, Uguz A, et al. Mucormycosis-associated fungal infections in patients with haematologic malignancies. Int J Clin Pract 2007 (epub ahead of print).

210. Bengel D, Susa M, Schreiber H, et al. Early diagnosis of rhinocerebral mucormycosis by cerebrospinal fluid analysis and determination of 16s rRNA gene sequence. Eur J Neurol 2007; 14:1067–1070.

211. Hosseini SM, Borghei P. Rhinocerebral mucormycosis: pathways of spread. Eur Arch Otorhinolaryngol 2005; 262:932–993.

212. Bongiovanni M, Ranieri R, Ferrari D, et al. Prolonged survival of an HIV infected subject with severe lymphoproliferative disease and rhinocerebral mucormycosis. J Antimicrobiol Chemother 2007; 60(1):192–193.

213. Ruoppi P, Dietz A, Nikanne E, et al. Paranasal sinus mucormycosis: a report of two cases. Acta Otolaryngol 2001; 121:948–952.

214. De Biscop J, Mondie JM, Venries de la Guillamie B, et al. Mucormycosis in an apparently normal host. J Cranio Max Fac Surg 1991; 19:275–278.

215. Parfrey N. Improved diagnosis and prognosis of mucormycosis. A clinicopathologic study of 33 cases. Medicine 1986; 65:113–123.

216. LaTouche CJ, Sutherland TW, Telling M. Histopathological and mycological features of a case of rhinocerebral mucormycosis (phycomycosis) in Britain. Sabouraudia 1963; 3:148–150.

217. Maiorano E, Favia G, Capodiferro S, et al. Combined mucormycosis and aspergillosis of the oro-sinonasal region in a patient affected by Castleman disease. Virchows Arch 2005; 446:28–33.

218. Kaufman L, Padhye AA, Parker S. Rhinocerebral zygomycosis caused by *Saksenaea vasiformis*. J Med Vet Mycology 1988; 26:237–241.

219. Ribes JA, Vanover-Sams CL, Baker DJ. Zygomycetes in Human Disease. Clin Microbiol Rev 2000; 13:236–301.

220. Okafor JI, Testrake D, Mushinsky HR, et al. A *Basidiobolus* sp. and its association with reptiles and amphibians in Southern Florida. Sabouraudia 1984; 22:47–51.

221. Gilbert EF, Khoury GH, Pore RS. Histologic identification of *Entomophthora* phycomycosis. Arch Pathol 1970; 90:583–587.

222. Prabhu RM, Patel R. Mucormycosis and entomophthoramycosis: a review of the clinical manifestations, diagnosis and treatment. Clin Microbiol Infect Supp 2004; 1:31–47.

223. Okafor BC, Gugnani HC. Nasal entomophthoromycosis in Nigerian Igbos. Trop Geograph Med 1983; 35:53–57.

224. Costa AR, Porto E, Pegas JRP, et al. Rhinofacial zygomycosis caused by *Conidiobolum coronatus*. Mycopatholog 1991; 115:1–8.

225. Castro E Souza Filho LG, Nico MMS, Salebian A, et al. Entomoftoromicose rinofacial por *Conidiobolus coronatus*. Registro de um caso tratado com sucesso pelo fluconazol. Rev Inst Med Trop Sao Paulo 1992; 34:483–487.

226. Dworzack DL, Pollack AS, Hodges GR, et al. Zygomycosis of the maxillary sinus and palate caused by *Basidobolus haptosporus*. Arch Intern Med 1978; 138:1274–1276.

227. Ghorpade A, Sarma PSA, Iqbal SM. Elephantine nose due to rhinoentomophthoromycosis. Eur J Dermatol 2006; 16:87–91.

228. Thammayya A. Zygomycosis due to Conidiobolus coronatus in west Bengal. Indian J Chest Dis Allied Sci 2000; 42:305–309.

229. Thomas MM, Bai SM, Jayaprakash C, et al. Rhinoentomophthoromycosis. Indian J Dermatol Venereol Leprol 2006; 72:296–299.

230. Valle ACF, Wanke B, Lazera MDS, et al. Entomophthoramycosis by *Conidiobolus coronatus*. Report of a case successfully treated with the combination of itraconazole and fluconazole. Rev Inst Med Trop S Paulo 2001; 43:233–236.

231. Jayamohan Y, Ribes JA. Pseudallescheriasis: a summary of patients from 1980–2003 in a tertiary care center. Arch Pathol Lab Med 2006; 130:1843–1846.

232. Tadros TS, Workowski KA, Siegel RJ, et al. Pathology of hyalohyphomycosis caused by Scedosporium apiospermum (Pseudallescheria boydii): an emerging mycosis. Hum Pathol 1998; 29:1266–1272.

233. Shear CL. Life histories and undescribed genera and species of fungi. Mycologia 1922; 15:120–131.

234. Travis LB, Roberts GD, Wilson WR. Clinical significance of *Pseudallescheria boydii*: a review of 10 years' experience. Mayo Clin Proc 1985; 60:531–537.

235. Kanafani ZA, Comair Y, Kanj SS. *Pseudallescheria boydii* cranial osteomyelitis and subdural empyema successfully treated with voriconazole: a case report and literature review. Eur J Clin Microbiol Infect Dis 2004; 23:836–840.

236. Bates DD, Mims JW. Invasive fungal sinusitis caused by Pseudallescheria boydii: case report and literature review. Ear Nose Throat J 2006; 85:729–737.

237. Sateesh CS, Makannavar JH. Chronic sino-naso-orbital fungal infection due to Pseudallescheria boydii in a nonimmunocompromised host–a case report. Indian J Pathol Microbiol 2001; 44:359–361.

238. Watters GW, Milford CA. Isolated sphenoid sinusitis due to Pseudallescheria boydii. J Laryngol Otol 1993; 107:344–346.

239. Meyer RD, Gaultier CR, Yamashita JT, et al. Fungal sinusitis in patients with AIDS: report of 4 cases and review of the literature. Medicine 1994; 73:69–78.

240. Bark CJ, Zaino LJ, Rossmiller K, et al. *Petriellidium boydii* sinusitis. JAMA 1978; 240:1339–1340.

241. Gluckman SJ, Ries K, Abrutyn E. *Allerscheria (Petriellidium) boydii* sinusitis in a compromised host. J Clin Microbiol 1977; 5:481–484.

242. Salitan M, Lawson W, Som PM, et al. *Pseudoallescheria* sinusitis with intracranial extension in a nonimmunocompromised host. Otolaryngol Head Neck Surg 1990; 102: 745–750.

243. Meyer RD, Gaultier CR, Yamashita JT, et al. Fungal sinusitis in patients with AIDS: report of 4 cases and review of the literature. Medicine 1994; 73:69–79.

244. Rippon JW, Carmicheal JW. Petriellidiosis (Allesheriosis): Four unusual cases and review of the literature. Mycopathologia 1976; 58:117–124.

245. Gilgado F, Serena C, Cano J, et al. Antifungal susceptibilities of the species of the *Pseudallescheria boydii* complex. Antimicrob Agents Chemo 2006; 50:4211–4213.

246. Revankar SG. Dematiaceous fungi. Mycoses 2007; 50: 91–101.

247. Silveira F, Nucci M. Emergence of black moulds in fungal disease: epidemiology and therapy. Curr Opin Infect Dis 2001; 14:679–684.

248. Nucci M, Akiti T, Barreiros G, et al. Nosocomial fungemia due to *Exophiala jeanselmei var. jeanselmei* and a *Rhinocladiella* species: newly described causes of bloodstream infection. J Clin Microbiol 2001; 39:514–518.

249. Fung F, Tappen D, Wood G. Alternaria-associated asthma. Appl Occup Environ Hyg 2000; 15:924–927.

250. Zieske LA, Kopke RD, Hamill R. Dematiaceous fungal sinusitis. Otolaryngol Head Neck Surg 1991; 105: 567–577.

251. Adam RD, Paquin ML, Petersen EA, et al. Phaeohyphomycosis caused by the fungal genera *Bipolaris* and *Exserohilum*. A report of 9 cases and review of the literature. Medicine 1986; 65:203–217.

252. Young CN, Swart JG, Ackermann D, et al. Nasal obstruction and bone erosion caused by *Drechslera hawaiiensis*. J Laryngol Otol 1978; 92:137–143.

253. Sobol SM, Love RG, Stutman HR, et al. Phaeohyphomycosis of the maxilloethmoid sinus caused by *Dreschlera spicifera*: A new fungal pathogen. Laryngoscope 1984; 94:620–627.

254. Alcorn JL. Generic concepts in *Drechslera, Bipolaris,* and *Exserohilum*. Mycotaxin 1983; 17:1–86.

255. Ambrosetti D, Hofman V, Castillo L, et al. An expansive paranasal sinus tumour-like lesion caused by *Bipolaris spicifera* in an immunocompetent patient. Histopathology 2006; 49:660–662.

256. Toul P, Castillo L, Hofman V, et al. A pseudo tumoral sinusitis caused by *Bipolaris* sp. J Infect 2006; 53:e235–e237.

257. Castelnuovo P, De Bernardi F, Cavanna C, et al. Invasive fungal sinusitis due to *Bipolaris hawaiiensis*. Mycoses 2004; 47:76–81.

258. Togitani K, Kobayashi M, Sakai M, et al. Ethmoidal sinusitis caused by *Exserohilum rostratum* in a patient with malignant lymphoma after non-myeloablative allogeneic peripheral blood stem cell transplantation. Transpl Infect Dis 2007; 9:137–141.

259. Lasala PR, Smith MB, McGinnis MR, et al. Invasive *Exserohilum* sinusitis in a patient with aplastic anemia. Pediatr Infect Dis J 2005; 24:939–941.

260. Colton R, Zeharia A, Karmazyn B, et al. *Exserohilum* sinusitis presenting as proptosis in a healthy adolescent male. J Adolesc Health 2002; 30:73–75.

261. Adler A, Yaniv I, Samra Z, et al. *Exserohilum*: an emerging human pathogen. Eur J Clin Microbiol Infect Dis 2006; 25:247–253.

262. Parva P, Rojas R, Palacios E. Unusual rhinosinusitis caused by *Curvularia* fungi. Ear Nose Throat J 2005; 84:270, 275.

263. Taj-Aldeen SJ, Hilal AA, Schell WA. Allergic fungal rhinosinusitis: a report of 8 cases. Am J Otolaryngol 2004; 25:213–218.

264. Safdar A. *Curvularia*–favorable response to oral itraconazole therapy in two patients with locally invasive phaeohyphomycosis. Clin Microbiol Infect 2003; 9:1219–1223.

265. Ebright JR, Chandrasekar PH, Marks S, et al. Invasive sinusitis and cerebritis due to *Curvularia clavata* in an immunocompetent adult. Clin Infect Dis 1999; 28:687–689.

266. Elliott JA. Taxonomic characteristics of the genera *Alternaria* and *Macrosporidium*. Am J Bot 1917; 4:439–476.

267. Meronuck RA, Steele JA, Mirocha CJ, et al. Tenuazonic acid, a toxin produced by *Alternaria alternaria*. Appl Microbiol 1972; 23:613–617.

268. Chen L, Thompson K, Taxy JB. Pathologic quiz case: a 56-year-old woman with anterior nasal pain and intermittent epistaxis. *Alternaria alternate* infection of the nasal sinus. Arch Pathol Lab Med 2004; 128:1451–1452.

269. Garau J, Diamond RD, Lagrotteria LB, et al. *Alternaria* osteomyelitis. Ann Inter Med 1977; 86:747–748.

270. Goodpasture HC, Carlson T, Ellis B, et al. Alternaria osteomyelitis. Evidence of specific immunologic tolerance. Arch Pathol Lab Med 1983; 107:528–530.

271. Shugar MA, Montgomery WW, Hyslop NE. *Alternaria* sinusitis. Ann Otol 1981; 90:251–255.

272. Wiest PM, Wiese K, Jacobs MR, et al. *Alternaria* infection in a patient with AIDS: case report and review of invasive *Alternaria* infections. Rev Infect Dis 1987; 9:799–803.

273. Cody DT, Neel HB, Ferreiro JA, et al. Allergic fungal sinusitis: The Mayo clinic experience. Laryngoscope 1994; 104:1074–1079.

274. Buzina W, Braun H, Freudenschluss K, et al. Fungal biodiversity – as found in nasal mucus. Med Mycol 2003; 41:149–161.

275. Dosa E, Doczi I, Mojzes L, et al. Identification and incidence of fungal strains in chronic rhinosinusitis patients. Acta Microbiol Immunol Hung 2002; 49:337–346.

276. Park AH, Muntz HR, Smith ME, et al. Pediatric invasive fungal rhinosinusitis in immunocompromised children with cancer. Otolaryngol Head Neck Surg 2005; 133: 411–416.

277. Brown JW, Nadell J, Sanders CV, et al. Brain abscess caused by *Cladosporium trichoides* (Bantianum): A case with paranasal sinus involvement. South Med J 1976; 69:1519–1521.

278. Brumpt E. Rhinosporidium. In: Precis de Parasitologie. 6th Ed. Paris, France: Masson et Cie Editeurs, 1949.

279. Nucci M, Anaissie E. Cutaneous infection by *Fusarium* species in healthy and immune compromised hosts: implications for diagnosis and management Clin Infect Dis 2002; 35:909–920.

280. Nucci M. Emerging moulds: Fusarium, Scedosporium and Zygomycetes in transplant recipients. Curr Opin Infect Dis 2003; 16:607–612.

281. Nucci M, Anaissie EJ, Queiroz-Telles F, et al. Outcome predictors of 84 patients with hematologic malignancies and Fusarium infection. Cancer 2003; 98:315–319.

282. Pino RV, Trinidad RG, Keituqwa YT, et al. Maxillary sinusitis by *Fusarium* sp. Report of a case and literature review An Otorrinolaringol Ibero Am 2004; 31:341–347.

283. Valenstein P, Schell WA. Primary intranasal *Fusarium* infection. Potential for confusion with rhinocerebral zygomycosis. Arch Pathol Lab Med 1986; 110:751–754.

284. Milgrim LM, Rubin JS, Rosenstreich DL, et al. Sinusitis in HIV infection: typical and atypical organisms. J Otolaryngol 1994; 23:450–453.

285. Rizk SS, Kraus DH, Gerresheim G, Mudan S. Aggressive combination treatment for fungal sinusitis in

immunecompromised patients. Ear Nose Throat J 2000; 79:278–280, 282, 284–285.

286. Chakrabarti A, Sharma SC. Paranasal sinus mycoses. Ind J Chest Dis Allied Sci 2000; 42:293–304.

287. Ramos-e-Silva M, Vasconcelos C, Carneiro S, et al. Sporotrichosis. Clin Dermatol 2007; 25:181–187.

288. Rosa AC, Scroferneker ML, Vettorato R, et al. Epidemiology of sporotrichosis: a study of 304 cases in Brazil. J Am Acad Dermatol 2005; 52:451–459.

289. Aarestrup FM, Guerra RO, Vieira BJ, et al. Oral manifestation of sporotrichosis in AIDS patients. Oral Dis 2001; 7:134–136.

290. Clay BM, Anand VK. Sporotrichosis: nasal obstruction in an infant. Am J Otolaryngol 1996; 17:75–77.

291. Morgan MA, Wilson WR, Neel HB, et al. Fungal sinusitis in healthy and immunocompromised individuals. Am J Clin Pathol 1984; 82:597–601.

292. Khabie N, Boyce TG, Roberts GD, et al. Laryngeal sporotrichosis causing stridor in a young child. Int J Pediatr Otorhinolaryngol 2003; 67:819–823.

293. Agger WA, Seager GA. Granulomas of the vocal cords caused by *Sporothrix schenckii*. Laryngoscope 1985; 95: 595–596.

294. Kumar R, Kaushal V, Chopra H, et al. Pansinusitis due to Sporothrix schenckii. Mycoses 2005; 48:85–88.

295. Gori S, Lupetti A, Moscato G, et al. Pulmonary sporotrichosis with hyphae in a human immunodeficiency virus-infected patient. A case report. Acta Cytol 1997; 41: 519–521.

296. Lii SL, Shigemi F. Demonstration of hyphae in human tissue of sporotrichosis, with statistics of cases reported from Tokushima. Tokushima J Exp Med 1973; 20:69–92.

297. Rodriguez G, Sarmiento L. The asteroid bodies of sporotrichosis. Am J Dermatopathol 1998; 20:246–249.

298. Choi SS, Lawson W, Bottone E, et al. Cryptococcal sinusitis: A case report and review of the literature. Otolaryngol Head Neck Surg 1988; 99:414–418.

299. Prendiville S, Bielamowicz SA, Hawrych A, et al. Isolated cryptococcal sphenoid sinusitis with septicemia, meningitis, and subsequent skull base osteomyelitis in an immunocompetent patient. Otolaryngol Head Neck Surg 2000; 123:277–279.

300. Malhotra R, Mikaelian D, Israel H. Cryptococcal sinusitis: A case report and review of the literature Otolaryngol Head Neck Surg 1995; 113:P182.

301. Day TA, Stucker FJ. Blastomycosis of the paranasal sinuses. Otolaryngology-Head Neck Surg 1994; 110:437–440.

302. Witzig RS, Quimosing EM, Campbell WL, et al. Blastomyces dermatitidis infection of the paranasal sinuses. Clin Infect Dis 1994; 18:267–268.

303. Norman WG. Rhinosporidiosis in Texas. Arch Otolaryngol 1960; 72:361–362.

304. Lasser A, Smith HW. Rhinosporidiosis. Arch Otolaryngol 1976; 102:308–310.

305. Jimenez JF, Young DE, Hough AJ. Rhinosporidiosis. A report of two cases from Arkansas. Am J Clin Pathol 1984; 82:611–615.

306. Rajam RV, Viswanathan GS, Rao AR, et al. Rhinosporidiosis–A study with report of a fatal case of systemic dissemination. In J Surg 1955; 17:269–298.

307. Naik RS, Siddiqui RS, Naik V. Urethronasal rhinosporidiosis. J Ind Med Assoc 1979; 72:238–239.

308. Ahluwala KB. Rhinosporidiosis: a study that resolves etiologic controversies. Am J Rhinol 1997; 11:1–5.

309. Herr RA, Ajello L, Taylor JW, et al. Phylogenetic analysis of Rhinosporidium seeberi's 18S small subunit ribosomal DNA groups this pathogen among members of the protoctistan Mesomycetozoa clade. J Clin Microbiol 1999; 37:2750–2754.

310. Arsecularatne SN. Rhinosporiodiosis: what is the cause? Curr Opin Infect Dis 2005; 8:113–118.

311. Ho MS, Tay BK. Disseminated rhinosporidiosis. Ann Acad Med 1986; 15:80–83.

312. Nayak S, Acharjya B, Devi B, et al. Disseminated cutaneous rhinosporidiosis. Indian J Dermatol Venereol Leprol 2007; 73:185–187.

313. Ashworth JH. On *Rhinosporidium seeberi* (Wernicke 1903) with special reference to its sporulation and affinities. Trans Royal Soc Edin 1923; 53:301–342.

314. Job A, Venkateswaran S, Mathan M, et al. Medical therapy of rhinosporidiosis with dapsone. J Laryngol Otol 1993; 107:809–812.

315. McClatchie S, Warambo MW, Bremner AD. Myospherulosis: A previously unreported disease? Am J Clin Pathol 1969; 51:699–704.

316. Kyriakos M. Myospherulosis of the paranasal sinuses, nose and middle ear. A possible iatrogenic disease. Am J Clin Pathol 1977; 67:118–130.

317. Rosai J. The nature of myospherulosis of the upper respiratory tract. Am J Clin Pathol 1978; 69:475–481.

318. Sindwani R, Cohen JT, Pilch BZ, et al. Myospherulosis following sinus surgery: pathological curiosity or impartant clinical entity? Laryngoscope 2003; 113: 1123–1127.

319. Syed SP, Wat BY, Wang J. Pathologic Quiz Case: A 55-year-old man with chronic maxillary sinusitis. Arch Pathol Lab Med 2005; 129:84–86.

320. Kuhnel TS, Kazikdas KC. Spherulocytosis of the maxillary sinus: A case report. Auris Nasus Larynx 2006; 33:461–463.

321. Sitheeque MAM, Samaranayake LP. Chronic hyperplastic Candidosis/Candidiasis (Candidal Leukoplakia). Crit Rev Oral Biol Med 2003;14:253–267.

322. Redding SW, Dahiya MC, Kirkpatrick WR, et al. Candida glabrata is an emerging cause of oropharyngeal candidiasis in patients receiving radiation for head and neck cancer. Oral Surg Oral Med Oral Pathol Oral Radiol Endod 2004; 97:47–52.

323. Zhang S, Farmer TL, Frable MA, et al. Adult herpetic laryngitis with concurrent candidal infection. Arch Otolaryngol Head Neck Surg 2000; 126:672–674.

324. Makitie AA, Back L, Aaltonen LM, et al. Fungal infection of the epiglottis simulating a clinical malignancy. Arch Otolaryngol Head Neck Surg 2003; 129:124–126.

325. Chemaly RF, Fox SB, Alkotob LM, et al. A case of zygomycosis and invasive candidiasis involving the epiglottis and tongue in an immunocompromised patient. Scand J Infect Dis 2002; 34:149–151.

326. DePasquale K, Sataloff RT. Candida of the larynx. Ear Nose Throat J 2003; 82:419.

327. Sharma N, Berman DM, Scott GB, et al. Candida epiglottitis in an adolescent with AIDS. Pediatr Infect Dis J 2005; 24:91–22.

328. Luo G, Samaranayake LP. *Candida glabrata*, an emergin fungal pathogen, exhibits superior relative cell surface hydrophobicity and adhesion to denture acrylic surfaces compared to *Candida albicans*. APMIS 2002; 110:601–610.

329. Soysa NS, Samaranayake LP, Ellepola ANB. Diabetes mellitus as a contributory factor in oral candidosis. Diabet Med 2005; 23:455–459.

330. Ajello L. Cocciodiodomycosis and histoplasmosis—a review of their epidemiology and geographical distribution. Mycopathol Mycol Appl 1971; 45:221–230.

331. Sunenshine RH, Anderson S, Erhart L, et al. Public health surveillance for coccidioidomycosis in Arizona. Ann N Y Acad Sci 2007 (epub ahead of print).

332. Drutz DJ, Catanzaro A. State of the Art: Coccidioidomycosis. Part I. Am Rev Resp Dis 1978; 117:559–585.

333. Dudley JE. Coccidioidomycosis and neck mass "single lesion" disseminated disease. Arch Otolaryngol Head Neck Surg 1987; 113:553–555.

334. Werner SB, Pappagianis D, Heindl I, et al. An epidemic of coccidiodomycosis among archeology students in Northern California. N Engl J Med 1972; 286:507–512.

335. Werner SB, Pappagianis D. Coccidioidomycosis in northern California—an outbreak among archeology students near Red Bluff. Calif Med 1973; 119:16–20.

336. Petersen LR, Marshall SL, Barton-Dickson C, et al. Coccidioidomycosis among workers at an archeological site, northeastern Utah. Emerg Infect Dis 2004; 10:637–642.

337. Crum-Cianflone NF. Coccidioidomycosis in the U.S. Military: A Review. Ann N Y Acad Sci. 2007 (epub ahead of print).

338. Pappagianis D. Epidemiology of Coccidioidomycosis. Curr Top Med Mycol 1988; 2:199–238.

339. Eckmann BH, Schaeffer GL, Huppert M. Bedside interhuman transmission of coccidioidomycosis via growth on fomites. An epidemic involving six persons. Am Rev Respir Dis 1964; 89:175–185.

340. Symmers W St. C. Cases of coccidioidomycosis seen in Britain. In: Ajello L, ed. Coccidioidomycosis. Tucson, Arizona: University of Arizona Press, 1967:13–22.

341. Sotgiu G, Corbelli G. Micosi rare: Osservazione dei primi due casi di isoteoplasmosi in Italia e di un caso di coccidioidomicosi. Bull Sci Med Bologna 1955; 127:85–92.

342. Van Bergen W, Fleury FJ, Cheatle EL. Fatal maternal disseminated coccidioidomycosis in a nonendemic area. Am J Obstet Gynecol 1976; 124:661–663.

343. Blair JE, Coakley B, Santelli AC, et al. Serologic testing for symptomatic Coccidioidomycosis in immunocompetent and immunosuppressed hosts. Mycopathologia 2006; 162:317–324.

344. Arnold MG, Arnold JC, Bloom DC, et al. Head and neck manifestations of disseminated coccidioidomycosis. Laryngoscope 2004; 114:747–752.

345. Verghese S, Arjundas D, Krishnakumar C, et al. Coccidioidomycosis in India: report of a second imported case. Med Mycol 2002; 40:307–309.

346. Fish DG, Ampel NM, Galgiani JN, et al. Coccidioidomycosis during HIV infection. A review of 77 patients. Medicine 1990; 69:384–390.

347. Jarvik JG, Hesselink JR, Wiley C, et al. Coccidioiomycotic brain abscess in an HIV-infected man. The Western J Med 1988; 149:83–86.

348. Hajare S, Rakmusan TA, Kalia A, et al. Laryngeal coccidioidomycosis causing airway obstruction. Ped Infect Dis J 1989; 8:54–56.

349. Boyle JO, Coulthard SW, Mandel RM; Laryngeal involvement in disseminated coccioidomycosis. Arch Otolaryngol Head Neck Surg 1991; 117:433–438.

350. Rodriguez RA, Konia T. Coccidioidomycosis of the tongue. Arch Pathol Lab Med 2005; 129:4–6.

351. Bialek R, Gonzalez GM, Begerow D, et al. Coccidioidomycosis and blastomycosis: Advances in molecular diagnosis. FEMS Immunology Med Microbiol 2005; 45:355–360.

352. Saubolle MA, McKellar PP, Sussland D. Epidemiologic, clinical, and diagnostic aspects of coccidioidomycosis. J Clin Microbiol 2007; 45:26–30.

353. Binnicker MJ, Buckwalter SP, Eisberner JJ, et al. Detection of Coccidioides species in clinical specimens by real-time PCR. J Clin Microbiol 2007; 45:173–178.

354. Galgiani J. Coccidiodomycosis: Changing perceptions and creating opportunities for its control. Ann N Y Acad Sciences 2007 (epub ahead of print).

355. Almeida SM. Central nervous system paracoccidioidomycosis: An overview. Braz J Infect Dis 2005; 9:126–133.

356. Sant'Anna GD, Mauri M, Arrarte JL, et al. Laryngeal manifestations of Paracoccidioidomycosis (South American Blastomycosis). Arch Otolaryngol 1999; 125:1375–1378.

357. Furtaldo T. Infection versus disease in South American blastomycosis. Int J Dermato 1975; 14:117–125.

358. Lazow SK, Seldin RD, Solomon MP. South American blastomycosis of the maxilla: Report of a case. J Oral Maxillofac Surg 1990; 48:68–71.

359. Paniago AMM, Freitas ACC, Aguilar ESA, et al. Paracoccidioidomycosis in patients with HIV review of 12 cases observed in an endemic region in Brazil. J Infect 2005; 51:248–252.

360. Sposto MR, Scully C, Almeida OP, et al. Oral paracoccidioidomycosis. A study of 36 South American patients. Oral Surg Oral Med Oral Pathol 1993; 75:461–465.

361. Almeida OP, Jorge J, Scully C, et al: Paracoccidioidomycosis of the mouth: An emerging deep mycosis. Crit Rev Oral boil Med 2003; 14: 268–274.

362. Bicalho RN, Santo MFD, Aguiar MCF, et al. Oral paracoccidioidomycosis: a retrospective study of 62 Brazilian patients. Oral Dis 2001; 7:56–60.

363. Castro LG, Muller AP, Mimura MA, et al. Hard palate perforation: an unusual finding in paracoccidioidomycosis. Int J Dermatol 2001; 40:281–283.

364. Ricci G, Da Silva ID, Sano A, et al. Detection of *Paracoccidioides brasiliensis* by PCR in biopsies from patients with paracoccidioidomycosis: correlation with the histopathological pattern. Pathologica 2007; 99:41–45.

365. Menezes VM, Soares BGO, Fontes CJF. Drugs for treating Paracoccidioidomycosis. Cochrane Database Syst Rev 2007; 3:CD004967 (review).

366. Klein BS, Vergeront JM, Weeks RJ, et al. Isolation of *Blastomyces dermatitidis* in soil associated with a large outbreak of blastomycosis in Wisconsin. New Engl J Med 1986; 314:529–534.

367. Lemos L, Guo M, Baliga M. Blastomycosis: Organ involvement and etiologic diagnosis. A review of 123 patients from Mississippi. Ann Diagn Pathol 2000; 4:391–406.

368. Dworkin MS, Duckro AN, Proia L, et al. The epidemiology of blastomycosis in Illinois and factors associated with death. Clin Infect Dis 2005; 41:107–111.

369. Centers for Disease control and Prevention (CDC). Blastomycosis—Wisconsin, 1986–1995 MMWR Morb Mortal Wkly Rep 1996; 45(28):601–603. Available at: www.cdc.gov/mmwr/preview/mmwrhtml/00043101.htm. Accessed July 2007.

370. MacDonald PDM, Langley RL, Gerkin SR, et al. Human and canine pulmonary blastomycosis, North Carolina, 2001–2002. Emerg Infect Dis (serial on the Internet). 2006. Available at: www.cdc.gov/ncidod/EID/vol12no08/05-0781.htm (accessed July 2007).

371. Baumgardner DJ, Steber D, Glazier R, et al. Geographic information system analysis of blastomycosis in northern Wisconsin, USA: waterways and soil. Med Mycol 2005; 43:117–125.

372. McCullough MJ, DiSalvo AF, Clemons KV, et al. Molecular epidemiology of Blastomyces dermatitidis. Clin Infect Dis 2000; 30:328–335.

373. Body BA. Cutaneous manifestations of systemic mycoses. Dermatol Clin 1996; 14:125–135.

374. Reder PA, Neel HB. Blastomycosis in otolaryngology: review of a large series. Laryngoscope 1993; 103:53–58.

375. Taxy JB. Blastomycosis; Contributions of morphology to diagnosis. A surgical pathology, cytopathology, and autopsy pathology study. Am J Surg Pathol 2007; 31:615–623.

376. Varkey B and Raugi GJ. Blastomycosis. Available at: www.emedicine.com/med/topic231.htm. Accessed July 2007.

377. Suen JY, Wetmore SJ, Wetzel WJ, et al. Blastomycosis of the larynx. Ann Otol 1980; 89:563–566.

378. Payne J, Koopman C. Laryngeal carcinoma - or is it laryngeal blastomycosis? Laryngoscope 1984; 94:608–611.

379. Dumich PS, Neel HB. Blastomycosis of the larynx. Laryngoscope 1983; 93:1266–1270.

380. Rose HD, Gingrass DJ. Localized oral blastomycosis mimicking actinomycosis. Oral Surg Oral Med Oral Pathol 1982; 54:12–14.

381. Cury PM, Pulido CF, Furtado VM, et al. Autopsy findings in AIDS patients from a reference hospital in Brazil: analysis of 92 cases. Pathol Res Pract 2003; 199:811–814.

382. Emmons CW: Prevalence of *Cryptococcus neoformans* in pidgeon habitats. Pub Health Rep (Washington) 1960; 75:362–364.

383. Nielsen K, De Obaldia AL Heitman J. *Cryptococcus neoformans* mates on pigeon guano: implications for the realized ecological niche and globalization. Eukaryotic Cell 2007; 6:949–959.

384. Nosanchuk JD, Shoham S, Fries BC, et al. Evidence of zoonotic transmission of *Cryptococcus neoformans* from a pet cockatoo to an immunocompromised patient. Ann Intern Med 2000; 132:205–208.

385. Benesova P, Buchta V, Cerman J, et al. *Cryptococcus* - a review of 13 autopsy cases from a 54-year period in a large hospital. APMIS 2007; 115:177–183.

386. Goldani LZ, Zavascki AP, Maia AL. Fungal thyroiditis: an overview. Mycopathologia 2006; 161:129–139.

387. Mehrabi M, Bagheri S, Leonard MK Jr. Perciaccante VJ: Mucocutaneous manifestation of cryptococcal infection: report of a case and review of the literature. J Oral Maxillofac Surg 2005; 63:1543–1549.

388. Bamba H, Tatemoto K, Inoue M, et al. A case of vocal cord cyst with Cryptococcal infection. Otolayrngol Head Neck Surg 2005; 133:150–152.

389. McGregor DK, Citron D, Shahab I. Cryptococcal infection of the larynx simulating laryngeal carcinoma. South Med J 2003; 96:74–77.

390. Shibuya K, Coulson WF, Wollman JS, et al. Histopathology of cryptococcosis and other fungal infections in patients with AIDS. Int J Infect Dis 2001; 5:78–85.

391. Bottone EJ, Wormser GP. Capsule-deficient cryptococci in AIDS. Lancet 1985; 2:553 (lettr).

392. Bottone EJ, Toma M, Johansson BE, et al. Capsule-deficient *Cryptococcus neoformans* in AIDS patients. Lancet 1985; 1:400 (lettr).

393. Ro JY, Lee SS, Ayala AG. Advantage of Fontana-Masson stain in capsule-deficient cryptococcal infection. Arch Pathol Lab Med 1987; 111:53–57.

394. Darling ST. A protozoon general infection producing pseudotubercles in the lungs and focal necrosis in the liver, spleen and lymph nodes. JAMA 1906; 46:1283–1285.

395. Feare C. The Starling. Oxford, England: Oxford University Press, 1984.

396. Chapman FM. Handbook of Birds in Eastern North America. New York, NY: Appleton, 1895.

397. Shakespeare W. The First Part of Henry IV. Act I, Scene 3, line 224.

398. Kaufman CA. Histoplasmosis: A clinical and laboratory update. Clin Microbiol Rev 2007; 20:115–132.

399. Furcolow ML, Tosh FE, Larsh HW, et al. The emerging pattern of urban histoplasmosis. Studies on an epidemic in Mexico, Missouri. New Engl J Med 1961; 264:1226–1230.

400. Tosh FE, Weeks RJ, Pfeiffer FR, et al. The use of formalin to kill *Histoplasma capsulatum* at an epidemic site. Amer J Epidem 1967; 85:259–265.

401. Parrott T, Taylor G, Poston M, et al. An epidemic of histoplasmosis in Warrenton, North Carolina. South Med J 1955; 48:1147–1150.

402. Wheat LJ, Conolly-Stringfield PA, Baker RL, et al. Disseminated histoplasmosis in AIDS: Clinical findings, diagnosis and treatment, and review of the literature. Med 1990, 69: 361–374.

403. Assi M, Sandid M, Baddour LM *et al:* Systemic Histoplasmosis. A 15-year retrospective institutional review of 111 patients. Medicine (Baltimore) 2007; 86:162–169.

404. Cunha VS, Zampese MS, Aquino VR, et al. Mucocutaneous manifestations of disseminated Histoplasmosis in patients with acquired immunodeficiency syndrome: particular aspects in a Latin-American population. Clin Dermatol 2007; 32:250–255.

405. Zain RB, Ling KC. Oral and laryngeal histoplasmosis in a patient with Addison's disease. Ann Dent 1988; 47:31–33.

406. Cobb CM, Shultz RE, Brewer JH, et al. Chronic pulmonary histoplasmosis with an oral lesion. Oral Surg Oral Med Oral Pathol 1989; 67:73–76.

407. Miller RL, Gould AR, Skolnick JL, et al. Localized oral histoplasmosis. A regional manifestation of mild chronic disseminated histoplasmosis. Oral Surg 1982; 53: 367–374.

408. Loh F, Yeo J, Tan W, et al. Histoplamosis presenting as hyperplastic gingival lesion. J Oral Pathol Med 1989; 18:533–536.

409. Ferreira OG, Cardoso SV, Borges AS, et al. Oral Histoplasmosis in Brazil. Oral Surg Oral Med Oral Pathol Oral Radiol Endod 2002; 93:654–659.

410. Larsen CG, Militsakh O, Fang F, et al. Histoplasmosis presenting as upper airway obstruction. Otolaryngol Head Neck Surg 2005;132:514–516.

411. Hernandez SL, De Blanc SAL, Sambuelli RH, et al. Oral Histoplasmosis associated with HIV infection: a comparative study. J Oral Pathol Med 2004; 33:445–450.

412. Bennett DE. Histoplasmosis of the oral cavity and larynx. Arch Intern Med 1967; 120:417–427.

413. Young LL, Dolan T, Sheridan PJ, et al. Oral manifestations of histoplamosis. Oral Surg 1972; 33:191–204.

414. Negroni P. Histoplasmosis. Diagnosis and Treatment. Springfield, Ill: Charles C Thomas, 1965.

415. Woods JP. Knocking on the right door and making a comfortable home: Histoplasma capsulatum intracellular pathogenesis. Curr Opin Microbiol 2003; 6:327–331.

416. Cobb CM, Shultz RE, Brewer JH, et al. Chronic pulmonary histoplasmosis with an oral lesion. Oral Surg Oral Med Oral Pathol 1989; 67:73–76.

417. Tsui WMS, Ma KF, Tsang DNC. Disseminated *Penicillium marneffei* infection in HIV-infected subject. Histopathol 1992; 20:287–293.

418. Wheat LJ. Current diagnosis of Histoplasmosis. Trends Microbiol 2003; 11:488–494.

419. Saxinger WC, Levine PH, Dean AG, et al. Evidence for exposure to HTLV-III in Uganda before 1973. Science 1985; 227:1036–1038.

420. Bygbjerg IC. AIDS in a Danish surgeon (Zaire 1976). Lancet 1983; i:925.

421. Vandepitte J, Verwilghen R, Zachee P. AIDS and cryptococcosis (Zaire 1977). Lancet 1983; i:925–926.

422. Kanki PJ, Alroy J, Essex M. Isolation of T-lymphotrophic retrovirus related to HTLV-III/LAV from wild-caught African green monkeys. Science 1985; 230:951–954.

423. Daniel MD, Letvin NL, King NW, et al. Isolation of T-cell trophic HTLV-III-like retrovirus from macaques. Science 1985; 228:1201–1204.

424. Kanki PJ, Barin F, M'Boup S, et al. New HTLV retrovirus related to STLV-IIIa.AGM. Science 1986; 232:238–243.

425. Siebert C. Smallpox is dead. Long live smallpox. New York Times 1994 August 21; 6:31–55.

426. Van de Perre P, Lepage P, Kestelyn P, et al. AIDS in Rwanda. Lancet 1984; ii:62–65.

427. Piot P, Taelman H, Mbendi N, et al. AIDS in a heterosexual population in Zaire. Lancet 1984; ii:65–69.
428. Clumeck N, Sonnet J, Taelman H, et al. AIDS in African patients. New Engl J Med 1984; 310:492–497.
429. Clumeck N, Robert-Guroff M, Van de Perre P, et al. Serological studies of HTLV-III antibody prevalence among selected groups of heterosexual Africans. JAMA 1985; 254:2599–2602.
430. Center for Disease Control. Opportunisitic infections and Kaposi's sarcoma among Haitians in the United States. MMWR 1982; 31:353–361.
431. Levy JA. HIV pathogenesis: knowledge gained after two decades of research. Adv Dent Res 2006; 19:10–16.
432. Marmor M, Laubenstein L, Wiliam DC, et al. Risk factors for Kaposi's sarcoma in homosexual men. Lancet 1982; i:1083–1087.
433. Centers for Disease control and Prevention (CDC). Available at: www.cdc.gov/hiv/resources/factsheets/At-A-Glance.htm. Accessed October 2007.
434. Centers for Disease control and Prevention (CDC). Available at: www.cdc.gov/hiv/topics/surveillance/resources/reports/2003report/default.htm. Accessed October 2007.
435. UNAIDS. 2004 Report on the global AIDS epidemic July 2004. Available at: www.unaids.org/bangkok2004/GAR2004_html/GAR2004_00_en.htm. Accessed October 2007.
436. Dalgleish A, Beverly PCL, Clapham PR, et al. The CD4 (T4) antigen is an essential component of the receptor for the AIDS retrovirus. Nature 1984; 312:763–767.
437. Chan DC, Fass D, Berger JM, et al. Core structure of gp41 from the HIV envelope glycoprotein. Cell 1997; 88:263–273.
438. Rosen CA, Soddroski JG, Haseltine WA. The location of cis-acting regulatory sequences in the human T-cell lymphotrophic virus type III (HTLV-II/LAV) long terminal repeat. Cell 1985; 41:813–823.
439. Gatignol A. Transcription of HIV: Tat and cellular chromatin. Adv Pharmacol 2007; 55:137–159.
440. Gibellini D, Vitone F, Schiavone P, et al. HIV-1 tat protein and cell proliferation and survival: a brief review. New Microbio 2005; 28:95–109.
441. Vogel J, Hinrichs SH, Reynolds RK, et al. The HIV tat gene induces dermal lesions resembling Kaposi's sarcoma in transgenic mice. Nature 1988; 335:606–611.
442. Vogel J, Hinrichs SH, Napoliani LA, et al. Liver cancer in transgenic mice carrying the HIV tat gene. Cancer Res 1991; 51:6686–6690.
443. Peruzzi F. The multiple functions of HIV-1 Tat: Proliferation versus apoptosis. Frontiers in Bioscience. 2006; 11:708–717.
444. Steffens CM, Hope TJ. Recent advances in the understanding of HIV accessory protein function. AIDS 2001; 15(suppl 5):S21–S26 (review).
445. Strebel K. Virus-host interactions: role of HIV proteins Vif, Tat, and Rev.AIDS 2003; 17(suppl 4):S25–S34.
446. Rhodes DI, Ashton L, Solomon A, et al. Characterization of three nef-defective HIV-1 strains associated with long-term nonprogression. Australian Long-Term Nonprogression Study Group. J Virol 2000; 74:10581–10588.
447. Bukrinsky M, Adzhubei A. Viral protein R of HIV-1. Rev Med Virol 1999; 9:39–49.
448. Levy JA. HIV Pathogenesis: Knowledge gained after two decades of research. Adv Dent Res 2006; 19:10–16.
449. Rabeneck L, Popovic M, Gartner S, et al. Acute HIV infection presenting with painful swallowing and esophageal ulcers. JAMA 1990; 263:2318–2322.
450. Reichart P. US1 HIV - changing patterns in HAART era, patients' quality of life and occupational risks. Oral Dis 2006; 12(suppl 1):3.
451. Palella FJ, Delaney KM, Moorman AC, et al. Declining morbidity and mortality among patients with advanced human immunodeficiency virus infection. HIV Outpatient Study Investigators. N Eng J Med 1998; 338:853–860.
452. Dybul M, Fauci AS, Bartlett JG, et al. Panel on clinical practices for the treatment of HIV. Guidelines for using antiretroviral agents among HIV-infected adults and adolescents. recommendations of the panel on clinical practices for treatment of HIV. MMWR Recomm Rep 2002; 51:1–55.
453. Thomas CF, Limper AH. Current insights into the biology and pathogenesis of Pneumocystis pneumonia. Nat Rev Microbiol 2007; 5:298–308.
454. Ng VL, Yajko DM, Hadley WK. Extrapulmonary pneumocystosis. Clin Microbiol Rev 1997; 10:401–418.
455. Edman JC, Kovacs JA, Masur H, et al. Ribosomal RNA sequence shows Pneumocystis carinii to be a member of the Fungi. Nature 1988; 334:519–522.
456. Miller RF, Ambrose HE, Wakefield AE. Pneumocystis carinii f. sp. hominis DNA in immunocompetent health care workers in contact with patients with P. carinii pneumonia. J Clin Microbiol 2001; 39:3877–3882.
457. Vargas SL, Ponce CA, Gigliotti F, et al. Transmission of Pneumocystis carinii DNA from a patient with P. carinii pneumonia to immunocompetent contact health care workers. J Clin Microbiol 2000; 38:1536–1538.
458. Oz HS, Hughes WT. Search for Pneumocystis carinii DNA in upper and lower respiratory tract of humans. Diagn Microbiol Infect Dis 2000; 37:161–164.
459. Nevez G, Magois, E, Duwat H, et al. Apparent absence of Pneumocystis jirovecii in healthy subjects. Clin Infect Dis 2006; 42:e99–e101.
460. Breda SD, Hammerschlag PE, Gigliotti FR, et al. Pneumocystis carinii in the temporal bone as a primary manifestation of the AIDS. Ann Otol Rhinol Laryngol 1988; 97:427–431.
461. Praveen CV, Terry RM, Elmahallawy M, et al. Pneumocystis carinii infection in bilateral aural polyps in a human immunodeficiency virus-positive patient. J Laryngol Otol 2002; 116:288–290.
462. Henneberry JM, Smith RRL, Hruban RH. Pneumocystis carinii infection of the external auditory canal. Arch Otolaryngol Head Neck Surg 1993; 119:466–469.
463. Coulman CU, Green I, Archibald RWR. Cutaneous Pneumocystosis. Ann Int Med 1987; 106:396–398.
464. Park S, Wunderlich H, Goldenberg RA, et al. Pneumocystis carinii infection in the middle ear. Arch Otolaryngol Head Neck Surg 1992; 118:269–270.
465. Sandler ED, Sandler JM, Le Boit PE, et al. Pneumocystis carinii otitis media in AIDS: a case report and review of the literature regarding extrapulmonary pneumocystosis. Otolaryngol Head Neck Surg 1990; 103:817–821.
466. Wasserman L, Haghighi P. Otic and ophthalmic pneumocystosis in AIDS. Arch Pathol Lab Med 1992; 116:500–503.
467. Feller L, Wood NH, Lemmer J. HIV-associated Kaposi's sarcoma: pathogenic mechanisms. Oral Surg Oral Med Oral Pathol Oral Radiol Endod 2007; 104:521–529.
468. Oettle AG. Geographic and racial differences in the frequency of Kaposi's sarcoma as evidence of environmental or genetic causes. Acta Unio Internat Contra Cancrum 1962; 18:330–363.
469. Wamburu G, Masenga EJ, Moshi EZ, et al. HIV - associated and non - HIV associated types of Kaposi's sarcoma in an African population in Tanzania. Status of immune suppression and HHV-8 seroprevalence. Eur J Dermatol 2006; 16:677–6682.
470. Darling M, Thompson I, Meer M. Oral Kaposi's sarcoma in a renal transplant patient: Case report and literature review. J Can Dent Assoc 2004; 70:617–620.

471. Chang Y, Cesarman E, Pessin MS, et al. identification of herpesvirus-like DNA sequences in AIDS-associated Kaposi's sarcoma. Science 1994; 266:1865–1869.
472. Ramos-da-Silva S, Elgui-de-Oliveira D, Borges L, et al. Kaposi's sarcoma-associated herpesvirus infection and Kaposi's sarcoma in Brazil. Braz J Med Biol Res 2006; 39:573–580.
473. Rezza G, Andreoni M, Dorrucci M, et al. Human herpesvirus 8 serpositivity and risk of Kaposi's sarcoma and other acquired immunedeficiency syndrome-related diseases. J Natl Cancer Inst 1999; 91:1468–1474.
474. Jacobson LP, Jenkins FJ, Springer G, et al. Interaction of human immunedeficiency virus type 1 and human herpesvirus type 8 infections on the incidence of Kaposi's sarcoma. J Infect Dis 2000; 181:1940–1949.
475. Larocca L, Leto D, Celesta BM, et al. Prevalence of antibodies to HHV-8 in the general population and in individuals at risk for sexually transmitted and blood-borne infections in Catania, Eastern Sicily. Infez Med 2005; 13:79–85.
476. Engels EA, Sinclair MD, Biggar RJ, et al. Latent class analysis of human herpesvirus 8 assay performance and infection prevalence in sub-saharan Africa and Malta. Int J Cancer 2000; 88:1003–1008.
477. Ziegler J, Newton R, Bourboulia D, et al. Risk factors for Kaposi's sarcoma: a case-control study of HIV-seronegative people in Uganda. Int J Cancer 2003; 103:233–240.
478. Klaskala W, Brayfield BP, Kankasa C, et al. Epidemiological characteristics of human herpesvirus-8 infection in a large population of antenatal women in Zambia. J Med Virol 2005; 75:93–100.
479. Mbulaiteye SM, Pfeiffer RM, Whitby D, et al. Human herpesvirus 8 infection within families in rural Tanzania. J Infect Dis 2003; 187:1780–1785.
480. Ablashi D, Chatlynne L, Cooper H, et al. Seroprevalence of human herpesvirus-8 (HHV-8) in countries of Southeast Asia compared to the USA, the Caribbean and Africa. Br J Cancer 1999; 81:893–897.
481. Gnamm JW, Pellett PE, Jaffe HW. Human herpesvirus 8 and Kaposi's sarcoma in persons infected with human immunodeficiency virus. Clin Infect Dis 2000; 30:S72–S76.
482. Whitby D, Luppi M, Barozzi P, et al. Human herpesvirus 8 seropositivity in blood donors and lymphoma patients from different regions in Intaly. J Natl Cancer Inst 1998; 9:395–397.
483. Widmer IC, Erb P, Grob H, et al. Human herpesvirus 8 oral shedding in HIV-infected men with and without Kaposi sarcoma. J Acquir Immune Defic Syndr 2006; 42:420–425.
484. Gnepp DR, Chandler W, Hyams V. Primary Kaposi's sarcoma of the head and neck. Ann Inter Med 1984; 100:107–114.
485. Bottler T, Kuttenberger J, Hardt N, et al. Non-HIV-associated Kaposi's sarcoma of the tongue. Case report and review of the literature. Oral Maxfac Surg 2007; 36(12):1218–1220.
486. Venizelos I, Andreadis C, Tatsiou Z. Primary Kaposi's sarcoma of the nasal cavity not associated with AIDS. Eur Arch Otorhinolaryngol 2008; 265(6):717–720.
487. Schiff NF, Annino DJ, Woo P, et al. Kaposi's sarcoma of the larynx. Ann Otol Rhinol Laryngol 1997; 106:563–567.
488. Mochloulis G, Irving RM, Grant HR, et al. Laryngeal Kaposi's sarcoma in patients with AIDS. J Laryngol Otol 1996; 110:1034–1037.
489. Fliss DM, Parikh J, Freeman JL. AIDS-related Kaposi's sarcoma of the sphenoid sinus. J Otolaryngol 1992; 21:235–237.
490. Baccaglini L, Atkinson JC, Patton LL, et al. Management of oral lesions in HIV-positive patients. Oral Surg Oral Med Oral Pathol Oral Radiol Endod 2007; 103(suppl):S50.e1–23.
491. Couderc LJ, D'Agay MF, Danon F, et al. Sicca complex and infection with HIV. Arch Intern Med 1987; 147:898–901.
492. Finfer MD, Schinella RA, Rothstein SG, et al. Cystic parotid lesions in patients at risk for AIDS. Arch Otolaryngol Head Neck Surg 1988; 114:1290–1294.
493. Shugar JM, Som PM, Jacobson AL, et al. Multicentric parotid cysts and cervical adenopathy in AIDS patients. A newly recognized entity: CT and MR manifestations. Laryngoscope 1988; 98:772–775.
494. Tunkel DE, Loury MC, Fox CH, et al. Bilateral parotid enlargement in HIV-seropositive patients. Laryngoscope 1989; 99:590–545.
495. Ryan JR, Ioachim HL, Marmer J, et al. AIDS-related lymphadenopathies presenting in the salivary gland lymph nodes. Arch Otolaryngol 1985; 111:554–556.
496. Schoidt M, Greenspan D, Levy JA, et al. Does HIV cause salivary gland disease? AIDS 1989; 3:819–822.
497. Ulirisch RC, Jaffe ES. Sjogren's syndrome-like illness associated with the AIDS-related complex. Hum Pathol 1987; 18:1063–1068.
498. D'Agay MF, de Roquancourt A, Peuchmaur M, et al. Cystic benign lymphoepithelial lesion of the salivary glands in HIV-positive patients. Virch Archiv A 1990; 417:353–356.
499. Vargas PA, Mauad T, Bohm GM, et al. Parotid gland involvement in advanced AIDS. Oral Dis 2003; 9:55–61.
500. Basu D, Williams FM, Ahn CW, et al. Changing spectrum of the diffuse infiltrative lymphocytosis syndrome. Arthr Rheum 2006; 55:466–472.
501. Rivera H, Nikitakis N, Castillo S, et al. Histopathological analysis and demonstration of EBV and HIV p-24 antigen but not CMV expression in labial minor salivary glands of HIV patients affected by diffuse infiltrative lymphocytosis syndrome. J Oral Pathol Med 2003; 32: 431–437.
502. McArthur CP, Subtil-DeOliveira A, Palmer D, et al. Characteristics of salivary diffuse infiltrative lymphocytosis syndrome in West Africa. Arch Pathol Lab Med 2000; 124:1773–1779.
503. Ihrler S, Zietz C, Riederer A, et al. HIV-related parotid lymphoepithelial cysts. Immunohistochemistry and 3-D reconstruction of surgical and autopsy material with special reference ro formal pathogenesis. Virch Arch 1996; 429:139–147.
504. Mandel L, Surattanont F. Regression of HIV parotid swellings after antiviral therapy: case reports with computed tomographic scan evidence. Oral Surg Oral Med Oral Pathol Oral Radiol Endod 2002; 94:454–459.
505. Olsen WL, Jeffrey RB, Sooy CD, et al. Lesions of the head and neck in AIDS patients: CT and MR findings. Am J Neuroradiology 1988; 9:693–698.
506. France AJ, Kean DM, Douglas RHB, et al. Adenoidal hypertrophy in HIV-infected patients. Lancet 1988; 2(8619):1076.
507. Desai SD. Seropositivity, adenoid hypertrophy, and secretory otitis media in adults—a recognized clinical entity. Otolaryngol Head Neck Surg 1992; 107:755–757.
508. Wenig BM, Thompson LD, Frankel SS, et al. Lymphoid changes of the nasopharyngeal and palatine tonsils that are indicative of human immunodeficiency virus infection. A clinicopathologic study of 12 cases. Am J Surg Pathol 1996; 20:572–287.
509. Malm G, Engman ML. Congenital cytomegalovirus infections. Sem Fetal Neonatal Med 2007; 12:154–159.
510. Centers for Disease control and Prevention (CDC). Available at: www.cdc.gov/cmv/facts.htm. Accessed November 2007.

511. Kylat RI, Kelly EN, Ford-Jones EL. Clinical findings and adverse outcome in neonates with symptomatic congenital cytomegalovirus (SCCMV) infection. Eur J Pediatr 2006; 165:773–778.

512. Steininger C. Clinical relevance of cytomegalovirus infection in patients with disorders of the immune system. Clin Microbiol 2007; 13:953–963.

513. Pescovitz MD. Benefits of Cytomegalovirus Prophylaxis in Solid Organ Transplantation. Transplantation 2006; 82: S4–S8.

514. Steininger C, Puchhammer-Stockl E, Popow-Kraupp T. Cytomegalovirus disease in the era of highly active antiretroviral therapy (HAART). J Clin Virol 2006; 37:1–9.

515. Kemper JH, Min YI, Freeman WR, et al. Risk of immune recovery uveitis in patients with AIDS and cytomegalovirus retinitis. Opthal 2006; 113:684–694.

516. Springer KL, Weinberg A. Cytomegalovirus infection in the era of HAART: fewer reactivations and more immunity. J Antimicrob Chemother 2004; 54:582–586.

517. Griffiths P. Cytomegalovirus infection of the central nervous system. Herpes 2004; 11(supp 2):A95–A104.

518. Lalwani AK, Snyderman NL. Pharyngeal ulceration in AIDS patients secondary to CMV infections. Ann Otol Rhinol Laryngol 1991; 100:484–487.

519. Kanas R, Jensen JL, Abrams AM, et al. Oral mucosal CMV as a manifestation of AIDS. Oral Surg Oral Med Oral Pathol 1987; 64:183–189.

520. Langford A, Kunze R, Timm H, et al. CMV associated oral ulcerations in HIV-infected patients. J Oral Pathol Med 1989; 19:71–76.

521. Imoto EM, Stein RM, Shellito JE, et al. Central airway obstruction due to CMV-induced necrotizing tracheitis in a patient with AIDS. Am Rev Resp Dis 1990; 142: 884–886.

522. Marelli RA, Biddinger PW, Gluckman JL. CMV infection of the larynx in the AIDS. Otolaryngol Head Neck Surg 1992; 106:296–301.

523. French PD, Birchall MA, Harris JR. Cytomegalovirus ulceration of the oropharynx. J Laryngol Otol 1991; 105:739–742.

524. Zemnick C, Asher ES, Wood N, et al. Immediate nasal prosthetic rehabilitation following cytomegalovirus erosion: A clinical report. J Prosthet Dent 2006; 95: 349–353.

525. Lopez-Amado M, Yebra-Pimentel MT, Garcia-Sarandeses A. Cytomegalovirus causing necrotizing laryngitis in a renal cardiac transplant recipient. Head Neck 1996; 18:455–457.

526. Small PM, McPhaul LW, Sooy CD, et al. CMV infection of the laryngeal nerve presenting as hoarseness in AIDS patients. Am J Med 1989; 86:108–110.

527. Redleaf MI, Bauer CA, Robinson RA. Fine-needle detection of CMV parotitis in a patient with AIDS. Arch Otolaryngol Head Neck Surg 1994; 120:414–416.

528. Vargas PA, Villalba H, Passos AP, et al. Simultaneous occurrence of lymphoepithelial cysts, cytomegalovirus and mycobacterial infections in the intraparotid lymph nodes of a patient with AIDS. J Oral Pathol Med 2001; 30:507–509.

529. Salzberger B, Myerson D, Boeckh M. Circulating cytomegalovirus (CMV)-infected endothelial cells in marrow transplant patients with CMV disease and CMV infection. J Infect Dis 1997; 176:778–781.

530. Davis MG, Kenney SC, Kamine J, et al. Immediate-early gene region of human CMV trans-activates the promoter of HIV. Proc Natl Acad Sci 1987; 84:8642–8646.

531. Griffiths PD. CMV as a cofactor enhancing progression of AIDS. J Clin Virol 2006; 35:489–492.

532. Margalith M, D'Aquila RT, Manion DJ, et al. HIV-1 DNA in fibroblast cultures infected with urine from HIV-seropositive cytomegalovirus (CMV) excretors. Arch Virol 1995; 140:927–935.

533. Skolnick PR, Kosloff BR, Hirsch MS: Bidirectional interactions between HIV Type 1 and CMV. J Infect Dis 1988; 157: 508–513.

534. Smith PD, Miyake Y, Rook AH, et al. CMV infection depresses monocyte production of interleukin-1. In: The Physiologic, Metabolic, and Immunologic Actions of Interleukin-1. Alan R Liss, 1985: 319–326.

535. Schrier RD, Rice GPA, Oldstone MBA. Supression of natural killer cell activity and T-cell proliferation by fresh isolates of human cytomegalovirus. J Infect Dis 1986; 153:1084–1091.

536. Looney RJ, Falsey A, Campbell D, et al. Role of cytomegalovirus in the T-cell changes seen in elderly individuals. Clin Immunol 1999; 90:213–219.

537. Khan N, Shariff N, Cobbold M, et al. Cytomegalovirus seropositivity drives the CD8 T-cell repertoire toward greater clonality in healthy elderly individuals. J Immunol 2002; 169:1984–1992.

538. Moss P, Khan N. CD8 T-Cell Immunity to Cytomegalovirus. Human Immunology. 2004; 65:456–464.

539. Epstein MA. Vaccination against EBV: Current progress and future stratagies. Lancet 1986; i:1425.

540. Moutschen M, Leonard P, Sokal E, et al. Phase I/II studies to evaluate safety and immunogenicity of a recombinant gp350 EBV vaccine in healthy adults. Vaccine 2007; 25:4697–4705.

541. Lung MI, Chang RS, Huang ML, et al. EBV genotypes associated with nasopharyngeal carcinoma in Southern China. Virology 1990; 177:44–53.

542. Adldinger HK, Delius H, Freese UK, et al. A putative transforming gene of Jijoye virus differs from that of EBV prototypes. Virol 1985; 141:221–234.

543. Zimber U, Adldinger HK, Lenoir GM, et al. Geographical prevalence of two types of EBV. Virology 1986; 154:56–66.

544. Sixbey JW, Chesney PJ, Shirley P, et al. Detection of a second widespread strain of EBV. Lancet 1989; 2:761–765.

545. Klemenc P, Marin J, Soba E, et al. Distribution of Epstein-Barr Virus genotypes in throat washings, sera, peripheral blood, lymphocytes and in EBV positive tumor biopsies from Slovenian patients with nasopharyngeal carcinoma. J Med Virol 2006; 78:1083–1090.

546. Srivastava G, Wong KY, Chiang AKS, et al. Coinfection of multiple strains of EBV in immunocompetent normal individuals: Reassessment of the viral carrier state. Blood 2000; 95:2443–2445.

547. Sculley C, Apolloni A, Hurren L, et al. Coinfection with A- and B-Type EBV in HIV-positive subjects. J Infect Dis 1990; 162:643–648.

548. Thorley-Lawson DA. EBV the prototypical human tumor virus—just how bad is it? J Allergy Clin Immunol 2005; 116:251–261.

549. Thorley-Lawson DA, Babcock GJ: A Model for persistent infection with EBV: The stealth virus of human B-cells. Life Sci 1999; 65:1433–1453.

550. Sixbey JW, Vesterinen EH, Nedrud JG, et al. Replication of EBV in human epithelial cells infected in vitro. Nature 1983; 306:480–483.

551. Young LS, Sixbey JW, Clark D, et al. EBV receptors on human pharyngeal epithelia. Lancet 1986; i:240–242.

552. Sixbey JW, Davis DS, Young LS, et al. Human epithelial cell expression of an EBV receptor. J Gen Virol 1987; 68:805–811.

553. Yao QY, Rickinson AB, Epstein MA. A re-examination of the EBV carrier state in healthy seropositive individuals. Int J Canc 1985; 35:35–42.

554. Tugizov SM, Berline JW, Palefksy JM. EBV infection of polarized tongue and nasopharyngeal epithelial cells. Nature Med 2003; 9:307–314.

555. Tugizov SM, Herrera R, Veluppillai P, et al. Epstein-Barr virus (EBV)-infected monocytes facilitate dissemination of EBV within the oral mucosal epithelium. J Virol 2007; 81: 5484–5496.

556. Hutt-Fletcher LM. EBV entry. J Virol 2007; 81:7825–7832.

557. Herrmann K, Frangou P, Middeldorp J, et al. EBV replication in tongue epithelial cells. J Gen Virol 2002; 83: 2995–2998.

558. Raab-Traub N. EBV in the pathogenesis of NPC. Canc Biol 2002; 12:431–441.

559. Yates JL, Warren N, Sugden B. Stable replication of plasmids derived from EBV in various mammalian cells. Nature 1985; 313:812–815.

560. Lindner SE, Sugden B. The plasmid replicon of EBV: Mechanistic insights into efficient, licensed, extrachromosomal replication in human cells. Plasmid 2007; 58:1–12.

561. Zimber-Stroble U, Strobl LJ. EBNA2 and Notch signaling in EBV mediated immortalization of B lymphocytes. Sem Canc Biol 2001; 11:423–434.

562. Radkov SA, Touitou R, Brehm A, et al. EBV nuclear antigen 3C interacts with histone deacetylase to repress transcription. J Virol 1999; 73:5688–5697.

563. Samanta M, Iwakiri D, Kanda T, et al. EB virus-encoded RNAs are recognized by RIG-I and activate signaling to induce type I IFN. EMBO 2006; 25:4207–4214.

564. Fok F, Friend K, Steitz JA. EBV noncoding RNAs are confined to the nucleus, whereas their partner, the human La protein, undergoes nucleocytoplasmic shuttling. J Cell Biol 2006; 173:319–325.

565. Yoshizaki T, Kazuhira Endo K, Ren Q, et al. Oncogenic role of EBV-encoded small RNAs (EBERs) in nasopharyngeal carcinoma. Auris Nasus Larynx 2007; 34:73–78.

566. Eliopoulos AG, Stack M, Dawson CW, et al. EBV-encoded LMP1 and CD40 mediate IL-6 production in epithelial cells via an NF-kappaB pathway involving TNF receptor-associated factors. Oncogene 1997; 14:2899–2916.

567. Kieser A, Kilger E, Gires O, et al. EBV latent membrane protein-1 triggers AP-1 activity via the c-Jun N-terminal kinase cascade. EMBO 1997; 16:6478–6485.

568. Huen DS, Henderson SA, Croom-Carter D, et al. The EBV latent membrane protein-1 (LMP1) mediates activation of NF-kappa B and cell surface phenotype via two effector regions in its carboxy-terminal cytoplasmic domain. Oncogene 1995; 10:549–560.

569. Longnecker R, Miller CL. Regulation of EBV latency by latent membrane protein 2. Trends Microbiol 1996; 4: 38–42.

570. Fahraeus R, Rymo L, Rhim JS, et al. Morphological transformation of human keratinocytes expressing the LMP gene of EBV. Nature 1990; 345:447–449.

571. Wang D, Liebowitz D, Kieff E. An EBV membrane protein expressed in immortalized lymphocytes transforms established rodenT-cells. Cell 1985; 43:831–840.

572. Niedobitek G, Fahraeus R, Herbst H, et al. The EBV encoded membrane protein (LMP) induces phenotypic changes in epithelial cells. Virch Archiv B Cell Pathol Incl Mol Pathol 1992; 62:55–59.

573. Dawson C, Rickinson AB, Young LS. EBV latent membrane protein inhibits human epithelial cell differentiation. Nature 1990; 344:777–780.

574. Fries KL, Miller WE, Raab-Traub N. Epstein–Barr virus latent membrane protein 1 blocks p53-mediated apoptosis through the induction of the A20 gene. J Virol 1996; 70:8653–8659.

575. Okan I, Wang Y, Chen F, et al. The EBV-encoded LMP1 protein inhibits p53-triggered apoptosis but not growth arrest. Oncogene 1995; 11:1027–1031.

576. Miller G. The switch between latency and replication of EBV. J Infect Dis 1990; 161:833–844.

577. Miller G, El-Guindy A, Countryman J, et al. Lytic Cycle Switches of Oncogenic Human Gammaherpesviruses. Adv Cancer Res 2007; 97:81–109.

578. Zhang Q, Gutsch D, Kenney S. Functional and physical interaction between p53 and BZLF-1: implications for EBV latency. Mol Cell Biol 1994; 14:1929–1938.

579. Cayrol C, Flemington EK. The EBV bZIP transcription factor Zta causes G0/G1 cell cycle arrest through induction of cyclin-dependent kinase inhibitors. EMBO J 1996; 15:2748–2759.

580. Mauser A, Saito S, Appella E, et al. The EBV immediate-early protein BZLF1 regulates p53 function through multiple mechanisms. J Virol 2002; 76:12503–12512.

581. Centers for Disease control and Prevention (CDC). Available at: www.cdc.gov/ncidod/disease/ebv.htm. Accessed November 2007.

582. Omori MS. Mononucleosis. Available at: www.emedicine.com/emerg/topic319.htm. Accessed November 2007.

583. Vetsika E, Callan M. Infectious mononucleosis and Epstein-Barr virus. Expert Rev Mol Med 2004; 6:1–16.

584. Madden BR, Werhaven J, Wessel HB, et al. Infectious mononucleosis with airway obstruction and multiple cranial nerve palsies. Otolaryngol Head Neck Surg 1991; 104:529–532.

585. Iwatsuki K, Yamamoto T, Tsuji K, et al. Spectrum of clinical manifestations caused by responses against EBV infections. Acta Medica Okayama 2004; 58:169–180.

586. Okano M, Kawa K, Kimura H, et al. Proposed guidelines for diagnosing chronic active EBV infection. Am J Hematol 2005; 80:64–69.

587. Okano M. Overview and problematic standpoints of severe chronic active EBV infection syndrome. Crit Rev Oncol Hematol 2002; 44:273–282.

588. Middeldorp JM, Brink AATP, van den Brule AJC, et al. Pathogenic roles for Epstein-Barr virus (EBV) gene product in EBV associated proliferative disorders. Crit Rev Oncol Hematol 2003; 45:1–36.

589. Niedobitek G, Meru N, Delecluse HJ. EBV infection and human malignancies. Int J Exp Pathol 2001; 82:149–170.

590. Okano M, Gross T. A Review of EBV infection in patients with immunodeficiency disorders. Am J Med Sci 2000; 319:392–396.

591. Ochs HD, Thrasher AJ. The Wiskott-Aldrich syndrome. J Allergy Clin Immunol 2006; 117:725–738.

592. Snapper SB, Rosen FR. A Family of WASPs. N Engl J Med 2003; 348:350–351.

593. Sebire NJ, Haselden S, Malone M, et al. Isolated EBV lymphoproliferative disease in a child with Wiskott-Aldrich syndrome manifesting as cutaneous lymphomatoid granulomatosis and responsive to anti-CD20 immunotherapy. J Clin Pathol 2003; 56:555–557.

594. de-The G, Geser A, Day NE, et al. Epidemiological evidence for causal relationship between EBV and Burkitt's lymphoma from Ugandan prospective study. Nature 1978; 274:756–761.

595. Orem J, Mbidde EK, Lambert B, et al. Burkitt's lymphoma in Africa, a review of the epidemiology and etiology. Afr Health Sci 2007; 7:166–175.

596. Whittle HC, Brown J, Marsh K, et al. T-cell control of EBV infected B-cells is lost during P. Falciparum malaria. Nature 1984; 312:449–450.

597. Aya T, Kinoshita T, Imai S, et al. Chromosome translocation and c-MYC activation by EBV and *Euphorbia tirucalli* in B lymphocytes. Lancet 1991; 337:1190.

598. Osato T, Imai S, Koizumi S, et al. African Burkitts's lymphoma and an EBV enhancing plant *Euphorbia tiruncalli*. Lancet 1987; ii:1257–1258.

599. Ito Y. Vegetable activators of the viral genome and the causation of Burkitt's lymphoma and nasopharyngeal

carcinoma. In: Epstein MA, Achong BG, ed. The EBV. Recent Advances. New York, NY: Wiley and Sons, 1986:207–236.

600. Weiss LM, Movahed LA, Warnke RA, et al. Detection of EBV genomes in Reed-Sternberg cells of Hodgkin's disease. N Engl J Med 1989; 320:502–506.

601. Wu TC, Mann RB, Charache P, et al. Detection of EBV gene expression in Reed-Sternberg cells of Hodgkin's disease. Int J Cancer 1990; 46:801–804.

602. Kapatai G, Murray P. Contribution of EBV to the molecular pathogenesis of Hodgkin lymphoma. J Clin Pathol 2007; 60:1342–1349.

603. Ambinder RF, Browning PJ, Lorenzana I, et al. EBV and childhood Hodgkin's disease in Honduras and the United States. Blood 1993; 81:462–467.

604. Armstrong AA, Alexander FE, Paes RP, et al. Association of EBV with pediatric Hodgkin's disease. Am J Pathol 1993; 42:1683–1688.

605. Chang KL, Albujar PF, Chen YY, et al. High prevalence of EBV in the Reed Sternberg cells of Hodgkin's disease occurring in Peru. Blood 1996; 81:496–501.

606. Weinreb M, Day PJR, Niggli F, et al. The consistent association between EBV and Hodgkin's disease in children in Kenya. Blood 1996; 87:3828–3836.

607. Armstrong AA, Alexander FE, Cartwright R, et al. EBV and Hodgkin's disease: further evidence for the three disease hypothesis. Leukemia 1998; 12:1272–1276.

608. Herndier BG, Sanchez HC, Chang KL, et al. High prevalence of EBV in the Reed-Sternberg cells of HIV-associated Hodgkin's disease. Am J Pathol 1993; 142:1073–1079.

609. Raab-Traub N. EBV in the pathogenesis of NPC. Canc Biol 2002; 12:431–441.

610. Sheng ZY, Sham JST, Tai OX, et al. Immunoglobulion A against viral capsid antigen of EBV and indirect mirror examination of the nasopharynx in the detection of asymptomatic nasopharyngeal carcinoma. Cancer 1992; 69:3–7.

611. Ho HC. Incidence of nasopharyngeal cancer in Hong Kong. UICC Bulletin 1971; 9:5.

612. Clifford P. Carcinoma of the nasopharynx in Kenya. East African Med J 1965; 42:373–396.

613. Lanier A, Bender T, Talbot M, et al. Nasopharyngeal carcinoma in Alaskan Eskimos, Indians and Aleuts: a review of cases and study of EBV, HLA, and environmental risk factors. Cancer 1980; 46:2100–2106.613.

614. Friborg J, Wohlfahrt J, Koch A, et al. Cancer susceptibility in NPC families—a population-based cohort study. Cancer Res 2005; 65:8567–8572.

615. Khabir A, Karray H, Rodriguez S, et al. EBV latent membrane protein 1 abundance correlates with patient age but not with metastatic behavior in North African nasopharyngeal carcinomas. Virol J 2005; 20:39–46.

616. Chang ET, Adami HO. The enigmatic epidemiology of nasopharyngeal carcinoma. Cancer Epidemiol Biomarkers Prev 2006; 15:1765–1777.

617. Jia WH, Collins A, Zeng YX, et al. Complex segregation analysis of nasopharyngeal carcinoma in Guangdong, China: evidence for a multifactorial mode of inheritance (complex segregation analysis of NPC in China). Eur J Hum Genet 2005; 13:248–252.

618. Chen DL, Huang TB. A case-control study of risk factors of nasopharyngeal carcinoma. Cancer Lett 1997; 117:17–22.

619. Jia WH, Feng BJ, Xu ZL, et al. Familial risk and clustering of nasopharyngeal carcinoma in Guangdong, China. Cancer 2004; 101:363–369.

620. Huang DP, Gough TA. Analysis for volatile nitrosamines in salt-preserved foodstuffs traditionally consumed by Southern Chinese. IARC Sci Pub 1978; 20:309–314, 620.

621. Huang DP, Ho JHC, Saw D, et al. Carcinoma of the nasal and paranasal regions in rats fed Cantonese salted marine fish. IARC Sci Pub 1978; 20:315–328.

622. Yu MC, Ho JHC, Lai SH, et al. Cantonese style salted fish as a cause of nasopharyngeal carcinoma: Report of a case control study in Hong Kong. Cancer Res 1986; 46:956–961.

623. Fong LYY, Ho JHC, Huang DP. Preserved foods as possible cancer hazards: Wa rats fed salted fish have mutagenic urine. Int J Can 1979; 23:542–546.

624. Fong YY, Walse EO'F. Carcinogenic nitrosamines in Cantonese salt-dried fish. Lancet 1971; ii:1032.

625. Fong YY, Chan WC. Bacterial production of Di-methyl nitrosamine in salted fish. Nature 1973; 243:421–422.

626. Nam JM, McLaughlin JK, Blot WJ. Cigarette smoking, alcohol, and nasopharyngeal carcinoma: a case-control study among U.S. whites. J Natl Cancer Inst 1992; 84:619–622.

627. Chow WH, McLaughlin JK, Hrubec Z, et al. Tobacco use and nasopharyngeal carcinoma in a cohort of US veterans. Int J Cancer 1993; 55:538–540.

628. West S, Hildesheim A, Dosemeci M. Non-viral risk factors for nasopharyngeal carcinoma in the Philippines: results from a case-control study. Int J Cancer 1993; 55:722–727.

629. Zhu K, Levine RS, Brann EA, et al. Cigarette smoking and nasopharyngeal cancer: an analysis of the relationship according to age at starting smoking and age at diagnosis. J Epidemiol 1997; 7:107–111.

630. Yuan JM, Wang XL, Xiang YB, et al. Non-dietary risk factors for nasopharyngeal carcinoma in Shanghai, China. Int J Cancer 2000; 85:364–369.

631. Zhu K, Levine RS, Brann EA, et al. Case-control study evaluating the homogeneity and heterogeneity of risk factors between sinonasal and nasopharyngeal cancers. Int J Cancer 2002; 99:119–123.

632. Clifford P, Beecher JL. Nasopharyngeal cancer in Kenya. Clinical and environmental aspects. Brit J Canc 1964; 18:25–43.

633. Hildesheim A, West S, DeVeyra E, et al. Herbal medicine use, EBV and risk of nasopharyngeal carcinoma. Cancer Res 1992; 52:3048–3051.

634. Osato T, Imai S, Koizumi S, et al. African Burkitts's lymphoma and an EBV enhancing plant *Euphorbia tiruncalli*. Lancet 1987; ii:1257–1258.

635. Ito Y. Vegetable activators of the viral genome and the causation of Burkitt's lymphoma and nasopharyngeal carcinoma. In: Epstein MA, Achong BG, ed. The EBV. Recent Advances. New York, NY. Wiley and Sons, 1986:207–236.

636. Zeng Y, Miao XC, Jaio B, et al. EBV activation in Raji cells with ether extracts of soil from different areas in China. Cancer Lett 1984; 23:53–59.

637. Chan JKC, Bray F, McCarron P, et al. Nasopharyngeal carcinoma. In: WHO Classification of Head and Neck Tumors. IARC press, 2005:85–91.

638. de-The G, Ambrosioni JC, Ho HC, et al. Lymphoblastoid transformation and presence of herpes-type viral particle in a Chinese nasopharygeal tumor cultured in vitro. Nature 1969; 221:770–771.

639. Raab-Traub N, Flynn K. The structure of the termini of the EBV as a marker of clonal proliferation. Cell 1986; 47:883–889.

640. Pathmanathan R, Prasad U, Sadler R, et al. Clonal proliferations of cells infected with EBV in preinvasive lesions related to nasopharyngeal carcinoma. N Engl J Med 1995; 333:693–698.

641. Niedobitek G, Hansmann ML, Herbst H, et al. EBV and carcinomas: undifferentiated carcinomas but not squamous cell carcinomas of the nasopharynx are regularly associated with the virus. J Pathol 1991; 165:17–24.

642. Niedobitek G, Agathanggelou A, Barber P, et al. p53 overexpression and EBV infection in undifferentiated and squamous cell nasopharyngeal carcinoma. J Pathol 1993; 170:457–461.

643. Fan H, Nicholls J, Chua D, et al. Laboratory markers of tumor burden in nasopharyngeal carcinoma: a comparison of viral load and serologic tests for EBV. Int J Cancer 2004; 112:1036–1041.

644. Lin JC, Wang WY, Chen KY, et al. Quantification of plasma EBV DNA in patients with advanced nasopharyngeal carcinoma. New Eng J Med 2004; 350:2461–2470.

645. Leung SF, Zee B, Ma BB, et al. Plasma Epstein-Barr viral deoxyribonucleic acid quantitation complements tumor-node-metastasis staging prognostication in nasopharyngeal carcinoma. J Clin Oncol 2006; 24:5414–5418.

646. To EWH, Chan KCA, Leung SF, et al. Rapid clearance of plasma EBV DNA after surgical treatment of nasopharyngeal carcinoma. Clin Canc Res 2003; 9:3254–3259.

647. Twu CW, Wang WY, Liang WM, et al. Comparison of the prognostic impact of serum anti-EBV antibody and plasma EBV DNA assays in nasopharyngeal carcinoma. Int J Radiat Oncol Biol Phys 2007; 67:130–137.

648. Albeck H, Henle W, Klein G, et al. EBV in nasopharyngeal and salivary gland carcinomas in Greenlanders. In: Harvald B, Hansen JPH, eds. Circumpolar Health 81: Report series 33. Oulu, Finland: Nordic Council for Artic Medical Research, 1982:257–277.

649. Krishnamurthy S, Lanier AP, Dohan P, et al. Salivary gland cancer in Alaskan natives. Hum Pathol 1987; 18:986–996.

650. Huang DP, Ng HK, Ho YH, et al. EBV-associated undifferentiated carcinoma of the parotid gland. Histopathology 1988; 13:509–517.

651. Raab-Traub N, Rajamanathanm P, Flynn K, et al. EBV infection in carcinoma of the salivary gland. J Virol 1991; 65:7032–7035.

652. Hamilton-Dutiot SJ, Therkildsen MH, Nielsen NH, et al. Undifferentiated carcinoma of the salivary gland in Greenlandic Eskimos: Demonstration of EBV DNA by *in-situ* nucleic acid hybridization. Human Pathol 1991; 22:811–815.

653. Saku T, Cheng J, Jen KY, et al. EBV infected lymphoepithelial carcinomas of the salivary gland in the Russia-Asia area: a clinicopathologic study of 160 cases. Arkh Patol 2003; 65:35–39.

654. Saqui-Salces M, Martinez-Benitez B, Gamboa-Dominguez A. EBV+ lymphoepithelial carcinoma of the parotid gland in Mexican Mestizo patients with chronic autoimmune diseases. Pathol Oncol Res 2006; 12:441–445.

655. Herbst H, Niedobitek G. Sporadic EBV-associated lymphoepithelial salivary gland carcinoma with EBV-positive low-grade myoepithelial component. Virchows Arch 2006; 448:648–654.

656. Greenspan D, Greenspan JS, Conant M, et al. Oral "hairy" leukoplakia in male homosexuals: evidence of association with both papillomavirus and a herpes-group virus. Lancet 1984; ii:831–834.

657. Greenspan D, Hollander H, Friedman-Kien A, et al. Oral hairy leukoplakia in two women, a haemophiliac, and a transfusion recipient. Lancet 1986; ii:978–979.

658. Syrjänen S, Laine P, Happonen R, et al. Oral hairy leukoplakia is not a specific sign of HIV-infection but related to immunosupression in general. J Oral Pathol Med 1989; 18:28–31.

659. Kanitakis J, Euvrands S, Lefrancois N. Oral hairy leukoplakia in HIV-negative renal graft recipient. Br J Dermatol 1991; 124;483–486.

660. Eisenberg E, Krutchkoff D, Yamase H. Incidental oral hairy leukeplakia in immunocompetent persons: report of two cases. Oral Surg Oral Med Oral Pathol 1992; 74:332–333.

661. Felix DH, Watret K, Wray D, et al. Hairy leukoplakia in an HIV-negative, nonimmunosuppressed patient. Oral Surg Oral Med Oral Pathol 1992; 74:563—566.

662. Milagres A, Dias EP, Tavares DS, et al. Prevalence of oral hairy leukoplakia and epithelial infection by EBV in pregnant women and diabetes mellitus patients-cytopathologic and molecular study. Mem Inst Oswaldo Cruz 2007; 102:159–164.

663. Moura MD, Guimarães TR, Fonseca LM, et al. A random clinical trial study to assess the efficiency of topical applications of podophyllin resin (25%) versus podophyllin resin (25%) together with acyclovir cream (5%) in the treatment of oral hairy leukoplakia. Oral Surg Oral Med Oral Pathol Oral Radiol Endod 2007; 103:64–71.

664. Moura MD, Grossmann SM, Fonseca LM, et al. Risk factors for oral hairy leukoplakia in HIV-infected adults of Brazil. J Oral Pathol Med 2006; 35:321–326.

665. Chattopadhuay A, Caplan DJ, Slade GD, et al. Incidence of oral Candidiasis and oral hairy leukoplakia in HIV-infected adults in North Carolina. Oral Surg Oral Med Oral Pathol Oral Radiol Endod 2005; 99:39–47.

666. Sandvej K, Krenacs L, Hamilton-Dutoit SJ, et al. EBV latent and replicative gene expression in oral hairy leukoplakia. Histopathology 1992; 20:387–395.

667. Walling DM, Ling PD, Gordadze AV, et al. Expression of EBV latent genes in oral epithelium: determinants of the pathogenesis of oral hairy leukoplakia. J Infect Dis 2004; 190:396–399.

668. Palefsky JM, Berline J, Greenspan D, et al. Evidence for trafficking of EBV strains between hairy leukoplakia and peripheral blood lymphocytes. J Gen Virol 2002; 83: 317–321.

669. Walling DM, Etienne W, Ray AJ, et al. Persistence and transition of EBV genotypes in the pathogenesis of oral hairy leukoplakia. J Infect Dis. 2004; 190:387–395.

670. Greenspan JSM, Greenspan D, Lennette ET, et al. Replication of EBV within the epithelial cells of oral "hairy" leukoplakia, an AIDS-associated lesion. N Engl J Med 1985; 313:1564–1571.

671. Loning T, Henke RP, Reichart P, et al. *In-situ* hybridization to detect EBV in oral tissue of HIV-infected patients. Virch Archiv 1987; 412:127–133.

672. Eversole LR, Stone CE, Beckamn AM. Detection of EBV and HPV DNA sequences on oral "hairy" leukoplakia by *in-situ* hybridization. J Med Virol 1988; 26:272–277.

673. Snijders PJF, Schulten EAJM, Mullink H, et al. Detection of HPV and EBV DNA sequences in oral mucosa of HIV-infected patients by PCR. Am J Pathol 1990; 137: 659–666.

674. Niedobitek G, Young LS, Lau R, et al. EBV infection in oral hairy leukoplakia: virus replication in the abscence of a detectable latent phase. J Gen Virol 1991; 72: 3035–3046.

675. Walling DM, Ray AJ, Nicols JE, et al. EBV infection of Langerhans cell precursors as a mechanism of oral epithelial entry, persistence, and reactivation. J Virol 2007; 81:7249–7268.

676. Shannon-Lowe CD, Neuhierl B, Baldwin G, et al. Resting B-cells as a transfer vehicle for EBV infection of epithelial cells. PNAS 2006; 103:7065–7070.

677. Feederle R, Neuhier B, Bannert H, et al. EBV B95.8 produced in 293 cells shows marked tropism for differentiated primary epithelial cells and reveals interindividual variation in susceptibility to viral infection. Int J Canc 2007; 121:588–594.

678. Brandwein M, Nuovo G, Ramer M, et al. EBV reactivation in hairy leukoplakia. Mod Pathol 1996; 9:298–303.

679. Harabuchi Y, Yamanaka N, Kataura A, et al. EBV in nasal T-cell lymphomas in patients with lethal midline granuloma. Lancet 1990; 335:128–130.

680. Mishima K, Horiuchi K, Kojya S, et al. EBV in patients with polymorphic reticulosis (lethal midline granuloma) from China and Japan. Cancer 1994; 73:3041–3046.

681. Jones JF, Shurin S, Abramowsky C, et al. T-cell lymphomas containing EBV DNA in patients with chronic EBV infections. NEJM 1988; 318:733–741.

682. Ho FCS, Srivastava G, Loke SL, et al. Presence of EBV DNA in nasal lymphomas of B and T-cell type. Hematol Oncol 1990; 8:271–281.

683. Arber DA, Weiss LM, Albujar PF, et al. Nasal lymphomas in Peru. High incidence of T-cell immunophenotype and EBV infection. Am J Surg Pathol 1993; 17:392–399.

684. Chan JKC, Yip TTC, Tsang WTM, et al. Detection of EBV RNA in malignant lymphomas of the upper aerodigestive tract. Am J Surg Pathol 1994; 18:938–946.

685. Kurniawan AN, Hongyo T, Hardjolikito ES, et al. Gene mutation analysis of sinonasal lymphomas in Indonesia. Oncol Reports 2006; 15:1257–1263.

686. Weiss LM, Gaffrey MJ, Chen YY, et al. Frequency of EBV DNA in "Western" sinonasal and Waldeyer's ring non-Hodgkin's lymphomas. Am J Surg Pathol 1992; 16:156–162.

687. Ott G, Kalla J, Ott MM, et al. The EBV in malignant non-Hodgkin's lymphoma of the upper aerodigestive tract. Diagn Mol Pathol 1997; 6:134–139.

688. Gaal K, Sun NC, Hernandez AM, et al. Sinonasal NK/T-cell lymphomas in the United States. Am J Surg Pathol 2000; 24:1511–1517.

689. Xu F, Sternberg MR, Kottiri BJ, et al. trends in HSV type 1 and type 2 seroprevalence in the United States. JAMA 2006; 296:964–973.

690. Whitley RJ, Roizman B. Herpes simplex virus infections. Lancet 2001; 357:1513–1518.

691. Knaup B, Schunemann S, Wolff MH. Subclinical reactivation of HSV type 1 in the oral cavity. Oral Microbiol Immunol 2000; 15:281–283.

692. Silva LM, Guimarães AL, Victória JM, et al. HSV type 1 shedding in the oral cavity of seropositive patients. Oral Dis 2005; 11:13–16.

693. Hyland PL, Coulter WA, Abu-Ruman I, et al. Asymptomatic shedding of HSV-1 in patients undergoing oral surgical procedures and attending for noninvasive treatment. Oral Dis 2007; 13:414–418.

694. Eversole LR. Viral infections of the head and neck among HIV-seropositive patients. Oral Surg Oral Med Oral Pathol 1992; 73:155–163.

695. Kawaguchi K, Inamura H, Abe Y, et al. Reactivation of HSV type 1 and varicella-zoster virus and therapeutic effects of combination therapy with prednisolone and valacyclovir in patients with Bell's palsy. Laryngoscope 2007; 117:147–156.

696. Lazarini PR, Vianna MF, Alcantara MP, et al. HSV in the saliva of peripheral Bell's palsy patients. Rev Bras Otorrinolaringol 2006; 72:7–11.

697. Abiko Y, Ikeda M, Hondo R. Secretion and dynamics of HSV in tears and saliva of patients with Bell's palsy. Otol Neurotol 2002; 23:779–783.

698. Langenberg AG, Corey L, Ashley RL, et al. A prospective study of new infections with HSV type 1 and type 2. Chiron HSV Vaccine Study Group. N Engl J Med 1999; 341:1432–1438.

699. Benedetti J, Corey L, Ashley R. Recurrence rates in genital herpes after symptomatic first-episode infection. Ann Intern Med 1994; 121:847–854.

700. Kim HN, Meier A, Huang ML, et al. Oral herpes simplex virus type 2 reactivation in HIV-positive and -negative men. J Infect Dis 2006; 194:420–427.

701. Ramasamy K, Lim ZY, Savvas M, et al. Disseminated HSV-2 infection with rhabdomyolysis and hemophagocytic lymphohistiocytosis in a patient with bone marrow failure syndrome. Ann Hematol 2006; 85:629–630.

702. Abbo L, Alcaide ML, Pano JR, et al. Fulminant hepatitis from HSV type 2 in an immunocompetent adult. Transpl Infect Dis 2007; 9:323–326.

703. Montalbano M, Slapak-Green GI, Neff GW. Fulminant hepatic failure from HSV: Post liver transplantation acyclovir therapy and literature review. Trans Proc 2005; 37:4393–4396.

704. Curley MJ, Hussein SA, Hassoun PM. Disseminated HSV and varicella zoster virus coinfection in a patient taking thalidomide for relapsed multiple myeloma. J Clin Microbiol 2002; 40:2302–2304.

705. Epstein JI, Ambinder RF, Kuhajda FP, et al. Localized *Herpes Simplex* lymphadenitis. Am J Clin Pathol 1986; 86:444–448.

706. Gaffey MJ, Ben Ezra JM, Weiss LM. *Herpes Simplex* lymphadenitis. Am J Clin Pathol 1991; 95:709–714.

707. Howat AJ, Campbell AR, Stewart DJ. Generalized lymphadenopathy due to HSV-1. Histopathol 1991; 19:563–564.

708. Wat PJ, Strickler JG, Myers JL, et al. HSV infection causing acute necrotizing tonsillitis. Mayo Clin Proc 1994; 69:269–271.

709. Gonen C, Uner A, Cetinkaya Y, et al. Tonsillar abscess formation due to HSV-1 in a severely immunocompromised stem cell transplant patient with chronic myeloid leukemia. Transpl Infect Dis 2006; 8:166–170.

710. Kimberlin DW. Neonatal Herpes Simplex infection. Clin Microbiol Rev 2004; 17:1–13.

711. Spear PG. HSV: receptors and ligands for cell entry. Cell Microbiol 2004; 6:401–410.

712. Rice SA, Long MC, Lam V, et al. RNA polmerase II is aberrantly phosphorylated and localized to viral replication compartments following HSV infection. J Virol 1994; 68:988–1001.

713. Kemp LM, Latchman DS. Induction and repression of cellular gene transcription during HSV infection are mediated by different viral IE gene products. Eur J Biochem 1988; 174:443–449.

714. Taddeo B, Roizman B. The virion host shutoff protein (UL41) of HSV-1 is an endoribonuclease with a substrate specificity similar to that of RNase A. J Virol 2006; 80:9341–9345.

715. Miller CS, Danaher RJ, Jacob RJ. Molecular aspects of HSV-1 latency, reactivation, and recurrence. Crit Rev Oral Biol Med 1998; 9:541–562.

716. Su L, Knipe DM. Herpes Simplex virus alpha protein ICP27 can inhibit or augment viral gene transactivation. Virol 1989; 170:496–504.

717. Randall RE, Dinwoodie N. Intranuclear localization of Herpes Simplex virus immediate early and delayed early proteins: evidence that ICP 4 is associated with progeny virus DNA. J Gen Virol 1986; 67:2163–2177.

718. McCusker CT, Bacchetti S. The responsiveness of HPV upstream regulatory regions to HSV IE proteins. Virus Res 1988; 11:199–207.

719. Albrecht MA, DeLuca NA, Byrn RA, et al. The HSV IE protein, ICP4 is required to potentiate replication of HIV in CD4 lymphocytes. J Virol 1989; 63:1861–1868.

720. Becker Y. HSV evolved to use the human defense mechanisms to establish a lifelong infection in neurons—a review and hypothesis. Virus Genes 2002; 24:187–196.

721. Farrell MJ, Dobson AT, Feldman LT. HSV latency-associated transcript is a stable intron. PNAS 1999; 88:790–794.

722. Gupta A, Gartner JJ, Sethupathy P, et al. Anti-apoptotic function of a microRNA encoded by the HSV-1 latency-associated transcript. Nature 2006; 446:82–85.

723. Henderson G, Peng W, Jin L, et al. Regulation of caspase 8- and caspase 9-induced apoptosis by the HSV type 1 latency-associated transcript. J Neurovirol 2002; 8(suppl 2):103–111.

724. Furniss CS, McClean MD, Smith JF, et al. HPV 16 and head and neck squamous cell carcinoma. Int J Cancer 2007; 120:2386–2392.

725. Kreimer AR, Clifford GM, Snijders PJ, et al. HPV16 semiquantitative viral load and serologic biomarkers in oral and oropharyngeal squamous cell carcinomas. Int J Cancer 2005; 115:329–332.

726. Medeiros LR, Ethur AB, Hilgert JB, et al. Vertical transmission of the HPV a systematic quantitative review. Cad Saude Publica 2005; 21:1006–1015.

727. Smith EM, Ritchie JM, Yankowitz J, et al. HPV prevalence and types in newborns and parents: concordance and modes of transmission. Sex Transm Dis 2004; 31:57–62.

728. Rintala MA, Grenman SE, Puranen MH, et al. Transmission of high-risk HPV between parents and infant: a prospective study of HPV in families in Finland. J Clin Microbiol 2005; 43:376–381.

729. Mant C, Kell B, Rice P, et al. Buccal exposure to HPV type 16 is a common yet transitory event in childhood. J Med Virol 2003; 7:593–598.

730. Quick CA, Krzyzek RA, Watts SL, et al. Relationship between condylomata and laryngeal papillomata. Clinical and molecular virological evidence. Ann Otol 1980; 89:467–471.

731. Silverberg MJ, Thorsen P, Lindeberg H, et al. Condyloma in pregnancy is strongly predictive of juvenile-onset recurrent respiratory papillomatosis. Obstet Gynecol 2003; 101:645–652.

732. Gerein V, Soldatski IL, Babkina N, et al. Children and partners with recurrent respiratory papillomatosis have no evidence of disease during long-term observation. Int J Ped Otorhinlaryngol 2006; 70:2061–2066.

733. Sisk J, Schweinfurth JM, Wang XT, et al. Presence of HPV DNA in tonsillectomy specimens. Laryngoscope 2006; 116:1372–1374.

734. Chen R, Sehr P, Waterboer T, et al. Presence of DNA of HPV 16 but no other types in tumor-free tonsillar tissue. J Clin Microbiol 2005; 43:1408–1410.

735. Mammas IN, Sourvinos G, Michael C, et al. HPV in hyperplastic tonsillar and adenoid tissues in children. Pediatr Infect Dis J 2006; 25:1158–1162.

736. Shope RE. Infectious papillomatosis of rabbits. J Exp Med 1933; 58:607–627.

737. Longsworth MS, Laimins LA. Pathogenesis of HPV in differentiating epithelia. Microbiol Molec Biol Rev 2004; 68:362–372.

738. Hebner CM, Laimins LA. HPV: Basic mechanisms of pathogenesis and oncogenicity. Rev Med Virol 2006; 16:83–97.

739. Stunkel W, Bernard HU. The chromatin structure of the long control region of HPV 16 represses viral oncogene expression. J Virol 1999; 73:1918–1930.

740. Archard HO, Heck JW, Stanley HR. Focal epithelial hyperplasia: An unusual oral mucosal lesions in Indian children. Oral Surg Oral Med Oral Pathol 1965; 20:210–212.

741. Cuberos V, Perez J, Lopez CJ, et al. Molecular and serological evidence of the epidemiological association of HPV 13 with focal epithelial hyperplasia: a case-control study. J Clin Virol 2006; 37:21–26.

742. Borborema-Santos CM, Castro MM, Santos PJ, et al. Oral focal epithelial hyperplasia: report of five cases. Braz Dent J 2006; 17:79–82.

743. Ledesma-Montes C, Vega-Memije E, Garces-Ortiz M, et al. Multifocal epithelial hyperplasia. Report of nine cases. Med Oral Patol Oral Cir Bucal 2005, 10:394–401.

744. Carlos R, Sedano HO. Multifocal papillomavirus epithelial hyperplasia. Oral Surg Oral Med Oral Pathol 1994; 77:631–635.

745. Jimenez C, Correnti M, Salma N, et al. Detection of HPV DNA in benign oral squamous epithelial lesions in Venezuela. J Oral Pathol Med 2001; 30:385–388.

746. Steinhoff M, Metze D, Stockfleth E, et al. Successful topical treatment of focal epithelial hyperplasia (Heck's disease) with interferon-beta. Brit J Dermatol 2001; 144:1067–1069.

747. Akyol A, Anadolu R, Anadolu Y, et al. Multifocal papillomavirus epithelial hyperplasia: successful treatment with CO2 laser therapy combined with interferon-alpha-2b. Int J Dermatol 2003; 42:733–735.

748. Greenspan D, Canchola AJ, MacPhail LA, et al. Effect of highly active antiretroviral therapy on frequency of oral warts. Lancet 2001; 357:1411–1412.

749. Anderson KM, Perez-Montiel D, Miles L, et al. The histologic differentiation of oral condyloma acuminatum from its mimics. Oral Surg Oral Med Oral Pathol 2003; 96:420–428.

750. Henley JD, Summerlin DJ, Tomich CE. Condyloma acuminatum and condyloma-like lesions of the oral cavity: a study of 11 cases with intraductal component. Histopathol 2004; 44:216–221.

751. Daley T, Birek C, Wysocki GP. Oral bowenoid lesions: Differential diagnosis and pathogenetic insights. Oral Surg Oral Med Oral Pathol Oral Radiol Endod 2000; 90:466–473.

752. Rinaggio J, Glick M, Lambert WC. Oral bowenoid papulosis in an HIV-positive male. Oral Surg Oral Med Oral Pathol Oral Radiol Endod 2006; 101:328–332.

753. Draganov P, Mateev G, Motev I, et al. Identification of multiple HPV genotypes in a patient with oral condylomata acuminate. Biotechnol and Biotechnol Eq 2006. Available at: www.diagnosisp.com (accessed July 2007).

754. Volter C, He Y, Delius H, et al. Novel HPV types present in oral papillomatous lesions from patients with HIV infection. Int J Cancer 1996; 66:453–456.

755. Adler-Storthz K, Newland JR, Tessin BA, et al. Identification of HPV types in oral verruca vukgaris. J Oral Pathol 1986; 15:230–233.

756. Padayachee A. HPV types 2 and 57 in oral verrucae demonstrated by in-situ hybridization. J Oral Pathol Med 1994; 24:413–417.

757. Padayachee A, Sanders CM, Maitland NJ. A PCR investigation of oral verrucae which contain HPV types 2 and 57 by in-situ hybridization. J Oral Pathol Med 1995; 24:329–334.

758. Soldatski I, Onufrieva EK, Steklov AM, et al. Tracheal, bronchial and pulmonary papillomatosis in children. Laryngoscope 2005; 115:1848–1854.

759. Ruparelia S, Unger ER, Nisenbaum R, et al. Predictors of remission in juvenile-onset recurrent respiratory papillomatosis. Arch Otolaryngol Head Neck Surg 2003; 129:1275–1278.

760. Byrne JC, Tsao MS, Fraser RS, et al. HPV-11 DNA in a patient with chronic laryngotracheobronchial papillomatosis and metastatic squamous cell carcinoma of the lung. N Eng J Med 1987; 317:873–878.

761. Zarod AP, Rutherford JD, Corbitt G. Malignant progression of laryngeal papilloma associated with HPV 6 DNA. J Clin Pathol 1988; 41:280–283.

762. Sidhu TS, Sharma AK, Sharma N, et al. Unusual malignant transformation of juvenile recurrent respiratory papillomatosis. Otolaryngol Head Neck Surg 2007; 136:321–323.

763. Lindeberg H, Syrjänen S, Karja J, et al. HPV 11 DNA in squamous cell carcinomas and pre-existing multiple laryngeal papillomas. Acta Otolaryngol 1989; 107: 141–149.

764. Ullman EV. On the aetiology of laryngeal papillomas. Acta Otolaryngol 1928; 5:317–338.

765. Steinberg BS, Topp WC, Schneider PS, et al. Laryngeal papillomavirus infection during clinical remission. N Engl J Med 1983; 308:1261–1264.

766. Vambutas A, DeVoti J, Pinn W, et al. Interaction of HPV 11 E7 protein with TAP-1 results in the reduction of ATP-dependent peptide transport. Clin Immunol 2001; 101:94–99.

767. Vambutas A, Bonagura VR, Steinberg BM. Altered expression of TAP-1 and major histocompatibility complex class I in laryngeal papillomatosis: correlation of TAP-1 with disease. Clin Diagn Lab Immunol 2000; 7:79–85.

768. Aaltonen LM, Cajanus S, Back L, et al. Extralaryngeal HPV infections in male patients with adult-onset laryngeal papillomatosis. Eur Arch Otorhinolaryngol 2005; 262:708–712.

769. Quiney RE, Hall D, Croft CB. Laryngeal papillomatosis: analysis of 113 patients. Clin Otolaryngol Allied Sci 1989; 143:217–225.

770. Naiman AN, Ayari S, Nicollas R, et al. Intermediate-term and long-term results after treatment by cidofovir and excision in juvenile laryngeal papillomatosis. Ann Otol Rhinol Laryngol 2006; 115:667–672.

771. Naiman AN, Abedipour D, Ayari S, et al. Natural history of adult-onset laryngeal papillomatosis following multiple cidofovir injections. Ann Otol Rhinol Laryngol 2006; 115:175–181.

772. Lee JH, Smith RJ. Recurrent respiratory papillomatosis: pathogenesis to treatment. Curr Opin Otolaryngol 2005; 13:354–359.

773. Ackerman LV. Verrucous carcinoma of the oral cavity. Surgery 1948; 23:670–678.

774. Lin JI. Occasional notes: Virchow's pathological reports on Frederick III's cancer. N Eng J Med 1984; 311:1261–1264.

775. Kraus FT, Perez-Mesa C. Verrucous carcinoma. Cinical and pathologic study of 105 cases involving oral cavity, larynx and genitalia. Cancer 1966; 19:26–38.

776. Noble-Topham SE, Fliss DM, Hartwick WJ, et al. Detection and typing of HPV in verrucous carcinoma of the oral cavity using PCR. Arch Otolaryngol Head Neck Surg 1993; 119:1299–1304.

777. Kasperbauer JL, O'Halloran GL, Espy MJ, et al. PCR identification of HPV DNA in verrucous carcinoma of the larynx. Laryngoscope 1993; 103:416–420.

778. Perez-Ayala M, Cabello FR, Esteban F, et al. Presence of HPV 16 sequences in laryngeal carcinomas. Int J Can 1990; 46:8–11.

779. Fliss DM, Noble-Topham SE, McLachlin M, et al. Laryngeal verrucous carcinoma: A clinicopathologic study and detection of HPV using PCR. Laryngoscope 1994; 104: 146–152.

780. Miller CS, Johnstone BM. HPV as a risk factor for oral squamous cell carcinoma: A meta-analysis, 1982-1997. Oral Surg Oral Med Oral Pathol, Oral Radiol Endod 2001; 91:622–635.

781. Mitsuishi T, Ohara K, Kawashima M, et al. Prevalence of HPV DNA sequences in verrucous carcinoma of the lip: genomic and therapeutic approaches. Canc Letters 2005; 222:139–153.

782. Shear M, Pindborg JJ. Verrucous hyperplasia of the oral mucosa. Cancer 1980; 46:1855–1862.

783. Shroyer KR, Greer RO. Detection of HPV DNA by in-situ hybridization and PCR in premalignant and malignant oral lesions. Oral Surg Oral Med Oral Pathol 1991; 71: 708–713.

784. Zakrzewska JM, Lopes V, Speight P, et al. Proliferative verrucous leukoplakia: a report of ten cases. Oral Surg Oral Med Oral Pathol Oral Radiol Endod 1996; 82:396–401.

785. Murrah VA, Batsakis JG. Proliferative verrucous leukoplakia and verrucous hyperplasia. Ann Otol Rhinol Laryngol 1994; 103:660–663.

786. Chen HM, Yu CH, Tu PC, et al. Successful treatment of oral verrucous hyperplasia and oral leukoplakia with topical 5-aminolevulinic acid-mediated photodynamic therapy. Lasers Surg Med 2005; 37:114–122.

787. Femiano F, Gombos F, Scully C. Oral proliferative verrucous leukoplakia (PVL); open trial of surgery compared with combined therapy using surgery and methisoprinol in papillomavirus-related PVL. Int J Oral Maxillofac Surg 2001; 30:318–322.

788. Kusiak RJ, Hudson WR. Nasal papillomatosis. South Med J 1970; 63:1277–1280.

789. Ogura H, Fujiwara T, Hamaya K, et al. Detection of HPV type 57 in a case of inverted nasal papillomatosis in Japan. Eur Arch Otorhinolaryngol 1995; 252:513–515.

790. Siivonen L, Virolainen E. Transitional papilloma of the nasal cavity and paranasal sinuses. Clinical course, viral etiology and malignant transformation. ORL J Otorhinolaryngol Relat Spec 1989; 51:262–267.

791. Bryan RL, Bevan IS, Crocker J, et al. Detection of HPV 6 and 11 in tumours of the upper respiratory tract using the PCR. Clin Otolaryngol Allied Sci 1990; 15:177–180.

792. Weber RS, Shilltoe, Robbins T, et al. Prevalence of HPV in inverted papillomas. Arch Otolaryngol Head Neck Surg 1988; 114:23–26.

793. Saegusa M, Nitta H, Hashimura M, et al. Down-regulation of p27Kip1 expression is correlated with increased cell proliferation but not expression of p21waf1 and p53, and HPV infection in benign and malignant tumours of sinonasal regions. Histopathology 1999; 35:55–64.

794. Kassim SK, Ibrahim SA, Eissa S, et al. Epstein Barr virus, HPV, and flow cytometric cell cycle kinetics in nasopharyngeal carcinoma and inverted papilloma among Egyption patients. Dis Markers 1998; 14:13–20.

795. Respler DS, Jahn A, Pater A, et al. Isolation and characterization of papillomavirus DNA from nasal inverting (Schneiderian) papillomas. Ann Otol Rhinol Laryngol 1987; 96:170–173.

796. Wu TC, Trujillo JM, Kashima HK, et al. Association of HPV with nasal neoplasia. Lancet 1993; 341:522–524.

797. Syrjänen S, Happonen RP, Virolainen E, et al. Detection of HPV structural antigens and DNA types in inverted papillomas and squamous cell carcinomas of nasal cavities and paranasal sinuses. Acta Otolaryngol (stockh) 1987; 104:334–341.

798. McLachlin CM, Kandel RA, Colgan TJ, et al. Prevalence of HPV in sinonasal papillomas: A study using PCR and in-situ hybridization. Mod Pathol 1992; 5:406–409.

799. Brandsma JL, Abramson AL, Scuibba J, et al. Papillomavirus infection of the nose. In: Steinberg BM, Brandsma JL, Taichman LP, eds. Cancer Cells 5: Papillomaviruses. Cold Spring Harbor, NY: Cold Spring Harbor Press, 1987:301.

800. Brandwein MS, Steinberg B, Thung S, et al. HPV 6/11 and 16/18 in Schneiderian inverted papillomas. Cancer 1989; 63:1708–1713.

801. Ishibashi T, Tsunokawa Y, Matsushima S, et al. Presence of HPV type-6-related sequences in inverted nasal papillomas. Eur Arch Otorhinolaryngol 1990; 247:296–299.

802. Judd R, Sherif RZ, Coffield LM, et al. Sinonasal papillomas and HPV: HPV 11 detected in fungiform Schneiderian papillomas by in-situ hybridization and PCR. Hum Pathol 1991; 22:550–556.

803. Furuta Y, Shinohara T, Sano K, et al. Molecular pathologic study of HPV infection in inverted papilloma and squamous cell carcinoma of the nasal cavities and paranasal sinuses. Laryngoscope 1991; 101:79–85.

804. Sarkar FH, Visscher DW, Kintanar EB, et al. Sinonasal Schneiderian papillomas: HPV typing by PCR. Mod Pathol 1992; 5:329–332.

805. Kashima HK, Kessis T, Hruban RH, et al. HPV in sinonasal papillomas and squamous cell carcinoma. Laryngoscope 1992; 102:973–976.

806. Tang AC, Grignon DJ, MacRae DL. The association of HPV with Schneiderian papillomas: a DNA in situ hybridization study. J Otolaryngol 1994; 23:292–297.

807. Buchwald C, Franzmann MB, Jacobsen GK, Lindeberg H. HPV in sinonasal papillomas: a study of 78 cases using in situ hybridization and PCR. Laryngoscope 1995; 105: 66–71.

808. Beck JC, McClatchey KD, Lesperance MM, et al. HPV types important in progression of inverted papilloma. Otolaryngol Head Neck Surg 1995; 113:558–563.

809. Macdonald MR, Le KT, Freeman J, et al. A majority of inverted sinonasal papillomas carries Epstein-Barr virus genomes. Cancer 1995; 75:2307–2312.

810. Gaffey MJ, Frierson HF, Weiss LM, et al. HPV and Epstein-Barr virus in sinonasal Schneiderian papillomas. An in situ hybridization and PCR study. Am J Clin Pathol 1996; 106:475–482.

811. Shen J, Tate JE, Crum CP, et al. Prevalence of HPV in benign and malignant tumors of the upper respiratory tract. Mod Pathol 1996; 9:15–20.

812. Caruana SM, Zwiebel N, Cocker R, et al. p53 alteration and HPV infection in paranasal sinus cancer. Cancer 1997; 79:1320–1328.

813. Bernauer HS, Welkoborsky HJ, Tilling A, et al. Inverted papillomas of the paranasal sinuses and the nasal cavity: DNA indices and HPV infection. Am J Rhinol 1997; 11: 155–160.

814. Hwang CS, Yang HS, Hong MK. Detection of HPV in sinonasal inverted papillomas using PCR. Am J Rhinol 1998; 12:363–366.

815. Mirza N, Montone K, Sato Y, et al. Identification of p53 and HPV in Schneiderian papillomas. Laryngoscope 1998; 108:497–501.

816. Weiner JS, Sherris D, Kasperbauer J, et al. Relationship of HPV to Schneiderian papillomas. Laryngoscope 1999; 109:21–26.

817. Kraft M, Simmen D, Casas R, et al. Significance of HPV in sinonasal papillomas. J Laryngol Otol 2001; 115:709–714.

818. Fischer M. Investigation of a broad-spectrum PCR assay for HPV in screening benign lesions of the upper aerodigestive tract. ORL J Otorhinolaryngol Relat Spec 2005; 67:237–241.

819. McKay SP, Gregoire L, Lonardo F, et al. HPV transcripts in malignant inverted papilloma are from integrated HPV DNA. Laryngoscope 2005; 115:1428–1431.

820. Katori H, Nozawat A, Tsukuda M. Relationship between p21 and p53 expression, HPV infection and malignant transformation in sinonasal-inverted papilloma. Clin Oncol (R Coll Radiol) 2006; 18:300–305.

821. Hoffman M, Klose N, Gottschlich S, et al. Detection of HPV DNA in benign and malignant sinonasal neoplasms. Cancer Lett 2006; 239:64–70.

822. Lawson W, Schlecht NF, Brandwein-Gensler M. The Role of the Human Papillomavirus in the Pathogenesis of Schneiderian Inverted Papillomas: A Systematic Review (in Progress).

823. Gillison ML, Koch WM, Capone RB, et al. Evidence for a causal association between HPV and a subset of head and neck cancers. J Natl Cancer Inst 2000; 92:709–720.

824. Mellin H, Friesland S, Lewensohn R, et al. HPV DNA in tonsillar cancer: clinical correlates, risk of relapse, and survival. Int J Cancer 2000; 89:300–304.

825. Schwartz SR, Yueh B, McDougall JK, et al. HPV infection and survival in oral squamous cell cancer: a population-based study. Otolaryngol Head Neck Surg 2001; 125:1–9.

826. Ringstrom E, Peters E, Hasegawa M, et al. HPV type 16 and squamous cell carcinoma of the head and neck. Clin Cancer Res 2002; 10:3187–3192.

827. Dahlstrom KR, Adler-Storthz K, Etzel CJ, et al. HPV type 16 infection and squamous cell carcinoma of the head and neck in never-smokers: a matched pair analysis. Clin Cancer Res 2003; 9:2620–2626.

828. El-Mofty SK, Lu DW. Prevalence of HPV type 16 DNA in squamous cell carcinoma of the palatine tonsil, and not the oral cavity, in young patients: a distinct clinicopathologic and molecular disease entity. Am J Surg Pathol 2003; 11:1463–1470.

829. Herrero R, Castellsague X, Pawlita M, et al. HPV and oral cancer: the International Agency for Research on Cancer multicenter study. J Natl Cancer Inst 2003; 95: 1772–1783.

830. Begum S, Cao D, Gillison M, et al. Tissue distribution of HPV 16 DNA integration in patients with tonsillar carcinoma. Clin Cancer Res 2005; 11:5694–5699.

831. El-Mofty SK, Patil S. HPV-related oropharyngeal non-keratinizing squamous cell carcinoma: characterization of a distinct phenotype. Oral Surg Oral Med Oral Pathol Oral Radiol Endod 2006; 101:339–345.

832. Hansson BG, Rosenquist K, Antonsson A, et al. Strong association between infection with HPV and oral and oropharyngeal squamous cell carcinoma: a population-based case-control study in southern Sweden. Acta Otolaryngol 2005; 125:1337–1344.

833. Ibieta BR, Lizano M, Fras-Mendivil M, et al. HPV in oral squamous cell carcinoma in a Mexican population. Oral Surg Oral Med Oral Pathol Oral Radiol Endod 2005; 99:311–315.

834. Koppikar P, deVilliers EM, Mulherkar R. Identification of HPV in tumors of the oral cavity in an Indian community. Int J Cancer 2005; 113:946–950.

835. Tachezy R, Klozar J, Salakova M, et al. HPV and other risk factors of oral cavity/oropharyngeal cancer in the Czech Republic. Oral Dis 2005; 11:181–185.

836. Licitra L, Perrone F, Bossi P, et al. High-risk HPV affects prognosis in patients with surgically treated oropharyngeal squamous cell carcinoma. J Clin Oncol 2006; 24: 5630–5636.

837. Nemes JA, Deli L, Nemes Z, et al. Expression of p16 (INK4A), p53, and Rb proteins are independent from the presence of HPV genes in oral squamous cell carcinoma. Oral Surg Oral Med Oral Pathol Oral Radiol Endod 2006; 102:344–352.

838. Weinberger PM, Yu Z, Haffty BG, et al. Molecular classification identifies a subset of HPV-associated oropharyngeal cancers with favorable prognosis. J Clin Oncol 2006; 24:736–747.

839. D'Souza G, Kreimer AR, Viscidi R, et al. Case-control study of HPV and oropharyngeal cancer. N Engl J Med 2007; 356:1944–1956.

840. Pintos J, Black MJ, Sadeghi N, et al. HPV infection and oral cancer: A case-control study in Montreal, Canada. Oral Oncol 2007 (epub ahead of print).

841. Smith EM, Ritchie JM, Pawlita M, et al. HPV seropositivity and risks of head and neck cancer. Int J Cancer 2007; 120:825–832.

842. Schlecht NF, Burk RD, Adrien L, et al. Gene expression profiles in HPV-infected head and neck cancer. J Pathol 2007; 213:283–293.

843. Mork J, Lie AK, Glattre E, et al. HPV infection as a risk factor for squamous-cell carcinoma of the head and neck. N Engl J Med 2001; 344:1125–1131.

844. Ritchie JM, Smith EM, Summersgill KF, et al. HPV infection as a prognostic factor in carcinomas of the oral cavity and oropharynx. Int J Ca 2003; 104:336–344.

845. Chen PC, Kuo C, Pan CC, et al. Risk of oral cancer associated with HPV infection, betel quid chewing, and cigarette smoking in Taiwan–an integrated molecular and epidemiological study of 58 cases. J Oral Pathol Med 2002; 31:317–322.

846. Correnti M, Rivera H, Cavazza ME. Detection of HPV of high oncogenic potential in oral squamous cell carcinoma in a Venezuelan population. Oral Dis 2004; 10:163–166.

847. Zhang ZY, Sdek P, Cao J, et al. HPV type 16 and 18 DNA in oral squamous cell carcinoma and normal mucosa. Int J Oral Maxillofac Surg 2004; 33:71–74.

848. Boy S, Van Rensburg EJ, Engelbrecht S, et al. HPV detection in primary intra-oral squamous cell carcinomas-commensal, aetiological agent or contamination? J Oral Pathol Med 2006; 35:86–90.

849. Sugiyama M, Bhawal UK, Kawamura M, et al. HPV-16 in oral squamous cell carcinoma: clinical correlates and 5-year survival. Br J Oral Maxillofac Surg 2007; 45: 116–122.

850. Balderas-Loaeza A, Anaya-Saavedra G, Ramirez-Amador VA, et al. HPV-16 DNA methylation patterns support a causal association of the virus with oral squamous cell carcinomas. Int J Cancer 2007; 120:2165–2169.

851. Torrente MC, Ampuero S, Abud M, et al. Molecular detection and typing of HPV in laryngeal carcinoma patients. Acta OtoLaryngol 2005; 125:888–893.

852. Almadori G, Cadoni G, Cattani P, et al. HPV infection and epidermal growth factor receptor expression in primary laryngeal squamous cell carcinoma. Clin Canc Res 2001; 7:3988–3993.

853. Brito H, Vassallo J, Altemani A. Detection of HPV in laryngeal dysplasia and carcinoma. An In-situ hybridization and signal amplification study. Acta Otolaryngol 2000; 120:540–544.

854. Koskinen WJ, Brondbo K, Mellin DH, et al. Alcohol, smoking and HPV in laryngeal carcinoma: a Nordic prospective multicenter study. J Canc Res Clin Oncol 2007 (epub ahead of print).

855. Oliveria DE, Bacchi MM, Macareneco RSS, et al. HPV and EBV infection, p53 expression and cellular proliferation in laryngeal carcinoma. Am Clin Pathol 2006; 126:284–293.

856. Venuti A, Manni V, Morello R, et al. Physical state and expression of HPV in laryngeal carcinoma and surrounding normal mucosa. J Med Virol 2000; 60:396–402.

857. Manjarrez M, Ocadiz R, Valle L, et al. Detection of HPV and relevant tumor suppressors and oncoproteins in laryngeal tumors. Clin Canc Res 2006; 12:6946–6951.

858. Szládek G, Juhász A, Kardos G, et al. High prevalence of genogroup 1TT virus and HPV is associated with poor clinical outcome of laryngeal carcinoma. J Clin Pathol 2005; 58:402–405.

859. Hawley-Nelson P, Vousden KH, Hubbert NL, et al. HPV16 E6 and E7 proteins cooperate to immortalize human foreskin keratinocytes. EMBO 1989; 8:3905–3910.

860. Munger K, Phelps WC, Bubb V, et al. The E6 and E7 genes of the HPV 16 together are necessary and sufficient for transformation of primary keratinocytes. J Virol 1989; 63: 4417–4421.

861. Werness BA, Levine AJ, Howley PM. Association of HPV 16 and 18 E6 proteins with p53. Science 1990; 248:76–79.

862. Scheffner M, Werness BA, Huibregtse JM, et al. The E6 oncoprotein encoded by HPV16 and 18 promotes the degradation of p53. Cell 1990; 63:1129–1136.

863. Scheffner M, Whitaker NJ. HPV-induced carcinogenesis and the ubiquitin-proteasome system. Sem Canc Biol 2003; 13:59–67.

864. Hiller T, Poppelreuther S, Stubenrauch F, et al. Comparative analysis of 19 genital HPV types with regard to p53 degradation, immortalization, phylogeny, and epidemiologic risk classification. Can Epidem Biomark Prev 2006; 15:1262–1267.

865. Mantovani F, Banks L. The HPV E6 protein and its contribution to malignant progression. Oncogene 2001; 20:7874–7887.

866. Nagasaka K, Nakagawa S, Yano T, et al. Human homolog of Drosophilia tumor suppressor Scribble negatively regulates cell-cycle progression from G1 to S phase by localizing at the basolateral membrane of epithelial cells. Canc Sci 2006; 97:1217–1225.

867. Dyson N, Howley PM, Munger K, et al. The HPV 16 E7 oncoprotein is able to bind the retinoblastoma gene product. Science 1989; 243:934–937.

868. Dyson N. The regulation of E2F by pRB-family proteins. Gene Dev 1998; 12:2245–2265.

869. Narisawa-Saito M, Kiyono T. Basic mechanism of high-risk HPV-induced carcinogenesis: Role of E6 and E7 proteins. Canc Sci 2007; 9:1505–1511.

870. Kamio M, Yoshida T, Ogata H, et al. SOC1 inhibits HPV-E7-mediated transformation by inducing degradation of E7 protein. Oncogene 2004; 23:3107–3115.

871. Schmitt A, Harry B, Rapp B. Comparison of the properties of the E6 and E7 genes of low- and high-risk cutaneous papillomaviruses revelas reveals strongly transforming and high-Rb-binding activity for the E7 protein of the low-risk human papillomavirus type 1. J Virol 1994; 68: 7051–7059.

872. Storey Al, Osborn K, Crawford L. Co-transformation by HPV types 6 and 11. J Gen Virol 1990; 71:165–171.

873. Braakhuis BJ, Snijders PJ, Keune WJ, et al. Genetic patterns in head and neck cancers that contain or lack transcriptionally active HPV. J Natl Cancer Inst 2004; 96:998–1006.

874. Koskinen WJ, Chen RW, Leivo I, et al. Prevalence and physical status of HPV in squamous cell carcinomas of the head and neck. Int J Canc 2003; 107:401–406.

875. Nelson BL, Thompson LD. Molluscum contagiosum. Ear Nose Throat J 2003; 82:560.

876. Dohil MA, Lin P, Lee J, et al. The epidemiology of molluscum contagiosum in children. J Am Acad Dermatol 2006; 54:47–54.

877. Mansur AT, Goktay F, Gunduz S, et al. Multiple giant molluscum contagiosum in a renal transplant recipient. Transpl Infect Dis 2004; 6:120–123.

878. Fornatora ML, Reich RF, Gray RG, et al. Intraoral molluscum contagiosum: a report of a case and a review of the literature. Oral Surg Oral Med Oral Pathol Oral Radiol Endod 2001; 92:318–320.

879. Henderson W. Notice of the molluscum contangiosum. Edinburgh Med and Surg J 1841; 56:213–218.

880. Paterson R. Cases and observations on the Molluscum Contagiosum of Bateman, with an account of the minute structure of the tumors. Edinburgh Med Surg J 1941; 56:279–288.

881. Centers for Disease control and Prevention (CDC). Available at: www.cdc.gov/ncidod/dvrd/molluscum/clinical_overview.htm. Accessed December 2007.

882. New York City Department of Health. The measles emergency. An epidemic alert. City Health Info 1991; 10:1.

883. Akang EEU, Ekweozor C, Pindiga HU, et al. Childhood infections in Nigeria: an autopsy study. J Trop Med and Hyg 1993; 96:231–236.

884. Monafo WJ, Haslam DB, Roberts RL, et al. Disseminated measles infection after vaccination in a child with congenital immunodeficiency. J Pediatr 1994; 124:273–276.

885. Stankovic KM, Mckenna MJ. Current research in otosclerosis. Curr Opin Otolaryngol Head Neck Surg 2006; 14: 347–351.

886. Kurihara N, Zhou H, Reddy SV, et al. Experimental models of Paget's disease. J Bone Miner Res 2006; 21(suppl 2):P55–P57.

887. Warthin AS. Occurrence of numerous large giant cells in the tonsils and pharyngeal mucosa in the prodromal stage of measles. Arch Pathol 1931; 11:864–874.

888. Finkeldey W. Uber Riesenzellbefunde in den gaumenmandeln zugleich ein beitrag zur histopathologie der mandelveranderungen im maserninkubationsstadium. Virch Archiv Pathol Anat 1931; 281:323–329.

889. Kjeldsberg CR, Kim H. Polykaryocytes resembling Warthin-Finkeldey giant cells in reactive and neoplastic lymphoid disorders. Human Pathol 1981; 12:267–272.

890. Peltola H, Kulkarni PS, Kapre SV, et al. Mumps outbreaks in Canada and the United States: time for new thinking on mumps vaccines. Clin Infect Dis 2007; 45:459–466.

891. Centers for Disease control and Prevention (CDC). Available at: www.cdc.gov/mmwr/preview/mmwrhtml/mm55e601a1.htm. Accessed November 2007.

892. Seifert G, Miehlke A, Haubrich J, et al. Diseases of the salivary glands. Pathology-Diagnosis-Treatment-Facial Nerve Surgery. New York, NY: George Thieme, 1986.

893. Nirasawa M, Sugaya N, Mitamura K, et al. Prethyroidal swelling in mumps. Ped J Infect Dis 1990; 9:855–856.

894. Alhaj S, Ozyylmaz I, Altun G, et al. Eyelid, facial and presternal edema in mumps. Pediatr Infect Dis J 2007; 7:661.

895. Ishida M, Fushiki H, Morijiri M, et al. Mumps virus infection in adults: three cases of supraglottic edema. Laryngoscope 2006; 116:2221–2223.

896. Shanley JD. The resurgence of mumps in young adults and adolescents. Cleve Clin J Med 2007; 74:42–44, 47–48.

897. Henson D, Siegel S, Strano A. Mumps virus sialoadenitis. Arch Pathol 1971; 92:469–474.

898. Jin L, Feng Y, Parry R, et al. Real-time PCR and its application to mumps rapid diagnosis. J Med Virol 2007; 79:1761–1767.

899. Frenkel JK. Pursuing toxoplasma. J Infect Dis 1970; 122:553–559.

900. Frenkel JK, Dubey JP. Toxoplasmosis and its prevention in cats and man. J Infect Dis 1972; 126:664–673.

901. Montoya JG, Liesenfeld O. Toxoplasmosis. Lancet 2004; 363:1965–1976.

902. Ruiz A, Frenkel JK, Cerdas L. Isolation of *Toxoplasma* from soil. J Parasitol 1973; 59:204–206.

903. Hadi U, Rameh C. Intraglandular toxoplasmosis of the parotid gland pre- or postoperative diagnosis? Am J Otolaryngol 2007; 28:201–204.

904. Hill D, Dubey JP. *Toxoplasma gondii*: transmission, diagnosis and prevention. Clin Microbiol Infect 2002; 8:634–640.

905. Hohlfeld P, Daffos F, Costa JM, et al. Prenatal diagnosis of congenital toxoplasmosis with a PCR test on amniotic fluid. N Engl J Med 1994; 331:695–699.

906. Eapen M, Mathew CF, Aravindan KP. Evidence based criteria for the histopathological diagnosis of toxoplasmic lymphadenopathy. J Clin Pathol 2005; 58:1143–1146.

907. Kardon DE, Thompson LD. A clinicopathologic series of 22 cases of tonsillar granulomas. Laryngoscope 2000; 110: 476–481.

908. Petersen E. Toxoplasmosis. Semin Fetal Neonatal Med 2007; 12:214–223.

909. Centers for Disease control and Prevention (CDC). Available at: www.cdc.gov/mmwr/preview/mmwrhtml/ss5206a1.htm. Accessed October 2007.

910. Dupouy-Camet J. Trichinellosis: a worldwide zoonosis. Vet parasitol 2000; 93:191–200.

911. Gajadhar AA, Gamble HR. Historical perspectives and currnet global challenges of *Trichinella* and trichinellosis. Vet Parasitol 2000; 93:183–189.

912. Feldmeier H, Bienzle U, Jansen-Rossek R, et al. Sequelae after infection with *Trichinella spiralis*: A prospective cohort study. Wien Klin Wochenschr 1991; 103:111–116.

913. Pozio E, Zarlenga DS. Recent advances on the taxonomy, systematics and epidemiology of Trichinella. Int J Parasitol 2005; 35:1191–1204.

914. Kociecka W. Trichinellosis: human disease, diagnosis and treatment. Vet Parasitol 2000; 93:365–383.

915. Akar S, Gurler O, Pozio E, et al. Frequency and severity of musculoskeletal symptoms in humans during an outbreak of trichinellosis caused by *Trichinella britovi*. J Parasitol 2007; 93:341–344.

916. Duran-Ortiz JS, de la Torre IG, Barocio GO. Trichinosis with severe myopathic involvement mimicking polymyositits. Report of a family outbreak. J Rheumatol 1992; 19:310–312.

917. Cvorovic L, Milutinovic Z, Kiurski M. *Trichinella spiralis* and laryngeal carcinoma: a case report. Eur Arch Otorhinolaryngol 2005; 262:456–458.

918. Pozio E. New patterns of *Trichinella* infection. Vet Parasitol 2001; 98:133–148.

919. Murray C. Trichinosis. Available at: www.emedicine.com/med/topic2306.htm#section~workup. Accessed October 2007.

920. Abdou N, NaPombejara C, Sagawa A, et al. Malakoplakia: evidence for monocyte lysosomal abnormality correctable by cholinergic agonist in vitro and in vivo. N Eng J Med 1977; 297:1413–1419.

921. Stanton MJ, Maxted W. Malacoplakia: a study of the literature and current concepts of pathogenesis, diagnosis, and treatment. J Urol 1981; 125:139–146.

922. Wagner D, Joseph J, Huang J, et al. Malakoplakia of the prostate on needle core biopsy: a case report and review of the literature. Int J Surg Pathol 2007; 15:86–89.

923. Pang LC. Pulmonary malakoplakia coexistent with tuberculosis of the hilar lymph node mimicking malignancy. Respiration 2005; 72:95–100.

924. Dale JC, Robinson RA. Malakoplakia of the parotid gland. J Laryngol Otol 1988; 102:737–740.

925. Love RB, Bernard A, Carpenter BF. Malakoplakia of the tongue—a case report. J Otolaryngol 1985; 14:179–182.

926. Salins PC, Triveldi P. Extensive malakoplakia of the nasopharynx: Management of a rare disease. J Oral Maxillofac Surg 1998; 56:483–487.

927. Vitellaro-Zuccarello L, Felletti V, Paizis G. et al. Ultrastructural study of granulomatous tissue in tonsillar malakoplakia. Histol Histopath 1987; 2:307–312.

928. Nayar RC, Garg I, Alapatt JJ. Malakoplakia of the temporal bone in a nine-month old infant. J Laryngol Otol 1991, 105:568–570.

929. Azadeh B, Dabiri S, Moshfegh I. Malakoplakia of the middle ear. Histopathol 1991; 19:276–278.

930. Larsimont D, Hamels J, Fortunati D. Thyroid-gland malakoplakia with autoimmune thyroiditis. Histopathol 1993; 23:491–494.

931. Simpson C, Strong NP, Dickinson J, et al. Medical management of ocular malakoplakia. Ophthal 1992; 99:192–196.

932. Akkuzu G, Aydin E, Bilezikci B, et al. Malakoplakia in nasal vestibule. Otolaryngol Head Neck Surg 2006; 135:636–637.

933. Kumar V, Coady MSE. Malakoplakia of the neck in an immunosuppressed patient. Plastic Reconstruct Surg 2005; 116:125e–127e.

934. Von Hansemann D. Uber Malakolaki der Harnblase. Virch Archiv fur Pathol Anat Physiol Klin Med 1903; 173:302–308.

935. Michealis L, Gutmann C. Ueber Einschlusse in Blasentumoren. Klin Med (Mosk) 1902; 47:208–215.

936. Rybicki BA, Iannuzzi MC. Epidemiology of sarcoidosis: Recent advances and future prospects. Sem Resp Crit Care Med 2007; 28:22–35.

937. Rybicki BA, Iannuzzi MC, Frederick MM, et al. Familial aggregation of sarcoidosis: A case-control etiologic study of sarcoidosis (ACCESS). Am J Respir Crit Care Med 2001; 164:2085–2091.

938. Shetty A, Gedalia A. Sarcoidosis. Available at: www .emedicine.com/ped/topic2043.htm (accessed July 2007).

939. Siltzbach LE. Editorial. Current thoughts on the epidemiology and etiology of sarcoidosis. Am J Med 1965; 39: 361–368.

940. Siltzbach LE. Sarcoidosis: Clinical features and management. Med Clin No Am 1967; 51:483–502.

941. Rottoli P, Bargagli E, Chidichimo C, et al. Sarcoidosis with upper respiratory tract involvement. Resp Med 2006; 100:253–257.

942. Gupta D, Agarwal R, Aggarwal A, et al. Molecular evidence for the role of mycobacteria in sarcoidosis: A meta-analysis. Eur Resp J 2007; 30(3):508–516 (epub 2007 May 30).

943. Almenoff PL, Johnson A, Lesser M, Mattman LH. Growth of acid fast L forms from the blood of patients with sarcoidosis. Thorax 1996; 51:530–533.

944. Brown ST, Brett I, Almenoff PL, et al. Recovery of cell wall-deficient organisms from blood does not distinguish between patients with sarcoidosis and control subjects. Chest 2003; 123:413–417.

945. Hiramatsu J, Kataoka M, Nakata Y, et al. Propionibacterium acnes DNA detected in bronchoalveolar lavage cells from patients with sarcoidosis. Sarcoidosis Vasc Diffuse Lung Dis 2003; 20:197–203.

946. Ishihara M, Ohno S, Ono H, et al. Seroprevalence of anti-Borrelia antibodies among patients with confirmed sarcoidosis in a region of Japan where Lyme borreliosis is endemic. Graefes Arch Clin Exp Ophthalmol 1998; 236:280–284.

947. Rosen Y. Pathology of sarcoidosis. Sem Resp Crit Care Med 2007; 28:36–52.

948. Schaumann J, Hallberg VL. Koch's bacilli manifested in the tissue of lymphogranulomatosis benigna (Schaumann) by using Hallberg's staining method. Acta Medica Scandinavica 1941; 152:499–501.

949. Schaumann J. On the nature of certain peculiar corpuscles present in the tissue of lymphogranulomatosis benigna. Acta Medica Scandinavica 1941; 151:239–253.

950. Hamazaki Y. Ueber ein neues säurefeste Substanz fuhrendes Spindle körperchen der menschlichen Lymphdrüsen. Virch Archiv fur pathol Anat und Physiol und fur Klin Med 1938; 301:490–522.

951. Wesenberg W. Ueber säurefeste "Spindlekörper Hmamzaki" bei Sakoidose der Lymphknoten und uber doppelichtbrechende Zelleinschlusse bei Sarkoidose der Lungen. Arch Klin Exp Dermatol 1966; 227:101–107.

952. Wallach J. Interpretation of Diagnostic Tests. 8th Ed. Philadelphia, PA: Lippincott Williams & Wilkins, 2007: 1050.

953. McCluggage WG, Bharucha H. Lymph node hyalinization in rheumatoid arthritis and systemic sclerosis. J Clin Pathol 1994; 47:138–142.

954. Coyne JD. Colonic carcinoma with granulomatous (sarcoid) reaction. J Clin Pathol 2002; 55:708–709.

955. Kovacs J, Varga A, Bessenyei M, et al. Renal cell cancer associated with sarcoid-like reaction. Pathol Oncol Res 2004; 10:169–171 (epub 2004 Sep 25).

956. Brincker H. Sarcoid reactions in malignant tumours. Cancer Treat Rev 1986; 3:147–156.

957. Baughman RP, Lower EE. Novel therapies for sarcoidosis. Sem Resp Crit Care Med 2006; 28:128–133.

26

Miscellaneous Disorders of the Head and Neck

Leon Barnes

Department of Pathology, University of Pittsburgh Medical Center,
Presbyterian-University Hospital, Pittsburgh, Pennsylvania, U.S.A.

I. GIANT CELL ARTERITIS

A. Introduction

Giant cell arteritis (GCA) is a granulomatous panarteritis that characteristically involves one or more craniofacial branches of the carotid arteries, especially the temporal. In some instances, there is also a concomitant systemic vasculitis that may or may not be clinically apparent.

Although the disease is also referred to by a variety of synonyms (temporal arteritis, cranial arteritis, Horton's disease, Hutchinson-Horton's disease), GCA is preferred, since it may also involve vessels other than the temporal artery, and this vessel can also be targeted by other forms of vasculitis (1–4).

B. Clinical Features

The disease is two times more common in women than in men and is distinctly uncommon in individuals younger than 50 years (5). The four cases of juvenile temporal arteritis reported by Lie et al., as occurring in three males and one female, aged 7 to 22 years, bear little resemblance to classic GCA and, as suggested by them, may represent a new entity (6). The frequency of GCA rises steadily with age. GCA shows a striking bias for the white population of Britain, northern European nations, and the northern regions of the United States (7). In Olmsted County, Minnesota, the annual age-specific incidence was 1.7 cases per 100,000 for the 50- to 60-year-old group, as compared with 55.5 cases for individuals older than 80 years (8). It is rare in blacks and in individuals of Latin or Oriental descent (7–9).

Symptoms are highly variable and often vague. They include headache, myalgia, fever, malaise, weight loss, fatigue, depression, anorexia, visual disturbances, tenderness of the scalp, dysphagia, masticatory claudication, hearing loss, various neurological disturbances, mucosal ulcers, infarcts, and glossitis. It is this constellation of seemingly nonspecific complaints that should alert the astute clinician to the correct diagnosis. Headaches, one of the most common manifestations, usually have an abrupt onset, are worse at night, and are unilateral in distribution. The pain is severe, boring, and throbbing, and tends to be localized to the temporal region, but may radiate widely over the scalp, face, jaws, and occiput. Forty to sixty percent of patients with GCA will also have polymyalgia rheumatica (PMR), a syndrome characterized by stiffness and pain of the muscles of the neck, shoulder, lower back, and thighs. Conversely, approximately 10% to 50% with PMR will have GCA (5,10–12). This association has led some to believe that these two conditions (GCA and PMR) are variations of the same disease. PMR can be detected several months to years before the diagnosis of GCA or can begin years after a positive temporal artery biopsy.

Claudication of the jaws accentuated by eating and talking and relieved by rest is virtually pathognomonic of GCA and is presumably due to progressive involvement of the facial artery. The scalp rarely ulcerates, but is exquisitely tender; paroxysms of pain can be triggered by simply wearing a hat, brushing the hair, or sleeping on a pillow. Fever is usually low grade, but sometimes may spike to 102°F to 103°F, resulting in the patients being hospitalized with a "fever of unknown origin." Blindness, either unilateral or bilateral, is the most serious complication of the disease and occurs in about 10% to 20% of all patients. It is irreversible and, if it occurs, tends to develop within the first year of the disease. Unfortunately, there are often no reliable premonitory signs or symptoms to forewarn of this tragedy.

The finding of clinically negative temporal arteries should not distract from a diagnosis of GCA, for they may harbor histological evidence of active disease. In fact, only 35% to 55% of patients actually present with temporal arteries that are palpable, nodular, pulseless, or painful (13).

The American College of Rheumatology (ACR) has developed guidelines for diagnosing GCA (14). These are displayed in Table 1. According to the ACR, a patient shall be said to have GCA if at least three of these five criteria are present. The presence of any three or more criteria yields a sensitivity of 93.5% and a specificity of 91.2%.

C. Angiography and Ultrasonography

GCA does not have a specific angiographic appearance and may involve arteries without causing any detectable changes. Hence, the use of selective temporal

Table 1 Criteria for the Classification of Giant Cell (Temporal Arteritis) (Traditional Format)[a]

Criterion definition	
1. Age at disease onset >50 yr	Development of symptoms or findings beginning at age ≥50
2. New headache	New onset of or new type of localized pain in the head
3. Temporal artery abnormality	Temporal artery tenderness to palpation or decreased pulsation, unrelated to arteriosclerosis of cervical arteries
4. Elevated erythrocyte sedimentation rate	Erythrocyte sedimentation rate >50 mm/hr by the Westergren method
5. Abnormal artery biopsy	Biopsy specimen with artery showing vasculitis characterized by a predominance of mononuclear cell infiltration or granulomatous inflammation, usually with multinucleated giant cells

[a]For purposes of classification, a patient shall be said to have giant cell (temporal) arteritis if at least three of these five criteria are present. The presence of any three or more criteria yields a sensitivity of 93.5% and a specificity of 91.2%.

arteriography to improve the yield of random biopsies has not been rewarding (15–17).

Color duplex ultrasonography, however, may be helpful in establishing the diagnosis. According to Schmidt et al., this is an excellent method of examining blood vessels, and there are characteristic signs of GCA that can be visualized (18). The most specific feature is a dark halo, which may be due to edema of the arterial wall. In patients with typical clinical signs and a halo on ultrasonography, it may be possible to make a diagnosis and begin treatment without performing a temporal artery biopsy.

D. Laboratory Tests

A striking elevation of the erythrocyte sedimentation rate (ESR) is the laboratory hallmark of GCA. Values are usually in the 75–100 mm/hr range. An abnormal ESR is so characteristic that, according to Fan et al., "one should be very suspicious of the diagnosis without an ESR exceeding 50 mm/hr" (7). A total of 15% to 30% of patients manifest a normochromic, normocytic, or hypochromic, microcytic anemia (hemoglobin values of usually 9–11 g) (10). The anemia does not respond to iron therapy, but will abate with control of the arteritis.

Abnormalities in liver function tests have also been observed. In 50% to 60% of patients, there is retention of sulfobromophtalein or an elevation of the serum alkaline phosphatase (19). The serum glutamic oxalacetic transaminase (SGOT) and bilirubin values tend to be normal. Liver biopsies, in these instances, have shown only nonspecific findings, such as fatty metamorphosis, "portal triaditis," or spotty hepatocyte necrosis (19).

Serological tests for rheumatoid factor and antinuclear antibodies are characteristically normal, whereas plasma protein levels are elevated, including

c-reactive protein. Electromyograms (EMGs) and tests for serum muscle enzymes (aldolase, creatine phosphokinase, and transaminases) performed on patients with both GCA and PMR have shown no abnormalities (5,20).

Studies of the human leukocyte antigen (HLA) complex indicate that both GCA and PMR are frequently associated with HLA-DRB1*04 and DRB1*01 alleles (21,22). Although an autoimmune mechanism has long been postulated, the etiology of GCA remains unclear. Immunofluorescent studies of arteries have not been consistent, some showing negative results and others, positive results. Attempts to identify serum antibodies to elastic tissue have not been rewarding.

More recently, Powers et al. studied 39 consecutive temporal artery biopsies in patients suspected of having GCA for the presence of herpes simplex DNA using the polymerase chain reaction. They found evidence of the virus in 88% of the specimens, raising the possibility that herpes simplex might be etiologically related to GCA (23).

E. Pathology

No matter how suspicious the clinical and laboratory data might be, the diagnosis of GCA can be established definitively only by biopsy of a diseased artery. Because of its high incidence of involvement and ease of accessibility, the temporal artery is the one most often selected. As unilateral involvement of the temporal arteries occurs in only 5% of patients with GCA, either artery may be sampled. Bilateral biopsies, however, do increase the yield by 5% to 10%. Both surgeons and pathologists should be aware that the disease may involve the artery only focally or segmentally in 18% to 28% cases (24,25). The frequency of "skin lesions" is greatest in those arteries that are normal to palpation. Klein et al. have recommended that a long segment of artery (3–7 cm) be removed and examined by frozen section at several levels. If the frozen sections are normal, then the authors suggest a biopsy of the contralateral artery (25). More recently, it has been shown that skip areas are rarely more than 1 mm in length and that a temporal artery biopsy of 0.5 cm in length is statistically sufficient to make a histological diagnosis (26).

Adequate histological examination requires that the entire biopsy, both cross and longitudinal sections, be evaluated. On pathological examination, the vessels exhibit a transmural infiltrate of mononuclear cells (lymphocytes, histiocytes, and plasma cells), disruption and fragmentation of the internal elastic lamina, fibrosis, thrombosis, and/or recanalization (Fig. 1). Giant cells, which may be of the Langerhans or foreign body type, often contain fragments of the internal elastic lamina within their cytoplasm (Fig. 2). Fibrinoid necrosis, neutrophils, and eosinophils are rare to absent. Veins are not affected. Although giant cells are not essential for diagnosis, one should be cautious in making a diagnosis in their absence, because the temporal artery may also be involved by other arteritides.

It now appears that GCA is a T-cell-mediated disease (27). Activation of CD-positive T cells occurs

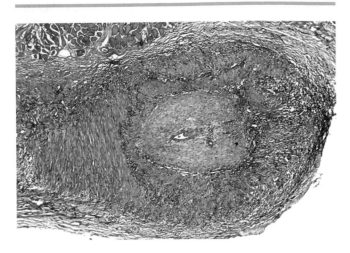

Figure 1 Marked narrowing and inflammation of the temporal artery in a patient with giant cell arteritis (H&E stain, 40×). *Abbreviation*: H&E, hematoxylin and eosin.

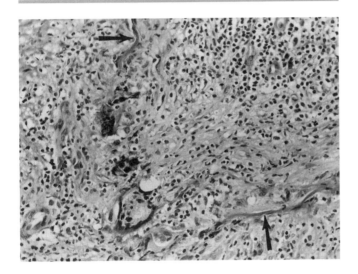

Figure 2 Giant cell arteritis. Giant cells are characteristically aligned along the partially destroyed internal elastic lamina (*arrows*) (H&E stain, 250×). *Abbreviation*: H&E, hematoxylin and eosin.

in the adventitia of the arterial well, which orchestrates macrophage differentiation. These cells infiltrate the vascular wall and ultimately mediate myofibroblastic proliferation with ultimate luminal stenosis and ischemia.

One should be aware that the histological changes may be altered by prior corticosteroid therapy. Ideally, a temporal artery biopsy should be obtained either before or within one to five days of starting therapy; however, data do indicate that the biopsy may still be diagnostic even after more than 14 days of corticosteriod therapy (28,29). In addition to previous corticosteroid therapy, other causes for negative temporal artery biopsies include (*i*) imprecise clinical

criteria for performing the procedure, (*ii*) small biopsies that may not include "skip areas," and (*iii*) failure to examine multiple histological levels.

Evidence suggests that a chronic low-grade axial synovitis may account for many of the symptoms of PMR, making the term "polymyalgia" somewhat of a misnomer because of the lack of true muscle involvement. Synovial biopsies in patients with PMR have shown vascular congestion, edema, and mild to moderate inflammation (30,31). Muscle biopsies are normal.

F. Differential Diagnosis

The changes of arteriosclerosis should not be confused with healed GCA. According to Lie et al., the two can be distinguished by the characteristic zonal arrangement of the intima (32). In arteriosclerosis, the intima is divided into an inner dense collagenous layer and an outer hyperplastic elastic layer. In healed GCA, several layers of circularly oriented smooth muscle cells with condensation of concentric elastic fibers form a narrow and compact inner zone, whereas the broader outer zone of the intima tends to be heavily collagenized. Patchy loss of internal elastic lamina occurs with advancing age and is not necessarily a sign of arteritis (33).

Corcoran et al. have also observed that patients with chronic perivascular inflammation but no arteritis are no more likely to have GCA on clinical grounds than similar patients without inflammation on biopsy (34).

G. Treatment and Prognosis

Corticosteroids are the most effective drug against the disease. With this medication, clinical symptoms are alleviated in 48 to 72 hours, followed in one to four weeks by normalization of the ESR. Treatment usually begins with 40 to 60 mg/day of prednisone for a period of four to six weeks, after which the dose is gradually tapered to a maintenance level that keeps the patient asymptomatic and the ESR within normal range. Although no consensus on duration of treatment exists, most patients require at least one year, possibly two years, of therapy (5,12,13). With prompt recognition and treatment, GCA is a rare cause of death. When fatalities do occur, they are most often due to cerebral and cardiac involvement or to ruptured aortic aneurysms (35).

II. PHARYNGOESOPHAGEAL (ZENKER'S) DIVERTICULUM

A. Introduction and Pathology

Esophageal diverticula represent an outward herniation of all or a portion of the esophageal wall from the lumen of the esophagus. Anatomically, they can be classified according to site of occurrence as (*i*) pharyngoesophageal or hypopharyngeal, (*ii*) midesophageal or thoracic, and (*iii*) epiphrenic or supradiaphragmatic. They can also be categorized as traction or pulsion, true or false, and congenital or acquired. Traction diverticula are usually due to the pull of extrinsic inflammatory adhesions and are most often found in the midesophagus adjacent to diseased bronchial lymph nodes. Pulsion diverticula, on the other hand, are the result of increased intraluminal pressure and occur at either end of the esophagus. True diverticula contain all layers normally present in the esophagus, whereas false diverticula lack the outer muscular wall. In this book, only the pharyngoesophageal diverticulum (PED) will be considered.

The PED (hypopharyngeal diverticulum, Zenker's diverticulum) is an acquired pulsion diverticulum of the false type that invariably arises from the posterior hypopharyngeal wall just to the left of the midline between the oblique fibers of the inferior pharyngeal constrictor and the horizontal fibers of the cricopharyngeal muscles, known as the triangle of Killian or Killian's dehiscence (Fig. 3) (1). Originally described by Ludlow in 1769 (2), it often bears the name of Zenker (3), who, along with von Ziemssen, studied the disease extensively in 1878.

Although the exact cause is unknown, attention has been focused on a possible obstructive role of the cricopharyngeal muscle. Normally, this muscle is in a state of contraction and serves as a sphincter between the hypopharynx and upper esophagus. With swallowing, coincident with pharyngeal muscular contraction, it relaxes to allow the bolus of food to pass. Various disorders have been ascribed to this sphincter, including inflammatory stenosis, spasm, premature contraction, delayed relaxation, and lack of relaxation, all of which could lead to elevated intraluminal pressure with mural herniation (4–13).

B. Clinical Features

The incidence of PED has been reported by Shallow and Clerf (14) as 1 in every 1400 hospital admissions and by Dorsey and Randolf as 1 in 800 upper gastrointestinal barium studies (7). It is twice as frequent in males as in females and characteristically occurs in individuals older than 50 years (15). Its rarity in children and in adults younger than 30 years has been used as evidence in support of the acquired, rather than congenital, basis of disease (7,16).

Symptoms, which vary according to the size of the diverticulum, include a choking sensation associated with food sticking in the throat, noisy swallowing or gurgling on swallowing, hoarseness, coughing spells, a constant desire to clear the throat, regurgitation, and weight loss. Because the mouth of the diverticulum lies above the superior esophageal sphincter, there is no barrier to prevent spontaneous pharyngeal reflux. Consequently, and especially at night, with changes in the position of the head and neck at various angles on the pillow, sudden unpredictable expulsion of sac contents occurs, often leading to repeated bouts of pneumonitis or even a lung abscess. As the diverticulum elongates, gravity pulls it downward toward the mediastinum, which results in the kinking of the esophageal lumen. This, as well as the extrinsic compressive effect of the sac on the esophageal wall, leads to dysphagia (Fig. 4). Another infrequent complication, presumably related to chronic irritation from food stagnation, is the development of squamous cell carcinoma within the pouch (17,18). The presence of blood-streaked secretions and radiographic evidence of a diverticular-filling defect

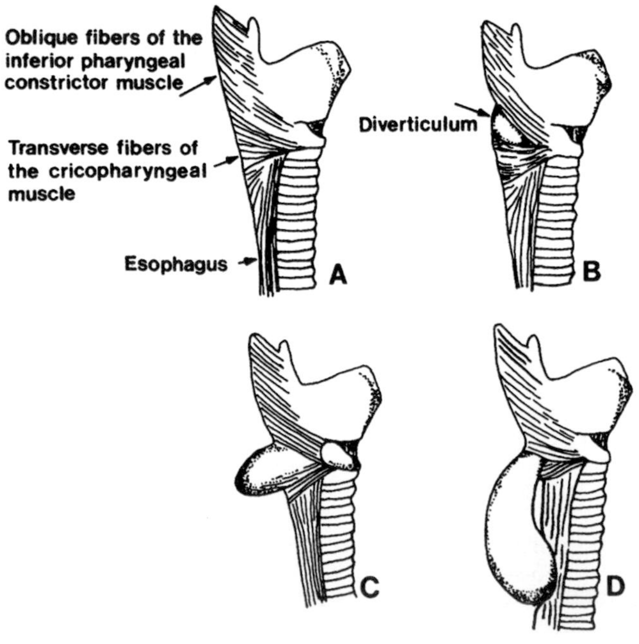

Figure 3 Developmental stages of a pharyngoesophageal diverticulum.

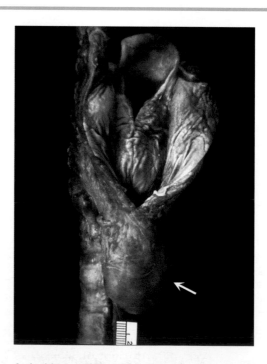

Figure 4 Incidental pharyngoesophageal (Zenker's) diverticulum discovered at autopsy (*arrow*). Note the diverticulum pressing on the cervical esophagus and the larynx above.

should always raise the possibility of superimposed carcinoma (10).

A total of 8% of patients with PED are noted to have additional esophageal diseases (15). Included among these are hiatal hernias, traction diverticula, varices, achalasia, and carcinomas. The diagnosis of a PED can be established by barium swallow. Esophagoscopy is generally not required in the preoperative evaluation and should be avoided if at all possible, because it carries the risk of perforation and the possibility of aspiration of stagnant sac contents. Shallow and Clerf, in their evaluation of 186 PED, observed that 30% were less than 2 cm in length, 43% were between 2.5 and 5.0 cm, and 27% more than 5 cm (14). Although the orifice of the pouch may measure as much as 5 or 6 cm in diameter, most are considerably less (15). About three-fourths exhibit clinical evidence of inflammation (14).

C. Treatment and Prognosis

Although dilation of the esophagus at the level of the diverticulum may result in relief in small lesions, surgical repair eventually becomes necessary in all PED (19). This may be accomplished through an external approach using a one- or two-stage procedure (10,11,14,20). Or, the pouch may be resected internally through an endoscope (6,7,15,21). A few of the smaller ones have also been effectively managed by simple cricopharyngeal myotomy (8). Depending on the surgical procedure employed, 2% to 10% of patients experience recurrence of their diverticulum (6,15). Recurrences are more common in individuals treated endoscopically, as opposed to an external approach. The most feared complication of surgery is mediastinitis; others include fistulas, recurrent

laryngeal nerve paralysis (which is often temporary), and esophageal stenosis. As many of the patients are of advanced age, often debilitated by their disease, and occasionally suffering from other organ dysfunctions, an operative mortality as high as 2% to 3% has been reported (7,14).

III. TUMORS OF THE PARAPHARYNGEAL SPACE

A. Anatomy

The parapharyngeal space (pterygomaxillary, pharyngomaxillary, or lateral pharyngeal space) is one of several potential recesses of the head and neck (Fig. 5). Its shape is roughly pyramidal, with its base corresponding to the base of the skull and its apex terminating at the greater cornu of the hyoid bone. The medial border is formed by the superior pharyngeal constrictor muscle and tonsillar fossa. Laterally, it is limited by the internal (medial) ptyerygoid, inner surface of the mandibular ramus, and deep lobe of the parotid gland. Anteriorly, it is bound by the pterygomandibular raphe, and, posteriorly, it is defined by the vertebral column and paravertebral muscles (1–7).

The space can be divided into three compartments: (*i*) prestyloid (anterior), (*ii*) retrostyloid (posterior), and (*iii*) retropharyngeal (medial). The prestyloid division contains the parotid gland, internal maxillary artery, and the inferior alveolar, lingual, and auriculotemporal nerves (1). The poststyloid compartment is the most important, as it houses the internal carotid artery; internal jugular vein; cranial nerves IX, X, XI, and XII; cervical sympathetic chain; paraganglionic system (vagal and carotid bodies); and a few lymph

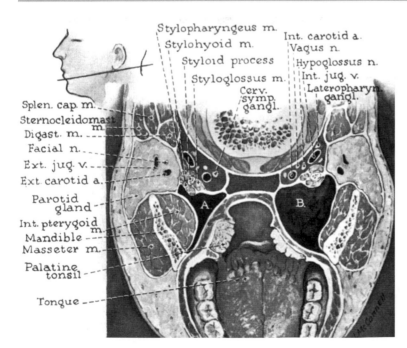

Figure 5 Sagittal section through the parapharyngeal spaces (**A** and **B**) at the level of the palatine tonsil. Tumors and abscesses originating in this space characteristically result in medial and downward displacement of the tonsil, soft palate, and lateral pharyngeal wall (**B** vs. **A**). *Source*: From section "Tumors of the Parapharyngeal Space," Ref. 13.

nodes. The retropharyngeal portion contains only lymph nodes, of which the most important is the lateral node of Rouviere, as it is often the first site of dissemination of nasopharyngeal carcinoma.

B. Clinical Features

Because three of its boundaries are composed of bones, the growth of parapharyngeal tumors is limited. They may extend toward the pharynx, producing a non-ulcerative medial and downward displacement of the tonsillar fossa, soft palate, and lateral pharyngeal wall (Fig. 5), or they may grow inferiorly and present as a cervical mass between the submandibular gland and tail of the parotid gland, or as a retromandibular lesion. Signs and symptoms that are related to the compressive effects of the neoplasm include unilateral serous otitis media with hearing loss, throat discomfort, dysphagia, voice change, and pain.

C. Pathology

Tumors of the parapharyngeal space are uncommon. They account for about 0.5% to 0.8% of all head and neck neoplasms (5). Of the tumors presenting in this space, 70% to 80% are benign and 20% to 30% malignant (4,5) (Table 2).

They can be either primary or secondary, the latter arising by direct extension or metastasis, and can be grouped into five major categories: (*i*) salivary, 41%; (*ii*) neural, 38%; (*iii*) lymphomas, 10%; (*iv*) soft tissue, 7%; and (*v*) miscellaneous, 4%. In descending order of frequency, the most common benign neoplasms are pleomorphic adenomas, schwannomas (neurilemomas), and paragangliomas, whereas the most prevalent malignant tumors are lymphomas, adenoid cystic carcinomas, and malignant schwannomas. Most of the pleomorphic adenomas develop from the deep lobe of the parotid gland and present in the space as either a circumscribed or "dumbbell-shaped" mass, the latter configuration resulting from extension of the tumor through the narrow stylomandibular tunnel. They rarely arise from the minor salivary glands of the adjacent pharynx. Schwannomas characteristically arise from either the vagus nerve or sympathetic chain and only infrequently from the glossopharyngeal, hypoglossal, or spinal accessory nerves.

D. Treatment and Prognosis

The tumor should be removed en bloc, using one of several external surgical approaches (2). Intraoral incisional biopsies are to be condemned, for they may result in uncontrolled bleeding, nerve damage, infection, or tumor "spillage" (8–10,12). Supplemental irradiation therapy may be warranted in the event that the tumor should be malignant.

The pleomorphic adenoma is the most common benign tumor of the parapharyngeal space. It is not uncommon during surgery that the tumor has to be excised in a piecemeal fashion or removed with less than the usual standard margins. In a review of 68 pleomorphic adenomas of the parapharyngeal space,

Table 2 Tumors of the Parapharyngeal Space: Histological Distribution of 256 Cases

Site	No. of cases (%)
Salivary gland	105 (41)
Pleomorphic adenoma	85
Adenoid cystic	12
Malignant mixed	4
Mucoepidermoid	1
Acinic cell	1
Primary epidermoid carcinoma	1
Adenocarcinoma, NOS	1
Neural	97 (38)
Schwannoma	57
Paraganglioma	22
Malignant schwannoma	7
Neurofibroma	5
Meningioma	2
Ganglioneuroma	2
Neuroblastoma	1
Malignant carotid body paraganglioma	1
Malignant lymphomas	26 (10)
Soft tissue	17 (7)
Hemangioma	4
Lymphangioma	2
Hemangiopericytoma	2
Hemangioendothelioma	1
Desmoid	1
Fibrosarcoma	1
Malignant fibrous histiocytoma	1
Lipoma	1
Hibernoma	1
Liposarcoma	1
Leiomyoma	1
Rhadomyosarcoma	1
Miscellaneous	11 (4)
Metastatic	3
Branchial cleft cyst	2
Hyperplastic lymph node	2
Aneurysm	1
Chordoma	1
Plasmacytoma	1
Teratoma	1

Source: From section "Tumors of the Parapharyngeal Space", Ref. 11.

Hughes et al. noted that only three (4%) recurred (median follow-up was 6.2 years) (6). Tumor rupture was reported in 10 of these pleomorphic adenomas, but recurrence was detected in only one case. The follow-up period for the remaining nine cases in whom the tumor had ruptured was from 1 day to 27.7 years (median 2.2 years). These data suggest that pleomorphic adenomas in this space are less prone to local recurrence than in other sites.

IV. THOROTRAST GRANULOMAS AND RELATED NEOPLASMS

A. Introduction

Thorotrast is a 25% colloidal solution of radioactive thorium dioxide suspended in an aqueous solution of dextrin. The thorium particles range in size from 3 to 10 μ, have a half-life of 1.4×10^{10} years, and emit 90% α, 9% β, and 1% γ rays (1). It was widely used as a radiographic contrast medium from about 1930 to the

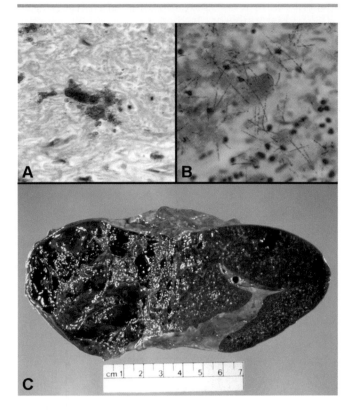

Figure 6 (**A**) Thorotrast granuloma composed of dense scar tissue with small granular deposits of Thorotrast (H&E stain, 400×). (**B**) Autoradiograph showing alpha tracts of Thorotrast. (**C**) Thorotrast-induced angiosarcoma of the liver. The multiple hemorrhagic nodules of various sizes represent tumor. *Abbreviation*: H&E, hematoxylin and eosin. *Source*: Courtesy of CD Bedetti, Forbes Regional Hospital, Pittsburgh, Pennsylvania, U.S.A.

early 1950s, but was subsequently banned because of its neoplastic and nonneoplastic side effects. It has been estimated that more than 50,000 patients have been injected with Thorotrast, mainly for arteriography, but also for hepatosplenography, retrograde pyelography, hysterosalpingography, and paranasal sinus visualization (2).

Thorotrast, following injection, is rapidly and preferentially concentrated in the reticuloendothelial cells of the liver, spleen, lymph nodes, and bone marrow. Because its half-life is so long and only minute amounts are ever excreted from the body, Thorotrast, once instilled, remains in the body permanently. With continual release of α rays, which have a range of 1 mm, contiguous tissues become progressively fibrotic and in some instances undergo malignant mutations (3) (Fig. 6).

B. Clinical Features

One of the most common complications of administering this agent has been the so-called Thorotrast granuloma (thorotrastoma), a tumorlike fibrotic mass caused by extravasation of the contrast medium into the area of injection (Fig. 6) (4). A total of 4% of all angiographic procedures, according to Blomburg et al., are associated with inadvertent extravascular injection or leakage (5). Because Thorotrast was used primarily for visualization of the carotid and cerebral blood vessels, most of these granulomas are found in the neck.

The symptomatology depends entirely on the amount of material extravasated, the extent of the granuloma, the time interval from administration, and the functional value of the structures involved (1). Symptoms have included dysphonia, hoarseness, dysphagia, cranial nerve palsies, Horner's syndrome, pain on movement, tracheal obstruction, asphyxia, fistulas, pharyngeal necrosis, repeated bouts of pneumonia, and spontaneous bleeding (3,4,6). Radiation may also produce stenosis of the carotid arteries and lead to cerebral vascular insufficiency or even encephalomalacia. Blomberg et al. studied 35 patients known to have had inadvertent cervical extravascular injections of Thorotrast (5). Of these 35 patients, 8 died of the cerebral disease that was being investigated by arteriography and 4 were lost to follow-up. Among the remaining 23 patients, 10 developed granulomas and 2 cervical sarcomas.

Another important issue, already alluded to, is that of Thorotrast-induced tumors. As of 1971, there were about 200 pathologically documented cases recorded in the literature (2). To qualify as such, the following criteria should be met: (*i*) Thorotrast particles should be found in the immediate vicinity of the neoplasm; (*ii*) the latency period should be sufficiently long, usually 18 to 25 years (range 10–35 years); and (*iii*) the radiation dose should be relatively high (4). The amount of Thorotrast injected in patients developing malignant tumors of the liver has usually been in excess of 30 mL (5).

C. Pathology

Grossly, the granulomas are hard, fibrotic, partially calcified, and adherent to surrounding tissues. On cut surface, they are white and chalky, often with areas of ischemic necrosis. By light microscopy, Thorotrast appears as a light brown to gray-black granular material that does not refract under polarized light (7). The deposits may lie free in the tissue or be contained within the cytoplasm of histiocytes.

Dahlgren divides Thorotrast-related neoplasms into three groups, according to their mode of origin: (*i*) those appearing at the site of injection following extravasation, (*ii*) those directly caused by Thorotrast deposited in hollow organs or cavities, and (*iii*) those caused by Thorotrast injected systematically and deposited in the reticuloendothelial system (1). Group I constitutes the rarest group. As of 1975, there were only about eight cases described in the literature, seven of which occurred in the neck and one in the axilla (7,8). These eight cases included two neurofibrosarcomas, two "spindle cell sarcomas," and one example each of fibrosarcoma, extraosseous chondrosarcoma, malignant hemangioendothelioma, and extraosseous osteosarcoma. Group II is the second most common category, with the kidney accounting for the majority of these. Among 31 renal tumors reviewed by Grampa, there were 23 transitional cell carcinomas, 6 hypernephomas, and 2 sarcomas arising in the pelvis (2). There have also been at least seven tumors arising in the paranasal sinuses (3 epidermoid carcinomas, 1 adenocarcinoma, 1 mucoepidermoid carcinoma, and 2 carcinomas of unknown type) (9). The overwhelming majority of Thorotrast-induced neoplasms fall into group III. Out of a total of 200 tumors related to Thorotrast, Grampa noted that over half occurred in the liver or extrahepatic bile ducts (31 hepatomas, 47 bile duct carcinomas, and 46 angiosarcomas) (Fig. 6) (2). Other studies of Thorotrast-related hepatic malignancies continue to show that bile duct carcinomas and angiosarcomas far outnumber hepatomas (10). Angiosarcomas of the spleen are also quite common. In addition, various hematological diseases have been described, including leukemia (usually acute myeloid), aplastic anemia, myelosclerosis, and agranulocytosis (2,11).

D.   Treatment and Prognosis

A clinical diagnosis of Thorotrast injection without a clear history rests on three prerequisites: (*i*) the presence of radiopaque deposits in the liver and spleen, (*ii*) physical detection of radioactivity in the body of the patient, and (*iii*) a biopsy confirmed by autoradiography (12). Following diagnosis, treatment becomes somewhat controversial and even has mediocolegal overtones. Owing to its carcinogenic potential, some have advocated a radial neck dissection (3). Because patients with cervical granulomas almost invariably have Thorotrast deposits in their liver and spleen, organs that are at significantly higher risk for developing malignancies than the neck, the rationale for such an extensive operative procedure is dubious. Futhermore, experience has consistently shown that the granulomas are almost impossible to excise completely and that attempts to do so are often accompanied by impaired or delayed healing of the operative wound (3,13). A much more reasonable approach, as suggested by Trible and Small, would be a biopsy for diagnosis and close follow-up of the patients for non–head and neck malignancies (13). In addition, they recommend angiography to determine the patency of the carotid system. If circulation is impaired without compensation, a vascular graft might be considered.

V.   CERVICAL THYMOMA

A.   Introduction

The thymus normally appears around the sixth week of gestation and is derived primarily from the third and, to a lesser extent, fourth branchial (pharyngeal) pouches (1,2). During the 7th through 10th weeks, the thymic primordia migrate caudally, fuse in the midline, and eventually, the organ occupies its final adult position in the anterior, superior mediastinum. It reaches its largest relative size close to three years of

age, but continues to grow, attaining its largest weight (20–40 g) at puberty. It then slowly involutes and weighs only about 15 g in the adult.

During embryogenesis, a variety of cervical thymic abnormalities may occur as a consequence of an arrest in descent, failure of involution, or sequestration of thymic tissue during migration. Among these disorders include cervical thymic cysts, cervical thymus, ectopic hamartomatous thymoma (EHT), and cervical thymoma.

Thymomas occur almost exclusively in the chest and are the most common tumors of the anterosuperior mediastinum (3,4). They have, however, been described in several unusual sites, such as the neck, lung, and thyroid (5–7).

B.   Clinical Features

Cervical thymomas are distinctly uncommon. Chan et al. reviewed 16 cases and observed them to be more common in males (88% of all cases), with age range of 11–71 years (average 42.7 years) (7).

The tumors have varied from 2 to 13 cm and are typically found in the anterolateral neck (usually deep to the sternomastoid muscle) or adjacent to the submandibular gland or thyroid (5,7–9). Most present as a swelling or result in some discomfort or swallowing. Only one case has possibly been associated with myasthenia gravis (7,10).

C.   Imaging

At least one cervical thymoma has been studied by magnetic resonance imaging. On T1-weighted imaging, the tumor was isotense to skeletal muscles, and on T2-weighted imaging, it had a slightly higher signal intensity than muscle and a lobulated internal structure separated by linear areas of low intensity (11).

D.   Pathology

The pathology is similar to that described for thymomas in the mediastinum (1,2). Of the 16 cases reviewed by Chan et al., 13 were encapsulated or circumscribed, 2 were invasive, and 1 was not further characterized (7) (Fig. 7). Residual ectopic "normal" thymus may be seen microscopically in areas adjacent to the tumor.

Because of their rarity and ectopic location, cervical thymomas are usually mistaken on fine needle aspiration and frozen sections for malignant lymphoma, metastatic carcinoma, follicular dendritic cell sarcoma, or Hashimoto's thyroiditis (8,9,11–13).

E.   Treatment and Prognosis

The natural history of cervical thymoma is largely unknown because of their rarity and limited follow-up. Complete surgical excision, however, appears to be curative for those that are circumscribed or encapsulated, whereas invasive ones may be at risk for local recurrence. At least one case of metastatic cervical

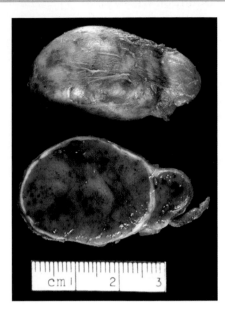

Figure 7 Encapsulated cervical thymoma removed from the left jugulodigastric area in a 37-year-old man.

thymoma has been described (14). The patient, a 51-year-old physician, had a 4-cm, right cervical thymoma associated with enlarged cervical lymph nodes. The tumor was excised along with a neck dissection. Metastatic thymoma was detected in 2 or 24 cervical lymph nodes (level III). Postoperative radiotherapy was administered, and he was reported as being without disease at last follow-up. One should also be aware that, in rare instances, mediastinal thymomas may metastasize to the head and neck and not confuse this event with a primary cervical thymoma (15).

VI. ECTOPIC HAMARTOMATOUS THYMOMA— BRANCHIAL ANLAGE MIXED TUMOR

A. Introduction

EHT is an exceptionally rare tumor of the neck. It was first described, simultaneously, in 1982, by Smith and McClune as an "unusual subcutaneous mixed tumor exhibiting adipose, fibroblastic, and epithelial components," and by Rosai et al. as a "spindle cell thymic anlage tumor" (1,2). Because the lesion exhibited features of both a hamartoma and a neoplasm, Rosai et al. in 1984 suggested the term "ectopic hamartomatous thymoma" as being more appropriate (3). Fetsch et al., however, in a detailed immunohistochemical analysis of 21 cases found no evidence of thymic differentiation and recommended that the lesion be classified as a "branchial anlage mixed tumor (BAMT)" (4).

The tumor is thought to arise from the third branchial pouch or sinus of His (3,5,6). As of to date, less than 50 cases have been described (4–11).

B. Clinical Features

EHT-BAMT has been reported in patients aged 26 to 79 years (average about 45–50 years) and exhibits a marked male predominance of greater than 10:1 (4,6). It occurs primarily in the supraclavicular or suprasternal area and may involve the superficial or deep soft tissue. Five cases have been described as involving the subcutaneous tissue and one attached to the periosteum of the clavicle (4). Otherwise, the tumors are not associated with the skin (dermis), bone, or thyroid.

EHT-BAMTs are slowly growing and typically present as asymptomatic masses often mistaken clinically for a cyst, enlarged lymph node, lipoma, or goiter.

C. Pathology

The tumors average about 5 cm (range 1.4–19 cm) and are circumscribed, but nonencapsulated, with a gray-white, tan, or pink cut surface, punctuated with small cysts (Figs. 8–10).

Microscopically, they are composed of four components: (*i*) spindle cells, (*ii*) epithelial cells, (*iii*) adipose tissue, and (*iv*) cysts. The proportion of these elements in any given tumor is highly variable, although the spindle element typically predominates. The spindle cells are arranged in short fascicles, or occasionally, in a storiform pattern. The nuclei are oval to elongated with fine chromatin and indistinct nucleoli, if seen at all. The cytoplasm varies from pale to eosinophilic.

The epithelial component consists primarily of squamous cells, either keratinizing or nonkeratinizing, arranged as solid islands, anastomosing cords, or cysts. Glands and/or cysts, ranging from microscopic up to 2 cm, are present in almost all cases, but form only a minor component.

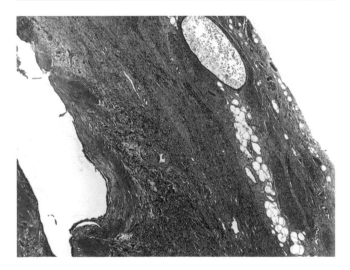

Figure 8 EHT-BAMT. Note the circumscription and spindle cells, adipose tissue, and cysts (H&E, 40×). *Abbreviations*: EHT, ectopic hamartomatous thymoma; BAMT, branchial anlage mixed tumor; H&E, hematoxylin and eosin.

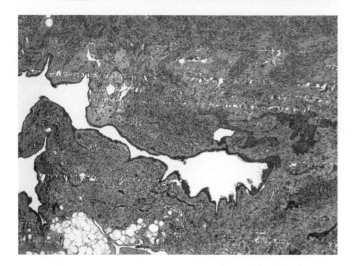

Figure 9 EHT-BAMT. Note the prominent cyst and islands of epithelium (H&E, 40×). *Abbreviations*: EHT, ectopic hamartomatous thymoma; BAMT, branchial anlage mixed tumor; H&E, hematoxylin and eosin.

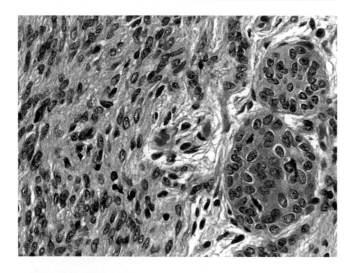

Figure 10 EHT-BAMT. Higher magnification of the spindle cells and epithelial islands (H&E, 400×). *Abbreviations*: EHT, ectopic hamartomatous thymoma; BAMT, branchial anlage mixed tumor; H&E, hematoxylin and eosin.

The amount of adipose tissue varies from insignificant to prominent. Mitoses are scant (0–7/50 high-power cells), and necrosis is not seen. Thus far, normal thymic tissue has not been observed either within or adjacent to the tumor.

Noteworthy, Michal et al. have described two EHT-BAMTs that allegedly contained foci of adenocarcinoma (9).

D. Imunohistochemistry

The epithelial cells stain for a variety of cytokeratins, while the spindle cells exhibit features of myoepithelial cells as evidenced by coexpression of cytokeratins (5, 5/6, and 14), α-smooth muscle actin, CD10, and, to a lesser extent, calponin (4).

E. Differential Diagnosis

Because of its biphasic appearance (spindle and epithelial cells), EHT-BAMT may be confused with a synovial sarcoma. Synovial sarcomas of the head and neck are mainly deep soft tissue lesions that usually present in the posterolateral neck at the level of the bifurcation of the common carotid artery and rarely in the suprasternal-supraclavicular area favored by EHT-BAMT. Moreover, synovial sarcomas usually do not contain a prominent component of squamous epithelium or adipose tissue. Synovial sarcomas also exhibit a characteristic X:18 translocation on cytogenetic analysis.

EHT-BAMT might also be mistaken for a cutaneous adnexal carcinoma, pleomorphic adenoma (mixed tumor) of salivary origin, spindle cell squamous carcinoma, and a teratoma. Cutaneous adnexal carcinoma, by definition, arises in the dermis. Although EHT-BAMT may rarely involve the subcutis, they do not originate in the dermis. Pleomorphic adenoma can arise in ectopic sites, but the suprasternal-supraclavicular would be most unusual. Pleomorphic adenoma also frequently contains chondroid or chondromyxoid areas, which are not seen in EHT-BAMT. EHT-BAMT does not exhibit the degree of pleomorphism or mitotic activity of a spindle cell squamous carcinoma nor contain tissues derived from all germ layers, as seen in a teratoma.

F. Treatment and Prognosis

With the possible exception of the two malignant cases described by Michal et al., EHT-BAMT is a benign lesion that is appropriately managed by simple excision (8). The presence of focal malignant change as observed by Michal et al., however, has not to date been shown to adversely affect patient outcome (4). Local recurrences following incomplete excision have been documented.

VII. CARNEY COMPLEX

Carney complex (CNC), first described in 1985, is a multiple neoplasia disorder characterized by spotty pigmentation, myxomas, endocrine tumors, and schwannomas (1–4). It should not be confused with Carney triad, also sometimes referred to as Carney syndrome, which is a nonfamilial disorder of unknown etiology that predilect young females consisting of gastrointestinal stromal tumors, pulmonary chondromas, and extra-adrenal paragangliomas (5).

CNC is inherited as an autosomal dominant trait, although sporadic cases do occur. Genetic-linkage studies have identified two distinct loci for the complex, one located on chromosome 2p16 (CNC2) and the other one on chromosome 17 q22-24 (CNC1, PRKAR1A gene) (3,6–9). Only about 500 cases have been registered as of 2007, and, of these, about 70% were familial (4). CNC occurs worldwide in all ethnic groups and is more common in females (57% vs. 43% males) (4,7).

The manifestations of CNC are variable and appear over many years. The median age at diagnosis is about 20 years. One of the most conspicuous and most common feature is the spotty pigmentation (lentigines, macules, ordinary and blue nevi, and café au lait spots) that usually appear around puberty and predilect the lips, eyelids, conjunctiva, ears, neck, and genital area. Oral mucosa pigmentation is uncommon (about 5% of cases) (2).

The myxomas are often multiple and may involve the skin, breasts, and heart. The cutaneous myxomas can occur at any site, but, in the head and neck, typically involve the eyelids, external auditory canal, scalp, cheek, and neck. The most serious and life-threatening myxomas are those that arise in the heart. Cardiac myxomas are found in about half of all patients with CNC (7). They may be single or multiple and occur in any chamber of the heart, especially the left atrium. The odontogenic myxoma is not associated with CNC.

CNC affects several endocrine organs, including the adrenal glands (pigmented nodular adenocortical disease with Cushing syndrome), pituitary gland (acromegaly), thyroid gland (nodules, adenomas, carcinoma), and testes (large cell-calcifying Sertoli cell tumors, which are frequently bilateral).

The schwannomas are of a special type referred to as psammomatous melanotic schwannomas, some of which are malignant.

Other less common manifestations possibly associated with CNC include ductal papillomas of breast, osteochondromyxomas, pilonidal sinuses, and cardiomyopathy (7,10).

The frequency of the above clinical manifestations of CNC at the time of diagnosis are as follows: spotty skin pigmentation (77%), cardiac myxoma (53%), cutaneous myxomas (33%), pigmented nodular adrenocortical disease (26%), large cell-calcifying Sertoli cell tumor (33% of male patients), acromegaly (10%), psammomatous melanotic schwannoma (10%), thyroid nodules or cancer (5%), and ductal adenoma of breast (3% of female patients) (7).

Criteria for diagnosis of CNC are shown in Table 3 (7).

The life span of patients with CNC is decreased with a 15% mortality. The most common cause of death is heart related, usually the result of a myxoma, followed by malignant psammomatous melanotic schwannomas (3).

VIII. MAZABRAUD SYNDROME

The association of fibrous dysplasia with intramuscular myxomas is referred to as Mazabraud syndrome

Table 3 Diagnostic Criteria for CNC[a]

1. Spotty skin pigmentation with a typical distribution (lips, conjunctiva and inner or outer canthi, and vaginal and penile mucosa)[b]
2. Myxoma (cutaneous and mucosal)
3. Cardiac myxoma[b]
4. Breast myxomatosis[b] or fat-suppressed magnetic resonance imaging findings suggestive of this diagnosis
5. PPNAD[b] or paradoxical positive response of urinary glucocorticosteroids to dexamethasone administration during Liddle test
6. Acromegaly due to GH-producing adenoma[b]
7. LCCSCT[b] or characteristic calcification on testicular ultrasonography
8. Thyroid carcinoma[b] or multiple, hypoechoic nodules on thyroid ultrasonography, in a young patient
9. Psammomatous melanotic schwannoma[b]
10. Blue nevus, epithelioid blue nevus (multiple)[b]
11. Breast ductal adenoma (multiple)[b]
12. Osteochondromyxoma[b]

Supplemental criteria:

1. Affected first-degree relative
2. Inactivating mutation of the PRKAR1A gene

[a]To make a diagnosis of CNC, a patient must either (*i*) exhibit two of the manifestations of the disease listed or (*ii*) exhibit one of these manifestations and meet one of the supplemental criteria (an affected first-degree relative or an inactivating mutation of the PRKAR1A gene).
[b]With histological confirmation.
Abbreviations: CNC, Carney complex; PPNAD, primary pigmented nodular adrenocortical disease; GH, growth hormone; LCCSCT, large cell calcifying Sertoli cell tumor.
Source: From Ref. 7.

(1–5). Although the disorder was first described by Henschen in 1926, it was Mazabraud et al. in 1967 who recognized it as a separate and distinct entity and not a fortuitous occurrence, and, in recognition, the syndrome now bears his name (6,7).

Mazabraud syndrome is uncommon with only 36 documented cases as of 1999 (2,3). It is two to three times more common in women and occurs in patients aged 17 to 82 years (mean 46 years). There is no known pattern of inheritance.

The myxomas are exclusively intramuscular and usually multiple (72% of cases) and, rarely, solitary (28%) (2,3). One patient has been described who had nine myxomas (8). The myxomas appear years to decades after discovery of the bone lesions and tend to occur in groups or clusters, often on the right side of the body near, but distinct from, the dysplastic bone (s). They average about 5 cm in greatest dimension but have been reported up to 25 cm (2). The large muscle groups of the thigh, buttocks, arms, shoulders, and chest are the sites of predilection.

The fibrous dysplasia is most often polyostotic (81% of all cases) rather than monostotic (19% of all cases) and, in at least 10 cases, the patients have had features of McCune-Albright syndrome (polyostotic fibrous dysplasia, endocrine disturbances, cutaneous pigmentation, and precocious sexual development) (2,3).

The intramuscular myxomas of Mazabraud syndrome are histologically identical to conventional intramuscular myxomas. Interestingly, all intramuscular myxomas, whether syndromic or nonsyndromic, share the same Gsα mutation as seen in fibrous dysplasia (9–11)

Mazabraud myxomas have no malignant potential. However, at least three cases of osteosarcomas have developed in 36 reported cases of Mazabraud syndrome for an incidence of 8.3%, which is higher than the 0.5% incidence of malignant transformation in nonsyndromic fibrous dysplasia (3). The osteosarcomas all developed in dysplastic bone, and none of the patients had a history of prior radiation. Patients who have both Mazabraud and McCune-Albright syndromes may be of even greater risk of developing a sarcoma (2 of 11 patients or 18.2%) (3).

IX.   GIANT CELL ANGIOFIBROMA

A.   Introduction

Giant cell angiofibroma (GCA) was first described in 1995 as a distinctive orbital tumor in adults (1). Subsequent reports, however, have indicated that the tumor has a wider anatomic distribution than initially recognized. While the orbit continues to be the most frequent location, GCA has also been described in extraorbital sites, including the buccal mucosa, nasolacrimal duct, scalp, retroauricular region, parotid gland, submandibular area, neck, forearm, back, axilla, hip, groin, vulva, mediastinum, and retroperitoneum (2–10).

It is currently thought that the tumor most likely represents a giant cell-rich variant of solitary fibrous tumor (5,11).

B.   Clinical

GCA has only been described in adults aged 18 to 81 years (mean 48 years) (10). In the orbit, males predominate, while extraorbital tumors are more common in females (1,5,6).

Orbital tumors present with swelling of the eyelids, proptosis, or diplopia, while extraorbital lesions typically manifest as a nonpainful mass.

C.   Pathology

Most tumors are less than 5 cm, well circumscribed and, on cut section, are gray to gray-pink with microcysts and small hemorrhagic areas. Microscopically, they are composed of a moderately cellular, patternless proliferation of spindle and giant cells alternating with hypocellular, often collagenized, areas. The giant cells are widely dispersed and contain multiple nuclei often peripherally arranged in a floret-like pattern. Blood vessels are prominent and vary from small to medium size with thick walls. Occasionally, pseudovascular spaces lined by giant cells are seen. Necrosis is sparse to absent, and mitoses never exceed 2 to 3 of 10 high-power fields (HPFs).

D.   Immunohistochemistry

The spindle and giant cells are uniformly positive for vimentin, CD34, CD99, and bcl-2, and may also focally decorate with smooth muscle actin and S-100 protein. Desmin, keratin, and epithelial membrane antigen are usually negative (5).

E.   Molecular-Genetic

Two cases of GCA have been examined cytogenetically. One tumor of the eyelid exhibited abnormalities of chromosome band 6q13, while one of the neck revealed a 12:17 translocation (4,12).

F.   Differential Diagnosis

The differential diagnosis includes giant cell fibroblastoma (GCFB), solitary fibrous tumor (SFT), and possibly a spindle-pleomorphic lipoma (SPL). GCFB is a variant of dermatofibrosarcoma protuberans, which occurs in the dermis-subcutis and predilects young children. In contrast to GCA, it has infiltrating margins and a less conspicuous vascular component. As previously indicated, GCA is now thought to be a variant of an SFT. The absence of giant cells and pseudovascular spaces separate a conventional SFT from GCA. Although SPLs may contain spindle and floret cells, the presence of a prominent component of adipose tissue distinguishes it from a GCA.

Although both GCA and nasopharyngeal angiofibroma share the term "angiofibroma," they are two discrete entities. Nasopharyngeal angiofibroma is always centered in the nasopharynx, occurs exclusively in adolescent males, lacks giant cells, and, other than blood vessels, is CD34-negative.

G.   Treatment

GCA has no malignant potential. Complete surgical excision is curative. Local recurrence is exceptional.

X.   NUCHAL FIBROCARTILAGINOUS PSEUDOTUMOR

Nuchal fibrocartilaginous pseudotumor (NFP) was first described in 1997 by O'Connell et al. as a distinctive soft tissue lesion associated with prior neck injury (1). In some instances, the history of cervical trauma may be remote, as illustrated by one patient of O'Connell et al. who experienced a neck injury 27 years prior to the appearance of NFP. Cases have also been described in patients with no history of trauma (2,3). Whether some degenerative diseases, such as osteoarthritis, and advanced age may also contribute to NFP is open to speculation.

The pathology takes place in the nuchal ligament, which is a fibroelastic structure that extends from the occipital bone to the spine of the seventh cervical vertebra. NFP involves the lower portion of the ligament at the level of C4 to C7 and manifests as a thickening or mass up to 3 cm in greatest dimension (2).

Microscopically, NFP consists of a poorly demarcated nodular proliferation of moderately cellular fibrocartilaginous tissue centered in the nuchal ligament, with occasional extension into the adjacent soft tissues (muscle and fascia). The chondrocytes have small hyperchromatic nuclei devoid of nucleoli. Mitoses and binucleated cells are not seen.

Immunohistochemistry has been performed on at least two cases (3). All cells were noted to express vimentin. S-100 protein positivity was restricted to the chondroid areas and was only focal or mild. CD34 was strongly positive in both chondroid and fibroblast-like cells. Actin, desmin, and CD99 were negative. On the basis of the finding of CD34 positivity in both spindle and chondroid cells, Zamecnik and Michal have speculated that NFP may represent a lesion of CD34-positive fibroblasts that have undergone cartilaginous metaplasia (3).

Although one case has been described in a 10-year-old girl, NFP primarily involves adults aged 22 to 53 years, with no significant gender difference (1–4). Signs and symptoms include a stiff neck, headache, dizziness, and an asymptomatic, sometimes tender, mass. Simple excision is curative. Recurrences have not been documented.

NFP is often confused with a soft tissue chondroma. A soft tissue chondroma, however, is more cellular than an NFP, often contains chondromyxoid areas, and is composed mainly of hyaline rather than fibrocartilage (3).

XI. RENAL CELL-LIKE SINONASAL ADENOCARCINOMA

Zur et al. and Storck et al. have described four unusual primary sinonasal tumors that are histologically indistinguishable from metastatic renal cell carcinoma (RCC) and, because of this similarity, they proposed the term "renal cell-like sinonasal adenocarcinoma (RCSA)" for these lesions (1,2).

The tumors occurred in three women and one man aged 22 to 69 years (mean 46 years). Three arose in the nasal cavity and one in the nasopharynx.

Histologically, RCSAs are composed of glycogen-rich, mucin-negative, cuboidal to polyhedral clear cells arranged in a solid or glandular pattern. No perineural/vascular invasion or necrosis is seen. They are positive for cytokeratin 7 and negative for vimentin and RCC antigen. Exceptionally, they may focally decorate with cytokeratin 20 and S-100 protein. Calponin and actin are negative.

No patient was found to have a RCC on extensive evaluation. Three patients were treated with surgery, two of whom also received adjuvant radiation. The fourth patient received primary radiation. All were found to be free of disease at two-, four-, five-, and eight-year follow-up.

The differential diagnosis includes metastatic RCC and salivary tumors with a prominent component of clear cells, namely, epithelial-myoepithelial carcinoma (EMEC), clear cell myoepithelial carcinoma (CMEC), and clear cell carcinoma (CCC). In contrast to RCSA, RCC is often positive for RCC antigen and negative for cytokeratin 7 and 20. EMEC and CMEC can be eliminated by their prominent component of myoepithelial cells, which thus far have not been observed in RCSA. CCC is more problematic. The presence of fibrous trabeculae (so-called hyalinizing CCC), absence of a glandular pattern, and variable staining for S-100 protein, glial fibrillary acidic protein, actin, and vimentin are more in favor of CCC (3). In uncertain cases, imaging evaluation of the kidneys is warranted.

XII. LOW-GRADE SINONASAL SARCOMA WITH NEURAL AND MYOGENIC FEATURES

Lewis et al. have described 15 low-grade sinonasal sarcomas with both neural and myogenic features, which occurred in 10 women and 5 men aged 24 to 74 years (mean 51 years) (1). None had a history of neurofibromatosis. All tumors involved either the ethmoid sinus (11 cases) and/or the nasal cavity (8 cases). Each had a prominent vascular pattern and frequently invaded bone, but the mitotic index was low, and there was no significant nuclear pleomorphism.

S-100 protein expression was spotty or patchy in all tumors. Smooth muscle actin was positive in 12 of 13 cases, muscle specific actin in 9 of 10 cases, and CD34 in 4 of 13 cases. Desmin and myogenin were negative in 10 and 8 cases, respectively.

Limited follow-up was available in eight cases. Multiple local recurrences were noted in five, but no patient developed metastasis or died of disease.

XIII. MIDLINE CARCINOMA WITH NUT REARRANGEMENT (NUT-TOMA)

A. Introduction

Midline carcinoma with NUT rearrangement (MCNUTR) is a recently recognized, highly lethal neoplasm defined by its characteristic chromosomal translocation, t (15:19) (1–9).

B. Clinical Features

It typically occurs in children and young adults and only infrequently in older individuals (8,9). As the name implies, it presents as a midline mass and arises almost exclusively in sites lined by respiratory epithelium (sinonasal tract, nasopharynx, trachea, lungs) or the thymus. Only a single case has been described thus far below the diaphragm; this involved the urinary bladder in a three-year-old boy (8).

C. Pathology

MCNUTR appears as an undifferentiated carcinoma, often with abrupt foci of squamous differentiation, and is usually mistaken for a sinonasal undifferentiated carcinoma or a poorly differentiated squamous cell carcinoma. Gland formation is not seen. Mitoses average 10 or more/10 HPFs.

D. Immunohistochemistry

The tumor is uniformly positive for cytokeratins (AE1/AE3, pankeratin, CAM 5.2) and often positive for p63 (80%) and CD34 (54%) (8,9). It is negative for placental alkaline phosphatase. Using a NUT polyclonal antibody, Stelow et al. observed that four of their five cases exhibited strong diffuse nuclear expression (9).

E. Molecular Genetic Data

The molecular signature of MCNUTR is a translocation involving chromosomes 15 and 19, resulting in a BRD4-NUT fusion product (8). In a review of 11 MCNUTRs, French et al. observed that eight (73%) tumors showed the characteristic BRD4-NUT product, while three (27%) were found to be fused to an oncogene other than BRD4 (8). They referred to these latter three tumors as NUT-variants. They also noted that the NUT-variant tumors tended to show more squamous differentiation than the BRD4-type.

F. Treatment and Prognosis

MCNUTRs are highly lethal neoplasms resistant to chemoradiation. Although the series is small, preliminary data indicate that the BRD4 tumors have a significantly worse prognosis than the NUT-variants, 28-week average survival for the former versus 96 weeks for the latter (8). Metastasis is usually vascular and only infrequently lymphatic.

XIV. TANGIER DISEASE

Tangier disease (TD) is a rare, autosomal recessive disorder characterized by excessive deposits of cholesterol esters in macrophages throughout the body (especially the tonsils, lymph nodes, spleen, liver, bone marrow, and intestinal mucosa) as well as in nerves (neuropathy) and blood vessel (atherosclerosis) (1–5).

The disease was first recognized in 1960 in a five-year-old boy and his sister from Tangier Island, Virginia (hence the name "Tangier disease"), who presented with enlarged, orange tonsils associated with an abnormal lipid profile. Although additional cases have since been identified in the United States (Missouri, Kentucky), Canada, Britain, Italy, Germany, and Chile, worldwide it is a very rare disorder.

Mutation of the cell membrane protein adenosine triphosphate–binding cassette transporter A1 (ABCAL1) on chromosome 9 is the underlying molecular defect in TD. This protein plays a pivotal role in reverse cholesterol transport, the pathway by which excellular cholesterol is transported via high-density lipoproteins (HDLs) back to the liver for excretion. The end result is an abnormal plasma lipoprotein profile characterized by virtual absence of HDL-cholesterol (HDL-C), reduced levels of low-density lipoprotein–cholesterol (LDL-C), and mild to moderately elevated levels of triglycerides. With absent HDL-C, the extracellular efflux and transport of cholesterol is impaired, resulting in prominent lipid-laden macrophages and massively enlarged, yellow/orange tonsils.

TD can be diagnosed by observing the enlarged, discolored tonsils and demonstrating absence of HDL-C in the patient and both parents. Treatment is largely symptomatic. Although the risk for early atherosclerosis and death is enhanced, this increase is not as dramatic as might be expected. Owing to its ability to deplete cells of cholesterol and to raise HDL levels, ABCA1, however, may be a potential therapeutic target.

REFERENCES

I. GIANT CELL ARTERITIS

1. Jennette JC, Falk RJ, Andrassy K, et al. Nomenclature of systemic vasultidies. Proposal of an international consensus conference. Arthritis Rheum 1994; 37:187–192.
2. Jennette JC, Falk RJ. Do vasculitis categorization systems really matter? Curr Rheumatol Rep 2000; 2:430–438.
3. Jennette JC, Falk FJ. Nosology of primary vasculitis. Curr Opin Rheumatol 2007; 19:10–16.
4. Narula N, Gupta S, Narula J. The primary vasculitidies. A clinicopathologic correlation. Am J Clin Pathol 2005; 124 (suppl 1):S84–S95.
5. Salvarani C, Cantini F, Boiardi L, et al. Polymyalgia rheumatica and giant cell arteritis N Engl J Med 2002; 347:261–271.
6. Lie JT, Gordon LP, Titus JL. Juvenile temporal arteritis. Biopsy study of four cases. JAMA 1975; 234:496–497.
7. Fan PT, Davis JA, Somer T, et al. A clinical approach to systemic vasculitis. Semin Arthritis Rheum 1980; 9:248–304.
8. Hauser WA, Ferguson RH, Holley KE, et al. Temporal arteritis in Rochester, Minnesota 1951 to 1967. Mayo Clin Proc 1971; 46:597–602.
9. Odom L, Goldman JA. Temporal artertitis in a black patient. South Med J 1980; 73:828.
10. Ortel RW. Polymyalgia rheumatica and giant cell arteritis. W V Med J 1981; 77:116–121.
11. Hunder GG, Davis JS IV. Giant cell arteritis and polymyalgia rheumatica. Hosp Pract 1992; 27:75–93.
12. Unwin B, Williams CM, Gilliland W. Polymyalgia rheumatica and giant cell arteritis. Am Fam Physician 2006; 74:1547–1554.
13. Goodman BW Jr. Temporal arteritis. Am J Med 1979; 67:839–851.
14. Hunder GG, Bloch DA, Michel BA, et al. The American College of Rheumatology 1990 criteria for the classification of giant cell arteritis. Arthritis Rheum 1990; 33:1120–1128.
15. Horwitz HM, Pepe PF. Johnsrude S, et al. Temporal arteriography and immunofluoresensce as diagnostic tools in temporal arteritis. J Rheumatol 1977; 4:76–85.
16. Layfer LF, Banner BF, Huckman MS, et al. Temporal arteriography. Analysis of 21 cases and review of the literature. Arthritis Rheum 1978; 21:780–784.
17. Sewell JR, Alison DJ, Tarin D, et al. Combined temporal arteriography and selective biopsy in suspected giant cell arteritis. Ann Rheum Dis 1980; 39:124–128.
18. Schmidt WA, Kraft HE, Vorpahl K, et al. Color duplex ultrasonography in the diagnosis of temporal arteritis. N Engl J Med 1997; 377:1336–1342.
19. Von Knorring J, Wasastjerna C. Liver involvement in polymyalgia rheumatica. Scand J Rheumatol 1976; 5:197–204.
20. Bruk MI. Articular and vascular manifestations of polymyalgia rheumatica. Ann Rheum Dis 1967; 26:103–116.
21. Weyand CM, Hunder NNH, Hicok KC, et al. HLA-DRB1 allele in polymyalgia rheumatica, giant cell arteritis, and rheumatoid arthritis. Arthritis Rheum 1994; 37:514–520.

22. Haworth S, Ridgeway J, Stewart I, et al. Polymyalgia rheumatica is associated with both HLA-DRB1*0401 and DRB*0404. Br J Rheumatol 1996; 35:632–635.

23. Powers JF, Bedri S, Hussein S, et al. High prevalence of herpes simplex virus DNA in temporal artery biopsy specimens. Am J Clin Pathol 2005; 123:261–264.

24. Albert DM, Ruchman MC, Keltner JL. Skip areas in temporal arteritis. Arch Ophthalmol 1976; 94:2072–2077.

25. Klein RG, Campbell RJ, Hunder CG, et al. Skip lesions in temporal arteritis. Mayo Clin Proc 1976; 51:504–510.

26. Mahr A, Saba M, Kambouchner M, et al. Temporal artery biopsy for diagnosing giant cell arteritis: The longer, the better? Ann Rheum Dis 2006; 65:826–828.

27. Ma-Krupa W, Kwan M, Goronzy JJ, et al. Toll-like receptors in giant cell arteritis. Clin Immunol 2005; 115:38–46.

28. Allison ML, Gallager PJ. Temporal artery biopsy and corticosteroid therapy. Ann Rheum Dis 1984; 43:416–417.

29. Achkar AA, Lie JT, Hunder GG, et al. How does previous corticosteroid therapy affect the biopsy findings in giant cell (temporal arteritis)? Ann Intern Med 1994; 120:987–992.

30. Healy LA. Long-term follow-up of polymyalgia rheumatica: evidence for synovitis. Semin Arthritis Rheum 1984; 13:322–328.

31. Chou CT, Schumacher HR. Clinical and pathologic studies of synovitis in polymyalgia rheumatica. Arthritis Rheum 1984; 27:1107–1117.

32. Lie JT, Brown AL Jr., Carter ET. Spectrum of aging changes in temporal arteries. Its significance in interpretation of biopsy of temporal artery. Arch Pathol 1970; 90:278–285.

33. Parker G, Healy LA, Wilske KR, et al. Light and electron microscopic studies on human temporal arteries with special references to alterations related to senescence, atherosclerosis, and giant cell arteritis. Am J Pathol 1975; 79:57–80.

34. Corcoran GM, Prayson RA, Herzog KM. The significance of perivascular inflammation in the absence of arteritis in temporal artery biopsy specimens. Am J Clin Pathol 2001; 115:342–347.

35. Cohle SD, Titus JL, Espinola A, et al. Sudden unexpected death due to coronary giant cell arteritis. Arch Pathol Lab Med 1982; 106:171–172.

II. PHARYNGOESOPHAGEAL (ZENKER'S) DIVERTICULUM

1. Killian G. Ueber den Mund der Speiserohre. Z Ohrenheilkd Krankheiten Luftwege 1908; 55:1–41.

2. Ludlow A. A case of obstructed deglutition from a preternatural dilatation bag formed in the pharynx. Medical Observations and Inquiries by a Society of Physicians in London, vol. 3. 2nd ed. 1969:85–101.

3. Zenker FA, Von Ziemssen H. Cyclopedia of the Practices of Medicine, vol 8. Baltimore, MD: William Wood 1878:1–214.

4. Ballenger JJ. Diseases of the Nose, Throat and Ear, 12 ed. In: Ballenger JJ, ed. Philadelphia, PA: Lea & Febiger, 1977:1062–1064.

5. Dohlman G. Mattson O. The role of the cricopharyngeal muscle in cases of hypopharyngeal diverticula. A cineroentgenographpic study. Am J Roentgenol Radium Ther Nucl Med 1959; 81:561–569.

6. Dohlman G. Mattson O. The endoscopic operation for hypopharyngeal diverticula. A roentgen cinematographic study. Arch Otolaryngol 1960; 71:744–752.

7. Dorsey JM, Randolf DA. Long term evaluation of pharyngoesophageal diverticulectomy. Ann Surg 1971; 173:680–685.

8. Ellis FH Jr, Schlegal JF, Lynch VP, et al. Cricopharyngeal myotomy for pharyngo-esophageal diverticulum. Ann Surg 1969; 170:340–349.

9. Kodicek J, Creamer B. A study of pharyngeal pouches. J Laryngol Otol 1961; 75:406–411.

10. Lahey FH. Pharyngo-esophageal divericulum: its management and complications. Ann Surg 1946; 124:617–636.

11. Negus VE. Pharyngeal diverticulua. Observations on their evolution and treatment. Br J Surg 1950; 38:129–146.

12. Negus VE. The etiology of pharyngeal diverticula. Bull Johns Hopkins Hosp 1957; 101:209–223.

13. Payne WS, Ellis FH Jr. Esophagus and diaphragmatic hernias. In: Schwartz SI, Shires T, Spencer FC, et al. eds. Principles of Surgery. 3rd ed. New York, NY: McGraw Hill, 1979.

14. Shallow TA, Clerf LH. One stage pharyngeal diverticulectomy. Improved technique and analysis of 186 cases. Surg Gynecol Obstet 1948; 86:317–322.

15. Holinger PH, Schild JA. The Zenker' (hypopharyngeal) diverticulum. Ann Otol Rhinol Laryngol 1969; 78:679–688.

16. Meadows JA Jr. Esophageal diverticula in infants and children. South Med J 1970; 63:691–694.

17. Zitsch RP, O'Brien CJ, Maddox WA. Pharyngoesophageal diverticulum complicated by squamous cell carcinoma. Head Neck Surg 1987; 9:290–294.

18. Kerner MM, Bates ES, Hernandez F, et al. Carcinoma-in-situ occurring in a Zenker's diverticulum. Am J Otolaryngol 1994; 15:223–226.

19. Tucker JA. Esophageal diverticula. In: Bockus Hl, ed. Gastroenterology, vol I, 3rd ed. Philadelphia: WB Saunders, 1974:319–328.

20. Clagett OT, Payne WS. Surgical treatment of pulsion diverticula of the hypopharynx: one-stage resection in 478 cases. Dis Chest 1960; 37:257–261.

21. Van Overbeek JJM. Meditation on the pathogenesis of hypopharyngeal (Zenker's) diverticulum and a report of endoscopic treatment in 545 patients. Ann Otol Rhinol Laryngol 1994; 103:178–185.

III. TUMORS OF THE PARAPHARYNGEAL SPACE

1. Heeneman H, Gilbert JJ, Rood SR. The Pharyngeal Space: Anatomy and Pathologic Conditions, with Emphasis on Neurogenous Tumors. Rochester, MN: American Academy of Otolaryngology, 1980.

2. Lawson VG, Leliever WC, Makerewich LA, et al. Unusual parapharyngeal lesions. J Otolaryngol 1979; 8:241–249.

3. Som PM, Biller HF, Lawson W. Tumors of the parapharyngeal space. Preoperative evaluation, diagnosis, and surgical approaches. Ann Otol Rhinol Laryngol Suppl 1981; 90:3–15.

4. Shoss SM, Donovan DT, Alford BR. Tumors of the parapharyngeal space. Arch Otolaryngol 1985; 111:753–757.

5. Carrau RL, Myers EN, Johnson JT. Management of tumors arising in the parapharyngeal space. Laryngoscope 1990; 100:583–589.

6. Hughes KV, Olsen KD, McCaffery TV. Parapharyngeal space neoplasms. Head Neck 1995; 17:124–130.

7. Pensak ML, Gluckman JL, Shumrick KA. Parapharyngeal space tumors: an algorithm for evaluation and management. Laryngoscope 1994; 104:1170–1173.

8. Heeneman H, Maran AGD. Review. Parapharyngeal space tumors. Clin Otolaryngol 1979; 4:57–66.

9. Work WP. Tumors of the parapharyngeal space. Trans Am Acad Ophthalmol Otolaryngol 1969; 73:389–394.

10. Work WP, Hybels RL. A study of tumors of the parapharyngeal space. Laryngoscope 1874; 84:1748–1755.

11. Barnes L, Gnepp DR. Miscellaneous disorders of the head and neck. In: Barnes L, ed. Surgical Pathology of the Head and Neck. New York, NY: Marcel Dekker, 1985:1823–1847.

12. Brandenburg JH. Symposium on malignancy. IV. Neurogenic tumors of the parapharyngeal space. Laryngoscope 1972; 82:1292–1305.

13. Ballenger JJ. Diseases of the Nose, Throat, and Ear. In: Ballenger JJ, ed. 12th ed. Philadelphia, PA: Lea & Febinger, 1977:282.

IV.   THOROTRAST GRANULOMAS AND RELATED NEOPLASMS

1. Dahlgren S. Thorotrast tumors. A review of the literature and report of two cases. Acta Pathol Microbiol Scand 1961; 53:147–161.

2. Grampa G. Radiation injury with particular reference to Thorotrast. Pathol Annu 1971; 6:147–169.

3. Chalat NI, Zane AI. Radical neck dissection for thorium dioxide granuloma. Arch Otolaryngol 166; 83:610–614.

4. Da Silva Horta J. Effects of colloidal thorium dioxide extravasates in the subcutaneous tissues of the cervical region in man. Ann N Y Acad Sci 1967; 145:776–785.

5. Blomberg R, Larsson LE, Lindell B, et al. Late effects of Thorotrast in cerebral angiography. Ann N Y Acad Sci 1967; 145:853–858.

6. Dickens JRE. Resident's page, pathologic quiz case 2, thorium dioxide-induced granuloma of the neck. Arch Otolaryngol 1978; 104:58–61.

7. Hasson J, Hartman KA, Milikow E, et al. Thorotrast-induced extraskeletal osteosarcoma of the cervical region. Report of a case. Cancer 1975; 36:1827–1833.

8. Fujikura T, Kawai S. Thorotrast tumors in Japan. Report of two cases with autopsy findings and a brief review of the literature. Acta Pathol Jpn 1973; 23:139–154.

9. Kligerman M, Lattes R, Rankow R. Carcinoma of the maxillary sinus following Thorotrast instillation. Report of 3 cases. Cancer 1960; 13:967–973.

10. Ito Y, Kojiro M, Nakasima T, et al. Pathomorphologic characteristics of 102 cases of Thorotrast-related hepatocellular carcinoma, cholangiocarcinoma, and hepatic angiosarcoma. Cancer 1988; 62:1153–1162.

11. Faber M, Johansen C. Leukemia and other hematological diseases after Thorotrast. Ann N Y Acad Sci 1967; 145:755–758.

12. Baserga R, Yokoo H, Henegar GC. Thorotrast-induced cancer in man. Cancer 1960; 13:1021–1031.

13. Trible WM, Small A. Thorium dioxide granuloma of the neck: a report of four cases. Laryngoscope 1976; 86:1633–1638.

V.   CERVICAL THYMOMA

1. Suster S, Rosai J. Histology of the normal thymus. Am J Surg 1990; 14:284–303.

2. Millman B, Pransky S, Castillo J III, et al. Cervical thymic anomalies. Int J Pediatr Otorhinolaryngol 1999; 47:29–39.

3. Verley JM, Hollmann KH. Thymoma. A comparative study of clinical stages, histologic features, and survival in 200 cases. Cancer 1985; 55:1074–1086.

4. Lewis JE, Wick MR, Scheithaur BW, et al. Thymoma. A clinicopathologic review. Cancer 1987; 60:2727–2743.

5. Martin JME, Randhawa G, Temple WJ. Cervical thymoma. Arch Pathol Lab Med 1986; 110:354–357.

6. Kung ITM, Loke SL, So SY, et al. Intrapulmonary thymoma: report of two cases. Thorax 1985; 40:471–474.

7. Chan JKC, Rosai J. Tumors of the neck showing thymic or related branchial pouch differentiation: a unifying concept. Hum Pathol 1991; 22:349–367.

8. Mourra N, Duron F, Parc R, et al. Cervical ectopic thymoma: a diagnostic pitfall on frozen section. Histopathology 2005; 46:583–585.

9. Bakshi J, Ghosh S, Pragache G, et al. Ectopic cervical thymoma in the submandibular region. J Otolaryngol 2005; 34:223–226.

10. Sease CI. Cervical thymoma, a case report. Va Med 1956; 83:345–346.

11. Nagasawa K, Takahashi K, Hoyashi T, et al. Ectopic cervical thymoma: MRI findings. Am J Roentgenol 2004; 182:262–263.

12. Ponder TB, Collins BT, Bee CS, et al. Diagnosis of cervical thymoma by fine needle aspiration biopsy with flow cytometry. A case report. Acta Cytol 2002; 46:1129–1132.

13. Chang ST, Chuang SS. Ectopic cervical thymoma: a mimic of T-lymphoblastic lymphoma. Pathol Res Pract 2003; 199:633–635.

14. Juarbe C, Conley JJ, Gillooley JF, et al. Metastatic cervical thymoma. Otolaryngol Head Neck Surg 1989; 100:232–236.

15. Barat M, Rybak LP, Dietrich J. Metastatic thymoma to the head and neck. Laryngoscope 1988; 98:418–421.

VI.   ECTOPIC HAMARTOMATOUS THYMOMA— BRANCHIAL ANLAGE MIXED TUMOR

1. Smith PS, McClure J. Unusual subcutaneous mixed tumour exhibiting adipose, fibroblastic, and epithelial components. J Clin Pathol 1982; 35:1074–1077.

2. Rosai J., Levine GD, Limas C. Spindle cell thymic anlage tumor: four cases of previously undescribed benign neoplasm of the lower neck (abstr). Lab Invest 1982; 46:70A.

3. Rosai J, Limas C, Husband EM. Ectopic hamartomatous thymoma. A distinctive benign lesion of the lower neck. Am J Surg Pathol 1984; 8:501–513.

4. Fetsch JF, Laskin WE, Michal M, et al. Ectopic hamartomatous thymoma. A clinicopathologic and immunohistochemical analysis of 21 cases with data supporting reclassification as a branchial anlage mixed tumor. Am J Surg Pathol 2004; 28:1360–1370.

5. Fetsch JF, Weiss SW. Ectopic hamartomatous thymoma. A distinctive benign lesion of the lower neck. Am J Surg Pathol 1984; 8:501–513.

6. Chan JKC, Rosai J. Tumors of the neck showing thymic or related branchial pouch differentiation: a unifying concept. Hum Pathol 1991; 22:349–367.

7. Saeed IT, Fletcher CDM. Ectopic hamartomatous thymoma containing myoid cells. Histopathology 1990; 17:572–574.

8. Armour A, Williamson JMS. Ectopic cervical hamartomatous thymoma showing extensive myoid differentiation. J Laryngol Otol 1993; 107:155–158.

9. Michal M, Zamecnik M, Gogora M, et al. Pitfalls in the diagnosis of ectopic hamartomatous thymoma. Histopathology 1996; 29:549–555.

10. Mentzel T, Kriegsmann J, Kosmehl H, et al. Ectopic hamartomatous thymoma. Case report with special reference to differential diagnosis. Pathologe 1995; 16:359–363.

11. Henderson CJA, Gupta L. Ectopic hamartomatous thymoma: A case study and review of the literature. Pathology 100; 32:142–146.

VII.   CARNEY COMPLEX

1. Carney JA, Gordon H, Carpenter PC, et al. The complex of myxomas, spotty pigmentation, and endocrine overactivity. Medicine 1985; 64:270–283.

2. Carney JA. Carney complex: the complex of myxomas, spotty pigmentation, endocrine overactivity, and schwannomas. Semin Dermatol 1995; 4:90–98.

3. Boikos SA, Stratakis CA. Carney complex: pathology and genetics. Neuroendocrinology 2006; 83:189–199.

4. Boikos SA, Stratakis CA. Carney complex: the first 20 years. Curr Opin Oncol 2007; 19:24–29.

5. Diment J, Tamborini E, Casali P, et al. Carney triad: case report and molecular analysis of gastric tumor. Hum Pathol 2005; 36:112–116.

6. Kirschner LS, Carney JA, Pack SD, et al. Mutations of the gene encoding the protein kinase A type 1-alpha subunit in patients with the Carney complex. Nat Genet 2000; 26:89–92.

7. Stratakis CA, Kirschner LS, Carney JA. Clinical and molecular features of the Carney complex: diagnostic criteria and recommendations for patient evaluation. J Clin Endocrinol Metab 2001; 86:4041–4046.

8. Matyakhina L, Pack S, Kirschner LS, et al. Chromosome 2 (2 p16) abnormalities in Carney complex tumors. J Med Genet 2003; 40:268–277.

9. Wilkes D, McDermott DA, Basson CT. Clinical phenotypes and molecular genetic mechanisms of Carney complex. Lancet Oncol 2005; 6:501–508.

10. Carney JA, Boccon-Gibbod L, Jarke DE, et al. Osteochondromyxoma of bone: a congenital tumor associated with lentigines and other unusual disorders. Am J Surg Pathol 2001; 25:164–176.

VIII.   MAZABRAUD SYNDROME

1. Sedmak DD, Hart WR, Belhobek GH, et al. Massive intramuscular myxoma associated with fibrous dysplasia of bone. Cleve Clin Q 1983; 50:469–472.

2. Cabral CEL, Guedes P, Fonseca T, et al. Polyostotic fibrous dysplasia associated with intramuscular myxomas: mazabraud's syndrome. Skeletal Radiol 1998; 27:278–282.

3. Lopez-Ben R, Pitt MJ, Jaffe KA, et al. Osteosarcoma in a patient with McCune-Albright syndrome and Mazabraud's syndrome. Skeletal Radiol 1999; 28:522–526.

4. Jhala DN, Eltoum I, Carroll AJ, et al. Osteosarcoma in a patient with McCune-Albright syndrome and Mazabraud's syndrome: a case report emphasizing the cytological and cytogenetic findings. Hum Pathol 2003; 34:1354–1357.

5. McLaughlin A, Stalley P, Magee M, et al. Correlative imaging in an atypical case of Mazabraud syndrome. AJR Am J Roentgenol 2007; 189:W353–W356.

6. Henschen F. Fall von ostitis fibrosa mit multiplen tumoren in der umgebenden muskurature. Verh Dtsch Ges Pathol 1926; 21:93–97.

7. Mazabraud A, Semat P, Rose R. A propos del l'association de fibromixomes des tissus mous a la dysplasie fibreuse des os. Presse Med 1967; 75:2223–2228.

8. Wirth WA, Leavitt D, Enzinger FM. Multiple intramuscular myxomas. Another extraskeletal manifestation of fibrous dysplasia. Cancer 1971; 27:1167–1173.

9. Weinstein LS, Shenker A, Gejman PV, et al. Activating mutations of the stimulatory G protein in the McCune—Albright syndrome. N Engl J Med 1991; 325:1688–1695.

10. Marie PJ, de Pollak C, Chanson P, et al. Increased proliferation of osteoblastic cells expressing the activating GS alpha mutation in monostotic and polyostotic fibrous dysplasia. Am J Pathol 1997; 150:1059–1069.

11. Okamoto S, Hisaoka M, Ushijima M, et al. Activating Gs alpha mutation in intramuscular myxomas with and without fibrous dysplasia of bone. Virchows Arch 2000; 437:133–137.

IX.   GIANT CELL ANGIOFIBROMA

1. De Tos AP, Seregard S, Calonje E, et al. Giant cell angiofibroma. A distinctive orbital tumor in adults. Am J Surg Pathol 1995; 19:1286–1293.

2. Rousseau A, Perez-Ordonez, B, Jordan RCK. Giant cell angiofibroma of the oral cavity: report of a new location for a rare tumor. Oral Surg Oral Med Oral Pathol Oral Radiol Endod 1999; 88:581–585.

3. Kintarak S, Natiella J, Aguirre A, et al. Giant cell angiofibroma of the buccal mucosa. Oral Surg Oral Med Oral Pathol Oral Radiol Endod 1999; 88:707–713.

4. Qian Y-W, Malliah R, Lee H-J, et al. A t (12; 17) in an extraorbital giant cell angiofibroma. Cancer Genet Cytogenet 2006; 165:157–160.

5. Guillou L, Gebhard S, Coindre JM. Orbital and extraorbital giant cell angiofibroma: a giant cell-rich variant of solitary fibrous tumor? Clinicopathologic and immunohistochemical analysis of a series in favor of a unifying concept. Am J Surg Pathol 200; 24:971–979.

6. Thomas R, Banerjee SS, Eyden BP, et al. A study of four cases of extra-orbital giant cell angiofibroma with documentation of some unusual features. Histopathology 2001; 39:390–396.

7. Mikami Y, Shimizu M, Hirokawa M, et al. Extraorbital giant cell angiofibromas. Mod Pathol 1997; 10:1082–1087.

8. Husek K, Vesely K. Extraorbital giant cell angiofibroma. Cesk Patol 2002; 38:117–120.

9. Sigel JE, Fisher C, Vogt D, et al. Giant cell angiofibroma of the inguinal region. Ann Diagn Pathol 2000; 4:240–244.

10. Keyserling H, Peterson K, Camacho D, et al. Giant cell angiofibroma of the orbit. Am J Neuroradiol 2004; 25:1266–1268.

11. Guillou L. Bridge. Giant cell angiofibroma. In: Fletcher CDM, Unni KK, Mertens F, eds. World Health Organization Classification of Tumours. Pathology and Genetics. Tumours of Soft Tissue and Bone. Lyon: IARC Press, 2002:79–80.

12. Sonobe H, Iwata J, Komatsu T, et al. A giant cell angiofibroma involving 6 q. Cancer Genet Cytogenet 2000; 116:47–49.

X.   NUCHAL FIBROCARTILAGINOUS PSEUDOTUMOR

1. O'Connell JX, Janzen DL, Hughes TR. Nuchal fibrocartilaginous pseudotumor: a distinctive soft-tissue lesion associated with prior neck injury. Am J Surg Pathol 1997; 21:836–840.

2. Laskin WB, Fetsch JF, Miettinen M. Nuchal fibrocartilaginous pseudotumor: a clinicopathologic study of five cases and review of the literature. Mod Pathol 1999; 12:663–668.

3. Zamecnik M, Michal M. Nuchal fibrocartilaginous pseudotumor: immunohistochemical and ultrastructural study of two cases. Pathol Int 2001; 51:723–728.

4. Nicholetti GF, Platania N, Cicero S, et al. Nuchal fibrocartilaginous pseudotumor. Case report and review of the literature. J Neurosurg Sci 2003; 47:173–175.

XI.   RENAL CELL-LIKE SINONASAL ADENOCARCINOMA

1. Zur KB, Brandwein M, Wang B, et al. Primary description of a new entity, renal cell-like carcinoma of the nasal cavity. Arch Otolaryngol Head Neck Surg 2002; 128:441–447.

2. Storck KI, Simpson RH, Ramer M, et al. Renal cell-like sinonasal adenocarcinoma. Arch Pathol Lab Med 2007; 131:1474–1475 (abstr).

3. Ellis G. Clear cell carcinoma, not otherwise specified. In: Barnes L, Eveson JW, Reichart P, et al. eds. World Health Organization Classification of Tumours. Pathology and Genetics. Head and Neck Tumours. Lyon: IARC Press, 2005:227–228.

XII. LOW-GRADE SINONASAL SARCOMA WITH NEURAL AND MYOGENIC FEATURES

1. Lewis JE, Oliveira AM, Lewis JT, et al. Low grade sinonasal sarcoma with neural and myogenic features: a distinct subset of primary sinonasal sarcomas. Mod Pathol 2007; 20(suppl 2):226A (abstr).

XIII. MIDLINE CARCINOMA WITH NUT REARRANGEMENT (NUT–TOMA)

1. Kubonishi I, Takehara N, Iwata J, et al. Novel t (15:19) (q 15: p 13) chromosome abnormality in a thymic carcinoma. Cancer Res 1991; 51:3327–3328.
2. Kees UR, Mulcahy MT, Willoughby ML. Intrathoracic carcinoma in an 11-year-old girl showing a translocation t(15:19). Am J Pediatr Hematol Oncol 1991; 13:459–464.
3. Lee AC, Kwong YI, Fu KH, et al. Disseminated mediastinal carcinoma with chromosomal translocation (15:19): a distinctive clinicopathologic syndrome. Cancer 1993; 72:2273–2276.
4. Dang TP, Gazdar AF, Virmani AK, et al. Chromosome 19 translocation, over-expression of Notch 3, and human lung cancer. J Natl Cancer Inst 2000; 92:1355–1357.
5. Vargas SO, French CA, Paul PN, et al. Upper respiratory tract carcinoma with chromosomal translocation 15;19: evidence for a distinct disease entity of young patients with a rapidly fatal course. Cancer 2001; 92:1195–1203.
6. French CA, Miyoshi I, Aster JC, et al: BRD4 bromodomain gene rearrangement in aggressive carcinoma with translocation t (15; 19), Am J Pathol 2001; 159:1987–1992.
7. Toretsky JA, Jenson J, Sun CC, et al. Translocation (11;15:19): a highly specific chromosome rearrangement associated with poorly differentiated thymic carcinoma in young patients. Am J Clin Oncol 2003; 26:300–306.
8. French CA, Kutok JL, Faquin WC, et al. Midline carcinoma of children and young adults with NUT rearrangement. J Clin Oncol 2004; 22:4135–4139.
9. Stelow EB, Bellizzi AM, Mills SE, et al. Undifferentiated carcinomas of the upper aerodigestive tract associated with NUT rearrangements. Mod Pathol 2008; 21(suppl 1):242A (abstr).

XIV. TANGIER DISEASE

1. Serfaty-Lacrosniere C, Civeira F, Lanzberg A, et al. Homozygous Tangier disease and cardiovascular disease. Atherosclerosis 1994; 10:85–98.
2. Remaley AT, Rust S, Rosier M, et al. Human ATP-binding cassette transporter 1 (ABC1): genomic organization and identification of the genetic defect in the original Tangier kindred. Proc Natl Acad Sci 1999; 96:12685–12690.
3. Lawn RM, Wade DP, Garvin MR, et al. The Tangier disease gene product ABC1 controls the cellular apolipoprotein-mediated lipid removal pathway. J Clin Invest 1999; 104: R25–R31.
4. Nelson BL, Thompson LDR. Tonsil with Tangier disease. Ear Nose Throat J 2003; 82:178.
5. Kolovou GD, Mikhailidis DP, Anagnostopoulos SS, et al. Tangier disease four decades of research: a reflection of the importance of HDL. Curr Med Chem 2006; 13:771–782.

Index